Cancer Imaging: Instrumentation and Applications

Cancer Imaging: Instrumentation and Applications

Volume 2

Edited by

M.A. Hayat

Distinguished Professor
Department of Biological Sciences
Kean University
Union, New Jersey

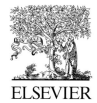

AMSTERDAM • BOSTON • HEIDELBERG • LONDON
NEW YORK • OXFORD • PARIS • SAN DIEGO
SAN FRANCISCO • SINGAPORE • SYDNEY • TOKYO

Academic Press is an imprint of Elsevier

Elsevier Academic Press
30 Corporate Drive, Suite 400, Burlington, MA 01803, USA
525 B Street, Suite 1900, San Diego, California 92101-4495, USA
84 Theobald's Road, London WC1X 8RR, UK

This book is printed on acid-free paper. ∞

Library of Congress Cataloguing-in-Publication Data
Cancer imaging: instrumentation and applications/edited by M.A. Hayat.
   p. ; cm.
  "Volume 2."
  Includes bibliographical references and index.
  ISBN 978-0-12-374183-7 (hardcover : alk. paper) 1.   Cancer–Imaging.
  2.   Cancer–Imaging–Instruments. I. Hayat, M. A., 1940-
  [DNLM: 1.   Neoplasms–diagnosis. 2.   Diagnostic Imaging–instrumentation.
  3.   Diagnostic Imaging–methods. QZ 241 C2144 2008]
  RC270.3.D53C36 2008
  616.99′40754–dc22   2007026695

British Library Cataloguing in Publication Data
A catalogue record for this book is available from the British Library

ISBN 13: 978-0-12-374183-7

For all information on all Elsevier Academic Press publications visit our Web site at www.books.elsevier.com

Printed in China
07 08 09 10 9 8 7 6 5 4 3 2 1

To

The men and women involved in the odyssey of deciphering the complexity of cancer initiation, progression, and metastasis, its diagnosis, cure, and hopefully its prevention.

Contents

Part I   Instrumentation

Part II   General Imaging Applications

Contents of Volume 1

Contributors

Agildere, A. Muhtesem
Department of Radiology
Baskent University Medical School
B. Evler
06490 Ankara
Turkey

Aiura, Koichi
Center for Diagnostic and Therapeutic Endoscopy
Keio University School of Medicine
35 Shinanomachi
Shinjuku-ku
Tokyo 160-8582
Japan

Akatsu, Tomotaka
Department of Surgery
Keio University School of Medicine
35 Shinanomachi
Shinjuku-ku
Tokyo 160-8582
Japan

Amendola, Marco A.
Department of Radiology
University of Miami
Miami, FL 33136

Anand, Vijay K.
Department of Otolaryngology
Weill Medical College of Cornell University
New York-Presbyterian Hospital
525 East 68th Street
New York, NY 10021

Anand, Vivek
Department of Nuclear Medicine
All India Institute of Medical Sciences
New Delhi 110029
India

Antoch, G.
Department of Diagnostic and Interventional
Radiology and Neuroradiology
University Hospital Essen
Hufelandstrasse 55
D-45122 Essen
Germany

Bacovsky, Jaroslav
IIIrd Internal Department
University Hospital
I.P. Pavlova 6
77200 Olomouc
Czech Republic

Bao, Ande
Department of Otolaryngology-Head and
Neck Surgery
University of Texas Health Science Center
7703 Floyd Curl Drive
San Antonio, TX 78229

Barentsz, Jelle O.
Department of Radiology
University Medical Center Nijmegen
Geert Grooteplein zuid 10
NL 6500HB Nijmegen
The Netherlands

Bathen, Tone F.
Department of Circulation and Medical Imaging
Norwegian University of Science and Technology
7491 Trondheim
Norway

Bazot, Marc
Service de Radiologie
Hopital Tenon
4 rue de la Chine
75020 Paris
France

Been, L.B.
Department of Surgical Oncology
University Medical Center Groningen
University of Groningen
9700 RB Groningen
The Netherlands

Belhocine, Tarik
Department of Diagnostic Radiology and Nuclear Medicine
Saint Joseph's Hospital
268 Grosvenor Street
London, Ontario N6A 4V2
Canada

Bergström, Mats
Department of Pharmaceutical Biosciences
Uppsala University
Lagerhyddsv 3
SE-751 85 Uppsala
Sweden

Bockisch, Andreas
Department of Nuclear Medicine
University Hospital Essen
Hufelandstrasse 55
D-45122 Essen
Germany

Brenner, Winfried
Department of Nuclear Medicine
University Medical Center Hamburg-Eppendorf
Martinistrasse 52
20246 Hamburg
Germany

Brianzoni, Ernesto
Nuclear Medicine Unit
Department of Oncology
Macerata Hospital Via S. Lucia 1
62100 Macerata
Italy

Bruhn, Harald
Charité Campus Virchow-Klinikum
University Medicine Berlin
Augustenburger Platz 1
13353 Berlin
Germany

Bygrave, Michael
Robarts Research Institute
University of Western Ontario
London, Ontario N64 5B9

Castellucci, Paolo
Department of Nuclear Medicine
Policlinico S. Orsola-Malpighi
University of Bologna
PAD 30 Via Massarenti 9
40139 Bologna
Italy

Chapman, D.
Anatomy and Cell Biology
University of Saskatchewan
101 Perimeter Road
Saskatoon, SK S7N 5E5
Canada

Chang, Kevin J.
Rhode Island Medical Imaging
20 Catamore Boulevard
East Providence, RI 02914

Chen, Antony K.
Department of Bioengineering
University of Pennsylvania
240 Skirkanich Hall
210 S. 33rd Street
Philadelphia, PA 19104

Chen, Yen-Kung
Department of Nuclear Medicine and
PET Center
Shin Kong Wu Ho-Su Memorial Hospital
and Fu Jen Catholic University
No. 95 Wen-Chang Road
Shih-Lin District
Taipei City 111
Taiwan (R.O.C.)

Cheng, Leo L.
Pathology Research, CNY-7
Mail Code: 149-7151
Massachusetts General Hospital
149 13th Street
Charlestown, MA 02129

Chin, Joseph L.
Urology Clinic
London Health Sciences Center
800 Commissioners Road E.
London, Ontario N6A 4G5
Canada

Cobben, D.C.P.
Department of Surgical Oncology
University Medical Center Groningen
University of Groningen
9700 RB Groningen
The Netherlands

Colagrande, Stefano
Sezione di Radiodiagnostica
Dipartimento di Fisiopatologia Clinica
Università degli Studi di Firenze
Azienda Ospedaliero-Universitaria Careggi
Viale Morgagni 85
50134 Firenze
Italy

Cova, Maria Assunta
Department of Radiology
University of Trieste
Ospedale di Cattinara
Strada di Fiume 447
34149 Trieste
Italy

Czupryna, Julie
Department of Bioengineering
University of Pennsylvania
240 Skirkanich Hall
210 S. 33rd Street
Philadelphia, PA 19104

Di Lollo, Simonetta
Dipartimento di Patologia Umana e Oncologia
Università degli Studi di Firenze
Azienda Ospedaliero-Universitaria Careggi
Viale Morgagni 85
50134 Firenze
Italy

Di Martino, Ercole
Children's Hospital "St Georg"
Delitzscher Strauss 141
D-04129 Leipzig
Germany

Driedger, Albert
Department of Diagnostic Radiology and
Nuclear Medicine
Saint Joseph's Hospital
268 Grosvenor Street
London, Ontario N6A 4V2
Canada

Drozd, Valentina
Department of Endocrinology
Belarussian Medical Academy of Postgraduate
Education
Brovki Street
Minsk 220013
Republic of Belarus

Elsinga, P.H.
Department of Surgical Oncology
University Medical Center Groningen
University of Groningen
9700 RB Groningen
The Netherlands

Endo, Masahiro
Department of Research Promotion
National Institute of Radiological Sciences
4-9-1 Anagawa
Inage-ku
Chiba-shi
Chiba 263-8555
Japan

Engel, Ahuva
Department of Medical Imaging
Rambam Medical Center
P.O. Box 9602
Haifa 31096
Israel

Even-Sapir, Einat
Department of Nuclear Medicine
Tel-Aviv Sourasky Medical Center
6 Weizman Street
Tel-Aviv 64239
Israel

Fanti, Stefano
Department of Nuclear Medicine
Policlinico S. Orsola-Malpighi
University of Bologna
PAD 30 Via Massarenti 9
40138 Bologna
Italy

Farsad, Mohsen
Department of Nuclear Medicine
Policlinico S. Orsola-Malpighi
University of Bologna
PAD 30 Via Massarenti 9
40138 Bologna
Italy

Fayad, Laura M.
Department of Radiology and Radiological Science
Johns Hopkins Medical Institutions
601 N. Wolfe Street
Baltimore, MD 21287

Fenster, Aaron
Robarts Research Institute
University of Western Ontario
London, Ontario N6A 5B9
Canada

Flamen, Patrick
Department of Nuclear Medicine
Jules Bordet Institute
Waterloolaan 121
B-1000 Brussels
Belgium

Franchi, Roberto
Department of Nuclear Medicine
Policlinico S. Orsola-Malpighi
University of Bologna
PAD 30 Via Massarenti 9
40138 Bologna
Italy

Freudenberg, Lutz
Department of Nuclear Medicine
University Hospital Essen
Hufelandstrasse 55
D-45122 Essen
Germany

Futawatari, Nobue
Department of Surgery
School of Medicine
Kitasato University
1-15-1 Kitasato
Sagamihara-shi
Kanagawa 228-8555
Japan

Fütterer, Jurgen J.
Department of Radiology
University Medical Center Nijmegen
Geert Grooteplein zuid 10
6500 HB Nijmegen
The Netherlands

Galons, Jean-Philippe
Department of Radiology
Arizona Cancer Center
1515 N. Campbell Avenue
Tuscon, AZ 85724

Gershater, Raziel
Department of Radiology
North York General Hospital
4001 Leslie Street
Toronto, Ontario M2K 1E1
Canada

Geus-Oei, Lioe-Fee de
Department of Nuclear Medicine
Radboud University
Nȳmegen Medical Center
P.O. Box 9101
6500 HB Nijmegen
The Netherlands

Ghersin, Eduard
Department of Diagnostic Imaging
Rambam Medical Center and B. Rappaport
Faculty of Medicine
Technion-Israel Institute of Technology
P.O. Box 9602
Haifa 31096
Israel
and
Department of Radiology
Leonard M. Miller School of Medicine
University of Miami
P.O. Box 016960 (R-109)
Miami, FL 33101

Gillies, Robert J.
Department of Biochemistry
Arizona Cancer Center
1515 N. Campbell Avenue
Tuscon, AZ 85724

Goerres, Gerhard W.
Institute of Diagnostic Radiology
Department of Medical Radiology
University Hospital
Raemistrasse 100
8091 Zürich
Switzerland

Gotthardt, Martin
Department of Nuclear Medicine
Radboud University
Nÿmegen Medical Center
P.O. Box 9101
6500 HB Nijmegen
The Netherlands

Gribbestad, Ingrid S.
Department of Circulation and Medical
Imaging
Norwegian University of Science and
Technology
7491 Trondheim
Norway

Hambrock, Thomas
Department of Radiology
P.O. Box 9101
University Medical Center Nijmegen
Geert Grooteplein zuid 10
6500 HB Nijmegen
The Netherlands

Hartmann, Dirk
Department of Medicine C (Gastroenterology)
Academic Teaching Hospital of the Johannes-
Gutenburg-University of Mainz Bremserstrasse 79
67063 Ludwigshafen
Germany

Hasnah, Moumen O.
Department of Math and Physics
University of Qatar
P.O. Box 2713
Doha
Qatar

Haubner, Roland
Universitätsklinik für Nuklearmedizin
Medizinische Universität Innsbruck
Anichstrasse 35
A-6020 Innsbruck
Austria

Hoffman, John M.
Utah Center for Advanced Imaging Research
Department of Radiology and Department of
Bioengineering CAMT
University of Utah
729 Arapeen Drive
Salt Lake City, UT 84108

Imaizumi, Akiko
Department of Oral and Maxillofacial
Radiology
Graduate School
Tokyo Medical and Dental University
Yushima 1-5-45
Bunkyo-ku
Tokyo 113-8549
Japan

Ishiwata, Kiichi
Positron Medical Center
Tokyo Metropolitan Institute of
Gerontology
1-1 Naka-cho
Itabashi-ku
Tokyo 173-0022
Japan

Ishiyama, Koichi
Department of Radiology
Akita University School of Medicine
1-1-1 Hondo
Akita City
Akita 010-8543
Japan

Iwata, Ren
CYRIC
Tohoku University
Aramaki
Aoba-ku
Sendai 980-8578
Japan

Iyer, Revathy B.
Department of Radiology
Unit 57
University of Texas M.D. Anderson
Cancer Center
1515 Holcombe Boulevard
Houston, TX 77030

Izawa, Jonathan I.
Urology Clinic
London Health Sciences Center
800 Commissioners Road E.
London, Ontario N6A 4G5
Canada

Jager, P.L.
Department of Surgical Oncology
University Medical Center Groningen
University of Groningen
9700 RB Groningen
The Netherlands

Jana, Suman
Division of Cardiovascular Medicine
University of Kentucky
900 South Limestone Street
Room 329 CTW Building
Lexington, KY 40536-0200

Jiang, Hongyi
Urology Research Laboratory
London Health Sciences Center
375 South Street
London, Ontario N6A 4G5
Canada

Jordan, Benedicte F.
Laboratory of Biomedical
Magnetic Resonance
Av. Mounier 73.40
1200 Brussels
Belgium

Jordan, Kate W.
Molecular Pathology/Radiology
Massachusetts General Hospital/Harvard Medical
School CNY
149 13th Street, Room 4022
Charlestown, MA 02129

Jung, Seung Eun
Department of Radiology
St. Mary's Hospital
College of Medicine
The Catholic University of Korea
62 Youido-dong
Youngdeungpo-gu
Seoul 150-713
South Korea

Kadrmas, Dan J.
Utah Center for Advanced Imaging Research
Department of Radiology and Department of
Bioengineering CAMT
729 Arapeen Drive
University of Utah
Salt Lake City, UT 84108

Khan, Gazala N.
Division of Hematology/Oncology
Department of Medicine
University of Michigan Comprehensive
Cancer Center
1500 E. Medical Center Drive
C369 Med Inn
P.O. Box 0848
Ann Arbor, MI 48109-0848

Kida, Mitsuhiro
Department of Gastroenterology
School of Medicine
Kitasato University
1-15-1 Kitasato
Sagamihara-shi
Kanagawa 228
Japan

Kikuchi, Shiro
Department of Surgery
School of Medicine
Kitasato University
1-15-1 Kitasato
Sagamihara-shi
Kanagawa 228-8555
Japan

Kim, Hyo-Cheol
Department of Diagnostic Radiology
Seoul National University Hospital
28 Yeongeon-dong
Jongno-gu
Seoul 110-744
South Korea

Kim, Seung Hyup
Department of Radiology
Seoul National University College of Medicine
28 Yongon-Dong
Chongno-Gu
Seoul 110-744
Korea

Kim, Sun Ho
Department of Radiology
Seoul National University College of Medicine
28 Yongon-Dong
Chongno-Gu
Seoul 110-744
Korea

Kitamura, Keishi
R&D Department
Medical Systems Division
Shimadzu Corporation
1 Nishinokyo-Kuwabara-cho Nakagyo-ku
Kyoto 604-8511
Japan

Ko, Sheung-Fat
Department of Diagnostic Radiology
Chang Gung Memorial Hospital
Linkou Medical Center
5 Fu-Shin Street
Kueishan
Taoyuan 333
Taiwan (R.O.C.)

Krohn, K.A.
Department of Radiation Oncology
Box 356113
University of Washington
Seattle, WA 98195

Kubota, Katsumi
Department of Radiology
School of Medicine
Kitasato University
1-15-1 Kitasato
Sagamihara-shi
Kanagawa 228-8555
Japan

Kubota, Kuzuo
Department of Radiology
Division of Nuclear Medicine
International Medical Center of Japan
1-21-1 Toyama
Shinjuku-ku
Tokyo 162-8655
Japan

Kumar, Rakesh
Department of Nuclear Medicine
All India Institute of Medical Sciences
New Delhi 110029
India

Kupelian, Patrick A.
Department of Radiation Physics
M.D. Anderson Cancer Center Orlando
1400 S. Orange Avenue
MP 730
Orlando, FL 32806

Kurabayashi, Tohru
Department of Oral and Maxillofacial
Radiology
Graduate School
Tokyo Medical and Dental University
Yushima 1-5-45
Bunkyo-ku
Tokyo 113-8549
Japan

Lacefield, James C.
Robarts Research Institute
University of Western Ontario
London, Ontario N6A 5B9
Canada

Lalich, Mihailo
The University of Wisconsin Hospital and
Clinics
600 Highland Avenue
Madison, WI 53792

Langen, Katja M.
Department of Radiation Physics
M.D. Anderson Cancer Center Orlando
1400 S. Orange Avenue
MP 730
Orlando, FL 32806

Lauenstein, Thomas C.
Department of Radiology
The Emory Clinic
1365 Clifton Road
Building A
Suite AT-627
Atlanta, GA 30322

Laufer, Ilya
Department of Neurosurgery
Weill Medical College of Cornell University
New York-Presbyterian Hospital
525 East 68th Street
New York, NY 10021

Lee, Jeong Min
Department of Diagnostic Radiology
Seoul National University Hospital
28 Yeongeon-dong
Jongno-gu
Seoul 110-744
South Korea

Leibovici, Dan
Department of Urology
The University of Texas
M.D. Anderson Cancer Center
1515 Holcombe Boulevard
Houston, TX 77030

Li, Allen
Department of Diagnostic Radiology
Tuen Mun Hospital
Tsing Chung Koon Road
Tuen Mun
New Territories
Hong Kong
SAR

Li, Hong
Department of Radiology
Kobe University Graduate School of Medicine
7-5-2, Kusunoki-cho
Chuo-ku
Kobe 650-0017
Japan

Li, Tianfang
Department of Radiation Oncology
Stanford University School of Medicine
Stanford, CA 94305

Liang, Jerome Zhengrong
Department of Radiology
School of Medicine 4L-120
Health Sciences Center
State University of New York
Stony Brook, NY 11794-8460

Lim, Jae Hoon
Samsung Medical Center
Department of Radiology
Sungkyunkwan University
School of Medicine
50 Ilwon-dong
Kangnam-ku
Seoul 135-710
Korea

Liu, Feng-Yuan
Department of Nuclear Medicine and Molecular
Imaging Center
Chang Gung Memorial Hospital
Chang Gung University College of Medicine
199 Dunhua N. Road
Taipei 10507
Taiwan (R.O.C.)

Liu, Glenn
Genitourinary Oncology and Developmental
Therapeutics
The University of Wisconsin Comprehensive
Cancer Center
600 Highland Avenue
Madison, WI 53792

Lyshchik, Andrej
Department of Radiology and
Radiological Sciences
Vanderbilt University Medical Center
CCC-1118 MCN
1161 21st Avenue South
Nashville, TN 37232

Massoud, Tarik
University of Cambridge
School of Clinical Medicine
Department of Radiology
Addenbrooke's Hospital
Box 219
Level 5 Hills Road
CB2 2QQ Cambridge
United Kingdom

Matsumoto, Keiichi
Department of Image-Based Medicine
Institute of Biomedical Research and Innovation
2-2 Minatojima-Minamimachi
Chuo-Ku
Kobe 650-0047
Japan

Mautner, Victor F.
Department of Maxillofacial Surgery
University Medical Center Hamburg-Eppendorf
Martinistrasse 52
20246 Hamburg
Germany

McShane, Teresa M.
Oncology Technology Lead
Global Clinical Technology
Pfizer Global Research and Development
Eastern Point Road
Groton, CT 06340

McQuade, Paul
Department of Imaging Research
Merck Research Laboratories
WP44C-2
West Point, PA 19486

Meeks, Sanford L.
Department of Radiation Physics
M.D. Anderson Cancer Center Orlando
1400 S. Orange Avenue
MP 730
Orlando, FL 32806

Menges, Marcus
Department of Internal Medicine II
Saarland University Medical Center
D-66421 Homburg
Germany

Miller, Frank R.
Department of Otolaryngology-Head and
Neck Surgery
University of Texas Health Science Center
7703 Floyd Curl Drive
San Antonio, TX 78229

Monetti, Francesco
Department of Radiology
National Institute for Cancer Research
Largo R. Benzi 10
16132 Genova
Italy

Morcos, Sameh K.
University of Sheffield
Department of Diagnostic Imaging
Northern General Hospital
Herries Road
S5 7AU Sheffield
United Kingdom

Mori, Shinichiro
Department of Radiation Oncology
Massachusetts General Hospital
100 Blossom Street
COX 3
Boston, MA 02114

Motoyama, Satoru
Department of Surgery
Akita University School of Medicine
1-1-1 Hondo
Akita City
Akita 010-8543
Japan

Moussa, Madeleine
Urology Research Laboratory
London Health Sciences Center
375 South Street
London, Ontario N6A 4G5
Canada

Muylle, Kristoff
Department of Nuclear Medicine
Jules Bordet Institute
Waterloolaan 121
B-1000 Brussels
Belgium

Myslivecek, Miroslav
Department of Nuclear Medicine
University Hospital
I.P. Pavlova 6
77200 Olomouc
Czech Republic

Nagino, Masato
Division of Surgical Oncology
Department of Surgery
Nagoya University Graduate School of Medicine
65 Tsurumai-cho
Showa-ku
Nagoya 466-8550
Japan

Nakamoto, Yuji
Department of Diagnostic Imaging and
Nuclear Medicine
Kyoto University Graduate School of Medicine
54 Shogoinkawahara-cho
Sakyo-Ku
Kyoto 606-8507
Japan

Nakamura, Takashi
Department of Radiology and Cancer Biology
Nagasaki University School of Dentistry
1-7-1 Sakamoto
Nagasaki 852-8588
Japan

Nariai, Tadashi
Department of Neurosurgery
Tokyo Medical and Dental University
1-5-45 Yushima
Bunkyo-ku
Tokyo 113-8519
Japan

Ng, Chaan S.
Department of Radiology
Unit 57
University of Texas M.D. Anderson
Cancer Center
1515 Holcombe Boulevard
Houston, TX 77030

Ng, Shu-Hang
Department of Diagnostic Radiology
Chang Gung Memorial Hospital
Linkou Medical Center
5 Fu-Shin Street
Kueishan
Taoyuan 333
Taiwan (R.O.C.)

Nimura, Yuji
Digestive Surgery
Aichi Cancer Center
1-1 Kanokoden
Chikusa-Ku
Nagoya 464-8681
Japan

Ogawa, Jun-ichi
Department of Surgery
Akita University School of Medicine
1-1-1 Hondo
Akita City
Akita 010-8543
Japan

Oyen, Wim J.G.
Department of Nuclear Medicine
Radboud University
Nȳmegen Medical Center
P.O. Box 9101
6500 HB Nijmegen
The Netherlands

Papathanassiou, Dimitri
Service de Médecine Nucléaire
Institut Jean Godinot
1 avenue du Général Koenig
BP 171
51056 Reims Cedex
France

Pinkernelle, Jens
Charité Campus Virchow-Klinikum
University Medicine Berlin
Augustenburger Platz 1
13353 Berlin
Germany

Pisters, Louis L.
Department of Urology-1373
The University of Texas M.D. Anderson
Cancer Center
1515 Holcombe Boulevard
Houston, TX 77030

Plukker, J.Th.M.
Department of Surgical Oncology
University Medical Center Groningen
University of Groningen
9700 RB Groningen
The Netherlands

Price, Pat
Academic Department of Radiation Oncology
The University of Manchester
Christie Hospital NHS Trust
Withington
M20 4BX Manchester
United Kingdom

Proietti, Alfredo
Radiotherapy Unit
Macerata Hospital Via S. Lucia 1
62100 Macerata
Italy

Rajendran, Joseph G.
Division of Nuclear Medicine
Department of Radiology
Box 356113
University of Washington
Seattle, WA 98195

Ravenel, James G.
Department of Radiology
Box 250322
Medical University of South
Carolina
169 Ashley Avenue
Charleston, SC 29425

Razifer, Pasha
GEMS PET Systems AB
Uppsala Applied Science Laboratory (UASL)
Husbyborg
752 88 Uppsala
Sweden

Reiser, M.
Department of Nuclear Medicine
University of Münich
Marchioninistr. 15
Münich 81377
Germany

Riemann, Juergen F.
Department of Medicine C
(Gastroenterology)
Academic Teaching Hospital of the
Johannes-Gutenburg-University of Mainz
Bremserstrasse 79
67063 Ludwigshafen
Germany

Rosenbaum, S.
Department of Nuclear Medicine
University Hospital Essen
Hufelandstrasse 55
D-45122 Essen
Germany

Rossi, Alexia
Department of Radiology
University of Trieste
Ospedale di Cattinara
Strada di Fiume 447
34149 Trieste
Italy

Rossi, Gloria
Medical Physic Unit
Macerata Hospital Via S. Lucia 1
62100 Macerata
Italy

Rozanes, Izzet
Department of Radiology
Istanbul University
Istanbul Faculty of Medicine
34390-Capa
Istanbul
Turkey

Rust, Thomas C.
Utah Center for Advanced Imaging Research
Department of Radiology and Department of
Bioengineering CAMT
729 Arapeen Drive
University of Utah
Salt Lake City, UT 84108

Sadrozinski, Hartnut F.–W.
Santa Cruz Institute of Particle Physics
University of California at Santa Cruz
Santa Cruz, CA 95064

Samnick, Samuel
Department of Nuclear Medicine
Saarland University Medical Center
D-66421 Homburg
Germany

Santoro, Lucia
Sezione di Radiodiagnostica
Dipartimento di Fisiopatologia Clinica
Università degli Studi di Firenze
Azienda Ospedaliero-Universitaria Careggi
Viale Morgagni 85
50134 Firenze
Italy

Sasaki, Mayumi
Department of Radiology
School of Medicine
Kitasato University
1-15-1 Kitasato
Sagamihara-shi
Kanagawa 228
Japan

Sashi, Ryuji
Department of Radiology
Akita University School of Medicine
1-1-1 Hondo
Akita City
Akita 010-8543
Japan

Satogata, Todd J.
Collider-Accelerator Department
Brookhaven National Laboratory
Upton, NY 11973

Schaefer, Niklaus G.
Institute of Diagnostic Radiology
Department of Medical Radiology
University Hospital
Raemistrasse 100
8091 Zürich
Switzerland

Scher, Bernhard
Department of Nuclear Medicine
University of Münich
Marchioninistr. 15
81377 Münich
Germany

Schindera, Sebastian T.
Abdominal Imaging Division
Department of Radiology
Duke University Medical Center
Box 3808
Erwin Road
Durham, NC 27710

Schlenker, B.
Department of Urology
University of Münich
Marchioninistr. 15
81377 Münich
Germany

Schmalbach, Cecelia E.
Department of Head and Neck Surgicial Oncology
Wilford Hall USAF Medical Center
2200 Bergquist Drive
Lackland AFB, TX 78236

Scholbach, Jakob
Children's Hospital "St Georg"
Delitzscher Strauss 141
D-04129 Leipzig
Germany

Scholbach, Thomas
Children's Hospital "St Georg"
Delitzscher Strauss 141
D-04129 Leipzig
Germany

Schuetze, Scott M.
Division of Hematology/Oncology
Department of Medicine
University of Michigan Comprehensive
Cancer Center
1500 E. Medical Center Drive
C369 Med Inn
P. O. Box 0848
Ann Arbor, MI 48109-0848

Schulte, Reinhard W.
Department of Radiation Medicine
Loma Linda University Medical Center
Loma Linda, CA 92354

Schwartz, Theodore H.
Department of Neurosurgery
Weill Medical College of Cornell University
New York- Presbyterian Hospital
525 East 68th Street
New York, NY 10021

Seitz, M.
Department of Urology
University of Münich
Marchioninistr. 15
81377 Münich
Germany

Sheir, Khaled Z.
Urology and Nephrology Center
Mansoura University
72 Elgomhoria Street
Mansoura
Dakahlia 35516
Egypt

Shibuya, Hitoshi
Tokyo Medical and Dental University
Department of Diagnostic Radiology
and Oncology
5-45, Yushima 1-chome
Bunkyo-ku
Tokyo 113-8519
Japan

Shimofusa, Ryota
Department of Radiology
Chiba University Hospital
1-8-1, Inohana, Chuo-ku
Chiba City
Chiba 260-8677
Japan

Shokeir, Ahmed A.
Urology and Nephrology Center
Mansoura University
72 Elgomhoria Street
Mansoura
Dakahlia 35516
Egypt

Sitter, Beathe
Department of Circulation and Medical Imaging
Norwegian University of Science and Technology
7491 Trondheim
Norway

Spiess, Philippe E.
Department of Urology
The University of Texas
M.D. Anderson Cancer Center
1515 Holcombe Boulevard
Houston, TX 77030

Stacul, Fulvio
Department of Radiology
University of Trieste
Ospedale di Cattinara
Strada di Fiume 447
34149 Trieste
Italy

Sugarbaker, Paul H.
Department of Surgical Oncology
Washington Cancer Institute
Washington Hospital Center
106 Irving Street, NW
Suite 3900
Washington, D.C. 20010

Sugihara, Ryo
Department of Radiology
Kobe University Graduate School of Medicine
7-5-2, Kusunoki-cho
Chuo-ku
Kobe 650-0017
Japan

Sugimura, Kazuro
Department of Radiology
Kobe University Graduate School of Medicine
7-5-2, Kusunoki-cho
Chuo-ku
Kobe 650-0017
Japan

Sumi, Misa
Department of Radiology and Cancer Biology
Nagasaki University School of Dentistry
1-7-1 Sakamoto
Nagasaki 852-8588
Japan

Tanaka, Yumiko Oishi
Department of Radiology
Graduate School of Comprehensive
Human Sciences
University of Tsukuba
1-1-1 Tennodai Tsukuba
Ibaraki 305-8575
Japan

Thomlinson, W.
Canadian Light Source Inc.
University of Saskatchewan
101 Perimeter Road
Saskatoon, SK S7N 0X4
Canada

Thompson, William M.
Department of Radiology
Duke University Medical Center
Box 3808
Erwin Road
Durham, NC 27710

Thorek, Daniel L.J.
Department of Bioengineering
University of Pennsylvania
240 Skirkanich Hall
210 S. 33rd Street
Philadelphia, PA 19104

Tiling, R.
Department of Nuclear Medicine
University of Münich
Marchioninistr. 15
81377 Münich
Germany

Tiseo, Marcello
Division of Medical Oncology
University Hospital of Parma
Via Gramsci 14
43100 Parma
Italy

Tomiguchi, Seiji
Diagnostic Radiology
Kumamoto University School of Health Sciences
Saiseikai Kumamoto
4-24-1 Kuhonji
Kumamoto 862-0976
Japan

Tomura, Noriaki
Department of Radiology
Akita University School of Medicine
1-1-1 Hondo
Akita City
Akita 010-8543
Japan

Tsourkas, Andrew
Department of Bioengineering
University of Pennsylvania
240 Skirkanich Hall
210 S. 33rd Street
Philadelphia, PA 19104

Turkmen, Cuneyt
Department of Nuclear Medicine
Istanbul University
Istanbul Faculty of Medicine
34390-Capa
Istanbul
Turkey

Uematsu, Takayoshi
Division of Diagnostic Radiology and Breast Care Unit
Shizuoka Cancer Center Hospital
Naga-izumi
Shizuoka 411-8777
Japan

Ulusan, Serife
Department of Radiology
Baskent University
Adana Teaching and Medical Research Center
Dadaloglu Mah Serinevier
Adana
Turkey

Utsunomiya, Daisuke
Diagnostic Imaging Center
Saiseikai Kumamoto Hospital
5-3-1 Chikami
Kumamoto 861-4193
Japan

Van Westreenen, H.L.
Department of Surgical Oncology
University Medical Center Groningen
University of Groningen
9700 RB, Groningen
The Netherlands

Veit-Haibach, Patrick
Department of Medical Radiology
Division of Nuclear Medicine
University Hospital Zürich
Ramistrasse 100
8091 Zürich
Switzerland

Villari, Natale
Università degli Studi di Firenze
Azienda Ospedaliero-Universitaria Careggi
Sezione di Radiodiagnostica
Dipartimento di Fisiopatologia Clinica
Viale Morgagni 85
50134 Firenze
Italy

Wagner, Thomas H.
Department of Radiation Physics
M.D. Anderson Cancer Center Orlando
1400 S. Orange Avenue
MP 730
Orlando, FL 32806

Watanabe, Masahiko
Department of Surgery
School of Medicine
Kitasato University
1-15-1 Kitasato
Sagamihara-shi
Kanagawa 228-8555
Japan

Wells, Paula
Department of Radiotherapy
St. Bartholomews' Hospital
West Smithfield
EC1A 7BE London
United Kingdom

Williams, David C.
Santa Cruz Institute of Particle Physics
University of California at Santa Cruz
Santa Cruz, CA 95064

Wirtzfeld, Lauren A.
Robarts Research Institute
University of Western Ontario
London, Ontario N6A 5B9
Canada

Xuan, Jim W.
Urology Research Laboratory
London Health Sciences Center
375 South Street
London, Ontario N6A 4G5
Canada

Yan, Tristan D.
University of New South Wales
Department of Surgery
St. George Hospital
Sydney
Australia

Yen, Tzu-Chen
Department of Nuclear Medicine
Chang Gung Memorial Hospital
Linkou Medical Center
5 Fu-Shin Street
Kueishan
Taoyuan 333
Taiwan (R.O.C.)

Yerli, Hasan
Department of Radiology
Baskent University
Zubeyde Hanim Training and Research
Center
6371 SK. No: 34 Bostanli/Karsiyaka
Izmir
Turkey

Yokoyama, Yukihiro
Division of Surgical Oncology
Department of Surgery
Nagoya University Graduate School of Medicine
65 Tsurumai-cho
Showa-ku
Nagoya 466-8550
Japan

Zeidan, Omar A.
Department of Radiation Physics
M.D. Anderson Cancer Center Orlando
1400 S. Orange Avenue
MP 730
Orlando, FL 32806

Zhong, Z.
National Synchrotron Light Source
Brookhaven National Laboratory
Upton, New York 19763

Zivian, Marilyn T.
Department of Psychology
Faculty of Health
York University
4700 Keele Street
Toronto, Ontario M3J 1P3
Canada

Preface

In developed countries, cancer is the second leading cause of death exceeded only by cardiovascular diseases. There are more than 100 types of cancers that can inflict any part of the body. In 2005, 7.6 million people died of cancer, which constitutes 13% of the 58 million deaths worldwide. Approximately, 1.3 million people are diagnosed each year with cancer in the United States, and ~ 1500 of them die every day.

Imaging plays an important role not only in the pretherapeutic assessment but also in monitoring the tumor after therapy. Imaging technology continues to progress at a rapid pace, providing important diagnostic and therapeutic information. Regardless of the speed of future advancements in imaging technologies, it is already accepted that many difficult, intriguing medical problems that could not have been previously addressed can now be solved. Exciting times are ahead in the investigation of anatomical, molecular, and functional aspects of cancer development and patient management, including diagnostic and therapeutic assessment and interventions, and even in potentially life-saving consequences. The ultimate goal is early detection and prevention of cancer and other diseases.

Deciphering the complexity of cancer diagnosis, therapy, and prognosis would not be possible without the wide spectrum of imaging technologies developed during the last three decades. Presently, the detection, surgical management, radiation planning, chemotherapeutic assessment, and follow-up evaluation of patients with cancer and other diseases are highly dependent on imaging technologies. These technologies include mammography, ultrasound and Doppler imaging, magnetic resonance imaging (MRI), computed tomography (CT), positron emission tomography (PET), single photon emission computed tomography (SPECT), electron paramagnetic resonance imaging, microwave imaging, and their variations and combinations. Applications, advantages, and limitations of most of the aforementioned and other imaging modalities are discussed in this and the first volume. It is difficult to imagine where disciplines of determination of cancer risk and intervention, cancer diagnosis and

treatment, radiation dose determination, and therapy assessment would be without these tools. These modalities are also beginning to be used for drug development and gene therapy, which are discussed in this series.

Briefly, the importance of prior laboratory prediction of individual drug response cannot be overestimated. Drug sensitivity is determined by multiple genes. The complexity of mechanisms involved in drug sensitivity becomes apparent, considering that gene expression profiles in response to drug exposure vary considerably among individuals even for the same drug or regimen. Therefore, determination of predictive marker genes for drug sensitivity is urgently needed, which will allow us to predict therapeutic response to drugs. This approach will identify patients who would benefit from a specific antitumor drug.

Because imaging has the capability to quantitate drug properties *in vivo* and for the aforementioned and other reasons, this technology is playing an important role in developing effective drugs. Drug discovery and development are accelerating owing to rapid synthesis of potential drugs and development of high-throughput *in vitro* tests. In fact, imaging is beginning to be used in all phases of drug discovery and development. A detailed discussion of such developments is presented by Janet C. Miller and colleagues in Volume 1, and by Mihailo Lalich and colleagues in this volume.

Predictive factors allowing an estimation of tumor prognosis and prediction of the response to specific drugs prior to the onset of treatment as well as post-treatment assessment are increasingly gaining importance in modern therapy designs in oncology, and imaging is playing a key role in achieving these goals. A pertinent example of this role is in chemotherapy. Chemotherapy plays an important role in the treatment of recurrent, metastatic, or nondissectible tumors. Selection and dosage of antitumor agent as well as the schedule of treatment are usually based on the personal experience of each doctor. However, the need of an evidence-based decision is apparent at least to optimize post-treatment schedule. Thus, early detection of tumor response to chemotherapy is of great importance for further treatment or change of treatment of tumors, and imaging evidence is helpful in the decision-making process.

Tumor gene therapy is beginning to be tested in clinical settings. To achieve the full potential of this therapy, the efficiency of this method needs to be assessed as early as possible. Imaging methods, such as magnetic resonance imaging and magnetic resonance spectroscopy, can assess early treatment response. In fact, these methods are capable of assessing different stages of therapy from transgene delivery to the final tumor eradication. This subject is discussed in detail by Kettunen and Grohn in Volume 1.

One of the important advancements in imaging instrumentation is the development of hybrid modalities. Multimodality image-guided diagnosis and therapy means acquisition and interpretation of multiple imaging modalities in order to attempt medical intervention. One of the hybrid modalities is PET/CT, which is considered to be a road map for imaging studies in oncology, with CT adding anatomical details to functional details provided by PET. This single schedule examination provides many clinical and workflow benefits. This combination makes CT almost a standard part of a PET purchase. Some of the combined imaging approaches that facilitate accurate spatial and temporal registration of information are discussed in this series.

As is true in the case of molecular genetics, imaging, especially molecular imaging, is revolutionizing the understanding of cancer. Imaging technology has advanced to diagnose not only at the whole-body, organ, tissue, and cell levels, but also at the molecular level *in vivo*. A relatively recent advance consists of molecular imaging that provides information on cellular processes and molecular pathways *in vivo*. Molecular imaging provides insight into the molecular mechanisms underlying carcinogenesis by chemical, physical, and biological agents and into inherited susceptibility to cancer. An example of the use of molecular imaging in the study of gene expression and high-throughput screening is discussed by Daniel L.J. Thorek and colleagues and Tarik F. Massoud in this volume.

Although anatomical imaging is in common use, functional imaging has the advantage of discerning the underlying biochemical pathways that confirm the presence or absence of pathology. In other words, molecular imaging advances our understanding of biology and medicine through noninvasive *in vivo* investigation of molecular events involved in normal and pathologic processes. In addition, the importance of molecular imaging in early diagnosis and assessment of therapy becomes apparent considering that alterations in molecular processes during treatment generally precede anatomical changes. Positron emission tomography is ideally suited to detect changes in molecular processes resulting, for example, from chemotherapy. The transition of molecular imaging from the animal-imaging environment to the clinical-human environment is progressing rapidly. An effort

has been made through these volumes to integrate molecular imaging into clinical radiology. It is not an exaggeration to say that we are observing the practice of medical imaging in an era of molecular medicine.

Advantages and adverse reactions of a number of tracers used for imaging are described in this volume. One of them is ^{18}F-fluorodeoxyglucose, which is an established imaging modality (FDG-PET) in oncology. High sensitivity and high-negative predictive value have led to its important role in cancer patients. Thus, the application of this tracer in the diagnosis of lung and breast cancers is discussed extensively in both Volume 1 and this volume. However, it should be noted that ^{18}F-FDG is also taken up by normal tissues as well as in inflamed conditions. Nevertheless, there is increasing uptake of ^{18}F-FDG with time, for example, in breast malignancies, whereas such uptake in inflammatory lesions and normal breast tissues decreases with time. In any case, it is necessary to be aware of normal variants, artifacts, and other causes of false-positive results.

Another PET tracer is 3′-deoxy-3′-^{18}F-fluorothymidine (^{18}F-FLT), which is thought to be a superior predictor, for example, of brain tumor progression and survival when compared with ^{18}F-FDG. FLT-PET is also thought to be a promising imaging modality monitoring the early effects of radiation therapy. It is a thymidine analog and is stable *in vivo* because it is a substrate for thymidine kinase but not for thymidine phosphorylase. FLT retention correlates with thymidine uptake, TK1 activity, and the percentage of cells in S phase; TK activity is very sensitive to ionizing radiation, and the changes in FLT uptake are thought to reflect the direct biological effect of radiation therapy. Therefore, this radiopharmaceutical has been proposed to be a promising imaging agent for monitoring early response to radiation therapy.

It is well established that early diagnosis is the key to cancer "cure." Prognosis is highly dependent on the stage of the disease. Thus, a simple and reliable screening method would be of tremendous advantage. For example, mammography and CT colonography have established a niche for imaging in cancer screening. Imaging techniques in clinical practice are used for the staging of tumors, detection of tumor recurrence, monitoring of efficacy of therapy, and differentiation between malignant and benign tissues. Imaging techniques, especially MRI, are playing a key role in the assessment of patients after treatment. In cases of local tumor recurrences, imaging has become the standard of care; even small local recurrences can be detected. Unfortunately, however, there are no or only a few associated early symptoms of some cancer types. Pancreatic and ovarian cancers and lymphoma are examples of malignancies difficult to diagnose at an early stage.

It cannot be overemphasized that careful training and thoughtful use of imaging technology undeniably enhance patient care. This technology enhances physical examination, can image the disease process, and bring to light new issues in patient management with greater clarity than patient history and conventional examination alone. Medical or surgical treatment plans can be modified according to the information extracted from imaging.

It is estimated that imaging testing would cost more than $100 billion in the year 2006 in the United States. This staggering amount of money would be spent because imaging is also a defensive medicine. Nevertheless, excessive use of imaging will exact a heavy toll on the available monetary resources.

Although whether or not exposure to medical radiation increases the incidence of cancer in the general population is controversial, but repeated exposure, for example, to mammography and computed tomography screening (depending upon the radiation dose), is known to be harmful to the patient. Therefore, imaging modalities introducing radiation should be used only when necessary. This subject is discussed in detail in this series. For example, medical radiation-induced cancer is discussed by Hitoshi Shibuya in this volume. In addition, the European Union has adopted a Directive cautioning against occupational exposure to electromagnetic fields produced by MRI; the caution applies only to workers, not to patients.

Three major topics discussed in this volume are imaging instrumentation, general imaging applications, and imaging of a number of human cancer types, including prostate, colorectal, ovarian, gastrointestinal, and bone cancers. Although cancer therapy is not the main subject of this series, the crucial role of imaging in selecting the type of therapy and its post-treatment assessment are discussed. The major emphasis in this volume is on cancer imaging; however, differentiation between benign tumors and malignant tumors is also discussed. Continued investment of time and expertise by researchers worldwide has contributed significantly to a greater understanding of the cancer process. In most cases the methodologies presented were either introduced or refined by the authors and routinely used in their clinical facilities. Some of the new topics that are at an experimental stage are also included for further testing and refinement. Each chapter provides unique individual practical knowledge based on the expertise of the author.

This volume has been developed through the efforts of 195 authors representing 25 countries. The high quality of each manuscript made my work as the editor an easy one. Strictly uniform style of manuscript writing has been accomplished. I am indebted to the contributors for their promptness in accepting my suggestions, and I appreciate their dedication and hard work in sharing their knowledge with the readers. The chapters contain the most up-to-date information, and it is my hope that the volume will be published expeditiously.

I am thankful to the Board of Trustees of Kean University and its president, Dr. Dawood Farahi, for recognizing the importance of scholarship in an institution of higher education, and providing resources to complete this project. I am thankful to Betsy Mathew, Ayesha Muzaffar, and Natalie DiTerlizzi for their expert help in preparing this volume.

M.A. Hayat
March 2007

Selected Glossary

ABI: Analyzer-based imaging

Ablation: Ablation consists of removal of a body part or the destruction of its function.

ACS: Autocalibrating signals

ACF: Autocorrelation function

ADC: Apparent diffusion coefficient is a measure of the mean-square displacement of an ensemble of molecules within a unit of time.

Adenocarcinoma: Adenocarcinoma is a malignant neoplasm of epithelial cells in a glandular or glandlike pattern.

Adenoma: Adenoma is a benign epithelial neoplasm in which the tumor cells form glands or glandlike structures. It does not infiltrate or invade adjacent tissues.

Adjuvant: Adjuvant is additional therapy given to enhance or extend the primary therapy's effect, as in chemotherapy's addition to a surgical regimen. It is a treatment added to a curative treatment to prevent recurrence of clinical cancer from microscopic residual disease.

Algorithm: Algorithm is a systematic process consisting of an ordered sequence of steps; each step depends on the outcome of the previous one. It is a step-by-step protocol management of a health-care problem.

Antibody: Antibody (immunoglobulin) is a protein produced by B-lymphocytes that recognizes a particular foreign antigenic determinant and facilitates clearance of that antigen; antigens can also be carbohydrates and even DNA.

APTI: Amide proton transfer imaging

ATR: Attenuated total reflection

BCT: Breast-conserving therapy

BOLD: Blood oxygen level-dependent

BPAS-MR: Basiparallel anatomic scanning-MR

Brachyradiotherapy: Brachyradiotherapy is radiotherapy in which the source of radiation is placed close to the surface of the body or within a body cavity.

CAD: Computer-aided detection

CADx: Computer-aided diagnosis

Cancer chemoprevention: Cancer chemoprevention is defined as the prevention of cancer or treatment of identifiable precancers; histopathologic or molecular intraepithelial neoplasia.

Carcinoma: Carcinoma is of various types of malignant neoplasm arising from epithelial cells, mainly glandular (adenocarcinoma) or (squamous cell). Carcinoma is the most common cancer and displays uncontrolled cellular proliferation, anaplasia, and invasion of other tissues, spreading to distant sites by metastasis. The origin of carcinoma in both sexes is in skin, and in prostate in men and in breast in women. The most frequent carcinoma in both sexes is bronchogenic carcinoma.

CBCT: Cone beam computed tomography

CCA: Conical correlation analysis

CCDC: Charge-coupled device camera

CDMAM: Contrast detectability mammography phantom

CDUS: Color Doppler ultrasonography

CECT: Contrast-enhanced computed tomography

CED: Convection-enhanced drug delivery

CE-MRA: Contrast-enhanced magnetic resonance angiography

CEUS: Contrast-enhanced ultrasound

CHARMED: Composite hindered and restricted model of diffusion

CIMS: Chemical imaging mass spectrometry provides both the chemical information of a mass spectrometer and the spatial organization of each component on a surface, including biological surfaces.

CISS: Constructive interference in a steady state.

Clinical Guidelines: Clinical guidelines are statements aimed to assist clinicians in making decisions regarding treatment for specific conditions. They are systematically developed, evidence-based, and clinically workable statements that aim to provide consistent and high-quality care for patients. From the perspective of litigation, the key question has been whether guidelines can be admitted as the evidence of the standard of expected practice, or whether this should be regarded as hearsay. Guidelines may be admissible as evidence in the United States if qualified as authoritative material or a learned treatise, although judges may objectively scrutinize the motivation and rationale behind guidelines before accepting their evidential value. The reason for this scrutiny is the inability of guidelines to address all the uncertainties inherent in clinical practice. However, clinical guidelines should form a vital part of clinical governance.

CMRI: Cardiac magnetic resonance imaging

CMT: Continuously moving table

CNB: Core needle biopsy

COX: Cyclooxygenase

CR: Computed radiography

CSI: Chemical shift imaging

CTA: Computed tomography arteriography

CTC: Computed tomography colonography

CTDI: CT dose index

CTF: Computed tomography fluoroscopy

CTHA: Computed tomography hepatic arteriography

CTLM: Computed tomography laser mammography

CTP: Computed tomography portography

CTV: Clinical target volume

CW-NMRI: Continuous wave NMR imaging

DBT: Digital breast tomosynthesis

DBTM: Digital breast tomosynthesis mammography

DCIS: Ductal carcinoma *in situ*

DEDM: Dual-energy digital mammography

DEI: Diffraction-enhanced imaging

DEPT: Distortionless enhancement by polarization enhancement

DFM: Dipolar field microscopy

DFS: Disease-free survival

Diagnosis: Diagnosis means the differentiation of malignant from benign disease or of a particular malignant disease from others. A tumor marker that helps in diagnosis may be helpful in identifying the most effective treatment plan.

DOP: Depth of penetration

DOT: Diffuse optical tomography

DPI: Doppler perfusion index

DSA: Digital subtraction angiography

DSC: Dynamic susceptibility contrast

DSE: Dobutamine stress echocardiography

DSR: Dynamic spatial reconstructor

DTI: Diffusion tensor imaging

DT-MRI: Diffusion tensor magnetic resonance imaging

DVH: Dose volume histogram

DWI: Diffusion-weighted imaging

DWMRI: Diffusion-weighted MRI

EBCT: Electron beam computed tomography

EBCTA: Electron beam computed tomographic angiography

EBP: Evidence-based practice

EBRT: External beam radiotherapy

EBT: Electron beam tomography

ECD: Electrochemical detector

ECGI: Electrocardiographic imaging

ECR: Equivalent cross-relaxation rate

ECRI: Equivalent cross-relaxation rate imaging

ECS: Echocontrast cystosonography

EEG/MEG: Electro- and magnetoencephalography

EFG: Electric field gradient

EGFR: Epidermal growth factor receptor

EPI: Echo-planar imaging

EPI: Echo-portal imaging

EPID: Electronic portal imaging device

EPR: Electron paramagnetic resonance

EPR: Enhanced permeation and retention

EPSI: Echo-planar imaging spectroscopic imaging

ERCP: Endoscopic retrograde cholangiopancreatography

ERUS: Endorectal ultrasound

ESFT: Ewing sarcoma family of tumors

EUS: Endoscopic ultrasonography

FA: Fractional anisotropy

FBP: Filter backprojection

FDG: ^{18}F-fluoro-2-deoxy-D-glucose

FDPM: Frequency-domain photon migration

FDTD: Finite difference time domain

FFDM: Full-field digital mammography

FFT: Fast Fourier transform

FIGO: Federation of International Gynecology and Obstetrics

FISP: Fast imaging with steady precession

FLAIR: Fluid attenuation inversion recovery

FLASH: Fast low angle shot

FLIM: Fluorescence lifetime imaging microscopy

FLIP: Functional lumen imaging probe

FLT: [^{18}F] 3'-deoxy-3'-fluorothymidine

FMISO: ^{18}F-fluoromisonidazole

fMRI: Functional magnetic resonance imaging

FMT: Fluorescence-mediated tomography

FNAB: Fine needle aspiration biopsy

FNH: Focal nodular hyperplasia

fNIRS: Functional near-infrared spectroscopy

FOV: Field-of-view

FOXs: Fields of excitation

FPA: Focal plane array

FPI: Flat-panel imager

FPI: Fluorescent protein imaging

FPT: Fast Padè transform

FRET: Fluorescence resonance energy transfer

FSCT: Fast-scan computed tomography

FSE: Fast spin echo

3D FSE: 3D T2-weighted fast spin echo

FSEI: Fast spin echo imaging

FTIR: Fourier transform infrared resonance

Gallium-68:   Gallium-68 (^{68}Ga) is a positron-emitting cyclotron-independent radionuclide with a short half-life of 68 min.

Gastritis: Gastritis refers to the inflammation, especially mucosal, of the stomach.

Gd-DTPA: Gd-diethylenetriaminepentaacetic acid

Gene Therapy: Gene therapy is defined as a therapy in which a gene(s) or gene-transducer cells are introduced to the patient's body for a therapeutic or gene-making purpose. Gene therapy by definition is not necessarily a molecular targeting therapy, but there are high expectations that the new mechanisms of cancer cell targeting can be integrated into therapy.

GIST: Gastrointestinal stromal tumor.

GRAPPA: Generalized autocalibrating partially parallel acquisition

HCC: Hepatocellular carcinoma

HCT: Helical computed tomography

HDR: High-dose rate

HGGT: High-grade glial tumor

HIPAA: Health Insurance Portability and Account Ability Act

HPLC: High-performance liquid chromatography

HRCT: High-resolution computed tomography

HRMAA: High-resolution melting amplicon analysis is used primarily to screen for mutationally activated proteins.

HT: Helical tomography

ICRP: International Commission on Radiological Protection

IGRT: Image-guided radiotherapy

Immunotherapy: Immunotherapy involves delivering therapeutic agents conjugated to monoclonal antibodies that bind to the antigens at the surface of cancer cells. Ideal antigens for immunotherapy should be strongly and uniformly expressed on the external surface of the plasma membrane of all cancer cells. Many solid neoplasms often demonstrate regional variation in the phenotypic expression of antigens. These regional differences in the immunophenotypic profile within the same tumor are referred to as intratumoral heterogeneity. Therapeutic agents that have been used include radioisotopes, toxins, cytokines, chemotherapeutic agents, and immunologic cells.

IMRT: Intensity-modulated radiation therapy is a special form of CFRT (conformal radiotherapy). The former is the delivery of radiation to the patient via fields that have nonuniform radiation fluence. However, it is fluence, not intensity, that is modulated.

IOC: Intraoperative cholangiogram

IRFSE: Inversion recovery fast spin echo

IRSE: Inversion recovery spin echo

IVM: Intravital microscopy

LDR: Low-dose rate

LGGT: Low-grade glial tumor

LINAC: Linear accelerator

LRRT: Loco-regional radiotherapy

LSI: Laser speckle imaging

LSS: Light scattering spectroscopy

Lymph: Lymph is the intracellular tissue fluid that circulates through the lymphatic vessels.

Lymphadenopathy: Lymphadenopathy is the enlargement of the lymph nodes.

Lymph nodes: Lymph nodes are small secondary lymphoid organs containing populations of lymphocytes, macrophages, and dendric cells that serve as sites of filtration of foreign antigens and activation of lymphocytes.

Lymphoma: Lymphoma is a cancer of lymphoid cells that tends to proliferate as solid tumors.

MADD: Maximum allowed dose difference

Malignant: Malignant tumors have the capacity to invade and alter the normal tissue.

MALT: Mucosa-associated lymphoid tissue

MBF: Myocardial blood flow

MCE: Myocardial contrast echocardiography

MCMLI: Multicolumn multiline interpolation

MCR-ALS: Multivariate curve resolution-alternating least square

MDCT: Multidetector row computed tomography

MDEFT: Modified driven equilibrium Fourier transform

Mediastinoscopy: Mediastinoscopy is an invasive procedure used for staging mediastinal lymph node metastases, which has a sensitivity of ~ 90%.

MEG: Magnetoencephalography

MEMRI: Manganese-enhanced magnetic resonance imaging

Metastasis: Initially, tumor growth is confined to the original tissue of origin, but eventually the mass grows sufficiently large to push through the basement membrane and invade other tissues. When some cells lose adhesiveness, they are free to be picked up by lymph and carried to lymph nodes and/or may invade capillaries and enter blood circulation. If the migrant cells can escape host defenses and continue to grow in the new location, a metastasis is established. Approximately more than half of all cancers have metastasized by the time of diagnosis. Usually it is the metastasis that kills the person rather than the primary (original) tumor.

Metastasis itself is a multistep process. The cancer must break through any surrounding covering (capsule) and invade the neighboring (surrounding) tissue. Cancer cells must separate from the main mass and be picked up by the lymphatic or vascular circulation. The circulating cancer cells must lodge in another tissue. Cancer cells traveling through the lymphatic system must lodge in a lymph node. Cancer cells in vascular circulation must adhere to the endothelial cells and pass through the blood vessel wall into the tissue. For cancer cells to grow, they must establish a blood supply to bring oxygen and nutrients; this usually involves angiogenesis factors. All of these events must occur before host defenses can kill migrating cancer cells.

If host defenses are to be able to attack and kill malignant cells, they must be able to distinguish between cancer and normal cells. In other words, there must be immunogens on cancer cells not found on normal cells. In the case of virally induced cancer-circulating cells, viral antigens are often expressed, and such cancer cells can be killed by mechanisms similar to those for virally infected tissue. Some cancers do express antigens specific for those cancers (tumor-specific antigens), and such antigens are not expressed by normal cells.

As already stated, metastasis is the principal cause of death in individuals with cancer, yet its molecular basis is poorly understood. To explore the molecular difference between human primary tumors and metastases, gene expression profiles of adenocarcinoma metastases of multiple tumor types have been compared with unmatched primary adenocarcinomas. A gene-expression signature that distinguished primary from metastatic adenocarcinomas was found. More importantly, it was found that a subset of primary tumors resembles metastatic tumors with respect to this gene-expression signature. The results of this study differ from most other earlier studies in that the metastatic potential of human tumors is encoded in the bulk of a primary tumor. In contrast, some earlier studies suggest that most primary tumor cells have low metastatic potential, and cells within large primary tumors rarely acquire metastatic capacity through somatic mutation. The emerging notion is that the clinical outcome of individuals with cancer can be predicted using the gene profiles of primary tumors at diagnosis.

MIP: Maximum-intensity projection

MITS: Matrix inversion tomosynthesis

Molecular Genetics: Molecular genetics is a subdivision of the science of genetics involving how genetic information is encoded within the DNA and how the cell's biochemical processes translate the genetic information into the phenotype.

Molecular Imaging: Molecular imaging is defined as the *in vivo* characterization and measurement of biological processes at the cellular and molecular levels. In other words, in contrast to conventional diagnostic imaging, molecular imaging probes the molecular abnormalities that are the basis of disease, including cancer, rather than image the end effects of these molecular alterations.

Monitoring: Monitoring means repeated assessment if there are early relapses or other signs of disease activity or progression. If early relapse of the disease is identified, a change in patient management will be considered, which may lead to a favorable outcome for the patient.

MPR: Multiplanar reconstruction

MRA: Magnetic resonance angiography

MRA: Magnetic resonance arthrography

MRCP: Magnetic resonance cholangiopancreatography

MRDSA: Magnetic resonance digital substraction angiography

MRE: Magnetic resonance elastography

MREIT: Magnetic resonance electrical impedance tomography

MRS: Magnetic resonance spectroscopy analyzes specific atomic nuclei and their compounds using the phenomenon of MR and chemical shift. This method provides information on the metabolism of organs and cells, biochemical changes, and quantitative analysis of compounds in humans, with no harm to the body.

MRSI: Multi-voxel magnetic resonance spectroscopic imaging

MSCT: Multislice computed tomography

MTC: Magnetization transfer contrast

MTD: Maximum tolerated dose

MTI: Microwave tomographic imaging provides quantitative maps of tissue dielectric properties that may correlate with tissue functional information.

MVCT: Megavoltage computed tomography

NDD: Normalized dose difference

NEC: Noise-equivalent quanta describe the equivalent number of quanta or counts required by an ideal imaging system to produce the same noise characteristics as does an actual system that is degraded by noise.

NECR: Noise-equivalent counting rate

Neoplasia: Neoplasia refers to the pathologic process that causes the formation and growth of an abnormal tissue.

Neoplasm: Neoplasm is an abnormal tissue that grows by cellular proliferation faster than normal and continues to grow.

NIOI: Near-infrared optical imaging

NIR: Near-infrared

NIRL: Near-infrared light

NIRS: Near-infrared spectroscopy

NMR: Nuclear magnetic resonance

NPV: Negative-predictive values

NSA: Number of signal averages

NTCP: Normal tissue complication probability

OAP: Oblique axial plane

OCT: Optical coherence tomography is based on imaging probes inserted into a body lumen or directly into a soft tissue through thin catheters. Such catheter-based OCT has been developed primarily for gastrointestinal and intravascular imaging.

ODT: Optical diffusion tomography

ODT: Optical Doppler tomography

OGTT: Oral glucose tolerance test

OHR: Optimized head and neck reconstruction

OIS: Optical imaging spectroscopy

OOSCC: Oropharyngeal squamous cell carcinoma

OPET: Optical positron emission tomography

OPSI: Orthogonal polarization spectral imaging

OPT: Optical projection tomography

OSEM: Ordered subsets expectation maximization

Palliative: Palliative treatment means reducing the severity of a disease; it denotes the alleviation of symptoms without curing the underlying disease.

PAM: Photoacoustic mammoscope

Pancreatitis: Pancreatitis refers to the inflammation of the pancreas. It can be caused by alcoholism, endocrine diseases, heredity, viral, parasitic, allergic, immunologic, pregnancy, drug effects, and abdominal injury.

PAT: Parallel acquisition technique

PAT: Photoacoustic tomography

PIT: Parallel imaging technique

PCA: Principal component analysis

PCM: Phase-contrast mammography

PCNA: Proliferating cell nuclear antigen

PCT: Perfusion computed tomography

PDT: Photodynamic therapy is a promising treatment for accessible tumors. It is localized to the tumor tissue by using photosensitive drugs, which may lead to tumor regression or even death.

PEDRI: Proton electron double resonance imaging

Phase contrast X-ray imaging: Phase contrast X-ray imaging utilizes refractive index variations (phase information) in addition to conventional absorption information with conventional X-ray absorption techniques. Phase contrast images can be recorded with a significantly lower dose than conventional images.

phMRI: Pharmacological MRI technique can be used to monitor the neurophysiological effects of central nervous system-active drugs.

PI: Parallel imaging

PMRI: Pharmacologic magnetic resonance imaging

PPI: Partially parallel imaging

PPILS: Partially parallel imaging with localized sensitivities

PPV: Positive-predictive values

Prognosis: Prognosis is defined as the prediction of how well or how poorly a patient is likely to fare in terms of response to therapy, relapse, survival time, or other outcome measures.

PSI: Probabilistic similarity index

PTC: Percutaneous transhepatic cholangiogram

RCT: Randomized controlled trial

RECIST: Response evaluation criteria in solid tumors

RET: Resonance energy transfer

RF: Radiofrequency

RGCT: Respiratory-gated CT scanning

ROCM: Receiver operating characteristic method

ROI: Region of interest

RP: Radical prostatectomy

Sarcoma: Sarcoma is a connective tissue neoplasm that is usually highly malignant. It is formed by proliferation of mesodermal cells.

Sarcomatoid: Sarcomatoid is a neoplasm that resembles a sarcoma.

SAR: Specific absorption ratio

SARs: Specific absorption rates

SCI: Spatial compound imaging

Scintigraphy: A diagnostic method consisting of the administration of a radionuclide having an affinity for the organ or tissue of interest, followed by photographic recording of the distribution of the radioactivity with a stationary or scanning external scintillation camera.

Screening: Screening is defined as the application of a test to detect disease in a population of individuals who do not show any symptoms of their disease. The objective of screening is to detect disease at an early stage, when curative treatment is more effective.

SEA: Single echo acquisition

SENSE: Sensitivity encoding

SFRT: Stereotactic fractionated radiation therapy

SIMS: Secondary ion mass spectrometry

SLEPI: Spin-locked echo-planar imaging

SLN: Sentinel lymph node

SLNB: Sentinel lymph node biopsy

SMART: Simultaneous modulated accelerated radiation therapy

SMASH: Simultaneous acquisition of spatial harmonics

SMRI: Stereotactic magnetic resonance imaging

SNB: Sentinel node biopsy

SNR: Signal-to-noise ratio

Specificity: Specificity is the capacity for discrimination between antigenic determinants by an antibody or lymphocyte receptor.

SPECT: Single photon emission computed tomography is a cross-sectional, quantitative functional imaging modality in routine use in oncology for the initial staging of the cancer.

SPI: Single-point imaging

SPIO: Superparamagnetic iron oxide

Sporadic: Sporadic is a multilocal genocopy, occurring irregularly. A disease occurring only rarely without regularity; extreme variability in the expression of a gene.

SPRITE: Single-point ramped imaging with T_1 enhancement

SSCT: Slow-scan computed tomography

SS-NMR: Solid-state nuclear magnetic resonance

STAT: Signal transducers and activators of transcription

STEAM: Stimulated echo acquisition mode

STIR: Short-T1 inversion recovery

STRAFI: Stray field imaging

SURLAS: Scanning ultrasound reflector linear array system

SUV: Standardized uptake value

SWI: Stiffness-weighted image

SWR: Standardized whole-body reconstruction

TACE: Transarterial chemoembolization

TACT: Tuned aperture computed tomography

TCP: Tumor control probability

TDI: Tissue Doppler imaging

TEE: Transesophageal echocardiography

TEM: Transverse electromagnetic

TERUS: Tracked endorectal ultrasound

TESO: Time-efficient slice ordering

TGC: Time gain compensation

THI: Tissue harmonic imaging is a gray-scale ultrasound mode that can provide images of higher quality than conventional sonography by using information from harmonics. Harmonics are generated by nonlinear wave propagation of ultrasound in tissue.

Tomography: Tomography is the making of a radiographic image of a selected plane by means of reciprocal linear or curved motion of the X-ray tube and film cassette; images of all other planes are out of focus and blurred.

TPPM: Two-pulse phase-modulated

TRAIL: Two reduced acquisitions interleaved

Transmit SENSE: Transmit sensitivity encoding

TTE: Transthoracic echocardiography

Tumor Microenvironment: Tumor microenvironment means the interaction between epithelial tumors and their stroma, including fibroblasts, blood vessels, and extracellular matrix. This definition is extended to interactions between potential tumor cells and the immediately surrounding cells of the same tissue type.

TVDT: Tumor volume doubling time

UHF: Ultrahigh magnetic field

US: Ultrasonography

USP: United States Pharmacopeia

VEGFR: Vascular endothelial growth factor receptor

XeCT: Xenon-enhanced computed tomography

XRF: X-ray fluoroscopy

I
Instrumentation

1

Proton Computed Tomography

Jerome Zhengrong Liang, Tianfang Li, Reinhard W. Schulte,
Todd J. Satogata, David C. Williams, and Hartnut F.-W. Sadrozinski

Introduction

This chapter presents the principles of proton computed tomography (pCT) and reviews its clinical applications. The emphasis is on image reconstruction from projected data along proton paths, which may not necessarily be straight lines through the object to be imaged.

The potential of pCT in medicine relies mainly on its role in improving proton beam therapy. Proton beams have distinct advantages compared to other radiation therapy options, such as X-rays and electron beams, because they deliver radiation energy in a quite precise manner while leaving the normal tissues around a targeted tumor mostly unharmed or undamaged. This is possible due to the characteristics of the dose distribution along the proton path inside the body: a relatively low dose along the entrance toward the path end and a high-dose peak at the end, called high-dose Bragg peak. Beyond the Bragg peak the dose falls off rapidly, that is, from 90 to 20% of the peak dose within a few millimeters. Positioning the peak inside the target delivers a maximum dose to the tumor with minimal damage to the surrounding tissues.

By contrast, when an X-ray beam of therapeutic energy (at MeV level) traverses the whole body, it delivers radiation energy along its entire path in a relatively uniform manner (see the chapter by Meeks in this volume: Megavoltage Computed Tomography Imaging). If a tumor is near a critical region like the spinal cord or the optic nerve, proton beams have a clear advantage by leaving the adjacent critical region unexposed regardless of the beam direction because of the Bragg peak, whereas X-ray beams can only avoid the critical structure if it is not on the beam path. Electron beams share a similar dose distribution as X-ray beams, except for a relatively shorter path. For example, by an X-ray beam of 6 MeV, a therapeutic dose can be delivered at a target ≥ 15 cm deep inside the body, while an electron beam of the same energy cannot effectively deliver a therapeutic dose beyond 5 cm (the effective path of electron beam is approximately half the energy quantity, i.e., 3 cm).

Because of the above advantages of proton beams, several medical proton accelerator facilities have been established during the past 15 years in the United States and Japan. Proton treatment facilities are now coming on line at major hospitals in the United States (e.g., Massachusetts General Hospital, Loma Linda University Medical Center, and University of Florida) and around the world. Over 100,000 patients have been benefited from these proton treatment centers.

In these existing proton treatment centers, the dose calculations are currently performed based on X-ray computed tomography (xCT; see the chapter by Bavenel in this volume: Multidetector Row Computed Tomography), and the patient is positioned with the help of X-ray radiographs. Hence, direct visualization of the three-dimensional (3D) patient anatomy in the treatment room is presently impossible, limiting the accuracy of proton therapy. It is technically challenging to integrate xCT in the treatment room for patient position. In addition, the accuracy of xCT for proton treatment planning is limited due to the difference in physical

3

interactions between photons and protons, which partially obviates the advantage of proton therapy. Using proton beam for the purposes of dose calculation and patient anatomy position in the treatment room would offer a great advantage in terms of convenience and cost effectiveness and would achieve more precise patient treatment. This is now recognized as the major motivation of developing pCT and also the major clinical application of proton beams for imaging.

Review of Prior Studies on Proton Imaging

Several early publications have demonstrated the feasibility of proton beams for imaging. In the late 1960s, Koehler (1968) showed that with parallel-sided objects with a thickness nearly equal to the path length or range of an incident 160 MeV proton beam, proton radiographic films could be produced with much greater image contrast than was possible with X-ray radiographs taken under the same conditions. Since that time, a number of publications about proton radiography (Koehler and Steward, 1974) and tomography (Cormack and Koehler, 1976) have appeared in the literature, which mainly addressed proton imaging as a diagnostic tool (Hanson et al., 1981, 1982). However, because most of the technological development efforts successfully went into improving the diagnostic xCT in those decades, the interest in developing medical pCT stagnated.

The situation changed with the development of medical proton gantries for delivery of proton beams, first at Loma Linda University Medical Center and now in several other proton treatment centers, resulting in an increasing number of patients treated with proton therapy. This new technical development and increase of patient number elevated the need for an accurate prediction of the proton dose distributions and verification of the patient position on the treatment table, and also demanded the development of accurate 3D imaging techniques. This has led to a renewed interest in proton imaging and the construction of a proton radiography system at the Paul Scherrer Institute in Switzerland (Schneider et al., 2004).

A pCT system utilizing a proton gantry and fast image reconstruction techniques has not yet been developed. However, a recently published design study has concluded that a pCT scanner should utilize instrumentation developed for high-energy physics such as silicon track detectors and crystal calorimeters equipped with fast readout electronics, allowing one-by-one registration of protons traversing the body during a full revolution of the proton gantry (Schulte et al., 2004). Different from proton beam therapy where the Bragg peak is positioned inside the targeted tumor inside the body, pCT may label each incident proton and detect that proton when it exits from the body by a high-energy detector where the high-dose Bragg peak will occur inside the detector. The pCT scanner will provide precise information on the proton's incident energy, location, and direc-

tion, as well as its exit energy, location, and direction. Another recently published study further concluded that a completely new image reconstruction paradigm is needed for pCT, which deals with the proton path of curves rather than the well-known X-ray path of straight lines in xCT (Li et al., 2006). An adequate image reconstruction algorithm shall utilize the pCT scanner measurements to map the energy loss along the proton trajectories through the body.

A successful implementation of pCT would avoid the ambiguities of mapping xCT Hounsfield Units (HU, which is related to the X-ray attenuation coefficients) to electron densities and would allow actual dose distribution as well as verification of patient position in the treatment room. In other words, the availability of pCT in the treatment room will predict very accurately the position of the Bragg peak within the patient's body, resulting in a maximum dose delivery to the targeted tumor and successful sparing of the surrounding normal tissues. Furthermore, a successful integration of pCT with proton therapy may lead to the ultimate form of image-guided 3D conformal radiation therapy, which has the potential to deliver the optimal dose to any point within the patient and provide arbitrarily shaped inhomogeneous dose distributions as desired (see the chapter by Yap in this volume, Cancer Therapy: Positron Emission Tomography/Computed Tomography). This is now recognized as the major potential of pCT in medicine. The image formation principles of proton beam are presented in this chapter. Hardware configuration and data acquisition for pCT will also be discussed. The emphasis will be on the issue of image reconstruction from projected data along proton trajectories through the body.

Image Formation Principles of Proton Computed Tomography

Image formation for pCT, similar to other imaging modalities, relies on the interaction of incident energy with the tissues inside the body. Knowledge of the interaction and the accuracy of measuring the difference of the exit energy from the incident energy determine the quality of the reconstructed image about the body internals.

Interactions of Protons with Atomic Components of the Tissues Inside the Body

When traversing the body, protons lose some of their energy via inelastic collisions with the outer electrons of the tissue atomic components leading to ionizations and excitations. Furthermore, they will be deflected by multiple small-angle scattering (i.e., multiple Coulomb scattering—MCS) from the nuclei of the tissue atomic components. These two main processes, occurring a great number of times along the macroscopic path length of the protons, lead to the macroscopic effects of the interaction of protons with the tissues inside the body: (1) loss of energy and (2) deflection from their original direction. As individual interaction events occur randomly, these two processes result in a statistical distribution of the following two principal quantities observed for proton imaging: (1) the amount of energy lost by each proton after traversing the body, and (2) the lateral and angular displacements of the proton from its incident position and direction. The amount of energy-loss variation (i.e., energy straggling, which is reflected by the variation of the Bragg peak width of a proton traversing along the same path through the same object) is the principal limitation for the intrinsic image contrast or density resolution of pCT (Satogata et al., 2003; Schulte et al., 2005). The variation of proton trajectory due to the random MCS, resulting in the lateral and angular displacements, is the principal limitation for the intrinsic image spatial resolution of pCT (Li et al., 2004, 2006). These two principal limitations will be discussed in more detail later.

In addition to the above two main processes of inelastic collisions with the outer atomic electrons and deflection from the atomic nuclei due to MCS, protons in the energy range (at the MeV level) used for pCT also undergo nuclear interactions, leading to reduction of proton transmission in a depth-dependent manner. Protons undergoing nuclear interactions mostly deposit their energies locally and hence contribute to the dose within the patient without contributing to the image formation. This would be a concern in developing pCT for clinical use. Below we will briefly discuss the magnitude of this effect as a function of the thickness of the absorbing object before introducing the fundamental image formation equation of pCT. More quantitative discussion on proton absorption will be given later.

Energy Requirement and Tissue Characterization for Proton Computed Tomography

The protons used for pCT must have sufficient energy to penetrate the body to be imaged. According to the NIST PSTAR database (National Institute for Standards and Technology, PSTAR database, www.physics.nist.gov/Phys RefData/Star/Text/PSTAR.html), the path depth or range in a continuous slowing-down approximation (CSDA) of 200 MeV protons in a tissue equivalent plastic is 25.8 cm, which is sufficient to penetrate an adult human skull (nominal width of 20 cm in anterior-posterior direction). For 250 MeV protons the range is 37.7 cm, sufficient to penetrate an adult trunk (nominal width of 34 cm, excluding arms). The relationship between the average range and the incident energy for water may be approximately expressed as (Satogata et al., 2003):

$$< R > = 4.90k^2 + 2.77 \, k \quad (1)$$

where R is in units of gram/cm², $k = E/100$[MeV], and E is the incident kinetic energy in units of MeV. Given an incident kinetic energy E in MeV, Equation (1) predicts the average range of the proton in the water. At energy levels greater than 200 MeV, protons are relativistic particles, and their energy-velocity relationship is described by

$$\beta^2(E) = 1 - \left(\frac{E_p}{E + E_p} \right)^2 \quad \text{and} \quad \beta = \frac{v}{c} \quad (2)$$

where c is the light velocity (2.998×10^{10} cm/s), v the proton velocity, and E_p the rest mass of protons (938.3 MeV). For example, for 250 MeV protons, the relativistic velocity ratio is $\beta = 0.61$, which shall be considered in quantitative analysis of the proton energy loss.

The energy loss of protons after traversing the body is a measure of the integrated electron density distribution along the proton path. More electrons are on the path, more interactions occur, and more energies are lost. The electron density of a medium is defined as the number of electrons/cm³. The relationship between the electron density ρ_e and the physical density ρ is given by

$$\rho_e = \rho N_A \left(\frac{Z_e}{A_e} \right) \quad (3)$$

where N_A is Avogadro's number (6.022×10^{23}), and Z_e and A_e are the effective atomic number and atomic weight of the traversed object, respectively. Human tissues are composed of atoms of relatively low atomic number (Z) and weight (A) (ICRU Report No. 44, 1989). Since the ratio Z_e/A_e for the human tissues is fairly constant, usually lying between 0.50 and 0.55, the electron density closely reflects the physical density of the tissues to be imaged. In other words, the intrinsic image contrast of pCT is somewhat directly related to the physical density contrast among the tissues. To avoid large numbers associated with absolute electron density values (at the order of 10^{23} electrons/cm³), it is advantageous to express the results in terms of relative electron density, defined as:

$$\eta_e = \frac{\rho_e}{\rho_{e,water}} \quad (4)$$

where $\rho_{e,water} = 3.343 \times 10^{23}$ electrons/cm³ is the electron density of water. For human soft tissues, the physical density ρ (or the relative electron density η_e) varies little between different tissues at the order of a few percentage points, and their density values scatter around that of water (ICRU Report No. 44, 1989). Thus, pCT for the distribution of η_e inside the human body is inherently relative low contrast, similar to the xCT for the distribution of attenuation coefficients of soft tissues.

Mean Energy Loss and Integral Equation for pCT Image Formation

In the important energy range for pCT $(10 - 250\,\text{MeV})$, the mean energy loss of protons per unit path length, also called stopping power dE/dr, is mainly due to the ionizations and atomic excitations and is well described by the Bethe Bloch theory. For protons in the stated energy range, corrections for density and shell effects are not required (Leo, 1994). In this case, the Bethe Bloch formula may be written in the following form, convenient for pCT image reconstruction:

$$-\frac{dE}{dr}(r) = \eta_e(r)F[I(r),E(r)] \qquad (5)$$

where η_e was defined before as the relative volume electron density to be reconstructed, and its dependence on the position vector r is a reminder that all quantities in equation (5) can vary with spatial position inside the body. The function $F[I(r), E(r)]$ can be expressed as:

$$F(I(r),E(r)) = K\frac{I}{\beta^2(E)}\left[\ln\left(\frac{2m_ec^2}{I(r)}\right.\right.$$
$$\left.\left.\times\frac{\beta^2(E)}{1-\beta^2(E)}\right) - \beta^2(E)\right] \qquad (6)$$

where m_ec^2 is the electron rest energy $(0.511\,\text{MeV})$, and $I(r)$ is the mean excitation potential of the material, which for water is about 75 eV (National Institute for Standards and Technology, Material Composition database, www.physics.nist.gov/cgi-bin/Star/compos.pl?ap). The constant K is defined as:

$$K = 4\pi\,r_e\,m_e\,c^2\rho_{e,water} = 0.170\,\frac{\text{MeV}}{\text{cm}} \qquad (7)$$

where r_e is the classical electron radius $(2.818 \times 10^{-13}\,\text{cm})$.

Note that Equation (5) is an approximation of the original Bethe Bloch equation, which contains a term W_{max}, the maximum energy transfer in a single collision (Bichsel et al., 1972). This approximation is valid if the mass of the incident projectile is large relative to the electron mass, which is the case for protons. The Bethe Bloch Equation (5) is a nonlinear first-order differential equation of the function $E(r)$. Since $I(r)$ is not known a priori, direct integration of this equation is intractable. However, for human tissues the variation of $I(r)$ is relatively small, and the dependence of the function $F(.)$ on $I(r)$ is relatively weak due to the logarithmic function in Equation (6). Therefore, it is reasonable to assume that $I(r)$ is independent of location and can be replaced by the mean ionization potential of water $I_{water} = 75$ eV. In this case, $F(.)$ is only a function of E, and Equation (5) can be integrated as:

$$\int_{E_{out}}^{E_{in}} \frac{dE}{F(I_{water},E)} = p(I_{water}) = \int_S \eta_e(r)dr \qquad (8)$$

where the integration on the left side can be calculated numerically, given the incident proton energy E_{in}, the exit proton energy E_{out} after traversing the body, and the complicated energy-dependent function $F(.)$ of Equation (6), as denoted by the notation $p(I_{water})$. The right-side integration is along the proton path S. The relative electron density distribution $\eta_e(r)$ can be reconstructed based on the derived projection data $p(I_{water})$ (from measurements). Equation (8) resembles the format of the Radon transform for xCT if the proton path S is assumed as a straight line. Image reconstruction in pCT is to invert the path integral for the relative electron density distribution $\eta_e(r)$. Unlike the inversion in xCT, the proton path is unknown in pCT due to MCS and must be estimated. This uniqueness of pCT renders a challenge for image reconstruction from the projection data along an unknown path. In addition to this challenge and the approximation made for Equation (5) from the original Bethe Bloch equation, it can be further noted that the integrated density along the proton path on the right side of Equation (8) is approximated by the water-equivalent length of the proton trajectories through the body because of the use of I_{water} for calculating the projection data $p(I_{water})$.

Equation (8) is the fundamental integral formula for image formation of pCT and is derived based on the energy interactions along the entire path through the body, ignoring the two main statistical processes of (1) energy-loss straggling and (2) proton path uncertainty due to MCS, and the third one of proton absorption due to nuclear interaction.

Energy-Loss Straggling

After traversing an object of certain thickness and density, monoenergetic protons will have experienced varying numbers of random collisions with the electrons along their paths. Furthermore, the energy transferred by a proton to the atoms (mainly to their outer electrons) of the tissues is also subject to statistical fluctuations. In consequence, a monoenergetic beam incident on the body will have an energy distribution after traversing the object, which was first described mathematically by Bohr (1948) and later by others.

For energy losses not exceeding 20% of the initial energy (> 20% loss will be discussed later), but large enough that the Central Limit Theorem applies, the energy-loss distribution is well described by a normal (Gaussian) distribution, for which only the first two moments of the distribution (i.e., mean and variance) are different from zero. For relativistic protons, the variance of the energy-loss distribution after passing through a layer of thickness d can then be described by Bohr's theory as:

$$\sigma_B^2(d) = \eta_e K$$

$$\times \int_0^d \frac{1 - \frac{1}{2}\beta^2(E(E_{in}, x))}{1 - \beta^2(E(E_{in}, x))} dx \qquad (9)$$

where $E(E_{in}, x)$ is the mean energy of protons of incident energy E_{in} after traversing a path length x inside the body, and η_e and K were defined above. For example, the spread of the energy loss after traversing the water of average range $<R>$ may be expressed by a root mean squares (RMS) measure as (Satogata et al., 2003):

$$\sigma_B(R) \Rightarrow \sigma_R[\text{MeV}] \approx 0.30 <R>^{1/2} \quad \text{or}$$

$$\sigma_R[\text{g}/\text{cm}^2] \approx 0.30(0.098k + 0.028) <R>^{1/2} \qquad (10)$$

where σ_R is in units of MeV, $<R>$ is given by Equation (1) and $k = E/100[\text{MeV}]$, with E being the incident kinetic energy in units of MeV as defined before. For example, an incident 200 MeV energy would have an RMS energy spread of about 1.5 MeV or an RMS range spread of 0.34 cm by Equation (10) at the end of its range of 25 cm in water. This intrinsic variation on the energy loss will ultimately affect the image contrast or density resolution of pCT as described below.

Successful implementation of pCT for applications in radiation therapy treatment planning requires that the relative electron density of the targeted tumor and surrounding normal tissues be determined with a high degree of accuracy (e.g., at the order of 1%), maintaining a sufficient degree of spatial resolution (e.g., at the order of 1 mm). The random noise in the energy measurement of outgoing protons will ultimately limit the ability to measure small density differences. Refer to xCT, where the principal noise limit is due to counting statistics of detected photons; pCT's principal noise limit is due to the energy-straggling statistics of protons traversing the object. As in xCT, the only way to improve measurement accuracy is to increase the number of protons (if inaccuracy of the detection system is not considered), thereby improving the statistics of the measurement. This will be at the cost of more radiation dosage. Therefore, it would be important to establish a dose-density discrimination relationship for a given density resolution (or image contrast) and voxel size, where the voxel size would reflect the proton beam flux as well as the spatial resolution. It is expected that the radiation dosage, image contrast, and image resolution (voxel size) will be interrelated. The following gives a qualitative description.

The density resolution or intrinsic image contrast of a pCT scanner may be defined as the one-sigma spread of the derived relative electron density value with respect to its mean value, which in pCT is usually close to unity. It is assumed that this value is derived from the energy-loss measurement of N protons traversing a given voxel of the object. Three main components contribute to the spread, (1) the energy-loss straggling, (2) the energy or momentum spread of the incident protons, and (3) the noise of the energy measurement detector. Because we are mainly concerned with the principal density resolution limitation of pCT, we will assume that only energy-loss straggling contributes to the pCT noise, and that the other two components can be neglected. In other words, we only consider the primary cause due to energy-loss straggling and we ignore the other secondary effects.

Let $\Delta\eta_e$ be the incremental variation of the relative electron density in a cubic voxel of size a. The corresponding mean increment in outgoing proton energy for a proton traversing this voxel can be expressed as (Schulte et al., 2005):

$$\Delta E_{out} = \frac{dE}{dx} \cdot \Delta\eta_e \cdot a \qquad (11)$$

where the stopping power dE/dx has to be evaluated at the location of the voxel. Assuming the relative electron density derivation is based on N protons traversing the voxel during the pCT scan, the energy-loss straggling of individual protons, σ_B, will lead to a spread in the derived relative electron density given by

$$\sigma_{\eta_e} = \frac{\sigma_B}{\sqrt{N} \cdot a \cdot \left(\frac{dE}{dx}\right)} \qquad (12)$$

where σ_B was defined before. Furthermore, the dose delivered to the object at the location of the voxel may be expressed as:

$$D = \frac{N}{a^2 \cdot \rho_e} \cdot \left(\frac{dE}{dx}\right) \qquad (13)$$

Solving Equation (13) for N and substituting N into Equation (12) give the following useful relationship between relative electron density resolution and radiation dosage:

$$\sigma_{\eta_e} = \frac{\sigma_B}{\sqrt{D \cdot a^4 \cdot \rho_e \cdot \left(\frac{dE}{dx}\right)}} \qquad (14)$$

Equation (14) reflects the dose dependence of the density resolution for a given object diameter as well as the dependence of the resolution on object diameter and incident proton energy for a given dose. For water medium, the number of needed protons N and the resulting dosage D can be estimated, for an object diameter equal to the energy range $<R>$ of Equation (1), by (Satogata et al., 2003):

$$N\sigma_{\eta_e}^2 a^2 \approx 0.28k(4.9k + 2.8)(0.10k + 0.03)^2 \qquad (15)$$

$$D\sigma_{\eta_e}^2 a^4 \approx 4.5 \times 10^{-11} k(4.9k + 2.8)(0.10k + 0.03)^2 \qquad (16)$$

For example, a single 200 MeV proton ($k = 2$) passing through a square pixel (or cubic voxel) of size 1 mm in water (of diameter 25 cm) delivers an average dose of about 7.2×10^{-8} Gy to the voxel. To achieve density resolution of $\sigma_{\eta e} = 1\%$ in voxel size of $a = 1$ mm, $N = 370{,}000$ protons are needed to pass through each voxel in water, and the surface dose is $D = 26$ mGy (Satogata *et al.*, 2003).

Multiple Coulomb Scatter and Proton Path Uncertainty

When passing through the object to be imaged, protons in the energy range used for pCT experience multiple small-angle deflections due to scattering at the nuclear potential of the target atoms leading to a macroscopic deviation from the original direction by up to a couple of degrees and a displacement of the exit point with respect to the entry point by up to a few millimeters. More specifically, assuming that the incident proton beam has zero size and zero angular spread (i.e., zero emittance), the transverse size of a 200 MeV beam acquires an RMS spread of transverse size of 0.65 cm at the end of its range of 25 cm in water (Satogata *et al.*, 2003). This is the physical root cause of the poor reputation that proton radiography has historically acquired, due to the inevitable blurring in simple transmission images. Fortunately, while MCS is the main limitation of the spatial resolution of proton imaging as discussed elsewhere (Schneider and Pedroni, 1994; Williams, 2004), it makes only a limited contribution to the energy-loss spread of the protons due to statistical variation in the path length of protons undergoing MCS in a layer of given thickness. Furthermore, with new detection technology development, the exit proton displacement and direction can be measured very accurately (Sadrozinski *et al.*, 2003). This proton-to-proton tracking measurement on a 200 MeV incident proton's entrance and exit positions can reduce the RMS spread of transverse size from 0.65 cm to less than 0.1 cm at the end of its path range of 25 cm in water (Satogata *et al.*, 2003). This retained 1 mm transverse size is due mainly to the proton path uncertainty inside the body, which is the intrinsic limitation of the spatial resolution of pCT (Williams, 2004; Li *et al.*, 2003, 2004, 2006).

Proton Loss Due to Nuclear Interactions

When imaging with protons, one has to account for the chance that protons will undergo nuclear interactions that may lead to an abrupt energy loss and/or large deflections. The probability of inelastic nuclear interactions of protons in the energy range used for pCT becomes significant above 100 MeV. Nuclear interactions result in a reduction of transmission with increasing thickness of the traversed object and thus contribute to unwanted patient dose. Janni (1982) tabulated the probability that a proton of a given initial energy will undergo at least one nuclear interaction

during its path length. For 250 MeV protons, which have a CSDA range of about 38 cm, this probability was given as 30%. The ICRU Report 49 (1993) lists probabilities of at least one nuclear interaction for protons with initial energies from 100 to 1000 MeV for different path lengths ranging from 1 to 100 cm. For example, the probability that a 200 MeV proton can be transmitted without undergoing a nuclear interaction is 92.2% for a water layer of 10 cm thickness and 83.6% for a layer of 20 cm thickness. Although the probability of that at least one nuclear interaction for a proton of 200 MeV can traverse a water layer of more than 20 cm thickness can be as high as 20%, the likelihood of the proton being absorbed inside the layer remains to be determined. If the proton is deflected and then escapes the absorption inside the body, its majority energy may not contribute to the dose to the body.

Detector Design and Data Acquisition for Proton Computed Tomography

As discussed earlier, the pCT system shall use the proton-to-proton tracking measurements to reduce the beam transverse spread due to the MCS. In the same time, the detector shall have an excellent energy resolution to measure accurately the energy loss after the proton exits from the body. A prototype system design for the proton-to-proton tracking measurements and high energy resolution is described next.

Design of a Proton Computed Tomography Scanner

Figure 1 illustrates our conceptual design of an ideal pCT system, which has the potential to label each incident proton and to measure its exit energy, location, and direction (Sadrozinski *et al.*, 2003; Schulte *et al.*, 2004). The object is traversed by a broad (ideally but not necessarily parallel) beam of protons of known energy E_{in}. By using an active proton beam scanning system, the incident energy E_{in} may be adjusted while scanning around the object, to optimize the density resolution according to spatial variations of the object thickness. A detector system is arranged on both sides of the object and records the exit energy E_{out} of individual protons, as well as their entrance and exit locations and directions with respect to the detector system.

Acquisition of Proton Radiography by the Proton Computed Tomography Design

Our initial experiment setup of Figure 1 was installed on the research beam line of the medical proton synchrotron at Loma Linda University Medical Center. A monochromatic 250 MeV proton beam was degraded by a 25.4-cm-thick (approximately cube-shaped) wax block ($\rho = 0{:}926$ gram/cm^2)

Figure 1 Schematic illustration of an idealized sin-gle-proton-tracking pCT scanner. Protons with known incident energy E_{in} are individually recorded by the four planes of position-sensitive silicon detectors that form the scanner reference system (t, u, v). These four planar detectors provide positions as well as azimuth and declination angles of the protons in front and behind the object. The exit energy E_{out} of each proton is recorded with a seg-mented calorimeter in coincidence with its position and angle information in planes 3 and 4. For a complete scan, the object is traversed by broad proton beams from many different projection angles ϕ. For parallel beam incidence, ϕ may go from 0 to 180°. For cone beam incidence (i.e., protons come from a point source), ϕ may go a full circle around the object. The resulting parallel- or cone beam data set allows reconstruction of the relative electron den-sity distribution inside the object reference system (x, y, z).

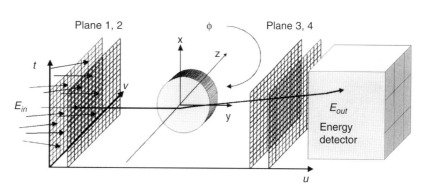

to a mean energy of about 130 MeV. At a distance of 25 cm downstream from the wax block, the beam encountered the image object, a 5.0-cm-long hollow aluminum cylinder $\rho = 2.7$ gram/cm² of outer diameter of 3.0 cm and inner diameter of 0.68 cm. Behind the object, protons were indi-vidually detected by two silicon detector modules, each con-sisting of a pair of single-sided silicon strip detectors (SSDs) with strips oriented at right angles to each other (see the four detector planes in Fig. 1). These detectors, located immedi-ately behind 27 cm downstream of the object, served to mea-sure the spatial coordinates (x and y), the exit angles, and the energy of the protons that passed or traversed the object.

The data collected in our experiment was comprised of x- and y-hit positions and time over threshold (TOT) values from the four silicon planes. Proton transmission images were calculated for each SSD module by averaging the pro-ton energy over a large number ($\approx 10^6$) of individual events, and were displayed as 2D maps of proton energy versus the x- and y-strip positions in the respective SSD module. It was found that the image measured with the downstream module (SSD planes 3 and 4) showed almost no object features. This can be explained by the effect of multiple scattering. The 2D plot in Figure 2 (left) shows the spatial distribution of average energy in the upstream module for proton energies averaged in four-by-four strip pixels ($\approx 0.8 \times 0.8$ mm²) or the proton energy averaged over pixels of 4×4 strips (pixel size $\approx 0.8 \times 0.8$ mm²). The image of the phantom projec-tion is clearly seen in the spatial energy distribution. Note that the coloring of the structure in Figure 2 (left) is directly proportional to the energy loss in the aluminum object and thus is proportional to the product of its length and density. Figure 2 (left) thus demonstrates the principle of image for-mation based on the proton-to-proton tracking spatial mea-surements of proton energy loss behind the image object. Future work will be devoted to improve the accuracy of the energy-loss and proton-to-proton tracking measurements.

To better understand the features of the proton transmis-sion images, we performed simulations using the GEANT4 Monte Carlo (MC) toolkit (Agostinelli *et al.*, 2003). Figure 2 (right) shows the measured and simulated angular distribu-tions of protons in two areas or regions of interest (ROIs) in the transmission image: area A contains only protons, which traverse the object in its entirety, while area B contains protons, which miss the object completely. The difference between the distributions was caused by the increased MCS inside the object. The agreement between data (symbols) and simulations (histograms) is good in both areas. Because of this good agreement of MC simulation with the experimental data, in the following studies the GEANT4 MC toolkit was used to simulate pCT projection data and investigate image reconstruction algorithm performance on the data.

Image Reconstruction Algorithms

Equation (8) is the mathematical expression of an image reconstruction problem in pCT, where the projected data $p(.)$ are derived from the measurements of the energy loss of each incident proton and of the lateral and angular displace-ments from its incident direction. Four different categories of image reconstruction algorithms are reviewed below.

Filtered Backprojection Reconstruction Algorithm

The filtered backprojection (FBP) reconstruction algo-rithm was established mathematically for the inversion of the Radon transform, widely used in xCT. A fundamental assumption in the Radon transform is that the integral path S in Equation (8) is a straight line. This assumption could be

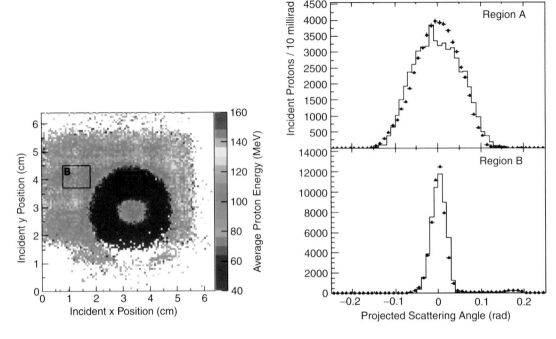

Figure 2 Spatial distribution of the average energy of protons hitting all four SSD planes (left). The image of the object can be clearly seen. Areas A and B are selected to compare with the results from the GEANT4 MC simulation. On the right is shown the comparison between experimental angular distributions (points) and GEANT4 MC simulated histograms) in areas A (through the object) and B (the wax degrader only).

satisfied by approximating the actual proton path inside the body as a line connecting the entry and exit positions (see the line *AB* in Fig. 3). This line is called the straight-line path (SLP). Here we limit our illustration to two dimensions. The third dimension normal to the *t-u* plane is not considered. At the scanning angle of zero degree (i.e., horizontal direction from left to right in Fig. 3), each proton may have a different path inside the body, resulting in a corresponding path line that may not be parallel to the line *AB*. Since we limit our illustration in the *t-u* plane, those lines that are not in the plane will not be considered. After rotating the incident proton beams over 180° counterclockwise, we would collect various path lines, which should span at least over 180° in the *t-u* plane and therefore satisfy the sampling requirement for inversion of the Radon transform. The inversion of these measurements along their SLPs gives the 2D distribution image of $\eta_e(t, u)$.

By interpolating these straight lines into M groups such that in each group the lines are parallel to each other and equally spaced on the *t*-axis, the image reconstruction becomes an inversion of the Radon transform from M projections (Li *et al.*, 2003). The inversion has been solved exactly and efficiently by FBP algorithm. Given the fundamental image formation Equation (8) for pCT, the FBP reconstruction is accurate up to the limit where the actual proton path can be approximated by straight lines. In reality, the approximation is not acceptable because the line could be off from the actual path curve by a few millimeters (see Fig. 3). If the

actual path is not a straight line, inversion of Equation (8) by a FBP-type algorithm remains an open problem to be solved. In the following, we explore alternative algorithms if the actual path curve can be estimated.

Estimation of Proton Path

Using a Gaussian approximation of MCS and a χ^2-formalism, researchers recently showed that it is possible to construct a closed-form expression for the most likely path (MLP) of a proton in a uniform material incorporating the effect of continuous energy loss when the entrance and exit positions and angles are measured by the pCT system of Figure 1 with good accuracy (Williams, 2004). This proton path estimate technique also provides estimates of the probability that the particle deviates from the MLP and could be utilized in image reconstruction (to be discussed later). It was also shown that the MLP predicts the true path to better than 1 mm despite the broadening of a needle beam to a size of several millimeters under typical pCT conditions. This prediction suggested the choice of 1 mm³ voxel size in our numerical calculations above. An example of MLP is shown in Figure 4. Another proton path estimate technique fits the smoothest curve by cubic spline as the proton path (called the cubic spline path—CSP) using the measured entry and exit positions and directions (Li *et al.*, 2006). This CSP does not assume that the object is made from a uniform material, but it also does not consider the physics of MCS; therefore, its

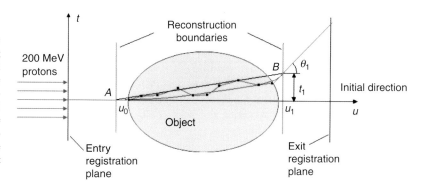

Figure 3 Schematic illustration of proton path for the pCT scanner of Figure 1. The path of protons traveling inside an object is determined by a multitude of individual scattering events leading to a zigzag path (red). Both the position and direction of entry and exit proton are registered. Given the object boundary, the intersecting points A and B of a proton with the object can be obtained. While the intersecting points are sufficient to estimate the straight-line path (black) of the proton, additional knowledge of the entry and exit directions permits estimation of the most likely path (blue line) (Williams, 2004).

accuracy could be potentially compromised. Given the estimated proton path, iterative algorithms are a choice to reconstruct the electron density distribution image $\eta_e(t, u)$. This is because iterative reconstruction algorithms trace the energy loss along the path for an estimate of the projection data and then utilize the difference of the estimated and actual measured projection data to refine the reconstruction iteratively until the difference becomes very small as defined by some criteria (Li *et al.*, 2004).

Algebraic Reconstruction Algorithm

The algebraic reconstruction technique (ART) is a typical example of iterative reconstruction algorithms and was specifically tailored for xCT tomographic image reconstruction. It can be mathematically expressed as:

$$\eta_e^{(n+1)} = \eta_e^{(n)} + \frac{\mathbf{H}^T[p - \mathbf{H}[\eta_e^{(n)}]]}{\mathbf{H}^T[\mathbf{H}[1]]} \tag{17}$$

where $\mathbf{H}[.]$ is the operator for forward projection and T denotes the transpose operation; that is, $\mathbf{H}^T[.]$ is the operator for backward projection. The denominator is the normalization constant relating to the projection operations. Index n is the iteration number. The notation η_e denotes, as already defined, the relative electron density vector to be reconstructed, and p denotes the projection data of the relative electron density derived from the measured energy loss using the right integral of Equation (8). The forward and backward projections are usually performed by weighted summation using the intersecting lengths of each path with the associated voxels on that path in the object. In other

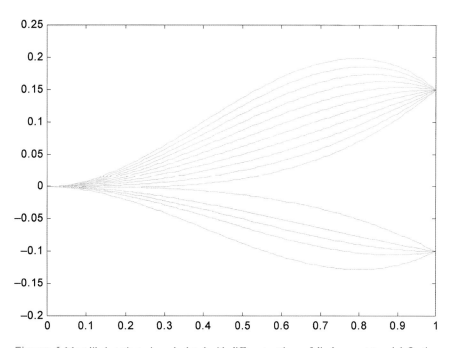

Figure 4 Most likely trajectories calculated with different settings of displacement t_1 and deflection angle θ_1 of Figure 3. The proton entries at $t = 0$. Two exit positions are assumed, where eleven exit directions are measured for one exit position and five directions are measured at another exit position.

words, the value of H_{ij} is the intersecting length of path i with image voxel j. The forward projection operator $\mathbf{H}[\eta_e^{(n)}]$ traces along path i through the nth iterated reconstruction $\eta_e^{(n)}$ in the image domain for an estimate of the projection data p_i. The difference $p_i \sim \mathbf{H}[\eta_e^{(n)}]_i$ is then backprojected by operator $\mathbf{H}^T[.]$ along path i and scaled by the corresponding denominator (or the normalization constant) before being added to the first term $\eta_e^{(n)}$ on the right of Equation (17) to obtain the $(n + 1)$th iterated estimate of all voxels on that path i, that is, those voxel values $\eta_e^{(n+1)}$ on path i. The forward and backward operators along each path i and the weighted update for the next iteration estimation along that path make a beautiful piece of art architecture for this ART algorithm for tomographic imaging. The iterative reconstruction process is terminated when the difference of successively iterated estimates satisfies a criterion (say less than 0.1%) or a preset maximum iteration number is reached.

An MC simulation study reported below shows the difference between FBP and iterative ART algorithms, as well as the difference of using different proton paths of MLP and CSP for the same iterative ART reconstruction algorithm. The phantom used for the pCT scan simulation is shown in Figure 5. For characterization of the spatial resolution, it contains two sets of line patterns (strips) arranged on a circle and embedded within a water phantom with elliptical cross section simulating the human head with a longitudinal diameter of 16 cm, a transverse diameter of 14 cm, and a height of 20 cm. The first set of strips has ICRU-compact bone density (ICRU Report No. 49, 1993), while the second set comprises strips with air density. The line-pair densities of each set of strip patterns are 2.0, 2.5, 3.0, 3.5, 4.0, 4.5, 5.0, and 6.0 line pairs per cm (lp cm^{-1}). The elliptical water phantom is surrounded by a 1-cm-thick shell of ICRU compact bone density, simulating the human skull.

Proton beams of 200 MeV were generated using the GEANT4 (version 6.2) for the pCT scanner of Figure 1, with 50,000 protons randomly distributed along the t-axis over a length of 24 cm at each projection angle. The incident beams were idealized parallel beams on the t-axis. The beams inside the object were idealized fan-type beams confined to the t-u plane for a 2D simulation for simplicity (see Fig. 3). (If a proton is scattered out from the t-u plane by MCS, it is ignored. If these scattered protons are considered, a full 3D reconstruction would be pursued. This is a future research topic.) A total of 180 projections were acquired, evenly distributed over 360°. The dose to the center of the phantom was estimated using the formalism to determine the proton dose to a circular water phantom described previously (Schulte et al., 2004). To adapt this formalism to the present phantom, the bone shell was converted to a shell of 1.9 cm water-equivalent thickness (WET), and the resulting uniform ellipse (ignoring inserts) was converted to a circular disk of identical area with a WET of 8.8 cm and a height of 1 mm. The dose at the center of the disk resulting from

the 180 projections with 50,000 protons per projection was calculated to be 3.5 mGy. The relevant entry and exit data of each proton, including the position in the (t, u) entry plane ($u = 0$ cm), exit energy and position in the (t, u) exit plane ($u = 30$ cm), and exit direction projected onto the (t, u) plane (see Fig. 3), were stored in the computer. The position and direction data were used to calculate the path estimates for each proton within a "virtual" circular object boundary of 22 cm diameter. Due to MCS, the exiting protons were no longer confined to the t-u plane. In order to limit the reconstruction to a 2D case, the coordinate in the direction vertical to the t-u plane was set to zero, that is, confining the exit protons in the t-u plane and ignoring those protons which were scattered out the t-u plane. The energy information for each proton was used to compute the energy lost in the object as well as the integrated relative electron density along each proton path by the use of Equation (8).

By the use of the FBP algorithm, the simulated pCT data of the elliptical phantom were first interpolated so that all the approximated SLPs were sampled into 180 parallel-beam projections evenly spaced over 360°. These interpolated data were then reconstructed by the FBP algorithm with the Ramp filter at the Nyquist cut-off frequency. The reconstructed image is shown on the top left of Figure 5. By the use of the iterative ART algorithm, three kinds of estimated proton paths were considered for the forward- and backward-projection operators. The first kind was the approximated SLPs of the 180 projections over 360° without the interpolation. The ART reconstruction is shown on the top right of Figure 5. The second kind was the estimated CSPs, and the reconstructed image is shown in the middle left of Figure 5. The third kind was the estimated MLPs assuming a uniform medium of water, and the reconstructed image is shown on the middle right of Figure 5.

A pixel size of 0.25 mm was used for all the reconstructions. The initial image for ART algorithm was set to be zero, and satisfactory reconstructions were obtained after 120 iterations in all cases. It is seen that the SLP-based reconstruction (by either FBP or ART algorithms) shows a considerable loss of spatial resolution, with a resolution of about 2.5 lp cm^{-1} for the air density pattern and about 2 lp cm^{-1} for the bone density pattern. The FBP reconstruction seems better than that of ART with SLPs. This difference is due to different algorithm performances. Due to the mismatch of assumed SLPs to the true proton paths, the ART may need much more iterations to achieve a good reconstruction, while FBP does not have this convergence problem. In comparison, tracing the proton paths with CSP or MLP for the ART reconstruction demonstrates observable improvement (over the SLP-based reconstructions) in spatial resolution to about 5.0 and 4.5 lp cm^{-1} for the air density pattern and the bone density patterns, respectively. The ART reconstruction with either the CSP estimate or the MLP estimate seems to generate similar image quality. This is understandable because the phantom is made mostly by water and the true proton path is

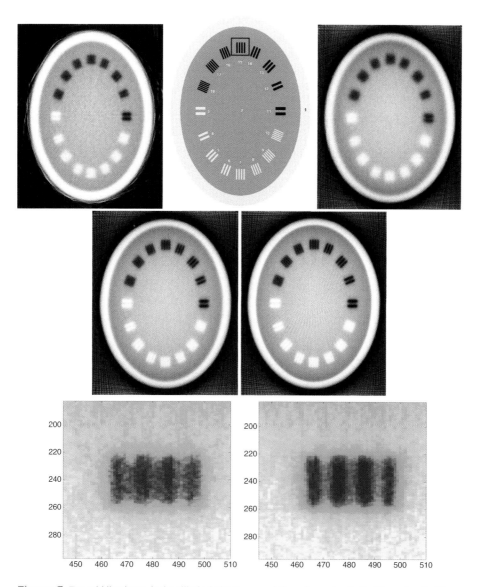

Figure 5 Top middle picture is the elliptical phantom consisting of an outer shell of bone density (1), an elliptical interior of water density (2), and two sets of strip patterns with either bone density (white) or air density (black). The strip densities of the patterns (listed by number) are: 2 lp cm⁻¹ (3, 11), 2.5 lp cm⁻¹ (4, 12), 3 lp cm⁻¹ (5, 13), 3.5 lp cm⁻¹ (6, 14), 4 lp cm⁻¹ (7, 15), 4.5 lp cm⁻¹ (8, 16), 5 lp cm⁻¹ (9, 17), and 6 lp cm⁻¹ (10, 18). The top right picture shows the FBP result after the SLPs were interpolated onto regular grids in sinogram space. The top right picture shows the ART result using the SLPs. Middle row pictures are the ART results by tracing the CSPs (left) and MLPs (right), respectively. Bottom pictures are the zoomed results of the strips of #15 in the ART results of the middle row. A square box indicates the strips of #15 in the phantom.

expected to be smooth except for small changes around the air and bone strips. However, some small difference can be seen from their zoomed strips on the bottom of Figure 5.

The ART algorithm seeks iteratively a solution that matches the estimated projection data (by the forward projection operator) with the measured data until a preset criterion is satisfied or a preset maximum iteration number is reached. It does not consider the data statistics. Statistical model-based image reconstruction algorithms model the data statistics and incorporate any other available constraint for a statistically opti-

mal solution (Liang *et al.*, 1989). This kind of statistics-based image reconstruction algorithms has not yet been explored for the pCT data of Figure 1. An example of statistics-based image reconstruction algorithms is given below.

Penalized Maximum Likelihood Reconstruction Algorithm

Given the approximated Gaussian distribution of energy loss due to the inelastic collision with atomic electrons (see the sections Interactions of Protons with Atomic Components and Energy-Loss Straggling), a penalized weighted least-squares (PWLS) approach would be a choice as a statistical model-based image reconstruction algorithm. The PWLS approach aims to minimize the cost function of

$$\Phi(\eta) = (p - H\eta)^T \Sigma^{-1}(p - H\eta) + \alpha Q(\eta) \qquad (18)$$

where η represents η_e and Σ is a diagonal matrix, with the diagonal value being the corresponding variance of a datum. The first term in Equation (18) is the weighted least-squares (WLS) measure of $\Phi(\eta) = (p - H\eta)^T \Sigma^{-1}(p - H\eta)$, which models the data statistics. The second term is a penalty that incorporates any other available constraint, where α is a smoothing parameter that controls the degree of agreement between the estimated and the measured data. The penalty is usually chosen as a quadratic form of

$$Q(\eta) = \eta^T Q \eta = \frac{1}{2} \sum_j \sum_{m \in N_j} w_{jm}(\eta_j - \eta_m)^2 \qquad (19)$$

where index j runs over all image elements in the image domain and, N_j represents the set of eight neighbors of the jth image pixel in two dimensions. In the 2D case, the parameter w_{jm} is equal to 1 for the vertical and horizontal first-order neighbors and 1/2 for the diagonal (second-order) neighbors. The task for PWLS image reconstruction is to estimate the electron density distribution map $\eta(.)$ from the derived measurements or projection data $p(.)$:

$$\eta = \arg \min_{n \geq 0} \Phi(\eta). \qquad (20)$$

Many numerical methods can be employed to calculate iteratively the solution of Equation (20). One would be the conjugate gradient method (Luenberger, 1984). A simple numerical method could be the Gauss-Seidel (GS) update strategy (Sauer and Bouman, 1993) or the well-known iterated conditional modes (ICM) strategy. A sophisticated iterative expectation maximization (EM) update strategy could be another choice for the data of Gaussian distribution (Dempster et al., 1977; Liang and Ye, 1994).

In the above statistical model-based image reconstruction, the proton path is estimated prior to the reconstruction. This implementation could be modified by adding an update of the proton path estimation into each iterative cycle of image reconstruction. In other words, after the nth iteration, we would have obtained both $\eta^{(n)}$ and $S^{(n)}$, where the initial $\eta^{(0)}$ is chosen as uniform and $S^{(0)}$ is given by the CSP or MLP estimate. From the current ($\eta^{(n)}$, $S^{(n)}$), the update for $S^{(n+1)}$ can be performed by, for example, by MC simulation. From the updated $S^{(n+1)}$ and current $\eta^{(n)}$, the forward and backward projection operators can be applied to obtain the update $\eta^{(n+1)}$. This interleaved approach had been explored for simultaneous image reconstruction and regions of interest (ROI) segmentation (Liang et al., 1991). In addition to the above four different categories of image reconstruction algorithms of (1) FBP with interpolated SLPs, (2) iterative ART, (3) statistics-based minimization, and (4) interleaved update of proton path and electron density distribution map, there may be other alternatives. One can be a joint minimization for both proton path and electron density distribution map.

Discussion and Conclusions

Proton radiation therapy is one of the most precise forms of noninvasive image-guided cancer therapy. At present, the potential of proton therapy cannot be fully exploited because the conversion of HU values, measured with xCT, to relative electron density values is not always accurate (Schaffner and Pedroni, 1998). The resulting range uncertainty is usually quoted to be between 3 and 10 mm, or 3% of the proton range in tissue, depending on the anatomical region treated and the penetration depth of the proton beam (Schneider and Pedroni, 1998). In the studies (Satogata et al., 2003; Schulte et al., 2005), we have explored the principal limitations of pCT image contrast (or density resolution) and spatial resolution due to energy-loss straggling and MCS in the body. Some results were reviewed in the section Image Formation Principles of Proton Computed Tomography. By use of the pCT system design of Figure 1, one may be able to reduce the range error in proton treatment planning and delivery to less than 3 mm without exceeding practical dose limits. Our results confirmed this expectation that with a dose of about 10 mGy, which is clinically acceptable, the desired density resolution of 1% in the center of a cylindrical object of 20 cm and the desired spatial resolution of 1 mm can, in principle, be achieved. This indicates the potential of pCT to improve current xCT-based treatment planning for proton therapy.

The use of cone beam xCT scanners utilizing the rotating gantry of a linear accelerator in the treatment room has become a major innovation for alignment verification and image-guided X-ray photon radiation therapy in recent years (Jaffray et al., 2002; Seppi et al., 2003). Patient exposure is an important consideration in this new technology (Groh et al., 2002). Both therapeutic megavoltage (MeV) radiation and kilovoltage (keV) X-ray tubes mounted on the accelerator gantry in combination with flat-panel imaging systems have been tested. Doses required to distinguish soft tissue structures in cylindrical phantoms are of the order of 1 cGy (10 mGy) for keV systems but are of one order of magnitude higher for MeV systems (due to the low-detection efficiency of photon detectors in the MeV energy range) (Groh et al., 2002). According to our results, the doses required for soft tissue density resolution with pCT will be similar to those for keV xCT. Proton CT, however, would have the advantage of using the same radiation modality for both treatment and imaging.

So far we have considered multiple Coulomb scatter (MCS) and energy-loss straggling as the only uncertainty components contributing to the density and spatial resolutions, thus neglecting external noise sources such as the momentum spread of the proton accelerator and the uncertainty of the energy detector. Some additional spread may be introduced by beam line detectors such as fluence and beam centering monitors. These effects seem small but need to be investigated. Our dose estimate did not take into account the loss of protons by nuclear interactions. In order to make up for these losses, one would need to increase the dose by corresponding amounts. The additional dose needed may be up to ~30% from what we have estimated if objects of 30 g cm^{-2} (equivalent to 30 cm of water) have to be penetrated and less for smaller objects. Thus the dose needed to reach 1% density resolution would increase from 10 mGy to 13% more for thick objects.

In Equation (8), which is central to the reconstruction of pCT images, we have replaced the mean excitation potential $l(r)$ of the material traversed with that of water as a tissue substitute. This simplification may lead to systematic errors in the estimation of the line integral of the relative electronic density when the object contains materials with mean excitation potentials very different from that of water. Mean excitation potentials of various tissues have been published by the ICRU (1989) and are available from the NIST material database (National Institute for Standards and Technology, Material Composition database, www.physics.nist.gov/cgi-bin/Star/compos.pl?ap). For example, for adipose tissue, muscle tissue, and compact bone, the mean excitation potentials are 63.2 eV, 74.7 eV, and 91.9 eV, respectively, while the value for water is 75 eV. Corresponding errors in the stopping power (dE/dx) resulting from using the water value instead of the true tissue-specific value can be calculated to be −2% for adipose tissue and +2% for compact bone, while for muscle tissue the error is practically zero (ICRU, 1993). This means that if the tissue evaluated with pCT consisted entirely of fat or bone, an additional density error of ±2% would be introduced. However, as most body sections contain a mixture of these tissues, the actual systematic error due to the use of the mean excitation potential for water will be smaller than 2%.

In inverting the path integral of Equation (8) for pCT, we have concluded that the approximation of the straight-line path (SLP) is not acceptable and that the proton path must be estimated. Two estimated proton paths of most likely path (MLP) and cubic spline path (CSP) have been implemented with similar improvement over the SLP. By carefully inspecting the ART reconstructed images from MLP and CSP, the result from MLP seems slightly better than that from CSP. This is assumed due to the consideration of the MCS physics in MLP estimation because CSP does not consider the internal interactions, except for the entry and exit positions and directions. This leads to the hypothesis

that tracing the proton path in a nonuniform media such as the human body would further improve the pCT reconstruction of Figure 5.

In addition to the possible improvement by tracing the proton path through the patient-specific tissue structure, another possible improvement may be obtained by statistical model-based image reconstruction. For example, for the PWLS reconstruction algorithm, the data variance contains the ground truth of the energy-loss straggling via Equation (9) when the energy loss is less than 20%. This can be further refined for cases of energy losses larger than 20% of the initial energy. For these cases, the theory of Tschalar (1968) would provide a more accurate description of the process than the Gaussian distribution. The variance of the energy-loss distribution in Tschalar's theory can be expressed by the differential equation as:

$$\frac{d}{dx}\sigma_T^2(x) = \kappa_2(x) - 2\left(\frac{d}{dE}\kappa_1(E(x))\right)\sigma_T^2(x) \qquad (21)$$

$$+ \text{ higher order terms}$$

where

$$\kappa_2(x) = \eta_e K \frac{1 - 1/2 \cdot \beta^2(E(E_{in,x}))}{1 - \beta^2(E(E_{in,x}))} \qquad (22)$$

and $\kappa_1(E(x))$ is identical to the stopping power given by the Bethe Bloch formula (5), and the higher-order terms contain higher-order derivations of $\kappa_1(E(x))$ with respect to energy.

In conclusion, pCT has a great clinical potential to improve the utility of current proton beam therapy practice. Despite several challenges in advancing pCT toward clinical use, such as hardware construction and fast image reconstruction development, we have performed several studies to demonstrate the pCT potential. One is the pCT design study (Schulte et al., 2004), which describes the needed hardware components to achieve the desired performance of pCT for proton therapy. The second one is the analysis of image contrast (or density resolution), spatial resolution, and dosage for the pCT design of Figure 1 (Satogata et al., 2003; Schulte et al., 2005). The third one is the pCT instrumentation progress (Sadrozinski et al., 2003). The last one is our development of sophisticated image reconstruction algorithms, which consider the data statistics and object-specific proton paths (Li et al., 2003, 2004, 2006). By these studies, we can conclude that a density resolution of 1 to 2% and a range uncertainty of the same order of magnitude (i.e., of 1 mm order) seem possible with proton doses of 10 mGy or less, which is comparable to doses stated for cone beam xCT with keV X-ray beams and an order of magnitude less than the dose required to resolve soft tissues with megavoltage X-ray photon radiation.

Acknowledgments

This work was supported in part by the NIH National Cancer Institute under Grant No. CA082402. The authors would like to thank all colleagues (S. Peggs, K. Mueller, A. Wroe) of the pCT collaboration for their encouragement and invaluable advice.

References

Agostinelli, S., Allison, J., Amako, K., Apostolakis, J., Araujo, H., Arce, P., Asai, M., Axen, D., Banerjee, S., and Barrand, G. 2003. GEANT4—a simulation toolkit. *Nucl. Instrum. Meth. Phys. Res. A 506*:250–303.

Bichsel, H., Groom, D.E., and Klein, S.R. 1972. *Passage of Charged Particles through Matter*. 42:188–189. New York: McGraw-Hill. (Coordinating Editor: D.E. Gray; American Institute of Physics Handbook).

Bohr, N. 1948. The penetration of atomic particles through matter. *K. Dan. Vidensk. Selsk, Mat. Fys. Med. 18*:1.

Cormack, A.M., and Koehler, A.M. 1976. Quantitative proton tomography: preliminary experiments. *Phys. Med. Biol. 21*:560–569.

Dempster, A., Laird, N., and Rubin, D. 1977. Maximum likelihood from incomplete data via the EM algorithm. *J. R. Stat. Soc. 39B*:1–38.

Groh, B.A., Siewerdsen, J.H., Drake, D.G., Wong, J.W., and Jaffray, D.A. 2002. A performance comparison of flat-panel imager-based MV and kV cone-beam CT. *Med. Phys. 29*:967–975.

Hanson, K.M., Bradbury, J.N., Cannon, T.M., Hutson, R.L., Laubacher, D.B., Macek, R.J., Paciotti, M.A., and Taylor, C.A. 1981. Computed tomography using proton energy loss. *Phys. Med. Biol. 26*:965–983.

Hanson, K.M., Bradbury, J.N., Koeppe, R.A., Macek, R.J., Machen, D.R., Morgado, R., Paciotti, M.A., Sandford, S.A., and Steward, V.W. 1982. Proton computed tomography of human specimens. *Phys. Med. Biol. 27*:25–36.

ICRU Report No. 44. 1989. *Tissue Substitutes in Radiation Dosimetry and Measurements*. International Commission on Radiation Units and Measurements, Bethesda, MD.

ICRU Report No. 49. 1993. *Stopping Powers and Ranges for Protons and Alpha Particles*. International Commission on Radiation Units and Measurements, Bethesda, MD.

Jaffray, D.A., Siewerdsen, J.H., Wong, J.W., and Martinez, A.A. 2002. Flat-panel cone-beam computed tomography for image-guided radiation therapy. *Int. J. Radiat. Oncol. Biol. Phys. 53*:1337–1349.

Janni, J.F. 1982. Proton range-energy tables. *Atomic Data and Nuclear Data Tables 27*:212–245.

Koehler, A.M. 1968. Proton radiography. *Science 160*:303–304.

Koehler, A.M., and Steward, V.W. 1974. Proton radiographic detection of strokes. *Nature 245*:38–40.

Leo, W.R. 1994. *Techniques for Nuclear and Particle Physics Experiments*. Berlin: Springer Verlag, p. 21.

Li, T., and Liang, Z. 2004. Reconstruction with most likely trajectory for proton computed tomography. *SPIE Medical Imaging: Image Processing 5370*:2067–2074.

Li, T., Liang, Z., Mueller, K., Heimann, J., Johnson, L.R., Sadrozinski, H.F.-W., Seiden, A., Williams, D.C., Zhang, L., Peggs, S., Satogata, T.J., Bashkirov, V., and Schulte, R.W. 2003. Reconstruction for proton computed tomography: a Monte Carlo study. *Conference Record of IEEE Nuclear Science Symposium and Medical Imaging Conference 5*, in CD-ROM (IEEE Publication).

Li, T., Liang, Z., Singanallur, J., Satogata, T.J., Williams, D.C., and Schulte R.W. 2006. Reconstruction for proton computed tomography by tracing proton trajectories—a Monte Carlo study. *Med. Phys. 33*:699–706.

Liang, Z., Jaszczak, R.J., and Greer, K.L. 1989. On Bayesian image reconstruction from projections: uniform and non-uniform *a priori* source information. *IEEE Trans. Med. Imag. 8*:227–235.

Liang, Z., Jaszczak, R.J., and Coleman, E.R. 1991. On reconstruction and segmentation of piecewise continuous images. *Inform. Proc. Med. Imag. 12*:94–104.

Liang, Z., and Ye, J. 1994. Reconstruction of object-specific attenuation map for quantitative SPECT. *Conference Record of IEEE Nuclear Science Symposium and Medical Imaging Conference 2*:1231–1235 (IEEE Publication).

Luenberger, D.G. 1984. *Linear and Nonlinear Programming*. Addison-Wesley, Reading, MA.

Sadrozinski, H.F.-W., Bashkirov, V., Bruzzi, M., Johnson, L.R., Keeney, B., Ross, G., Schulte, R.W., Seiden, A., Shahnazi, K., Williams, D.C., and Zhang, L. 2003. Issues in proton computed tomography. *Nucl. Instrum. Methods Phys. Res. A. 511*:275–281.

Satogata, T.J., Sadrozinski, H.F.-W., Dilmanian, A., Peggs, S., and Ruggiero, A. 2003. Dose/Sensitivity in Proton Computed Tomography. *Conference Record of IEEE Nuclear Science Symposium and Medical Imaging Conference 5*, in CD-ROM (IEEE Publication).

Sauer, K., and Bouman, C. 1993. A local update strategy for iterative reconstruction form projections. *IEEE Trans. Sig. Proc. 41*:534–548.

Schaffner, B., and Pedroni, E. 1998. The precision of proton range calculations in proton radiotherapy treatment planning: experimental verification of the relation between CT-HU and proton stopping power. *Phys. Med. Biol. 43*:1579–1592.

Schneider, U., and Pedroni, E. 1994. Multiple Coulomb scattering and spatial resolution in proton radiography. *Med. Phys. 21*:1657–1663.

Schneider, U., Besserer, J., Pemler, P., Dellert, M., Moosburger, M., Pedroni, E., and Kaser-Hotz, B. 2004. First proton radiography of an animal patient. *Med. Phys. 31*:1046–1051.

Schulte, R.W., Bashkirov, V., Li, T., Liang, Z., Mueller, K., Heimann, J., Johnson, L.R., Keeney, B., Sadrozinski, H.F.-W., Seiden, A., Williams, D.C., Zhang, L., Li, Z., Peggs, S., Satogata, T.J., and Woody, C. 2004. Conceptual design of a proton computed tomography system for applications in proton radiation therapy. *IEEE Trans. Nucl. Sci. 51*:866–872.

Schulte, R.W., Bashkirov, V., Klock, M., Li, T., Wroe, A., Evseev, I., Williams, D.C., and Satogata, T.J. 2005. Density resolution of proton computed tomography. *Med. Phys. 32*:1035–1046.

Seppi, E.J., Munro, P., Johnsen, S.W., Shapiro, E.G., Tognina, C., Jones, D., Pavkovich, J.M., Webb, C., Mollov, I., Partain, L.D., and Colbeth, R.E. 2003. Megavoltage cone-beam computed tomography using a high-efficiency image receptor. *Int. J. Radiat. Oncol. Biol. Phys. 55*:793–803.

Tschalar, C. 1968a. Straggling distributions of large energy losses. *Nucl. Instrum. Methods 61*:141–156.

Tschalar, C. 1968b. Straggling distributions of extremely large energy losses. *Nucl. Instrum. Methods 64*:237–243.

Williams, D.C. 2004. The most likely path of an energetic charged particle through a uniform medium. *Phys. Med. Biol. 49*:2899–2911.

2

Multidetector Computed Tomography

James G. Ravenel

Introduction

For the past two decades, computed tomography (CT) has served as the workhorse of anatomical imaging for the detection, staging, and follow-up of neoplasms. Rapid improvements in technology have occurred more recently with the development of multidetector computed tomography (MDCT) scanners. These scanners have the ability to provide true isotropic data, allowing for exquisite anatomic detail in any plane necessary to display the findings to best clinical advantage. Even as molecular diagnosis and imaging become more engrained, MDCT will be needed to place the findings in anatomic context, as can be seen with the current generation of combined positron emission tomography (PET) with MDCT.

Evolution of Computed Tomography

The guiding principle of CT is the reconstruction of many two-dimensional X-ray beams to create an image of a three-dimensional object. In the 1910s the foundations for image reconstruction were first addressed by an Austrian mathematics professor named Johann Radon. He was the first to present mathematical equations to convert a number of two-dimensional projections into a three-dimensional object, but it was not until the 1960s that Allan Cormack at Tufts University modified equations, taking into account tissue inhomogeneities (Cormack, 1963). While this information was necessary for

the development of CT, it is unclear what influence these contributions had on the invention of CT by Godfrey Hounsfield at EMI Central Research laboratory in 1972. The first clinical scanner was limited to imaging the head (Ambrose and Hounsfield, 1973). This first scanner had a single detector to acquire information, and due to the extremely slow rotation (requiring 4½ min rotation time for each axial image), only motionless structures could be imaged. Subsequently, additional detectors were added, making the system more efficient, and technology progressed rapidly such that tube rotation time was decreased to 18 sec by 1975, opening up the technology to imaging the chest, abdomen, and pelvis (Evens, 1976). Scanners from this era still required simultaneous rotation of both the X-ray tube and detectors. In the end, the fourth generation of axial CT scanners had a complete ring of detectors in the gantry so that only the X-ray rotated. However, the scan mode was still limited to a "step-and-shoot" axial approach that required each image to be acquired individually rather than the continuous approach to come with helical scanners. Thus, the entire chest or abdomen had to be collected over several breaths.

The next major development took place with the creation of slip-ring technology. This development, along with high-power X-ray tubes and new computer algorithms to interpolate complex nonlinear data, allowed for continuous data acquisition along the z-(head to toe) axis (Kalender *et al.*, 1990). These so-called helical or spiral scanners were designed so that the patient could pass through the CT gantry as the data were being collected; therefore, an acquisition of the entire thorax or abdomen could be obtained in a single breath hold. While this advance was clearly revolutionary, the available tube speed, collimation, and detector efficiency limited the applications, particularly as they applied to multiplanar and three-dimensional images. This problem was solved with the development of multislice scanners that provided an array of detectors with variable width and improved resolution along the z-axis. The first iteration, dual-slice scanners, appeared in 1993, and by 1998 the predominant scanner could acquire four slices (usually 2.5 or 5 mm) simultaneously. At the same time, gantry rotation times of 0.5 sec allowed for more rapid scanning. However, there was still a trade-off between speed and z-axis resolution. It was not until the development of 16-detector array scanners that isotropic volumes with sub-millimeter spatial resolution could be realized (Flohr et al., 2005). To compare speeds, a single-slice helical scanner with a rotation time of 1 sec and 10 mm collimation would take 30 to 40 sec (a difficult breath hold even for healthy individuals) to cover the entire thorax, whereas a 16-slice scanner with a rotation time of 0.5 sec and 1.25 mm collimation could scan the same volume in 10 sec or less. Today, multidetector CT is the standard at almost all institutions with 64-detector array scanners with 0.625–0.75 mm collimation as the state-of-the-art. Future developments are less clear. Are 64-detector arrays sufficient? Are 256-detector arrays necessary? Is a true isotropic system with rotating flat panels feasible or clinically useful? For the practice of cancer imaging, future developments may not be critical in clinical practice but may be quite valuable for small-animal imaging in the laboratory.

Basic Physics of Multidetector Computed Tomography and Image Quality

Regardless of scanner type, the fundamental approach of CT is to create a map of attenuation measurements through a given thickness (slice) of tissue. Tissue attenuation is based on the amount of the X-ray beams that reach the detector (ray sum). Tissue can then be broken up into defined volume elements (voxels); the image reconstruction process can calculate the attenuation average based on the ray sums that intersect each individual voxel. In CT, this is generally performed by a process called filtered backprojection. In essence, ray sums are collected into groups (which may be as many as 500 to 1000) to create a single projection, and each voxel is viewed from many different directions. Backprojection is then the process of adding the value of each ray back through the reconstruction matrix, and a mathematical filter smoothes out the blurriness (Mahesh, 2002). The specific attenuation value is based on the density of the tissue and is termed the Hounsfield Unit (HU). An HU of zero is equal to water, and attenuation values can then be compared to water as either more dense (> 0) or less dense (< 0). The actual HU

of any given tissue will vary depending on the manufacturer and scan settings.

The last step is to display the image in shades of gray depending on the HU. The image itself can have different appearances depending on the window and level settings. The level expresses the midpoint of the window and is displayed as gray. The window then accounts for the number of shades of gray, and everything outside the bottom of the window is displayed as black, whereas everything above the window is displayed as white. A typical abdominal window and level setting is 400 and 40, meaning the shades of gray are displayed from −160 to 240 and all voxels below −160 are displayed as black and those above 240 are displayed as white. Other typically viewed window and level settings include lung windows (W/L 1500/−600) and bone windows (W/L 1600/400). Tissue contrast can be enhanced by narrowing the window and is sometimes referred to as a liver window. Similarly, the brain is usually viewed with a narrow window to enhance the contrast between gray and white matter.

For a CT, the in-plane spatial resolution is essentially fixed and independent of radiographic technique factors; however, other settings, such as tube voltage (kilovoltage peak-kVp), tube current (milliamperes per second-mAs), and pitch, will impact image quality, particularly contrast and noise. The tube voltage, tube current, and pitch can all be set at the CT console and individualized for a given patient. In general, CT excels at low-contrast resolution and can be enhanced by modifying the display contrast of CT images by adjusting the display window and level settings interactively at a workstation (e.g., liver window). As a result, lesion detection in CT images is generally not limited because of inadequate image contrast. Most manufacturers set kVp at 120 with an available range from 80 to 140. Increasing kVp will increase the mean photon energy while at the same time reducing image contrast.

Tube current accounts for the number of X-rays emitted passing through the subject. Noise or quantum mottle is a reflection of the number of X-rays that reach the detector; the fewer the rays, the greater the graininess or mottle of the image. At a given kV and mA, noise will vary in different parts of the body, increasing in conspicuity in areas of increased soft tissue such that more noise will be visible in a region of the shoulder girdle when compared to the mid-thorax. Thus, image mottle can be reduced by increasing mAs, kV, and slice thickness, and can be minimized by the use of various reconstruction filters.

Image quality, then, depends on the contrast-to-noise ratio (CNR), and the choice of technique factors (kVp and mAs) will therefore affect both the image contrast and the level of mottle (noise). Because CT is most limited by noise, CNR may be most easily adjusted by modifying the mAs, decreasing noise by increasing mAs. At a fixed X-ray tube voltage, doubling the mAs will increase image CNR by 41.2% (Huda et al., 2002). Increasing the X-ray tube voltage will reduce image contrast because of the increase in average photon energy and will also reduce mottle due to the increased number of photons transmitted through the patient. In CT, the reduction in contrast with increasing kVp is generally accompanied by a greater reduction in image noise. Low-density structures (soft tissue and fat) benefit to a greater extent from increasing kVp than high-density structures (bone or iodinated contrast), as increasing the photon energy for high-density materials results in a much greater loss of contrast.

The concept of pitch was relatively simple for single-slice CT and defined as the beam width in millimeters (W) divided by the distance traveled by the table in a single gantry rotation (T) or T/W. With the development of MDCT, the concept of pitch becomes more difficult and is compounded by different manufacturers using different definitions. Because pitch now has a component of detector width and detector number, it is best defined by detector pitch, the detector width (D) divided by distance travelled (T), and the beam pitch reflects the detector pitch divided by the number of detectors (Mahesh *et al.*, 2001). The higher the pitch, the more rapidly the patient passes through the scanner. Thus, there is a trade-off between pitch and noise. The choice of pitch also influences the *z*-axis resolution that can be achieved, with higher PR values reducing spatial resolution performance.

Artifacts in Multidetector Computed Tomography

Clearly, the image quality of MDCT is an advance over earlier technology, and many of the difficulties associated with SDCT are mitigated by MDCT. Nevertheless, it remains important to be aware that potential artifacts may impact diagnostic performance. These include physic-based (beam hardening and partial volume effects), patient-based (metallic materials and motion), and scanner-based artifacts (Barrett and Keat, 2004).

Beam Hardening

Because the X-ray beam is made up of an array of photon energies, as the beam passes through a patient the lower energy photons will be absorbed more rapidly resulting in a higher energy or "harder" beam. This results in two important changes. First, because the beam reaching the detector is of higher energy than expected, the resulting attenuation values differ from actual attenuation. Second, streaks may run across the image depending on the attenuation of the object through which the beam passes. Examples are most readily apparent when the beam passes through dense contrast, osseous structures, and metallic prostheses. With current scanners, these artifacts are minimized by beam filtration, which removes some of the low-energy beams before reaching the

patient, calibration of detectors, and reconstruction algorithms designed to remove the streak effects.

Partial Volume

There are two separate partial-volume effects one should be aware of: (1) partial-volume averaging and (2) artifacts of an off-axis object being partial, detected by the diverging photon beam. The first occurs due to the averaging of all attenuation values with a voxel. Its practical effect is to make attenuation measurements of small objects unreliable. For example, a small cyst in the liver may be averaged with normal liver parenchyma, resulting in a higher attenuation value for the lesion and possibly misclassification as a non-cyst. The second artifact may result from shading artifacts around the intervening object. Both of these effects can be minimized by using thin collimation.

Metallic Materials

As already discussed, metallic materials, including orthopedic prostheses, spinal fusion hardware, and pacemakers, will all harden the X-ray beam and can compound partial-volume effects. Strategies for reducing this artifact include excluding the object from the scan by collimation, increasing kV, and using thin collimation. Software corrections for beam hardening are also effective at reducing artifacts from metallic objects.

Patient Motion

Patient motion and/or breathing is less of a problem with rapid scan times, but in some cases is unavoidable. The effect of this motion is to cause misregistration of anatomic structures and create blurring of the image. Patient preparation, including putting the patient at ease, practicing breath-holding, and immobilization and sedation as needed can minimize motion, as can decreasing scan time through tube rotation or limiting the area of scanning.

Helical Artifacts

With MDCT, the interpolation of helical data as it is reconstructed into an axial image will affect the appearance of anatomic structures and can occasionally be mistaken for disease. This problem is more pronounced in regions where the anatomy changes rapidly (ex. dome of liver) and is caused by the inherent difficulties of approximating the edges of tissues with different attenuation. Similarly, the cone beam artifact that may result in partial-volume effects can also occur and is more pronounced with increasing detector rows. These effects are limited in practice by using different reconstruction techniques. With multiplanar imaging, artifacts may occur along the *z*-axis, including stair-step artifact and zebra artifact. These bands or stripes result from the helical interpolation and are more severe with thick collimation and nonoverlapping slices. With overlapping thin collimation and 16- or 64-detector row scanners, these are now relatively uncommon in clinical practice.

Radiation Dose Considerations

The patient dose for any CT study is directly proportional to the selected mAs value and the scan length. For example, increasing the mAs or the scan length by 50% will increase the patient effective dose by 50%. For single body examinations, routine CT application doses are typically between 4 and 6 mSv in the chest and abdomen, or approximately double the natural background radiation dose received by an individual in the United States in one year (3 mSv) (Huda et al., 2002). Current estimates are that an effective dose of 5 mSv (500 mrem) corresponds to a risk of developing a fatal cancer of 2.5 per 10,000 (ICRP report, 1991), and it is generally accepted that radiation risks at CT doses do truly exist and are not based solely on extrapolation from higher doses (Pierce and Preston, 2000). While this may be a moot issue for an older patient with cancer, even a single CT of the thorax may increase the lifetime risk for developing breast cancer in females under the age of 20. For example, a breast-absorbed dose of 50 mSv would result in a relative risk of 1.68 for the development of breast cancer by age 35 (Hurwitz et al., 2006). Absorbed breast doses in chest CT range from 17 to 66 mSv, depending on technique factors (Hurwitz et al., 2006; Hohl et al., 2006).

The ability to generate thinner images over a greater region has implications for the radiation dose imparted to the patient. As noise increases with thinner collimation, mA is usually increased to provide the same image quality as would be found at thicker collimation. Furthermore, multiphasic examinations (e.g., arterial and portal venous phase liver) of the abdomen are sometimes necessary for optimal lesion detection. Fortunately, the addition of detector elements (16- or 64-slice) improves tube output utilization, compared with 4-slice systems, and reduces the radiation dose that does not contribute to the final image (Flohr et al., 2002).

Several strategies are available to reduce radiation dose. The most important is to closely monitor technique factors and appropriately lower the mA to the lowest possible setting to maintain good image quality. In general, this should be lower than the manufacturer's settings and adapted for the size of the patient and diagnostic information required. Use of a soft tissue or other noise reduction filters also helps to reduce the conspicuity of mottle in low-dose CT examinations. In general, increasing pitch will decrease radiation dose; however, the relationship of pitch ratio to dose is much more complex with MDCT than with single-slice helical scanners. Moreover, when changing pitch on MDCT, care

must be exercised because on some systems a change in pitch is accompanied by an automatic proportional increase in tube current to maintain image quality and thus does not truly change dose (Mahesh et al., 2001).

The current generation of MDCT scanners is available with various forms of tube current modulation. Akin to automatic exposure control in conventional radiography, the CT projection radiograph used for procedure planning is also used with the computer to take an attenuation-based measurement of the variability to approximate the number of X-rays reaching the detector. Two forms of tube current modulation are used; angular and longitudinal (McCollugh et al., 2006). Angular (x- and y-axis) tube current modulation is based on changing tube current as the tube rotates around the patient. By doing so, the number of photons is adjusted to ensure that a relatively similar number of photons reach the detector in all projections. Using the shoulder girdle as an example, we see that many fewer photons are required in the generally antero-posterior projection relative to the lateral projection to maintain the same image quality. Longitudinal (z-axis) tube current modulation allows for variation of tube current along the long axis of the patient. Again using the shoulder girdle as an example, we find that the mA to maintain image quality and CNR at that location is much greater than at mid-thorax to attain the same image quality. These dose-modulation features can be used alone (either angular or longitudinal) or together. It is still incumbent on the imager to set the amount of noise he or she feels is acceptable to maintain image and diagnostic quality. Based on the amount of noise accepted and the maximum mA selected, tube current is then adapted on the fly by the computer such that mA is changed to allow the same number of photons to reach the detector for each slice. Thus, these automated systems allow for dose reduction up to 20–50% without compromising overall image quality (McCullough et al., 2006).

Electrocardiogram-Gated Multidetector Computed Tomography

Although initially available on 4-slice scanners, state-of-the-art ECG-gated CT is performed with 64-slice CT scanners and provides an unmatched combination of speed and spatial resolution for noninvasive cardiac imaging. Two ECG-gating techniques are available. Prospective gating allows the selection of a single point (often diastole) in the cardiac cycle to be used for imaging. The main advantage of this technique is the reduction of radiation exposure as the radiation beam is only on for a short burst. With regards to cancer imaging, prospective gating is useful for "freezing" cardiac motion, allowing for a better delineation of cardiac structures. The main application would then be critical analysis of pericardial, cardiac, or vascular invasion in circumstances where involvement is not clear by nongated techniques and has therapeutic implications (Fig. 1), although it is not sufficiently robust for imaging the coronary arteries.

Retrospective ECG gating requires slow table motion and simultaneous recording of the ECG tracing; it is used to link scan data to the appropriate phase of the cardiac cycle (Ohnesorge *et al.*, 2000). Multiphasic information allows for the optimal selection of images for reconstruction, thus improving overall image and diagnostic quality, and permits multiple reconstructions to be performed when separate important structures are optimally visualized at different phases of the cycle. By summing the phases together, cine motion of the cardiac chambers can be visualized, and chamber size at both diastole and systole can be directly measured. For these reasons, a retrospectively ECG-gated acquisition with the thinnest possible overlapping reconstruction is the preferred method for contrast-enhanced high-spatial-resolution imaging of small cardiac structures, especially the coronary arteries. There is little data regarding the use of retrospective ECG-gating in cancer patients, but one could envision it as a way to noninvasively image the coronary arteries following radiation therapy, potentially monitor cardiac function in selected cases (although it is doubtful that it would ever replace radionuclide ventriculography or echocardiography in the evaluation of cardiac toxicity related to chemotherapy), or evaluate the size, functional effect, and significance of intracardiac tumors, including myxomas.

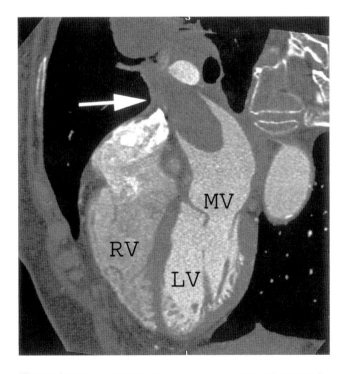

Figure 1 ECG-gated MDCT of lung cancer growing into pulmonary vein. Long axis view in diastole better delineates relationship of tumor to mitral valve (MV). Note absence of motion of mitral valve leaflets. LV = left ventricle; RV = right ventricle.

Current scanners have a 330 msec gantry rotation time and can provide a consistent temporal resolution of 150 msec for all heart rates. This allows for motion-free data in the majority of patients with low and moderate heart rates (< 80 bpm). For rates > 80 bpm, beta blockers are often utilized in clinical practice for rate reduction.

The use of retrospective cardiac gating can significantly increase dose due to the need for increased sampling to fully acquire the necessary data. Like the tube current modulation strategies described previously, additional dose-reduction techniques are available for ECG-gated examinations (Jakobs *et al.*, 2002). Since the images are most likely to be reconstructed in diastole, the tube output is maximized only during this phase of the cycle and is substantially reduced throughout the rest of the cardiac cycle. Depending on the heart rate, it should be possible to reduce the radiation exposure for CT coronary angiography to a level of 5–7 mSv. ECG-gated dose modulation is best used in patients with steady heart rates and in patients whose time point of the diastolic image reconstruction interval can be predicted with some certainty.

Use of Intravenous Contrast in Multidetector Computed Tomography Oncologic Imaging

Iodinated intravenous contrast material is frequently used in oncologic imaging. Benefits of contrast include an increase in conspicuity of lesions in solid organs, improved lesion detection, and delineation of relationships to vascular structures. There are several ways a contrast bolus can be timed and structured. For most routine applications in the chest and abdomen, imaging begins after a set delay after initiation of the contrast bolus. When a higher rate of injection is required, particularly for arterial phase imaging, bolus tracking is often applied. Bolus tracking allows the technologist to place a region of interest over the target of interest, usually the aorta, and periodic low-dose scans are taken at a single level. When the attenuation value meets a set threshold, scanning begins.

Deciding on the timing of intravenous contrast depends on knowledge of the primary tumor (Johnson and Fishman, 2006). In general, imaging may occur during the arterial phase (20 sec after start of bolus) or during the portal venous phase (60–70 sec after start of bolus), or it may be delayed (2–5 min after bolus) (Fig. 2). Slight adjustments may be necessary to optimally evaluate the pancreatic parenchyma (35 sec after bolus). The rapid scanning of MDCT allows for thin-section evaluation of solid organs such that multiple phases can be imaged with one bolus. Arterial phase imaging is optimal for assessing the relationships of lesions to major arteries as well as hypervascular liver lesions. Certain tumors, such as hepatocellular carcinoma and occasionally metastases from

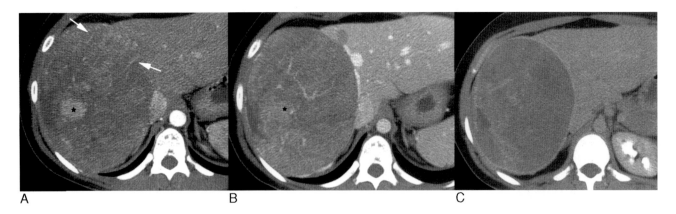

Figure 2 Multiphase imaging of hepatic adenoma. (**A**) Arterial phase reveals small arterial vessels in the periphery of the tumor (arrows) and hypervascular nodule (*). (**B**) During portal venous phase, peripheral arterial vessels are isodense to the mass, nodule is only faintly visible (*), and hepatic veins are now seen in normal hepatic parenchyma. (**C**) Delayed phase imaging reveals no discernible vascular structures, and the hypervascular nodule cannot be detected.

breast and neuroendocrine tumors, may only be detected during the arterial phase as the lesions become isodense to liver after the portal venous bolus arrives. Similarly, in the kidney the complete evaluation of a renal cell carcinoma may require arterial/corticomedullary phase imaging to define the arterial anatomy, including accessory arteries, nephrographic phase to define the maximum size of the tumor, and excretory phase to assess the relationship to the collecting system (Ueda *et al.*, 2006).

Three-Dimensional and Multiplanar Reformations

Two-Dimensional Multiplanar Reconstruction (2D-MPR)

While images are usually displayed in the transverse plane, with isotropic resolution the data can be displayed along any axis without significant loss of image quality. Although any slice thickness can be used, to take full advantage of the data, axial slice collimation of 1.25 mm or less can be used to avoid significant artifacts of reconstruction in other planes. This also allows the physician to interactively view images at robust workstations and quickly work out how best to display a structure to communicate the relevant anatomy for staging or planning interventions.

As previously noted, data acquired at MDCT are a three-dimensional data set made up of individual voxels. Given a z-axis resolution equal to x-y resolution, a ray passed through the volume at any angle can be used to make the image. The simplest reformation is to display a different plane in two dimensions, typically the coronal (Fig. 3) or sagittal plane (perpendicular to the axial image). As relationships become

more complex or are not suited to the anatomic region, the plane of section can be modified in any obliquity in an interactive fashion until the desired image is created. For example, evaluation of vascular invasion by a pancreatic neoplasm may be best displayed by an oblique coronal plane along the axis of the superior mesenteric artery. For objects that are not linear structures, curved reformatted images allow a structure to be traced out and displayed as if it lay along a single axis. The interactive process allows the user to deposit points along a structure of interest and have it displayed as if it were straight. While this is used more frequently for vascular imaging applications, decreasing errors in the sizing of stenoses, it can also be used to better display an entire organ on one image such as the colon in virtual colonoscopy.

Maximum (MIP), Minimum (minIP), and Average Intensity Projection (AIP)

Maximum (MIP) and minimum intensity projection (minIP) images are created in a similar fashion and can be obtained either as an entire volume or slab of tissue with a predefined thickness, often 5–10 mm. An MIP image is generated by analyzing individual pixel elements within a given volume and displaying the volume at the attenuation value equal to the highest pixel value (rather than an average of all pixel values). Conversely, an minIP image is generated in the same way, only displaying the entire voxel volume as the lowest pixel value. Three-dimensional images are then, in essence, displaying the entire volume rather than a predefined slab. Using this algorithm, ~90 to 95% of original data are lost (Dalrymple *et al.*, 2005). MIP images do not contain surface shading or other depth cues, which make assessment of spatial relationships difficult. In general, full-volume three-dimensional structures are of limited value such

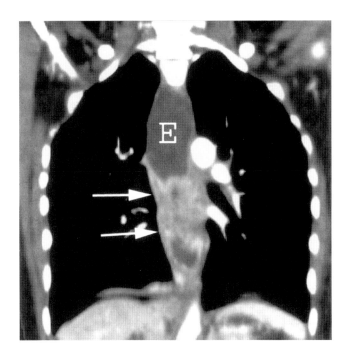

Figure 3 Esophageal cancer. Coronal contrast-enhanced CT reveals the actual length of tumor extent in cranio-caudal dimension (arrows), a difficult assessment to make with axial images. Note fluid-filled esophageal lumen (E) due to obstruction.

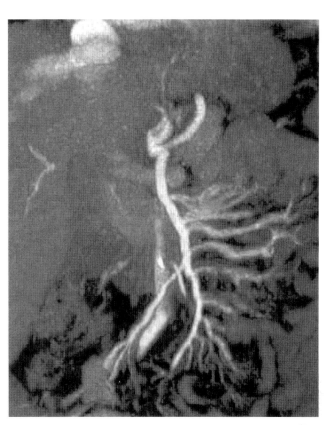

Figure 4 Maximum intensity projection image (15-mm-thick slab) along the axis of the superior mesenteric artery shows normal arborization of vascular tree.

that "slabs" of varying thickness (sliding thick slab-STS) are used to view individual structures (Napel *et al.*, 1993). Like 2D reformations, these slabs can be displayed in any projection to show the relevant anatomy (Fig. 4). Not surprisingly, the loss of pixel data except for the highest (or lowest) value can result in a misrepresentation of structures. While this may be most notable in vascular imaging underestimating or overestimating vessel size or stenosis, practically for oncologic imaging, an MIP may spuriously suggest vascular invasion where none exists. Therefore, MIP projections alone are insufficient for analysis of structural relationships, and careful attention should also be paid to the source data.

Average intensity projection (AIP) is an additional algorithm available. Through use of this technique, the data of thin sections can be "thickened" and displayed with an appearance similar to a traditional thicker section. The advantage is the maintenance of low-contrast resolution while decreasing image noise. Applications of this technique include analysis of solid organs and the walls of hollow structures such as bowel (Dalrymple *et al.*, 2005).

Three-Dimensional Volume Rendering

Three-dimensional volume rendering (3D VR) has the advantage over 3D MIP images of using all of the acquired data to create the final image. Each voxel is summed and displayed as a composite image on the monitor (Calhoun *et al.*, 1999). By choosing different parameters (often defined by the software manufacturer), the data can be segmented by attenuation values to display the desired structure such as the airway, blood vessels, or chest wall. Because volume rendering is less user-dependent, measurements, particularly in those structures perpendicular to the axial plane, are more accurately obtained. Volume rendering enables the user to change opacity and shading characteristics, so that one can assign different color characteristics to different attenuation values, "see through" closer structures to those farther away, and use lighting effects to accentuate spatial relationships (Dalrymple *et al.*, 2005) (Fig. 5). This technique can be used to road map the approach to the lesion and show the intervening structures that might be in the path in a more intuitive manner. The user also has the ability to "cut away" structures and display only the organ of interest. As an example, the chest wall can be cut away to display only the heart and great vessels.

While 3D VR is often performed with an external perspective, looking at the surface of structures, the data can also be displayed from an internal perspective allowing the user to "fly through" hollow structures. This produces images similar to those obtained at endoscopy and can be useful for planning endoscopic procedures (Rubin *et al.*, 1996). Examples of this technique include virtual colonoscopy and virtual bronchoscopy (Fig. 6).

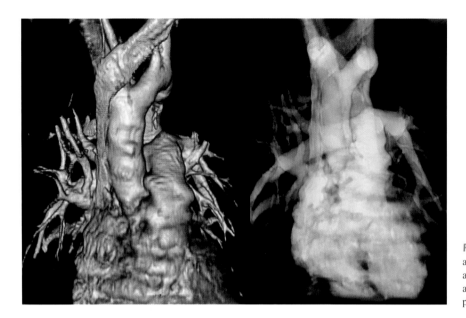

Figure 5 Volume rendered views of double aortic arch performed with different shading characteristics. Note on left image ability to see right arch through superior vena cava as well as right pulmonary artery passing behind aorta.

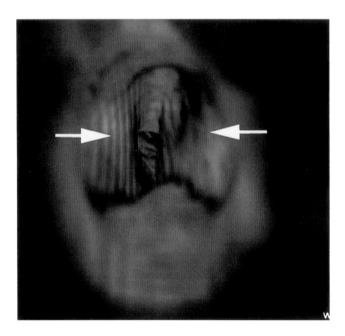

Figure 6 Virtual bronchoscopy. Perspective volume rendered image presents a view of stenosis related to extrinsic compression by lymphoma (arrows) similar to that a bronchoscopist would see and can aid in planning interventions.

Volumetric Analysis of Lesions

One difficulty in the management of cancer patients involves the accuracy and reproducibility of tumor measurements (Erasmus *et al.*, 2003). As a result, the current criteria for progression or regression require relatively significant changes in size (Therasse *et al.*, 2000). New software allows for the automated or semiautomated analysis of lesion volume. These measurements are highly reproducible and can be performed on even the smallest pulmonary nodules. However, there are several pitfalls limiting utility in current practice. Segmentation relies on the differentiation of high-contrast objects and thus has been reliably performed only in the lung. For lesions close to a vessel, the computer may include vascular structures as part of the lesion, spuriously increasing volume and introducing a new variable for follow-up examinations. For consistency, studies need to maintain the same (preferably thin) slice collimation. In some circumstances, these vessels can be edited manually; however, this adds a new source of measurement variability.

Because both Response Evaluation Criteria in Solid Tumors (RECIST) and World Health Organization (WHO) criteria for response or progression require the addition of all metastatic lesions, volumetric analysis, currently able to measure pulmonary metastases, is not necessarily a panacea for whole-body staging and comparisons to traditional staging measures. Relatively low-contrast lesions are not good targets for automated segmentation at this time. Therefore manual segmentation is required, a time-consuming process with great variability, and volumetric measurements may be discordant with traditional criteria in up to one-third of cases (Prasad *et al.*, 2002). Similarly, many of the intrinsic problems associated with linear measurements persist with volumetric analysis (Jaffe, 2006). Adjacent inflammatory change, effects of contrast materials, and adjacent structures that obscure tumor boundaries will all lead to relative inaccuracies in tumor volume.

Perhaps a better use of volumetric analysis is the follow-up of the small indeterminate pulmonary nodule. While morphologic features (lobular or spiculated margins) can help stratify nodules into potentially benign or malignant categories (Erasmus et al., 2000), it is often difficult to appreciate these characteristics in nodules < 1 cm in diameter. Current management of these nodules requires CT follow-up every three to six months for at least two years to document stability. However, precise measurement of small nodules on serial CT examinations can be quite difficult. For instance, a 5 mm nodule need only increase in diameter by 1.25 mm in order to double in volume. It is thus often difficult to accurately determine growth in small nodules by serial CT. 3D volumetric evaluation may solve these limitations by providing an accurate total volume measurement, a more precise doubling time, and a better prediction of asymmetric growth (Kostis et al., 2004). Both in vivo and in vitro analysis of small nodules with 3D volumetric CT have shown that analysis of doubling time can be performed, and early repeat CT with thin sections can show growth in nodules as small as 5 mm in as little as one month; eccentric growth and subtle volume change are more easily visualized with the 3D models (Yankelevitz et al., 2000). In the future, it is hoped that volume rendering of pulmonary nodules will allow for rapid categorization into benign and malignant categories, with greater accuracy in screened populations. The ultimate goal is to determine whether a small indeterminate pulmonary nodule represents a metastasis in patients with an extrathoracic malignancy prior to definitive therapy with a short interval follow-up.

Computer-Aided Detection

Another challenge facing the radiologist is the detection of small pulmonary nodules both in screening for lung cancer and in detecting small pulmonary metastases. Even in the best of circumstances the ability to detect nodules is not perfect. Using computer-generated nodules, sensitivity and specificity for nodules < 7 mm are around 60% and 80%, respectively (Naidich et al., 1993). Not surprisingly, performance was best when nodules were larger and peripheral. Maximum intensity projected (MIP) images described previously are one way to increase nodule conspicuity and may allow the detection of more potential metastases (Gruden et al., 2002). However, in clinical practice, these will generally be less than 1 cm (nonmeasurable disease by RECIST criteria), and the incremental value of detecting more small lesions may not be of great clinical benefit. Thus, computer-aided detection (CAD) has been touted as an effective second reader to help the radiologist detect subtle nodules.

Many different CAD algorithms have been developed to improve the radiologist's accuracy when performing nodule detection. Overall, these studies show an augmentation of

reader sensitivity of 5 to 10% and also suggest an improvement in reader confidence (Wormanns et al., 2002; McCulloch et al., 2004). Most studies, however, have lacked the statistical significance and rigorous testing to clearly demonstrate clinical efficacy. As a result, comparing and assessing the merits of these differing approaches based on the published results are extremely difficult. Nonetheless, most publications have concluded that CAD methods show potential to improve the radiologist's performance. Unfortunately, the sensitivity of CAD alone is rather poor and therefore is not a substitute for careful analysis of the CT.

All CAD systems produce over an order of magnitude more false positives than does an experienced radiologist. While many false-positive marks can be easily dismissed as vessel branch points, other marks may be problematic for less experienced readers. The overall effect of false positives on studies has not been formally addressed. A well-conceived CAD algorithm should enhance the radiologist's ability by detecting lesions that would otherwise be difficult to perceive because of distracting structures and allow for earlier detection and categorization into benign and malignant diseases (Krupinski, 2004).

CAD may also be suitable for detecting other high-contrast lesions. Thus, a second potential application is in the detection of polyps at virtual colonoscopy. Much of the early work is generally positive, with CAD alone sensitivities ranging from 70 to 100% for polyps > 6 mm and anywhere from 1 to 15 false positives per patient. Similar to CAD for pulmonary nodules, CAD polyp detection increases reader sensitivity approximately 10% (Yoshida and Dachman, 2005).

MDCT continues to evolve and adapt to the ever-needed changes in imaging. In the foreseen future, MDCT will continue to be the backbone of anatomical imaging and will increasingly be fused with physiologic imaging techniques provided by nuclear medicine and positron emission tomography. It is hoped that further refinements will allow for robust computer-aided detection techniques that will help detect not only high-contrast but also low-contrast lesions.

References

Ambrose, J., and Hounsfield, G. 1976. Computerized transverse axial tomography. *Brit. J. Rad. 46*:148–149.

Barrett, J.F., and Keat, N. 2004. Artifacts in CT: recognition and avoidance. *RadioGraphics 24*:1679–1691.

Calhoun, P.S., Kuszyk, B.S., Heath, D.G., Carley, J.C., and Fishman, E.K. 1999. Three-dimensional volume rendering of spiral CT data: theory and method. *RadioGraphics 19*:745–764.

Cormack, A.M. 1963. Representation of a function by its line integrals, with some radiological application. *J. Appl. Physiol. 34*:2722–2727.

Dalrymple, N.C., Prasad, S.R., Freckleton, M.W., and Chintapalli, K.N. 2005. Introduction to the language of three-dimensional imaging with multidetector CT. *RadioGraphics 25*:1409–1428.

Erasmus, J.J., Connolly, J.E., McAdams, H.P., and Roggli, V.L. 2000. Solitary pulmonary nodules: part 1. Morphologic evaluation for differentiation of benign and malignant lesions. *RadioGraphics 20*:43–58.

Erasmus, J.J., Gladish, G.W., Broemeling, L., Sabloff, B.S., Truong, M.T., Herbst, R.S., and Munden, R.F. 2003. Interobserver and intraobserver variability in measurement of non-small-cell carcinoma lung lesions: implications for assessment of tumor response. *J. Clin. Oncol. 21*:2574–2582.

Evens, R.G. 1976. New frontier for radiology: computed tomography. *AJR 126*:1117–1129.

Flohr, T., Bruder, H., Stierstorfer, K., Simon, J., Schaller, S., and Ohnesorge, B. 2002. New technical developments in multislice CT, part 2: submillimeter 16-slice scanning and increased gantry rotation speed for cardiac imaging. *Rofo. 74*:1022–1027.

Flohr, T.G., Schaller, S., Stierstorfer, K., Bruder, H., Ohnesorge, B.M., and Schoepf, U.J. 2005. Multi-detector row CT systems and image reconstruction techniques. *Radiology 235*:756–773.

Gruden, J.F., Ouanounou, S., Tigges, S., Norris, S.D., and Klausner, T.S. 2002. Incremental benefit of maximum-intensity-projection images on observer detection of small pulmonary nodules revealed by multidetector CT. *AJR 179*:149–157.

Hohl, C., Wildberger, J.E., Sub, C., Thomas, C., Muhlenbruch, G., Schmidt, T., Honnef, D., Gunther, R.W., and Mahnken, A.H. 2006. Radiation dose reduction to breast and thyroid during MDCT: effectiveness of an in-plane bismuth shield. *Acta Radiol. 47*:562–567.

Huda, W., Ravenel, J.G., and Scalzetti, E.M. 2002. How do radiographic techniques affect image quality and patient doses in CT. *Seminars Ultrasound, CT, MRI 23*:411–422.

Hurwitz, L.M., Yoshizumi, T.T., Reiman, R.E., Paulson, E.K., Frush, D.P., Nguyen, G.T., Toncheva, G.I., and Goodman, P.C. 2006. Radiation dose to the female breast from 16-MDCT body protocols. *AJR 186*:1718–1722.

International Commission on Radiologic Protection. 1991. 1990 recommendations of the ICRP. In: *Annals of the ICRP 21*, nos. 1–3. ICRP publication 60. Oxford, England.

Jaffe, C.C. 2006. Measures of response: RECIST, WHO, and new alternatives. *J. Clin. Oncol. 24*:3245–3251.

Jakobs, T.F., Becker, C.R., Ohnesorge, B., Flohr, T., Suess, C., Schoepf, U.J., and Reiser, M.F. 2002. Multislice helical CT of the heart with retrospective ECG gating: reduction of radiation exposure by ECG-controlled tube current modulation. *Eur. Radiol. 12*:1081–1086.

Johnson, P.T., and Fishman, E.K. 2006. IV contrast selection for MDCT: current thoughts and practice. *AJR 186*:406–415.

Kalender, W.J., Seissler, W., Klotz, E., and Vock, P. 1990. Spiral volumetric CT with single breath-hold technique, continuous transport, and continuous scanner rotation. *Radiology 176*:181–183.

Kostis, W.J., Yankelevitz, D.F., Reeves, A.P., Fluture, S.C., and Henschke, C.I. 2004. Small pulmonary nodules: reproducibility of three-dimensional volumetric measurement and estimation of time to follow-up CT. *Radiology 231*:446–452.

Krupinski, E.A., 2004. Computer-aided detection in clinical environment: benefits and challenges for radiologists. *Radiology 231*:7–9.

Mahesh, M., Scatarige, J.C., Cooper, J., and Fishman, E.K. 2001. Dose and pitch relationship for a particular multi-slice CT scanner. *AJR 177*:1273–1275.

Mahesh, M. 2002. Search for isotropic resolution in CT from conventional through multiple-row detector. *RadioGraphics 22*:949–962.

McCulloch, C.C., Kaucic, R.A., Mendonca, P.R., Walter, D.J., and Avila, R.S. 2004. Model-based detection of lung nodules in computed tomography exams. Thoracic computer-aided diagnosis. *Acad Radiol. 11*:258–266.

McCollough, C.H., Bruesewitz, M.R., and Kofler, J.M. 2006. CT dose reduction and dose management tools: overview of available options. *RadioGraphics 26*:503–512.

Naidich, D.P., Rusinek, H., McGuinness, G., Leitman, B., McCauley, D.I., and Henschke, C.I. 1993. Variables affecting pulmonary nodule detection with computed tomography: evaluation with three-dimensional computer simulation. *J. Thorac. Imaging. 8*:291–299.

Napel, S., Rubin, G.D., and Jeffrey, R.B. 1993. STS-MIP: a new reconstruction technique for CT of the chest. *J. Comput. Assist. Tomogr. 17*:832–838.

Ohnesorge, B., Flohr, T., Becker, C., Kopp, A.F., Schoepf, U.J., Baum, U., Knez, A., Klingenbeck-Regn, K., and Reiser, M.F. 2000. Cardiac imaging by means of electrocardiographically gated multisection spiral CT: initial experience. *Radiology 217*:564–571.

Pierce, D.A., and Preston, D.L. 2000. Radiation related-cancer risks at low doses among atomic bomb survivors. *Radiation Research 154*:178–186.

Prasad, S.R., Jhaveri, K.S., Saini, S., Hahn, P.F., Halpern, E.F., and Sumner, J.E. 2002. CT tumor measurement for therapeutic response assessment: comparison of unidimensional, bidimensional, and volumetric techniques initial observations. *Radiology 225*:416–419.

Rubin, G.D., Beaulieu, C.F., Argiro, V., Ringl, H., Norbash, A.M., Feller, J.F., Dake, M.D., Jeffrey, R.B., and Napel, S. 1996. Perspective volume rendering of CT and MR images: applications for endoscopic imaging. *Radiology 199*:321–330.

Therasse, P., Arbuck, S.G., Eisenhauer, E.A., Wanders, J., Kaplan, R.S., Rubinstein, L., Verweij, J., Van Glabbeke, M., van Oosterom, A.T., Christian, M.C., and Gwyther, S.G. 2000. New guidelines to evaluate the response to treatment in solid tumors. European Organization for Research and Treatment of Cancer, National Cancer Institute of the United States, National Cancer Institute of Canada. *J. Natl. Cancer Inst. 92*:205–216.

Ueda, T., Mori, K., Minami, M., Motoori, K., and Ito, H. 2006. Trends in oncologic CT imaging: clinical application of multidetector-row CT and 3D CT imaging. *Int. J. Clin. Oncol. 11*:268–277.

Wormanns, D., Fiebich, M., Saidi, M., Diederich, S., and Heindel, W. 2002. Automatic detection of pulmonary nodules at spiral CT: clinical application of a computer-aided diagnosis system. *Eur. Radiol. 12*:1052–1057.

Yankelevitz, D.F., Reeves, A.P., Kostis, W.J., Zhao, B., and Henschke, C.I. 2000. Small pulmonary nodules: volumetrically determined growth rates based on CT evaluation. *Radiology 217*:251–256.

Yoshida, H., and Dachman, A.H. 2005. CAD techniques, challenges, and controversies in computed tomographic colonography. *Abdom. Imaging. 30*:26–41.

3

Megavoltage Computed Tomography Imaging

Omar A. Zeidan, Sanford L. Meeks, Katja M. Langen, Thomas H. Wagner, and Patrick A. Kupelian

Introduction

The main purpose of computed tomography (CT) imaging in radiation therapy is to get a pretreatment volumetric estimate of the region of the patient that needs to be treated. Because patient anatomy can change between treatment fractions (intrafraction motion), it is important to monitor regions of interest in order to maximize the tumor exposure to radiation with minimal side effects on the regions at risk (i.e., achieving organ sparing). Ideally, the patient should be set up in a reproducible position for each fraction of the treatment. This is achieved by aligning the patient in the treatment position using external markers. For example, skin tattoos are aligned with the lasers inside the treatment room. However, several studies have shown that there could be significant intrafraction organ motion that is site and patient dependent (Langen and Jones, 2001). Daily alignment to patient external marks does not necessarily guarantee accurate positioning of the clinical target volume (CTV). Hence, it is critical to determine the precise location of the CTV during every fraction of treatment to achieve this goal and minimize geometrical uncertainties during radiation therapy.

The need for improved treatment precision has spawned the development of image-guided radiotherapy (IGRT), in which a real-time imaging device that is registered with the treatment unit is used to acquire images immediately prior to/and potentially during radiation therapy. IGRT techniques have been developed using the most common imaging modalities, including electronic portal imaging, kilovoltage X-ray imaging, ultrasound, and computed tomography (CT). While each of these imaging modalities has unique strengths and weaknesses for use in IGRT, CT is the most comprehensive database for IGRT; CT provides a spatially consistent three-dimensional imaging database with sufficient contrast resolution to appreciate a large amount of anatomic detail. Jaffray et al. (2002) describe a cone beam CT (CBCT) scanner in which a kV X-ray tube and a flat panel detector are mounted on the C-arm of a linear accelerator. The detector and array were mounted on an SL-20 linear accelerator (Elekta Oncology Systems). Another major manufacturer of radiation therapy systems, Varian Medical Systems, has started using on-board CBCT imaging using a flat-panel portal imager with source-detector geometry similar to Elekta's. A conventional CT may be introduced inside the treatment room if space permits. The first commercial CT-linac system in the United States was installed in 2000 in Morristown Memorial Hospital, New Jersey (Wong et al., 2001). The system consists of a Siemens medical linac (Siemens Medical Solutions) and a movable Siemens CT scanner that can slide along a pair of rails. In addition, Siemens has recently introduced MVision™ as the first commercial implementation of CBCT technology using a standard radiotherapy treatment beam rather than kV beams for volumetric imaging. The premise is to use these imaging devices for daily image guidance (IG) to improve daily target position reproducibility.

Megavoltage CT (MVCT) has some distinct advantages over previously mentioned kVCT modalities in that it uses the linac-emitted MV photons as the photon source rather than a separate X-ray source. This efficient use of radiation source reduces the cost of mounting a kVCT unit on existing radiation therapy devices. In addition, the elimination of the kVCT imaging components reduces the treatment room clutter. The earliest prototype of an MVCT system for radiotherapy IG was developed in the early 1980s at the University of Arizona (Simpson *et al.*, 1982; Swindel, 1983; Swindel *et al.*, 1983). Since then it has gone through several stages of development. The major problem with the use of MVCT was that the imaging process is too slow due either to slow reconstruction and data acquisition, or simply to the slow mechanical rotation of the imaging components. At least one complete rotation is necessary to reconstruct a 3D CT image. Because the MV beam is on continuously during a full rotation, these older models delivered several cGy of dose per rotation even at low-dose rates (Mosleh-Shirazi *et al.*, 1998). At the University of Wisconsin, a system was developed in 1999 that collected MV transmission beams using a CT detector placed opposite the treatment linac (Mackie, 1999). The UW tomotherapy machine could detect contrast better than 2% with doses ~8 cGy, which compares favorably with other MVCT systems found in the literature to that date. A brief history of the development of MVCT on a tomotherapy system is outlined by Ruchala *et al.* (1999).

The most successful integration of MVCT imaging with radiation therapy devices is the TomoTherapy™ Hi-ART (TomoTherapy, Inc., Madison, Wisconsin). It is currently the only type of patient treatment in which MVCT imaging is integrated as part of the treatment device itself. The Hi-ART II system can generate CT images from the same megavoltage X-ray beam it uses for treatment. These megavoltage CT (MVCT) images offer verification of the patient position prior to and potentially during radiation therapy. For the remaining part of this chapter, we will focus on the general characteristics of MV images and their successful clinical applications in the tomotherapy modality.

Fundamentals of Megavoltage Imaging

The kinds of physical interactions in tissue for kV and MV beams are slightly different. For a 120 kV tomography scan, the mean photon energy is 60 keV, and Compton interactions account for nearly 88% of all interactions in soft tissue, while photoelectric interactions make up 12%. The probability of photoelectric interaction is proportional to Z^3, where Z is the atomic number of the medium. Because bone has a high concentration of high-Z elements ($Z_{equivalent}$ = 12.31) compared to muscle tissue ($Z_{equivalent}$ = 7.64), the photoelectric effect will be more pronounced in bone than in soft tissue. This is clinically desirable as it leads to better distinction between soft tissue and bone. Megavoltage photons interact primarily through Compton scattering and pair production. In the case of MV beams, the Compton and pair production

interactions are less sensitive to differences in Z. Thus, bone and soft tissue are not as clearly distinguishable, based on these interactions, as the photoelectric interactions. Accordingly, soft tissue contrast will depend on the physical densities of the medium. A common artifact in conventional kVCT imaging is caused by metal objects in the imaged medium. The high-Z metal attenuates the kV beam in a nonlinear fashion due to the photoelectric effect. The basic assumption in conventional CT image reconstruction is that each detector, at every position will observe some transmitted radiation. If a high-density material severely reduces the transmission, the detector may record no transmission. This violates the basic assumption, and the reconstruction algorithm will not account for such a violation. Consequently, streaks will appear in the reconstructed image. In MVCT images, the artifacts are much less pronounced because the photon beams are penetrating enough to eliminate artifacts. Figure 1 shows the difference between MVCT and kVCT images for patients with dental fillings and hip prosthesis. Notice that the streak artifacts in the kVCT images (top) do not appear in the MVCT images (bottom).

The primary purpose of MV imaging is to verify radiotherapy treatments by determining the position of the patient's internal anatomy at the time of treatment. Therefore, it is essential that MVCT images have high-contrast detectability because the tissue of interest generally has low contrast. The kV photons have higher mass attenuation coefficients in water than MV photons (by nearly one order of magnitude). However, their mass energy attenuation coefficients are similar. Therefore, for equivalent fractions of kV and MV photons, MV photons will deposit greater dose in tissue. To achieve comparable doses to kV imaging, the number of MV photons must be reduced. Although MV photons are much more penetrating than kV photons, the reduction of detectable MV photons will decrease the signal-to-noise ratio in the detection elements and degrade the tissue contrast. For example, patient thickness plays a significant role in image contrast due to photon exponential attenuation along the photon path, which is energy dependent. For the same patient thickness, kV photons attenuate much more than MV photons owing to their lower energy, which will lead to lower contrast since fewer kV photons penetrate the patient and reach the detector element. However, there are other factors, such as detector efficiency, that affect image contrast and tend to decrease with increasing energy. When combining these factors, it is found that diagnostic energy CT can offer better contrast for smaller patients (diameter < 20 cm), given equivalent doses. When imaging larger patients (diameter > 40 cm) using an efficient MV detector, MVCT can actually offer comparable and even superior contrast at equivalent doses. This effect is further accentuated in the presence of metallic or high-Z objects that cause photon starvation. One should keep in mind that the ability to perform fast, efficient, and low-dose scans is limited by the need to balance dose

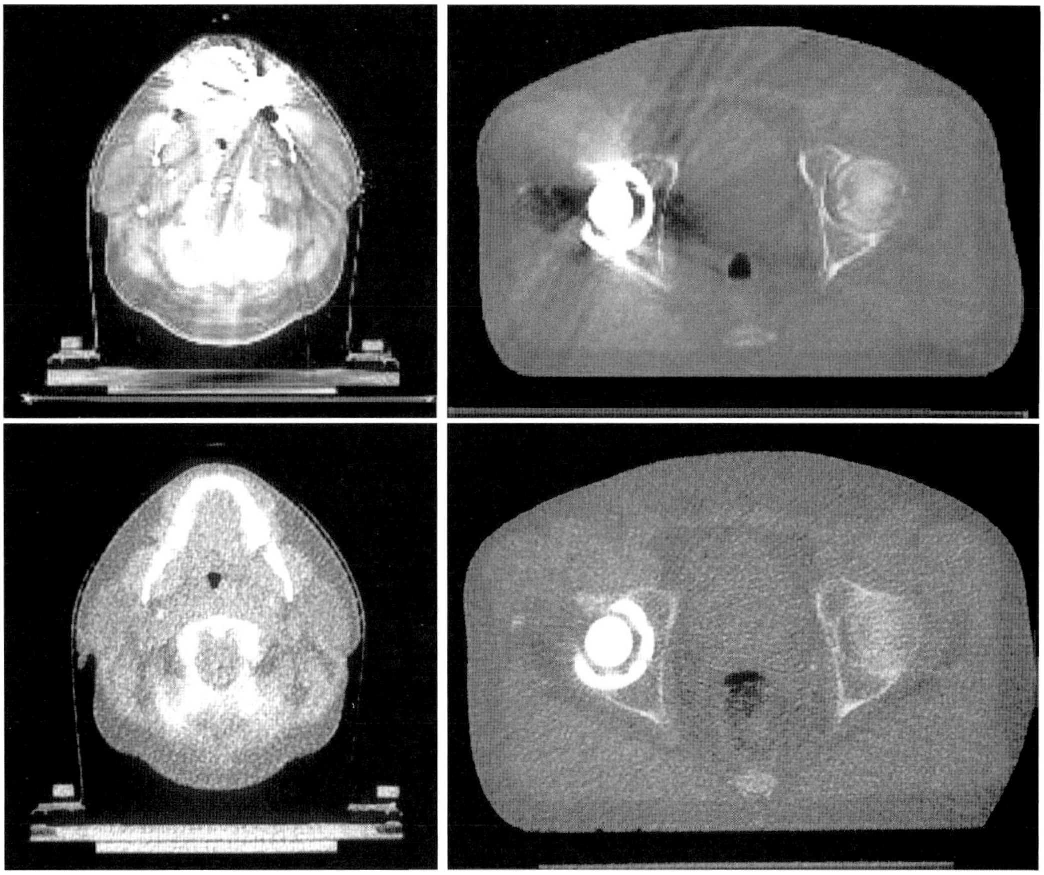

Figure 1 Comparison of kVCT (top) and MVCT (bottom) images.

and image quality. For a quantitative analysis of the above discussion, the reader is referred to (Ruchala *et al.*, 1999).

Megavoltage CT images should supply information that is directly proportional to the attenuation of the photon beam in order to be used for dose planning. Tomotherapy MVCT images were shown (Langen *et al.*, 2005) to have a linear relationship between electron density and CT number and to be reproducible and stable with time. A series of phantom-based end-to-end tests of the MVCT recalculation chain was performed at our institution. Those results show that the MVCT images can be used for dose calculations and that the accuracy of these calculations is similar to that of the initial dose calculations based on kVCT images.

Design and Performance Characteristics of Tomotherapy Megavoltage Computed Tomography

The TomoTherapy Hi-ART II imaging system consists of a ring gantry with a detector chamber array mounted opposite to the radiation source (Mackie *et al.*, 2003). The linear

accelerator that emits the imaging photons is the same MV photon source that is also used for patient treatment. However, when tomotherapy is operated in the imaging mode, the nominal photon energy is reduced from 6.0 MV in treatment mode to 3.5 MV for the imaging mode (Jeraj *et al.*, 2004). This change in the photon energy spectrum results in better imaging characteristics (better contrast per given dose).

Helical tomotherapy is analogous to helical CT imaging, where the gantry and the couch are in simultaneous motion. Like helical CT, helical tomotherapy uses slip rings to pass power and communications to the rotating gantry, allowing continuous radiation delivery. The images are acquired in helical mode as the gantry rotates continuously while the patient is translated through the bore. The operator has control over the pitch, which relates to the thickness of the image slice. The pitch is defined as table translation per gantry rotation divided by the field length at isocenter. If the beam is collimated to 25 mm at the isocenter, a pitch 1 means that the table moves 25 mm per gantry rotation; a pitch of 0.3 means that the table moves 7.5 mm per gantry rotation. An increase in pitch value results in a reduction of image resolution in the superior/inferior direction, while the absorbed dose decreases. The MVCT field-of-view (FOV) is limited to a diameter of ~ 40 cm.

Figure 2 is a schematic of the hardware components inside of a tomotherapy unit showing the position of imaging components with respect to the MV fan beam on the gantry. The characteristics of the Hi-ART II detector system are described in detail by Keller *et al.* (2002). The detection system consists of an arc of pressurized xenon gas detectors. The detector array consists of 738 detector cells, each comprising two gas cavities divided by a thin tungsten septal plate. A voltage of +300 volts is applied to these cells. The effective cell size is 1.28 mm (perpendicular to the beam direction). A thin aluminum plate is mounted in front (upstream) of the detector to filter contaminate electrons. The front face of the detector is placed 129.2 cm away from the photon source. The high-Z tungsten plates have a high cross section for MV photons. The electrons liberated from the interaction of photons with the tungsten plates are collected in the xenon gas cavity after gain is applied. The total energy deposited in the xenon gas is a measure of the detector signal. The combination of a high-Z material together with a gas as the active detection medium leads to a very high efficiency for megavoltage radiation detection (Keller, 2002).

A good practice for accurate daily image reconstruction is to collect an air-scan MVCT image where no obstruction (such as the treatment couch) is in the beam path. This is important for image reconstruction since the measured transmission signal needs to be normalized by the incident fluence vector, which is a measurement of the signal in each detector with the beam on but no attenuation material in place (Ruchala, 2000). The image data reconstruction looks at the collected data for that procedure and uses it for image reconstruction for all images taken on that day. This procedure helps eliminate intra-daily detector response differences and their effect on image reconstruction quality.

The performance characteristics of MVCT images on a helical tomotherapy unit were recently investigated (Meeks *et al.*, 2005). Typical noise standard deviations were nearly 2 to 4% (percentage of the linear attenuation coefficient of water corrected for the scanner contrast scale), indicating that the MVCT image noise characteristics are slightly worse than those of a commonly utilized CT simulator. For an equivalent reconstruction matrix of 512 × 512 pixels and pitch value of 1.0, the noise is approximately twice as large for the MVCT as in the CT simulator. As expected, the noise increases with matrix size and shows a slight increase with increasing collimator pitch. Spa-

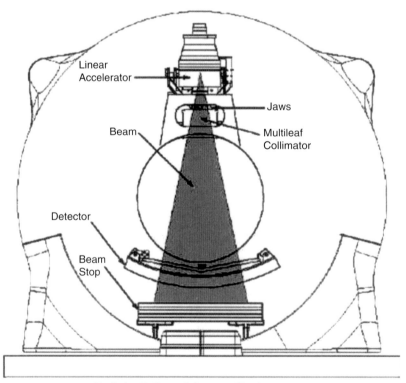

Radiation Delivery Subsystem Hardware

Figure 2 A schematic of the Tomography system.

tial resolution measurements using a high-contrast resolution pattern indicates that the visible resolution is ~ 1.25 mm for the 512 × 512 images and 1.00 mm for the 768 × 768 images. In their investigation of MVCT image contrast resolution, the relatively low-dose MVCT scans provided sufficient contrast to delineate many soft tissue structures; the electron density difference between muscle and fat is 8 to 10%, and the contrast-detail curves indicate that objects as small as 4 mm should be resolvable at this level of contrast. Hence, MVCT images are not only useful for verifying the patient's position at the time of therapy, but are also sufficient for delineating certain anatomy.

The amount of integral dose (total dose in tissue) that the patient receives during MVCT images is dependent on the MVCT slice thickness and total length of the imaged region. A recent study (Meeks *et al.*, 2005) has shown that the dose delivered at the center of a solid water phantom of 20 cm diameter from an MVCT scan of 5 mm thickness on a tomotherapy machine ranges between 0.4 cGy for a pitch value of 2.4 (coarse resolution) and 1.05 cGy for a pitch value of 1.0 (fine resolution). The dose delivered from a normal resolution scan was nearly 0.65 cGy for a pitch value of 1.6. Hence, for example, if this phantom were to resemble a patient, for a typical prostate treatment of 39 fractions with daily imaging at fine resolution, the total dose delivered would be ~ 1.05 × 39 = 41 cGy, which is only 0.5% of the total therapeutic dose.

Clinical Implementation of Megavoltage Computed Tomography

Image Acquisition and Registration

To establish proper patient positioning, the MVCT images need to be registered with the kVCT images. Once the MVCT images are acquired and reconstructed, the radiation therapist (RTT) has the option to use either automatic or manual registration, with the kVCT data set as the primary data set. Axial, sagittal, and coronal views are available on the treatment console to assist the operator during the manual registration process. Once the registration is complete, a set of couch shifts are calculated and displayed on the screen for the operator. Those shifts are consequently applied by the RTT before the start of the radiation treatment session. Figure 3a is a snapshot of an image registration process in which a checkerboard technique is used to align the MV and kV images on an axial cut in the cervical region. There are currently three different available MVCT scanning modes: coarse, normal, and fine, which correspond to MVCT image slice thicknesses of 6.0, 4.0, and 2.0 mm, respectively. Since the gantry speed is fixed during the scanning process (currently set to 10 sec or 6 rotations/min), the length of each scanning procedure can then be easily calculated. The current imaging procedure in our clinic takes on average of 3 to 5 min to acquire the daily MVCT scan and ~ 5 min for reconstruction and registration.

The registration of real patient images rarely constitutes a rigid body problem. More likely, the operator is faced with a deformed body registration. Both the rearrangement of internal anatomy and the change in body contours can influence the doses received by the target and normal tissue structures. For example, the influence of tumor regression in the head and neck (H&N) region can be seen in Figure 3a. Over the course of the treatment, the tumor volume on the right side of the patient regressed and a systematic deformation of the anatomy can be observed. The MVCT (darker image) was taken on the last day of treatment. The kVCT (lighter image) is the initial planning CT.

The protocol for best patient alignment depends on the treatment site. The H&N region is fairly rigid, such that a bony anatomy alignment is expected to yield reasonable results. However, in H&N cases the bony anatomy itself is frequently deformed, and not all bony anatomy structures can be equally well aligned. Figure 3b shows such an example. A registration of the base of skull (a) results in a misalignment of the lower spinal cord region (b). In this case, priority is given to the bony structures that are closest to the high-dose region. Different registration techniques can be used in clinical practice to guide the registration of the MVCT with kVCT images. Langen *et al.* (2005a) have compared the following three techniques for prostate patients with implanted fiducial markers: (1) *Fiducial marker-based registration*: using three small gold markers (3 mm in length), which are clearly visible in both kVCT and MVCT scans. (2) *Anatomy-based registration*: the prostate was used in their study as their registration surrogate and markers were ignored. (3) *Contour-based registration*: the contoured rectum, bladder, and prostate on the kVCT set were overlaid onto the MVCT images and were used for image registration. Their study indicates that for prostate treatments, bony anatomy alignment is not sufficient because the prostate can move relative to the bony anatomy. An alignment of the gland itself is required. However, the identification of soft tissue structures is somewhat subjective, and the use of implanted fiducial markers may reduce this subjectivity. The study shows that the use of fiducial marker-based registration has the least interuser variability of the three registration techniques. Next, we will explore the implementation of MVCT image guidance for site-specific applications and consequent dosimetric evaluations.

Use of Megavoltage Computed Tomography for Daily Alignment: Head and Neck Cancers

Targets in the head and neck region are, in general, assumed to be fairly rigidly attached to bony anatomy, and the main source of uncertainty in positioning these patients is setup error. Typically, the setup uncertainty is minimized with head or head and shoulder masks that help to reposition and immobilize the patient. The improvement in setup accuracy that

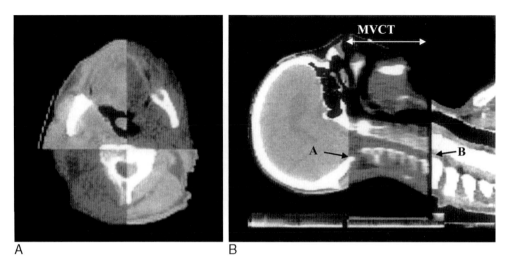

Figure 3 An illustration of kVCT and MVCT image registration in the head and neck.

can be achieved for immobilized head and neck patients with daily IG was recently investigated in our institution (Zeidan *et al.*, 2006). The acceptability of the reduced setup accuracy and precision that is due to infrequent use of image guidance depends on treatment margins and the proximity of sensitive structures. If target structures are in close proximity to critical sensitive structure, image guidance should be used daily.

Using the daily alignment data from 24 head and neck tomotherapy patients in our institution (a total of 804 fractions), seven protocols were retrospectively replayed. The patient's daily MV images were registered with kVCT images using bony anatomy alignment. The protocols range from using no IG to using IG with every other fraction. The three-dimensional setup error is the vector calculated from the remaining setup errors in the three principal anatomic directions: anterior-posterior, lateral, and superior-inferior. The residual setup errors quantify the improvement in setup accuracy that can be achieved with daily image guidance for this class of patients. The main findings of the investigation show that reducing IG frequency from daily to 50% results in 11% of all treatments being subject to a misalignment error of at least 5 mm. Approximately one-third of all treatments are subject to a ≥ 5-mm misalignment if protocols are used with IG on a weekly basis. The effect of these misalignments on the target coverage can be mitigated if appropriate planning target volume (PTV) margins are used. For patients with target volumes in close proximity to critical structures, PTV margins may have to be small. In these cases daily IG should be used. Less frequent use of image guidance will reduce the associated costs at the expense of reduced setup accuracy. The gain in setup accuracy that is expected with the daily use of image guidance will depend on the nature and magnitude of setup and organ motion uncertainties.

Adaptive Image Guidance: Lung Cancers

With the advent of in-room soft tissue imaging techniques such as MVCT imaging with a helical tomotherapy unit, daily documentation of the status of a grossly visible targeted tumor becomes possible. Kupelian *et al.* (2005) retrospectively analyzed a total of 274 MVCT images sets obtained from 10 patients with non-small cell lung cancers. The tumors were readily visualized on the MVCT images, and their corresponding volumes can be calculated from daily MVCT image sets as contoured by the physician. The rate of regression was found to be relatively consistent across the 10 patients, with an average of 1.2% per day. The decrease in volume was observed at a relatively constant rate throughout the treatment. This clinical information was not previously possible due to lack of daily imaging that yields volumetric 3D CT information. Ramsey *et al.* (2005) have used the same patient data of the previous study to adjust the PTV and reduce excessive irradiation of the lung tissue if the PTV were left unchanged throughout the treatment course. The MVCT images were of sufficient quality to allow for daily tumor alignment with the planning kVCT to ensure proper patient positioning before treatment. By reducing the value of the PTV during the course of treatment due to tumor reduction as seen by daily MVCT images, the absolute volume of the ipsilateral lung receiving 20 Gy dose was reduced by ~ 21% by adapting the treatment delivery. MVCT images show that fixed treatment margins effectively become larger as the target decreases in volume. Hence, MVCT images can feasibly be used for image-guided adaptive radiation therapy.

Image-Based Volumetric Dose Calculations: Prostate Cancer

A retrospective study of tissue-specific cumulative dose throughout the course of prostate treatments was recently carried out on helical tomotherapy (Kupelian *et al.*, 2006). The aim of this work was to study the variations in delivered doses to the prostate, rectum, and bladder during a full course of image-guided external beam radiotherapy. The daily alignment of MVCT images with the kVCT planning set was done on implanted prostate markers. The ability to distinguish soft tissue in MVCT images with a reasonable soft tissue contrast in the male pelvis allowed the physician to contour the bladder, rectum, and prostate on MVCT images (total of 390 scans) that were acquired daily on prostate patients (total of 10). Daily dosimetric analysis was performed with dose recalculation. The main study findings were that unlike the prostate doses, there were significant daily variations in the rectal and bladder doses. The most significant variation was found during a particular fraction for one of the patient's treatments in whom the prostate D95 (dose to the 95% of the prostate volume) dropped to 1.79 Gy, versus the planned 2.0 Gy. This was the result of significant rectal distention and deformation of the prostate gland, to the extent that the planned delivery geometry could not fit the prostate shape on that particular day, thus causing partial coverage of the gland. The bladder and rectal partial volumes receiving the prescription dose of 2.0 Gy varied considerably from one patient to the other post-alignment. For some patients, intrafraction changes were as large as 65 cc (maximum) to 1 cc (minimum) for the rectum and as large as 38 cc (maximum) to 1 cc (minimum) for the bladder. Figure 4 (left) displays the bladder, rectum, and prostate contours on the kVCT planning image set. These kVCT contours are overlaid on the contours drawn on a daily MVCT data set (right). These CT scans clearly show deformations of the prostate, rectum, and bladder that result in variation in delivered doses. This study demonstrates the impact of daily evaluation of delivered doses through the use of daily MVCT images, thereby providing a more complete picture of the dose delivery compared with relying only on the initial treatment plan.

Image-Based Volumetric Dose Calculations: Intracavitary Brachytherapy

Unlike most teletherapy planning situations, the practitioner finds that, in attempting CT-based brachytherapy planning, many brachytherapy applicators are not CT compatible, owing to the large degree of attenuation of the kV X-ray CT beam by the metal components of many applicators. Without CT-compatible applicators, most practitioners utilize some variety of 2D dosimetry planning techniques, usually based on plane radiographs. The doses to the rectum and bladder are determined as single-dose points from orthogonal plane radiographs. With planar point reconstruction, no dose volume histograms or 3D dose distributions can be calculated or visualized. Hence, the practitioner lacks the 3D dose picture that is normally provided by external beam therapy treatment planning systems.

Our institution has recently begun an investigation of an MVCT imaging technique using a helical tomotherapy treatment unit for patients with high-Z intracavitary temporary implants. The high energy of the MVCT imaging beam permits CT imaging of non-CT compatible (high-Z metallic objects) with less reconstruction artifact. Figure 5 (left) shows a conventional CT (120 kVp) image of a patient with the standard Fletcher-Suit applicator implanted during the first of two implants. Figure 5 (right) shows a tomotherapy MVCT image of the same patient and applicator during the second of two implants. The MVCT images were of sufficient

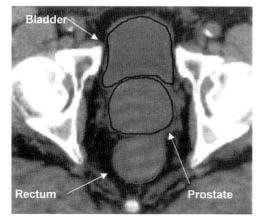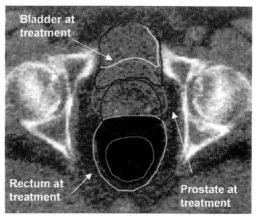

Figure 4 Imaging of a brachytherapy Fletcher-Suit applicator using kVCT imaging (left) and MVCT imaging (right).

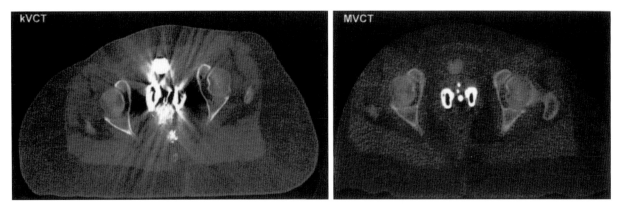

Figure 5 A kVCT image of a Fletcher-Suit applicator (left) and an image of the same applicator using MVCT (right).

quality for use in 3D, MVCT-based dosimetry (Langen, *et al.*, 2005b). The dose points for bladder and rectum can be located on the planar radiographs based on specific geometrical rules. These points are commonly referred to as the standard ICRU (International Commission on Radiation Units) points (ICRU, 1985). Dose rates at the ICRU points are used by the radiation oncologist to determine the amount of time or total dose that the brachytherapy source would remain inside of the patient to deliver the required therapeutic dose. Dose distributions from Cs-137 tube sources (3M Model 6500, 2 cm physical length and 1.4 cm active length) were calculated on the MVCT images for 15 insertions (total of 10 patients), and dose points were intercompared with the same dose points from standard planar radiographs of these patients. The 3D dose data indicate that the maximum 3D bladder dose was higher than the ICRU bladder point dose by a factor of as high as 2.3, and the maximum 3D rectal dose was higher than the ICRU rectal point dose by a factor of as high as 1.59. The 3D maximum bladder and rectal point doses differed significantly from the corresponding ICRU reference point doses ($p < 0.001$). In addition, the 3D data provide volumetric information regarding the rectal and bladder volumes exceeding the desired dose. Helical tomotherapy MVCT imaging facilitates the use of 3D dosimetry for gynecological brachytherapy, without the need for CT-compatible brachytherapy applicators. Volumetric point dose information can be reported based on dose calculations on MVCT image sets.

In this chapter we have outlined MVCT-based technology and its clinical implementation in the field of radiation oncology through its currently successful integration with the tomotherapy modality. A broad comparison between the widely used conventional kVCT and MVCT was presented. MVCT generally yields a poorer image quality than kVCT partially due to differences in the nature of the physical interactions in tissue and beam characteristics. In many cases, however, the MVCT image contrast resolution is of sufficient quality that soft tissue differentiation is possible. Similar to kVCT images, MVCT images can be suitable for dose calculations. The unique properties of MVCT allow the suppression of high-Z metal artifact commonly observed in conventional CT. The implementation of daily MVCT for IG was presented for different disease sites. There is currently significant interest in radiation oncology to extend the use of MVCT for daily imaging to other disease sites and implement it as a routine IG tool. It is early to draw conclusions on the clinical benefits of daily MVCT implementation. However, daily dose-delivery evaluation based on MVCT complements image guidance can be done. Ultimately, such daily dose evaluation will lead to the transition from image-guided radiotherapy to dose-guided radiotherapy, in which actual positioning of the patient is performed on the basis of dosimetric assessments rather than image registration alone.

References

ICRU, ICRU Report 38: Dose and volume specification for reporting intracavitary brachytherapy in gynecology. 1985. Bethesda, MD: International Commission on Radiation Units and Measurements.

Jaffray, D.A., Siewerdsen, J.H., Wong, J.W., and Martinez, A.A. 2002. Flat panel cone-beam computed tomography for image guided radiation therapy. *Int. J. Radiat. Oncol. Biol. Phys. 53*:1337–1349.

Jeraj, R., Mackie, T.R., Balog, J., Olivera, G., Pearson, D., Kapatoes, J., Ruchala, K., and Reckwerdt, P. 2004. Radiation characteristics of helical tomotherapy. *Med. Phys. 31*:396–400.

Keller, H., Glass, M., Hinderer, R., Ruchala, K., Jeraj, R., Olivera, G., and Mackie, TR. 2002. Monte Carlo study of a highly efficient gas ionization detector for megavoltage imaging and image-guided radiotherapy. *Med. Phys. 29*:165–175.

Kupelian, P.A., Ramsey, C.R., Meeks, S.L., Willoughby, T.R., Forbes, A., Wagner, T.H., and Langen, K.M. 2005. Serial megavoltage CT imaging during external beam radiotherapy for non-small cell lung cancer: observations on tumor regression during treatment. *Int. J. Radiat. Oncol. Biol. Phys. 63*:1024–1028.

Kupelian, P.A., Langen, K.M., Zeidan, O.A., Meeks, S.L., Willoughby, T.R., Wagner, T.H., Jeswani, S., Ruchala, K.J., Haimerl, J., and Olivera, G.H. 2006. Daily variations in delivered doses in patients treated with radiotherapy for localized prostate cancer. *Int. J. Radiat. Oncol. Biol. Phys.* 66:876–872.

Langen, K.M., and Jones, D.T. 2001. Organ motion and its management. *Int. J. Radiat. Oncol. Biol. Phys.* 50:265–278.

Langen, K.M., Zhang, Y., Andrews, R.D, Hurley M.E., Meeks, S.L., Poole, D.O., Willoughby, T.R., and Kupelian, P.A. 2005a. Initial experience with megavoltage (MV) CT guidance for daily prostate alignments. *Int. J. Radiat. Oncol. Biol. Phys.* 62:1517–1524.

Langen, K.M., Meeks, S.L., Poole, D.O., Wagner, T.H., Willoughby, T.R., Kupelian, P.A., Ruchala, K.J., Haimerl, J., and Olivera, G.H. 2005b. The use of megavoltage images for dose recompilations. *Phys. Med. Biol.* 50:4259–4276.

Mackie, T.R. 1999. Tomotherapy. *Semin. Radiat. Oncol. 9*:108–117.

Mackie, T.R., Balog, J., Ruchala, K., Shepard, D., Aldridge, S., Flitchard, E., Reckwerdt, P., Olivera, G., McNutt, T., and Mehta, M. 2003. Helical tomotherapy intensity-modulated radiation therapy. *The State of the Art. AAPM Summer School Proceedings*. Madison, WI: Medical Physics Publishing.

Meeks, S.L., Harmon J.F., Langen K.M., Willoughby, T.R., Wagner, T.H., and Kupelian P.A. 2005. Performance characterization of megavoltage computed tomography imaging on helical tomotherapy unit. *Med. Phys.* 32:2673–2681.

Mosleh-Shirazi, M.A., Evans, P.M., Swindell, W., Webb, S., and Partridge, M. 1998. A cone-beam megavoltage CT scanner for treatment verification in conformal radiotherapy. *Radiother Oncol. 48*: 319–328.

Ramsey, C.R., Langen, K.M., Kupelian, P.A., Scaperoth, D.D., Meeks, S.L., Mahan, S.L., and Rebecca, M.S. 2005. A technique for adaptive image-guided helical tomotherapy for lung cancer. *Int. J. Radiat. Oncol. Biol. Phys. 64*:1237–1244.

Ruchala, K.J., Olivera, G.H., Scholoesser, E.A., and Mackie, T.R. 1999. Megavoltage CT on a tomotherapy system. *Phys. Med. Biol.* 44:2597–2621.

Ruchala, K.J., Olivera, G.H., Kapatoes, J.M., Scholoesser, E.A., Reckwerdt, P.J., and Mackie, T.R. 2000. Megavoltage CT image reconstruction during tomotherapy treatments. *Phys. Med. Biol.* 45:3545–3562.

Simpson, R.G, Chen, C.T., Grubbs, E.A., and Swindell, W. 1982. A 4-MV CT scanner for radiation therapy: the prototype system. *Med. Phys. 9*:574–579.

Swindell, W. 1983. A 4-MV CT scanner for radiation therapy: spectral properties of the therapy beam. *Med. Phys. 10*:347–351.

Swindell, W., Simpson, R.G., and Oleson, J.R. 1983. Computed tomography with a linear accelerator with radiotherapy applications. *Med. Phys. 10*:416–420.

Wong, J.R., Cheng, C.W., Grimm, L., and Uematsu, M. 2001. Clinical implementation of the world's first Primatom, a combination of CT scanner and linear accelerator, for precise tumor targeting and treatment. *Physica Medica 17*:271–276.

Zeidan, O.A., Langden, K.M., Meeks, S.L., Manon, R.R., Wagner, T.H., Willougby, T.R., Jenkens, D.W., and Kupelian, P.A. 2007. Evaluation of image-guidance protocols in the treatment of head and neck cancers. *Int. J. Radiat. Oncol. Biol. Phys. 67*:670–677.

4

Integrated SET-3000G/X Positron Emission Tomography Scanner

Keishi Kitamura and Keiichi Matsumoto

Introduction

Positron emission tomography (PET) provides qualitative as well as quantitative information about the distribution over space and time of a given radiotracer within the human body (Phelps, 2000). Currently, one of the most widespread applications of PET is the measurement of glucose metabolism by using ^{18}F-fluorodeoxyglucose (^{18}F-FDG). The ability of ^{18}F-FDG PET to detect tumors via changes in glucose metabolism has had a major impact on the diagnosis, staging, and follow-up of oncologic patients. In particular, the whole-body technique, which effectively extends the axial field of view of the PET scanner by moving the bed in steps through the tomograph, offers the potential to monitor the malignant spread of disease in many areas of the body. This technique requires a high-performance PET camera that can both reduce the amount of tracer activity needed for the examination and shorten image acquisition time, while maintaining a high signal-to-noise ratio (SNR) in reconstructed images. This is especially true in Japan where cancer screening of symptom-free subjects with ^{18}F-FDG PET is becoming more popular (Yasuda et al., 2000), making PET units with low ^{18}F-FDG dosages and high throughput desirable.

However, several physical effects can influence quality and throughput during PET whole-body imaging. Most significant of these effects are the limitation of the number of events that can be acquired and the photon attenuation of gamma rays. The former leads to a long-duration scan, whereas the latter requires an additional transmission scan in order to obtain attenuation maps. Thus, when developing PET cameras that enable high patient throughput, two major strategies are increased sensitivity in three-dimensional (3D) emission scans and shortening transmission scan times.

During 3D acquisition, a large increase in sensitivity can be obtained by removing all interplane shielding and thus collecting all possible lines of gamma-ray response. However, in conventional whole-body scans, due to cylindrical detector geometry, acquiring data at distinct bed positions and overlapping several slices result in a sensitivity profile with axial variations.

A new acquisition and reconstruction method for continuous 3D scanning can improve the sensitivity of whole-body studies (Dahlbom et al., 2001). This acquisition mode has significant advantages, including uniform axial sensitivity and uniform axial resolution, reduced noise from detector normalization, and reduced sensitivity to slight patient movements. Also, one earlier work (Kitamura et al., 2002) has shown that continuous 3D scanning can be implemented without large amounts of computer memory or hard disk space, and requires only a minimum of time for offline data processing, which helps to increase study throughout.

Performing a transmission scan for attenuation correction is widely used in PET imaging for accurate quantitation to eliminate distortions in lesion size and shape and to make image interpretation easier. However, when transmission measurement uses positron or gamma-ray sources, count-limited transmission data can lead to statistical errors in attenuation correction factors. This prevents the shortening of transmission scan times and reduces scanner throughput, especially with whole-body studies. Ideally, transmission data are acquired simultaneously with emission data, utilizing a dedicated hardware design. Simultaneous emission and transmission (SET) would both ensure perfect spatial registration of the two measurements and shorten the length of the study. Previous work has shown that SET scanning is feasible using fully extended rod sources and electronic rod windowing (Meikle et al., 1995). However, an SET scan precludes 3D emission data acquisition and high photon source flux due to deadtime and the contamination of the emission data by random coincidences. In addition, most currently available PET/CT systems use CT for attenuation correction. The significantly higher source strength used to acquire a CT image reduces photon statistical noise at the cost of an increased radiation dose.

Recently, however, a new high-resolution and high-sensitivity PET camera (SET-3000G/X) was developed by Shimadzu Corporation (Kyoto, Japan). This PET camera features a new technique called continuous emission and spiral transmission (CEST), which allows high-throughput scanning with transmission-based attenuation correction and the administration of a reduced radiation dose. With this method, 3D emission and single-transmission data can be obtained simultaneously by moving the patient bed continuously through both the emission and the dedicated transmission scanners, which are separated axially by a lead shield. Separation of the transmission source mechanism leads to a high photon flux due to the elimination of deadtime and random coincidences in emission data. The CEST scan design's separation of the transmission source mechanism leads to a smaller emission ring diameter, producing high sensitivity in 3D emission studies. The CEST scan method can also be applied to a PET/CT system, without using CT scans for attenuation correction. In this chapter, we describe acquisition and reconstruction methods for CEST scanning and discuss the advantages of these methods, specifically in comparison with current PET/CT scanners.

System Description

Figure 1 shows a schematic of the SET-3000G/X, where a 3D emission scanner is combined with a transmission scanner, and both are separated axially by a lead shield. Details of this system were described in previous reports (Kitamura et al., 2005; Matsumoto et al., 2006) and are summarized in Table 1. In brief, this PET camera uses cylindrically arranged germanium oxyorthosilicate (GSO) [$Gd_2Sio_5(Ce)$] crystals for dedicated 3D emission scanning, and a ring of bismuth germanate (BGO) ($Bi_4Ge_3O_{12}$) crystals with a ^{137}Cs point source for transmission scanning. These scanners are coaxially attached and separated by a lead shield for CEST scanning (Fig. 1).

In the PET camera's GSO scanner, small (2.45 × 5.1 mm²), long (30 mm) crystals are arranged in blocks (23 × 52 mm²) to produce high-resolution and high-count rates. The detector ring has a large solid angle with an aperture of 664 mm, axial coverage of 260 mm, and a patient port diameter of 600 mm. The transmission scanner consists of 6-ring BGO block detectors (diameter: 798 mm, axial width: 23 mm), and a rotating ^{137}Cs point source of 740 MBq collimated both axially and transaxially with a tungsten collimator. Transmission count rate is almost 3 Mcps, and the rotation speed of the source is 3 sec per rotation. Since the emission and transmission sections are separated by a 32.5-mm-thick lead shield and the point source is axially highly collimated, the background coincidence rate of the emission scanner due to the transmission source is considered to be negligible. Axial collimation also decreases the scatter fraction of the transmission data and provides more accurate attenuation values.

This design reduces total scanning time by allowing simultaneous emission and transmission scanning using a high-flux transmission source, a goal that is usually difficult when the same detector is used for both purposes. Because there is no transmission source within the emission scanner, the diameter of the emission detector can be reduced to only 664 mm, which increases the solid angle and sensitivity. The GSO scintillator allows the use of small-size crystals for high spatial resolution, while maintaining scintillating light output. The GSO also has a high-count rate, which allows 3D data acquisition using a large solid angle. Furthermore, even though it contains two scanners and all their electronics, including signal processing and coincidence circuits, the small-ring diameter enables a relatively small-size gantry.

A performance evaluation of this product based on the NEMA NU2-2001 protocols was described in a previous report (Matsumoto et al., 2006). The main performance results are summarized as follows:

The measured spatial resolution near the center of the field-of-view (FOV) is 3.5 mm, a value superior to any reported for commercially available whole-body PET cameras for clinical use. Absolute sensitivity is 18.2 cps/kBq, more than two times higher than current scanners. In addition, this unit's high-count rate produces a maximum noise equivalent count (NEC) rate of 62.3 kcps at activity levels of 9.8 kBq/ml. In typical clinical situations, where soft tissue (ex. liver) activity concentration is assumed to be 3 kBq/ml, this NEC rate is 41.1 kcps, a value high enough to provide images with high SNR ratios.

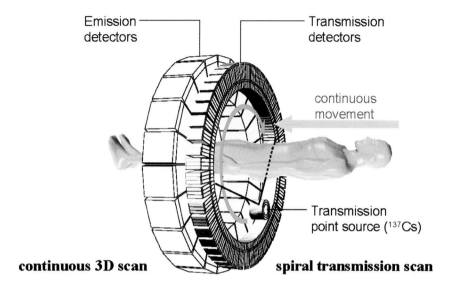

Figure 1 SET-3000G/X schematic design.

Continuous Emission and Spiral Transmission Scanning

During CEST acquisition, the patient bed moves continuously through the emission and transmission scanners in a single pass. After all scan protocol settings are entered, the bed is automatically moved to a starting point beyond the transmission scanner and the transmission source begins rotating, irradiating the patient. The patient is first scanned through the transmission scanner, and simultaneously emission data can be acquired in continuous 3D mode. In a whole-body study, bed speed is calculated according to the time used to acquire the axial scan range. In order to obtain completely uniform axial sensitivity, the extended scan's length must be equal to the axial length of both the transmission and emission scanners, while the extra length equivalent to

the transmission scanner is sufficient to obtain attenuation-corrected images.

During CEST scanning, the emission scanner is run in coincidence mode while the transmission scanner is run in singles mode, and, as described in Table 1, the energy windows used by these scanners are different. All acquisition data are transferred to the host PC as list mode data and separated in real time into transmission and emission sinograms. The report stream of the bed and point source position data, sent from the gantry and from the bed controller, are merged into the event stream as tag packets. Tag insertion is then handled completely by the event-sorting process.

Single-transmission data can be acquired as fan-beam data using a spiral motion. Correction for contamination from the emission detector to the transmission detector is performed by masking and measuring the background counts

Table 1   SET-3000G/X Scanner Specifications

	Emission Scanner	Transmission Scanner
Scintillation crystal	GSO	BGO
Crystal size	2.45 × 5.10 × 30 mm^3	6.25 × 3.8 × 30 mm^3
Number of crystals	39,600	2304
Number of detector blocks	88/ring	48/ring
Number of detector rings	50	6
Detector ring diameter	664 mm	798 mm
Axial field-of-view	260 mm	23.1 mm
Transverse field-of-view	600 mm	600 mm
Target gamma-ray energy	511 keV	662 keV
Energy window	400–700 keV	600–800 keV
Coincidence time window	6 ns	—

of the off-collimation detectors. During the rotation of the transmission source, the singles count obtained by one detector element will change, while the emission signal count rate remains almost constant, except for the source position, where the collimator is in front of the detector. Collimator penetration components of the off-collimation detectors can be measured in advance using a blank scan. Then, the emission contamination (EC) count is subtracted from the transmission data obtained in the front view area, assuming that the emission component is uniformly distributed. After correction for all detector elements is completed, transmission data are stored on a hard disk drive.

This method allows us to accurately correct EC components in transmission data without increasing scan time. Over a range of clinical activity and after correction for emission contamination, the attenuation coefficient obtained from transmission data for a cylindrical phantom was an average of $0.095 \, cm^{-1}$ (standard deviation of $0.02 \, cm^{-1}$), and was not different from the value obtained for a cold phantom. Furthermore, no significant increase in image noise was observed using this correction method (Kitamura *et al.*, 2005).

Transmission data corrected for emission contamination are sequentially rebinned into transaxial slices, according to the spiral pitch (i.e., bed and rotation speed). Axial (z) direction filtering is performed with several data sets. This z-filtering method is almost the same method used in a multislice helical CT (Taguchi and Aradate, 1998). After z-filtering is completed, to improve the image's SNR ratio, direct slice data perpendicular to the scanner axis are reconstructed using a statistical reconstruction method. These images are subsequently scaled to match attenuation coefficients for the annihilation gamma-ray energy (511 keV) and are then forward-projected to estimate 3D attenuation correction.

Emission coincidence events are sorted into sinograms (histogram format) according to reports of the actual bed position. Sinograms for a pair of rings are added to sinograms of the incremented ring pairs in real time by moving the bed axially (Kitamura *et al.*, 2002). This provides uniform sensitivity over most of the axial FOV using all ring pair data, up to the maximum ring differences. After histogram creation, normalization correction is performed on the emission sinograms to correct for detector efficiency, and normalized data are summed into oblique sinograms using the same histogram creation parameters as are used for the emission data. A normalization table is then obtained for each oblique sinogram by averaging all axial planes of a bed position. Since the patient is first scanned through the transmission scanner, a precalculated attenuation table can be applied to emission sinograms immediately after normalization. These sinograms are subsequently rebinned into transaxial sinograms at each axial sampling. Rebinned sinograms are reconstructed using a statistical reconstruction method to minimize noise propagation from projection data to the reconstructed image. In CEST scanning, both transmission and emission data can be processed in a pipeline fashion, according to bed movement. Pipeline-style processing eliminates the need to handle large amounts of data at the same time and improves data processing efficiency.

In the previous work (Matsumoto *et al.*, 2006), the spatial resolution was measured at a stationary bed arrangement according to the NEMA NU 2-2001 standard (3.49 mm FWHM transverse, 5.04 mm FWHM axially at 1 cm off center, 3.82 mm FWHM tangentially, 5.14 mm FWHM radially, and 5.40 mm FWHM axially at 10 cm off center). Similar results were obtained with the CEST data acquisition mode regardless of the bed velocity (3.62 mm FWHM transverse, 5.47 mm FWHM axially at 1 cm off center, 3.93 mm FWHM tangentially, 5.29 mm FWHM radially, and 6.07 mm FWHM axially at 10 cm off center). Therefore, the CEST mode does not degrade spatial resolution.

PET/CT System with cEST Scanning

The great advantage of a PET/CT scanner is its ability to produce fused PET/CT images; as a result, these units are rapidly replacing dedicated PET cameras in the market. Most of the currently available PET/CT systems use CT for attenuation correction. In these systems, the CT scan must be acquired for the entire axial length of the PET scan in order to acquire attenuation correction data and may include areas for which fused images are not requested. This, in turn, results in increased radiation exposure. In many cases, however, minimization of radiation exposure is essential, especially in cancer screenings using ^{18}F-FDG PET with symptom-free subjects or during serial studies of the same patient where only the time course of tracer uptake is of interest.

Because the PET camera described in this chapter uses the CEST technique, which provides attenuation data without requiring additional scanning time and with little additional radiation exposure from the transmission scan, if the PET camera is incorporated into a PET/CT system a CT scan is not required for attenuation correction. Based on this idea, a new PET/CT scanner, the SET-3000GCT, has also been developed by Shimadzu Corporation. This new PET/CT system can acquire CT scans only in areas for which fusion images are requested and does not require an entire axial length scan.

Unlike conventional PET/CT scanners, this new scanner's PET tomograph unit is located in the front of the gantry and the CT tomograph unit is in the rear. Both tomograph units are housed in a single gantry, which has a bore of 60 cm and an axial length of 168 cm. The CT scanner is single slice, with both axial or helical acquisition modes and different rotation speeds, allowing PET scans to be acquired using the CEST technique for both emission and transmission data in whole-body studies.

A typical PET/CT protocol usually first acquires a CT scout scan, followed by a CT scan and a PET scan. With the SET-3000GCT, a PET scan is first acquired using the CEST technique, which obtains both emission and transmission data simultaneously. Raw PET emission data are then reconstructed using the single-transmission images for attenuation correction. Instead of the CT scout view, PET emission or transmission images with sagittal, coronal, or maximum intensity projection (MIP) views are used to define the starting and ending locations of the actual CT acquisitions, and the CT scan is acquired over the range defined on the PET scan. Rather than acquiring the entire axial length, it is possible to acquire a CT scan only in consecutive or discrete areas for which fusion images are required. During cancer screening of a symptom-free subject using PET, not acquiring any CT scan is a possible choice if no malignancies are found on the PET images.

Computed tomography scans can be obtained using various imaging protocols for each scan area depending on the targeted organ. Upon completion of the definition of CT scan range, the bed is automatically moved to position the patient in the field-of-view of the CT scanner. The patient is positioned so that the CT scan will cover the area of interest. After the CT scan, CT raw data are then reconstructed, and both PET and CT images can be displayed either side by side or overlaid, as shown in Figure 2.

Discussion

Shimadzu Corporation has developed PET and PET/CT systems using the CEST scan method; these are the first systems in the world to provide spiral single-transmission and continuous 3D emission images simultaneously from a single bed movement. The design of these emission scanners is based on large-aperture cylindrical detectors, which extends axial range and reduces scanner diameter, creates a large solid angle of acceptance and, as a result, a high geometric sensitivity that leads to higher sensitivity per unit detector volume as well as cost efficiencies. Continuous bed movement can provide uniform sensitivity and resolution over a wide axial range for both transmission and emis-

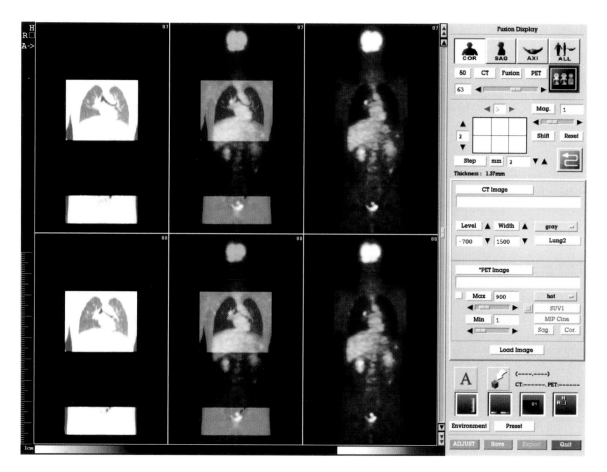

Figure 2 Sample PET/CT images acquired using SET-3000GCT.

sion images. In addition, use of *z*-filtering and continuous 3D rebinning methods ensures that all data are efficiently utilized in the transmission and emission data reconstruction processes.

Although continuous bed movement requires an extended scan range to cover the same area obtained by a conventional scan, the CEST scan eliminates the need for additional bed movement time, as well as the source extension and retraction between discrete bed positions required with conventional PET scanners. Furthermore, these units' on-the-fly reconstruction minimizes the time required for offline data processing and helps to increase throughput in whole-body studies.

The combination of CEST technology in a PET scanner together with a CT scanner allows the elimination of CT data for attenuation correction of PET emission data, without compromising patient throughput. Computed tomography-based transmission can reduce transmission acquisition time significantly; however, the radiation doses required to do so were much higher than those observed with gamma-ray transmission. To overcome this problem, most of the currently available PET/CT systems perform a CT scan for attenuation correction by lowering the X-ray tube current, which results in a much lower dose of radiation than that of a high-quality CT scan, at the expense of image quality. During CEST scanning, use of a strong transmission source and the statistical reconstruction method is sufficient to decrease transmission image noise. Nevertheless, when compared even with current PET/CT scanners using a low-radiation mode scan for attenuation correction, this unit's highly collimated transmission source results in a much lower radiation dose (Shimizu *et al.*, 2005).

In addition, with a PET/CT unit using CEST scanning, most commonly seen PET/CT image artifacts can be avoided due to the use of a PET transmission scan, instead of a CT scan for attenuation correction of the PET data. Artifacts in PET emission images that are commonly corrected for attenuation using a CT scan often are the result of positional mismatches caused by patient motion or respiration differences between the PET and CT scans, or by incorrect calculation of attenuation coefficients for CT contrast agents or metallic implants (Kinahan *et al.*, 2003).

A CT scan is usually acquired during a specific stage of the patient's breathing cycle. Conversely, because of the long acquisition time required for a PET scan, it is usually acquired while the patient is breathing freely. Thus, the final image is an average of many breathing cycles. This difference in respiratory motion between PET scans and CT scans causes breathing artifacts on PET/CT images. In CEST scanning, even though the axial range of the transmission scanner is much shorter than that of the emission scanner, in contrast to a CT scan it can average a number of breathing cycles as a result of slow bed movement, which helps minimize respiratory motion artifacts.

If the CT scan is used to estimate attenuation maps for 511 keV gamma rays, contrast agent can be easily confused with bone tissue because of its high atomic number. This can result in overestimation of PET attenuation coefficients and, consequently, radiotracer concentration. The same situation occurs when the patient has metallic implants, which results in high CT values and generates streaking artifacts on CT images, due to their high photon absorption. When transmission scans are acquired with ^{137}Cs sources (662 keV gamma rays), attenuation maps show small differences between regions of high- and low-contrast agent concentration and prevent artifacts due to metallic implants.

Continuous emission and spiral transmission scans also have the following advantages:

Emission and transmission scanners using the same transaxial FOV prevent truncation artifacts, while keeping the patient's arms in the FOV. Low operation costs due to using a 30-year half-life source eliminate the need to replace the transmission source as it decays. Simultaneous acquisition minimizes misalignments of emission and transmission data caused by patient motion.

In summary, a new technology named CEST scanning was developed for whole-body PET studies requiring low radiation dosages and high patient throughput. With this method, 3D emission and single-transmission data can be obtained simultaneously by moving the patient bed continuously through the emission and the dedicated transmission scanners, which are separated axially by a lead shield. This technology has led to a new type of PET-CT scanner that can perform CT scanning only for localized areas of cancer, areas that were previously determined by whole-body PET scanning. This technology also outperforms current scan acquisition methods, especially for cancer screening, and can reduce radiation dose without compromising patient throughput.

References

Dahlbom, M., Reed, J., and Young, J. 2001. Implementation of true continuous 2D/3D whole body PET scanning. *IEEE Trans. Nucl. Sci.* 48:1465–1469.

Kinahan, P.E., Hasegawa. B.H., and Beyer, T. 2003. X-ray-based attenuation correction for positron emission tomography/computed tomography scanners. *Semin. Nucl. Med.* 33:166–179.

Kitamura, K., Tanaka, K., and Sato, T. 2002. Implementation of continuous 3D whole body PET scanning using on-the-fly Fourier rebinning. *Phys. Med. Biol.* 47:2705–2712.

Kitamura, K., Takahashi, S., Tanaka, A., Ishikawa, A., Mizuta, T., Tanaka, K., Amano, M., Matsumoto, K., Yamamoto, S., Nakamoto, Y., Sakamoto, S., and Senda, M. 2005. 3D Continuous emission and spiral transmission scanning for high-throughput whole-body PET. *IEEE Nucl. Sci. Symp. Med. Imag. Conf. Rec.* 2004:M3-2.

Matsumoto, K., Kitamura, K., Mizuta, T., Tanaka, K., Yamamoto, S., Sakamoto, S., Nakamoto, Y., Amano, M., Murase, K., and Senda, M. 2006. Performance characteristics of a new 3-dimensional continuous-emission and spiral-transmission high-sensitivity and high-resolution PET camera evaluated with the NEMA NU 2-2001 standard. *J. Nucl. Med. 47*:83–90.

Meikle, S.R., Bailey, D.L., Hooper, P.K., Eberl, S., Hutton, B.F., Jones, W.F., Fulton, R.R., and Fulham, M.J. 1995. Simultaneous emission and transmission measurements for attenuation correction in whole-body PET. *J. Nucl. Med. 36*:1680–1688.

Phelps, M.E. 2000. PET: the merging of biology and imaging into molecular imaging. *J. Nucl. Med. 41*:661–681.

Shimizu, K., Matsumoto, K., and Kitamura, K. 2005. Radiation exposure caused by transmission measurement in clinical whole body PET: comparison with four types of PET scanners and CT scanner [abstract]. *Eur. J. Nucl. Med. Mol. Imaging 32(Suppl.)*:S253.

Taguchi, K., and Aradate, H. 1998. Algorithm for image reconstruction in multi-slice helical CT. *Med. Phys. 25*:550–561.

Yasuda, S., Ide. M., Fujii, H., Nakahara, T., Mochizuki, Y., Takahashi, W., and Shohtsu, A. 2000. Application of positron emission tomography imaging to cancer screening. *Br. J. Cancer. 83*:1607–1611.

5

High-Resolution Magic Angle Spinning Magnetic Resonance Spectroscopy

Beathe Sitter, Tone F. Bathen, and Ingrid S. Gribbestad

Introduction

Various human diseases have been explored by magnetic resonance spectroscopy (MRS) for more than two decades, and this research has contributed to the understanding of different biological processes in conditions of health and disease. Cancerous tissue differs from its healthy counterparts in numerous ways—for instance, by increased cell proliferation and degree of cell differentiation. Cell processes involve chemical reactions, which may be altered in cancerous cells. Such alterations can be observed by MRS. It is likely that we are looking for the same metabolites as normally present, but in abnormal proportions (Ross, 1992). Another possible contribution to observed differences between cancerous and normal tissue is the altered physiology. Alterations in blood and substrate supply, tumor necrosis, and nutritional disturbances in the host are all factors likely to contribute.

Magnetic resonance spectroscopy gives a description of the studied material on a molecular level, providing a molecular image of the studied object. *In vivo* spectra of patients are performed at low magnetic field strengths (from 1 to 4 Tesla). These relatively low field strengths and the fixed positions of molecules in the tissue put limitations on the spectral resolution, and only a small number of metabolites can be observed. *Ex vivo* analyses of tissue specimens can

be performed at much higher field strengths (from 7 to 21 Tesla), providing spectra with enhanced resolution. Traditionally, tissue samples have been analyzed by two different approaches: either by acquiring MR spectra from an intact sample or from an extract of the tissue. Magnetic resonance spectra of intact samples are of low resolution, and the biochemical information is thereby limited. Magnetic resonance spectra of tissue extracts provide detailed information on chemical composition, but at the cost of tissue destruction and possibly modified composition. The technique called high-resolution magic angle spinning (HR MAS) MRS decreases the restrictions caused by the fixed position of molecules, providing further resolved spectra comprising numerous metabolites. HR MAS MRS has been applied in studies of intact tissue specimens since 1996 (Cheng *et al.*, 1996).

Molecules in tissue have very limited mobility compared to molecules in solutions. The lack of molecular mobility leads to anisotropic interactions, imposing a spin orientation dependence on the MR frequency (Andrew, 1996), and the result is broad MR lines. Andrew *et al.* (1958) and Lowe (1959) first described the narrowing of MR lines when solids were spun at the magic angle. Line broadening in solids can be reduced by spinning the sample rapidly about an axis inclined 54.7° to the direction of the static magnetic field (Fig. 1). The spinning splits the broad resonance into a narrow line at the isotropic resonance frequency and spinning sidebands (Mehring, 1983). All spin interactions become time-dependent, and sidebands appear at integer multiples of the spinning rate. The time-independent part of the anisotropic interactions is dependent on $(3\cos^2\theta-1)$ and is canceled by the choice of the magic angle, $54.7°$. The time-dependent anisotropic interactions average over a rotor period. If the spinning rate is much larger than the anisotropic spin interaction, the sidebands are well separated from the central line and their intensity decreases with increasing spinning rate. As a consequence, anisotropic interactions are averaged to their isotropic value, resulting in substantial line narrowing.

Samples

Samples analyzed by MAS are usually in the range of 10 to 50 mg. Spectra of sufficient signal-to-noise can be obtained by smaller samples, and tissue samples of 0.5 mg have been analyzed with respect to biochemical composition (Martinez-Granados *et al.*, 2006). Breast cancer tissue samples can be obtained from the surgically removed tumor by a needle biopsy or a fine-needle aspirate, and all types should be suitable for MAS analysis. So far, only MAS studies on breast cancer tissue samples from surgically removed tumor have been published (Cheng *et al.*, 1998; Sitter *et al.*, 2006). Needle biopsies have been analyzed successfully on liver tissue (Martinez-Granados *et al.*, 2006). Analyses of needle biopsies or fine-needle aspirates could provide a method to directly monitor treatment effects prior to surgery

and possibly predict patient treatment response (Gribbestad *et al.*, 2006).

Excised tissue is no longer under the control systems of the body, and the chemical components in biopsy samples change due to enzymatic and chemical processes. Because we want to portray the original chemical composition of the biopsy, the treatment of samples is crucial for preserving this information. The temperature should be kept as low as possible during sample storage, preparation, and MR analysis. Tissue should be frozen immediately after excision. A thermos containing liquid nitrogen in the operating room allows the samples to be frozen within minutes after excision. Tissue should be stored at $-80°C$ or colder to limit degradation. Samples usually need to be stored for practical reasons, but the freezing and thawing processes may have an impact on the MAS spectra. The effect on prostate tissue has been examined by Wu *et al.* (2003). They analyzed fresh and frozen samples from the same patients and reexamined the fresh sample after freezing. The resulting spectra showed that peak intensities were affected by freeze-thaw processes and for two of the metabolites; also the resonance linewidths were affected. The freezing of kidney tissue has reportedly led to increased amounts of amino acids and decreased contents of choline, glycerophosphocholine, glucose, *myo*-inositol, trimethylamine *N*-oxide (TMAO), and taurine (Middleton *et al.*, 1998; Waters *et al.*, 2000).

The effects of additives to biopsy samples need thorough consideration. Tissue rinsing prior to HR MAS analysis is reported in numerous publications (e.g. Rooney *et al.*, 2003). Tissue rinsing has been applied in order to remove residual blood (Garrod *et al.*, 2001) and improve water suppression (Tomlins *et al.*, 1998; Barton *et al.*, 1999). This tissue perfusion by an aqueous solution leads to a washout of water-soluble metabolites (Sitter *et al.*, 2002). Samples are usually immersed in a fluid (buffer) in the MAS rotor. A small amount of excess fluid is lost in the rotor assembly, which probably contains extracted metabolites. Studies have been presented where the sample has been analyzed without any additives to the MAS rotor (Cheng *et al.*, 1998). However, this procedure for sample preparation introduces air bubbles into the sample volume, and the large susceptibility differences of air and tissue can make it difficult to obtain highly resolved MR spectra.

During MAS analysis, samples are spun at high speeds, at several kHz. Spinning speeds are usually chosen to ensure that the spinning sidebands appear outside the spectral region of interest (5 kHz spinning speed for a 14.7 Tesla magnet, 600 MHz operating frequency for protons). The effect of high and low spinning speed on prostate tissue has been compared (Taylor *et al.*, 2003). Slow spinning requires MR acquisition methods to remove the spinning sidebands, whereas high-speed spinning can lead to destruction of tissue structure. Prostate tissue was found to have distorted ductal structures after high-speed spinning. However, only macro-

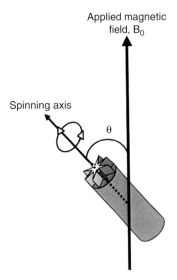

Figure 1 Schematic presentation of an MAS rotor in a magnetic field. θ is the magic angle, $54.7°$, B_0 is the static magnetic field.

structures were affected by the spinning, and the pathologist could clearly differentiate cell types. Our group has found that 82 of 85 breast tumor samples could be evaluated by microscopy after HR MAS analysis (Sitter *et al.*, 2006). Early on Smith *et al.* (1991) suggested that other types of tissue dilute the information from cancer cells metabolism in the spectra. The tissue being intact after MAS analysis provides a unique possibility to compare the chemical profile to other characteristics of the same tissue sample. A histopathological evaluation of the sample after MAS analysis will also reassure that actual tumor tissue is being investigated.

Spectral Analysis

Specific characteristics of the sample are to some extent selected by how the MR spectroscopy is performed. One-dimensional spectroscopy is used for correlations to clinical parameters. The resulting spectra can contain more than one hundred peaks, and sometimes two-dimensional spectroscopy is used in addition to resolve and identify overlapping peaks observed in one-dimensional spectra. Various pulse sequences can be applied to simplify one-dimensional spectra. As human tissues contain large amounts of water (60%), the water peak can dominate the spectrum completely and is usually suppressed in order to reveal the metabolite peaks. Large molecules, such as polypeptides and lipids, appear as broad signals. In studies where smaller molecules such

as amino acids and choline-containing compounds are of interest, the broad signals from macromolecules can be suppressed by a spin-echo sequence (Cheng *et al.*, 1998). Figure 2 illustrates the elimination of lipid signals and the revealing of the lactate resonance by spin-echo acquisition. Other techniques for acquisition of spectra have been applied in MAS MRS, including diffusion measurements to examine the cellular environments of tissue metabolites (Rooney *et al.*, 2003) and measurements of nuclear Overhauser effect (nOe) to observe interactions between molecules (Chen *et al.*, 2006).

Biological samples comprise a vast amount of MR detectable compounds, and the resulting proton MR spectra can be very complex. Different approaches are used to investigate MR spectra. Spectral characteristics can be explored by examining peak intensities or peak areas. Metabolites of interest can be quantified by comparing peak areas to an internal reference like water (Cheng *et al.*, 1997, 2001) or to an added reference (Ala-Korpela *et al.*, 1996). Peak-by-peak investigations have been useful in many studies and make direct comparison between chemical and biological features possible (Delikatny *et al.*, 1993; Leach *et al.*, 1998). Because of the complexity involved concerning biological MR spectra, multivariate analyses are often used to extract the information. Multivariate spectral analyses can be applied to entire data sets. They can be used to reduce the complexity in the data and to generate and test scientific hypotheses (Lindon *et al.*, 2001). An often used method for analyses of MR spectroscopic data is principal component analysis

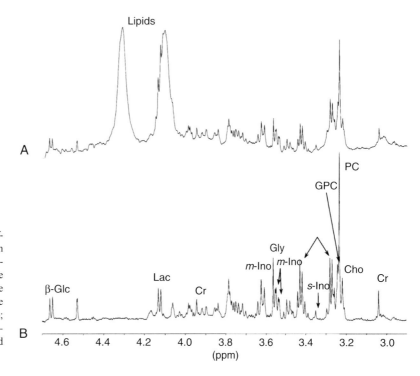

Figure 2 Spectral region 4.70 to 2.90 ppm from two different spectra from breast cancer tissue. (**A**) MAS spectrum of breast cancer sample acquired using a standard pulse-acquired sequence. (**B**) MAS spectrum from the same sample as in A recorded using a spin-echo sequence. Some peak assignments are given; the following abbreviations are used: β-Glc; β-glucose, Lac; lactate, Cr; creatine, *m*-Ino; *myo*-inositol, Gly; glycine, Tau; taurine, *s*-Ino; *scyllo*-inositol, GPC; glycerophosphocholine, PC; phosphocholine, and Cho; choline.

(PCA) (el Deredy, 1997; Hagberg, 1998). Principal component analysis creates linear combinations from the original spectra based on the variance, leading to a reduced set of independent variables, principal components (PCs), describing the original data set. It is a method for visualization of complex data and for reduction of data input before classification (el Deredy, 1997). Application of PCA on MR spectra has resulted in sample grouping based on score values for the PCs (Garrod et al., 1999; Tate et al., 2000). Principal component analysis uses solely the spectral characteristics of the samples and is a so-called unsupervised method. In order to develop methods for classification and prediction, supervised methods have proven efficient (Lindon et al., 2000). Such methods use a training set of MR spectra to construct a mathematical model, in which the spectra are related to a known class or clinical parameter. To determine the robustness of the model, validation using a testset of spectra and clinical parameters is performed. In cases with few samples, cross validation may be used instead. Further evaluation of the classification potential can be performed with a blind set, in which the clinical properties of samples are blinded for the model and the operator. Typical examples of supervised methods are partial least squares regression (PLS), regression extension of PCA, and artificial neural networks.

Results

The first study on MAS MRS of breast cancer biopsies was presented by Cheng et al. (1998), describing a possible method for discriminating invasive ductal carcinomas of different grading. They analyzed tissue samples from breast cancer patients (18 invasive ductal carcinomas and 1 ductal carcinoma in situ) and from one healthy patient. The MAS spectra were analyzed with respect to metabolite ratios (lactate/choline and phosphocholine/choline) and T_2 relaxation times. The results showed that an increase in lactate/choline ratio correlated with an increase in tumor grade. They also found that an increase in T_2 relaxation times of the phosphocholine resonance may differentiate grade II from grade III ductal carcinomas. Also, alterations in T_2 relaxation times among lipid components may be used to distinguish normal from carcinomas and between carcinoma grades.

The first study on MAS of breast cancer tissue from our group was presented by Sitter et al. (2002). This publication was based on MAS spectra from 10 samples and focused on spectral assignment. The spectra were related to spectra from perchloric acid extracts of breast cancer tissue. It was demonstrated that the spectral resolution of the MAS spectra, and the biochemical information obtained, was comparable to the spectrum from tissue extract. More than 30 different metabolites were identified from the intact tissue samples. Lipids, amino acids, and choline-containing compounds dominated the MAS spectra.

In a larger study, we investigated how MAS spectra of biopsies from breast cancer patients correlated to clinical parameters (Sitter et al., 2006). Spectra were acquired of tumor samples ($n = 85$) from breast cancer patients and of noninvolved adjacent tissue ($n = 18$) from the same patients. Tissue metabolite concentrations were estimated by relating metabolite peak to the internal standard TSP and sample wet weight. Concentrations of β-glucose, glycine, myo-inositol, taurine, glycerophosphocholine, phosphocholine, choline, and creatine were correlated to clinical and histopathological findings. Significant higher tissue concentrations of choline and glycine were found for tumors > 2 cm (0.78 and 3.09 μmol per gram tissue) compared to smaller tumors (0.69 and 2.34 μmol per gram tissue). Furthermore, the fraction of tumor cells was found to have an impact on the HR MAS spectra. Samples without cancer cells contained lower concentrations of choline and creatine compared to samples positively comprising cancer cells. Correlation between metabolic pattern and tissue composition was also found by PCA. Samples containing similar fractions of cancer cells showed similar scores for the PCs, and a high content of cancer cells was correlated to elevated levels of glycine and phosphocholine.

Samples from breast cancer patients with spread to lymph nodes could generally not be classified based on PCA. However, when using only spectra from patients diagnosed with invasive ductal carcinoma ($n = 73$), half of the spectra from lymph node negative patients separated from lymph node positive. Furthermore, when spectra from samples containing fat tissue were excluded, a near separation of samples from lymph node positive and negative patients was obtained ($n = 43$), shown in Figure 3. Samples from node-positive patients showed increased content of glycine and reduced taurine compared to node-negative patients.

In a recent study from our group (Bathen et al., 2006), spectra were obtained from patients ($n = 89$) diagnosed with invasive ductal carcinomas (grades 1, 2, and 3). The purpose was to use different multivariate methods to establish classification models for prediction of grade, lymphatic spread, and hormone receptor status, based on the MAS spectra. Only spectra obtained from biopsies containing at least 5% tumor cells were included. Twelve of the spectra were chosen to compose a blind data set and were kept outside all training (model construction). Verification of models by blind sample testing showed that hormone status was well predicted by both probabilistic neural network (PNN) and PLS (11 out of 12 correct), that lymphatic spread was best predicted by PLS (8 out of 12 correct), and that grade was best predicted by PLS uninformative variable elimination (PLS-UVE) PNN (9 out of 12 correct).

Discussion

The correlation of MAS spectral profiles to patient diagnosis verifies that the biochemical profiles obtained by the HR

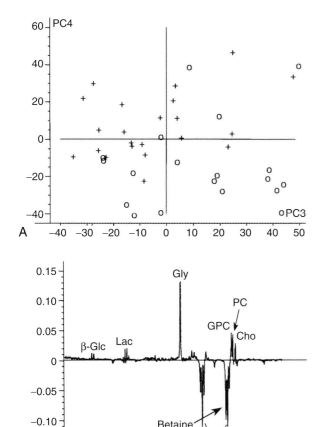

Figure 3 (**A**) Score plot of PC3 and PC4 from PCA of spin-echo spectra ($n = 41$) of samples from patients with invasive ductal carcinoma. The principal components PC3 and PC4 describe 11% and 10% of the variation in the spectra, respectively. + denotes samples from patients with lymphatic spread and o from lymph node negative patients. (**B**) Loading profile of PC4 from A in which most samples from patients with lymphatic spread showed high score. The loading profile corresponds to the spectral region 4.8 to 2.9 ppm, excluding the residual glycerol backbone signals from 4.4 to 4.2 ppm. Abbreviations: β-Glc; β-glucose, Lac; lactate, Cr; creatine, Gly; glycine, Tau; taurine, GPC; glycerophosphocholine, PC; phosphocholine, and Cho; choline. (Part of an illustration found in Sitter, B., Lundgren, S., Bathen, T.F., Halgunset, J., Fjosne, H.E., and Gribbestad, I.S. 2006. Comparison of HR MAS MR spectroscopic profiles of breast cancer tissue with clinical parameters. *NMR Biomed. 19*:30–40. Copyright © 2006 John Wiley & Sons Ltd.)

MAS technique correspond to pathological changes. Cheng *et al.* (1998) found that lactate/choline metabolic ratio and T_2 relaxation times possibly correlated to histological grading. These findings have not been confirmed by later studies by Sitter and coworkers. (2006). These authors found that breast tissueshowed elevated levels of numerous metabolites, probably connected to general increased cellular activity. Glycine was

elevated in samples from large breast tumors and was furthermore important in the characterization of samples from lymph node positive breast cancer patients. Ductal carcinomas are in part characterized by large fractions of connective tissue (Crum *et al.*, 2003), and high levels of glycine in tissue from such tumors might be connected to collagen synthesis.

Taurine was found to be important in the possible discrimination of samples from lymph node positive patients. Increased taurine levels have been found in malignant compared to noninvolved tissue studies of breast (Beckonert *et al.*, 2003), pancreatic (Kaplan *et al.*, 1997), colon (Moreno *et al.*, 1993), and prostate cancer (Swanson *et al.*, 2003). The roles of taurine are not fully understood, and it appears to have different functions in different tissues (Stapleton *et al.*, 1998).

Sitter *et al.* (2006) also found choline and phosphocholine to correlate to tumor size. In cancer studies using MRS, the altered pattern of choline compounds has added important diagnostic information (Nelson, 2003). Numerous studies confirm the altered pattern of choline metabolites in tumors (Podo, 1999), but the mechanisms are not fully understood. Enhanced choline transport and increased synthesis of betaine and phosphocholine were found to be dominant pathways responsible for increased levels of cholines in malignant mammary cell lines (Katz-Brull *et al.*, 2002). Choline kinase activity is increased in lung, prostate, and colon (Nakagami *et al.*, 1999; Ramirez de Molina *et al.*, 2002a) and breast carcinomas (Ramirez de Molina *et al.*, 2002b).

The strongest prognostic factor for breast cancer patients is their axillary lymph node status (Noguchi, 2002). Approximately, one-third of breast cancer patients die because of metastasis (Jones and McAdam, 2003). Negative findings of tumor spread in the axillary lymph nodes of breast cancer patients are associated with good prognosis for the patient. Still, ~ 25% of these patients experience systemic recurrence or spread of their breast cancer (Noguchi, 2002). A method that could provide a higher level of confidence in predicting patients with high probability of recurrence or metastasis would make a profound effect for the large number of women affected by the disease. Magic angle spinning spectra of breast cancer tissue have shown good correlation with lymph node status (Bathen *et al.*, 2006). A previous study using conventional MR spectroscopy on breast cancer tissue by Mountford *et al.* (2001) also found a possible connection between breast tumor biochemical profile and lymph node status. This method of lymph node prediction and the results from PCA of MAS spectra (Fig. 3) were restricted to samples without fat tissue. However, in the exploration of different classification models (Bathen *et al.*, 2006), the exclusion criterion was low content of tumor cell (< 5%), demonstrating that lymph node prediction can also be performed on spectra from samples containing fat tissue. If the HR MAS analysis of breast cancer tissue is to become a routine clinical tool, the analysis should be fast and kept as simple as possible. The protocols we have established require approximately 30 min totally. It is also important to establish a method of classification involving multivariate analysis, providing an automated analysis of the MAS MR spectra. The potential of this method can be evaluated retrospectively by comparing the HR MAS findings to patient 5-year survival. In the possible discrimination of MAS spectra from lymph node negative and positive patients by PCA (Fig. 3), 8 of the 19 samples from negative lymph node patients showed metabolic profiles comparable to samples from patients with lymph node spread. In the study exploring classification models (Bathen, 2006), 3 of the 12 blind samples actually defined as lymph negative by the sentinel node method are classified as lymph positive by all three prediction models. A comparison of patient outcome for all patients in the lymph node predictions will be performed to evaluate the prognostic potential of MAS analysis.

To further develop and evaluate MAS of breast cancer samples as a prognostic tool, a large number of samples need to be analyzed. If the method is to become a prognostic tool in diagnosis and treatment of breast cancer patients, the sample population has to be adjusted. There is a nonrepresentative high fraction of large tumors in bio-banks (McGuire, 1991), because all material in small tumors frequently is needed for routine clinical histological analysis. To make the results more representative, sampling should be stratified according to the tumor size of the breast cancer patient population. Also, samples from patients diagnosed with breast cancers other than the most common (invasive ductal carcinomas) should be included in further studies. The results should also be reproduced by other research centers.

References

Ala-Korpela, M., Posio, P., Mattila, S., Korhonen, A., and Williams, S.R. 1996. Absolute quantification of phospholipid metabolites in brain-tissue extracts by ^{1}H NMR spectroscopy. *J. Magn. Reson. B 113*:184–189.

Andrew, E.R., 1996. Magic angle spinning. In: *Encyclopedia of Nuclear Magnetic Resonance*, pp. 2891–2901.

Andrew, E.R., and Newing, R.A. 1958. The narrowing of nuclear magnetic resonance spectra by molecular rotation in solids. *Phys. Soc. 72*:959–972.

Barton, S.J., Howe, F.A., Tomlins, A.M., Cudlip, S.A., Nicholson, J.K., Bell, B.A., and Griffiths, J.R. 1999. Comparison of *in vivo* ^{1}H MRS of human brain tumours with ^{1}H HR-MAS spectroscopy of intact biopsy samples *in vitro*. *MAGMA 8*:121–128.

Bathen, T.F., Jensen, L.R., Sitter, B., Fjösne, H.E., Halgunset, J., Axelson, D.E., Gribbestad, I.S., and Lundgren, S. 2006. MR-determined metabolic phenotype of breast cancer in prediction of lymphatic spread, grade and hormone status. Epub: DOI: 10.1007/s10549-006-9400-z. *Breast Cancer Res. Treat.*

Beckonert, O., Monnerjahn, J., Bonk, U., and Leibfritz, D. 2003. Visualizing metabolic changes in breast-cancer tissue using ^{1}H-NMR spectroscopy and self-organizing maps. *NMR Biomed. 16*:1–11.

Bollard, M.E., Garrod, S., Holmes, E., Lindon, J.C., Humpfer, E., Spraul, M., and Nicholson, J.K. 2000. High-resolution ^{1}H and ^{1}H-^{13}C magic angle spinning NMR spectroscopy of rat liver. *Magn. Reson. Med. 44*:201–207.

Bourne, R., Dzendrowskyj, T., and Mountford, C. 2003. Leakage of metabolites from tissue biopsies can result in large errors in quantitation by MRS. *NMR Biomed. 16*:96–101.

Chen, J.H., Sambol, E.B., Decarolis, P., O'connor, R., Geha, R.C., Wu, Y.V., and Singer, S. 2006. High-resolution MAS NMR spectroscopy detection of the spin magnetization exchange by cross-relaxation and chemical exchange in intact cell lines and human tissue specimens. *Magn. Reson. Med. 55*:1246–1256.

Cheng, L.L., Chang, I.-W., Smith, B.L., and González, R.G. 1998. Evaluating human breast ductal carcinomas with high-resolution magic-angle spinning proton magnetic resonance spectroscopy. *J. Magn. Reson. 135*:194–202.

Cheng, L.L., Lean, C.L., Bogdanova, A., Wright, S.C., Jr., Ackerman, J.L., Brady, T.J., and Garrido, L. 1996. Enhanced resolution of proton NMR spectra of malignant lymph nodes using magic-angle spinning. *Magn. Reson. Med. 36*:653–658.

Cheng, L.L., Ma, M.J., Becerra, L., Ptak, T., Tracey, I., Lackner, A., and González, R.G. 1997. Quantitative neuropathology by high resolution magic angle spinning proton nuclear magnetic resonance spectroscopy. *Proc. Natl. Acad. Sci. USA 94*:6408–6413.

Cheng, L.L., Wu, C., Smith, M.R., and González, R.G. 2001. Non-destructive quantification of spermine in human prostate tissue samples using HR MAS ^{1}H NMR spectroscopy at 9.4 T. *FEBS Lett. 494*:112–116.

Crum, C.P., Lester, S.C., and Cotran, R.S. 2003. The female genital system and breast. In: Kumar, V., Robbins, S., and Cotran, R.S. (Eds.), *Robbins Basic Pathology, 7th ed*, pp. 679–718. St. Louis: Saunders.

Delikatny, E.J., Russell, P., Hunter, J.C., Hancock, R., Atkinson K.H., van Haaften-Day C., and Mountford, C.E. 1993. Proton MR and human cervical neoplasia: *ex vivo* spectroscopy allows distinction of invasive carcinoma of the cervix from carcinoma *in situ* and other preinvasive lesions. *Radiology 188*:791–796.

el Deredy, W. 1997. Pattern recognition approaches in biomedical and clinical magnetic resonance spectroscopy: a review. *NMR Biomed. 10*:99–124.

Garrod, S., Humpfer, E., Connor, S.C., Connelly, J.C., Spraul, M., Nicholson, J.K., and Holmes, E. 2001. High-resolution $_1$H NMR and magic angle spinning NMR spectroscopic investigation of the biochemical effects of 2-bromoethanoamine in intact renal and hepatic tissue. *Magn. Reson. Med. 45*:781–790.

Garrod, S., Humpfer, E., Spraul, M., Connor, S.C., Polley, S., Connelly, J., Lindon, J.C., Nicholson, J.K., and Holmes, E. 1999. High-resolution magic angle spinning ^{1}H NMR spectroscopic studies on intact rat renal cortex and medulla. *Magn. Reson. Med. 41*:1108–1118.

Gribbestad, I.S., Sitter, B., Lundgren, S., and Bathen, T.F. 2006. Metabolic MR spectroscopic profiles correlate to clinical parameters in breast cancer specimens. Poster at *ISMRM MR of Cancer Study Group Workshop*, Proco Manor, PA, USA, October 13–16.

Hagberg, G. 1998. From magnetic resonance spectroscopy to classification of tumors: a review of pattern recognition methods. *NMR Biomed. 11*:148–156.

Jones, A., and McAdam, K. 2003. Medical therapy of advanced disease. In: Rayter, Z., and Mansi, J. (Eds.), *Medical Therapy of Breast Cancer*, pp. 283–308. Cambridge: Cambridge University Press.

Kaplan, O., Kushnir, T., Askenazy, N., Knubovets, T., and Navon, G. 1997. Role of nuclear magnetic resonance spectroscopy (MRS) in cancer diagnosis and treatment: ^{31}P, ^{23}Na, and ^{1}H MRS studies of three models of pancreatic cancer. *Cancer Res. 57*:1452–1459.

Katz-Brull, R., Seger, D., Rivenzon-Segal, D., Rushkin, E., and Degani, H. 2002. Metabolic markers of breast cancer: enhanced choline metabolism and reduced choline-ether-phospholipid synthesis. *Cancer Res. 62*:1966–1970.

Leach, M.O., Verrill, M., Glaholm, J., Smith, T.A., Collins, D.J., Payne, G.S., Sharp, J.C., Ronen, S.M., McCready, V.R., Powles, T.J., and Smith, I.E. 1998. Measurements of human breast cancer using magnetic resonance spectroscopy: a review of clinical measurements and a report of localized ^{31}P measurements of response to treatment. *NMR Biomed.* 11:314–340.

Lindon, J.C., Holmes, E., and Nicholson, J.K. 2001. Pattern recognition methods and applications in biomedical magnetic resonance. *Prog. Nucl. Magn. Reson. Spectrosc.* 39:1–40.

Lindon, J.C., Nicholson, J.K., Holmes, E., and Everett, J.R. 2000. Metabonomics: metabolic processes studied by NMR spectroscopy of biofluids. *Concepts Magn. Resonan.* 12:289–320.

Lowe, I.J. 1959. Free induction decays of rotating solids. *Phys. Rev. Lett.* 2:285–287.

Martinez-Granados, B., Monleon, D., Martinez-Bisbal, M.C., Rodrigo, J.M., del, O.J., Lluch, P., Ferrandez, A., Marti-Bonmati, L., and Celda, B. 2006. Metabolite identification in human liver needle biopsies by high-resolution magic angle spinning ^{1}H NMR spectroscopy. *NMR Biomed.* 19:90–100.

McGuire, W.L. 1991. Breast cancer prognostic factors: evaluation guidelines. *J. Natl. Cancer. Inst.* 83:154–155.

Mehring, M. 1983. Nuclear spin interactions in solids. In: Mehring, M. (Ed.), *Principles of High Resolution NMR in Solids*, pp. 8–62. Berlin, Heidelberg, New York: Springer-Verlag.

Middleton, D.A., Bradley, D.P., Connor, S.C., Mullins, P.G., and Reid, D.G. 1998. The effect of sample freezing on proton magic-angle spinning NMR spectra of biological tissue. *Magn. Reson. Med.* 40:166–169.

Millis, K., Weybright, P., Campbell, N., Fletcher, J.A., Fletcher, C.D., Cory, D.G., and Singer, S. 1999. Classification of human liposarcoma and lipoma using *ex vivo* NMR spectroscopy. *Magn. Reson. Med.* 41:257–267.

Moreno, A., Rey, M., Montane, J.M., Alonso, J., and Arus, C. 1993. ^{1}H NMR spectroscopy of colon tumors and normal mucosal biopsies; elevated taurine levels and reduced polyethyleneglycol absorption in tumors may have diagnostic significance. *NMR Biomed.* 6:111–118.

Mountford, C.E., Somorjai, R.L., Malycha, P.L., Gluch, L., Lean, C.L., Russell, P., Barraclough, B.H., Gillett, D.J., Himmelreich, U., Dolenko, B., Nikulin, A.K., and Smith, I.C.P. 2001. Diagnosis and prognosis of breast cancer by magnetic resonance spectroscopy of fine-needle aspirates analysed using a statistical classification strategy. *Brit. J. Surg.* 88:1234–1240.

Nakagami, K., Uchida, T., Ohwada, S., Koibuchi, Y., Suda, Y., Sekine, T., and Morishita, Y. 1999. Increased choline kinase activity and elevated phosphocholine levels in human colon cancer. *Jpn. J. Cancer. Res.* 90:419–424.

Nelson, S.J. 2003. Multivoxel magnetic resonance spectroscopy of brain tumors. *Mol. Cancer Ther.* 2:497–507.

Noguchi, M. 2002. Therapeutic relevance of breast cancer micrometastases in sentinel lymph nodes. *Brit. J. Surg.* 89:1505–1515.

Podo, F. 1999. Tumour phospholipid metabolism. *NMR Biomed.* 12:413–439.

Ramirez de Molina, A., Rodriguez-Gonzalez, A., Gutierrez, R., Martinez-Pineiro, L., Sanchez, J., Bonilla, F., Rosell, R., and Lacal, J. 2002a. Overexpression of choline kinase is a frequent feature in human tumor-derived cell lines and in lung, prostate, and colorectal human cancers. *Biochem. Biophys. Res. Commun.* 296:580–583.

Ramirez de Molina, A., Gutierrez, R., Ramos, M.A., Silva, J.M., Silva, J., Bonilla, F., Sanchez, J.J., and Lacal, J.C. 2002b. Increased choline kinase activity in human breast carcinomas: clinical evidence for a potential novel antitumor strategy. *Oncogene* 21:4317–4322.

Rooney, O.M., Troke, J., Nicholson, J.K., and Griffin, J.L. 2003. High-resolution diffusion and relaxation-edited magic angle spinning ^{1}H NMR spectroscopy of intact liver tissue. *Magn. Reson. Med.* 50:925–930.

Ross, B.D. 1992. The biochemistry of living tissues: examination by MRS. *NMR Biomed.* 5:215–219.

Sitter, B., Lundgren, S., Bathen, T.F., Halgunset, J., Fjosne, H.E., and Gribbestad, I.S. 2006. Comparison of HR MAS MR spectroscopic profiles of breast cancer tissue with clinical parameters. *NMR Biomed.* 19:30–40.

Sitter, B., Sonnewald, U., Spraul, M., Fjosne, H.E., and Gribbestad, I.S. 2002. High resolution magic angle spinning MRS of breast cancer tissue. *NMR Biomed.* 15:327–337.

Smith, T.A., Glaholm, J., Leach, M.O., Machin, L., and McCready, V.R. 1991. The effect of intra-tumour heterogeneity on the distribution of phosphorus containing metabolites within human breast tumours: an *in vitro* study using ^{31}P NMR spectroscopy. *NMR Biomed.* 4:262–267.

Stapleton, P.P., O'Flaherty, L., Redmond, H.P., and Bouchier-Hayes, D.J. 1998. Host defense—a role for the amino acid taurine? *J. Parenter. Enter. Nutr.* 22:42–48.

Swanson, M.G., Vigneron, D.B., Tabatabai, Z.L., Males, R.G., Schmitt, L., Carroll, P.R., James, J.K., Hurd, R.E., and Kurhanewicz, J. 2003. Proton HR-MAS spectroscopy and quantitative pathologic analysis of MRI/3D-MRSI-targeted postsurgical prostate tissues. *Magn. Reson. Med.* 50:944–954.

Tate, A.R., Foxall, P.J.D., Holmes, E., Moka, D., Spraul, M., Nicholson, J.K., and Lindon, J.C. 2000. Distinction between normal and renal carcinoma kidney cortical biopsy samples using pattern recognition of ^{1}H magic angle spinning (MAS) NMR spectra. *NMR Biomed.* 13:64–71.

Taylor, J.L., Wu, C.L., Cory, D., Gonzalez, R.G., Bielecki, A., and Cheng, L.L. 2003. High-resolution magic angle spinning proton NMR analysis of human prostate tissue with slow spinning rates. *Magn. Reson. Med.* 50:627–632.

Tomlins, A.M., Foxall, P.J.D., Lindon, J.C., Lynch, M.J., Spraul, M., Everett, J.R., and Nicholson, J.K. 1998. High resolution magic angle spinning ^{1}H nuclear magnetic resonance analysis of intact prostatic hyperplastic and tumour tissues. *Anal. Commun.* 35:113–115.

Waters, N.J., Garrod, S., Farrant, R.D., Haselden, J.N., Connor, S.C., Connelly, J., Lindon, J.C., Holmes, E., and Nicholson, J.K. 2000. High-resolution magic angle spinning ^{1}H NMR spectroscopy of intact liver and kidney: optimization of sample preparation procedures and biochemical stability of tissue during spectral acquisition. *Anal. Biochem.* 282:16–23.

Waters, N.J., Holmes, E., Waterfield, C.J., Farrant, R.D., and Nicholson, J.K. 2002. NMR and pattern recognition studies on liver extracts and intact livers from rats treated with alpha-naphthylisothiocyanate. *Biochem. Pharmacol.* 64:67–77.

Wu, C.L., Taylor, J.L., He, W., Zepeda, A.G., Halpern, E.F., Bielecki, A., Gonzalez, R.G., and Cheng, L.L. 2003. Proton high-resolution magic angle spinning NMR analysis of fresh and previously frozen tissue of human prostate. *Magn. Reson. Med.* 50:1307–1311.

6

Spatial Dependency of Noise and Its Correlation among Various Imaging Modalities

Pasha Razifar and Mats Bergström

Introduction

Imaging modalities such as positron emission tomography (PET), computed tomography (CT), PET/CT, and single photon emission computed tomography (SPECT) are noninvasive tomographical tools used for creating two-dimensional (2D) cross-sectional images of three-dimensional (3D) objects or patients. Images generated by PET and SPECT can provide information about functional or biochemical properties of tissues by recording the kinetic behavior of administered radiolabeled molecules, while CT provides information about X-ray density in tissues in the body. Dual-imaging modality, PET/CT tomography combines two state-of-the-art imaging modalities—PET and CT—which generate fused images providing both functional and anatomical information.

Images generated by these types of imaging techniques contain noise with different magnitude, spatial dependence, and correlation, which is of high enough magnitude to significantly impair the visualization and affect the precision of quantification in the generated images. It is therefore essential to understand the properties of noise in these imaging techniques and how they influence the results when using these techniques.

This chapter focuses on spatial dependence of noise, its correlation, and the impact of different reconstruction methods.

Variance images are used to illustrate the spatial distribution of noise, and the autocorrelation function (ACF) is used as a tool to illustrate noise correlation and its isotropic or non-isotropic behavior in images generated by PET, CT, PET/CT, and SPECT. This is done separately with one of either of the most common reconstruction methods, iterative or filtered backprojection, to indicate the major impact of the reconstruction method.

Impact of Noise in Images

Noninvasive imaging has become a prime method for supplying information for the clinical handling of oncology patients. Imaging is used for diagnosis, differential diagnosis, staging, and treatment monitoring of solid tumors, where the specific modality—computed tomography (CT), magnetic resonance tomography (MRT), positron emission tomography (PET), or single photon emission computed tomography (SPECT)—is chosen depending on indication, tumor type and location, availability, and cost. The most available methods are CT and MRI where their use can be exemplified by MRI scanning for the diagnosis of brain tumors, CT scanning of the chest for lung tumors, SPECT imaging with antibodies for diagnosis of specific tumors, and PET with fluorodeoxyglucose (FDG) for diagnosis of soft tissue lesions.

The clinical tasks are in most cases either of the following: identification of a tumor, assessment of tumor extent and relation to neighboring organs, or assessment of tumor grade and evaluation of tumor response. This means that in most cases the diagnostic task is either to visualize the extent of the tumor or to obtain a quantitative value of the tumor with respect to the properties given by the imaging modality. For example, in PET it is desirable to see the tumor and discriminate it from the background, as well as to obtain a quantitative value of FDG uptake, which in turn can be indicative of tumor grade and/or be used to assess treatment effect.

Among the imaging modalities, PET and SPECT are especially affected by a high level of noise. This noise impairs the potential to detect and discriminate the tumor in relation to the background (Fig. 1), and because of its specific properties with correlation and spatial dependence it is important to understand its appearance in the images. The noise also impairs the ability to obtain quantitative values, so it is important to understand the limitations imposed on the precision of values.

Noise

Image noise is usually defined as statistical uncertainties or variations (errors) of the measured values of the image elements or pixels. In PET, CT, SPECT, and PET/CT, noise is categorized into structured and unstructured noise. Structured noise or artifacts refer to nonrandom variations or disturbing patterns in the images, usually caused by inadequate performance of the detector and imaging system or by patient movements. Unstructured, random, or statistical noise is one of the most disturbing factors in reconstructed images, and derives from random statistical variation in the counting rate (Poisson counting noise), modulated by applied corrections and the reconstruction algorithm (Razifar, 2005). Statistical noise is typically nonstationary, implying that noise properties such as correlation and magnitude depend on the position within the image (Zaidi *et al.*, 2002). In the following sections, common sources of the noise in data generated by PET, CT, PET/CT, and SPECT scanners are briefly described, followed by noise variation and correlation in reconstructed images.

Noise in Raw Data

The background to the image noise is best understood in relation to the raw sinogram data acquired by these imaging modalities. Common to all of these modalities is the measurement and counting of photons by nuclear detectors. The random process of detecting photons generates a variation in

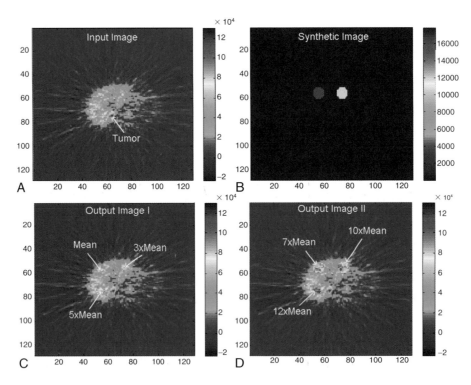

Figure 1 PET simulation study illustrates how the magnitude of noise disturbs and impairs the detection of tumors in a whole-body PET investigation. A slice through the liver containing a tumor was chosen **(A)**. Figure 1B shows a synthetic image containing three objects with different intensity. Figure 1C shows the image generated by adding Figure **B** to 1A, where the defined intensity value of pixels within each object is equal to the mean value of the image, 3 and 5 times the mean value, respectively. Figure 1**D** shows the image generated by adding Figure 1B to 1A, where the defined intensity value of pixels within each object is equal to 7, 10, and 12 times the mean value.

the counts, a variation that is described as Poisson distribution. If at a certain instance 100 photons are counted, a repetition of the measurement will likely give a new value that differs from the first one within ~10%. It is this variability that is the main cause of noise.

The magnitude of noise in a certain detection channel is affected by factors such as its flux of photons, type of scan, scan duration, out-of-field counts, normalization, random coincidences, deadtime, and scattered radiation counts. It is further modified by different corrections applied, such as random and scatter correction plus the major correction in emission tomography being attenuation correction (Razifar, 2005). The levels of contribution of these sources are different depending on acquisition mode. For instance, in PET both the signal and the noise are increased when data are acquired in 3D acquisition mode due to retraction of the interplane septa with increased detected count rate and sensitivity. Because the noise is approximately proportional to the square root of the counts, increasing the number of counts leads to a reduction of the noise fraction, defined as the ratio of noise and signal.

Noise Variation

Variation of the radioactive measurements obeys a Poisson distribution. Therefore, noise in the acquired data (not corrected) is nonstationary but retains a Poisson nature. Because of corrections prior to reconstruction and preprocessing or data transformation of the data, the noise in projections no longer obeys the Poisson distribution. Sometimes the magnitudes of the noise are amplified in acquired projections by factors of 10 or even 100 because of these corrections (Rowe and Dai, 1992). Noise variation and propagation in the reconstructed images are dependent on the utilized tomograph, applied acquisition mode, scan duration, amount of administered tracer, geometry of tracer distribution, applied correction methods, radioactive decay, choice of reconstruction algorithm, number of iterations, and type of convolution kernel (filter cut-off) (Razifar, 2005).

To study the variation of the noise and for further illustration of differences in noise behavior, variance images are generated from PET, SPECT, CT, and PET/CT images reconstructed by both analytical filtered backprojection (FBP) and iterative, ordered subsets expectation maximization (OSEM) methods (Fig. 2).

Images generated using the same type of reconstruction method express similar features independent of the used imaging modality. In PET and PET/CT images reconstructed with FBP, the noise variance gradually decreased from inside to outside of the phantom, whereas with OSEM the noise decreased rapidly at the border of the object. The noise variations are similar for SPECT (data not shown).

The variance across the CT image field shows a broad maximum at the center of the object, which gradually decreased toward the edge. Computed tomography data from a PET/CT show similar behavior as data acquired using stand-alone CT tomographs. It is noticeable that the magnitude of the noise in images generated by CT is markedly lower compared with images generated by the other modalities.

Noise Correlation

An essential aspect of these modalities, especially PET, PET/CT, and SPECT, is their ability to obtain quantitative values for regions of interest (ROIs) within the images. These values by themselves can have important diagnostic value, and can give insights into the physiology of normal versus diseased tissues, or can provide important information regarding drug distribution or its interaction with target systems. However, it is important to realize that noise is correlated within the images. A consequence of this is that the variations in between pixels cannot be used in simple statistics to estimate precision in the average over pixels. Hence, it is a difficult task to obtain an estimate of the precision of a ROI measurement.

Noise in raw data (not corrected) generated by these modalities is not correlated. Noise correlation is caused essentially by the recording system (Tsui *et al.*, 1981), applied correction algorithms followed by applied reconstruction algorithms, which contain filtering of the projections for generation of images. Further correlation can be induced by interpolations during reconstruction (Hoffman *et al.*, 1979; Demirkaya, 2002) or during manipulations of the image, such as correction for patient movement. Different degrees of filtering postreconstruction lead to different appearance and correlation of noise in the reconstructed images.

Filtered backprojection with lower filter cut-off frequencies creates images in which the noise is correlated over relatively long distances, and iterative reconstruction at lower iterations generates images in which the noise is correlated over shorter distances compared to FBP (Wilson and Tsui, 1993). It is shown that noise correlation is damaging the visual perception of lesion detection, and it reduces an observer's ability to detect cold spots in an image (Judy and Swensson, 1981; Myers *et al.*, 1985). Furthermore, inherent correlation caused by filtering limits the ability of extracting useful quantitative information from images (Inuma and Nagai, 1967). Correlation between the pixels within images affects the quality in images and also the potential to estimate precision in the quantitative measurements. Image quality, in its simplest form characterized by pixel signal-to-noise ratio (SNR), becomes an inadequate measurement when different types of noise correlation exist between the pixels within the images. Therefore, noise correlation should not be ignored (Myers *et al.*, 1985).

In PET and PET/CT, application of 3D acquisition mode for collecting data introduces axial correlation and degrades the spatial resolution in the reconstructed images. This is caused by the performed filtering in the reconstruction

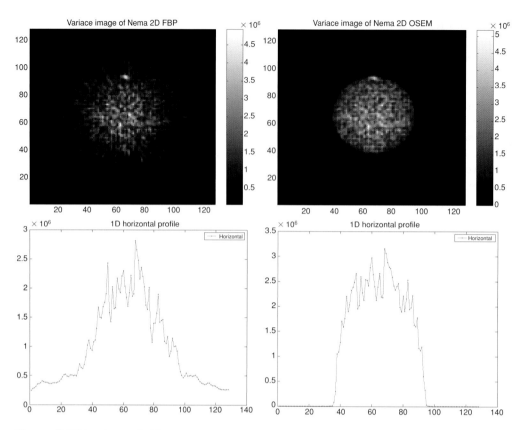

Figure 2 PET study on cylindrical NEMA phantom. Variance images generated from images reconstructed using FBP (upper left) and OSEM (upper right). Corresponding 1D horizontal profile through the variance image reconstructed using FBP (lower left) and OSEM (lower right).

algorithm, especially in FBP and retraction of the interplane septa leading to increased crystal solid angles and broadening the point spread function. Despite degrading of the spatial resolution in 3D acquired images, axial correlation in 3D acquired images is similar to 2D, at matched axial resolution (Pajevic *et al.*, 1998). 3D PET images contain strong and complex correlation between the values in adjacent pixels compared with 2D images (Blomqvist *et al.*, 1995). The correlation is modeled as a function of distance in conjunction with relative orientation of the pixels, particularly those pixels that are positioned away from the center or edge pixels (Carson *et al.*, 1993; Tanaka and Hurayama, 1982).

In the next section, autocorrelation function (ACF) is used to illustrate the correlation pattern of the noise in images generated by these modalities and reconstructed both analytically and iteratively.

Autocorrelation Function

Correlation means measuring the similarity of one signal to another in signal processing. In the field of image analysis, correlation indicates similarity between the pixels at different time points or different positions. Autocorrelation function can be used as a means to study the similarity between images or image parts (Papoulis, 1991) and is defined as a cross-correlation function of an image or part of an image with itself. 2D ACF is used to show how surrounding pixels affect the middle pixel within a single image. The correlation pattern is illustrated as a 2D image that can be used for further exploration. Here this method is used to study noise correlation within the image and to illustrate the performance of the reconstruction algorithm used for reconstruction of data generated using different imaging modalities (Razifar, 2005).

The spatial equation is based on 2D cross-correlation of the matrix a_{ij} with resolution of $i \times j$ with itself (b_{ij}) using the lags (time shifting) k and l

$$Corr(k,l) = \sum_{i=1}^{m} \sum_{j=1}^{n} a_{i,j} b_{i+k,j+l} \qquad (1)$$

where k and l refer to lags of the function and

$$\max(1, 1-k) \le i \le \min(m, m-k)$$

and

$$\max(1, 1-l) \le j \le \min(n, n-l)$$

Noise Correlation in Various Modalities

In this section, ACF has been used to illustrate noise correlation within 2D images, which are reconstructed either analytically or iteratively. A uniform Nema (NEMA, 2001) and a uniform, cylindrical, and elliptical Torso phantom were used as two objects for this purpose. Autocorrelation function was applied on the center part of each image of the object, and ACF images were generated. These ACF images were used to illustrate the pattern of noise correlation in images generated by different modalities and 1D profiles through the ACF images plotted to further exploration.

Positron Emission Tomography and PET/CT

Figures 3 and 4 illustrate as ACF images the noise-correlation pattern in PET images. These images show that the correlation is rotation symmetric or isotropic, independent of object shape when images are reconstructed using OSEM. This is not the case, however, in images reconstructed using FBP when the shape of phantom is not circular. When the radioactivity distribution is nonsymmetric, as in an elliptic phantom or with nonrotational symmetric activity distribution within a rotational symmetric object, and images are reconstructed with FBP, the correlation is nonrotational symmetric.

Noise correlation in PET/CT images shows similar behavior as in pure PET images. Noise in PET/CT images is identical independent of the magnitude of applied X-ray dose in the transmission part (CT), since the noise from the emission part (PET part) is dominant (Kamel *et al.*, 2002; Razifar *et al.*, 2005a, b). It is suggested that a lower X-ray dose to the patient could be used without impairment of image quality in PET/CT human studies.

Computed Tomography

Noise in CT images reconstructed by FBP has a nonisotropic pattern when the shape of the object is not circular (data not shown). This nonisotropic behavior depends on the way data are acquired in CT. The X-ray tube rotating around

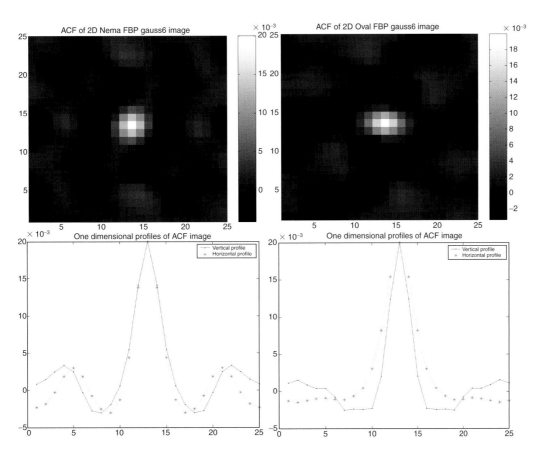

Figure 3 PET study of NEMA and Torso phantoms. ACF images obtained from images reconstructed using FBP on Nema (upper left) and Torso (upper right). 1D horizontal profile through the corresponding ACF image of Nema (lower left) and Torso (lower right).

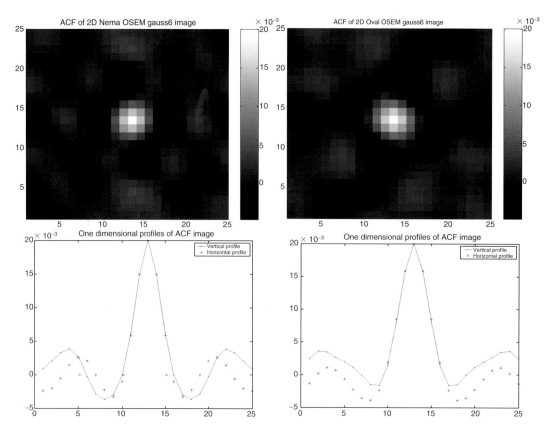

Figure 4 Same data as in Figure 4 but with images reconstructed using OSEM on Nema (upper left) and Torso (upper right). 1D horizontal profile through the corresponding ACF image of Nema (lower left) and Torso (lower right).

the object emits X-rays, which are observed by detectors that are placed as a block on the opposite side of the tube. The number of photons detected is highly dependent on the thickness of the object, and the relative noise is hence larger in the direction of the object with the largest thickness when the object is not circular. These differences in noise variation are, as indicated above earlier, handled by the FBP algorithm such that a nonisotropic noise correlation is given in the images. The reader is referred to the study by Razifar *et al.* (2005b) for further information regarding the other factors that might or not affect the noise correlation such as slice thickness and applied care dose.

Single Photon Emission Computed Tomography

In SPECT studies, the correlation pattern is still close to isotropic in images obtained from an elliptical object and independent of the reconstruction methodology used (data not shown). This behavior occurs because in SPECT the number of detected counts in different directions in the study on either circular or elliptical phantom is almost the same if there is a uniform distribution of radioactivity. The reason is

based on the way radioactivity is sensed, with a detector that records the superficial activity and not that deep inside the object. Because attenuation is a dominant factor with respect to the recording of radioactivity, the number of counts will become relatively similar for a uniform elliptic phantom. On the other hand, a focal radioactivity not centered in the phantom will instead give highly variable counts in different detectors. In addition, the detector sensitivity is significantly affected by distance from the detector.

Discussion

Despite the similarity in the underlying principle of tomographic imaging devices, the fact that the acquisition of detector data and modes of reconstruction differ can lead to differences in the expression of noise in the images. Computed tomography is based on measurement of transmitted X-ray photons from the X-ray tube through the object and to the detectors. Positron emission tomography is based on the simultaneous measurement of two annihilation photons that emerge from the body and hit each of two detectors on opposite sides of the object. Single photon emission tomography is based on recording single photons that emerge from the body and acquisition of a large number of projections by sequential rotation of the detector system around the body. For these techniques the measured data, typically organized in projections, are subjected to different corrections, where especially in PET and SPECT the attenuation correction is dominant. After performing the different corrections, the projection data are utilized in a reconstruction algorithm for the generation of images. The reconstruction part can be similar for the three devices, with the predominant methods being FBP or iterative reconstruction.

By using ACF, it is possible to illustrate the differences in noise correlation between images reconstructed using different types of reconstruction algorithms (such as FBP and OSEM) generated utilizing different imaging modalities. An asymmetric noise correlation for asymmetric objects in combination with noise variation across the image field considerably complicates the interpretation of the images when statistical methods are used, such as with statistical estimates of precision in average values, or when statistical parametric mapping methods and multivariate image analyses are used. These variations in the properties of noise are significantly reduced when images are reconstructed by iterative techniques; hence, iterative reconstruction methods are favorable for such applications. However, it is possible to calculate the noise analytically in images reconstructed by FBP, by following the mathematical processes applied from raw sinogram data to final image. It is not possible to do the same calculation in images reconstructed by iterative methods. Therefore, for performing statistical methods of analysis that depend on knowing the noise in raw data, it is a valid concept to generate a parallel route to FBP reconstruction whereby the influence of noise on images and quantitative values is evaluated (Huesman, 1984).

The methods described in this chapter for the characterization of noise in images are suitable for uniform objects but cannot readily be applied to describe noise in a complex patient study. For such cases, an analytical technique based on a parallel noise reconstruction would be applicable. Otherwise, more indirect methods have to be applied. This includes the generation of a large set of dynamic images, fitting of kinetic curves to the data, and describing variability as deviations from an ideal kinetic curve. A method that performs similarly without implicit use of kinetic curves is to apply principal component analysis for extracting kinetic behavior and use the higher components that contain only noise for an appropriate description of noise properties. In summary, we wish to indicate the complicated aspects of noise in reconstruction tomography in order to show that there are no simple methods that can avoid noise influence or that can be used to describe its impact on numerical values.

References

Blomqvist, G., Eriksson, L., and Rosenqvist, G. 1995. The effect of spatial correlation on the quantification in positron emission tomography. *Neuroimage 2*:2.

Carson, R.E., Ya, Y., Daube-Witherspoon, M.E., Freedman, N., Bacharach, S.L., and Herscovitch, P. 1993. An approximation formula for the variance of PET region-of-interest value. *IEEE Trans. Med. Imag. 12*:240–250.

Demirkaya, O. 2002. Anisotropic diffusion filtering of PET attenuation data to improve emission images. *Phys. Med. Biol. 47*:N271–N278.

Hoffman, E.J., Huang, S-C., and Phelps, M.E. 1979. Quantitation I positron emission computed tomography: 1. Effect of object size. *J. Comp. Ass. Tomog. 3*:299–308.

Huesman, R.H. 1984. A new fast algorithm for the evaluation of regions of interest and statistical uncertainty in computed tomography. *Phys. Med. Biol. 29*:543–552.

Iinuma, T.A., and Nagai T. 1967. Image restoration in radioisotope imaging systems. *Phys. Med. Biol. 12*:501–509.

Judy, P.F., and Swensson, R.G. 1981. Lesion detection and signal-to-noise ration in CT images. *Med. Physics 8*:12–23.

Kamel, E., Hany, T.F., Burger, C., Treyer, V., Lonn, A.H.R., Schulthess, G.K.V., and Buck, A. 2002. CT vs ^{68}Ge attenuation correction in a combined PET/CT system-evaluation of the effect of lowering the CT tube current. *Eur. J. Nucl. Med. 29*:346–350.

Myers, K.J., Barret, H.H., Borgsrom, M.C., Patton, D.D., and Seeley, G.W. 1985. Effect of noise correlation on detectability of disk signals in medical imaging. *J. Opt. Society of America A. 2*:1752–1759.

NEMA NU-2001. Performance standards of positron emission tomographs. National Electronics Manufacturers Association.

Pajevic, S., Daube-Witherspoon, M.E., Bacharach, S.L., and Carson, R.E. 1998. Noise characteristics of 3-D and 2-D PET images. *IEEE Trans. Med. Imag. 17*:9–23.

Papoulis, A. 1991. *Probability, Random Variables and Stochastic Processes*. New York: McGraw-Hill.

Razifar, P. 2005. Novel approaches for application of principal component analysis on dynamic PET images for improvement of image quality and clinical diagnosis. Ph.D. thesis, Centre for Image Analysis, University of Uppsala, Sweden. ISBN 91-554-6387-8.

Razifar, P., Lubberink, M., Schneider, H., Långström, B., Bengtsson, E., and Bergström, M. 2005a. Non-isotropic noise correlation in PET data reconstructed by FBP but not by OSEM demonstrated using autocorrelation function. *BMC Med. Imag. 5*:3.

Razifar, P., Sandström, M., Schneider, H., Långström, B., Maripuu, E., Bengtsson, E., and Bergström, M. 2005b. Noise correlation in PET, CT, SPECT and PET/CT data evaluated using autocorrelation function. *BMC Med. Imag. 5*:5.

Rowe, R.W., and Dai, S. 1992. A pseudo-Poisson noise model for simulation of positron emission tomographic projection data. *Med. Physics 19*:1113–1119.

Tanaka, E., and Hurayama, H. Properties of statistical noise in positron emission tomography. 1982. *Proceeding International Workshop Physics Engineering of Med. Imag.* New York, IEEE 158–164.

Tsui, B.M.W., Beck, R.N., Doi, K., and Metz, C.E. 1981. Analysis of recorded image noise in nuclear medicine. *Phys. Med. Biol. 26*:883–902.

Wilson, D.W., and Tsui, B.M.W. 1993. Noise properties of filtered-backprojection and ML-EM reconstruction emission tomographic image. *IEEE Trans. Nucl. Sci. 40*:1198–1203.

Zaidi, H., Gomez, M.D., Boudraa, A., and Slosman, D.O. 2002. Fuzzy clustering-based segmented attenuation correction in whole-body PET imaging. *Phys. Med. Biol. 47*:1143–1160.

7

Computed Tomography Scan Methods Account for Respiratory Motion in Lung Cancer

Shinichiro Mori and Masahiro Endo

Introduction

Continuing rapid progress in computer hardware and software has led to better radiation therapy planning and dramatic improvements in delivery. New types of conformal planning and delivery technology, of which intensity-modulated radiation therapy (IMRT) is a prominent example, have the potential to achieve a much higher degree of target conformity and normal tissue sparing than existing treatment techniques. These improvements, in turn, raise the need to minimize target margin. Organs in the thorax and abdomen, however, move with respiratory motion, complicating the treatment of tumors in these locations and raising the concern of many clinicians. Voluntary or imposed breath-holding techniques have been proposed as one way of reducing or eliminating the effects of respiratory motion during both imaging and radiotherapy treatment, but many patients cannot tolerate holding their breath.

Against this background, computed tomography (CT) technology has undergone dramatic changes over the past few years. Recent advances in multislice CT (MSCT) now allow the acquisition of > 200 contiguous images within a single breath-hold period, greatly improve multiplanar image reconstruction, and provide favorable three-dimensional (3D)

images of various structures (with expansion to four-dimensional [4D] imaging now realized). In this chapter we summarize research topics in CT scan methods for lung cancer. We first compare fast scan CT (FSCT) and slow scan CT (SSCT), and then (4D computed tomography) and respiratory-gated CT (RGCT). Finally, we introduce two newer technologies, volumetric cine CT (VCCT) and respiratory-gated segment CT (RSCT).

Slow Scan Computed Tomography vs. Fast Scan Computed Tomography

There are two scan modes in CT scanning: axial scan and helical scan (spiral scan). In axial scanning, images are acquired with the table position kept stable. When volume data are acquired, the CT makes a single axial scan, moves the couch to the next position, and then repeats the process until the entire volume is covered. This method is relatively inefficient compared to helical scanning, mentioned below, but is used in some institutions in radiotherapy planning.

Helical scanning was first presented in 1989 at the annual meeting of the Radiological Society of North America (RSNA) by Kalender *et al.* (1989) following practical development

61

and patenting by Mori (1986). The helical scan method uses continuous scanning with simultaneous table movement, allowing volume data to be imaged successfully, and is now used routinely for diagnosis in most hospitals. Because the images obtained differ over time at each couch position, however, the acquisition of time-based information is restricted.

Most commercial CTs allow the operator to optimize CT images by selecting from among a number of scan parameters, such as tube voltage, tube current, scan time, and slice collimator. Furthermore, rotation time and patterns can be selected. State-of-the-art rotation times as fast as 0.33 sec and temporal resolutions of < 0.25 sec have significantly improved diagnostic information, particularly in cardiac imaging.

Two types of gantry rotation scan are available in clinical use: combination with axial scan or helical scan. Fast scan computed tomography is defined as scanning with fast gantry rotation (~ 1.0 sec). Many hospitals use this method routinely for diagnostic purposes, and its high temporal resolution reduces motion artifacts. However, high-speed rotation scanning requires a large tube current to maintain signal-to-noise ratio, which is closely dependent on mAs value. To avoid the need to move anatomical sites such as the head, some hospitals scan with slow gantry rotation to increase mAs value. In the radiotherapeutic field, however, SSCT is used with slow gantry rotation for the unique purpose of capturing the whole respiratory cycle in one rotation (de Koste et al., 2003; Lagerwaard et al., 2001). SSCT is typically defined as a 4-sec rotation, based on the fact that the average human respiratory cycle is ~ 4 sec in length, which allows the scan to detect the range of tumor motion and shape throughout normal respiratory movement. Slow scan computed tomography for this purpose is recommended for lung tumors that are not involved with either the mediastinum or chest wall only.

As an example in a free-breathing patient, FSCT at peak exhalation and SSCT images are shown in Figures 1A and 1B, respectively (provided by Helen A Shin). Tumor positions are shown in green for FSCT at peak inhalation, in purple for FSCT at peak exhalation, and in yellow for SSCT. Some investigators have reported reproducible tumor volume definition by SSCT under free-breathing conditions. Lagerwaard et al. (2001) reported that the mean ratio of clinical target volume (CTV) to planning CT and SCCT was 88.8% ± 5.6%. In other words, target volumes are larger using SSCT than FSCT, but have good reproducibility. This finding indicates that a planning target volume (PTV) derived from an SSCT scan should carry an additional margin to ensure coverage of the "optimal" PTV. Additional interesting analysis has been done by Helen et al. (2004), who evaluated methods for defining internal margins beyond the gross tumor volume (GTV) to account for expected physiologic movement and summarized the required internal margins.

A number of quantitative and physical questions about SSCT require answering, however. Specifically, given that SSCT using conventional CT in the cranio-caudal direction images an apparent rather than the actual target volume, further physical evaluation is required to optimize dosage to the target volume using a phantom of known size, shape, movement direction, and so on.

Recently, Gagné and Robinson, (2004) reported the impact on motion artifacts of changes in CT rotation time and movement cycles in phantom and simulation studies. Furthermore, Mori et al. (2006b) also compared these variables using the 256-slice CT. Images for FSCT and SSCT in axial section are shown in Figures 1C and 1D, respectively. An acrylic ball of 30 mm diameter was moved to mimic respiratory motion in an oblique (left-right + cranio-caudal) direction, with a movement distance of 45 mm and a time period of 4 sec. The original phantom form could not be identified in the resulting SSCT images due to severe distortion, and accurate determination of the phantom edge was not possible. The direction of motion of this artifact is associated with the ray tube position at the start of reconstruction (Gagné and Robinson, 2004). Furthermore, the SSCT images were observed as separate objects. Moreover, the present results showed that radiation therapy planning using SSCT scanning results in underdosing compared with doses obtained in actual clinical planning, and thus also results in the exposure of normal tissue to harmful doses due to the excessively large contouring on SSCT images with unacceptable motion artifacts. Therefore, the optimum margin should be added to the GTV when SSCT images are used in radiotherapy planning.

Four-Dimensional Computed Tomography

The 4DCT scan method allows the incorporation of organ motion directly into diagnostic and therapeutic applications. This scanning method is performed in cine mode, which operates the scanner without couch movement using respiratory signals from surrogate systems to obtain all respiratory phases at each couch position, moves the couch to the next position, and sorts CT images at the same respiratory phase. As a result, 3DCT images can be obtained at each respiratory phase. This method has been integrated into commercial CT scanners, and many hospitals presently use it for radiotherapy planning. The acquisition of one respiratory cycle at each couch position is slower than conventional CT scanning, and a 4DCT scan requires ~ 1 min of scanning time with the 16MSCT.

Although there are two types of sorting variable, displacement and phase, most hospitals generally use phase sorting. Respiratory phase sorting methods for the 4DCT technique have been introduced. Low et al. (2003) proposed the tidal volume sorting method, which relies on quantitative spirometry,

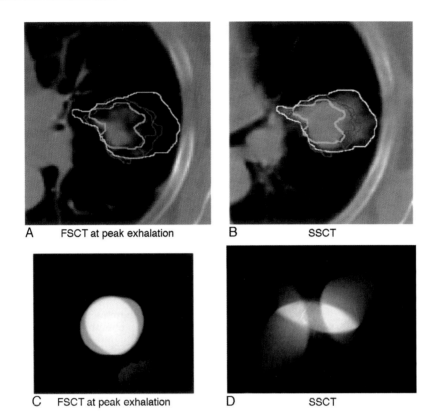

Figure 1 Variable tumor positions at different respiratory phases in axial section. Patient study under free breathing for (**A**) fast scan CT (FSCT) at peak exhalation and (**B**) slow scan CT (SSCT) (provided by Helen). Contours of tumors: red: FSCT at quiet free breathing, green: FSCT at peak inhalation, purple: FSCT, peak exhalation, yellow: SSCT at quiet free breathing. Phantom study (acrylic ball) for (**C**) FSCT at peak exhalation and (**D**) SSCT.

whereas Pan *et al.* (2004) described the internal or external sorting method, an internal sorting method in which data are registered according to total CT number in the regions of interest (ROIs) to depict respiratory motion and the correlation of anatomy in CT images in consecutive respiratory cycles.

The human respiratory cycle is not strictly regular, however, but rather varies in amplitude and period from one cycle to the next. Many authors have reported the limitations of the abdomen as an external surrogate for the respiratory phase, namely, that longer CT scanning time under free breathing and the placement of the marker conspire to produce inconsistency between the position of the marker and internal anatomy motion (Vedam *et al.*, 2003). Lujan *et al.* (2003) have reported that the motion of the diaphragm due to respiration is predominantly in the cranio-caudal direction and is periodic but asymmetric, with more time spent at the end of exhalation than at the end of inhalation. This may lead to erroneous prediction of the dose delivered to the patient and, when examination time is prolonged, may result in the degradation of 4DCT image quality.

To visualize the tumor-encompassing volume using 4DCT data, two image-processing methods—4DCT image average (4DIA) (Mori *et al.*, 2006b; Underberg *et al.*, 2005) and 4DCT

image maximum intensity projection (4DMIP) (Underberg *et al.*, 2005)—have been integrated into commercial CT scanner and visualization workstations. 4D Image Average is averaged from each pixel value on the volumetric CT data along the time axis, and 4DIM is the selected maximum value at the same pixel location along the time axis.

Figure 2 shows 4DCT, 4DIA, and 4DIM images obtained by the 256MSCT. Axial images at the edge of the tumor are shown for the position marked by the dotted line in the coronal image. The advantage of 4DIA is that it makes it easy to observe the time-average tumor position, which is derived from the probability density function (Fig. 2B). Although 4DCT captured the edge of the tumor (Fig. 2A), it is difficult to observe the tumor in the 4DIA images due to the decrease in CT number from the original. Thus, 4DIA may cause the underestimation of target definition.

The advantages of 4DIM are that the motion artifact due to patient breathing is greatly reduced and the edge of the tumor is visualized. However, 4DIM emphasizes pulmonary vessels, making it difficult to distinguish the tumor from normal lung, in lung fibrosis honeycomb in particular. When using 4DIM in radiotherapy planning, consideration should be given to the possibility that 4DIM may cause dose

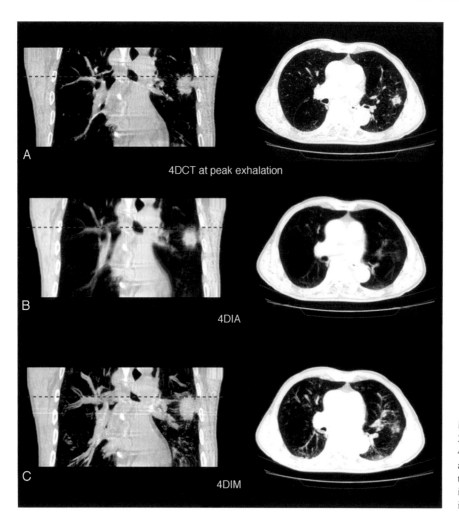

Figure 2 Coronal and axial images using 256MSCT for (**A**) 4DCT at peak exhalation, (**B**) 4DIA and (**C**) 4DIM. 4DIA and 4DIM were generated using one respiratory cycle. Axial image positions are marked by the dotted line in the coronal image. The tumor is marked by an arrow in axial images. Slice thickness is 0.5 mm.

prescription error. The concept of 4DIA and 4DIM is based on reconstructed image processing; however, calculation time is reduced by generating processes in projection data.

Respiratory Gating Computed Tomography

Respiratory gating is currently under investigation in a number of hospitals to account for respiratory motion during radiotherapy in thoracic and abdominal sites. Radiotherapy planning CT is necessary and essentially the same as in the treatment phase; in other words, imaging and treatment are synchronized with the respiratory cycle. One solution to the acquisition of representative CT scans is RSCT, a scan method similar to 4DCT, which differs in that scanning is done only at the most stable point of the gated respiratory cycle, usually peak exhalation (Sontag, 1999). Representa-

tive scan computed tomography provides wide cranio-caudal coverage beyond the CT detector width without image gaps during free breathing, significantly improving target definition. RGCT images are therefore the same as those with 4DCT at exhalation.

Since higher target conformity requires accurate target definition, RGCT has been adapted to radiotherapy treatment using charged particle beams as well as photon beams. Recently, several hospitals have undertaken gated charged particle beam treatment and demonstrated improvements in radiotherapy by determining the optimum gating window (beam irradiation phase).

Volumetric Cine Computed Tomography

Current high-end CT scanners at selected institutions employ up to 64 segments with a segment size of 0.5 to

0.625 mm at the center of rotation. Although the 64 MSCT represents a marked improvement over conventional MSCT, its cranio-caudal coverage without gantry movement is typically only 20 to 40 mm, which limits the width of coverage on cine imaging in the cranio-caudal direction. 4D computed tomography was developed to be able to provide 3DCT images at each respiratory phase. However, because these images are imaged from different respiratory cycles at consecutive couch positions, as in conventional 4DCT, many of the problems mentioned above remain.

Much effort has been devoted to adapting cone beam CT (CBCT) to the diagnostic and radiotherapy fields. Cone beam computed tomography is useful in the acquisition of a wide cranio-caudal range in a single rotation, facilitating CT scanning in patients who cannot tolerate holding their breath for long. However, since its rotation speed is a relatively long several minutes, it produces respiratory motion-induced motion artifacts and cannot accurately capture tumor position at each respiratory phase.

To overcome these disadvantages, slice counts of 256 and higher remain an active area of research. An example of such dedicated work is the 256MSCT developed by Toshiba Medical Systems and installed at the National Institute of Radiological Sciences in Japan in 2002 (Endo et al., 2003). The 256MSCT provides a 128-mm scan coverage with a 0.5 mm slice thickness in a single rotation (= 0.5 s/rot), allowing for reconstructions in multiple planes that can also be displayed in a cine loop, a hitherto impossible characteristic that is useful in reducing the uncertainties seen with 4DCT. Since all of the relevant anatomy is imaged during the same respiratory cycle, the need to patch together different CT slices from different respiratory cycles is obviated. The short total acquisition time (~6 s) allows a single respiratory cycle to be obtained satisfactorily, minimizing the above problems; neither sorting image nor respiratory sensing system errors occur across the 128 mm coverage. This characteristic is considered to differentiate the new technique (volumetric cine CT: VCCT) from the conventional 4DCT method.

Volumetric cine computed tomography images, which achieve an effective temporal resolution of 250 ms by adapting half-scan reconstruction, capture each respiratory phase exactly. The margins of the liver and pulmonary vessels are clearly seen (Fig. 3). The artifacts around the edge of the scan region in the cranio-caudal direction represent incomplete data sets (missing volumes) resulting from the cone angle (marked arrows in Fig. 3) and are an artifact characteristic of CBCT. VCCT significantly improves the observation of tumor displacement and overcomes some of the limitations of the present 4DCT method. Owing to its accurate determination of the margin, VCCT is a useful complement to current irradiation methods.

Respiratory-Correlated Segment Computed Tomography

Owing to its low temporal resolution, 4DCT does not remove motion artifacts completely in fast respiratory phases such as mid-inhalation and -exhalation, particularly if a relatively slow rotation CT speed is used, such as 1.0 sec. Moreover, it is unable to track the respiratory motion of an organ. RSCT was developed to improve this temporal resolution. Its essential concept is to sort projection data (= sinogram) in the same respiratory phase, rather than CT images. The segment reconstruction algorithm is widely used in combination with the electrocardiogram (ECG) signal to delineate coronary arteries with intravenous injection of contrast agent (Grass et al., 2003; Kachelriess et al., 2004).

Several investigators have reported the use of a segment reconstruction algorithm with the respiratory signal using MSCT (Lu et al., 2005) or CBCT (Sonke et al., 2005). Since RSCT considers both respiratory phase and projection angle, it is somewhat complex. And because respiratory movement is slower than cardiac motion, RSCT has not been adopted for routine clinical use.

As an example of the merit of RSCT, Sonke et al. (2005) reported the use of RSCT, with CBCT integrated with a linear accelerator. Since their rotation speed of approximately 4 min is relatively long, respiratory motion-induced motion artifacts occur and tumor position at each respiratory phase cannot be accurately captured. As part of their study, these researchers evaluated image quality and captured lung tumors showing regular and irregular respiratory motions.

The benefit of increasing temporal resolution is found not only in improved image quality but also in better dose distribution in radiotherapy. In particular, because the typical depth distribution of charged particles exhibits a strong Bragg peak at the very end of the maximum distance traveled by the particle (range), beyond which the dose very rapidly falls to zero, tumor shape has a greater effect on treatment accuracy in charged particle beam than photon beam therapy.

In clinical settings, where tumor geometry is more complex, motion generally results in variations in positional shift, which in turn lead to more complex motion artifacts. 4D computed tomography images are therefore not an actual but rather an apparent target if motion artifact is included. However, the planning system results in optimum beam parameters for apparent target. Figure 4 shows carbon beam dose distribution using a moving acrylic ball as an example (Mori et al., 2006a). Beam parameters and dose distributions were calculated using 4DCT images (Fig. 4A). Greater than 90% of the intended dose was delivered accurately with 4DCT, and the carbon beam stops correctly at the distal edge of the target

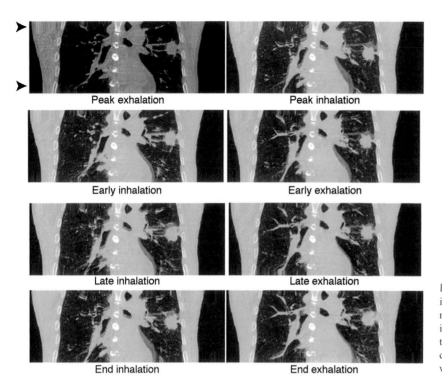

Peak exhalation   Peak inhalation

Early inhalation   Early exhalation

Late inhalation   Late exhalation

End inhalation   End exhalation

Figure 3 Free-breathing lung cancer patient images in coronal section were obtained with the 4DCT method using the 256MSCT. Cranio-caudal distance is 128 mm, and slice thickness is 0.5 mm. Effective temporal resolution is 250 ms with the half-scan reconstruction algorithm. Feldkamp artifact is marked with arrows at peak exhalation.

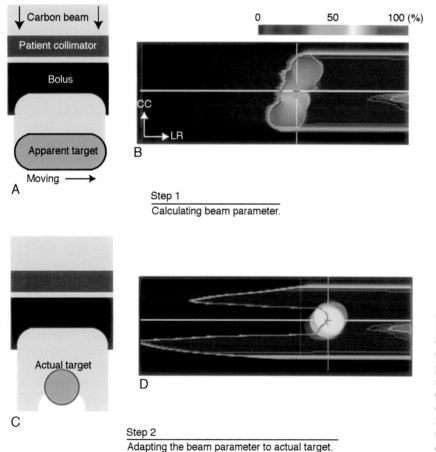

Step 1
Calculating beam parameter.

Step 2
Adapting the beam parameter to actual target.

Figure 4 Carbon beam dose calculation procedures to assess dose delivery accuracy in the planning system and in actual use. The left-right and cranial-caudal directions are denoted as LR and CC, respectively. Step 1: (**A**) Calculation of beam parameters (bolus design, range, beam field, and so on) and dose distribution using 4DCT images. (**B**) Dose distribution of the moving phantom in an oblique direction as obtained with 4DCT using the 256MSCT. Step 2: (**C**) Calculation of dose distribution using RSCT images with the beam parameters of 4DCT. (**D**) Dose distribution with RSCT.

(Fig. 4B). It is understood that this 4DCT image did not show the actual shape of the phantom. Dose distribution was then calculated using RSCT images with the beam parameters obtained for 4DCT (Fig. 4C). The delivered dose was clearly insufficient, and considerable dose leakage around the target is seen (Fig. 4D). Since the high temporal resolution of RSCT provides images that are nearly equivalent to the actual target, these planning methods can assess dose delivery accuracy in planning systems and in actual treatment.

The usefulness of RSCT is due to the reduction in motion artifacts it achieves by dividing the 2π projection data into a number of sections. As a result, temporal resolution increases in proportion to the number of sections, as, however, does total acquisition time. Furthermore, the restricted temporal resolution of this algorithm makes it necessary to control any related devices in order to avoid synchronization with the respiratory cycle. Moreover, as the period shifts between respirations, errors in the sorting process may lead to incorrect classification of the projection data into the wrong projection data section, and thereby result in image artifacts in the resultant RSCT. The same problem is seen in cardiac imaging with ECG gating (Dhanantwari et al., 2001). In this case, compensation of the projection data must be done by extending or shortening the range of the quadrant in both quadrant sections.

Moreover, it should be remembered that a tumor located in a lower lobe of the lung has a greater range of tumor motion than one in an upper lobe due to proximity to the diaphragm (Hoisak et al., 2004). This may also impact RS-FDK in clinical use and require correction of the correlation between respiration and target motion, such as by control of the patient's breathing by operator guidance (Balter et al., 1998; Hanley et al., 1999; Mageras et al., 2001) or by means of an occlusion valve (Dawson et al., 2001; Stromberg et al., 2000; Wong et al., 1999). It will be necessary to control for this time dependency of respiratory asymmetry through suitable correction methods.

As already mentioned, further investigation of these problems is necessary before clinical use. In summary, CT scanners play an important role in radiotherapy. Selecting the optimum scan method for each radiotherapy strategy will provide the additional information required to minimize margins and increase the accuracy of dose distribution to account for respiratory motion.

References

Balter, J.M., Lam, K.L., McGinn, C.J., Lawrence, T.S., and Ten Haken, R.K. 1998. Improvement of CT-based treatment-planning models of abdominal targets using static exhale imaging. *Int. J. Radiat. Oncol. Biol. Phys.* *41*:939–943.

Dawson, L.A., Brock, K.K., Kazanjian, S., Fitch, D., McGinn, C.J., Lawrence, T.S., Ten Haken, R.K., and Balter, J. 2001. The reproducibility of organ position using active breathing control (ABC) during liver radiotherapy. *Int. J. Radiat. Oncol. Biol. Phys.* *51*:1410–1421.

de Koste, J., Lagerwaard, F., de Boer, H., Nijssen-Visser, M., and Senan, S. 2003. Are multiple CT scans required for planning curative radiotherapy in lung tumors of the lower lobe? *Int. J. Radiat. Oncol. Biol. Phys.* *55*:1394–1399.

Dhanantwari, A.C., Stergiopoulos, S., Zamboglou, N., Baltas, D., Vogt, H.G., and Karangelis, G. 2001. Correcting organ motion artifacts in X-ray CT systems based on tracking of motion phase by the spatial overlap correlator. II. Experimental study. *Med. Phys.* *28*:1577–1596.

Endo, M., Mori, S., Tsunoo, T., Kandatsu, S., Tanada, S., Aradate, H., Saito, Y., Miyazaki, H., Satoh, K., Matsusita, S., and Kusakabe, M. 2003. Development and performance evaluation of the first model of 4D CT-scanner. *IEEE Trans. Nucl. Sci.* *50*:1667–1671.

Gagné, I.M., and Robinson, D.M. 2004. The impact of tumor motion upon CT image integrity and target delineation. *Med. Phys.* *31*:3378–3392.

Grass, M., Manzke, R., Nielsen, T., Koken, P., Proksa, R., Natanzon, M., and Shechter, G. 2003. Helical cardiac cone beam reconstruction using retrospective ECG gating. *Phys. Med. Biol.* *48*:3069–3084.

Hanley, J., Debois, M.M., Mah, D., Mageras, G.S., Raben, A., Rosenzweig, K., Mychalczak, B., Schwartz, L.H., Gloeggler, P.J., Lutz, W., Ling, C.C., Leibel, S.A., Fuks, Z., and Kutcher G.J. 1999. Deep inspiration breathhold technique for lung tumors: the potential value of target immobilization and reduced lung density in dose escalation. *Int. J. Radiat. Oncol. Biol. Phys.* *45*:603–611.

Helen, A.S., Steve, B.J., Khaled, M.A., Karen, P.D., and Noah, C.C. 2004. Internal target volume determined with expansion margins beyond composite gross tumor volume in three-dimensional conformal radiotherapy for lung cancer. *Int. J. Radiat. Oncol. Biol. Phys.* *60*:613–622.

Hoisak, J.D., Sixel, K.E., Tirona, R., Cheung, P.C., and Pignol, J.P. 2004. Correlation of lung tumor motion with external surrogate indicators of respiration. *Int. J. Radiat. Oncol. Biol. Phys.* *60*:1298–1306.

Kachelriess, M., Knaup, M., and Kalender, W.A. 2004. Extended parallel backprojection for standard three-dimensional and phase-correlated four-dimensional axial and spiral cone-beam CT with arbitrary pitch, arbitrary cone-angle, and 100% dose usage. *Med. Phys.* *31*:1623–1641.

Kalender, W.A., Seissler, W., and Vock, P. 1989. Single-breath hold spiral volumetric CT by continuous patient translation and scanner rotation. *Radiology 173(P)*:414.

Lagerwaard, F.J., Van Sornsen de Koste, J.R., Nijssen-Visser, M.R., Schuchhard-Schipper R.H., Oei, S.S., Munne, A., and Senan, S. 2001. Multiple "slow" CT scans for incorporating lung tumor mobility in radiotherapy planning. *Int. J. Radiat. Oncol. Biol. Phys.* *51*:932–937.

Low, D.A., Nystrom, M., Kalinin, E., Parikh, P., Dempsey, J.F., Bradley, J.D., Mutic, S., Wahab, S.H., Islam, T., Christensen, G., Politte, D.G., and Whiting, B.R. 2003. A method for the reconstruction of four-dimensional synchronized CT scans acquired during free breathing. *Med. Phys.* *30*:1254–1263.

Lu, W., Parikh, P.J., Hubenschmidt, J.P., Politte, D.G., Whiting, B.R., Bradley, J.D., Mutic, S., and Low, D.A. 2005. Reduction of motion blurring artifacts using respiratory gated CT in sinogram space: a quantitative evaluation. *Med. Phys.* *32*:3295–3304.

Lujan, A.E., Balter, J.M., and Ten Haken, R.K. 2003. A method for incorporating organ motion due to breathing into 3D dose calculations in the liver: sensitivity to variations in motion. *Med. Phys.* *30*:2643–2649.

Mageras, G.S., Yorke, E., Rosenzweig, K., Braban, L., Keatley, E., Ford, E., Leibel, S.A., and Ling, C.C. 2001. Fluoroscopic evaluation of diaphragmatic motion reduction with a respiratory gated radiotherapy system. *J. Appl. Clin. Med. Phys.* *2*:191–200.

Mori, I. 1986. Computerized tomographic apparatus utilizing a radiation source. United States Patent Number 4630202.

Mori, S., Endo, M., Kohno, R., Asakura, H., Kohno, K., Yashiro, T., Komatsu, S., Kandatsu, S., and Baba, M. 2006a. Respiratory correlated segment reconstruction algorithm toward four-dimensional radiation therapy using carbon ion beams. *Radiat. Oncol.* *80*:341–348.

Mori, S., Kanematsu, N., Mizuno, H., Sunaoka, M., Endo, M. 2006b. Physical evaluation of CT scan methods for radiation therapy planning: comparison of fast, slow and gating scan using the 256-detector row CT scanner. *Phys. Med. Biol. 51*:587–600.

Pan, T., Lee, T.Y., Rietzel, E., and Chen, G.T. 2004. 4D-CT imaging of a volume influenced by respiratory motion on multi-slice CT. *Med. Phys. 31*:333–340.

Sonke, J., Zijp, L., Remeijer, P., and Herk, M. 2005. Respiratory correlated cone beam CT. *Med. Phys. 32*:1176–1186.

Sontag, M. 1999. Respiratory gated radiotherapy. *Med. Phys. 26*:1112.

Stromberg, J.S., Sharpe, M.B., Kim, L.H., Kini, V.R., Jaffray, D.A., Martinez, A.A., and Wong, J.W. 2000. Active breathing control (ABC) for Hodgkin's disease: reduction in normal tissue irradiation with deep inspiration and implications for treatment. *Int. J. Radiat. Oncol. Biol. Phys. 48*:797–806.

Tarver, R.D., Conces, D.J., and Godwin, J.D. 1988. Motion artifacts on CT simulate bronchiectasis. *Am. J. Roentogenol. 151*:1117–1119.

Underberg, R., Lagerwaard, F., Slotman, B., Cuijpers, J., and Senan, S. 2005. Use of maximum intensity projections (MIP) for target volume generation in 4DCT scans for lung cancer. *Int. J. Radiat. Oncol. Biol. Phys. 63*:253–260.

Vedam, S.S., Kini, V.R., Keall, P.J., Ramakrishnan, V., Mostafavi, H., and Mohan, R. 2003. Quantifying the predictability of diaphragm motion during respiration with a noninvasive external marker. *Med. Phys. 30*:505–513.

Wong, J.W., Sharpe, M.B., Jaffray, D.A., Kini, V.R., Robertson, J.M., Stromberg, J.S., and Martinez, A.A. 1999. The use of active breathing control (ABC) to reduce margin for breathing motion. *Int. J. Radiat. Oncol. Biol. Phys. 44*:911–919.

8

Respiratory Motion Artifact Using Positron Emission Tomography/ Computed Tomography

Dimitri Papathanassiou

Introduction

The technology of hybrid positron emission tomography/computed tomography (PET/CT) devices recently led to unquestionable advantages in the clinical practice of PET. Besides the rapid acquisition of a relatively less noisy attenuation map necessary for correction purposes, it offers a direct fusion of anatomical and metabolic information, allowing more accurate localization of lesions and possible use of CT information for more comprehensive disease assessment. However, any technique suffers from its own artifacts, and PET/CT is accompanied by some specific artifacts in the nuclear medicine practice (Bockisch *et al.*, 2004), including those due to dual modality acquisition and combination.

The respiratory motion artifact is one of the most prominent artifacts (if not the most important) encountered with the use of PET/CT. It has been reported to be as frequent as in 84% (Osman *et al.*, 2003b) or 98% (Beyer *et al.*, 2003) of PET/CT studies performed without respiratory protocol. It results in mismatch of the position of organs or lesions in PET and CT images, and in alteration in quantification of tracer uptake. Potentially, it may lead to misinterpretation due to lesion mislocalization, or reduced sensitivity of PET/CT.

In this chapter, the sole effects of the artifact in oncology imaging will be considered, but the same respiratory motion artifact also has obvious consequences in myocardium nuclear imaging, with specific issues and attempts to reduce its effects. One of the main described effects in the myocardium imaging field is underestimation of tracer uptake in the anterior and lateral walls, leading to false results in defects assessment. On account of its frequency and potential consequences, different methods are used to minimize the artifact, with their own feasibility or efficiency. Besides the description of the artifact and its effects, those methods will be presented in this chapter.

Origin of the Artifact

The respiratory motion artifact arises from the motion of the thorax and the abdomen during the respiratory cycle, which does not have the same consequences during PET and CT imaging. The position of a tumor or an organ in the thorax or below the diaphragm is not static during respiration. The PET image is acquired during many respiratory cycles (typically 3 to 5 min), which leads to an average position of the diaphragm and surrounding organs or lesions on the final image. On the other hand, the spiral CT acquisition is much faster than the PET acquisition (a few seconds). The former is able to capture the diaphragm and the thoraco-abdominal structures in a single position, which may be different from the average position imaged in PET, or while their position varies from one slice to another if the patient breathes during the CT acquisition. The rise of the artifact depends on the characteristics of the CT device: it is less frequent or less marked with faster CT (Beyer *et al.*, 2005).

The difference in acquisition speed between PET and CT, together with the sequential nature of the PET/CT procedure, may lead to different aspects of the same organ on the two types of images. The first consequence of this phenomenon is the misregistration of organs or lesions. But besides this obvious effect, it also provokes a wrong attenuation correction, owing to the principle of CT-based attenuation correction. The latter effect essentially arises in regions in the body where a great difference in attenuation coefficients exists. This is the case if an anatomical volume, which is a radioactive source in PET image and has a tissue attenuation coefficient, is bordering on (as for instance with the liver) or surrounded by (as, for instance, with a pulmonary nodule) normal lung parenchyma, whose attenuation coefficient is lower.

Because of different positions during acquisition of the two images, the volume occupied by the source in PET image (with tissue attenuation coefficient in the patient) is partly or entirely replaced in CT image by a part of the lung (with lower attenuation coefficient). Therefore, the low attenuation coefficient wrongly attributed to a volume with a certain radioactivity causes undercorrection of attenuation and then underestimation of tracer uptake. This leads to artifactual cold areas in some organs with normal uptake or decreases (on corrected images) apparent signal corresponding to lesions with abnormally high uptake. Another effect of respiratory motion, important in the scope of nuclear imaging, appears—that is, the blurring due to motion during the relatively long time of acquisition. This damages both resolution and tracer uptake quantification. However, this effect of motion is not especially related to PET/CT and will not be extensively discussed in this chapter because it essentially focuses on the consequences of motion in dual modality imaging.

Appearance of the Artifact

The experienced physician observing the PET/CT images is able to recognize the respiratory motion artifact in most cases, and then suspects its consequences. Different signs, related to misregistration and abnormal cold areas, indicate that the phenomenon exists. However, the tiniest the motion, the most difficult the detection of the artifact. During the respiratory cycle, when a patient in a supine position breathes in, the ribcage moves upward and outward, but the main motion is for the diaphragm. It contracts, moving downward and becoming flatter. Abdominal organs move downward and outward, and the anterior abdominal wall moves ahead.

When the patient breathes out, the movements take the opposite direction. Those diverse movements are the origin of the artifacts that will be dealt with in the following paragraphs. Besides the impaired fusion of PET and CT images, or the deformation of the organ shapes, indirect clues may suggest that the artifact is present. Among these, an irregular anterior border of the thorax or of the abdomen on sagittal CT images indicates that CT slices were not acquired during the same respiratory condition. A default in attenuation correction in the anterior chest wall is another consequence of the respiratory motion described as possibly visible.

Impaired Superposition of Organs or Lesions

Similar to the gross artifacts consecutive to patient motion between CT acquisition and PET acquisition, as head or limb movement, a difference in the position of inner structures may be directly observed on the fusion of PET and CT images. This essentially occurs with high-uptake areas, such as myocardium or hyperactive lung tumor, corresponding to well-delineated dense areas on CT images. The borders of the areas obviously do not have the same position on the two images. In the same way, a hypodense lesion in the liver or the spleen, or a recognizable lesion (lymph node, abnormal adrenal gland) on the CT image, may not be fused with a high-uptake area on the PET image. The hot spots localized in renal cavities, or the tracer present in intestinal tract in the upper abdomen (as visible on PET images) may have a position different from the corresponding organs on CT images.

Due to the motion of the ribcage and to the consequences of the diaphragm contraction, the anterior border of the thorax and abdomen is sometimes wrongly superposed on the fusion image. In some cases, it may be easier to detect such phenomena by inspecting the CT images fused with the uncorrected PET images rather than erroneously corrected PET images.

Those rather easily detected abnormalities indicate that the respiratory motion artifact exists, but it must be borne in mind that sometimes this aspect is less clear or more disconcerting. Indeed, image acquisition during different phases of the respiratory cycle for the two modalities is not the sole origin of artifacts, and without breath-hold techniques, organ position varies while CT slices are acquired. It is, therefore, possible for the same organ to be viewed while moving in the same direction as the spiral CT acquisition (for instance, during inspiration) and afterward in the opposite direction (for instance, during expiration), the spiral CT acquisition keeping its own same speed and direction. As a result, the apparent size of organs may be slightly reduced or increased on the CT coronal or sagittal images, further hindering correct superposition of organs using the two image modalities. In such a case the manual displacement of one image set in order to fit it to the other one could improve the superposition only on a small part of the volume. The motion during CT acquisition may also make a tumor lose its shape, for example, lengthening its cranio-caudal dimension on CT images. In this case, it is possible that only part of the apparent tumor on the CT demonstrates an abnormal tracer uptake on PET.

Peri-Diaphragmatic Deformations

Many types of deformations can occur owing to respiratory motion artifact, as a result of a particular combination of respiratory motion amplitude, table speed, pitch, rotation time, and table direction in relation to diaphragm motion. Some patterns are relatively frequent, and may be rather easily recognized (Fig. 1). Upper abdomen organ deformations are visible on CT images and propagate in the CT-based attenuation-corrected PET images, where they eventually cause visible cold areas. When the diaphragm is lower on CT image than its average position during PET acquisition, or when the CT captures the diaphragm in such a low position during a relatively slow

movement, the respiratory motion artifact produced on CT-based attenuation-corrected PET images is a curvilinear cold area (so-called banana artifact) in the upper part of the liver, which may be accompanied by a similar effect in the spleen.

When the diaphragm movement is relatively faster, the upper part of the liver is caught by CT spiral, but the inspiration process shifts the liver downward and the posterior part of the liver is more displaced than the anterior part. The motion is often more notable in the liver closest to the rachis (that is, near the diaphragm crura). As a consequence, on subsequent slices, there is always a part of the liver (in the anterior part), but the posterior (and often posterior-interior) part of the liver is not included on the CT image. This leads to a cold area entering the liver, with a variable angle on the sagittal CT-based corrected PET images.

When the diaphragm movement is even faster as compared to the CT spiral, under the upper CT slice encompassing the liver dome, some slices capture a smaller part of the liver, because this organ moved downward and ahead, and

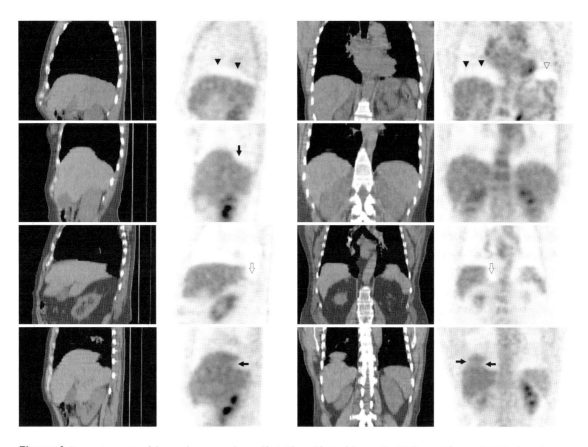

Figure 1 Frequent aspects of the respiratory motion artifact. The artifact arising on the CT image (*first and third columns*) propagates in the CT-corrected PET image (*second and fourth columns*). *Left*: sagittal slice through the liver; *right*: coronal slice. *Top row*: an upper curvilinear cold area is visible in the liver (arrowheads) and the spleen (open arrowhead) on the PET image. *Second row*: the cold area entering the liver causes a concave shape (vertical arrow) in place of the convex dome on the sagittal view. *Third row*: the cold area has a nearly vertical limit in the posterior and internal part of the liver (open arrow). *Fourth row*: the cold area enters under the upper part of the visible liver (horizontal arrows).

the artifactual cold area seems to enter the liver under the dome (leading to the so-called mushroom artifact on coronal slices). The maximal effect is an interruption between the top and the rest of the liver on CT images.

These effects producing a cold area seeming to enter the liver may often be combined with those yielding an upper cold area. The diverse cold areas obviously may also impact the aspect of the spleen or the stomach. However, artifacts are not necessarily equally prominent on both sides of the upper abdomen. Some investigators have observed a higher frequency of severe artifact on the left side (Osman *et al.*, 2003b). Such a discrepancy will be particularly expected if the top of the spleen is not situated at the same level as the top of the liver, and has not the same relation to the spiral progression. A less usual shape of the cold artifact can be encountered, displaying a cold area entering the anterior upper border of the liver.

An opposite effect to that described above is possible when the patient breathes out more during the CT acquisition than in his normal respiratory cycle. In this case, the liver on the CT is situated above its position during PET acquisition. A wrong correction of the attenuation leads, on CT-based corrected PET images, to an excessive liver volume above its actual limit in PET emission image. Such an effect is often unsuspected because the upper liver may have a classical shape and no cold area is visible. As stated above, it must be kept in mind that homogeneous global displacement is not expected when respiratory motion occurs. Instead, there is a variable association of deformations, especially lengthening and shortening in the cranio-caudal dimension, at different levels in the same subject, depending on the combination of the varying diaphragm motion and the constant table speed; these deformations are more or less perceptible. The appearance and the importance of the artifact depend on the speed of the CT.

Consequences of the Artifact

The respiratory motion causes deformations not only on CT images but also therefore on CT-based corrected PET images. The blurring in PET decreases the resolution and the standardized uptake value (SUV), and the motion decreases CT sensitivity for small lesions. However, the mislocalizations on PET/CT fused images and the decrease in the measured SUV due to erroneous attenuation correction (and thereby the reduced PET sensitivity) are principally dealt with in the following because they are particular consequences of respiratory motion in PET/CT (Fig. 2).

Errors in Anatomical Localization

Several investigators have quantitatively studied lung lesion motion. The motion during the respiratory cycle

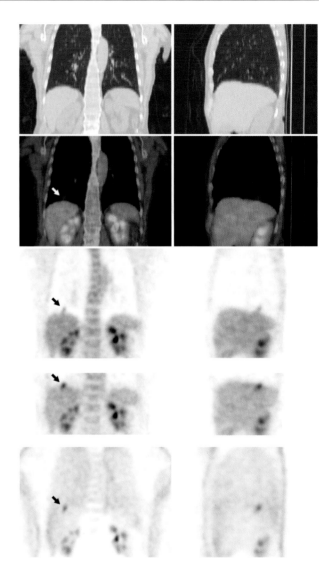

Figure 2 Example of the consequences of the respiratory motion artifact. Coronal (*left*) and sagittal (*right*) slices through a liver lesion. On the CT-based corrected PET image (*third row*) and the fusion image (*second row*), the lesion (arrow on the coronal slice) appears as lying in the lung base, but on the CT image (*first row*), no corresponding lung lesion is visible. On the cesium-based corrected PET image (*fourth row*), the lesion is accurately localized in the liver dome, and its apparent tracer uptake is greater than on the CT-based corrected PET image. The uncorrected PET image (*bottom row*) displays a tracer uptake focus more easily visible than on the CT-based corrected PET image.

using gated acquisition (which allows achieving images corresponding to diverse phases of a respiratory cycle) or the difference between the position of the lesion-related abnormality on PET and CT images could be used for these measurements. Table 1 summarizes representative values available from diverse studies. According to those studies, it appears that the motion of lung lesions usually ranges from 4 mm to 2.5 cm. The displacement of the lesion volume was observed to range from 24 to 93%, depending on the lesion size (Erdi *et al*., 2004).

The motion amplitude varies depending on the localization of the lesion. Several authors observed that the average distance was greater in the lower lung than in the upper lung. Movements of lower lung tumors appear to be more important in the cranio-caudal direction than movements in the anterior-posterior direction, which were themselves more than in the left-right direction (Beyer *et al*., 2005). The motion of a lung lesion seems to be often < 1 cm. Misregistration of a malignant lesion by a few millimeters in most of the cases would be unlikely to cause misinterpretations. Nevertheless, for lesions near the lung base, the mislocalization of lesions between the lung and liver may cause problems. A misregistration may also hinder the precise localization of a peripheral lesion in the lung parenchyma or in the chest wall.

Errors in anatomical localization occurring in the abdomen were also investigated. Table 1 shows several quantitative results from diverse studies. The coronal extent of the CT artifact in the liver (that is, a potential error in localization of lung versus liver) and the position of organs have been studied. The comparison of images corrected for attenuation using an external source with those obtained using CT-based correction also allowed assessment of the severity of artifact or accuracy of fusion and lesion localization (Nakamoto *et al*., 2003; Osman *et al*., 2003a, 2003b; Goerres *et al*., 2003b). With this technique in 300 patients, only 2% were found to exhibit mislocalization of lesions with clinical relevance; all six patients presented a liver lesion falsely located in the lung base on PET/CT (Osman *et al*., 2003a). Such a malpositioning of the liver dome lesion in the right lower lung due to respiratory motion artifact was also observed by others (Sarikaya *et al*., 2003). The possible but more rarely stated occurrence of the liver situated on the CT above its position during PET acquisition (if the patient breathes out enough during the CT acquisition) leads to another error. The related risk is to observe an abnormal uptake in an artificial liver dome on CT-based corrected PET images, while the pathological source is located in the lung base. In this case, a corresponding lung nodule would likely be apparent above the liver dome on the CT, without any metabolic hyperactivity visible on the fusion image. As the first consequence of respiratory motion artifact, errors in anatomical localization have no doubt been evidenced, but their impact on interpretation in a clinical setting seems to remain rather poor.

Underestimation of Tracer Uptake and Lesion Metabolism

Accurate quantification of tracer concentration has implications in characterizing lesions, guiding biopsies, allowing reproducibility during follow-up, and evaluating response to therapies. It has been shown with respiratory-gated PET that respiratory motion during PET acquisition reduced the measured SUVs in lung tumors because of image blurring. The reduction in the lesion volume when analyzing only one out of the phases of a gated study resulted in an increase of maximum SUV (ranging from 7 to 159%) (Nehmeh *et al*., 2002). A phantom study reproducing conditions of gated PET suggested that SUV may be underestimated by 21 to 45% because of respiratory blurring, depending on the lesion size (Boucher *et al*., 2004).

To this intrinsic PET problem related to respiratory motion, the mismatch between PET and CT adds a source of inaccuracy of SUV in PET/CT by degrading the quality of attenuation correction. As mentioned earlier, the misalignment of the attenuation map and the emission volume leads to the cold or relatively cold areas encountered in organs in the vicinity of the diaphragm. The same effect also reduces the intensity in the PET signal corresponding to hypermetabolic lesions on attenuation-corrected images. Several studies demonstrated a difference between count densities obtained with attenuation correction based on CT and those based on external source, without respect to respiratory motion (also stated in Kamel *et al*., 2002, and Nakamoto *et al*., 2002). But the respiration-induced artifact increased the difference. In this way, a bias in SUV has been found in normal tissues (lung, mediastinum, heart) and up to 51% in lung lesions. The bias was found to be greater when CT was acquired during inspiration. Table 2 gives results from several studies dealing with SUV modification due to respiratory motion.

Additional information was obtained from the CT-gated acquisition technique, which allowed studying the SUV or lesion volume variability depending on the phase of the respiratory cycle chosen for the CT data obtained with PET/CT. When the motion was ~ 10 mm, SUV changed on the order of 20%. The changes could be attributed to a combination of lesion size and motion amplitude, but this amplitude appeared to the investigators to be the major cause (Erdi *et al*., 2004). In another study using gated CT, the different phases of the CT data sets have been averaged to obtain a temporal resolution of CT similar to that of the PET. Misalignments between PET and CT were reduced, and the attenuation correction improved. The lesion SUVs, measured on PET corrected from averaged CT, and those obtained from the CT with mid-expiration breath hold, exhibited differences that were sometimes > 50% (Pan *et al*., 2005).

Besides the effect on lung tumors, respiratory motion has also been proven to alter SUV in liver lesions. In a study in which CT attenuation correction was compared with correction using a transmission map acquired with a cesium external source, the SUV in some liver metastases lying in the liver dome differed between the two correction methods (Papathanassiou *et al*., 2005a). The mean ratio of lesion

Table 1 **Displacement of Lung Lesions and Sub-Diaphragmatic Organs Due to Respiratory Motion**

Study		Breathing Instruction	Measurement	Value (mm)
Cohade and Wahl (2003)	PET/CT 36 patients 48 lesions	None	Distance between center of lung lesion in PET and CT	range: 0–26.2 mean: 7.55 upper lung: 6.67 middle lung: 6.94 lower lung: 10.2
Erdi *et al.* (2004)	Gated CT 5 patients 8 lesions	Customized verbal	Lung lesion displacement during cycle	range: 5.4–24.7 6/8 lesions < 11
Goerres *et al.* (2002b)	PET/CT 37 patients	Shallow breathing	Distance between lung lesion center of gravity in PET and CT	range: 1.7–14.7 mean: apical: 4.4 central: 4 peripheral: 6.5 base: 8.2
	38 patients	Breath hold at the end of normal expiration	Distance between lung lesion center of gravity in PET and CT	range: 0.5–11.4 mean: apical: 3 central: 3.3 peripheral: 6 base: 6.2
Beyer *et al.* (2003)	PET/CT 24 patients 19 patients	None Breath hold	Average coronal extent of the artifact in liver on CT image	69 33
Boucher *et al.* (2004)	Gated PET	None	Motion amplitude Right kidney Left kidney	range: 6.96–18.8 mean: 12 range: 3.5–17.1 mean: 11.1
Goerres *et al.* (2002a)	PET/CT 28 patients	Normal expiration Free breathing Maximal inspiration	Movement of the diaphragmatic dome on CT	range: − 24.7 to 18.9 mean: 0.4 range: − 29.1 to 18.9 mean: − 11.6 range: − 82.9 to 8.7 mean: − 44.4
Goerres *et al.* (2003b)	68Ge- and CT-based attenuation-corrected PET	Free breathing Maximal inspiration	Liver and spleen upper and lower borders, upper pole of the kidneys	mean: 5 to 10 mean: 15 to 40
Nakamoto *et al.* (2003)	68Ge- and CT-based attenuation-corrected PET	None	Upper margin of the liver or lower margin of the spleen	10% of the cases > 20 80% of the cases < 10
Pan *et al.* (2005)	PET/CT 100 patients	CT with mid-expiration breath hold	Cold area in right lower thorax	range: 0–70 50% of the cases > 10 34% of the cases > 20

SUV to normal liver SUV was 0.81 with CT and 1.51 with cesium for those lesions situated in the cold area due to the artifact, while it was 1.76 and 1.97, respectively, for other liver lesions. This represents a rather different problem from the lung lesions. The underestimation of SUV not only is due to misregistration of lesions on the two image modalities, but also relates to the more extended area of erroneous attenuation correction provoked by the mismatch between the diaphragm position during PET and during CT acquisition. Such an underestimation may reduce the sensitivity of PET, especially for small lesions exhibiting mild hypermetabolism (Papathanassiou *et al.*, 2005b).

Avoiding the Effects of the Artifact

Because of the degradation of image quality as well as the adverse effects of inaccurate lesion localization or impaired lesion detection or tumor activity estimation, minimizing the consequences of the artifact has been attempted in clinical practice. Different approaches are proposed or considered for this purpose. Examination of uncorrected PET images and transmission-based attenuation correction of PET images avoids the consequences of the erroneous CT-based attenuation correction. Breathing protocols are aimed at reducing the frequency of the inadequate diaphragm position during CT,

Table 2   Decrease Observed in Values Obtained during Different Respiratory Conditions

Study		Breathing Instruction	Measurement	Decrease
Erdi *et al.* (2004)	Gated CT 5 patients 8 lesions	Customized verbal	Lung lesion SUV during respiratory cycle	maximum 30%
Goerres *et al.* (2003a)	^{68}Ge- and CT-based attenuation-corrected PET	Inspiration during the CT acquisition	CT-based compared with ^{68}Ge-based	
			Heart SUV	range : 8–78% mean : 35%
			Lung SUV	range : 22–83% mean : 51%
			Lung lesion SUV	range : 25–49% mean : 37%
Pan *et al.* (2005)	PET/4D CT 8 patients 13 lesions	CT with mid-expiration breath hold	CT-based compared with averaged 4D CT-based lung lesion SUV	> 50% in 4/13 cases maximum 97.4%
Pevsner (2005)	PET/CT with body phantom	Body phantom at rest or moving during CT	Activity concentration in phantom spheres	maximum 75%

whereas synchronization with respiration allows acquiring adequate information despite respiratory motion. Software-based image registration is a postprocessing technique to remedy the varying position of the organs during respiration.

Examination of Uncorrected Positron Emission Tomography Images

Using the emission images without attenuation correction is the simplest way to avoid many of the consequences of the respiratory motion artifact in PET/CT. This possibility remains available when breathing protocols are inefficient. It is recommended to carefully inspect uncorrected images in PET (Bockisch *et al.*, 2004; Delbeke *et al.*, 2006). Among other reasons related to the resolution of issues arising from the CT-based attenuation-correction procedure, this is expected to reduce the risk of false-negative study.

The ability to detect lung hypermetabolic lesions with PET is known to decrease with the tumor size. The inaccurate registration of attenuation and emission data, whose probability is greater for small uptake foci, is likely to be involved in this phenomenon. Higher visibility of small lung lesions on nonattenuation-corrected images has indeed been observed (Reinhardt *et al.*, 2006). On the other hand, erroneous attenuation correction in the upper abdomen has been reported to lead to underestimation of the activity of some lesions encompassed in the cold area (Papathanassiou *et al.*, 2005a); uncorrected images showed abnormalities in most cases.

Nevertheless, even if uncorrected images may limit the reduction of the PET sensitivity, when a large diaphragmatic motion occurs during the CT acquisition, the correct superposition of organs on the CT and PET images is impossible, and a major advantage of PET/CT is then lost. Precise local-ization of a near-diaphragmatic hypermetabolic focus may be difficult with the uncorrected images only. However, if CT abnormalities exist, they may be helpful to draw conclusions of the PET/CT concerning this issue in the clinical practice.

Transmission-Based Attenuation Correction of Positron Emission Tomography Images

The attenuation correction performed using the attenuation map obtained with an external (^{68}Ge, germanium or ^{137}Cs, cesium) source is an alternative to CT-based attenuation correction. It is assumed to be free of the respiratory motion artifact because the temporal resolution of the transmission images is the same as that of emission images. Therefore, the diaphragm has the same average position on both images, and the correction is valid. For this reason, the transmission technique was chosen as a reference in several studies, as stated in other parts of this chapter. The acquisition of a transmission map covering the lower thorax and the upper abdomen is simple, and the additional absorbed dose or duration is still limited related to the whole PET/CT procedure.

Nevertheless, despite the theoretical maximal matching of emission and attenuation maps, the possibility of different average diaphragm position (e.g., because of variable respiratory frequency) could not be definitely ruled out with this technique. Moreover, the advantages of the spatial CT image properties are not brought in the corrected image. In addition, a correct fusion of the transmission-based corrected PET image and the CT image remains impossible, and the anatomical localization is still sometimes difficult. The potential of this technique is that the PET-corrected images are less disturbed than those with CT-based attenuation correction, and that the PET sensitivity is not reduced as when the artifact impairs the metabolism quantification. However, manufacturers currently propose only PET/CT models without the former conventional transmission source option, and this possibility is likely to disappear.

Breathing Protocols

Many authors dealing with artifacts or techniques in PET/CT mention diverse breathing techniques intended to minimize respiratory motion during CT acquisition (Cohade *et al.*, 2003; Cook *et al.*, 2004; Beyer *et al.*, 2004; Bockisch *et al.*, 2004; Coleman *et al.*, 2005; Delbeke *et al.*, 2006). While end-inspiration breath-holding is commonly rejected as a suitable protocol in PET/CT (contrary to the diagnostic CT scan technique), no optimal protocol has become standard. Besides normal or shallow breathing, holding the breath at the end of a normal expiration is the most often proposed protocol. A normal tidal breathing for both PET and CT acquisitions is sometimes preferred, being feasible for heavily debilitated patients (Cohade *et al.*, 2003). Some reports indicate that quantification is not excessively disturbed with normal breathing. Lesion SUVs have been found to be similar when the CT was acquired during normal breathing or during breath hold with expiration. In contrast, the breath hold with inspiration led to values clearly different from those obtained using a conventional transmission method (more different than the normal breathing or the breath hold with expiration) (Visvikis *et al.*, 2003).

Instructions to patients are helpful in order to optimize image quality. A patient breathing freely, without any instruction, might deeply inspire during critical seconds of the CT scanning. If patients are cautioned regarding this point and try to avoid large thoracic motion during this part of the procedure, the severity of the artifact will be reduced. Such a shallow breathing is an achievable condition by a large number of the patients and may be proposed in the case of patients unable to perform more elaborate techniques. Maintaining the diaphragm in an intermediate position is somewhat uneasy (because it is not an intuitive approach for many patients) and not easily reproducible. Furthermore, it is questionable whether such a position during the CT acquisition would match in all cases the average diaphragm position during PET acquisition. In such a protocol, the breath may be held at an even deeper inspiration than normal end-inspiration in free-breathing state. In a study where patients were asked to hold their breath in mid-expiration, a misalignment between CT and PET existed in 50 out of 100 subjects, exceeding 2 cm in 34 subjects (Pan *et al.*, 2005).

Goerres and colleagues recommended holding the breath at the end of a normal expiration and studied the impact of this protocol. They found no statistical difference in the abdominal organ movements between normal breathing and normal expiration (Goerres *et al.*, 2003b), but a notable difference was found when CT was acquired under breath hold with maximum inspiration (Table 1). During their investigations, they found that maintaining breath hold in maximum expiration was the least comfortable position (no patient kept it during the CT scan of ~ 22.5 sec). Analyzing the coregistration in the thorax, they compared different conditions: normal expiration breath-hold protocol, normal breathing, maximum inspiration, and maximum expiration. They found that normal expiration protocol led to the best results, concerning the similarities in measurements of determined distances (anatomical reference points or lung lesions) (Goerres *et al.*, 2002a), as well as frequency and severity of the curvilinear artifact (De Juan *et al.*, 2004), or distance of the tumor center of gravity between PET image and CT image (Goerres *et al.*, 2002b). However, the difference in the average latter distance between shallow breathing and holding in normal expiration position was small (~ 1 or 2 mm). They also studied the measured activity concentrations in lung and heart, and reported that the attenuation correction with CT acquired during maximum inspiration was significantly worse than that with the ^{68}Ge-based technique, but there was no difference between ^{68}Ge-based correction and the one using CT acquired under normal expiration condition (Goerres *et al.*, 2003a).

The latter result corroborates the conclusions of other studies regarding the superiority of the expiration condition over inspiration (Visvikis *et al.*, 2003), but does not prove its superiority over normal breathing condition. In spite of this reservation, theoretically breath-holding is preferable to normal breathing for attenuation-correction purposes. Because the CT image is altered by motion (Aquino *et al.*, 2006), breath-holding also allows limiting the degradation of the CT image for its own use in the analysis of the PET/CT study. One justification for preferring normal expiration condition during CT scanning is that during PET the upper abdominal organs and the lower mediastinum are mainly in a position close to that of expiration because in normal human breathing most of the time is spent in the expiration phase of the respiratory cycle.

However, holding the breath in the normal expiration position is not feasible throughout the CT scanning for every patient; this protocol would be more achievable with very fast CT devices. Therefore, a limited breath-hold protocol is possible, as proposed by Beyer and colleagues. Patients maintained normal breathing during the entire scanning except for the time the CT covered the lower thorax and upper abdomen (typically < 15 sec). They were asked to hold their breath (in normal expiration) only for that part of the scanning. The frequency of severe artifacts in the area of the diaphragm was observed as being reduced by half with this technique, and the spatial extent of artifacts by at least 40% compared with the acquisition without breathing instructions (Beyer *et al.*, 2003).

Nevertheless, in spite of being considered as an easily applicable method (depending on the patient's ability) to reduce respiratory motion artifact, breath-hold techniques do not fully overcome inaccurate matching between PET and CT, nor do they account for breathing artifacts in the PET scan such as blurring and contrast degradation.

Synchronizing Images with Respiration

Current techniques or concepts regarding respiratory gating in the topic of respiratory motion artifact in PET/CT are in part derived from the gating for radiotherapy planning purposes. Indeed, among other consequences of the artifact, the blurring in PET and the tumor shape distortion in CT provoke an uncertainty in the lesion volume, which necessitates the expansion of the margin around the tumor while defining the target. The respiratory gating implies the acquisition of data over a complete respiratory cycle for the volume studied and the sorting of the data corresponding to different phases (typically 8 to 10 phases) of the cycle. With this aim, a respiratory signal, such as an external signal (markers on the abdominal surface allowing the tracking of its vertical motion using a CCD camera) or lung volume (recorded using a spirometer) or breathing airflow (monitored with a thermometer in the airflow of the patient), is acquired together with images. For PET, a gated procedure, as an adapted version of the better known cardiac gating mode of the scanner, might be used. For CT, the acquisition time of the CT data may be used to stamp CT images, for retrospective image selection. Audio or visual coaching may allow ensuring reproducibility of the breathing cycle.

The gating technique requires additional tracking hardware. An alternative has been proposed with PET images acquired in consecutive short (1 sec) frames, with a point source attached to the patient's abdomen (Nehmeh et al., 2003). The PET frames corresponding to a particular position of the source are selected retrospectively and summed. This avoids tracking hardware but implies more computer memory and postprocessing time, and a worst time resolution than in the PET-gated acquisition mode. The respiratory gating for PET has been shown to reduce the image smearing and leads to more accurate delineation of the lesion and improved measurement of metabolic activity (Nehmeh et al., 2002; Boucher et al., 2004). To resolve the problem of the mismatch between the two modalities, only the PET frame corresponding to the position of the diaphragm during a nonsynchronized CT may be used. The delineation of small lesions with low tracer uptake may become difficult in a single-gated image where count statistics decrease and noise increases. However, the reduction of the smearing may still improve the signal-to-noise ratio.

For the so-called 4D CT (3D-CT image sets acquired over a breathing cycle: acquisition of repeated axial CT images for a specified period of time, at each table position), the technique is limited by the design features of the device (requiring multi-row detectors and sufficient speed of the gantry).

It also implies a trade-off between the temporal resolution and the delivered dose. The respiratory gating for CT was shown to lead to a better definition of the lesion volume on the CT images, and a better congruence of emission and attenuation data also provided a better estimation of metabolic activity in PET after attenuation correction (Erdi et al., 2004). Rendering the temporal resolution of CT similar to that of the PET by averaging the different phases of the CT data sets has been proposed (Pan et al., 2005), but this application of 4D CT is expected to degrade resolution in CT, and it does not take complete advantage of the possibilities offered by respiratory gating.

The full exploitation of the synchronization would be using 4D mode in both PET and CT. An additional advantage is that 4D CT also takes into account the motion during the attenuation map acquisition, while usually gating PET is only for the emission acquisition and not for the transmission. Because even with stand-alone PET and CT scanners 4D imaging seems useful to accurately combine images from both modalities (Wolthaus et al., 2005), PET/CT hybrid scanners are expected to allow maximal exploitation of the advantages of 4D imaging. Using 4D mode in both CT and PET with combined PET/CT, many of these advantages were again shown (Nehmeh et al., 2004): co-registration between 4D-PET and CT lesions improved; 4D PET reduced the blurring; the attenuation correction with 4D CT led to different lesion volumes in PET; tumor volume in CT was modified; and 4D PET/CT resulted in an increase in the SUV, compared to measurements from 4D PET corrected with nongated CT. When improvements of 4D modes in CT and PET were combined, the maximal SUV increased for all patients, up to 16%.

Presently, 4D CT or gated PET is not yet a standard procedure. With these techniques the session is noticeably lengthened. Due to an increase in absorbed dose owing to the 4D-CT technique, it should be suitable for radiotherapy planning but not for a standard diagnostic investigation. Absorbed dose would also increase if more FDG were used in order to obtain better information on PET-gated images. Moreover, the effects of respiratory motion could not be overcome for the whole thorax and upper abdomen in each patient, because such gated acquisitions cover only part of the body (e.g., the lower thorax and upper abdomen) and are used in addition to a conventional technique for the remaining body examined in the PET/CT session.

Software-Based Image Registration

Registration consists of a transformation of the coordinates from one image space into another. Combined PET/CT scanners reduced the need for rigid transformation to align the images of the two modalities, but did not rule out the software-based registration method for the nonrigid misalignments. Rigid or affine transformations are inadequate for data where different organs move in different directions and amplitudes. Deformable registration is required. Many methods exist and are subject to research in progress. Voxel-based methods, especially methods based on mutual information, appear to be the most accurate and robust image registration techniques currently available. Methods using mutual information (statistical measures not expecting direct correlation of intensities in homologous regions) apply to multimodality registration and have potential for whole-body elastic PET/CT registration. The registration of CT images obtained in a single breath hold and PET images obtained with the usual protocol, improved by the nonrigid warping method, leads to more accurate attenuation correction.

An algorithm using a variant of mutual information has been reported to enhance the alignment of PET/CT scans obtained from a combined scanner, with promising results (Shekhar et al., 2005). The reported application time was from 45 to 75 min, but the method could be further accelerated through hardware evolution. Indeed, besides the ability to deal with deformable anatomy, for clinical use, a whole-body CT and PET image registration method should be automatic and fast. Furthermore, such software-based image registration techniques may be combined with gating. PET images corresponding to each part of the respiratory cycle may then be transformed to match one position, and then merged before attenuation correction (Dawood et al., 2006). This technique both overcomes the loss of statistics in a single frame obtained with gated PET and reduces the effects of motion.

In conclusion, respiratory motion artifact using PET/CT is frequent. Its potential implications in lesion localization or PET/CT sensitivity are challenging, but misinterpretations remain rare. Being aware of its possibility, situation, and diverse effects, together with using simple methods such as examination of uncorrected PET images, notably reduce the risk of misleading interpretation. Breathing protocols may be used when possible, depending on the patient. Sophisticated techniques exist and are likely to develop for selected applications. In the future, the techniques for processing acquired data (such as synchronization with respiration) and image processing (such as morphing) are expected to become widely available to overcome the respiratory motion artifact, but as yet they are not a part of routine practice.

References

Aquino, S.L., Kuester, L.B., Muse, V.V., Halpern, E.F., and Fischman, A.J. 2006. Accuracy of transmission CT and FDG-PET in the detection of small pulmonary nodules with integrated PET/CT. Eur. J. Nucl. Med. Mol. Imaging 33:692–696.

Beyer, T., Antoch, G., Blodgett, T., Freudenberg, L.F., Akhurst, T., and Mueller, S. 2003. Dual-modality PET/CT imaging: the effect of respiratory motion on combined image quality in clinical oncology. Eur. J. Nucl. Med. Mol. Imaging 30:588–596.

Beyer, T., Antoch, G., Muller, S., Egelhof, T., Freudenberg, L.S., Debatin, J., and Bockisch, A. 2004. Acquisition protocol considerations for combined PET/CT imaging. J. Nucl. Med. 45 Suppl. 1:25S–35S.

Beyer, T., Rosenbaum, S., Veit, P., Stattaus, J., Muller, S.P., Difilippo, F.P., Schoder, H., Mawlawi, O., Roberts, F., Bockisch, A., and Kuhl, H. 2005. Respiration artifacts in whole-body (18)F-FDG PET/CT studies with combined PET/CT tomographs employing spiral CT technology with 1 to 16 detector rows. Eur. J. Nucl. Med. Mol. Imaging 32:1429–1439.

Bockisch, A., Beyer, T., Antoch, G., Freudenberg, L.S., Kuhl, H., Debatin, J.F., and Muller, S.P. 2004. Positron emission tomography/computed tomography—imaging protocols, artifacts, and pitfalls. Mol. Imaging Biol. 6:188–199.

Boucher, L., Rodrigue, S., Lecomte, R., and Benard, F. 2004. Respiratory gating for 3-dimensional PET of the thorax: feasibility and initial results. J. Nucl. Med. 45:214–219.

Cohade, C., and Wahl, R.L. 2003. Applications of positron emission tomography/computed tomography image fusion in clinical positron emission tomography-clinical use, interpretation methods, diagnostic improvements. Semin. Nucl. Med. 33:228–237.

Coleman, R.E., Delbeke, D., Guiberteau, M.J., Conti, P.S., Royal, H.D., Weinreb, J.C., Siegel, B.A., Federle, M.F., Townsend, D.W., and Berland, L.L. 2005. Concurrent PET/CT with an integrated imaging system: intersociety dialogue from the joint working group of the American College of Radiology, the Society of Nuclear Medicine, and the Society of Computed Body Tomography and Magnetic Resonance. J. Nucl. Med. 46:1225–1239.

Cook, G.J., Wegner, E.A., and Fogelman, I. 2004. Pitfalls and artifacts in 18FDG PET and PET/CT oncologic imaging. Semin. Nucl. Med. 34:122–133.

Dawood, M., Lang, N., Jiang, X., and Schafers, K.P. 2006. Lung motion correction on respiratory gated 3-D PET/CT images. IEEE Trans. Med. Imaging 25:476–485.

De Juan, R., Seifert, B., Berthold, T., von Schulthess, G.K., and Goerres, G.W. 2004. Clinical evaluation of a breathing protocol for PET/CT. Eur. Radiol. 14:1118–1123.

Delbeke, D., Coleman, R.E., Guiberteau, M.J., Brown, M.L., Royal, H.D., Siegel, B.A., Townsend, D.W., Berland, L.L., Parker, J.A., Hubner, K., Stabin, M.G., Zubal, G., Kachelriess, M., Cronin, V., and Holbrook, S. 2006. Procedure guideline for tumor imaging with 18F-FDG PET/CT 1.0. J. Nucl. Med. 47:885–895.

Erdi, Y.E., Nehmeh, S.A., Pan, T., Pevsner, A., Rosenzweig, K.E., Mageras, G., Yorke, E.D., Schoder, H., Hsiao, W., Squire, O.D., Vernon, P., Ashman, J.B., Mostafavi, H., Larson, S.M., and Humm, J.L. 2004. The CT motion quantitation of lung lesions and its impact on PET-measured SUVs. J. Nucl. Med. 45:1287–1292.

Goerres, G.W., Kamel, E., Heidelberg, T.N., Schwitter, M.R., Burger, C., and von Schulthess, G.K. 2002a. PET-CT image co-registration in the thorax: influence of respiration. Eur. J. Nucl. Med. Mol. Imaging 29:351–360.

Goerres, G.W., Kamel, E., Seifert, B., Burger, C., Buck, A., Hany, T.F., and von Schulthess, G.K. 2002b. Accuracy of image coregistration of pulmonary lesions in patients with non-small cell lung cancer using an integrated PET/CT system. J. Nucl. Med. 43:1469–1475.

Goerres, G.W., Burger, C., Kamel, E., Seifert, B., Kaim, A.H., Buck, A., Buehler, T.C., and von Schulthess, G.K. 2003a. Respiration-induced attenuation artifact at PET/CT: technical considerations. Radiology 226:906–910.

Goerres, G.W., Burger, C., Schwitter, M.R., Heidelberg, T.N., Seifert, B., and von Schulthess, G.K. 2003b. PET/CT of the abdomen: optimizing the patient breathing pattern. Eur. Radiol. 13:734–739.

Kamel, E., Hany, T.F., Burger, C., Treyer, V., Lonn, A.H., von Schulthess, G.K., and Buck, A. 2002. CT vs 68Ge attenuation correction in a combined PET/CT system: evaluation of the effect of lowering the CT tube current. Eur. J. Nucl. Med. Mol. Imaging 29:346–350.

Nakamoto, Y., Osman, M., Cohade, C., Marshall, L.T., Links, J.M., Kohlmyer, S., and Wahl, R.L. 2002. PET/CT: comparison of quantitative tracer uptake between germanium and CT transmission attenuation-corrected images. J. Nucl. Med. 43:1137–1143.

Nakamoto, Y., Tatsumi, M., Cohade, C., Osman, M., Marshall, L.T., and Wahl, R.L. 2003. Accuracy of image fusion of normal upper abdominal organs visualized with PET/CT. *Eur. J. Nucl. Med. Mol. Imaging 30*:597–602.

Nehmeh, S.A., Erdi, Y.E., Ling, C.C., Rosenzweig, K.E., Schoder, H., Larson, S.M., Macapinlac, H.A., Squire, O.D., and Humm, J.L. 2002. Effect of respiratory gating on quantifying PET images of lung cancer. *J. Nucl. Med. 43*:876–881.

Nehmeh, S.A., Erdi, Y.E., Rosenzweig, K.E., Schoder, H., Larson, S.M., Squire, O.D., and Humm, J.L. 2003. Reduction of respiratory motion artifacts in PET imaging of lung cancer by respiratory correlated dynamic PET: methodology and comparison with respiratory gated PET. *J. Nucl. Med. 44*:1644–1648.

Nehmeh, S.A., Erdi, Y.E., Pan, T., Pevsner, A., Rosenzweig, K.E., Yorke, E., Mageras, G.S., Schoder, H., Vernon, P., Squire, O., Mostafavi, H., Larson, S.M., and Humm, J.L. 2004. Four-dimensional (4D) PET/CT imaging of the thorax. *Med. Phys. 31*:3179–3186.

Osman, M.M., Cohade, C., Nakamoto, Y., Marshall, L.T., Leal, J.P., and Wahl, R.L. 2003a. Clinically significant inaccurate localization of lesions with PET/CT: frequency in 300 patients. *J. Nucl. Med. 44*:240–243.

Osman, M.M., Cohade, C., Nakamoto, Y., and Wahl, R.L. 2003b. Respiratory motion artifacts on PET emission images obtained using CT attenuation correction on PET-CT. *Eur. J. Nucl. Med. Mol. Imaging 30*:603–606.

Pan, T., Mawlawi, O., Nehmeh, S.A., Erdi, Y.E., Luo, D., Liu, H.H., Castillo, R., Mohan, R., Liao, Z., and Macapinlac, H.A. 2005. Attenuation correction of PET images with respiration-averaged CT images in PET/CT. *J. Nucl. Med. 46*:1481–1487.

Papathanassiou, D., Becker, S., Amir, R., Meneroux, B., and Liehn, J.C. 2005a. Respiratory motion artefact in the liver dome on FDG PET/CT: comparison of attenuation correction with CT and a caesium external source. *Eur. J. Nucl. Med. Mol. Imaging 32*:1422–1428.

Papathanassiou, D., Liehn, J.C., Bourgeot, B., Amir, R., and Marcus, C. 2005b. Cesium attenuation correction on the liver dome revealing hepatic lesion missed with computed tomography attenuation correction because of the respiratory motion artifact. *Clin. Nucl. Med. 30*:120–121.

Pevsner, A., Nehmeh, S.A., Humm, J.L., Mageras, G.S., and Erdi, Y.E. 2005. Effect of motion on tracer activity determination in CT accentuation corrected PET images: a lung phantom study. *Med. Phys. 32*:2358–2362.

Reinhardt, M.J., Wiethoelter, N., Matthies, A., Joe, A.Y., Strunk, H., Jaeger, U., and Biersack, H.J. 2006. PET recognition of pulmonary metastases on PET/CT imaging: impact of attenuation-corrected and non-attenuation-corrected PET images. *Eur. J. Nucl. Med. Mol. Imaging 33*:134–139.

Sarikaya, I., Yeung, H.W., Erdi, Y., and Larson, S.M. 2003. Respiratory artefact causing malpositioning of liver dome lesion in right lower lung. *Clin. Nucl. Med. 28*:943–944.

Shekhar, R., Walimbe, V., Raja, S., Zagrodsky, V., Kanvinde, M., Wu, G., and Bybel, B. 2005. Automated 3-dimensional elastic registration of whole-body PET and CT from separate or combined scanners. *J. Nucl. Med. 46*:1488–1496.

Visvikis, D., Costa, D.C., Croasdale, I., Lonn, A.H., Bomanji, J., Gacinovic, S., and Ell, P.J. 2003. CT-based attenuation correction in the calculation of semi-quantitative indices of [18F]FDG uptake in PET. *Eur. J. Nucl. Med. Mol. Imaging 30*:344–353.

Wolthaus, J.W., van Herk, M., Muller, S.H., Belderbos, J.S., Lebesque, J.V., de Bois, J.A., Rossi, M.M., and Damen, E.M. 2005. Fusion of respiration-correlated PET and CT scans: correlated lung tumour motion in anatomical and functional scans. *Phys. Med. Biol. 50*:1569–1583.

9

Gadolinium-Based Contrast Media Used in Magnetic Resonance Imaging: An Overview

Allen Li

Introduction

Gadolinium-based contrast media are the dominant types of contrast agents used in magnetic resonance imaging (MRI). This class of contrast media has wide clinical applications, is well established in the diagnostic work-up of a vast majority of disease processes, and has an expanding role in various morphological and functional imaging studies.

Mechanism of Action

Gadolinium is a member of the lanthanide group of elements, which all possess partially filled inner shells of electrons. In its native state, gadolinium is paramagnetic and has seven unpaired electrons in its 4f orbital, more than any other element. Electrons have a large charge-to-mass ratio and exert strong magnetic moments. Gadolinium ion, therefore, produces a strong magnetic moment even when it is chelated to a ligand such as diethylenetriamine pentaacetic acid (DTPA) (Hendrick and Haacke, 1993). At the molecular level, the strong magnetic moment of gadolinium reduces the relaxation times of the surrounding protons. Shortening of the relaxation time of tissues produces an increase in contrast between the lesion and its background in MRI. The enhanced contrast between pathological and normal anatomical structures facilitates the detection, characterization, and assessment of the extent of the disease. Other major applications of gadolinium-based contrast media include contrast-enhanced magnetic resonance angiography and perfusion studies, which have been developed to provide information regarding flow-related abnormalities and organ perfusion, respectively (Mathur-De et al., 1995). Gadolinium, in its native ionic form, is extremely toxic to the body. The gadolinium-based contrast agents currently available for clinical use are all chelates. The gadolinium ion is bound by a ligand to form a stable molecule that reduces its toxicity.

Classification

Gadolinium-based contrast media used in magnetic resonance imaging can be classified (Table 1) according to the distribution inside the body (nonspecific extracellular vs. targeted contrast media); the ligands chelated to the gadolinium ion (linear vs. cyclic); and the net overall charge on the gadolinium-containing molecule in solution (ionic vs. nonionic) (Tweedle, 1991).

Nonspecific extracellular gadolinium-based contrast media constitute the vast majority of MRI contrast agents currently used in clinical practice. Gadopentetate dimeglumine, the prototype, was the first gadolinium-based contrast agent approved by the Food and Drug Administration for clinical use in the United States (1988). These agents are hydrophilic molecules that do not bind to proteins or receptors. Because of their small size, after intravenous administration, the contrast media rapidly equilibrate between the intravascular and interstitial spaces in the body, and is subsequently excreted unmetabolized by passive glomerular filtration. Within the interstitial space, these agents diffuse freely with the exception of the central nervous system and the testes—the blood-brain barrier and blood-testis barrier are impermeable to these agents. The biodistribution of these agents is, therefore, nonspecific (Roberts and Roberts, 1999; Bellin et al., 2003).

Targeted MRI contrast media are designed to direct the agent to specific body compartments, intravascular space, tissues, or cells. Most of these agents are still in the experimental stages or early clinical trials. Hepatocyte-selective contrast agents have been introduced for clinical use as the prototype of targeted MRI contrast media. By modifying the functional groups of the ligands to increase the lipophilicity of the molecules, these agents are partially taken up by normal hepatocytes, positively enhancing the signal from the healthy liver. This increase in signal intensity leads to an improvement of lesion-to-liver contrast because tumors either do not contain hepatocytes or the functioning of intratumoral hepatocytes is hampered. Gadobenate dimeglumine and gadoxetic acid disodium are gadolinium-based contrast media that have both hepatocyte selectivity and nonspecific extracellular biodistribution (Unger, 1999; Reimer et al., 2004).

Ligands chelating the gadolinium ion can be classified into linear (DTPA) or cyclic forms (HPDO3A as in gadoteridol). The ligands are designed to tightly bind the gadolinium ion, preventing the release of the toxic gadolinium ion into the body. Theoretically, the cyclic gadolinium chelates are structurally more stable than the linear chelates. However,

for practical purposes and at the recommended dose, none of the commercial compounds releases significant amounts of toxic gadolinium ion into the body (Dawson and Blomley, 1994; Runge, 2000).

Nonionic gadolinium chelate molecules, when compared to their ionic counterparts, have reduced osmolality at the same concentration. For example, gadopentetate dimeglumine, whose formula is $Gd (DTPA)^{2-} (dimeglumine)^{2+}$, exists as three ions in solution, which contributes to its osmolality. In contrast, Gd DTPA-BMA, which is a neutral nonionic molecule, exists as only a molecule in solution (Tweedle, 1991). The clinical relevance of osmolality among different agents is negligible because generally only a small volume of contrast media is used. Theoretically, an agent with high osmolality may have a disadvantage in terms of pain and degree of tissue necrosis following accidental extravascular injection.

Clinical Safety

Gadolinium-based contrast media used in MRI are well tolerated by the vast majority of patients. At the recommended dose, these agents could be considered a safer alternative to iodinated contrast media used in computed tomography. Anaphylactoid reactions including death have been reported but are rare. The reported incidence of such a life-threatening event appears to be ~ 0.01% (Murphy et al., 1996; Shellock and Ranal, 1999; Li et al., 2006). For reference, the incidence of a life-threatening event with iodinated contrast media was reported to be 0.031% for low osmolarity and 0.157% for ionic contrast media (Caro et al., 1992). Patients with prior adverse reactions to iodinated or gadolinium-based contrast media, asthma, and various allergies are at a greater risk of developing adverse reactions to gadolinium-based contrast media (Nelson et al., 1995). Most of the adverse reactions encountered with gadolinium-based contrast agents are minor side effects such as nausea, urticaria, and headache. A meta-analysis of data obtained for 13,439 patients enrolled in Phase IIIb–IV studies, who received 0.1 or 0.2 mmol/kg of Gd-DTPA, showed an adverse event rate of 1.15%. In patients

Table 1   Current Gadolinium–Based Contrast Media Available in the International Market for Clinical Use

| Trade name | Generic name | Classifications | | |
		Type	Structure	Biodistribution
Magnevist®	Gadopentetate dimeglumine (Gd-DTPA)	Ionic	Linear	Extracellular
Dotarem®	Gadoterate meglumine (Gd-DOTA)	Ionic	Cyclic	Extracellular
Omniscan®	Gadodiamide (Gd-DTPA BMA)	Nonionic	Linear	Extracellular
Prohance®	Gadoteridol (Gd-HP-DO3A)	Nonionic	Cyclic	Extracellular
Multihance®	Gadobenate dimeglumine (Gd-BOPTA)	Ionic	Linear	Extracellular and hepatic
Primovist®	Gadoxetic acid disodium (Gd-EOB-DTPA)	Ionic	Linear	Extracellular and hepatic

Remarks: Approval status for clinical use of each individual drug is subject to local governing parties.

with a known history of allergy, the incidence of adverse events was found to be 2.6% (Niendorf *et al.*, 1993).

Gadolinium-based contrast media are safe for use in both children and adults. There are safety concerns for administering gadolinium-based contrast media to a pregnant woman because the contrast media are able to cross the blood-placenta barrier. The safe use of the contrast media during pregnancy has not been proven, and it should be administered only after well-documented and in-depth analysis shows that the potential benefits to the patient and/or fetus clearly outweigh the risk of exposure to the gadolinium ion (Kanal *et al.*, 2004).

Gadolinium-based contrast media, at the recommended dose, are not nephrotoxic compared with iodinated contrast media used in radiographic exams and computed tomography. The contrast media are efficiently cleared by glomerular filtration, and studies support that they are well tolerated in patients with renal insufficiency (Haustein *et al.*, 1992; Yoshikawa and Davies, 1997). However, it may be prudent to use these agents with caution in patients with severely impaired renal function, especially in high-dose applications such as contrast-enhanced magnetic resonance angiography. As recent reports have suggested possible gadolinium-associated nephrogenic systemic fibrosis is patients with advanced renal failure (Marckmann *et al.*, 2006; Grobner, 2006).

Other Applications

In addition to intravenous administration, gadolinium-based contrast media can also be given parenterally in abdominal MRI. The agent acts as a positive enhancer and helps to differentiate the bowel from the adjacent organs or pathological structures. Magnetic resonance arthrography has been successfully tried using direct intra-articular injection of diluted gadolinium-based contrast media to increase the sensitivity of lesion detection (Steinbach *et al.*, 2002). With improving hardware technology, coil design, field strength, software versatility, and parallel imaging technique, the dynamic perfusion and functional studies of the body are not only available as research tools but also for clinical use. With further refinements and developments, assessment of perfusion and functional MRI studies utilizing gadolinium-based contrast media may be possible in any vascular bed. In conclusion, gadolinium-based contrast media are considered to be safe and well tolerated by the vast majority of patients. This group of contrast media continues to have a well-established role in clinical medicine. Although clinical trials of a newer category of agents (blood-pool and targeted MRI contrast agents) are underway, the indications and clinical applications of these existing agents are expanding.

References

Bellin, M.F., Vasile, M., and Morel-Precetti, S. 2003. Currently used non-specific extracellular MR contrast media. *Eur. Radiol.* 13:2688–2698.

Caro, J.J., Trindade, E., and McGregor, M. 1992. The cost-effectiveness of replacing high-osmolarity with low-osmolarity contrast media. *AJR Am. J. Roentgenol.* 159:869–874.

Dawson, P., and Blomley, M. 1994. Gadolinium chelate MR contrast agent. Editorial. *Clin Radiol.* 49:439–442.

Grobner, T. 2006. Gadolinium—a specific trigger for the development of nephrogenic fibrosing dermopathy and nephrogenic systemic fibrosis? *Nephrol. Dial. Transplant* 21:1104–1108.

Haustein, J., Niendorf, H., and Krestin, G. 1992. Renal tolerance of gadolinium-DTPA dimeglumine in patients with chronic renal failure. *Invest. Radiol.* 27:153–156.

Hendrick, R.E., and Haacke, E.M. 1993. Basic physics of MR contrast agents and maximization of image contrast. *J. Mag. Reson. Imaging.* 3:137.

Kanal, E., Borgstede, J.P., Barkovich, A.J., Bell, C., Bradley, W.G., Etheridge, S., Felmlee, J.P., Froelich, J.W., Hayden, J., Kaminski, E.M., Lester, J.W., Jr., Scoumis, E.A., Zaremba, L.A., and Zinninger, M.D., American College of Radiology. 2004. American College of Radiology White Paper on MR Safety: 2004 update and revisions. *AJR Am. J. Roentgenol.* 82:1111–1114.

Li, A., Wong, C.S., Wong, M.K., Lee, C.M., and Au Yeung, M.C. 2006. Acute adverse reactions to magnetic resonance contrast media-gadolinium chelates. *Br. J. Radiol.* 79:368–371.

Marckmann, P., Skov, L., Rossen, K., Dupont, A., Damholt, M.B., Heaf, J.G., and Thomsen, H.S. 2006. Nephrogenic systemic fibrosis: suspected causative role of gadodiamide used for contrast-enhanced magnetic resonance imaging. *J. Am. Soc. Nephrol.* 17:2359–2362.

Mathur-De Vre, R., and Lemort, M. 1995. Biophysical properties and clinical applications of magnetic resonance imaging contrast agents. *Br. J. Radiol.* 68:225–247.

Murphy, K.J., Brunberg, J.A., and Cohan, R.H. 1996. Adverse reactions to gadolinium contrast media: a review of 36 cases. *AJR* 167:847–849.

Nelson, K.L., Gifford, L.M., Lauber-Huber, C., Gross, C.A., and Lasser, T.A. 1995. Clinical safety of gadopentetate dimeglumine. *Radiology.* 2:439–443.

Niendorf, H.P., Alhassan, A., Haustein, J., Clauss, W., and Cornelius, I. 1993. Safety and risk of gadolinium-DTPA: extended clinical experience after more than 5,000,000 applications. *Adv. MRI Contrast* 2:12–19.

Reimer, P., Schneider, G., and Schima, W. 2004. Hepatobiliary contrast agents for contrast enhanced MRI of the liver: properties, clinical development and applications. *Eur. Radiol.* 14:559–578.

Roberts, T.P.L, and Roberts, H.C. 1999. Macromolecular contrast agents. In: Dawson, P., Cosgrove, D.O., and Grainger, R.G. (Eds.), *Textbook of Contrast Media*. Oxford: Isis Medical Media Ltd., p. 355.

Runge, V.M. 2000. Safety of approved MR contrast media for intravenous injection. *J. Magn. Reson. Imaging.* 12:205–213.

Shellock, F.G., and Kanal, E. 1999. Safety of magnetic resonance imaging contrast agents. *J. Magn. Reson. Imaging.* 10:477–484.

Steinbach, L.S., Palmer, W.E., and Schweitzer, M.E. 2002. Special focus session. MR arthrography. *Radiographics* 22:1223–1246.

Tweedle, M.F. 1991. Non-ionic or neutral? *Radiology* 178:891.

Unger, E.C. 1999. Targeted MR contrast agents. In: Dawson, P., Cosgrove, D.O., and Grainger, R.G. (Eds.), *Textbook of Contrast Media*. Oxford: Isis Medical Media Ltd., pp. 379–407.

Yoshikawa, K., and Davies, A. 1997. Safety of ProHance in special population. *Eur. Radiol.* 7:246–250.

10

Molecular Imaging of Cancer with Superparamagnetic Iron-Oxide Nanoparticles

Daniel L. J. Thorek, Julie Czupryna, Antony K. Chen, and Andrew Tsourkas

Introduction

The field of molecular imaging has been defined as the noninvasive, quantitative, and repetitive imaging of biomolecules and biological processes in living organisms. Among its potential uses, molecular imaging strives to allow for more accurate, earlier detection of diseases and hopes to usher in an age of personalized medicine. Magnetic resonance (MR) is a particularly attractive platform for molecular imaging due to the ability of MR instruments to acquire high-resolution anatomical images, merely by relying on inherent differences between tissues and tissue states. It is envisioned that by combining conventional MR imaging with various molecular imaging contrast agents, MR may be used to gather both anatomic and molecular information simultaneously.

Contrast agents are seen as essential to the task of molecular imaging to increase both the sensitivity and specificity of imaging. Garnering great interest for more than a decade, superparamagnetic iron-oxide (SPIO) nanoparticles are spin-spin relaxation (T2) enhancers. Typically they are comprised of an iron-oxide core enveloped in a polysaccharide or synthetic polymer coating. SPIOs are expedient contrast agents thanks to their ease of synthesis, low cost, capacity for

derivatization to targeting molecules, and small size (which contributes both beneficial *in vivo* properties and nanoscale-dependent material properties).

A plethora of molecular imaging applications, both *in vivo* and *in vitro*, has been developed to facilitate the use of SPIO for the purposes of diagnostics. Because much of the literature on the utilization of SPIO is directed towards cancer-related imaging, this chapter will encompass much of the broad range of topics within the field. Following a discussion of their general makeup, physical and chemical properties, along with a brief summary of their synthesis, we will discuss the use of SPIO as both a passive and an active targeting imaging agent. Finally, we will examine several emerging applications for SPIO, including high-throughput screening and activatable contrast schemes.

Terminology

There are many forms of SPIO MR contrast agents in academic and clinical use, to the extent that classification of the different embodiments is necessary in order to dispel any confusion. Categories of SPIO, as defined by their overall hydrated diameter, are noted in the literature as Oral-SPIO at 300 nm to 3.5 μm, Standard-SPIO (SSPIO) at 60–150 nm,

Ultrasmall-SPIO (USPIO) of approximately 5–40 nm, and monocrystalline iron-oxide nanoparticles (MION—a subset of USPIO) ranging from 10 to 30 nm. A prevalent derivatization of MION, consisting of a chemically cross-linked polysaccharide shell, is referred to as CLIO (cross-linked iron oxide). Molecular imaging of cancer will generally require use of the smaller agents. As such, SPIO will be used herein to refer to SSPIO, MION, CLIO, and USPIO, unless otherwise noted.

The trade names given SPIO products are also often confusing. This is because different names are used for the same product, depending on their regional market. Ferumoxsil or AMI-121, an ~ 400 nm Oral-SPIO, is also known as Gastro-MARK (USA) and Lumirem (EU, Brazil). This agent is approved for use in Europe to distinguish between abdominal tissues and the bowels. Larger Oral-SPIO such as OMP (also known as Abdoscan) has a larger hydrated diameter at 3.5 μm. More relevant for the molecular imaging of cancer are the smaller agents; Ferumoxide or AMI-25 (also known as Feridex IV [USA] and Endorem [EU]) are FDA-approved SSPIO for liver imaging and are 80 to 150 nm in diameter. Ferumoxtran or AMI-227 (also known as Sinerem [EU] and Combidex [USA]) are dextran-coated USPIO (of between 20 and 30 nm) currently in late-phase clinical trials for detection of lymph node metastases. Ferucarbotran, Ferrixan, or SHU 555 (Resovist [EU and Japan]), is a carboxydextran coated SPIO of ~ 60 nm hydrodynamic diameter approved for use in Europe. Table 1 presents a concise listing of SPIOs, their alternate names, approval status, and size.

bulk ferromagnetic material, magnetic domains (so-called Weiss domains) are aligned at short range and separated by a transition region called a Bloch wall. At the nanometer scale (~ 14 nm and below), the formation of Bloch walls becomes thermodynamically unfavorable, resulting in single-domain crystals. Magnetite crystals at this scale exhibit strong paramagnetic behavior, lending them the name "superparamagnetic." Unlike ferromagnetic materials, which maintain the induced magnetization after an external field has been removed, paramagnetic and superparamagnetic materials exhibit no such remnant magnetization. Superparamagnetic iron-oxide agents possess large susceptibilities, affect the local magnetic field, and, like most MR contrast agents, the visualization of the agent is through its effect on the surrounding hydrogen nuclei or protons. The large susceptibilities affected by the agent are a result of the alignment of the entire crystal with the applied field.

When SPIO agents are placed in an external magnetic field, their moments align in the direction of the field and enhance the magnetic flux. When the field is removed, no remnant magnetization is carried by the particles, as thermal energy is strong enough to randomize the orientations of the SPIO colloid, keeping the particles from aggregating. In a field, the large magnetic moments lead to rapid dephasing of the surrounding protons. Superparamagnetic iron-oxide agents possess both high T1 and T2 relaxivities. Despite the fact that the majority of imaging and labeling studies investigate the T2-weighted contrast generated by the particles, several examinations have also demonstrated that there exists sufficient spin-lattice (T1) contrast for imaging in this regime.

Iron Oxide Core and Superparamagnetism

The two basic components of SPIO contrast agents are the exterior coating material and the magnetic iron-oxide core. The core is composed of inverse spinel crystal magnetite (Fe_3O_4) and/or maghemite (γFe_2O_3). The two materials have similar crystal structures and magnetic properties, although maghemite does have a lower saturation magnetization.

The magnetic properties of ferromagnetic materials arise from the alignment of unpaired spins of electrons. In a typical

Synthesis and Coating

Superparamagnetic iron oxide agents, with distinct sizes, physical properties, coatings, and distribution profiles, can be produced following a wide variety of production methods. The most commonly applied methods are co-precipitation and microemulsion of nanoscale iron, while lesser utilized techniques include ultrasound irradiation (or sonochemical synthesis), thermal decomposition, layer-by-layer deposition, and spray and laser pyrolysis. Although these latter methods

Table 1 Examples and Properties of Commercial SPIO Agents (Updated from Wang et al. (2001)

Class	Agent	Trade Name	Status	Mean Particle Size
Oral SPIO	AMI-121 (Ferumoxsil)	Lumirem, Gastromark	Approved	> 300 nm
	OMP	Abdoscan	Approved	3.5 μm
SSPIO	AMI-25 (Ferumoxide)	Endorem Feridex	Approved	80–150 nm
	SHU555A (Ferucarbotran or Ferrixan)	Resovist	Phase III complete	62 nm
USPIO	AMI-227 (Ferumoxtran)	Sinerem, Combidex	Phase III	20–40 nm
	NC100150	Clariscan	Phase III	20 nm
	CODE 7228	Advanced Magnetics	Phase II	18–20 nm

can provide finer distributions and sizes of nanoparticles, as well as more complex core/shell structures, they often require advanced equipment and expertise.

In the most widely adopted procedure, co-precipitation, ferric and ferrous salts in solution are precipitated by bringing the mixture to high pH, usually through the addition of concentrated base. The formation of these iron particles can be conducted either in water or in the presence of a surface coating material such as polyethylene glycol (PEG), dextran, or polyvinyl alcohol (PVA). Bare SPIO (those precipitated in the absence of a polymer solution) can subsequently be coated in monomers, silica, or polymers. Production using this technique offers great flexibility and control over the properties of the final product through relatively straightforward chemical means. The advantages of co-precipitation synthesis are somewhat offset by wide SPIO size distributions. Strict size selection, usually by filtration and centrifugation, are subsequently required.

In the microemulsion technique, it is possible to achieve greater control of size and shape of the nanoparticles (Pileni, 1993). Customarily a water-in-oil approach is pursued that sees "nanodroplets" of aqueous iron salts dispersed and coated in a surfactant-organic solution. This agent is then precipitated in these reverse micelles through the addition of an alkaline solution. This method is able to produce populations of particles with very tight distributions. However, a significant trade-off is that iron precipitates below 5 nm have been found to possess amorphous (noncrystalline) iron oxides (Ayyub et al., 1988) and might therefore lack uniform magnetic properties throughout a population of probes. Furthermore, the method generally requires greater knowledge and control over the synthesis conditions in order to generate satisfactory SPIO.

The use of (typically hydrophilic) surface complexing agents is often required to achieve stability and to enhance solubility of the colloid in physiological conditions, a requirement for use of SPIO in biomedical applications. In many cases, microemulsion-produced SPIO agents are not soluble in aqueous solvents, making chemical surface alterations necessary. Another goal of surface complexing agents is to avoid quick opsonization (Mornet et al., 2004). The surface groups are also useful in that they can be derivatized with transfection or targeting agents and can be conjugated to other imaging media, both optical and nuclear. Furthermore, the coating properties are important when considering the biodistribution of the agent. Carbohydrate or polymer-coated SPIO agents typically vary from ~20 to above 100 nm in hydrodynamic diameter (controlled by synthesis parameters such as the iron-to-dextran ratio), with iron-oxide core sizes between ~2 and 15 nm (Shen et al., 1993). The effect of particular coatings on SPIO pharmacokinetics is the fundamental reason behind the wide variety of different materials that have been tested as SPIO exteriors.

Biocompatibility and Biodistribution

The biocompatibility and metabolism of SPIO have been widely investigated since their introduction into the field of medical imaging (Weissleder et al., 1989). Given that iron is an essential element for human beings and is critical for the delivery of oxygen and the proliferation/survival of all cells, it is no surprise that SPIO can enter the body's normal iron metabolism cycle following uptake by the reticuloendothelial system (RES) (Runge, 2000). In fact, SPIO probes were originally developed as a ferritin substitute to treat anemia. The iron contained in SPIO, entering the cell independent of the transferrin pathway, has produced concerns that toxic levels of non-chelated iron may build up. This has the potential to produce radical oxygen species. Studies have shown, however, that the breakdown of magnetite in cells leads to ferric (rather than ferrous) iron release. This iron ion is efficiently chelated by citrate and rendered nontoxic.

Extensive research has been carried out on the impact of SPIO on cell viability and function. A recent study showed, in vitro, that SPIO enters the cell through endocytosis and can then either be released back into the extracellular space or shuttled into low pH environments in lysosomes, where they break down over the course of several days. Immortalized fibroblasts, when incubated with PEG-coated SPIO, showed no discernible changes in cell adhesion behavior or morphology (Gupta et al., 2004), and the same was reported for T-cells labeled with SPIO (Zhao et al., 2001). Transfection agents such as the HIV tat peptide, polyarginine and protamine, as well as many small molecules, have been conjugated or complexed with SPIO in order to achieve greater cellular uptake. The use of these agents alongside SPIO has also been found to have minimal cellular toxicity revealing no significant effects on cell viability (Arbab et al., 2004), clonogenic efficiency, biodistribution, or immunophenotypic changes; for example, macrophages are not activated upon uptake (Phelps, 1991).

While previous studies generally assert the indifferent response of cells to the presence of the probes, further work is required to validate their use in specific applications and the limitations therein. A recent study found no impact of SPIO on mesenchymal stem-cell viability, proliferation, adipogenesis, or osteogenesis; however, chondrogenesis was found to be inhibited in a dose-dependent manner (Bulte et al., 2004).

Upon intravenous administration of SPIO, anaphylactic-like reactions and hypotension have been noted. Adverse events from SPIO are, however, usually mild and short in duration (Anzai et al., 2003). The most common complaints included headache, back pain, vasodilation, and hives. Once introduced, the pharmacokinetics of each embodiment of SPIO is dependent primarily on the size and surface characteristics of the agent. The spleen and liver are able to screen SPIO that are ~ 200 nm or above, mainly through mechanical filtration. SPIO probes below ~ 10 nm are removed through extravasation and renal clearance. Agents with a diameter in the region of 30–50 nm have demonstrated longer plasma half-life, especially when coated in amphiphilic polymers including dextran, PEG, or PVA. In the case of targeted SPIO agents, longer circulation time can be equated with an enhanced probability of the probe binding its ligand. This is also true for nontargeted applications that seek to avert quick clearance by the liver and spleen. It should also be noted that large particle size may prevent effective extravasation and reduce diffusion of the agent through the interstitium; this is an important consideration for many SPIO imaging objectives such as lymph node imaging. This is generally less of a concern for the imaging of the vascular endothelium or tumor sites possessing leaky vasculature, where particles have routine access and tend to accumulate naturally.

Cell Tracking

Cells of any particular type may be loaded with nanoparticles *ex vivo* and have their movements (both initial distribution and secondary migration) followed once planted *in vivo*. The ability to track cells post-implantation is considered valuable in many fields, including cancer therapies involving, among others, dendritic cells, stem cells, T-lymphocytes, and natural killer (NK) cells.

Dendritic cells are able to stimulate or inhibit immune responses. The important role this phenotype plays in marshaling the body's defenses has made it attractive as a means to augment the native immune response against malignant cells. A reputed problem with this therapeutic approach has been that the cells do not always localize or migrate to target organs as desired. It is envisioned that *in vivo* imaging of dendritic cell migration may substantially aid in the design and administration of dendritic cell-based therapy. Initial studies have already shown that when dendritic cells, intended as a cancer vaccine for melanoma, were loaded with SSPIO via phagocytosis there was no unfavorable effect on phenotype, migration patterns, or antigen-presenting functions (de Vries *et al.*, 2005). Moreover, this study displayed the utility of tracking as few as 1.5×10^5 cells simultaneously with the high anatomical resolution normally provided via MR imaging.

Similar to dendritic cells, T-lymphocytes have been used to treat and image several classes of malignancies. However, unlike the phagocytic immature dendritic cell, delivery strategies must be employed in order to label the T-lymphocytes with SPIO. This can be accomplished in several ways including electroporation, lipofection agents, and cell-permeating peptides (CPP). Peptides such as HIV tat, protamine, and polyarginine have been used to greatly enhance cellular

uptake, allowing for greater loading of SPIO in cells. For example, the iron concentration per mesenchymal cell rose from undetectable (with unlabeled SSPIO) to 10 pg/cell using protamine-labeled SSPIO (Arbab *et al.*, 2004). CLIO-HD, a tat-conjugated SPIO with high T-lymphocyte uptake, has been used in a system where CD8+ T-cells were able to specifically target an antigen-expressing tumor on which it could be clearly delineated by MR imaging. Furthermore, T-lymphocytes labeled with CLIO-HD did not lose their ability to kill cells both *in vitro* and *in vivo*.

NK cells also hold promise for cell-based therapies as they exhibit high cytotoxic activity on multiple malignancy types, while sparing normal cells. A novel molecular imaging study used SPIO carried in a genetically modified NK-92 cell line, NK-92-scFv(FRP5)-ζ, which was directed against malignant cells overexpressing HER2/neu (a receptor found overexpressed in many human cancers, notably breast cancer). In this study, the MR monitoring of lipofected NK cells with SSPIO led to distinct and long-lasting recognition of HER2/neu-positive NIH 3T3 mammary tumors in mice (Daldrup-Link *et al.*, 2005). Persistent labeling and detection by MR was evident for at least 5 days.

Finally, stem cells have received enormous attention for their potential use as therapeutics. Stem cells possess the ability to both maintain themselves in an undifferentiated state and to differentiate into any mature cell type. Tracking of these cells using MR could help refine administration of this therapy, as it would be possible to monitor cellular distribution to specific organs and disease sites. SPIO labeling has already helped elucidate some of the difficulties inherent in stem-cell homing following intravenous injection (Bos *et al.*, 2004). Significant work has also been done on tracking the cerebral distribution of cells administered for ischemic therapy and in glioma models. As mentioned earlier, the impact, if any, of the presence of SPIO on stem-cell function and the ability to differentiate is currently under contention (Bulte *et al.*, 2004).

Organ-Specific/Passive Targeting

In many instances in both the literature and clinical practice, SPIO probes *without* targeting moieties have been used to image cancerous lesions. The mechanisms by which the particles are differentially situated include nontargeted cellular uptake, enhanced retention in leaky tumor vasculature, and accumulation in the reticuloendothelial system (RES). The local accumulation of SPIO is a critical factor in enhancing the T2 relaxation effect; thus, intracellular accumulation, typically through endocytosis, is critical for contrast enhancement of nontargeted SPIO. However, without an affinity ligand conjugated to the nanoparticle, the pharmacokinetics of the SPIO are the primary means with which differential distribution of the nanoparticles can occur. The hydrodynamic radius and the surface charge of the coating are factors that weigh heavily on the distribution of the contrast agent, altering the circulation time and opsonization, tissue accessibility, penetration of the capillary endothelium, and cell-type uptake. Imaging of a tumor requires that nanoparticle uptake between it and the surrounding bodily structure differ. This requires one of two strategies to generate contrast. In the first, nanoparticles locally accumulate at the site of a growth. The leaky vasculature of tumors and macrophage uptake at a cancerous lesion are the main contributors to this type of contrast enhancement. In the inverse case, contrast is generated because SPIO agents do not accumulate at tumor sites, thereby indicating the presence of a malignancy. This inverse contrast enhancement is often seen in the liver, bone metastasis, and lymph nodes.

Liver and Splenic Imaging

Imaging of the liver is a principal application of SPIO. Larger nanoparticles (~ 150 nm hydrodynamic radius) such as the dextran-coated SSPIO AMI-25 nonspecifically accumulate in Kupffer cells in the liver. Kupffer cells are members of the RES whose primary function is to recycle and accumulate iron from red blood cells that are no longer functional. The absence of normally functioning Kupffer cells in malignancies has been exploited to allow for enhanced accuracy in distinguishing between healthy and diseased tissue in T2-weighted images. This is a significant improvement over conventional non–contrast-enhanced imaging of hepatic tumors. It has been reported that non–contrast-agent enhanced imaging is limited to detection of lesions greater than 3 cm; however, MR imaging of 1 cm growths is possible with SPIO-enhanced contrast (Ward *et al.*, 2003).

The half-life of SPIO in the liver is typically < 3 days, and the amount administered is typically 8–15 μmol Fe/kg (Karabulut and Elmas, 2006), < 2% of the physiological iron stores (Bach-Gansmo, 1993). Upon administration, 80% of the SSPIO are sequestered by the liver and 10% by the spleen (Wang *et al.*, 2001). The SSPIO-enhanced MR imaging has shown the ability to distinguish between benign and malignant lesions with a sensitivity and accuracy for metastatic lesion detection > 90% (Bach-Gansmo *et al.*, 1993). Furthermore, MR of carboxydextran-coated SPIO can provide dynamic information on the vascularity of solid lesions. Admission or exclusion of SPIO to liver metastases and the characteristics of accumulation allow for T1-weighted insight into lesion classification (Reimer and Balzer, 2003).

Lymph Node Imaging

Smaller nanoparticles (< 50 nm) coated in amphiphilic substances such as dextran have longer half-lives and greater vascular persistence. This allows for broadening of SPIO distribution into lymph nodes and bone marrow via extravasation. The leakage of blood and SPIO into the interstitial space and subsequent transport to the lymph nodes via the lymphatic vessels allow for exquisite lymph node imaging. Systemically injected particles gain access to the interstitium and are drained through the lymphatic vessels, where the particles accumulate. The absence of SPIO in the nodes correlates with disturbances in node flow or architecture due to the presence of metastases, lending accuracy to the diagnosis of node metastases. For example, the sensitivity of MR increased (on a patient-by-patient basis) from 45.4 to 100%, with a sensitivity of 95.7% (Harisinghani *et al.*, 2006).

Bone Imaging

The contrast between bone marrow and metastasis was improved following injection of USPIO in a tibial metastasis rabbit cancer model (Seneterre *et al.*, 1991). Again, enhanced detection of malignancies is through the accumulation of USPIO in surrounding healthy tissue. Blood pooling of USPIO and phagocytic uptake of particles by bone marrow lead to a concomitant selective decrease in bone marrow intensity with T2-weighted imaging. Distinction between bone metastasis and marrow inflammation using SPIO can also reduce misdiagnosis. Similar results were obtained when testing larger diameter SSPIO (80–150 nm) (Vande Berg *et al.*, 1999).

Macrophage Imaging

Cellular accumulation of SPIO through phagocytic internalization allows for the MR imaging of inflammatory and degenerative disorders associated with high-macrophage and monocyte activity. Preferential uptake of SPIO by macrophage is likely borne through the scavenger function of this cell type; however, their surfaces contain a dextran receptor that may lend a degree of molecular sensitivity to dextran-coated SPIO for macrophage imaging. Regions of upregulated macrophage activity include sites of atherosclerotic plaque and transplant rejection as well as at the periphery and within tumors. The definition provided at tumor margins by USPIO-labeled macrophages (Enochs *et al.*, 1999) highlights the potential of SPIO for use in preoperative planning.

Brain Imaging

The role of macrophages in pathological tissue alterations also provides an opportunity for SPIO imaging in the central nervous system (CNS). Diverse examples from the imaging of strokes, multiple sclerosis, brain tumors, and carotid atherosclerotic plaques foreshadow more robust CNS imaging in the future. The blood-brain barrier (BBB) is a considerable hindrance to particulate accessibility. Accordingly, only low levels of MION dosage are found in the brain 24 hr post-administration (as little as 0.2% [Zimmer *et al.*, 1995]). However, this has been found sufficient for many imaging applications.

Degradation of the BBB in several neuropathologies does provide greater SPIO admission to the brain. Prolonged delineation of brain tumors has been demonstrated in such cases, whereby USPIO is localized through extravasation at the tumor site and surrounding cell uptake. In other diseases such as neuroinflammatory afflictions, the macrophage uptake of SPIO can even be used as a metric of disease progression. Under nonpathological conditions (unaccompanied by BBB degradation), it has been possible to image brain tissues using amino-polyvinly alcohol (PVA)-coated SPIO (30 nm) through uptake by cerebral cells (Cengelli *et al.*, 2006). This is significant due to the highly compartmentalized nature of the brain, which makes delivery of imaging and therapeutic agents difficult. Derivatized PVA-SPIO could be used in the future to deliver these agents to remote brain structures.

Active Targeting

Passive targeting relies on exploitation of natural pharmacokinetic and phagocytic mechanisms to localize and accumulate SPIO particulates. Although this is sufficient for some applications, active targeting provides a means to image the presence and localization of an immense library of biomedically relevant molecules. Information on the location and expression level of various molecular markers could allow for the early detection of a disease as well as more accurate pathological staging. Molecularly specific targeting of SPIO requires that the probes be functionalized with relevant biomolecules. This is usually accomplished through mild chemical conjugation strategies that attach chemical linkers to the surface coatings of the SPIO. The choice between different conjugation routes usually depends on the reactive moieties present on the surface coating as well as those present on the biomolecule of interest. Numerous studies have already demonstrated the ability to reveal early markers of cancer through MR by actively targeting SPIO.

Several different imaging approaches can be used to actively image cancer. For tumor site imaging, sufficient accumulation of SPIO generally requires that the ligands of interest be overexpressed. The most widely established approach is to bind SPIO to markers either specifically expressed or highly overexpressed on cancerous cells such as transferrin, folate, and uMuc-1. This provides for a high degree of specificity when appropriate ligands and targeting molecules are selected. While cancerous cells, themselves are often the objects of interest, other cells and cell states, such as apoptotic cells, can also provide important information about the tumor. Alternatively,

healthy cells can be selectively labeled, thereby inversely revealing cancerous cells.

Because of the intrinsically low signal of SPIO-enhanced MR imaging (as one forms contrast through a loss of signal), augmented SPIO accumulation with the purpose of achieving greater contrast within or on the surface of cells is often necessary. One commonly used approach to amplify the SPIO signal involves specifically targeting rapidly internalizing receptors. An internalizing receptor is a preferred target because following SPIO internalization the receptor can be recycled to the cell surface and used to internalize additional SPIO. Therefore, a single receptor can effectively be used to localize a large number of SPIO agents to the target site. Another approach borrowed from positron emission tomography (PET) studies is known as prelabeling and uses staggered injection of two populations of probes. The first probe targets a specific ligand, while the second (i.e., SPIO) only has an affinity for the first, not for any endogenous marker. This approach allows for improved contrast because the initial targeting agent typically possesses several high-affinity sites for the SPIO probe, effectively allowing multiple SPIO to bind each cell ligand. The aggregation of SPIO on the cell surface and intracellular accumulation have both been extensively validated.

Targeting Cancer Cell-Specific Ligands

There are many clinically relevant cancer cell-specific targets, and the list continues to expand. In order to develop the most likely successful imaging agents, this section details pertinent targets that have been validated as being overexpressed in cancers, *with low background signal in the body*. The transferrin receptor is one such example. The transferrin-receptor is overexpressed on a variety of cancer cell types, most notably breast cancer, as well as in glioblastomas. Transferrin is an abundant plasma protein required for intracellular iron ion delivery. Cells with accelerated metabolisms, particularly those that undergo rapid division, have been identified as having upregulated transferrin receptors due to their need for additional resources. Cancer cells, particularly from highly malignant lesions, have long been known to possess this aberration. SPIO conjugated to transferrin accumulate intracellularly following transferrin-receptor mediated endocytosis (Hogemann *et al.*, 2000). One study revealed a 40% decrease in tumor signal intensity when transferrin-USPIO was injected into rats bearing a mammary carcinoma, compared with only a 10% decrease with unlabeled USPIO (Kresse *et al.*, 1998).

Another well-studied target for cancer imaging is the folate receptor. This receptor is usually exposed at low levels on epithelia, but is overexpressed on many rapidly dividing cancer cells because folate is required for the production of new cells. Using a parallel approach to the transferrin work,

USPIO conjugated to folate experienced rapid and efficient uptake by tumor cells overexpressing the folate receptor (Antony, 1996). *In vivo* MR imaging revealed an average T2 intensity decrease of 38% with USPIO-folate, compared to precontrast images of a folate receptor expressing tumor (Choi *et al.*, 2004). Another clinically relevant, overexpressed target is the Her-2/neu tyrosine kinase receptor. This well-researched marker is found in human mammary luminal epithelial cells with very strong implications for breast cancer development, to the point of its being used as a progression metric. The breast cancer drug Herceptin functions by targeting this receptor. Thus, SPIO-herceptin is able to localize to the Her-2/neu receptor (Artemov *et al.*, 2003) and provides detailed imaging of difficult-to-detect growths.

Nonreceptor ligands have also been imaged. Underglycosylated MUC-1 tumor antigen (uMUC-1), a ligand found in numerous epithelial cell adenocarcinomas, 90% of all breast cancers, and a majority of pancreatic, colorectal, lung, prostate, and gastric cancers, has been targeted. Here an affinity peptide, EPPT1, for the antigen was bound to CLIO and successfully targeted to uMUC-1 expressing tumors in mice (Moore *et al.*, 2004).

Polyethylene glycol-coated SPIO conjugated to chlorotoxin (a scorpion-derived neurotoxin known to target gliomas) exhibited increased uptake in glioma cells and may prove to be an effective method to image brain tumors (Veiseh *et al.*, 2005). There is a growing library of other ligands that may be of interest to MR detection via the facile conjugation to SPIO. In some cases, little knowledge of the ligand itself is required; for example, an antibody bound SSPIO was able to bind an unknown ligand expressed in colorectal cancers (Toma *et al.*, 2005).

Targeting Healthy Cells

Using the inverse strategy to that of localizing nanoparticles to cancerous cells, SPIO accumulation specifically in healthy cells allows for malignant cells to appear in positive contrast in T2-weighted imaging. This is a similar strategy as that pursued in the passive imaging of tumor lesions using SPIO. In one example, tumors in the pancreas were effectively visualized by targeting CholecystokininA (CCKA) receptors that are expressed only on healthy acinar cells. When SPIO was labeled with CCK, a hormone produced by the small intestine that binds to CCKA-receptors, it generated a significant reduction in T2 relaxation of healthy pancreatic tissues, leading to the clear delineation of pancreatic tumors (Reimer *et al.*, 1994). More recently, malignancies in the pancreas have been detected through targeting of the bombesin (BN) receptor. Bombesin receptors are absent in human pancreatic ductal adenocarcinomas (PDAC). CLIO-BN were found to accumulate strictly in healthy pancreatic tissues, developing sufficient contrast between cancerous and healthy tissues (Montet *et al.*, 2006). The results showed

reduced T2-signal of the normal pancreas and enhanced the visualization of an implanted tumor in rats.

The ability to identify lesions in the liver has also been investigated by targeting healthy cells. Storage of glycogen is a critical function performed by the liver, and it has been noted that asialoglycoprotein (ASG) receptors are absent on cells in primary malignant or metastatic hepatic tumors. To image these growths, arabinogalactan (a polysaccharide ligand of ASG) conjugated MION was developed. Enhanced tumor-liver contrast was seen in rats (Reimer *et al.*, 1994) as the particles were only taken up by normally functioning hepatocytes.

Apoptosis

Apoptosis, or programmed cell death, plays an important role in the pathology of cancer, neurodegeneration, acute myocardial infarction, and chronic inflammation. It has been suggested that the ability to image apoptosis could provide insight into cancer progression/regression and can thus be used to determine the efficacy of different treatment options. As many cancer therapies act by inducing apoptosis, namely, chemotherapeutics, adequate imaging of apoptosis is highly desirable to evaluate the success of any prescribed regimens. By targeting SPIO to apoptotic cells, high spatial resolution imaging by MR can map tumor regression and treatment success as well as offer insight into other disease trajectories.

One method of targeting apoptotic cells involves the conjugation of the first C_2 domain of synaptotagmin I to SPIO (Zhao *et al.*, 2001). This domain binds phosphatidylserine (PS), a lipid that is known to redistribute from the inner to the outer leaflet of the plasma membrane early in apoptosis, following phosphorylation. After induction of apoptosis in EL4 and CHO-K1 cells, it was demonstrated that SPIO-C_2 could mark these dying cells. *In vivo* work demonstrated SPIO-C_2 enabled specific detection of apoptotic cells. Recently, a similar approach was taken by conjugating Annexin V (AnxV) to CLIO to target apoptotic cells (Schellenberger *et al.*, 2004a). AnxV is also known to bind exposed PS. The CLIO-AnxV added to a mixture of healthy and apoptotic Jurkat T-cells allowed for magnetic separation of healthy and apoptotic cells *in vitro*. Most recently, Zn(II) di-2-picolylamine (DPA) complexed to CLIO was shown to bind to phosphorylated-PS (Quinti *et al.*, 2006). This is significant because multiple DPAs are able to bind a single PS molecule on the surface of a cell undergoing apoptosis, thereby increasing the signal that may be generated as a result of the site-specific agglomeration of nanoparticles.

Magnetic Relaxation Switches

A unique magnetic property of SPIO is the dramatic reduction in the T2-relaxation time that is observed upon nanoparticle self-assembly. The physical explanation of the process centers around the iron-oxide cores of the SPIO probes working in a cooperative fashion when complexed together, thereby more efficiently dephasing surrounding nuclei. This effect manifests itself as a decrease of signal over the bulk signal. The term *magnetic relaxation switches* (MRS) refers to the switching between high or low T2-signal following SPIO self-assembly (or disassembly) as provoked by some molecular interaction. The self-assembly of SPIO, and in some cases their dissociation, has already been used to indicate the activity, presence, or absence of a wide variety of target biomolecules. Ligands that have been used to trigger SPIO self-assembly (or disassembly) include oligonucleotides (ON), enzymes, proteins, and enantiomers. A unique advantage of MRS over many alternative detection technologies is that changes in T2 can easily be measured in turbid media, whole-cell lysates, and potentially *in vivo*. The extension of MRS *in vivo* could provide an efficient, highly sensitive, and extremely multifarious targeting diagnostic agent.

Oligonucleotide Detection

One of the first applications utilizing the MRS scheme was for the detection of nucleic acid targets. To produce the MRS effect, close proximity of SPIO is needed. This required two populations of SPIO-ON probes to be synthesized, the sequences for each designed so that they hybridized to adjacent sites on the target nucleic acid (Josephson *et al.*, 2001). In these studies, a reduction in T2 was used to indicate the presence of a complementary target strand as SPIO-ON were forced into close proximity upon hybridization. In the case of addition of a noncomplementary ON target, no MRS was observed. The changes in signal occurred rapidly and were reversible upon melting the double-stranded nucleic acid complexes through temperature cycling. A lower detection limit of < 500 attomoles, the small sample requirements, and detection of signal changes within minutes render this assay appealing for a variety of diagnostic and biological applications. For example, in one application MRS was used in a high-throughput scheme to detect telomerase activity, which has been correlated to the genetic instability of a cell, in various cell-line lysates. Specifically, CLIO-ON assemblies were directed to hybridize to 30-bp target telomeric sequence repeats (TTAGGG) as a means of detecting telomerase activity at very low levels, without the use of PCR amplification (Grimm *et al.*, 2004). Bound CLIO probes were arranged linearly along the repeats. Detection was possible using as little as 10–100 attomoles of telomerase-synthesized DNA. This astounding lower detection limit is most likely due to the presence of multiple adjacent binding sites within the telomere, creating a multi-SPIO aggregate, augmenting the MRS effect.

In addition to detecting nucleic acid hybridization, MRS has also been used to monitor the efficacy of DNA cleaving (restriction) enzymes. Here, the reverse switch was detected—that of an increase in T2 signal upon the severance of CLIO-ON assemblies from target nucleic acids (Perez *et al.*, 2002). It was found that T2-signal rises to pre-target-hybridization levels when the assemblies are cleaved. Furthermore, it was shown that the methylation status of the target ON can play a role in restriction endonuclease function, as indicated by differential signal intensity change after the switch.

Protein Interactions and Molecular Detection

The MRS technique has also been used to detect proteins (Sun *et al.*, 2006a). One novel application used virus-surface-specific antibody-CLIO to detect low levels of virus particles in solution (Perez *et al.*, 2003). Similar to the detection of nucleic acids, assemblies of functionalized SPIO form in the presence of a protein target. A demonstration of the utility of this technique involved the sensitive and rapid detection of herpes simplex virus and adenovirus in a small volume (Perez *et al.*, 2003). CLIO-antibody conjugates against each virus allowed for specific detection of each target virus, respectively. As few as 5 viral particles in a volume of 10 uL (in 25% protein solution) could be detected, and no change in T2 was recorded when the off-target virus was used.

Another application of MRS with possible pharmacologic impact is the detection of enantiomeric impurities (Tsourkas *et al.*, 2004). D- and L-enantiomers of pharmaceuticals can sometimes induce drastically different effects *in vivo*, and thus the high-throughput detection of impurities in a stock solution is often required. In a proof-of-concept study, antibodies against D-Phe (i.e., the impurity) were used to trigger self-assembly and to cause a T2-drop in solutions containing SPIO-D-Phe, owing to the bivalent nature or antibodies. Subsequently, samples of L-Phe with various levels of D-Phe impurities were added to the SPIO sample in very low amounts. The presence of D-Phe impurities in the racemic mixture caused an increase in the T2 time. It was found that D-Phe enantiomeric impurities could be detected even in the presence of enantiomeric excesses of 99.998%.

Although MRS has not yet been used for *in vivo* applications, one potential application is in the detection of myeloperoxidase (MPO) activity. Myeloperoxidase is an enzyme associated with atherosclerosis and inflammation. In a recent study it was found that SPIO-serotonin could be used to detect MPO, where serotonin cross-linking resulted in a decrease in the T2-signal in a concentration-dependent manner. Cross-linking of the conjugate nanoparticles was specific to the enzyme, as detected by a clinical 1.5T scanner (Perez *et al.*, 2004). It should be noted that while MRS holds great promise for *in vivo* applications, a significant hindrance to the use of these techniques in living subjects is the possibility of the nonspecific aggregation of probes. Any accumulation of SPIO that is not the result of target binding may relay a false decrease in signal. Therefore, precautions must be taken when making conclusions from these types of experiments.

Imaging of Gene Expression

The ability to noninvasively monitor the expression of a transgene used in gene therapy (*in vivo*) would be of significant academic and clinical utility. Visualization can be accomplished through the coupling of a transgene to a reporter (in the optical modality, for example, green fluorescent protein). A myriad of approaches, using several different modalities (nuclear and optical), to image transgene expression have been put forward. However, the use of MR is unique in that it offers both high spatial and anatomical resolution and ease of use in an *in vivo* setting. It has been demonstrated that constitutive active overexpression of an engineered human transferrin receptor (hTfR) leads to accumulation of transferrin functionalized MION (MION-Tf) within cells. The receptor-mediated uptake of MION-Tf was specific and produced signal intensity changes that could be detected by MR imaging (Moore *et al.*, 1998). *In vivo*, transgene expression was visualized noninvasively, potentially validating engineered hTfR as a universal MR marker, which in conjunction with SPIO, allows for monitoring of gene therapy (Weissleder *et al.*, 2000). Further studies have shown that multiple transgenes from a single gene therapy vector can be correlated and monitored using the SPIO-engineered hTfR reporter system (Ichikawa *et al.*, 2002), making this an attractive means to measure gene transfer both *in vivo* and *in vitro*.

High-Throughput Screening

The nanoscale nature of SPIO makes it amenable to high-throughput strategies for determining appropriate targeting moieties. The attachment of antibodies and other large targeting proteins and biomolecules does provide more than adequate homing capabilities to the probes, but includes the drawbacks of decreased SPIO mobility (because of large protein size), specialized chemical conjugation strategies, and the need for extensive molecular biology work to isolate low-yield proteins. The generation of libraries of multivalent surface-modified CLIO and generalized conjugation strategies (Sun *et al.*, 2006b) will increase both the speed at which new targeting molecules are found and the rate of development of novel SPIO contrast agents. This model was validated when a small molecule screen conjugated to CLIO was able to reveal a macrophage-specific targeting molecule. Here, a

wide range of molecules were bound to CLIO through the use of six generalized conjugation strategies (Sun *et al.*, 2006a). The surface modified nanoparticles were subsequently incubated over U937 macrophages, and uptake was determined by fluorescence. In an extension of the above work, a combined peptide and small-molecule functionalized CLIO screen over apoptotic cells was used to produce a novel CLIO-based apoptotic sensor (Schellenberger *et al.*, 2004b). In the near future, the use of small-molecule and peptide/phage library scanning will greatly expand the number of biomarkers that is discovered by and for SPIO.

In conclusion, both in academic development and current practice, SPIO continues to sit on the cutting edge, balanced in the interdisciplinary space between nanotechnology, biology, and molecular medicine. Applications as diverse as cell tracking, gene detection, and enzymatic reactions are being observed through MR imaging of SPIO probes. As the techniques and probes themselves continue to mature, it is hoped that some of the limitations inherent in MR imaging, such as low sensitivity and long imaging times, can be overcome. Site-directed imaging by both active and passive targeting mechanisms has been shown to be a powerful tool for *in vitro* and *in vivo* imaging. Impressively, despite the wide number of markers and diverse applications that SPIOs have been directed against, the depth of the field will only increase as the library of molecules and pathways of interest continue to expand. Superparamagnetic iron oxide for use in molecular imaging has considerable future use for the study of the etiology, prevention, diagnosis, pathogenesis, and treatment of cancer.

References

Antony, A.C. 1996. Folate receptors. *Annu. Rev. Nutr. 16*:501–521.

Anzai, Y., Piccoli, C.W., Outwater, E.K., Stanford, W., Bluemke, D.A., Nurenberg, P., Saini, S., Maravilla, K.R., Feldman, D.E., Schmiedl, U.P., Brunberg, J.A., Francis, I.R., Harms, S.E., Som, P.M., and Tempany, C.M. 2003. Evaluation of neck and body metastases to nodes with ferumoxtran 10-enhanced MR imaging: Phase III safety and efficacy study. *Radiol. 228*:777–788.

Arbab, A.S., Yocum, G.T., Kalish, H., Jordan, E.K., Anderson, S.A., Khakoo, A.Y., Read, E.J., and Frank, J.A. 2004. Efficient magnetic cell labeling with protamine sulfate complexed to ferumoxides for cellular MRI. *Blood 104*:1217–1223.

Artemov, D., Mori, N., Okollie, B., and Bhujwalla, Z.M. 2003. MR molecular imaging of the her-2/neu receptor in breast cancer cells using targeted iron oxide nanoparticles. *Magn. Reson. Med. 49*:403–408.

Ayyub, P., Multani, M., Barma, M., Palkar, V.R., and Vijayaraghavan, R. 1988. Size-induced structural phase-transitions and hyperfine properties of microcrystalline Fe2O3. *J. Phys. C-Solid State Phys. 21*:2229–2245.

Bach-Gansmo, T. 1993. Ferrimagnetic susceptibility contrast agents. *Acta Radiol. Suppl. 387*:1–30.

Bach-Gansmo, T., Dupas, B., Gayet-Delacroix, M., and Lambrechts, M. 1993. Abdominal MRI using a negative contrast agent. *Br. J. Radiol. 66*:420–425.

Bos, C., Delmas, Y., Desmouliere, A., Solanilla, A., Hauger, O., Grosset, C., Dubus, I., Ivanovic, Z., Rosenbaum, J., Charbord, P., Combe, C., Bulte, J.W.M., Moonen, C.T.W., Ripoche, J., and Grenier, N. 2004. *In vivo* MR imaging of intravascularly injected magnetically labeled mesenchymal stem cells in rat kidney and liver. *Radiol. 233*:781–789.

Bulte, J.W.M., Kraitchman, D.L., Mackay, A.M., Pittenger, M.F., Arbab, A.S., Yocum, G.T., Kalish, H., Jordan, E.K., Anderson, S.A., Khakoo, A.Y., Read, E.J., and Frank, J.A. 2004. Chondrogenic differentiation of mesenchymal stem cells is inhibited after magnetic labeling with ferumoxides. *Blood 104*:3410–3413.

Cengelli, F., Maysinger, D., Tschudi-Monnet, F., Montet, X., Corot, C., Petri-Fink, A., Hofmann, H., and Juillerat-Jeanneret, L. 2006. Interaction of functionalized superparamagnetic iron oxide nanoparticles with brain structures. *J. Pharmacol. Exp. Ther. 318*:108–116.

Choi, H., Choi, S.R., Zhou, R., Kung, H.F., and Chen, I.W. 2004. Iron oxide nanoparticles as magnetic resonance contrast agent for tumor imaging via folate receptor-targeted delivery. *Acad. Radiol. 11*:996–1004.

Daldrup-Link, H.E., Meier, R., Rudeliu, M., Piotek, G., Piert, M., Metz, S., Settles, M., Uherek, C., Wels, W., Schlegel, J., and Rummeny, E.J., 2005. *In vivo* tracking of genetically engineered, anti-HER2/neu directed natural killer cells to HER2/neu positive mammary tumors with magnetic resonance imaging. *Eur. Radiol. 15*:4–13.

de Vries, I.J., Lesterhuis, W.J., Barentsz, J.O., Verdijk, P., van Krieken, J.H., Boerman, O.C., Oyen, W.J., Bonenkamp, J.J., Boezeman, J.B., Adema, G.J., Bulte, J.W., Scheenen, T.W., Punt, C.J., Heerschap, A., and Figdor, C.G. 2005. Magnetic resonance tracking of dendritic cells in melanoma patients for monitoring of cellular therapy. *Nat. Biotech. 23*:1407–1413.

Enochs, W.S., Harsh, G., Hochberg, F., and Weissleder, R. 1999. Improved delineation of human brain tumors on MR images using a long-circulating, superparamagnetic iron oxide agent. *J. Magn. Reson. Imag. 9*:228–232.

Grimm, J., Perez, J.M., Josephson, L., and Weissleder, R. 2004. Novel nanosensors for rapid analysis of telomerase activity. *Cancer. Res. 64*:639–643.

Gupta, A.K., and Curtis, A.S. 2004. Surface modified superparamagnetic nanoparticles for drug delivery: interaction studies with human fibroblasts in culture. *J. Mater. Sci. Mater. Med. 15*:493–496.

Harisinghani, M.G., Saksena, M.A., Hahn, P.F., King, B., Kim, J., Torabi, M.T., and Weissleder, R. 2006. Ferumoxtran-10-enhanced MR lymphangiography: does contrast-enhanced imaging alone suffice for accurate lymph node characterization? *Am. J. Roentgenol. 186*:144–148.

Hogemann, D., Josephson, L., Weissleder, R., and Basilion, J.P. 2000. Improvement of MRI probes to allow efficient detection of gene expression. *Bioconj. Chem. 11*:941–946.

Ichikawa, T., Hogemann, D., Saeki, Y., Tyminski, E., Terada, K., Weissleder, R., Chiocca, E.A., and Basilion, J.P. 2002. MRI of transgene expression: correlation to therapeutic gene expression. *Neoplasia 4*:523–530.

Josephson, L., Perez, J.M., and Weissleder, R. 2001. Magnetic nanosensors for the detection of oligonucleotide sequences. *Angew. Chem.-Int. Ed. 40*:3204–3206.

Karabulut, N., and Elmas, N. 2006. Contrast agents used in MR imaging of the liver. *Diagn. Interv. Radiol. 12*:22–30.

Kresse, M., Wagner, S., Pfefferer, D., Lawaczeck, R., Elste, V., and Semmler W. 1998. Targeting of ultrasmall superparamagnetic iron oxide (USPIO) particles to tumor cells in vivo by using transferrin receptor pathways. *Magn. Reson. Med. 40*:236–242.

Montet, X., Weissleder, R., and Josephson, L. 2006. Imaging pancreatic cancer with a peptide-nanoparticle conjugate targeted to normal pancreas. *Bioconj. Chem. 17*:905–911.

Moore, A., Basilion, J., Chiocca, E.A., and Weissleder, R. 1998. Measuring transferrin receptor gene expression by NMR imaging. *Biochim. et Biophys. Acta 1402*:239–249.

Moore, A., Medarova, Z., Potthast, A., and Dai, G. 2004. *In vivo* targeting of underglycosylated MUC-1 tumor antigen using a multimodal imaging probe. *Cancer Res. 64*:1821–1827.

Mornet, S., Vasseur, S., Grasset, F., and Duguet, E. 2004. Magnetic nanoparticles design for medical diagnosis and therapy. *Bioconj. Chem. 14*:2161–2175.

Perez, J.M., O'Loughin, T., Simeone, F.J., Weissleder, R., and Josephson, L. 2002. DNA-based magnetic nanoparticle assembly acts as a magnetic relaxation nanoswitch allowing screening of DNA-cleaving agents. *J. Am. Chem. Soc. 124*:2856–2857.

Perez, J.M., Simeone, F.J., Saeki, Y., Josephson, L., and Weissleder, R. 2003. Viral-induced self-assembly of magnetic nanoparticles allows the detection of viral particles in biological media. *J. Am. Chem. Soc. 125*:10192–10193.

Perez, J.M., Simeone, F.J., Tsourkas, A., Josephson, L., and Weissleder, R. 2004. Peroxidase substrate nanosensors for MR imaging. *Nano Lett. 4*:119–122.

Phelps, M.E. 1991. PET: a biological imaging technique. *Neurochem. Res. 16*:929–940.

Pileni, M.P. 1993. Reverse micelles as microreactors. *J. Phys. Chem. 97*:6961–6973.

Quinti, L., Weissleder, R., and Tung, C.-H. 2006. A fluorescent nanosensor for apoptotic cells. *Nano Lett. 6*:488–490.

Reimer, P., and Balzer, T. 2003. Ferucarbotran (resovist): a new clinically approved RES-specific contrast agent for contrast-enhanced MRI of the liver: properties, clinical development, and applications. *Eur. Radiol. 13*:1266–1276.

Reimer, P., Weissleder, R., Shen, T., Knoefel, W.T., and Brady, T.J. 1994. Pancreatic receptors: initial feasibility studies with a targeted contrast agent for MR imaging. *Radiol. 193*:527–531.

Runge, V.M. 2000. Safety of approved MR contrast media for intravenous injection. *J. Magn. Reson. Imag. 12*:205–213.

Schellenberger, E.A., Sosnovik, D., Weissleder, R., and Josephson, L. 2004a. Magneto/optical annexin V, a multimodal protein. *Bioconj. Chem. 15*:1062–10167.

Schellenberger, E.A., Reynolds, F., Weissleder, R., and Josephson, L. 2004b. Surface-functionalized nanoparticle library yields probes for apoptotic cells. *ChemBioChem. 5*:275–279.

Seneterre, E., Weissleder, R., Jaramillo, D., Reimer, P., Lee, A.S., Brady, T.J., and Wittenberg, J. 1991. Bone marrow: ultrasmall superparamagnetic iron oxide for MR imaging. *Radiol. 179*:529–533.

Shen, T., Weissleder, R., Papisov, M., Bogdanov, A., and Brady, T.J. 1993. Monocrystalline iron-oxide nanocompounds (MION): physiochemical properties. *Magn. Res. Med. 29*: 599–604.

Sun, E.Y., Josephson, L., Kelly, K.A., and Weissleder, R. 2006a. Development of nanoparticle libraries for biosensing. *Bioconj. Chem. 17*:109–113.

Sun, E.Y., Josephson, L., and Weissleder, R. 2006b. "Clickable" nanoparticles for targeted imaging. *Mol. Imag. 5*:122–128.

Toma, A., Otsuji, E., Kuriu, Y., Okamoto, K., Ichikawa, D., Hagiwara, A., Ito, H., Nishimura, T., and Yamagishi, H. 2005. Monoclonal antibody A7-superparamagnetic iron oxide as contrast agent of MR imaging of rectal carcinoma. *Br. J. Cancer 93*:131–136.

Tsourkas, A., Hofstetter, O., Hofstetter, H., Weissleder, R., and Josephson, L. 2004. Magnetic relaxation switch immunosensors detect enantiomeric impurities. *Angew. Chem. Int. Ed. Engl. 43*:2395–2399.

Vande Berg, B.C., Lecouvet, F.E., Kanku, J.P., Jamart, J., Van Beers, B.E., Maldague, B., and Malghem, J. 1999. Ferumoxides-enhanced quantitative magnetic resonance imaging of the normal and abnormal bone marrow: preliminary assessment. *J. Magn. Reson. Imag. 9*:322–328.

Veiseh, O., Sun, C., Gunn, J., Kohler, N., Gabikian, P., Lee, D., Bhattarai, N., Ellenbogen, R., Sze, R., Hallahan, A., Olson, J., and Zhang, M. 2005. Optical and MRI multifunctional nanoprobe for targeting gliomas. *Nano Lett. 5*:1003–1008.

Wang, Y.X., Hussain, S.M., and Krestin, G.P. 2001. Superparamagnetic iron oxide contrast agents: physicochemical characteristics and applications in MR imaging. *Eur. Radiol. 11*:2319–2331.

Ward, J., Guthrie, J.A., Wilson, D., Arnold, P., Lodge, J.P., Toogood, G.J., Wyatt, J.I., and Robinson, P.J. 2003. Colorectal hepatic metastases: detection with SPIO-enhanced breath-hold MR Imaging—comparison of optimized sequences. *Radiol. 228*:709–718.

Weissleder, R., Stark, D.D., Engelstad, B.L., Bacon, B.R., Compton, C.C., White, D.L., Jacobs, P., 0and Lewis, J. 1989. Superparamagnetic iron oxide: pharmacokinetics and toxicity. *Am. J. Roentgenol. 152*:167–173.

Weissleder, R., Moore, A., Mahmood, U., Bhorade, R., Benveniste, H., Chiocca, E.A., and Basilion, J.P. 2000. *In vivo* magnetic resonance imaging of transgene expression. *Nat. Med. 6*:351–354.

Zhao, M., Beauregard, D.A., Loizou, L., Davletov, B., and Brindle, K.M. 2001. Non-invasive detection of apoptosis using magnetic resonance imaging and a targeted contrast agent. *Nat. Med. 7*:1241–1244.

Zimmer, C., Weissleder, R., O'Connor, D., LaPointe, L., Brady, T., and Enochs, W. 1995. Cerebral iron oxide distribution: *in vivo* mapping with MR imaging. *Radiol. 196*:521–552.

11

Adverse Reactions to Iodinated Contrast Media

Sameh K. Morcos

Introduction

Iodinated contrast media (CM) are routinely used to enhance imaging of neoplastic lesions. They are crucial for accurate depiction of the tumor, monitoring response to treatment, and assessing possible recurrence of malignant lesions. Unfortunately, there are potential risks associated with the administration of CM, and adverse reactions may occur. In addition, CM may interact with some of the drugs and clinical tests used in the management of patients with oncological disease (Morcos et al., 2005). Reactions to CM can be divided into general and renal adverse effects. General reactions are subdivided into acute (those that develop within one hour of CM administration) and delayed (those that develop after one hour but less than a week after CM administration) (Morcos and Thomsen, 2001).

Acute General Adverse Reactions to Contrast Media

Acute reactions to CM are often unpredictable and not dose related. They are observed after intravenous or intra-arterial injection but may also develop after alimentary or intracavitary administration as some of the CM particles may be absorbed into the circulation. These reactions are labeled anaphylactoid since they have all the features of anaphylaxis but are IgE negative in most cases. They usually develop within 5 to 30 minutes after exposure to CM.

Acute reactions can be divided into minor, intermediate, and severe life-threatening reactions. The *minor reactions* include flushing, nausea, arm pain, pruritus, vomiting, headache, and mild urticaria. These effects are usually mild in severity, of short duration, self-limiting, and generally require no specific treatment. The incidence of these reactions to high osmolar CM (HOCM) is probably between 5–15% and 1–3% with low osmolar nonionic CM. *Intermediate reactions* include more serious degrees of the above symptoms: moderate degrees of hypotension and bronchospasm. They usually respond readily to appropriate therapy. The incidence of these reactions to HOCM is about 1–2% and around 0.2% with low osmolar nonionic CM (Morcos, 2005). *Severe life-threatening reactions* include severe manifestation of minor and intermediate reactions, convulsions, unconsciousness, laryngeal edema, severe bronchospasm, pulmonary edema, severe cardiac dysrhythmias and arrest, and cardiovascular and pulmonary collapse. In a large series of over 330,000 patients, Katayama et al. found that the incidence of severe and very severe reactions following intravascular administration of HOCM was 0.22 and 0.04%, respectively, and 0.04 and 0.004%, respectively, after low osmolar nonionic CM (Katayama et al., 1990). Thus, these data clearly demonstrate that the use of low osmolar nonionic CM reduces the incidence of all types of acute general reactions, particularly the severe and very severe reactions, which are reduced by a factor of 10 in comparison to HOCM. However, no difference was observed in the incidence of fatal reactions to both types of contrast media, which were exceedingly rare (1:170,000) (Katayama *et al.*, 1990). Other large surveillances of CM reactions also reported similar observations (Morcos, 2005).

Risk Factors of Acute General Reactions

There is a sixfold increase in reactions to both ionic and nonionic CM in patients with a history of previous severe adverse reaction to a contrast agent. Asthma is also an important risk factor with a reported six- to tenfold increase in the risk of a severe reaction in such patients. Patients with a strong history of allergic reactions to different substances, including those with a history of troublesome hay fever, are also at risk of acute adverse reactions to CM (Morcos, 2005). Race could also be a predisposing factor for CM reactions. Incidence of contrast reactions among patients of Indian origin and patients of Mediterranean origin in the United Kingdom was significantly higher in comparison to the endogenous white population (Ansell *et al.*, 1980). There is no clear explanation for the racial differences in the incidence of contrast reactions. Malignant tumors may also increase the incidence of anaphylactoid reactions. This could be due to an increase in histamine release in tumor patients (Celik *et al.*, 1999). In addition, patients treated with ß-adrenergic blockers or interleukin-2 (IL-2) are at increased risk of acute adverse reactions to CM (details are provided in the section of interaction between CM with drugs and clinical tests). Important risk factors for acute serious reactions to CM are presented in Table 1.

Prevention of Acute General Reactions to Contrast Media

All precautions should be considered in high-risk patients (those with a history of previous moderate or severe contrast reactions, allergic conditions that require treatment, or bronchial asthma) when CM administration is deemed essential. Imaging procedures that do not require the administration of iodinated CM should be considered first, but if the administration of iodinated CM is deemed essential, nonionic contrast media should be used. The potential risks of the procedure should be explained to the patient, and the resuscitation team should be present when the CM is given. Adequate provision to treat any reaction should be available. The prophylactic administration of corticosteroids (32 mg methyl prednisolone orally 12 hours and one hour before CM administration) in these patients has been recommended by several authors. However, the use of steroids as premedication has not received wide support, and some authors have concluded that nonionic agents should be used in patients

with definable risk factors and that the value of corticosteroid prophylaxis is not proven and may reasonably be abandoned. Antihistamines (H1 and H2) and ephedrine have also been advocated for high-risk patients often in combination with corticosteroids. However, the use of antihistamine H1 and H2 receptor antagonists as well as ephedrine to decrease the prevalence of adverse reactions to CM has not gained wide acceptance (Morcos, 2005).

It is important to emphasize that severe life-threatening reactions, or even fatality, may still occur in patients who receive premedication and low osmolar CM. Prompt recognition and treatment of adverse side effects to CM can be invaluable in blunting the response and may prevent a reaction from becoming severe or even life threatening. The patient should never be left alone for at least 20 minutes after CM injection, and the venous access should be left in place. Knowledge, training, and preparation are crucial in guaranteeing appropriate and effective therapy in the event of a contrast-related reaction (Morcos, 2005).

The Contrast Media Safety Committee of the European Society or Urogenital Radiology (ESUR) has produced simple guidelines on prevention of generalized reactions to CM (Table 1) (Morcos *et al.*, 2001).

Emergency Administration of Contrast Media in High-Risk Patients

Emergency administration of CM in patients at high risk of severe reaction to CM, particularly those with a history of previous serious reaction to CM requiring essential procedures, precludes prolonged prophylaxis pretreatment with corticosteroids. In these patients, in addition to the use of low osmolar nonionic CM pretreatment with hydrocortisone, 200 mg intravenously, immediately, and every 4 hours until the procedure is completed, and diphenhydramine, 50 mg intravenously before the procedure and the use of low osmolar nonionic CM has been recommended (Greenberger *et al.*, 1986).

Treatment of Acute Severe General Reactions to Contrast Media

The vast majority of patients with acute severe reactions to CM recover if they are treated quickly and appropriately. The first-line drugs and equipment should be readily available in rooms in which contrast material is injected. A list of recommended drugs and equipment is given in Table 2. Important first-line management includes establishment of an adequate airway, oxygen supplementation, administration of intravascular physiological fluids, and measure of the blood pressure and heart rate (Thomsen *et al.*, 2004).

Adrenaline is an effective drug for treating certain serious contrast reactions. It increases blood pressure, reverses

Table 1   European Society of Urogenital Radiology (ESUR) Guidelines on Prevention of Generalized Contrast Medium Reactions in Adults

A. Risk factors for reactions
Previous generalized contrast medium reaction, either moderate (e.g., urticaria, bronchospasm, moderate hypotension) or severe (e.g., convulsions, severe bronchospasm, pulmonary edema, cardiovascular collapse)
Asthma
Allergy requiring medical treatment

B. To reduce the risk of generalized contrast medium reactions
Use nonionic agents.

C. Premedication is recommended in high-risk patients (defined in A)
When ionic agents are used.
When nonionic agents are used, opinion is divided about the value of premedication.
Recommended premedication:
Corticosteroids.
Prednisolone 30 mg orally or methylprednisolone 32 mg orally 12 and 2 hours before contrast medium.
Corticosteroids are not effective if given less than 6 hours before contrast medium.
Antihistamines H1 and H2 may be used in addition to corticosteroids, but opinion is divided.
Remember for all patients:
Have a trolley with resuscitation drugs in the examination room.
Observe patients for 20 to 30 minutes after contrast medium injection.
Extravascular administration
When absorption or leakage into the circulation is possible, take the same precautions as for intravascular administration.

Source: Morcos *et al.*, 2001.

Table 2   First-Line Emergency Drugs and Instruments That Should Be in the Room Where Contrast Medium Is Injected

Drugs/instruments
Oxygen
Adrenaline 1:1000
Antihistamine H1—suitable for injection
Atropine
ß-2-agonist metered dose inhaler
I.V. fluids—normal saline or Ringer's solution
Anticonvulsive drugs (diazepam)
Sphygmomanometer
One-way mouth "breather" apparatus

Source: Thomson *et al.*, 2004.

peripheral vasodilatation, decreases angioedema and urticaria, reverses bronchoconstriction, and produces positive inotropic and chronotropic cardiac effects. Adrenaline should be avoided when possible for treating the pregnant patient with a severe contrast reaction and hypotension. Only one concentration (1:1000) of adrenaline should be available in the radiology department. Intramuscular injection of 0.5 ml of 1:1000 adrenaline preparation is recommended in preference to intravenous administration in management of acute anaphylaxis/anaphylactoid reaction. Intravenous injection of adrenalin requires careful ECG monitoring and should be administered very slowly, ideally by people experienced in its use. According to the

UK's Project Team of the Resuscitation Council, adrenaline 1:1000 should never be used intravenously because of the risk of arrhythmia, and subcutaneous administration is not helpful in acute life-threatening situations (Morcos, 2005).

Antihistamines H1 receptor blockers are used primarily to reduce symptoms from skin reactions. Compared with adrenaline, the first-response medication of acute anaphylaxis, antihistamines have a slow onset of action, and they cannot block events that occur subsequent to histamine binding to its receptors. The administration of H2-antagonists is not essential in the management of anaphylaxis/anaphylactoid reactions (Thomsen *et al.*, 2004).

Intravenous injection of high-dose corticosteroids may have an immediate stabilizing effect on the cell membrane and could be used in the second-line treatment. Standard doses can be effective in reducing delayed recurrent symptoms, which can be observed for as long as 48 hours after an initial reaction (Thomsen *et al.*, 2004).

Inhaled ß-2-adrenergic agonists such as albuterol, metaproterenol, and terbutaline deliver large doses of bronchodilating ß-2-agonist drugs directly to the airways with minimal systemic absorption and therefore minimal cardiovascular effects.

Atropine blocks vagal stimulation of the cardiac conduction system. Large doses of atropine (0.6–1.0 mg) are indicated, since low doses (e.g., less than 0.5 mg) of atropine can be detrimental to the treatment of bradycardia associated with contrast media-induced vagal reactions.

Guidelines for treatment of serious reactions to CM are presented in Table 3 (Thomsen *et al.*, 2004).

Delayed General Adverse Reactions to Contrast Media

A delayed reaction to intravascular contrast medium is defined as a reaction that occurs 1 hour or later after contrast medium injection. Most of the delayed reactions are not serious or life threatening and include flu-like illness, parotitis, nausea and vomiting, abdominal pain, and headache. Delayed allergy-like reactions with skin manifestation have also been observed. The majority of delayed adverse reactions resolve by 7 days. The pathophysiology of late reactions is still unclear, but it appears that many delayed reactions, particularly those with skin manifestations, are T-cell mediated (Christiansen *et al.*, 2000). The skin reactions often show the features of delayed hypersensitivity reactions, including exanthematous rash, positive skin test, lympho-cytic infiltrate together with eosinophils on skin biopsy (Webb *et al.*, 2003).

Frequency

Several studies suggest that the incidence of the different delayed reactions in the 1- to 24-hour period after CM administration is 4% or less and late skin reactions 1–3% over a period of 7 days. There do not appear to be significant differences in the incidence of delayed reactions between ionic and nonionic monomers or between the different nonionic monomers. No significant differences have been found between the nonionic monomers and the ionic dimer ioxaglate either. However, the incidence of late reactions is more common with the nonionic dimers, and skin reactions tend to be more severe (Webb *et al.*, 2003).

Predisposing Factors

A previous reaction to contrast medium is an important predisposing factor increasing the risk by a factor of 1.7 to 3.3.

Table 3   Simple Guidelines for First-Line Treatment of Acute Severe Reactions to Contrast Media

---

Bronchospasm
1. Oxygen by mask (6–10 l/min)
2. ß-2-agonist metered dose inhaler (2–3 deep inhalations)
3. Adrenaline
-Normal blood pressure
Intramuscular: 1:1000, 0.1–0.3 ml (0.1–0.3 mg; use smaller dose in a patient with coronary artery disease or elderly patient)
In pediatric patients: 0.01 mg/kg up to 0.3 mg maximum
-Decreased blood pressure
Intramuscular: 1:1000, 0.5 ml (0.5 mg; in pediatric patients: 0.01 mg/kg intramuscularly)

Laryngeal edema
1. Oxygen by mask (6–10 l/min)
2. Intramuscular adrenaline (1:1000), 0.5 ml (0.5 mg) for adults, repeat as needed

Isolated hypotension
1. Elevate patient's legs
2. Oxygen by mask (6–10 l/min)
3. Intravenous fluid: rapidly, normal saline or lactated Ringer's solution
4. If unresponsive: adrenaline: 1:1000, 0.5 ml (0.5 mg) intramuscularly, repeat as needed

Hypotension and bradycardia (vaso-vagal reaction)
1. Elevate patient's legs
2. Oxygen by mask (6–10 l/min)
3. Atropine 0.6–1.0 mg intravenously, repeat if necessary after 3–5 min, to 3 mg total (0.04 mg/kg) in adults.
   In pediatric patients give 0.02 mg/kg intravenously (maximum 0.6 mg per dose), repeat if necessary to 2 mg total
4. Intravenous fluids rapidly, normal saline or lactated Ringer's solution

Generalized anaphylactoid reaction
1. Call for resuscitation team
2. Suction airway as needed
3. Elevate patient's legs if hypotensive
4. Oxygen by mask (6–10 l/min)
5. Intramuscular adrenaline (1:1000), 0.5 ml (0.5 mg) in adults. Repeat as needed
   In pediatric patients 0.01 mg/kg to 0.3 mg maximum dose
6. Intravenous fluids (e.g., normal saline, lactated Ringer's)
7. H1-blocker (e.g., diphenhydramine 25–50 mg intravenously)
8. ß-2-agonist metered dose inhaler for persistent bronchospasm: 2 or 3 inhalations

---

Source: Thomson *et al.*, 2004.

However, no apparent relationship exists between the occurrence of immediate and delayed reactions. A history of allergy is a further risk factor increasing the likelihood of a reaction by approximately two times. A seasonal variation in the incidence of delayed skin reactions has been described, with 45% of reactions occurring in the period April to June in Finland. A relation to the pollen season and/or to the possible photosensitizing effect of contrast media has been postulated. Females are more likely to develop delayed adverse reactions than males. Japanese are more predisposed to develop late reactions than Europeans. Coexisting diseases also appear to predispose to delayed reactions, especially renal disease, but also cardiac and liver disease and diabetes mellitus. Some of the most severe skin reactions reported occurred in patients with systemic lupus erythematosus or patients who were taking hydralazine, which induces a lupus-like syndrome. There is increased incidence of delayed reactions to contrast media in patients who have received interleukin-2 (IL-2) (details are provided in the section of interaction between CM with drugs and clinical tests) (Webb *et al.*, 2003).

Contrast Media-Induced Nephrotoxicity

Patients suffering from reduced renal function or conditions causing reduction of renal perfusion may develop contrast media nephrotoxicity (CMN) (an increase in serum creatinine by more than 25% or 0.5 mg/dl [44 μmol/l] from baseline that occurred within 3 days following contrast media injection) (Morcos, 2005).

Incidence

The incidence of CMN in patients with normal renal function prior to injection of CM is low (< 10%) but may increase to 25% or more in patients with risk factors. The majority of patients with CMN tend to be nonoliguric except those with preexisting advanced chronic renal failure. The clinical course of CMN in most cases is benign and resolves within one to two weeks. However, CMN may increase the incidence of in-hospital morbidity and mortality (Morcos, 2005). A fifteen-fold increase in major adverse cardiac events (MACE) was observed in patients who developed CMN after percutaneous coronary angioplasty (Mehran *et al.*, 2004).

Risk Factors of Contrast Media Nephrotoxicity

One risk factor is *preexisting renal impairment* (serum creatinine >1.5 mg/dl [130 μmol/l]), particularly when the reduction in renal function is associated with *diabetes mellitus*.

The degree of renal insufficiency present before the administration of CM determines to a great extent the severity of CMN. Creatinine clearance of 30 ml/min or less markedly increases the incidence and severity of CMN (McCullogh *et al.*, 1997).

The *type and dose of CM* is an important risk factor for the development of CMN. It is well recognized now that low osmolar CM (LOCM) are less nephrotoxic in comparison to high osmolar CM (HOCM) in patients with preexisting renal impairment (Morcos, 2005). It has been suggested recently that the iso-osmolar nonionic dimer iodixanol is less nephrotoxic in comparison to LOCM (Aspelin *et al.*, 2003). However, low incidence of CMN with iodixanol was not confirmed in other studies. Patients with preexisting renal insufficiency are at high risk of CMN with all classes of CM, including the iso-osmolar dimer (Morcos, 2005).

The nephrotoxic effect of CM is dose dependent, and the higher the dose the higher the risk of CMN. *Multiple injections of CM within 72 hours* in patients with renal impairment are also likely to increase the risk of CMN.

Other risk factors for CMN may include dehydration, congestive cardiac failure, multiple myeloma, concurrent use of nephrotoxic drugs, hypertension, hyperuricemia, or proteinuria. Multiple myeloma has been considered in the past as a risk factor for CMN. However, if dehydration is avoided, LOCM administration rarely leads to CMN in patients with myeloma.

Concurrent use of nephrotoxic drugs, such as nonsteroidal anti-inflammatory drugs (NSAID) and aminoglycosides, is likely to exaggerate the nephrotoxic effects of CM. Nephropathy is found more frequently in patients with *hypertension, hyperuricemia, or proteinuria* than in patients without these factors, and these patients are likely to be more vulnerable to the renal effects of CM (Morcos, 2005; Morcos *et al.*, 1999).

Methods to Reduce the Risk of Contrast Media Nephrotoxicity

Ideally, intravascular administration of iodinated CM should be avoided in patients at high risk of CMN. Consideration should be given to alternative imaging techniques that do not require injection of iodinated CM. The use of gadolinium-based CM has been suggested for radiographic examinations as an alternative to iodinated CM in patients with renal impairment. However, clinical, toxicological, and experimental data raise concern about renal tolerance of these agents, particularly at doses above 0.3 mmol (0.6 ml)/kg body weight (Morcos, 2005). The report of the Contrast Media Safety Committee (CMSC) of the European Society of Urogenital Radiology (ESUR) concluded that gadolinium-based CM should not be given intravascularly at a dose above 0.3 mmol/kg body weight because it may induce nephrotoxicity in patients with preexisting renal impairment (Thomsen *et al.*, 2002). In addition, gadolinium-based CM is not approved by the drug-licensing authorities for intra-arterial administration or radiographic examinations (Morcos, 2005).

If iodinated CM administration is deemed necessary in high-risk patients, the lowest possible dose of a low osmolar or iso-osmolar nonionic CM should be used. In addition, volume expansion with intravenous administration of normal saline should be implemented. The administration of nephrotoxic drugs such as gentamicin and nonsteroid anti-inflammatory drugs (NSAIDs) (NB: small doses of aspirin as antithrombotic therapy is unlikely to worsen the reduction of renal perfusion induced by CM) should be stopped for at least 48 hours prior to CM injection (Morcos *et al.*, 1999; Morcos, 2005). In the following section, the use of extracellular volume expansion and pharmacological manipulation in the prevention of CMN is discussed.

- *Extracellular volume expansion:* Volume expansion [normal saline given IV at the dose of 1 ml/kg body weight for 8–12 hours before and after CM administration] offers protection against CMN through the combination of diuresis, dilution of the CM, and vasoconstrictive mediators in circulation, downregulating the tubulo-glomerular feedback (TGF) response and decreasing the activity of the renin-angiotensin system and antidiuretic hormone (ADH). Fluid infusion starting only at the time of the procedure does not offer any protection. Oral hydration (1000 mL clear liquid over 10 hours), followed by 6 hours of IV hydration (0.45% saline solution at 300 mL/hour) beginning just before contrast exposure, is a suitable alternative for outpatient cases (Morcos, 2005).
- *Volume expansion has some limitations:* it is not suitable for patients with cardiac failure, and it is of limited use in emergency situations since it requires fluid administration for several hours prior to CM exposure.
- *Pharmacological Manipulation:* The prophylactic administration of drugs such as renal vasodilators (atrial natriuretic peptide, calcium antagonists, dopamine, dopamine-1 receptor agonist "fenoldopam" or prostaglandin E-1), receptor antagonists of intrarenal vasoactive mediators (adenosine, or endothelin), the antioxidant acetylecystine, or infusion of sodium bicarbonate have been investigated in the prevention of CMN. Unfortunately, the results have been mixed, with some studies reporting a protective effect, while others failed to detect any benefit (Morcos, 2004). This chapter focuses only on the use of fenoldopam, acetylcysteine, and sodium bicarbonate infusion because their use is still receiving some support. The use of other drugs is no longer considered useful in the prevention of CMN.
- *Selective dopamine-1 receptor agonist (fenoldopam):* Fenoldopam has the advantage over dopamine in

increasing both the cortical and medullary renal blood flow, and its vasodilatory effect is six times more potent than that of dopamine. Fenoldopam also increases GFR and induces diuresis. However, the protective effect of fenoldopam infusion [0.1 µg/kg/min starting 15–20 minutes prior to CM injection and continued for 6 hours after the procedure] against CMN was not consistent. Furthermore, fenoldopam has several disadvantages. It has to be given by intravenous infusion, it induces hypotension, and it requires regular monitoring of blood pressure to adjust the dose according to the state of the blood pressure. Increasing the dose of fenoldopmam above 0.1 µg/kg/min to enhance the renoprotective effect is likely to increase the risk of hypotension, with resultant intrarenal vasoconstriction (Morcos, 2005).

- *Acetylcysteine:* Acetylcysteine is an antioxidant and scavenger of oxygen-free radicals. It also enhances the biological effect of the endogenous vasodilator nitric oxide. The results of studies evaluating the protective effect of oral acetylcysteine against CMN are mixed. However, a double dose of oral acetylcysteine (1200 mg b.d. for 2 days starting 24 hours before CM administration) was reported to offer better protection than the standard dose (600 mg b.d. for 2 days starting 24 hours before CM administration), especially when a large volume of CM (>140 ml) was used. Acetylcysteine intravenously [acetylcysteine 150 mg/kg in 500 ml normal saline over 30 min immediately before the procedure followed by acetylcysteine 50 mg/kg in 500 ml normal saline over 4 hours] was also found in one study to offer protection against CMN in emergency angiographic procedures. Considering all the published studies, including the meta-analysis reports, consistent protection of acetylcysteine against CMN has not been proven (Morcos, 2005; Zegler *et al.*, 2006). Although acetylcysteine has several attractive advantages, including its low cost, easy administration, and has limited side effects, further studies are required before its routine use can be endorsed unreservedly. Acetylcysteine also has certain disadvantages, including pharmacological activity varying between oral products and the noxious smell and taste of the liquid preparations of the drug.
- *Sodium bicarbonate infusion:* Pretreatment with sodium bicarbonate will lead to an increase in the pH of urine and renal medulla, which reduces the generation of free radicals and protects the kidney from oxidant injury that can be associated with CMN. Sodium bicarbonate infusion (154 mEq/L) given as a bolus of 3 ml/kg per hour for 1 hour before CM, followed by an infusion of 1 ml/kg body weight per hour for 6 hours after the procedure, offered significantly better protection against CMN compared with hydration with sodium chloride (Merten *et al.*, 2004). However, further studies are required to establish the consistency of sodium bicarbonate in reducing the

Table 4   Simple Guidelines to Avoid Contrast Medium Nephrotoxicity

Definition		Contrast medium nephrotoxicity is a condition in which an impairment in renal function (an increase in serum creatinine by more than 25% or 44 µmol/l) occurs within 3 days following the intravascular administration of a contrast medium (CM) in the absence of an alternative etiology.
Risk factors	Look for	• Raised S-creatinine levels, particularly secondary to diabetic nephropathy. • Dehydration. • Congestive heart failure. • Age over 70 years old. • Concurrent administration of nephrotoxic drugs, (e.g., nonsteroid anti-inflammatory drugs).
In patients with risk factor(s)	Do	• Make sure that the patient is well hydrated [give at least 100 ml (oral (e.g., soft drinks) or intravenous (normal saline) depending on the clinical situation) per hour starting 4 hours before to 24 hours after contrast administration—in hot climates increase the fluid volume]. • Use low- or iso-osmolar contrast media. • Stop administration of nephrotoxic drugs for at least 24 hours. • Consider alternative imaging techniques, which do not require the administration of iodinated contrast media.
	Do not	• *Give high osmolar contrast media.* • Administer large doses of contrast media. • Administer mannitol and diuretics, particularly loop-diuretics. • Perform multiple studies with contrast media within a short period of time.

Source: Morcos *et al.,* 1999.

incidence of CMN in high-risk patients. Guidelines on prevention of CMN are presented in Table 4.

Contrast Media Interactions with Other Drugs and Clinical Tests

Although contrast agents are not highly active pharmacologically, interaction with other drugs may occur, with possible serious consequences to the patient. In this section the interactions are grouped together according to clinical importance and the body system involved. In addition, the effects of contrast media on isotope studies and biochemical assays of body fluids are highlighted.

Drug-Induced Reduction in Renal Function

Contrast media may interfere with the pharmacokinetics (distribution, metabolism, and elimination of the drug) of other drugs, particularly those that are eliminated from the body through the kidneys. Iodinated contrast media can cause reduction of renal function, particularly in patients with preexisting reduced renal function. This leads to retention of drugs that are excreted exclusively through the kidneys. A good example is the indirect interaction between contrast media and metformin (Thomsen *et al.,* 1999). The potential reduction in renal function induced by CM may cause retention of metformin in the body, which can lead to the serious complication of lactic acidosis. Guidelines on the administration of CM

in patients receiving metformin are presented in Table 5 (Thomsen *et al.,* 1999).

Drug-Enhanced Renal Effects of Contrast Media

Nephrotoxic drugs such as nonsteroidal anti-inflammatory drugs (NSAIDs) have the potential to increase the renal effects of contrast media. This class of drugs inhibits the intrarenal synthesis of vasodilatory prostaglandins augmenting the renal vasoconstrictor effect of iodinated contrast media, and may facilitate the development of contrast media nephrotoxicity. Other nephrotoxic drugs such as gentamicin, cyclosporine, and cisplatin may also augment the nephrotoxic effects of contrast media. Diuretics such as acetazolamide, furosemide, and spironolactone may augment the diuretic effect of contrast media, particularly those of high osmolality, leading to dehydration, increased risk of contrast medium nephropathy, electrolyte imbalance, and hypotension (Morcos *et al.,* 2005).

Drug-Enhanced Reactions to Contrast Media

Patients receiving β-receptor blockers, interleukins, or interferons have an increased tendency to develop allergy-like reactions following the administration of contrast media. Delayed reactions to contrast media are more likely to develop in patients who receive interleukin-2 (IL-2) treatment (Choyke *et al.,* 1992). In addition, patients on hydralazine treatment, which can induce a syndrome like systemic lupus erythematosus

(SLE), may develop cutaneous vasculitis several hours after intravascular administration of nonionic iodinated contrast medium. It has been suggested that injection of iodinated contrast media should be avoided in patients receiving hydralazine as they may provoke severe reactions (Morcos *et al.*, 2005).

β-Blockers

Patients on β-blockers, including the ophthalmic preparations, who are given iodinated contrast media are three times more likely to have an anaphylactoid reaction than matched controls. There is also increased risk of contrast media-induced bronchospasm, particularly in asthmatics. Anaphylaxis-like reaction in these patients is more refractory to conventional treatment because of low reactivity to emergency medication. Adrenaline may be ineffective or may promote undesired α-adrenergic or vagal effects. Anaphylaxis associated with β-blockers was nine times more likely to result in hospitalization than in matched controls (Lang *et al.*, 1993).

Interleukin-2

Interleukin-2 (IL-2) can induce partial or complete responses in more than 20% of patients with advanced melanoma or renal cell carcinoma. In a prospective study of patients undergoing CT who had received IL-2 and intravenous nonionic low-osmolar or oral ionic high-osmolar contrast media, or both, there were immediate urticarial reactions in 1.8% of the patients within an hour of contrast administration. No acute reactions were observed in a control group who received contrast media but had not been treated with IL-2. Delayed reactions (erythema, rash, fever, flushing, pruritis, and flu-like symptoms) developed in 12% of IL-2 patients and in only 4% of the control group. Two of the IL-2 patients required admission to the hospital. The mean onset of symptoms was 4.5 hours after injection of contrast media, and the mean duration of reaction was 16.4 hours. The patients had no risk factor for delayed reactions other than IL-2 therapy, and all had had previous uneventful exposure to contrast media. None of the patients with immediate reactions developed delayed reactions. The average time since IL-2 therapy was 6 months (range 24 days to 2.4 years). Previous contrast media reaction in an IL-2 patient should be considered a relative contraindication to further contrast media administration. An increased risk of contrast reactions may remain for two years after stopping IL-2 treatment (Choyke *et al.*, 1992).

The administration of contrast media may also precipitate IL-2 toxicity. Fever, diarrhea, nausea, and vomiting have been observed 2 to 4 hours after CT scanning enhanced with nonionic low-osmolar contrast media. The exact mechanism is not clear and immunologic interactions are probable. Contrast media may generate the release of endogenous IL-2 or reactivate the IL-2 receptors. Patients who develop these reactions should avoid further exposure to contrast media, and imaging techniques such as MRI or CT without contrast media injection should be considered for monitoring response to treatment (Morcos *et al.*, 2005).

Drug-Interference Hematological Effects of Contrast Media

Both ionic and nonionic iodinated contrast media can prolong clotting time and may exaggerate the effects of anticoagulant and antiplatelet drugs. In addition, clotting tests will be falsely elevated after the administration of CM and should only be performed 6 hours or more after CM have been given.

Contrast media may also impede fibrinolysis and delay the onset of lysis by recombinant tissue-type plasminogen activator (rt-PA), urokinase, and streptokinase (Morcos *et al.*, 2005).

Table 5   Guidelines for the Administration of Contrast Media to Diabetics Taking Metformin

---

1. Serum creatinine level should be measured in every diabetic patient treated with biguanides prior to intravascular administration of contrast media. Low-osmolar contrast media should always be used in these patients.
2. <u>Elective studies</u>
a. *If the serum creatinine is normal*, the radiological examination should be performed and intake of metformin stopped from the time of the study. The use of metformin should not be resumed for 48 hours and should only be restarted if renal function/serum creatinine remains within the normal range.
b. *If renal function is abnormal*, the metformin should be stopped and the contrast study should be delayed for 48 hours. Metformin should only be restarted 48 hours later, if renal function/serum creatinine is unchanged.
3. <u>Emergency cases</u>
a. *If the serum creatinine is normal*, the study may proceed as suggested for elective patients.
b. *If the renal function is abnormal (or unknown)*, the physician should weigh the risks and benefits of contrast administration. Alternative imaging techniques should be considered. If contrast media administration is deemed necessary, the following precautions should be implemented:
• Metformin therapy should be stopped.
• The patient should be hydrated (e.g., at least 100 ml per hour of soft drinks or intravenous saline up to 24 hours after contrast medium administration. In hot climates more fluid should be given).

Source: Thomson *et al.*, 1999.

Contrast Media Effects on Isotope Studies and Treatment

The administration of iodinated contrast media interferes with both diagnostic scintigraphy and radioiodine treatment. The reduced uptake of the radioactive tracer is caused by the free iodide in the contrast medium solution. A delay before undertaking scintigraphy of 4–6 weeks for water soluble and 12 weeks for cholangiographic contrast media is advocated, depending on the indication for scintigraphy and on whether the patient is euthyroid or hyperthyroid. The administration of iodinated CM should be avoided in patients considered for radioiodine treatment (Morcos et al., 2005).

Intravascular administration of CM shortly after injection of isotope material (^{99m}Tc-pyrophosphate) for bone imaging can interfere with the body distribution of the ^{99m}Tc-pyrophosphate. Increased uptake of the isotope material in kidneys and liver with low uptake in bones was observed. The diuretic effect of CM may increase the elimination of the isotope material in urine, so that less is available for deposition in the skeleton. The increased uptake in the liver is not fully explained (Morcos et al., 2005).

Intravascular administration of CM may also interfere with red blood cell labeling with isotope material. ^{99m}Tc labeling of red blood cells should not be performed within 24 hours after CM injection. How CM interferes with red blood cell labeling is not fully understood (Morcos et al., 2004).

Contrast Media Effects on Biochemical Assays

Measurements of clotting time and other coagulation factors can be falsely increased after the intravascular administration of CM. Therefore, clotting tests should be avoided for 6 hours or more after injection of CM. Iodinated CM in the urine may also interfere with some of the protein assay techniques leading to false-positive results. Care must be exercised in interpreting tests for proteinuria for 24 hours post-CM injection (Morcos et al., 2004).

Iodinated CM may interfere with determination of bilirubin, cubber, iron, phosphate, and proteins in blood. Therefore, biochemical assays are better performed before CM injection or delayed for at least 24 hours afterwards or longer in patients with renal impairment. Urgent laboratory tests performed on specimens collected shortly after CM injection should be carefully assessed. Accuracy of unexpected abnormal results should be questioned and discussed with colleagues from the hospital laboratories.

Conclusion

Serious or fatal reactions to a contrast medium (CM) are unpredictable but fortunately rare. History of serious reaction to CM, bronchial asthma, or multiple allergies increases the incidence of serious reactions by at least a factor of 5. Avoiding CM administration in patients at high risk of serious reaction is advisable, but if the administration is deemed essential, all precautions should be implemented and measures to treat serious reactions should be readily available. Oxygen supplementation, intravenous administration of physiological fluids, and intramuscular injection of 0.5 ml adrenalin (1:1000) should be considered in the first-line management of acute anaphylaxis. Delayed reactions to CM include nonspecific symptoms such as headache, musculoskeletal pains and aches, fever, pyrexia, and enlargement of the salivary glands. Allergy-like skin reactions are well-documented delayed side effects of CM, with incidence around 2%. The prevalence is higher by a factor of 2 with nonionic dimers. Most delayed reactions are self-limiting and resolve within 7 days. Patients in treatment with interleukin-2 and patients having had a previous reaction to contrast media should be warned about the possibility of a delayed reaction.

Contrast media nephrotoxicity (CMN) remains an important complication of intravascular administration of CM. Prevention of CMN is important to avoid substantial morbidity and even mortality that can be associated with this condition. Identifying risk factors of CMN (preexisting renal impairment, dehydration, congestive heart failure, old age [over 70 years], concurrent administration of nephrotoxic drugs) through the use of screening questionnaires and renal function measurement before CM administration is crucially important. Patients at risk of CMN should receive the smallest possible dose of either nonionic iso-osmolar dimeric or nonionic low-osmolar monomeric CM and volume expansion with intravenous infusion (1 ml/kg body weight/hour) of 0.9% saline starting at least 4 hours before CM injection and continuing for 8–12 hours afterward. Pharmacological manipulation with a variety of drugs, including the renal vasodilator fenoldopam (selective dopamine-1 receptor agonist) or the antioxidant acetylcysteine, does not offer consistent protection against CMN, and the value of these drugs in prevention of CMN remains uncertain. Sodium bicarbonate infusion offers a new, promising approach for prevention of CMN, but further studies are required to confirm its protective effect. Contrast media may interact with other drugs and interfere with isotope studies and biochemical measurements. Awareness of these interactions is important to avoid potential hazards.

References

Ansell, G., Tweedie, M.C., West, C.R., Evans, P., and Couch, L. 1980. The current status of reactions to intravenous contrast media. *Invest. Radiol.* 15:S32–S39.

Aspelin, P., Aubry, P., Fransson, S.G., Strasser, R., Wellinbrock, R., and Berg, K.J. 2003. Nephrotoxic effects in high-risk patients undergoing angiography. *N. Engl. J. Med.* 348:491–499.

Celik, I., Hoppe, M., Lorenz, W., Sitte, H., Ishaque N., Jungraithmayr, W., Kapp, B., Schmiedel E., and Klose, K.J. 1999. Randomised study comparing a non-ionic with an ionic contrast medium in patients with malignancies: first answer with a new diagnostic approach. *Inflamm. Res. 48 (Suppl.1)*:S47–S48.

Choyke, P.L., Miller, D.L., Lotze, M.T., Whiteis, J.M., Ebbitt, B., and Rosenberg, S.A. 1992. Delayed reactions to contrast media after interleukin-2 immunotherapy. *Radiology. 183*:111–114.

Christiansen, C., Pichler, W.J., and Skotland, T. 2000. Delayed allergy-like reactions to X-ray contrast media: mechanistic considerations. *Eur. Radiol. 10*:1965–1975.

Greenberger, P.A., Halwig, J.M., Patterson, R., and Wallemark, C.B. 1986. Emergency administration of radiocontrast media in high-risk patients. *J. Allergy. Clin. Immunol. 77*:630–634.

Katayama, H., Yamaguchi, K., Kozuka, T., Takashima, T., Seez, P., and Matsuura, K. 1990. Adverse reactions to ionic and nonionic contrast media. *Radiology 175*:621–628.

Lang, D.M, Alpern, M.B., Visintainer, P.F., and Smith, S.T. 1993. Elevated risk of anaphylactoid reaction from radiographic contrast media is associated with both beta-blocker exposure and cardiovascular disorders. *Arch. Intern. Med. 153*:2033–2040.

Levy, E.M., Viscoli, C.M., and Horwitz, R.I. 1996. The effect of acute renal failure on mortality, a cohort analysis. *JAMA 257*:1489–1494.

McCullough, P.A., Wolyn, R., Rocher, L.L., Levin, R.N., and O'Neill, W.W. 1997. Acute renal failure after coronary intervention: incidence, risk factors and relationship to mortality. *Am. J. Med. 103*:368–375.

Mehran, R., Aymong, E.D., Nikolsky, E., Lasic, Z., Iakovou, I., Fahy, M., Mintz, G.S., Lansky A.J.,Moses, J.W., Stone, G.W., Leon, M.B., and Dangas, G. 2004. A simple risk score for prediction of contrast-induced nephropathy after percutaneous coronary intervention: development and initial validation. *JACC 44*:1393–1399.

Merten, G.J., Burgess, W.P., Gray, L.V., Holleman, J.H., Roush, T.S., Kowalchuk, G.J., Bersin, R.M., Moore A.V., Simonton, C.A., Rittase, R.A., Norton, H.J., and Kennedy, T.P. 2004. Prevention of contrast-induced nephropathy with sodium bicarbonate: a randomized controlled trial. *JAMA 291*:2328–2334.

Morcos, S.K., Thomsen, H.S., and Webb, J.A.W., and members of Contrast Media Safety Committee of European Society of Urogenital Radiology 1999. Contrast-media-induced nephrotoxicity: a consensus report. *Eur. Radiol. 9*:1602–1613.

Morcos, S.K., Thomsen, H.S., and Webb, J.A.W., and members of the Contrast Media Safety Committee of European Society of Urogenital Radiology (ESUR). 2001. Prevention of generalized reactions to contrast media consensus report and guidelines. *Eur. Radiol. 11*:1720–1728.

Morcos, S.K., and Thomsen, H.S. 2001. Adverse reactions to iodinated contrast media. *Eur. Radiol. 11*:1267–1275.

Morcos, S.K. 2004. Prevention of contrast media nephrotoxicity—the story so far. *Clin. Radiol. 59*:381–389.

Morcos, S.K. 2005. Prevention of contrast media nephrotoxicity following angiographic procedures. *JVIR 16*:13–23.

Morcos, S.K. 2005. Acute serious and fatal reactions to contrast media; our current understanding. *Br. J. Radiol. 78*:686–693.

Morcos, S.K., Thomsen, H.S., Exley, C.M., and Contrast Media Safety Committee of the European Society of Urogenital Radiology. 2005. Contrast media: interactions with other drugs and clinical tests. *Eur. Radiol. 15*:1463–1468.

Thomsen, H.S., Morcos, S.K., and members of Contrast Media Safety Committee of European Society of Urogenital Radiology (ESUR). 1999. Contrast media and metformin. Guidelines to distinguish the risk of lactic acidosis in non-insulin dependent diabetics after administration of contrast media. *Eur. Radiol. 9*:738–740.

Thomsen, H.S., Almén, T., Morcos, S.K., and members of Contrast Media Safety Committee of European Society of Urogenital Radiology (ESUR). 2002. Gadolinium-containing contrast media for radiographic examinations: a position paper. *Eur. Radiol. 12*:2600–2605.

Thomsen, H.S., Morcos S.K., and members of Contrast Media Safety Committee of European Society of Urogenital Radiology (ESUR). 2004. Management of acute adverse reactions to contrast media. *Eur. Radiol. 14*:476–481.

Webb, J.A.W., Stacul, F., Thomsen, H.S., Morcos, S.K., and members of Contrast Media Safety Committee of European Society of Urogenital Radiology (ESUR). 2003. Late adverse reactions to intravascular iodinated contrast media. *Eur. Radiol. 13*:181–184.

Zagler, A., Azadpour, M., Mercado, C., and Hennekens, C.H. 2006. N-acetylcysteine and contrast-induced nephropathy: a meta-analysis of 13 randomized trials. *Am. Heart. J. 151*:140–145.

II

General Imaging Applications

1

The Accuracy of Diagnostic Radiology

Marilyn T. Zivian and Raziel Gershater

Introduction

Measures of diagnostic accuracy attempt to answer the following questions: "How well does this test distinguish disease from nondisease?" (Sunshine and Applegate, 2004) and/or "Does this test do a better job of distinguishing disease from nondisease than another test?" The present chapter describes commonly used measures of accuracy, including their inherent advantages and shortcomings, and highlights possible interactions between research design and measures of accuracy. These interactions will be discussed within the context of screening mammography and computer-aided detection (CAD) in screening mammography. Whenever possible, the authors' aim is to reach radiologists who may not be well versed in statistical and empirical methods. To that end we will try to present information about measures of accuracy and research design in ways that alleviate the usual quantitative and conceptual demands of these topics.

Traditional Methods of Measuring Diagnostic Accuracy

Proportions and Probability Estimates

Proportions and probability estimates form the basis for assessing the accuracy of diagnostic radiology; however

their use in the assessment of diagnostic radiology should not be taken for granted. Like all methods of assessment, the assessment of diagnostic accuracy reflects theoretical preconceptions and assumptions (McFall, 1999). The assumption underlying the use of proportions and probability estimates in assessing diagnostic radiology is that events in nature, including (1) human disease, (2) human judgments about the presence vs. the absence of disease, and (3) a technology's ability to spot disease are probabilistic, not deterministic (McFall, 1999). There will always be error. The goal of diagnostic radiology is to provide information that is accurate enough to improve our estimates of the probability of disease.

Conditional Probabilities and the 2 × 2 Contingency Table

Simple probabilities (e.g., the number of women with breast cancer divided by the total number of women in a population) do not contain enough information for assessing diagnostic accuracy. Conditional probabilities do. Conditional probabilities tell us that given a particular condition (e.g., the number of women who were screened who have breast cancer), what proportion was correctly diagnosed (true positive) or incorrectly diagnosed (false negative), and given the number of women who were screened who did not have breast cancer, what proportion was correctly diagnosed (true negative) or incorrectly diagnosed (false positive).

Conditional probabilities cannot be compared using one-dimensional models; multidimensional models are needed. The simplest multidimensional model is the 2 × 2 contingency table—a model with two dimensions and two categories on each dimension (Langlotz, 2003; McFall, 1999). For screening mammography, one of the dimensions consists of the radiologist's decisions divided into the following two categories: "Yes, I see evidence of breast cancer," vs. "No, I do not see evidence of breast cancer." Normally, the dimension consisting of the radiologist's decisions is represented on the horizontal axis, that is, from left to right. The second dimension, represented on the vertical axis, that is, from top to bottom, consists of two categories of the disease status in the screened women: yes, these women have breast cancer vs. no, these women do not have breast cancer (Table 1). Note that in each cell in Table 1, there are two labels for the cell frequency. One set consists of the usual labels used in diagnostic radiology—true positive, false positive, false negative, and true negative. The corresponding set of labels—hit, false alarm, miss, and correct rejection—is widely used outside of diagnostic radiology. The second set of labels will be used in this chapter because (1) we believe they describe the data in each cell more intuitively, accurately, and vividly, (2) they are shorter, and (3) they are the descriptive labels used in signal detection theory, the contemporary theoretical basis for measuring diagnostic accuracy (McFall, 1999).

Sensitivity, Specificity, and Overall Accuracy

Note also that each cell in Table 1 contains a joint frequency. For example, the top left cell of Table 1 contains the joint frequency of the number of women who actually have breast cancer and for whom the radiologist correctly diagnosed breast cancer, the radiologist's hits. The relevant conditional probabilities are obtained by dividing the frequency in each cell by the marginal total for each level of the conditional variable. The number of the radiologist's hits divided by the total number of patients who have breast cancer (the radiologist's hits + misses) is a measure of the radiologist's *sensitivity* when doing screening mammography (Black and Welch, 1997). Sensitivity is a measure of how well a diagnostic

test such as screening mammography performs in a sample of sick patients (Black and Welch, 1997; Langlotz, 2003). Similarly, the number of the radiologist's correct rejections divided by the total number of patients who did not have breast cancer (the radiologist's correct rejections + false alarms) is a measure of the radiologist's *specificity* when doing screening mammography (Black and Welch, 1997). Specificity is a measure of how well a diagnostic test performs in a sample of well patients.

Sensitivity and specificity are basic measures of the accuracy of diagnostic tests (Langlotz, 2003; Obuchowski, 2003a). They also appear to be the most popular indices of diagnostic accuracy in the radiological literature. They are diagnostic accuracy descriptors that do not vary greatly among patient populations (Langlotz, 2003). However, they can vary greatly among radiologists. A radiologist's individual sensitivity and specificity will depend on the cut-point at which he or she is willing to say, "Yes, I see disease" vs. "No, I do not see disease" (Black and Welch, 1997). Unfortunately from the standpoint of diagnostic radiology, cut-points are implicit; they exist in the mind of the radiologist (Obuchowski, 2003a). Cut-points depend on many factors, some of which vary reliably, such as a radiologist's belief in which diagnostic technique is more reliable, to others which vary randomly, such as being tired. Often, cut-points depend on which of the two possible errors, misses or false alarms, the radiologist believes it is more important to avoid.

In situations where misses are less desirable than false alarms (e.g., when evaluating women with a history of breast cancer), a diagnostic technique that is highly sensitive is more valuable than one that is highly specific (Langlotz, 2003). In order to minimize misses, radiologists may lower their thresholds (i.e., change their cut-points) for perceiving disease. This will increase the likelihood of their correctly perceiving an abnormality. Their number of hits will increase, and their number of misses will decrease. Their sensitivity will increase. In contrast, in situations where false alarms are less desirable than misses (e.g., radiologists may want to avoid unnecessarily recalling women with no history of breast cancer for further examinations); a diagnostic technique that is highly specific is more valuable than one that is highly sensitive. In order to minimize

Table 1   Standard 2 × 2 Contingency Table Used for Assessing Diagnostic Accuracy in Screening Mammography

Radiologist's Decision	Patient		Total
	Breast cancer present	Breast cancer absent	
"Yes, I see breast cancer."	Hit (true positive)	False Alarm (false positive)	Hits + False Alarms
"No, I don't see breast cancer."	Miss (false negative)	Correct Rejection (true negative)	Misses + Correct Rejections
Total	Hits + Misses	False Alarms + Correct Rejections	*N*

false alarms, radiologists may raise their thresholds for perceiving disease. This will decrease the likelihood of their incorrectly perceiving an abnormality. Their number of false alarms will decrease, and their number of correct rejections, increase. Their specificity will increase. From this it can be seen that sensitivity and specificity tend to be related; as one increases, the other generally decreases (Black and Welch, 1997).

Overall accuracy is also a popular index of diagnostic accuracy in the radiological literature, though perhaps somewhat less popular than sensitivity and specificity. The overall accuracy of a diagnostic test is calculated by adding hits and correct rejections and dividing by the total number of patients tested ([hits + correct rejections]/N). Like sensitivity and specificity, overall accuracy changes with changes in cut-point (Harvey, 2003).

The following extreme examples demonstrate how overall accuracy, sensitivity, and specificity may be misleading indicators of diagnostic accuracy when cut-points are changed to take into account the prevalence of disease in a population. Consider someone, like the first author of this chapter (MTZ), who knows nothing about reading X-rays, except that 90% of the people being X-rayed for a particular disease, let us call it disease A, are healthy. In order to maximize her performance, it is important for MTZ in this situation to avoid false alarms and obtain the highest possible specificity score. To accomplish this, her best strategy is to set her cut-point or threshold for "seeing" an abnormality as high as possible and always say, "No, I do not see any disease." Table 2a contains the cell frequencies in her 2 × 2 contingency table for this particular situation. Her overall accuracy would be 90% ([hits + correct rejections]/N—[0 + 180]/200), and her specificity (correct rejections/[correct rejections + false alarms]—180/[180 + 0]) would be 100%. Note that her overall accuracy is high (90%) and that she obtained the highest possible specificity score (100%) and the lowest possible number of false alarms (zero). In this particular example, neither specificity nor overall accuracy reflects the skill of the reader or the adequacy of the technology. Someone walking along the street, pointing at people randomly, and saying, "You do not have disease A," would, by chance, get the same specificity and overall accuracy scores as MTZ.

Sensitivity and overall accuracy, on the other hand, may be misleading indicators of diagnostic accuracy when the prevalence of disease in the population is high. Now, say that the only thing MTZ knows is that 75% of the people are likely to have disease A. Here, in order to maximize her performance, it is important for her to avoid misses and obtain the highest possible sensitivity score. She would set her cut-point or threshold for "seeing" an abnormality as low as possible and always say, "Yes, I see disease." Table 2b contains the cell frequencies of her 2 × 2 contingency table for her new strategy. Her sensitivity (hits/[hits + misses]) would be 100% (150/[150 + 0]), and her overall accuracy ([hits + correct rejections]/N) would be 75% ([0 + 150]/200). Note that now,

her overall accuracy is still good (75%) and that she obtained the highest possible sensitivity score (100%) and the lowest possible number of misses (zero). But again, her diagnostic accuracy is no better than what would be expected by chance.

Although these examples are extreme, they show how sensitivity, specificity, and overall accuracy shift with changes in a radiologist's cut-point or threshold for what is a normal vs. an abnormal finding. They also show how the choice of a cut-point interacts with the base rate (prevalence) of disease in a population, compounding the problems with sensitivity, specificity, and overall accuracy as measures of diagnostic accuracy. When the prevalence of disease is high, radiologists are more likely to lower their thresholds for perceiving disease. By chance, they will have more hits, as well as more false alarms. Their sensitivity will increase as their specificity decreases. When the prevalence is low, they are more likely to raise their thresholds for perceiving disease. By chance, they will have more correct rejections and more misses. Their specificity will increase as their sensitivity decreases. What is needed is a measure of diagnostic accuracy that is not affected by radiologists' changes in cut-points. If it also detects chance performance when it occurs, that would be an added advantage.

Signal Detection Theory

Engineers originally developed receiver operating characteristic (ROC) analysis to quantify how well an electronic receiver detects electronic signals in the presence of noise. The analysis acquired its name from its application to radar detection problems during World War II (McFall, 1999).

Similar to the traditional measures of diagnostic accuracy, signal detection theory relies on the raw frequencies

Table 2   MTZ's 2 × 2 Contingency Tables

a

MTZ's Decision	Patient		
	Unhealthy	Healthy	Total
"Unhealthy"	0	0	0
"Healthy"	20	180	200
Total	20	180	200

b

MTZ's Decision	Patient		
	Unhealthy	Healthy	Total
"Unhealthy"	150	50	200
"Healthy"	0	0	0
Total	150	50	200

in a basic, simple 2 × 2 contingency table. (See Table 3 for an example of the signal detection theory 2 × 2 contingency table [Heeger, 2003].) However, unlike the traditional measures of diagnostic accuracy, signal detection theory provides a metric and a graphic notation for quantifying diagnostic accuracy that is independent of cut-points or prevalence rates. Signal detection theory partitions the data produced by diagnostic tests into two independent components: a perceptual component and a decisional component (Harvey, 2003). The perceptual index is a measure of diagnostic accuracy. It represents, quantitatively, how well the test discriminates between patients with disease vs. patients without disease. The decisional index, in contrast, represents quantitatively the position of the cut-off score, or criterion, employed to arrive at the discriminations.

Receiver Operating Characteristic (ROC) Curves

Signal detection theory estimates diagnostic accuracy by analyzing the receiver (or relative) operating characteristic. Receiver operating characteristic curves are obtained by plotting hit rate [hits/(hits + misses)] on the *y*-axis and false alarm rate [false alarms/(correct rejections + false alarms)] on the *x*-axis of a two-dimensional graph. Each point on the ROC curve corresponds to a pair of hit and false alarm rates that result from use of a specific cut-off value. In the language of diagnostic radiology, the ROC curve is a plot of sensitivity (on the *y*-axis) against 1-specificity (on the *x*-axis) at all possible cut-points (Obuchowski, 2003a). A single graph captures all the cut-points a radiologist (or radiologists) could possibly have at a particular level of accuracy.

Figure 1 shows a set of five (including the diagonal) ROC curves, each representing a diagnostic test that differs in accuracy from the others. All ROC curves are anchored at (0,0) and (1,1) (Harvey, 2003). For any reasonable cut-point, the hit rate should always be larger than the false alarm rate, bowing the ROC curve upward (Heeger, 2003). The more bowed toward the upper left-hand corner the ROC curve, the more accurate the diagnostic test. Curves below the diagonal indicate a diagnostic procedure that is doing more poorly than chance. Hit and false alarm rates that fall on the main diagonal indicate that an individual is operating at the level of chance (Harvey, 2003).

As one moves along a specific ROC curve from the lower left corner (where hit and false alarm rate are both 0.0) to

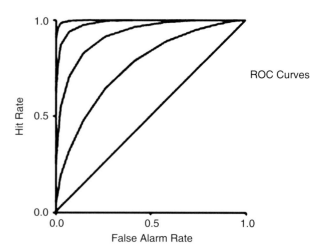

Figure 1 Receiver operating characteristic curves.

the upper right corner (where both are 1.0), the cut-point varies from maximally conservative (having a threshold or cut-point so high that one never perceives an abnormality) to maximally liberal (having a threshold or cut-point so low that one always perceives an abnormality) (Langlotz, 2003; McFall, 1999). A ROC curve can be thought of either as a series of points, each of which represents different radiologists with different thresholds or cut-points, or as a series of points, each of which represents a single radiologist moving along the ROC curve point by point from (0,0) to (1,1), lowering his or her cut-point while simultaneously increasing his or her hit and false alarm rates. By taking into account all possible cut-points, a ROC analysis, unlike sensitivity, specificity, and overall accuracy, is not affected by either changes in the cut-points of individual radiologists or differences in the cut-points of different radiologists.

Moreover, the ROC analysis, unlike sensitivity, specificity, and overall accuracy, would accurately assess the chance performance of MTZ. When the prevalence of disease in the population was very low, MTZ's hit rate [hits/(hits + misses)] and false alarm rate [false alarms/(correct rejections + false alarms)] would both have been 0.0, placing her at the lowest left-hand corner of the ROC graph (0,0), on the chance diagonal. When the prevalence of disease in the population was very high, MTZ's hit rate [hits/(hits + misses)] and false alarm rate [false alarms/(correct rejections + false alarms)] would have both been 1.0, placing her at the highest right-hand corner of the ROC graph (1,1) again, on the chance diagonal.

Finally, unlike sensitivity, specificity, and overall accuracy, ROC curves cannot be obtained from a single data set. They can, however, be generated in a variety of ways: (1) multiple pairs of hit and false alarm rates can be calculated from a single data set by asking radiologists to deliberately vary their cut-points; (2) diagnostic assessment methods can

Table 3   *General Signal Detection Table*

	Signal	
Observer's response	Present	Absent
"Yes"	Hit	False Alarm
"No"	Miss	Correct rejection

be used repeatedly with different decision criteria (i.e., from conservative to liberal) employed on a number of occasions, each occasion providing a different set of hit and false alarm rates; and (3) rating scale methods may used, in which raters classify images into one of two categories (disease absent vs. disease present) and also indicate their confidence level for the accuracy of their classification, typically on a 5-point scale (e.g., from "not at all confident" to "extremely confident"). In the latter case, multiple pairs of hit and false alarm rates can be obtained by treating each confidence level as a separate cut-point value (McFall, 1999); or (4) ROC curves can be constructed from objective measures of a diagnostic test (e.g., the five-category Breast Imaging Reporting and Data System, BI-RADS, used for mammography results). The only requirement is that the choices can be meaningfully ranked in magnitude.

Area under the ROC Curve (AUC)

Receiver operating characteristic curves enable a direct visual comparison of two or more diagnostic tests at all possible cut-points, and hit and false alarm rates can be easily read from the graph (McFall, 1999; Obuchowski, 2003a). Currently, the area under the ROC curve (AUC) is the preferred and most popular signal detection theory index of accuracy (McFall, 1999). The values for AUC can range from 0.0 (when the ROC curve passes from the lower left corner through the lower right corner to the upper right corner) to 1.0 (when the ROC curve passes from the lower left corner through the upper left corner to the upper right corner). A ROC curve with an area equal to 1.0 reflects perfect diagnostic accuracy. In contrast, a ROC curve with an area equal to 0.0 reflects perfect diagnostic inaccuracy. The diagonal line segment from (0,0) to (1,1), the chance diagonal, has an area of 0.5, indicating chance performance, for practical purposes the lower bound for diagnostic accuracy (McFall, 1999; Obuchowski, 2003a). Generally speaking, the greater the AUC, the better the accuracy of the diagnostic procedure (Langlotz, 2003). Computer programs exist that can be used to calculate AUC values. Statistical analyses (*t*-tests, etc.) may then be used to test whether one assessment measure (e.g., mammography without CAD) is significantly better than another (e.g., mammography with CAD) at discriminating between women with and without breast cancer.

Measures of AUC have several interpretations: (1) the average value of sensitivity for all possible values of specificity, (2) the average value of specificity for all possible values of sensitivity, and (3) the probability that a randomly selected patient with disease will have a test result that indicates a greater suspicion of disease than a randomly chosen patient without disease (Obuchowski, 2003a).

The usefulness of a diagnostic test in a practical setting is a function of the hit rate, false alarm rate, and prevalence of the disease. Radiologists must consider all three when choosing a cut-off. There is no true and unique optimal cut-point value. One approach for selecting optimal cut-off values that incorporate hit rate, false alarm rate, and prevalence of the disease combines signal detection theory analysis with a utility-based decision theory. That, however, is beyond the scope of the present chapter; for further information, see McFall (1999).

In Summary:

Both (1) the reliability (will a person [e.g., a radiologist] make the same decision [disease vs. no disease] to the same stimuli [e.g., a mammogram] over time) and (2) the validity (does the test measure what we think it measures) of the traditional indices of diagnostic accuracy (sensitivity, specificity, and overall accuracy) are affected by radiologists' cut-points or thresholds for diagnosing the presence or absence of disease. Furthermore, the prevalence of disease in the population may interact with radiologists' cut-points or thresholds, casting additional doubt on the indices' reliability and validity. In contrast, by taking into account radiologists' cut-points or thresholds, the indices based on signal detection theory (ROC curves and AUCs) provide a clear and significant advance over the traditional indices of diagnostic accuracy (McFall, 1999).

Threats to the accuracy of signal detection theory indices do exist, however. But they are not due to any weakness of signal detection theory itself (McFall, 1999). Rather they are due to weaknesses in experimental design. In mammography these include, but are not limited to: (1) inconsistent definitions of misses and false alarms, (2) systematic differences in radiologists' and/or pathologists' skill, and (3) a lack of knowledge about the instructions that radiologists and pathologists taking part in studies are following.

Mammography Screening: Misses and False Alarms

Different definitions of false alarms and misses result in different false alarm and hit rates, potentially raising or lowering AUC values. In some studies of diagnostic accuracy, all women who were recalled for any additional assessment but for whom no further evidence of malignancy was found are included in the false alarm count; in other studies, just women who have had negative biopsies are included. If only women who were recalled for biopsies are included, false alarm rates will be much lower than if women who are recalled for additional mammographic views are also included in the false alarm count (Black and Welch, 1997).

The definition of a miss depends on the length of the interval between a diagnosis of breast cancer and the prior screening mammogram. Some studies of diagnostic accuracy use the American College of Radiology's (ACR) definition of a miss as a diagnosis "of cancer within 1 year of a mammographic examination with normal or probably benign findings, BI-RADS 1 (negative), 2 (benign), or 3 (probably benign)". Other studies (e.g., Destounis *et al.*, 2004) use the Rules of the Mammography Quality Standard Act, which require that "Facilities must also include in their [systematic practice] audit any patients they become aware of who were subsequently found to have cancer that was not detected through their mammogram." According to the latter definition, the length of the interval between a diagnosis of breast cancer and the prior screening mammogram may be greater than 1 year.

An additional three months can have a significant impact on measures of diagnostic accuracy. Pisano *et al.* (2005) assessed the sensitivity [(hits/(hits + misses)] of film and digital mammography for the same patients after 455 days (1 year 3 months) and after 365 days (1 year). In the additional three months, the sensitivity of film mammography decreased from 0.66+/−0.03 to 0.41+/−0.03. (The results for digital mammography were comparable.) A total of 254 breast cancers were diagnosed within 365 days of the original screening mammography; an additional 81, between 365 and 455 days after study entry. All women who had been classified as correct rejections at their original screening mammogram, but had cancer at their follow-up mammogram, were reclassified as misses, accounting for probably most of the reduction in sensitivity at 455 days. The data make it clear that "estimates of sensitivity depend upon the definition used" for what constitutes a miss (Pisano *et al.*, 2005 p. 1779).

Since their values depend on hit and false alarm rates, ROC curves and their corresponding AUCs are not immune to differences in the definitions of misses and false alarms. Adopting standard definitions for both misses and false alarms would eliminate this threat to the reliability and validity of ROC curves and their corresponding AUCs as measures of diagnostic accuracy.

Mammography Screening: Radiologists and Pathologists

Without more precise descriptions of radiologists' and pathologists' skill levels and their instructions, study findings are difficult to interpret and compare. Most studies of the diagnostic accuracy of screening mammography contain rather complete descriptions of the patients (e.g., inclusion and exclusion criteria, recruitment, and sampling methods). Descriptions of the radiologists are often much less complete, and descriptions of the pathologists are mostly nonexistent. This is surprising since the radiologists, pathologists, and ultrasound readers (if any) directly determine diagnostic accuracy. They are the true subjects in the experiment. The patients supply their health status; they are the stimuli in the experiment.

The variability in radiologists' hit rate, false alarm rate, accuracy (as indicated by individual AUCs), and diagnos-

tic consistency has been well documented (Beam *et al.*, 1996; Elmore *et al.*, 1994). Unfortunately, the information that is provided about radiologists in studies of diagnostic accuracy (e.g., general descriptions of standards, accreditation, etc.) often does not indicate their level of skill. In one of the studies reviewed for the present chapter, radiologists who had met Mammography Quality Standard Act qualification standards and were asked to interpret mammograms and determine whether there was evidence of an "actionable lesion" had to be replaced because their sensitivity and/or specificity for a set of test mammograms was less than 50% (Burhenne *et al.*, 2000).

In addition, studies often do not report how the radiologists and/or pathologists were selected for a particular study. If (1) they were self-selected and if (2) systematic differences existed between those who volunteered and those who did not, measures of diagnostic accuracy are likely to be biased. The same, of course, would be true if there were systematic differences in how the radiologists and/or pathologists were selected by the study's researchers (Obuchowski, 2003b).

Furthermore, it seems that, although radiologists and pathologists are the subjects in experiments on diagnostic accuracy, they are rarely, if ever, given any explicit instructions, or at least, not any that are reported. If they are not following explicit instructions, they must be following implicit instructions. Consider the following: when radiologists are using computer-aided detection (CAD) programs for reading mammograms, the protocol requires that they must first interpret the mammograms without using CAD. They then review the same mammogram using CAD and may or may not change their interpretation. (Initial decisions to recall patients may not be reversed.) Gur *et al.* (2004) have voiced the concern that in studies where the protocol is followed, hit rates may be inflated because mammographic interpretations without and with CAD are reported on the same cases. Their hypothesis is that the radiologists may have a lower level of vigilance when first interpreting the mammograms because they know that they will be reviewing the films again with the use of CAD. If this is, in fact, what the radiologists are doing, it would make the diagnostic accuracy of CAD look better than it is. On the other hand, Birdwell *et al.* (2005) hypothesized that the opposite might be going on; that is, that radiologists will be overly vigilant when making their original interpretations because they know that anything they miss, which is then found when using CAD, will be recorded. If this is, in fact, what the radiologists are doing, the diagnostic accuracy of CAD would not be inflated. Either hypothesis may be true. We cannot choose between the two because we have no way of knowing which set of implicit instructions the radiologists are following. We do know, however, that their implicit instructions could be biasing measures of CAD's diagnostic accuracy.

In Summary:

All the indices of diagnostic accuracy, including the signal detection indices, are directly affected by differences in radiologists' and/or pathologists' skill. They may also be affected by biases in how radiologists and/or pathologists are recruited to take part in studies, as well as by the implicit instructions radiologists and pathologists may be following. Standard methods for (1) accurately and realistically assessing radiologists' and/or pathologists' levels of skill, (2) recruiting radiologists and/or pathologists to take part in studies, and (3) determining the explicit or implicit instructions they are following would eliminate these threats to ROC curves and their corresponding AUCS as reliable and valid measures of diagnostic accuracy.

Screening Mammography with Computer-Aided Detection (CAD)

Screening is the systematic testing of asymptomatic individuals for preclinical disease. The goal is to detect signs of breast cancer before there is any evidence of disease (e.g., a palpable mass) (Elmore and Carney, 2002) and to prevent or delay the development of advanced disease through early detection and treatment (Black and Welch, 1997).

Missed or late diagnoses of breast cancer are the leading cause of radiology malpractice lawsuits in the United States (Elmore and Carney, 2002). Approximately 25 to 30% of visible cancers are missed when mammograms are read by one reader (Freer and Ulissey, 2000). Even though cancer detection rates increase by 4.6 to 15% (Destounis et al., 2004; Taplin et al., 2000), as many as 25% of interval cancers and 19% of incident round cancers with detectable lesions are still missed when mammograms are double read (Keen, 2005).

It is thought that the following factors contribute to radiologists' failure to diagnose breast cancer: (1) the necessity of viewing a large number of images to detect a small number of cancers (just two to six cases of breast cancer are typically detected per 1000 mammograms in a screened population), (2) the complex radiographic structure of the breast, (3) the subtle nature of many mammographic characteristics of early breast cancer, and (4) radiologist fatigue or distraction. In addition, technical errors and limitations of the mammography technique itself may make it impossible to see a lesion.

Computers do not tire, do not forget, and do not get bored or distracted. Software able to decipher the complex structure of the breast and detect the subtle nature of many mammographic characteristics of early breast cancer could be a valuable adjunct to screening mammography. The ImageChecker 1000 series (R2Technology, 2006), reviewed below, consists of pattern recognition software that marks suspicious-looking regions on mammograms and brings them to a radiologist's attention. An asterisk indicates a pattern suggestive of a mass or an architectural distortion, and a solid triangle indicates an area of clustered bright spots suggestive of microcalcifications. The goal is to avoid misses without unduly increasing the number of false alarms (Castellino, 2005).

Computer-aided detection is not meant to replace the imaging technology; rather, it is an adjunct to mammography, an interpretive aid to be used during image review. When following the protocol, radiologists activate the CAD software only after having first interpreted a mammogram without using CAD. They then reevaluate the marked area(s) and issue a final report. The radiologist is responsible for making the diagnosis and deciding whether further diagnostic evaluation is warranted. If, on his or her initial reading, the radiologist identifies an abnormal area and that area is not marked by CAD, the radiologist is to still interpret the mammogram as abnormal and to recall the patient for further work-up (Castellino, 2005; Tec, 2002).

Mammography screening with CAD is not 100% sensitive; it misses some cancers. And it appears to be better at detecting malignant microcalcifications than malignant masses (Tec, 2002). Nor is mammography screening with CAD 100% specific. Current CAD systems generate many more false CAD marks than true CAD marks (Castellino, 2005). On average CAD places about one false mark per image (Tec, 2002). The ultimate responsibility for any finding lies with the radiologist. He or she is always the final judge.

The ImageChecker 1000 series (R2Technology, 2006) has been evaluated in retrospective, prospective, and historical studies with single or with double reading. In retrospective studies, first the membership of a group is defined. Then, the disease status of the group's members is determined from medical records produced prior to the beginning of the study (Sistrom and Garvan, 2004). In retrospective studies, it is difficult to simulate what is likely to occur when a new technology is actually introduced into everyday radiological practice. Decisions that would naturally occur in the normal course of interpreting screening mammograms are made by committees of radiologists, presumably to simulate differences in radiologists' skill, accuracy, and cutpoints. Most of the retrospective studies cited below used sets of different radiologists to judge whether an abnormality was visible in a prior mammogram or whether a lesion was actionable.

In historical studies, the disease status of a consecutive series of patients from a current clinical population is compared to historical controls. Generally speaking, comparing the diagnostic accuracy of an imaging technology in a current patient population to that in a historical control patient population is questionable. There is always the danger that the patient population in a historical control may be different (Sunshine and Applegate, 2004). In prospective studies, investigators follow up patients after the study's inception to collect information about the development of a disease (Sistrom and Garvan, 2004). Prospective studies are considered to be optimal for assessing the accuracy of a diagnostic test.

The studies reviewed for the present chapter included five retrospective studies: two single reading, Burhenne *et al.* (2000) and Vyborny *et al.* (2000) and three double reading (adding a second mammogram reader), Karssemeijer *et al.* (2003), Destounis *et al.* (2004), and CADET (Keen, 2005); two historical studies, both single reading, Gur *et al.* (2004) and Cupples *et al.* (2005); and four prospective studies: three single reading, Freer and Ulissey (2001), Morton *et al.* (2002), and Birdwell *et al.* (2005), and one double reading, Khoo *et al.* (2005).

The two single-reading, retrospective studies show that CAD has the potential to reduce the miss rate in screening mammography. Burhenne *et al.* (2000) determined that CAD would have detected 89 (77%) of 115 cancers that had been missed by the original radiologist, reducing the number of misses from 115 to 26, and Vyborny *et al.* (2000) showed that CAD was able to correctly mark 322 (86%) of the 375 masses interpreted by three radiologists to be spiculated on at least one view and 464 (79%) of the 585 masses that were classified as spiculated by at least one radiologist on one view.

The three double-reading, retrospective studies provide evidence that single reading with CAD in screening mammography may be as sensitive as double reading. Karssemeijer *et al.* (2003) used a special version of ImageChecker M1000 V2.0 that combined computer-aided detection with computer-aided diagnosis to compare single reading to independent double reading. The special version assigned a level of suspicion roughly corresponding to the probability that a region marked by CAD is cancerous. Hit rates for single reading without CAD, single reading with CAD, and double reading were 39.4%, 46.4%, and 49.4%, respectively. Unfortunately, the design of the experiment made it impossible for CAD to aid in avoiding misses. Even so, the data suggest that the addition of CAD may improve the hit rate of a single reader well enough to replace the second reader in double reading. Destounis *et al.* (2004) found that CAD has the potential to decrease miss rate at double reading by more than one-third (from 31 to 19%), and preliminary results (75% complete) presented at the 2004 Seventh International Workshop on Digital Mammography of the Computer Aided Detection Evaluation (CADET) study found that single reading with CAD detected significantly more cancers than double reading, but also produced a higher recall rate (Keen, 2005). Of the retrospective studies, the CADET study most closely simulates what can be expected to occur when CAD is actually introduced into everyday screening mammography.

One of the two studies using historical controls appears to show that CAD does what it is designed to do, and the other, that it does not. The Cupples *et al.* (2005) study found that the addition of CAD increased the cancer detection rate by 16.1% and the recall rate by 8.1%. Gur *et al.* (2004) found no difference in breast cancer detection rates or recall rates with or without the use of CAD. Both studies compared cancer detection rates with CAD in large samples of current patients to cancer detection rates without CAD in large samples of past patients (19,402 with CAD vs. 7872 without CAD in Cupples *et al.* [2005]; 56,432 with CAD vs. 59,139 without CAD in Gur *et al.* [2004]). Although it is unlikely, given such large numbers in the Gur *et al.* (2004) study, that there will be significant differences between the before-CAD and after-CAD groups, it is still possible that differences in the populations could account for the lack of an observed increase in cancer detection rates with CAD. Typically, the prevalence of cancer in patients being screened for the second and third time is lower than in patients undergoing mammography for the first time. The percentage of women who were screened for the first time decreased from approximately 40 to 30% in the Gur *et al.* (2004) study, but no adjustment was made for this confounding factor (Feig *et al.*, 2004). In addition to possible population differences, it learned improvement in screening ability over time could account for the observed increase in the cancer detection rates with CAD in the Cupples *et al.* (2005) study. Furthermore, neither study presented the data needed to calculate hit rates [hits/(hits + misses)]. Gur *et al.* (2004) presented no data at all on the number of misses, and although Cupples *et al.* (2005) reported that there were fewer misses with CAD, we do not know how many additional misses ultimately occurred among the current patients.

The results of the three single-reading prospective studies—Freer and Ulissey (2001), Morton *et al.* (2002), and Birdwell *et al.* (2005)—all appear to show that CAD does what it was designed to do. Freer and Ulissey (2001) found that the use of CAD increased (1) the number of cancers detected by 19.5%, (2) the proportion of early-stage malignancies detected, from 73 to 78%, and (3) the recall rate, from 6.5 to 7.7%. Morton *et al.* (2002) found that the use of CAD increased (1) the breast cancer detection rate by 6.46%, (2) the detection of early stage breast cancers from 73 to 79.37%, and (3) the recall rate from 9.82 to 10.89%. And Birdwell *et al.* (2005) reported that the use of CAD increased (1) the number of cancers detected by 7.4% and (2) the patient recall rate by just 0.79%.

It has been estimated that the double reading of screening mammograms increases sensitivity by 7 to 15% (Tec, 2002). The improvements in cancer detection, 19.5%, 6.5%, and 7.4%, reported by Freer and Ullisey (2001), Morton *et al.* (2002), and Birdwell *et al.* (2005), respectively, indicate that the addition of CAD could bring the sensitivity of single reading inline with that of double reading. However, the one prospective study comparing single reading with CAD to double reading, Khoo *et al.* (2005), appears to show that single reading with CAD is significantly less accurate than double reading. Sensitivities (calculated as a proportion of the total number of cancers detected by double reading with CAD) for single reading without CAD, single reading with CAD, and double reading without CAD were 90.2%, 91.5%, and 98.4%, respectively. The addition of CAD increased the recall rate by 5.8%.

The CAD algorithms are heavily biased toward sensitivity (avoiding misses) and less concerned about specificity (avoiding false alarms). For the first 5204 mammograms that Freer and Ulissey (2001) screened using CAD, a total of 14,214 computer marks were recorded, 368 (2.6%) of which were ultimately deemed actionable and 13,846 (97.4%) were dismissed. In the Khoo et al. (2005) study, 12 cancers were missed on single reading. Nine were correctly marked by CAD, but seven were overruled by the reader. Khoo et al. (2005) argued that the low specificity of CAD markings may explain why readers are more likely to ignore correct prompts. If the seven correct CAD prompts had not been ignored, the sensitivity of single reading with CAD (calculated as a proportion of the total number of cancers detected by double reading with CAD) would have come close to approximating that of double reading without CAD.

The ImageChecker M1000 series has a cut-point or threshold that maximizes hit rate at the expense of false alarm rate. If, however, radiologists' cut-points are set to avoid false alarms, they would be more likely to ignore and/or overrule a greater number of CAD markings than radiologists whose cut-points more closely match CAD's. Radiologists are the final arbiters of all radiological findings. A mismatch between the cut-points of the radiologists and the cut-point of CAD could account for the poorer diagnostic accuracy of screening mammography with CAD in the Khoo et al. (2005) study.

The results of the prospective studies appear promising; however they do not measure the diagnostic accuracy of adding CAD to mammography screening. We do not know how many interval misses, if any, ultimately occurred among the patients. Only Freer and Ulissey (2001) stated that they plan to follow their study group in order to identify and report any remaining misses.

Finally, by following the CAD protocol, the results of all the prospective studies may be biased in favor of CAD. When two tests, A (screening mammography without CAD) and B (screening mammography with CAD), are performed on the same patient and interpreted by the same reader, images that are read last will tend to be more accurately interpreted than images read first (Obuchowski, 2003b). In radiology, this is known as the reading order bias; in psychology, it is called the practice effect. Gur et al.'s (2004) fears about images being read twice by the same reader are well founded. However, an experiment that tests how well CAD (with the usual protocol) measures up to the accuracy of one reader simply reading every screening mammogram twice is a more direct way

of dealing with reading-order bias than Gur et al.'s (2004) solution of using historical controls. Straightforward prospective studies appear, too, not to be optimal for assessing the diagnostic accuracy of screening mammography with the addition of CAD.

Conclusion

In the first part of this chapter we described signal detection theory, a theory-based method of quantifying the accuracy of diagnostic systems. We showed that ROC curves and their corresponding AUCs provide a way of measuring diagnostic accuracy that is independent of changes in prevalence rates and radiologists' thresholds or cut-points. To the best of our knowledge there are no other methods that are as powerful.

In the second part of the chapter we demonstrated how (1) different definitions of false alarms and misses, (2) biases in the recruitment of radiologists and pathologists, (3) differences in radiologists' and pathologists' individual levels of accuracy, and (4) lack of knowledge about the instructions radiologists and pathologists are following in studies of mammography screening might affect measures of diagnostic accuracy, including ROC curves and their corresponding AUCs.

In the third, and final, part of the chapter we reviewed a number of studies and showed that the evidence is not good enough to demonstrate that the addition of CAD improves the diagnostic accuracy of mammography screening. If a practice effect or reading-order bias is operating, then the increases found in the number of cancers detected may not be due to the addition of CAD. Furthermore, because neither the historical nor the prospective studies have followed up their study populations to identify any interval misses, hit rates cannot be calculated, making it impossible to use signal detection theory. Weaknesses in research design will always undermine measures of diagnostic accuracy, no matter how powerful they are.

References

Beam, C.A., Layde, P.M., and Sullivan, D.C. 1996. Variability in the interpretation of screening mammograms by US radiologists: findings from a national sample. *Arch. Intern. Med. 156*:209–213.

Birdwell, R.L., Bandodkar, P., and Ikeda, D.M. 2005. Computer-aided detection with screening mammography in a university setting. *Radiology 236*:451–457.

Black, W.E., and Welch, H.G. 1997. Screening for disease. *Am. J. Radiol. 168*:3–11.

Burhenne, L.J.W., Wood, S.A., D'Orsi, C.J., Feig, S.A., Kopans, D.B., O'Shaughnessy, K.F., Sickles, E.A., Tabar, L., Vyborny, C.J., and Castellino, R.A. 2000. Potential contribution of computer-aided detection to the sensitivity of screening mammography. *Radiology 215*:554–562.

Castellino, R.A. 2005. Computer-aided detection (CAD): an overview. *Cancer Imag. 5*:17–19.

Cupples, T.E., Cunningham, J.E., and Reynolds, J.C. 2005. Impact of computer-aided detection in a regional screening mammography program. *Am. J. Radiol. 185*:944–950.

Destounis, S.V., DiNitto, P., Logan-Young, W., Bonaccio, E., Zuley, M.L., and Willison, K.M. 2004. Can computer-aided detection with double reading of mammograms help decrease the false-negative rate? Initial experience. *Radiology 232*:578–584.

Elmore, J.G., and Carney, P.A. 2002. Does practice make perfect when interpreting mammography? *J. Natl. Cancer Inst. 94*:321–323.

Elmore, J.G., Wells, C.K., Lee, C.H., Howard, D.H., and Feinstein, A.R. 1994. Variability in radiologists' interpretations of mammograms. *N. Engl. J. Med. 331*:1493–1499.

Feig, S.A., Sickles, E.A., Evans, W.P., and Linver, M.N. 2004. Re: changes in breast cancer detection and mammography recall rates after the introduction of a computer-aided detection system. *J. Natl. Cancer Inst. 96*:1260–1261.

Freer, T.W., and Ulissey, M.J. 2001. Screening mammography with computer-aided detection: prospective study of 12,860 patients in a community breast center. *Radiology 220*:781–786.

Gur, D., Sumkin, J.H., Rockette, H.E., Ganott, M., Hakim, C., Hardesty, L., Poller, W.R., Shah, R., and Wallace, L. 2004. Changes in breast cancer detection and mammography recall rates after the introduction of a computer-aided detection system. *J. Natl. Cancer Inst. 96*:185–190.

Harvey, L.O. 2003. Detection sensitivity and response bias. http://psych.colorado.edu/~lharvey/P4165_2003-Fall/2003_Fallpdf/P4165_SDT.pdf.

Heeger, D. 2003. Signal detection theory. http://www.cns.nyu.edu/david/sdt/set/html.

Karssemeijer, N., Otten, J.D.M., Verbeek, A.L.M., Groenewoud, J.H., de Koning, H.J., Hendriks, J.H.C.L., and Holland, R. 2003. Computer-aided detection versus independent double reading of masses on mammograms. *Radiology 227*:192–200.

Keen, C. 2005. Jury is still out on U.K. CAD utilization. *Women's imaging digital community*, Aunt Minnie.com. Accessed October 4, 2005.

Khoo, L.A.L., Taylor, P., and Given-Wilson, R.M. 2005. Computer-aided detection in the United Kingdom National Breast Screening Programme: prospective study. *Radiology 237*:444–449.

Langlotz, C.P. 2003. Fundamental measures of diagnostic examination performance: usefulness for clinical decision making and research. *Radiology 228*:3–9.

McFall, R.M. 1999. Quantifying the information value of clinical assessments with signal detection theory. *Ann. Rev. Psychol. 50*:215–241.

Morton, M., Amrami, K., Brandt, K., and Whaley, D. 2002. The effects of computer-aided detection (CAD) on a local/regional screening mammography program: prospective evaluation of 12,646 patients. *RSNA 2002*, 88th Scientific Assembly and Annual Meeting, Chicago, IL.

Obuchowski, N.A. 2003a. Receiver operating characteristic curves and their use in radiology. *Radiology 229*:3–8.

Obuchowski, N.A. 2003b. Special topics III: bias. *Radiology 229*:617–621.

Pisano, E.D., Gatsonis, C., Hendrick, E., Yaffe, M., Baum, J.K., Acharyya, S., Conant, E.F., Fajardo, L.L., Bassett, L., D'Orsi, C., Jong, R., and Rebner, M. for the Digital Mammographic Imaging Screening Trial (DMIST) Investigators Group. 2005. Diagnostic performance of digital versus film mammography for breast-cancer screening. *N. Engl. J. Med. 353*:1773–1783.

R2Technology. 2006. http://www.r2tech.com/main/home/index.php.

Sistrom, C.L., and Garvan, C.W. 2004. Proportions, odds, and risk. *Radiology 230*:12–19.

Sunshine, J.H., and Applegate, K.E. 2004. Technology assessment for radiologists. *Radiology 230*:309–314.

Taplin, S.H., Rutter, C.M., Elmore, J.G., Seger, D., White, D., and Brenner, R.J. 2000. Accuracy of screening mammography using single versus independent double interpretation. *Am. J. Radiol. 174*:1257–1262.

Technology Evaluation Center (Tec). 2002. Computer-aided detection (CAD) in mammography. BlueCross BlueShield Association Assessment Program, *17*(17):1–34.

Vyborny, C.J., Doi, T., O'Shaughnessy, K.F., Romsdahl, H.M., Schneider, A.C., and Stein, A.A. 2000. Breast cancer: importance of spiculation in computer-aided detection. *Radiology 215*:703–707.

2

Diffraction-Enhanced Imaging: Applications to Medicine

Moumen O. Hasnah, Z. Zhong, W. Thomlinson, and D. Chapman

Introduction

X-rays are one of the most commonly used forms of radiation in medical diagnostic imaging because of their ability to penetrate the body and yield quantitative morphological information. Although several interactions may occur, as the X-ray photons traverse the subject being radiographed, all of the common X-ray imaging techniques are based on absorption contrast. Soft tissues have density values that vary by 1 to 5%. The fact that the density variations of these tissues are small makes visualization of the difference between these tissues very difficult with conventional X-ray techniques. A number of imaging modalities of clinical relevance have been developed to address the problem of soft tissue imaging. These modalities typically use alternate methods of visualization based on sound propagation (ultrasound), proton density (magnetic resonance imaging: MRI), and others. In addition, enhancements to the X-ray technique include computed tomography (computed axial tomography: CAT) that has more sensitivity to tissue density, phase contrast methods relying on the phase of the traversing X-rays, and refraction methods such as diffraction-enhanced imaging (DEI).

Of these techniques, ultrasound, MRI, and CAT scans are presently common clinical techniques that are used to assist in the diagnosis and isolation of lesions in tissue. Diffraction-enhanced imaging is an emerging X-ray radiography technique based on monoenergetic X-rays (usually from a synchrotron X-ray source) that introduces two new sources of contrast to radiography besides the absorption. Because of the multiple sources of contrast, DEI is one of the most promising of the new X-ray imaging methods that has been shown to be clinically relevant.

Diffraction-Enhanced Imaging System

The diffraction-enhanced imaging system has several components (Fig. 1). We will focus on and introduce the major additional component, the crystal analyzer. The additional gain in contrast in DEI modality is derived from adding crystal diffraction optics (crystal monochrometer-analyzer), with the crystal analyzer placed between the sample and the detector. Only X-rays aligned within the angular acceptance of the crystal analyzer will be diffracted onto the detector. The angular acceptance is called the rocking curve of the crystal (Zachariasen, 1945). The width of this curve is a few microradians (Fig. 2). The crystal analyzer rejects all the photons that fall out of its angular acceptance, and within the acceptance, the intensity is modulated by the angle according to the shape of the rocking curve.

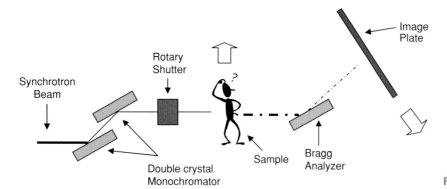

Figure 1 Schematic representation of the DEI setup.

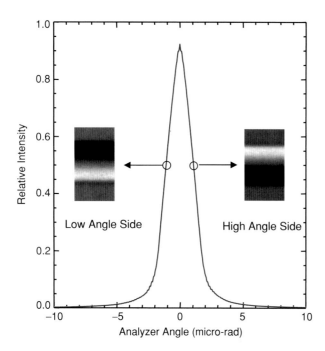

Figure 2 The Si(3,3,3) analyzer calculated rocking curve at 30 keV. considering the effects of the beam diffracted by the double Si(3,3,3) crystal monochromator. An image of nylon fiber is taken on each side of the rocking curve. The intensity is varied due to the slope of the rocking curve.

Principles of Diffraction-Enhanced Imaging

In DEI, an imaging beam is prepared by diffracting a polyenergetic beam from a crystal to create a very nearly monoenergetic imaging beam (Chapman *et al.*, 1997). This beam is then passed through the object being imaged. A matching crystal is placed between the object and the detector (Fig. 1). This crystal is set at or near the peak of the Bragg diffraction angle. Since the condition for diffraction from the analyzer crystal limits the X-rays that can be diffracted into

the detector, a high degree (microradians) of scatter rejection can result in improved image contrast. Such a high degree of scatter rejection is well beyond the capabilities of conventional antiscatter techniques, such as slit collimation and grids. The scatter that is rejected falls into a category referred to as small and ultra-small angle scattering (Zhong *et al.*, 2000). This type of scattering arises from structures with dimensions of a micron size and generally adds background noise that degrades contrast in a conventional radiograph. This scattering intensity is rejected in DEI, and thus image contrast is enhanced to reveal structural information that relates to ultra-small angle scattering. This scatter-rejection contrast is called extinction contrast, a term drawn from optics and X-ray diffraction to describe intensity loss due to diffraction and scattering. Therefore, in DEI, the image that represents the absorption of the object by X-rays is referred to as the apparent absorption image because it has contrast derived from both absorption and scatter rejection (extinction).

The analyzer rocking curve shape also introduces sensitivity to refraction occurring within the object when the crystal's angular orientation is detuned from the peak position. Density, thickness, and/or material variations in an object will refract the X-rays as they traverse the material. These small angular variations are generally in the submicroradian range. The steep sides of the reflectivity curve will convert these subtle angle variations into intensity variations, thus making refraction effects visible in an image. By acquiring an image pair with the analyzer set to diffract on each side of the rocking curve (on the low-angle side, θ_L, and the high-angle side, θ_H), we can separate refraction effects from combined absorption and extinction effects (Chapman *et al.*, 1997). The intensity of the images taken on the low-angle side, θ_L, and the high-angle side, θ_H, of the rocking curve is

$$I_L = I_{DEI} \left[R(\theta_L) + \frac{dR}{d\theta}(\theta_L)\Delta\theta_Z \right] \qquad (1)$$

$$I_H = I_{DEI} \left[R(\theta_H) + \frac{dR}{d\theta}(\theta_H)\Delta\theta_z \right] \qquad (2)$$

The expressions for I_L and I_H can then be used to derive two separate expressions for I_{DEI} and $\Delta\theta_z$, which describe the apparent absorption and refraction images (Fig. 3).

$$I_{DEI} = \frac{I_L R'(\theta_H) - I_H R'(\theta_L)}{R(\theta_L)R'(\theta_H) - R(\theta_H)R'(\theta_L)} \quad \begin{array}{l}\text{(Apparent}\\ \text{absorption}\\ \text{image)}\end{array} \qquad (3)$$

$$\Delta\theta_z = \frac{I_H R(\theta_L) - I_L R(\theta_H)}{I_L R'(\theta_H) - I_H R'(\theta_L)} \quad \text{(Refraction image)} \qquad (4)$$

where $R' = \frac{dr}{d\theta}$

In reviewing these DEI equations, it is clear that a number of parameters may play a role in the images obtained: specifically, the type of monochromator-analyzer, the lattice planes used in those crystals, the imaging energy, and the location of the analyzer when the images were acquired.

Thus, besides X-ray attenuation, DEI technique has introduced two additional sources of image contrast to X-ray radiography: refraction and extinction.

Diffraction-Enhanced Imaging Contrast Mechanisms

The additional sources of contrast from refraction and extinction have extended the usefulness of the radiography to a wide class of new systems including soft tissues in biological systems. It is of fundamental importance that the mechanisms of the new contrast sources be understood. The refraction contrast mechanism is well understood from an optical point of view extended to the X-ray wavelength range. At the X-ray energy typically used in medical imaging (17 to 100 keV), the absorption mechanism arises mainly from the photoelectric interaction. Refraction occurs primarily from variations in the projected electron density in the media. In both cases, contrast will arise from differences in absorption and refraction across the subject. Extinction contrast arises from the rejection of small-angle-scattering of X-rays by the object at the microradian level.

Absorption Contrast

Absorption contrast arises from the thickness of the target object, differences in density, and mass attenuation coefficient.

In the simple case where a single material object is embedded in a matrix material, the absorption contrast can be expressed as

$$\frac{\Delta I}{I} \cong \left(\frac{\mu_2}{\rho_2}\rho_2 - \frac{\mu_1}{\rho_1}\rho_1 \right)t \qquad (5)$$

where and μ_1/ρ_1 and ρ_1 and μ_2/ρ_2 and ρ_2 are the mass attenuation coefficients and densities for the two materials, respectively, and t is the thickness of the embedded object. The factors that affect the absorption contrast are therefore the thickness of the "embedded" object and the difference in the mass attenuation coefficients and the density.

Diffraction-enhanced imaging visualizes absorption contrast like the normal radiograph. However, DEI images are almost free of scatter because the scattered photons are rejected by the crystal analyzer. The combination of a well-defined incident beam and the angular and wavelength restrictions imposed by the analyzer prevent many of the photons that are widely scattered (photons that fall out of its angular acceptance of a few microradians) from being transmitted through to the detector.

Refraction Contrast

Like all other electromagnetic waves, X-rays refract at interfaces between different media. For most materials X-rays exhibit a refraction index slightly less than unity, typically ranging between $1-10^{-6}$ and $1-10^{-4}$. Therefore, they do not refract very much through materials, but pass right through with only small deviation from the original direction of propagation. The refraction angle $\Delta\theta_z$ that arises as the X-ray beam crosses two materials is closely approximated by Hasnah et al. (2002):

$$\Delta\theta_z \cong \frac{1}{4\pi} r_e \frac{\lambda^2}{m_n} (\rho_2 - \rho_1) \frac{dt}{dz} \qquad (6)$$

where r_e is the classical electron radius, λ is the X-ray wavelength, ρ is the material density, m_n is the nucleon mass, and dt/dz is the thickness gradient of the embedded object in the direction perpendicular to the beam direction.

This angular deviation of the X-ray photons from their original direction is too small to be directly measured, but is translated into intensity variations according to the analyzer rocking curve (Zachariasen, 1945). This intensity variation is the origin of refraction contrast. The factors that affect the refraction contrast are therefore the difference in densities and the gradient of the thickness of the embedded object. Diffraction-enhanced imaging visualizes refraction contrast as

$$\frac{\Delta I}{I} = C\lambda\Delta\rho\frac{dt}{dz} \qquad (7)$$

where C is a constant proportional to the slope of the rocking curve shoulder that depends on the diffraction planes, and the type of the crystal analyzer.

Extinction Contrast

Extinction for DEI means the loss of intensity due to scattering of the beam through angles comparable to the rocking curve width. This is typically caused by subvisible (specifically, subpixel dimension) features, occurring as the beam traverses the subject. For example, this can occur from small embedded spheres in a matrix material of differing density that scatter the beam. The intensity lost from the direct beam due to this scattering can be characterized with linear extinction coefficient χ_2. Then extinction contrast in terms of intensity is

$$E = \frac{I_0 - I_0 e^{-\chi_2 t}}{I_0} = 1 - e^{-\chi_2 t} \cong \chi_2 t \qquad (8)$$

where $\chi_2 = \rho_s \dfrac{d\sigma_s}{d\Omega}$, and ρ_s is the density of scatters per unit volume.

So, the factors that affect the extinction contrast are seen to be the thickness of the target and the extinction coefficient. It should be pointed out that the extinction contrast mechanism is characteristic of the DEI technique and requires a somewhat detailed investigation.

Diffraction-Enhanced Imaging Contrast Mechanisms in Breast Cancer Specimens

Screening mammography for breast cancer has generated considerable controversy in recent years. One of the controversial aspects of the procedure is the high incidence of false positives that puts the patient through a great deal of uncertainty and stress while other more invasive diagnostic methods are used to evaluate suspicious lesions. Even though screening mammography is the best tool for early detection of breast cancer, radiologists do not detect all cancers that are visible on images in retrospect. One reason for missed detections is the low contrast of the features that typically indicate a cancerous subject. A method to uniquely determine the presence of cancer with higher degree of certainty would be of great benefit in improving the diagnostic ability of mammography.

Compared with the absorption contrast of conventional radiography, DEI holds the promise of making features in objects more visible by one or some combination of its additional contrast mechanisms. It has been shown that DEI can improve visualization of the spiculations that are frequent features of cancer in breast tissue specimens and thus potentially might be useful for the early detection of that disease (Pisano *et al.*, 2000). These results indicate that features in DEI refraction images correlate histologically with cancer or

with fibrosis in the surrounding tissue. One of the key points of the analysis was the use of the DEI refraction images. These images show very clearly the boundaries of the cancerous tissues (Fig. 3).

Diffraction-Enhanced Imaging Conventional Radiography: Comparison of Contrast Mechanisms in Breast Cancer Specimens

To compare the contrast mechanisms of DEI and conventional radiography, a brief analysis of the absorption, refraction, and extinction contrasts is in order. For a structured object comprising two materials (material #2 is embedded in material #1 and has a thickness t_2 along the beam propagation direction, y), it can be shown that the refraction angle of X-rays traversing the object is (Hasnah *et al.*, 2002):

$$\Delta\theta_z \cong \left(\alpha_2 - \alpha_1\right)\frac{dt_2}{dz} \cong \Delta\alpha_{DEI}\frac{dt_2}{dz} \qquad (9)$$

Here $\Delta\alpha_{DEI}$ is the difference in refractive index between the two materials, and $\dfrac{dt_2}{dz}$ is the gradient of the thickness of material #2. The density change $\Delta\rho$ can be:

$$\Delta\rho \cong 2\pi \frac{m_n}{r_e \lambda^2}\Delta\alpha_{DEI} \qquad (10)$$

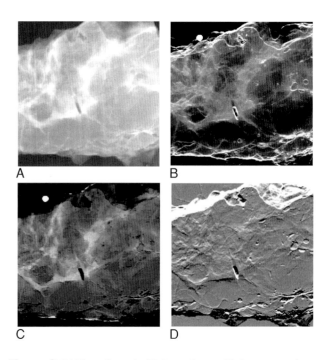

Figure 3 (**A**) The radiograph, (**B**) the top image, (**C**) the apparent absorption image, (**D**) the refraction image.

Absorption contrast can be shown to depend on the density of the two materials as well. For a two-component system in which the material #2 is embedded in material #1 and material #2 is thin ($\mu_2 t_2 \ll 1$) with thickness t_2:

$$\left(\frac{\Delta I}{I}\right)_{RAD} \cong (\mu_2 - \mu_1)t_2 \equiv \Delta\mu_{RAD}t_2 \qquad (11)$$

Here $\Delta\mu_{RAD}$ is the difference in the linear attenuation coefficients between the two materials. I is the intensity or photon counts obtained in a pixel for a radiograph and ΔI is the difference in intensity between two pixels, one with material #2 and one without it.

For cancer in soft tissue, we can model the absorption difference between the tissues as a density difference with an average $\frac{\mu}{\rho}$. The cancerous tissue is assumed to have a thickness of t_2. The contrast is then:

$$\left(\frac{\Delta I}{I}\right)_{RAD} \cong \frac{\overline{\mu}}{\rho}(\rho_2 - \rho_1)t_2 \cong \frac{\overline{\mu}}{\rho}\Delta\rho t_2 \qquad (12)$$

A comparison of Equations (9), (10), and (12) shows that the DEI refraction image and the radiograph share the same dependence on the density variations to visualize embedded objects that are different in density with respect to their surroundings. However, the mechanism of visualization is significantly different. The refraction image depends on the gradient in the thickness of the embedded object, a feature that strongly highlights the edges of the object, while the absorption image depends on the thickness of the embedded object. Therefore, there is a complementary behavior between these two images in terms of feature visualization.

The scatter-loss contrast mechanism (extinction) can be defined in a similar manner as the linear absorption coefficient. This parameter will be referred to as χ. A similar equation to that of Equation (11) can be derived for the change in intensity due to rejection of this scattering:

$$\left(\frac{\Delta I}{I}\right)_{ext} \cong (\chi_2 - \chi_1)t_2 \qquad (13)$$

Here $\left(\frac{\Delta I}{I}\right)_{ext}$ is the contrast of material #2 relative to the surroundings due to extinction alone. It should be noted that this intensity loss would depend on the setting of the analyzer crystal because the scattering has an angular dependence, as opposed to the linear absorption coefficient. Therefore, Equation (13) is approximate, and the values of χ will depend strongly on the analyzer setting while the image is being taken. Therefore, we expect that the value of this contrast will be higher when images are taken near the peak of the transmitted beam (TOP location) than the images acquired at the ½ peak locations used for the DEI refraction angle analysis (DEI locations) (Zhong *et al.*, 2000).

Since the extinction contrast appears in a similar manner to that of the absorption contrast, the DEI apparent absorption image (DEI subscript) and the DEI top image (TOP subscript) will have the combined contrast,

$$\left(\frac{\Delta I}{I}\right)_{DEI,TOP} \approx \left[(\mu_2 - \mu_1) + (\chi_2 - \chi_1)\right]t_2 \qquad (14)$$
$$\equiv \Delta\mu_{DEI,TOP}t_2$$

$\left(\frac{\Delta I}{I}\right)_{DEI,TOP}$ is the contrast of material #2 relative to its surroundings when it is imaged with the DEI system for the two situations, either from the DEI apparent absorption image (DEI subscript) or the DEI top image (TOP subscript). $\Delta\mu_{DEI,TOP}$ is the difference in the linear attenuation coefficient for these two DEI imaging situations.

A quantitative comparison study was done on DEI and conventional radiograph images of breast cancer specimen that contains invasive lobular carcinoma to investigate the above analysis. Figure 4 shows a radiograph of a breast specimen that contains invasive lobular carcinoma. This sample has undergone histologic evaluation to confirm that the fibrils in the box correspond to fingers of tumor extending from the surface of the tumor. The region is shown in an expanded view in Figures 4B–E. These expanded views represent the images obtained with radiography (4B) and the DEI technique (refraction image, (4C), apparent absorption, (4D), and top of the rocking curve image, (4E). In these expanded views, one can easily see the difference that each visualizes. Each expanded view is marked with a number of vertical lines in which the analysis is applied.

The results for the boxed region indicated in Figure 4 are given in Table 1. The rows correspond to data taken from the region indicated in the figures. The $\Delta\mu_{RAD}$ column is the result of the data shown in the radiograph, Figure 4B; $\Delta\alpha_{DEI}$ is from the DEI refraction, Figure 4C; $\Delta\mu_{DEI}$ is from the DEI apparent absorption, Figure 4D; and $\Delta\mu_{TOP}$ is from the DEI "top" image, Figure 4E. The density change across the fibril, $\Delta\rho$, is derived from the refractive index change $\Delta\alpha_{DEI}$ from the DEI refraction image using Equation (9). The $\Delta\rho$ derived from the DEI images is used to estimate the increase in contrast that will occur in absorption due to density variations. This estimated absorption contrast is calculated using Equation (12). This value can be compared with the measured absorption contrast of radiography, $\Delta\mu_{RAD}$. The $\Delta\mu_{DEI}$ is given for the same region in Table 1. Note that the values obtained from the apparent absorption are significantly larger than those found by radiography and are also larger than expected from a density variation alone. This indicates that the fibrils have a significant extinction component.

To verify this interpretation, a final column of measured data is taken from the DEI system top image. The analysis of these data is indicated in the $\Delta\mu_{TOP}$ column of Table 1. Again notice that these values are still larger than the apparent

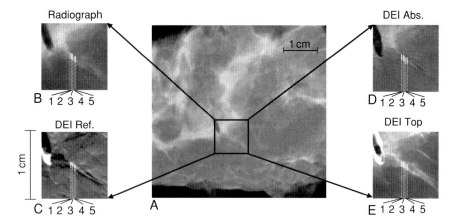

Figure 4 Breast tissue sample with invasive lobular carcinoma. Figure **A** is a synchrotron radiograph of the sample. Figures **B**, **C**, **D**, and **E** are expanded views of the box. The vertical lines are the regions analyzed. Figure **B** is an expanded view of the conventional radiograph; **C** is the DEI refraction image, **D** is the DEI apparent absorption image, and **E** is the DEI top image.

absorption and radiography values. Because both $\Delta\mu_{DEI}$ and $\Delta\mu_{TOP}$ contain combined extinction and absorption effects, an estimate of the extinction component can be found by subtracting $\Delta\mu_{RAD}$ from them. A normalized contrast gain is defined as:

$$Contrast\ Gain_{DEI,TOP} = \frac{\Delta\mu_{DEI,TOP} - \Delta\mu_{RAD}}{\Delta\mu_{RAD}}$$
$$= \frac{\Delta\chi_{DEI,TOP}}{\Delta\mu_{RAD}} \quad (15)$$

These contrast gain values are indicated in the last two columns of Table 1 for both the DEI apparent absorption image and the top image. Note that the contrast gain for DEI is several times that of the radiographic value (~ 8-fold higher). This is due entirely to the presence of extinction (or scatter-rejection) contrast from the fibrils. Also, the DEI top images of the same regions have a further enhancement of this contrast mechanism. The contrast gain is approximately another factor of 2 higher than the DEI values (~ 12-fold).

In conclusion, results show that both DEI refraction image and conventional X-ray absorption contrast depend on the density difference between the two materials (fibrils and normal tissue) as would be expected. This implies that

they share the same physical mechanism, the increased density of the cancerous fibril tissue. However, the refraction angle depends on the gradient of the thickness. This property of the refraction image makes it very sensitive to the edges of embedded objects, while the absorption image is most sensitive to the thick region of the object. This complementary behavior of the refraction angle image and the absorption image is an advantage of the DEI technique in determining the boundaries of cancerous tissues.

In comparison, the contrast of the DEI apparent absorption far exceeds that due to a density increase alone. The implication is that an additional contrast mechanism is present (i.e., that of extinction). As further proof of this mechanism, the analysis was also applied to the image taken at the top of the rocking curve where extinction will have the largest effects. The contrast obtained from the image at the top of the rocking curve has the highest value of all (from 8-fold higher contrast compared to the conventional radiograph).

We conclude that extinction plays a major role in the DEI contrast of fibrils in breast tissues. It appears from these limited measurements that spiculations, a sign present due to cancer itself or to the fibrotic response of the host to the cancer, has extinction as a dominating contrast mechanism when

Table 1   Results of Analysis for Lines Crossing Fibrils shown in Figure 4 for the Specimen Containing Invasive Lobular Carcinoma (The Bottom Row Contains the Averages for the Lines in these Boxes)

Line	$\Delta\alpha_{DEI}$ (10^{-6})	$\Delta\rho$ (g/cm³)	$\Delta\mu_{RAD}$ (cm⁻¹)	$\Delta\mu_{CALC}$ (cm⁻¹)	$\Delta\mu_{DEI}$ (cm⁻¹)	$\Delta\mu_{TOP}$ (cm⁻¹)	Contrast Gain (DEI)	Contrast Gain (TOP)
1	0.0149 ± 0.001	0.0232	0.025 ± 0.004	0.0229	0.179 ± 0.01	0.24 ± 0.07	6.16	8.72
2	0.0137 ± 0.001	0.0214	0.023 ± 0.002	0.0211	0.172 ± 0.03	0.24 ± 0.05	6.47	9.52
3	0.0170 ± 0.002	0.0181	0.019 ± 0.001	0.0178	0.164 ± 0.02	0.23 ± 0.07	7.63	10.94
4	0.0124 ± 0.001	0.0194	0.016 ± 0.002	0.0191	0.174 ± 0.01	0.25 ± 0.04	9.87	14.43
5	0.0127 ± 0.001	0.0200	0.016 ± 0.003	0.0197	0.157 ± 0.03	0.26 ± 0.01	8.81	15.50
Avg.	0.014	0.020	0.020	0.020	0.169	0.24	7.8	11.8

imaged with the DEI system. This leads to the possibility that the combination of DEI contrast mechanisms may allow this important feature to be more evident to the reader of diffraction-enhanced mammograms. This might permit for the earlier detection of the underlying malignancy, because spiculations are the most pathognomonic sign of malignancy, either when they are associated with a mass itself or when the mass is not obvious but there is architectural distortion in the surrounding breast tissue (Tabar and Dean, 1985).

References

Chapman, D., Thomlinson, W., Johnson, R.E., Washburn, D., Pisano, E., Gmur, N., Zhong, Z., Menk, R., Arfelli, F., and Sayers, D. 1997. Diffraction enhanced X-ray imaging. *Phys. Med. Biol. 42*:2015–2025.

Hasnah, M., Zhong, Z., Oltulu, O., Pisano, E., Johnston, R., Sayers, D., Thomlison, W., and Chapman, D. 2002. Diffraction enhanced imaging contrast mechanisms in breast cancer specimens. *Med. Phys. 29*:2216–2221.

Pisano, E.D., Johnston, R.E., Chapman, D., Geradts, J., Iacocca, M.V., Livasy, C.A., Washburn, D.B., Sayers, D.E., Zhong, Z., Kiss, M.Z., and Thomlinson, W. 2000. Diffraction enhanced imaging of human breast cancer specimens: improved conspicuity of lesion detail with histologic correlation. *Radiology 214*:895–901.

Tabar, L., and Dean, P.B. 1985. *The Mammographic Teaching Atlas.* New York: Georg Thieme Verlag.

Zachariasen, W.H. 1945. *Theory of X-Ray Diffraction in Crystals.* Chapter 4. New York: John Wiley & Sons.

Zhong, Z., Thomlinson, W., Chapman, D., and Sayers, D. 2000. Implementation of diffraction enhanced imaging experiments at the NSLS and APS. *Nucl. Instrum. Methods. Phys. Res. 450*:556–567.

3

Role of Imaging in Drug Development

Mihailo Lalich, Teresa M. McShane, and Glenn Liu

Introduction

The practice of oncology has evolved from the use of cytotoxic compounds that nonselectively inhibit cells actively engaged in the cell cycle toward newer targeted agents that can block particular pathways important for neoplastic transformation, growth, and metastasis. The ultimate hope is that individualized drugs can induce tumor regression (or prevent progression) while avoiding the common toxicities attributed to conventional cytotoxic chemotherapy. Within the last 10 years, the approval of several targeted agents has led some to believe that our current system for drug development is adequate. Examples of such successes include the anti-HER-2/*neu* antibody trastuzumab in HER-2 overexpressing breast cancer; the c-Kit tyrosine kinase inhibitor imatinib in gastrointestinal stromal tumors (GISTs) and chronic myelogeneous leukemia; the epidermal growth factor receptor (EGFR) inhibitors erlotinib in lung cancer and cetuximab in colon cancer; the proteosome inhibitor bortezomib in multiple myeloma; and more recently the multitargeted tyrosine kinase inhibitors sorafenib in kidney cancer and sunitinib in kidney cancer and GISTs. However, this ignores the considerable costs in financial expenditures, large numbers of patients, and time required for the development of these agents. While the goal of drug development has remained the same (e.g., bring promising new drugs to the patients in need), for every 5000 compounds currently in preclinical development, only five agents enter clinical trials. The overall average cost of a drug approved by the Food and Drug Administration is ~ \$802 million (DiMasi *et al.*, 2003). With the wealth of new agents being discovered, the current drug development paradigm is being challenged. It is clear that there are limitations in financial and human resources, and thus there is a demand for more efficient mechanisms of studying these newer drugs. For information related to this subject, see the chapter by Miller and colleagues in the first volume of this series.

This chapter will focus on the emerging role of novel radiographic imaging in the drug development process. Our goal is to provide an overview for the current understanding of how imaging can facilitate drug development. A number of examples of imaging applications used in clinical trials, placed in perspective with the traditional conduct of trials, will help to illustrate the prospects of these techniques. Recommendations for the need to incorporate functional imaging into future trials will be made, with an emphasis placed on technical considerations, trial design, and practical issues. Lastly, barriers and limitations in the use of imaging in drug development will be discussed.

Drug Development

Historical Perspective

Although the practice of medicine has been ongoing for hundreds of years, the field of oncology is still in its infancy.

The era of chemotherapy began with initial observations of the effects of mustard gas and folates on hematopoietic cells, leading to the development of alkylating agents and antifolates in the 1940s. The 1950s brought forth widespread screening of the diverse plant and marine compounds found in nature and, fueled by programs at the National Cancer Institute, yielded several important drug classes, including the taxanes, camptothecans, and vinca alkaloids. Although these efforts were successful, progress was slow. By the 1970s and 1980s, on average, only four to five new oncology drugs per five-year period were being approved by the FDA. The pace quickened by the early 1990s, when increased understanding of cell biology introduced thousands of potential new drug targets (Chabner and Roberts, 2005). This resulted in some new challenges. With the growing field of oncology and hundreds of combinations of cytotoxic chemotherapy regimens being concocted by investigators worldwide, uniformity in reporting results was needed.

Defining Benefit

Early chemotherapy trials focused on palliative benefits in symptomatic patients. Palliative end points that have significance for patients include relief of pain, maintenance of performance status, changes in quality of life scores, and improvements in body weight. Approval of drugs based primarily on palliative outcomes is now uncommon, but examples from the modern chemotherapy era include gemcitabine for pancreatic cancer and mitoxantrone for prostate cancer. While symptom palliation is a noble goal, it is a subjective end point that can be greatly influenced by patient selection.

The gold standard measure of benefit in clinical trials is improvement in survival. Overall survival is the benchmark by which most Phase III studies are evaluated. It is subject to the least amount of ambiguity in interpretation or measurement, and provides a definitive framework against which a new drug can be assessed. The main disadvantage of using survival as a primary end point, however, is that compared with other measures of drug activity, it requires the longest follow-up period. Depending on the natural history and stage of the cancer being studied, it may take many years to reach survival end points. While reasonable in a setting where there are limited treatment options, with newer regimens and agents available, this end point can be difficult to assess as crossover to other experimental therapies may diminish the survival benefit observed with a new drug (Schilsky, 2002). What was needed was an intermediate, or surrogate, end point that could more quickly predict benefit with a level of confidence acceptable to clinicians and patients.

Since the earliest chemotherapy trials, the ability of drugs to reduce tumor size has been equated with benefit, and thus radiologic imaging has served as an important measure of response. The introduction of computed tomography (CT) in the 1970s dramatically improved spatial resolution and broadened the role of imaging in assessing response to therapy. The universal availability, short acquisition time, and applicability to most tumor types have made CT the current mainstay of response evaluation in clinical trials. The World Health Organization (Miller *et al.*, 1981) called for standardized reporting of tumor responses as part of all clinical trials in the late 1970s. These criteria were more recently updated and revised into the Response Evaluation Criteria in Solid Tumors (RECIST) guidelines (Therasse *et al.*, 2000) in which a minimum percentage decrease (or increase) in measurable tumor lesions was required in order to characterize a patient as either a treatment responder or progressor. This minimum change took into account technical considerations (CT quality and acquisition slice width) as well as subjective measurements from the radiologist or investigator, and thus provided as best as possible a standard for the reporting of objective tumor responses.

Clinical Trials

Phase I trials: Testing of novel agents in humans begins in Phase I studies. The conduct of a traditional oncology Phase I trial typically entails the enrollment of 15 to 40 patients into cohorts that receive a fixed dose of the experimental drug. The dose level continues to escalate until the maximum tolerated dose (MTD) of the drug is found. This dose-escalation schema assumes that there will be a dose-response relationship with the drug, such that the highest dose of the drug given will result in the greatest antitumor effect. The goals of Phase I studies are to evaluate the safety of the new drug and to define the proper dose for subsequent trials. *Phase II trials*: Phase II studies aim to establish benefit in a given tumor type. They typically involve a population of 30 to 100 patients with the same tumor type. Although various end points including symptom palliation, time to progression, and survival can be used, the most common modern end point is the radiographic response rate. Further refinements of the dose or dosing schedule of the drug may be made, and additional toxicity and correlative data collected. The ultimate goal of Phase II studies is to select therapies with sufficient promise, in terms of both efficacy and safety, to justify ongoing testing in a Phase III trial. *Phase III trials*: The largest and most definitive trials are the Phase III studies. The experimental drug is compared in a randomized manner to the standard treatment, which serves as a control. The primary aim is to establish clinical benefit, so these trials are ideally powered to demonstrate prolongation in survival or time to progression. In general, hundreds to thousands of patients are required.

Food and Drug Administration Approval

The ultimate aim of the clinical trial process is to bring promising new drugs to the public. Every step in drug development is undertaken in view of the regulatory requirements that will eventually need to be satisfied for FDA approval. The FDA requires that the drug shows an acceptable safety profile and adequate clinical benefit in a defined patient population. Safety is demonstrated in Phase I and II studies, and it is unusual for new or unanticipated safety concerns to appear in Phase III. However, Phase III provides the longest duration of follow-up, and continued proof of safety remains a prerequisite for FDA approval. Clinical benefit can be expressed by a variety of measures; therefore, the main question becomes how much and what type of benefits are necessary for FDA approval. In the early 1980s, the FDA declared that improvements in survival or symptoms were necessary for oncology drug approval. To this day, demonstration of a survival benefit remains the most secure means of obtaining drug acceptance. While improvement in symptoms or quality of life has earned drug approval in the past, it currently is used mainly to complement survival data or other primary end points.

Limitations in achieving survival end points in Phase III studies have introduced a need for other suitable end points. In 1992, the FDA adopted the "accelerated approval" process. These rules allow for drug approval based on surrogate end points, such as time to progression, progression-free survival, or tumor response, which are reasonably likely to predict clinical benefit. New agents meeting these conditions may be approved with the caveat that a subsequent Phase IV study will be completed to confirm clinical benefit. If such postmarketing studies are not done, the FDA has the authority to withdraw drug approval. Between 1992 and 2004, 22 agents have been granted accelerated approval. The majority was approved based on an improvement in response rate, often demonstrated in uncontrolled Phase II trials. Of interest, only six of these agents have undergone confirmatory Phase IV testing (Abrams *et al.*, 2005). A prominent example of a novel agent granted such accelerated approval is imatinib for unresectable GISTs.

Current Status and Issues

The traditional drug development system has been based on the development of cytotoxic chemotherapeutic agents, an era characterized by sluggish drug development and small increments of progress. While this system has served us well for a number of years, the shift toward less toxic, predominantly cytostatic agents renders the existing paradigm inadequate. This inadequacy is seen throughout the entire drug development process. For example, the notion of dosing to the "maximal tolerated dose" in the Phase I setting may not be appropriate, especially for agents with little or no toxicity. During the Phase II process, assessing for objective radiologic responses, especially for a drug with presumed cytostatic activity, may lead to the abandonment of many agents with potential activity that cannot be recognized by

routine imaging with CT or magnetic resonance imaging (MRI). Specifically, spatially defined tumor responses serve only as a surrogate marker for more definitive measures of therapeutic benefit, such as overall survival. However, they may fail to account for measures of antitumor activity that are not reflected in tumor shrinkage, such as those seen with cytostatic agents (Therasse, 2002). Similarly, for Phase III testing, the length of time required, patient resources, and expenditures necessary to prove a benefit in overall survival are difficult to accept.

The total cost (in year 2000 dollars) of developing one new drug for FDA approval is ~ $802 million. This represents an inflation-adjusted increase from $318 million in 1991 and $138 million in 1979, or an annual rate increase of 7.4%. These expenditures include the costs of drugs that failed and were abandoned during testing (DiMasi *et al.*, 2003). The average cost of completing a single Phase III trial alone is estimated to be $10–20 million for an industry-sponsored drug, and $1 million for an NCI-sponsored drug (Roberts *et al.*, 2003). Concomitant with the high drug costs are the high failure rates of agents entering Phase II and III trials. It is estimated that only one in ten new drugs brought into clinical trials will eventually proceed to FDA approval. As Phase II trials seek to establish a preliminary response rate for the first time in humans, it is not surprising that many drugs are halted at this stage for failure to show sufficient activity. Evidence of prior activity *in vitro* or in animal models may translate poorly to activity in humans. Also, failure to adequately prove appropriate biologic responses (i.e., the drug is effective against its intended target) in Phase I studies may lead to attrition in Phase II. Even when drugs are apparently successful in Phase II, their value may still be inflated. The select, nonrandomized groups of patients and surrogate end points used in Phase II account for some of the bias introduced in these trials. Consequently, failure to achieve adequate efficacy in Phase III is also commonplace. An analysis of trials published between 1998 and 2003 showed that among positive Phase II studies, only 28% translated into a positive Phase III study using an identical regimen (Zia *et al.*, 2005). It is these late failures, laden with prior investment, that are particularly detrimental to the drug development process.

Limited patient resources are an additional barrier to current drug development. The present clinical trial system requires the treatment of hundreds to thousands of patients with a new drug, primarily in Phase III trials. Considering the extraordinary surge in the invention of new drugs and that only 2 to 5% of patients nationally participate in clinical trials, there are clearly not enough patients to satisfy the needs for efficient drug development within the existing system. Therefore, in order to optimize the development of novel agents, improved methods of assessing promising drugs in all phases of drug development are needed.

On the whole, the traditional design and conduct of Phase I–III trials are not ideal in the current era, in which large numbers of molecular targets and agents (Table 1) are redefining the standards of research and clinical practice. Can we use imaging to define a "biologically active dose" in Phase I, instead of focusing on the maximally tolerated dose? For Phase II studies, can imaging be used to identify a "pharmacodynamic response" instead of the objective response measured by tumor shrinkage? Can imaging be used in Phase III trials to accurately predict who will or will not show an early response to a given agent, thus allowing preselection of patients most likely to respond for a given treatment, or rapidly excluding those unlikely to benefit so they may opt for other treatment options? These issues will be discussed in more detail.

Role of Imaging

Biomarkers

Generally, a biomarker is an objectively measurable end point that provides insight into the biology or behavior of a cancer. In practice, a biomarker should predict some clinical end point acceptable to the clinical community and regulating bodies. Biomarkers commonly used in oncology include circulating tumor antigens such as prostate-specific antigen (PSA), CA-125, and carcinoembryonic antigen (CEA), surface growth factor receptors such as HER-2/*neu*, estrogen and progesterone receptor status, and molecular changes such as the presence of a c-kit mutation or *bcr-abl* translocation. A biomarker needs to be precise and reproducible, independent of operator or site differences. A common purpose of many of these biomarkers is to assist in the refinement of treatment decisions. A useful biomarker may aid in understanding which patients need treatment, predict which patients will respond to a specific treatment, and/or define which patients are responding to treatment. In the last-named capacity, a validated biomarker acts as a surrogate marker for clinical benefit. In the current era of targeted cancer therapies, the utility of biomarkers in the drug development process, especially as surrogate end points, is exploding. Suggested roles include validation of new targets or pathways, optimization of lead agents, selection of enriched patient populations for therapy, determination of drug dose and schedules, prediction of resistance and toxicity, and rapid discrimination of responders from nonresponders to therapeutic intervention (Park *et al.*, 2004).

Current Imaging Roles

Use of routine imaging during diagnosis and staging is common and is familiar to all clinicians. Depending on the tumor type and location, anatomic imaging using CT, MRI, or bone scintigraphy is the standard in most cases for delineating the size and extent of malignancy. While CT and MRI are excellent for identifying lesions, they alone cannot definitively label these lesions as cancer. Similarly, bone scintigraphy has the ability to identify areas of osteoblastic activity, but whether these areas are due to active cancer, healing bone, trauma, or inflammation is interpreted in the clinical context for which it is performed. In other words, the routine use of these imaging modalities is more *qualitative* than quantitative due to the subjectivity in interpretation among radiologists and clinicians. As a result, for diseases with primarily bony metastasis such as prostate cancer, assessing radiographical response has been difficult at best, with bone scintigraphy primarily used to evaluate for evidence of progression. Having some improved imaging modality to assess for response in bone metastasis would be of great value toward drug development for these types of diseases.

The subsequent use of CT and MRI scans for following disease status can be considered quantitative, and it is now routine to report tumor measurements in two dimensions so that a clinician can determine in a binary fashion whether or not patients are continuing to benefit from their current therapy (stable or shrinking lesions) or not benefiting (new or progressive lesions). These techniques suffer from a number of limitations, foremost being the dependence on changes in size for determining response. Reduction in tumor size may be a relatively late indicator of response from a drug, usually requiring at least two to three cycles (or 6 to 8 weeks) of therapy before meaningful changes can be expected. Similarly,

Table 1   Classes and Examples of Targeted Agents Currently in Clinical Trials

Molecular Target	Therapeutic Inhibitor
Angiogenesis	
VEGF	Bevacizumab (MoAb)
VEGF-R	Sunitinib (TKI)
Integrins	ATN-161
Endothelial cell	Combretastatin
Growth Factor Receptor	
EGFR	Erlotinib (TKI) Cetuximab (MoAb)
HER-2	Lapatinib (TKI) Trastuzumab (MoAb)
Signal Transduction	
Ras	Lonafarnib (FTI)
Raf	Sorafenib (Raf kinase)
MEK	PD0325901 (MEK kinase)
m-TOR	CCI-779 (mTOR inhibitor)
G-protein	Atrasentan (ETA inhibitor)
Apoptosis	
Bcl-2	G3139 (anti-sense RNA)
TRAIL	HGS-ETR2 (MoAb)
Cell Cycle	
Proteosome	Bortezomib (Prot inhibitor)
Cyclin-dependent kinase	Seliciclib (CDK inhibitor)
Histone deacetylase	SAHA (HDA inhibitor)
Oncogene	
Bcr-Abl	Imatinib (TKI)

some changes, such as tumor necrosis, may be present, suggesting potential benefit despite no apparent change in the lesion size as shown by CT/MRI imaging. Cavitary, cystic, and conglomerate (e.g., carcinomatosis) lesions also present difficulty in quantitative radiologic assessment using these standard imaging modalities. In addition, changes in size may not reflect the activity of antiproliferative (or cytostatic) targeted agents, which may inhibit their target without causing appreciable alterations in tumor mass. In summary, the current status of quantitative radiology is not without its limitations, yet we have accepted its role as a surrogate marker in clinical trials to date. As a result of these deficiencies, newer imaging methods, which assess physiologic changes (not simply changes in tumor size), are increasingly being investigated. Valuable information can be obtained by using functional and/or molecular imaging.

Functional and Molecular Imaging

Functional imaging is simply the use of imaging techniques for detecting molecular signals that indicate the presence of biochemical activity and changes, such as cell growth or death. Molecular imaging is a form of functional imaging that uses specific probes to visualize specific molecular targets or processes. Perhaps the most universally available technology for molecular imaging is 2-^{18}F-fluoro-2-deoxy-D-glucose (FDG)-PET. This technology relies on the fact that tumor cells utilize glycolysis for energy under both aerobic and anaerobic conditions. FDG is actively taken up and accumulates in cancer cells, and thus its specific uptake is reflective of tumor metabolism (glucose uptake in sites of "active" cancer). FDG-PET is now approved by the Centers for Medicare and Medicaid Services for staging of cancers of non-small cell lung, breast, esophageal, colorectal, head and neck, and cervix, melanoma and lymphoma, as well as for monitoring the response to treatment in breast cancer (Juweid and Cheson, 2006). It has been an invaluable tool in the treatment planning of these and other cancers. The potential of FDG-PET for assessing early subclinical responses has long been acknowledged, and standardized response criteria for using PET in clinical trials have been previously published (Young et al., 1999).

Using the same imaging platform, if one changes the molecular probe from FDG to 3′-deoxy-3′fluorothymidine (FLT), a complementary set of new information can be generated. The nucleoside thymidine is incorporated into deoxyribonucleic acid (DNA) during DNA synthesis, as well as through a salvage pathway during cell proliferation. As a result, by labeling thymidine with a positron-emitting nuclide, one can quantitatively assess the tumor proliferation rate using a PET scanner. In addition, using oxygen-15 (^{15}O) PET, one can begin to measure additional factors such as blood flow. When combined with CT or MRI technique, one can now obtain specific physiologic information in a spatial context.

Dynamic contrast-enhanced magnetic resonance imaging (DCE-MRI) has been used as a method to evaluate the microenvironment occurring within tumors. In this case, the use of a paramagnetic metal cation like gadolinium can quantitate changes in tumor vascular parameters such as perfusion and permeability. Similarly, the use of dynamic contrast-enhanced computed tomography (DCE-CT) can be used to assess tumor perfusion, especially in areas such as the lung where CT images are clearly superior to MRI methods. Lastly, the use of single photon emission computed tomography (SPECT) has gained momentum as the variety of available SPECT ligands has increased. Depending on the ligand used, information on tumor apoptosis, changes in receptor expression, and the presence of multidrug resistance (MDR) transporters can be quantified.

It is clear that functional imaging has the potential to better characterize specific changes in the tumor that may be even more reflective of a given drug's activity than conventional anatomic imaging alone. Ultimately, the goal of using any of these newer techniques in clinical trials is to establish functional imaging as a biomarker that meets criteria for surrogate end points, and thus could expedite the drug development process. Are we ready to adopt these techniques as part of the standard of care? In order for these applications to be successful, they must be able to influence decision making regarding the continued advancement of a novel agent in clinical trials. Presently, such a decisive role for functional imaging, with a few exceptions, is still exploratory. However, a number of clinical trials have incorporated functional imaging techniques and have displayed proof-of-concept in support of their use in the decision-making process.

There are several examples of clinical trials with targeted agents in which functional imaging has confirmed pharmacodynamic changes, and in some cases contributed to dose selection (Table 2). Among the benchmark trials, Morgan et al. (2003) published one of the first clinical studies showing the value of DCE-MRI as a biomarker for assessing anti-angiogenic response. Twenty-six patients with liver metastases from colorectal cancer receiving treatment with PTK787/ZK 222584 (PTK), an oral VEGFR-1 and -2 tyrosine kinase inhibitor, in two Phase I dose escalation studies were evaluated with DCE-MRI at baseline, day 2 of therapy, and at the end of each of the first two 28-day cycles. The primary imaging end point was the percentage change in baseline bidirectional transfer constant (Ki), a measure of tumor vascularity, blood flow, and vascular permeability. The authors found a rapid decrease in Ki within 26 to 33 hr following the first dose. The reduction in enhancement was significantly negatively correlated with increasing doses and plasma levels of PTK, both at day 2 and at the end of cycle 1. More importantly, among 12 nonprogressors, the reduction in Ki was significantly greater on day 2 compared with 9 progressors. This relationship was maintained through at least the end of cycle 1. This supports a link between DCE-MRI

Table 2 Clinical Trials with Targeted Therapy Incorporating Functional Imaging End Points

Drug	Author	Imaging Method	Trial Type	Patient Population	N	Result
PTK787/ ZK 22584	Morgan et al., 2003	DCE-MRI	Phase I	Colorectal liver metastases	26	• Significant decline in Ki by day 2 • Inverse correlation of Ki with drug levels • Greater reduction in Ki among nonprogressors • Supports Phase II dose selection
AG-013736	Liu et al., 2005	DCE-MRI	Phase I	Advanced solid tumors	26	• Significant decline in K^{trans} and IAUC by day 2 • Inverse correlation of K^{trans} and IAUC with drug levels • Phase II dose supported by K^{trans} and IAUC decrease of $\geq 50\%$
Imatinib	Demetri et al., 2001	FDG-PET	Phase II	Unresectable or metastatic GIST	64	• Marked decrease in FDG uptake in all tumors (as early as 24 hours) showing subsequent response on CT or MRI • Increased FDG uptake in all patients with progression
	Stroobants et al., 2003	FDG-PET	Phase I/II	Advanced soft tissue sarcoma or GIST	21	• PET response correctly predicted CT response in 18/21, median of 7 weeks before CT response • PET response in 6/6 with symptom reduction, PET progression in 7/8 with deterioration in PS • 1-year PFS 92% vs. 12% in PET responders vs. nonresponders, respectively
Sunitinib	Demetri et al., 2003	FDG-PET	Phase I/II	Refractory GIST	39	• Early FDG-PET response rate of 72% allowed confidence to proceed with Phase III trial
HuMV833 (anti-VEGF Ab)	Jayson et al., 2002	DCE-MRI	Phase I	Progressive solid tumors	20	• Substantial decrease in K_{fp}* at 48 hours in all patients • Inverse correlation of K_{fp} with drug concentration, but not dose
Combre-tastatin A4 phosphate (endothelial tubulin inhibitor)	Stevenson et al., 2003	DCE-MRI	Phase I	Refractory solid tumors	10	• Decrease in K^{trans} in 8 of 10 patients at day 5 • Greatest decrease in K^{trans} in tumors with highest enhancement at baseline • Inverse correlation between K^{trans} and plasma level of active metabolite at day 5
	Galbraith et al., 2003	DCE-MRI	Phase I	Refractory solid tumors	18	• Significant reduction in K^{trans} at 4 or 24 hours in 6 of 16 patients treated at $\geq 52\,mg/m^2$; no reduction in patients treated at $\leq 40\,mg/m^2$ • Significant inverse correlation between maximum reduction in K^{trans} and serum drug concentration • Supports Phase II dose of $52\,mg/m^2$
	Anderson et al., 2003	$H_2{}^{15}O$ and $C^{15}O$ PET	Phase I	Advanced solid tumors	13	• Significant dose-dependent reduction in tumor perfusion and blood flow at 30 minutes • Significant reduction in tumor perfusion at 24 hours for doses $\geq 52\,mg/m^2$ • Supports Phase II dose of $52-66\,mg/m^2$
ZD6126 (endothelial tubulin inhibitor)	Evelhoch et al., 2004	DCE-MRI	Phase I	Liver metastases of mixed primary solid tumor origin	9	• Decreased IAUC at 6 hours in all patients • Significant dose-response relationship with decreased IAUC • IAUC calculation reproducible in patients
DMXAA (anti-vascular, TNF-α induction)	Galbraith et al., 2002	DCE-MRI	Phase I	Refractory solid tumors	16	• Significant reduction in AUC in 9 of 16 patients 24 hours after first dose • No dose-response relationship with any vascular parameter
Endostatin (angio-genesis inhibitor)	Herbst et al., 2002	$H_2{}^{15}O$ and FDG PET	Phase I	Advanced solid tumors	21	• Nonlinear but dose-dependent changes in tumor metabolism and blood flow at 4 and 8 weeks • Supports Phase II dose of $180\,mg/m^2/day$
	Thomas et al., 2003	MRI, PET, CT, US	Phase I	Refractory solid tumors	21	• No consistent effect on tumor vasculature by any imaging modality

*K_{fp}: estimation of K^{trans} and relative tumoral blood volume from measurements made during first pass of contrast bolus.

changes with clinical outcome and confirms the pharmaco-dynamic response of PTK with its target. They also showed a threshold for the biologic effect of PTK at 1000 mg, with little change in Ki at higher doses. Combined with the pharmacokinetic data from Phase I, these DCE-MRI findings were used to assist with dose selection for a Phase III trial (Ellis, 2003).

A multi-institutional Phase I trial by Liu *et al.* (2005) evaluated the pharmacodynamic response to the oral anti-angiogenesis agent AG-013736 on tumor vasculature using DCE-MRI. AG-013736 is a multitargeted tyrosine kinase inhibitor of all known vascular endothelial growth factor receptors (VEGFR), platelet-derived growth factor receptor (PDGFR)-β, and c-Kit. DCE-MRI was performed on 26 patients at baseline and at day 2 of treatment, at the estimated C_{max}. Primary DCE-MRI end points included the mean change in volume transfer constant (K^{trans}) and initial area under the concentration time curve (IAUC), both measurements of tumor perfusion and vascular permeability. Data acquisition followed a standardized protocol with central image analysis. A total of 17 patients with complete data treated at various doses and schedules of AG-013736 were included in the analysis. Findings from this trial showed a rapid decrease in K^{trans} and IAUC at day 2 of AG-013736 dosing, with a strong and statistically significant dose-response relationship between mean steady-state drug concentrations and changes in K^{trans} and IAUC. Selecting a cut-off for a meaningful vascular response as a decrease in K^{trans} or IAUC of 50% or more, the serum concentrations obtained with the dosage recommended for Phase II study by conventional criteria were well within the range of AG-013736 exposure necessary to obtain a vascular response by DCE-MRI. Although only one patient with a confirmed clinical response was also evaluable by DCE-MRI, decreases in K^{trans} and IUAC in this patient were significant. Interestingly, all patients who had clinical benefit or objective changes in their tumors (decreased size or signs of tumor necrosis/cavitation) showed changes in their tumor vascular parameters (when obtainable) consistent with anti-angiogenic activity by day 2 of treatment. This would suggest that results from DCE-MRI scans could provide an early prediction of a clinically meaningful response from this type of therapy, and thus allow us to potentially steer patients without any signs of a vascular response by day 2 of therapy toward other therapeutic agents. These findings supported the use of DCE-MRI in confirming a biologically active dose and defining the mechanism of action of this new agent. While validation of the response end points is certainly needed, this study showed that performing serial DCE-MRI in a multi-institutional setting was feasible.

A good example of the utility of FDG-PET can be illustrated by a study using imatinib, a c-KIT, ABL, and PDGFR tyrosine kinase inhibitor, in patients with GISTs. A landmark international trial reported by Demetri *et al.* (2002) included FDG-PET evaluation of tumor response in 64 of the 147 patients. Positron emission tomography scanning

was performed at baseline and at various time points, even as early as 24 hr after starting treatment to complement CT imaging. The results of the trial were markedly positive, with 54% of patients achieving a partial response and another 30% maintaining stable disease on CT, leading to accelerated FDA approval of imatinib. In all cases with PET data, changes in FDG uptake correctly predicted tumor response, often at an earlier time point than with conventional imaging. These promising results were confirmed in a Phase I/II trial by the European Organization for Research and Treatment of Cancer (EORTC), in which FDG uptake was additionally able to predict symptom relief and progression-free survival in patients (Stroobants *et al.*, 2003).

While these trials have established a role for functional imaging in drug development, the most compelling demonstration of the effectiveness of these techniques in facilitating drug approval has emerged from the recent development of sunitinib, a multitargeted tyrosine kinase inhibitor of the VEGFR, PDGFR, and KIT, in refractory GISTs. A Phase I/II study of sunitinib in patients with GIST refractory to or intolerant of imatinib was initiated in April 2002. Patients were followed simultaneously for response by CT and FDG-PET imaging. Positron emission tomography scans were repeated after 1 week of therapy and at the beginning of cycle 2, whereas CT scans were repeated at the end of cycles 1 and 2. As of May 2003, 39 patients were evaluable by PET, with a PET response rate of 72%. Among the 33 evaluable patients by CT at the same time point, the CT partial response rate was 6% and the stable disease rate was 30% (Demetri *et al.*, 2003). Based largely on the PET findings, there was enough confidence to take this drug forward into a Phase III trial. By January 2005, significantly positive results in the Phase III study led to termination of the trial by the independent data and safety monitoring board and ultimately to FDA approval of sunitinib in refractory GIST in January 2006. In total, less than 4 years elapsed from the time the first dose of sunitinib was taken by a patient with GIST until it reached FDA approval, and this process was facilitated by the use of PET.

Functional Imaging as a Biomarker

The pharmaceutical industry is actively pursuing these new imaging technologies as biomarkers in drug development. Despite this interest, several barriers remain that limit their use. First, these imaging techniques can be complex and thus available only in specialized centers of research, such as those with an on-site cyclotron to generate appropriate nuclides. Second, the lack of standardization in equipment and methods among these specialized centers results in variable data making comparison between groups difficult. Lastly, validation of the biomarker is time-consuming and costly, but without validation, the results will not be acceptable to regulating bodies. Although these barriers are formidable, the advantages that functional imaging provides may certainly be worth investing in drug development.

Technical Considerations

The potential for a variety of non-invasive clinical imaging procedures to impact the speed and efficiency with which we develop new cancer therapies requires that we regard these procedures as quantitative, rather than merely qualitative, data. As such, the science behind cancer imaging as a tool for drug development must address a range of questions based on the intended use of the results. Selection of a specific imaging technique or test begins with "proof of technical concept." This refers to the linkage of a technical approach to biological/pathological correlates in animal models and/or human disease. Once established, the next phase of research must address proof of clinical concepts, or demonstrate the relationship between the signals measured using an imaging test and the clinical realities of the patient's disease. The quantitative aspects of the imaging test should allow for extraction of meaningful information from the images and demonstrate that the information is accurate and reproducible.

Proof of Concept

One of the most exciting applications for emerging quantitative imaging approaches is the ability to use them as a direct or indirect measure of the mechanism of action of an investigational new cancer drug. This is only possible when a clear direct or indirect link between the results of a specific imaging test is understood relative to the purported mechanism of action for the anticancer agent being tested. The practical application to evaluating a new cancer therapy is then based on predefined decision-making criteria based on results of the imaging test(s). First, a certain comfort level associated with use of data from an individual patient is necessary to conclude that a change in signal is a true reflection of pharmacology affecting that patient's disease. Second, a summary of such results from a cohort of patients, or a dose-escalation study, is often necessary to litigate the risk of testing an experimental drug in larger definitive clinical trials.

Statistics

None of the above assurances are possible without the appropriate use of statistical modeling. The selection of appropriate statistical tests is needed in order to (1) extract meaningful information as end points from the collected set of images; (2) appropriately use statistical variability to design and power a clinical study; and (3) summarize the results of image-based end points from a clinical study based on interpretation of the statistical analysis of the end points in context of the clinical picture.

When designing a clinical drug study, such as one to demonstrate proof-of-mechanism of an investigational new drug,

one must keep in mind that these studies are typically underpowered for any statistical conclusions; in practice, they are used to generate logical hypotheses to be tested in larger clinical studies that can be statistically powered to draw more definitive conclusions. Regardless of whether studies are designed to determine the development path of an investigational new drug or to understand the utility of alternative end points for managing patient care, there must be a high level of confidence in the results.

If a particular imaging test has been successfully used as a tool to measure drug mechanism, the logical next step might be to consider linking results of imaging to a clinical question regarding patient management. Did the results of the imaging test predict how that patient would later respond to the selected therapy? Does the imaging test provide a better tool to guide the management of each patient's disease? Is there an overall benefit to the information that imaging can provide in terms of accurate selection of therapeutic options, and is it cost effective relative to standard of care? These are the larger questions that research networks, practice networks, regulatory agencies, payers, pharmaceutical companies, and others will ultimately want to address in this new era of cancer therapies and diagnostic technologies.

Reproducibility

Statistical variables associated with imaging test-based end points are complex and not fully understood by the majority of end users for these approaches. Patient preparation, image acquisition procedures, readers, instrumentation, and methods of analysis typically differ to varying degrees across clinical imaging centers. Among the most important issues that first need to be addressed is the test-retest variability, in order for new end points to be used for guiding clinical study interpretation. This is critical for study design and sample size estimates in any investigation using a baseline test. A better understanding of the reproducibility of parameters derived from procedures such as FDG-PET (standardized uptake values) and DCE-MRI (IAUC, K^{trans}, etc.) obtained using standard defined protocols in a clinical setting is clearly needed to guide future trial design for testing objective responses to experimental oncology drugs in the minimal number of clinical subjects.

Preliminary data on reproducibility for FDG-PET have been published (Weber et al., 1999). In a study of 16 patients participating in Phase I studies of novel anti-neoplastic compounds, FDG-PET was performed twice within 10 days with no therapeutic intervention in between. Standardized uptake values, FDG net influx constants [Ki], glucose normalized SUVs [SUV(gluc)], and influx constants [K(i,gluc)]; were determined for 50 identified and separate lesions with precision of repeated measurements determined on a lesion-by-lesion and a patient-by-patient basis. None of the parameters showed a significant increase or decrease at the two examinations, suggesting that FDG-PET had highly reproducible quantitative parameters of tumor glucose metabolism.

Preliminary reproducibility data are also available for DCE-MRI. Dynamic contrast-enhanced MRI time series were acquired at two imaging centers from a group of patients with abdominal tumors and a group with gliomas. At both imaging centers, precontrast T(1) was calculated using a variable flip angle three-dimensional spoiled gradient-echo acquisition that could quantify tissue contrast agent concentration. A comparison of reproducibility showed that there was no statistically significant difference in reproducibility between IAUC(60) and K^{trans}, although there was a trend toward better reproducibility for K^{trans} ($p = 0.0782$). The 95% confidence intervals (CIs) for individual changes showed that for IAUC(60) and K^{trans}, changes in excess of 47% and 31%, respectively, are outside the range of normal variability (Roberts *et al.*, 2006).

The importance of reproducibility can be illustrated by any other clinical test used routinely for monitoring a patient's clinical status such as blood chemistries. There are standard procedures for processing the blood sample, calibrating the instrumentation, applying internal standards and replicates, and analyzing the results with an expected level of rigor in order to have confidence in comparing the results from a baseline measure to a follow-up test. It is this level of confidence in assay performance that allows clinicians to interpret the results of a second test relative to a baseline test and know if their approach to managing the case is working. Quantitative imaging "tests" should not be different in this regard. There is the desperate need for standard approaches ranging from preparation of the patient, calibration of the scanner or device, settings and timing of image acquisition, and the selection of algorithms and statistical analyses used in extracting results from the image-based data. Until more recently, the current approaches used in the majority of radiology practices have relied heavily on relatively subjective interpretation of images. Only in a relatively few specialized settings has there been an emphasis on improving our understanding of the more objective information extracted from images using advanced image analysis algorithms. This is an emerging field of research that is expected to enhance radiologists' and oncologists' ability to extract additional objective information from clinical images for interpretation in the context of each patient's disease.

Validation

Validation of imaging biomarkers for predicting clinical benefit of a therapeutic intervention and linkage to overall survival poses a significant challenge in that a large number of cases representing a range of responses tested using standard procedures are required to fully elucidate this. Efforts are increasing to better define guidelines for these types of studies. In recognizing the overall value as well as expense of this type of research, coordinated efforts across clinical research groups, funding agencies, industry sponsors, and regulatory agencies will be the formula for success in validating imaging-derived surrogate end points. In the meantime, testing biological efficacy is attainable in relatively small trials involving appropriate imaging tests.

Financial Considerations

There is a long list of "business drivers" that often influence a sponsor's decision to include imaging-based tests in a clinical trial protocol for testing an investigational new drug: How can we use a new test with *confidence* to *discontinue* the clinical development of an investigational new drug? Does it *really* allow us to reduce risk of investments in Phases II and III? Will it help oncologists select the right drug for their patients? What will be the clinical trial and clinical program budgetary impacts? How do we know if this is a good return on investment? Will there be an impact on patient accrual? Are these risks acceptable relative to the value of the data?

Sponsors of clinical trials are aware of the costs of making the correct development decisions, as these will have immediate cost savings by discontinuing a program early in development, and long-term benefit by shifting resources to programs with high likelihood of success. They are also aware that there is a cost to making the wrong development decisions, and this cost may result in discontinuing the development of a promising new drug, or investing in further development of a drug destined to fail in larger expensive definitive trials. Beyond the decisions surrounding the investment of further development are other commercial business drivers, such as how the approaches used may allow for the differentiation of new drugs from each other. Will a new test allow clinicians to prospectively select one product over another for their patient? Will it allow clinicians to select a specific product most likely to benefit patients relatively quickly in the treatment of their disease? Confidence in what the results of an imaging test can provide in terms of patient management equates to overall value to the oncology community, as well as direct and indirect benefits to the commercial success of an approved drug.

Standardization

Presently, the imaging approaches most commonly studied and used in the context of drug development include CT (1D, 2D, 3D, morphometrics), MRI (DCE-, diffusion, spectroscopy), PET (FDG-, FLT-, other specialized radiotracers), and PET/CT combined. Regardless of the imaging modalities and procedures employed, there are certain key standardization requirements to achieve reproducible imaging tests in a clinical trial setting: technical aspects of data acquisition; instrumentation; procedures and protocols impacting patient management and care; development of radiology and nuclear medicine facility workflow to ensure identical procedures are used at baseline and follow-up scans; image data configuration and handling for central archiving when sponsored clinical trials are concerned, with third-party central reads and analyses; and detailed patient records. For example, there has been sufficient experience to know that the results of DCE-MRI analysis are reproducible in a cancer center radiology department setting if appropriate planning has taken place. Data are emerging for guiding the standardization of imaging procedures and for better guiding clinical trial design involving imaging-based end points in clinical studies for investigational drugs.

Impact on Accrual

One drawback to consider is that the inclusion of a procedure such as DCE-MRI or FDG-PET in Phase I and II protocols is likely to decrease accrual rates relative to studies that are limited to routine CT scans for assessment of disease progression. Accrual rates are an important factor in the time it takes in Phases I and II to determine whether a Phase III program is warranted. Fast accrual rates in Phase III are particularly important in order to provide necessary data for regulatory agencies to review when applying for a new drug application. Better trial designs based on newer end points, together with rapid accrual rates, will increase the speed with which we get new drugs to the patients who need them. Imaging is expected to play a significant role in this critical path to new drug approvals.

Although there is not sufficient data to predict the impact imaging procedures will have on clinical trial accrual rates, early anecdotal observations suggest that as many as 20% of patients qualifying for a Phase I clinical trial based on routine RECIST inclusion criteria for "measurable disease" may not meet the lesion selection criteria for DCE-MRI where lung and liver lesions are concerned (McShane, unpublished observations). It will be important to track this type of information in order to provide clear guidance to clinical researchers involved in drug development. Accrual efforts will need to take this into consideration relative to the value of collecting these data. If the end points are able to test certain questions related to mechanism of action of an investigational drug, and statistical guidelines allow for smaller studies during shorter timeframes, then the advantages may outweigh the risks.

Feasibility

In the context of patient populations qualifying for Phase I and II clinical trials, common sites of metastatic disease are the liver and lungs. These sites are particularly challenging to evaluate using MRI or CT dynamic imaging because of motion from breathing, and are likely subject to variability in quantifying perfusion parameters. Thus, it is important to consider the technical and practical feasibility of each approach in a clinical trial setting.

Challenges and Needs

In oncology, the best strategy for patient care has always been a multidisciplinary approach, as it takes into consideration information regarding a given disease in the context of the complexities of an individual. The use of functional imaging in drug development also requires a team approach. Leading this team should be an investigator with knowledge of the relevant clinical question being asked, as well as keen insight in tumor biology and drug mechanisms. In addition, a quantitative radiologist with appropriate support (trained technicians, medical physicists, etc.) is required to properly supervise data acquisition and interpretation of the imaging performed. A statistician with expertise in analytical methods and study design is very important, as the quality of the data reported needs to meet appropriate statistical criteria. Lastly, appropriate resources are required to support commitments from each member necessary to conduct a successful trial and meet the significant challenges of this endeavor.

Applications

Drug Development

Functional imaging will play a key role in drug development. Most large drug companies now have established internal research programs as well as collaboration with academic centers and diagnostic imaging companies. Indeed, with the development of micro-CTs, micro-PET, optical imager scanners, and novel probes, it is likely that functional imaging will be used increasingly in the preclinical assessment of all new drugs in order to define biologic activity and better assess agents that will most likely succeed once allowed for clinical development. Early preclinical and clinical testing can utilize molecular imaging as a biomarker to confirm pharmacological effect or biochemical mechanism of action. This is invaluable information as it provides proof-of-mechanism within the tumor itself. Demonstrating pharmacodynamic activity related to the mode of action of a drug can include assessment of changes in metabolic activity, perfusion, proliferation rate, apoptosis, and differentiation. Finally, a biomarker may mature to the point where it is used to predict a clinical outcome. These are typically extensively evaluated in multiple trials as surrogate markers of activity, although not yet widely accepted as validated markers of benefit by the FDA (Floyd and McShane, 2004; Ludwig and Weinstein, 2005).

Innovative Trial Designs

Recognizing the need to facilitate and prioritize the role of imaging in laboratory and clinical cancer research, the NCI founded the Biomedical Imaging Program (now Cancer Imaging Program, or CIP) in 1996. In 2003 alone, the CIP administered more than $170 million in grant support for cancer imaging research. Although increasing emphasis has been placed on inclusion of functional imaging end points in clinical trials, the proportion of studies taking advantage of these technologies is sill woefully small. In an analysis of 60 recently published Phase I trials of targeted noncyto-toxic agents, only 6 included functional imaging studies. In only 1 of these 6 was the imaging data used to help make a decision on Phase II dosing (Parulekar and Eisenhauer, 2004). Acknowledging that our current clinical trial system is inadequate for efficiently studying and advancing novel targeted agents, how can the trial designs move forward to incorporate functional imaging as surrogate end points? To answer this question, one must again consider the goals of using imaging biomarkers in clinical trials (to move promising agents to the public more quickly, with less expense and fewer patient resources), in the context of the goals of the studies at each particular phase of development.

The testing of any new drug in clinical studies will first and foremost require safety and dose-finding evaluation in Phase I. There is ongoing debate regarding the ideal Phase I design; intrapatient and rapid dose-escalation schemes, and pharmacologically based dose escalation are among suggested strategies to efficiently reach the Phase I end point. One of the greatest challenges during the era of targeted therapy is defining the appropriate end point for dose selection. Dose escalation to maximal tolerated dose (MTD) may be less meaningful, and in some cases unreachable, for agents that tend to produce less toxicity. In addition, these drugs may achieve a "plateau effect" due to saturation kinetics of the target itself, thereby interrupting any strict dose-response relationship. As a result, a more relevant end point for targeted agents in Phase I is the optimal biologic dose. In other words, the dose selected is not that reached by escalation to MTD, but that reached by titration to optimal biologic response. In this scenario, assessment of biologic response requires a validated biomarker, and functional imaging with PET and DCE-MRI is particularly well suited for this role. K^{trans} or IAUC in DCE-MRI (Leach et al., 2005) and SUV in PET (Young et al., 1999) provide reproducible, quantitative measures that can be reliably compared between baseline and post-treatment scans.

Selection of the most appropriate imaging modality depends primarily on anticipated mechanism of drug action. The effects of antivascular and anti-angiogenic drugs may be best assessed by perfusion studies such as DCE-MRI and $H_2^{15}O$ PET, while other antiproliferative agents may be better evaluated with metabolic imaging. In all cases, scans prior

to treatment are required to provide baseline measurements. Timing of repeat scans should include one assessment after acute dosing when drug levels are near maximal, as well as a second time point at the end of the first cycle. This later time point is useful for assessing steady-state response and dosing schedule for drugs administered continuously and cyclically, respectively. Imaging should be performed during cycle 1 for each dose level, during which time most of the pharma-cokinetic (PK) and initial toxicity data are collected. Therefore, imaging changes are available for correlation with PK and toxicity outcomes. The minimal change in the imaging parameters indicative of a meaningful biologic response (i.e., the margin of imaging response, which indicates target inhibition and not baseline variability in scan reproducibility) is defined prior to the trial based on prior animal and clinical experience. For example, changes in FDG-PET of greater than 25% have been proposed as significant (Young et al., 1999), and decreases in K^{trans} and IUAC of at least 45 to 50% were chosen for significance in prior studies (Liu et al., 2005; Morgan et al., 2003), although the latter estimates may be overly conservative. In the end, a combination of all three variables of biologic response, toxicity, and PK data will be needed to determine optimal biologic dose.

As the dose is escalated, biologic responses can be counted as events and thus feed back into the dose-escalation scheme. If a set proportion of patients at a particular dose level experience a plateau in biologic response before reaching any dose-limiting toxicity, then that level would be expected to define the *optimal biologic dose*. In other circumstances, toxicity may be limiting, and imaging would function more to define a *minimum efficacious dose*, and thus potentially allows the use of a lower dose to avoid toxicity. In cases where biologic responses are minimal, even at drug levels expected to cause target inhibition, functional imaging can also demonstrate lack of a pharmacodynamic response. The inability of a drug to hit its target may indicate the absence of the target in humans, or even that the proposed mechanism of the drug is not valid in humans. Such information is invaluable in influencing decisions to advance agents to higher phase studies. Ultimately, by complementing the data obtained by PK and toxicity analysis, functional imaging can refine the search for optimal biologic dosing, thereby exposing fewer patients to ineffective or unnecessary dose levels, and shortening the time required for Phase I testing.

In contrast to Phase I, the primary goal of Phase II studies is to determine whether a drug provides some signs of activity or clinical benefit in a defined patient population. Traditionally, this assessment of benefit is equated with responses on conventional imaging or other surrogates of survival such as time to disease progression. Because cytostatic agents may not cause reductions in tumor size, anatomic imaging may be inadequate for study of these agents. In this capacity, functional imaging can provide a more accurate characterization of response rate. This, in turn, would minimize the chances of erroneously rejecting a drug due to apparent lack of activity. Also, because the physiologic changes in tumors can often be measured within days of initiation of treatment, functional imaging provides a unique opportunity to identify patient groups enriched for the target that are most likely to benefit from investigational treatment.

In order to determine whether changes in functional imaging can act as a surrogate marker for benefit, patients in Phase II trials should be followed simultaneously for functional imaging and traditional end points. Comparisons can then be made to distinguish if functional imaging adds to the ability to predict which patients benefit from treatment. Conceivably, increasing the accuracy or shortening the time interval to response assessment is a potentially favorable outcome of incorporating functional imaging into Phase II. This was demonstrated by FDG-PET in Phase II trials using imatinib for GIST, in which early response on PET was highly predictive of later objective response on CT and progression-free survival. Once these end points are established in Phase II, they can be validated in subsequent Phase II or III studies.

Aside from the rare drugs with unquestionable activity for disease states with limited therapeutic options, Phase III studies will still be required for approval of most novel compounds. Up to this point, functional imaging has not played a prominent role in advancing targeted agents through the Phase III trial process. It is possible that the greatest impact of these technologies on Phase III will be in helping to select the optimal agents for entry into randomized trials, thus cutting back on the number of agents with marginal activity in late clinical testing. Because Phase III trials generally are measured by survival end points, the role of functional imaging as a surrogate marker in this setting is less valuable. Alternatively, enrichment of patient populations with the desired target may represent a more useful role. The paradigm of population enrichment with a target of interest was proven successful with trastuzumab for the treatment of HER-2-*neu* positive metastatic and resectable breast cancer. In an analogous fashion, selection of patients with a marked response on DCE-MRI or PET after acute dosing with a study drug could identify enriched patient populations. Randomization and treatment of only these patients in a Phase III trial could significantly widen the treatment effect, thus facilitating approval of an agent. Such an enrichment strategy could also be utilized in the adjuvant setting, with the initial dosing (or screening period) done prior to definitive treatment. A summary of the proposed role for functional imaging in clinical trials and drug development is shown in Figure 1.

Discussion

Although functional imaging in drug development is currently in its infancy, its applications in clinical trials are

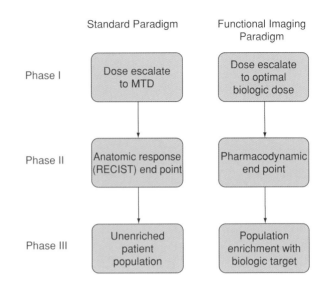

Figure 1 Proposed role for functional imaging in clinical trials.

likely to expand as additional experience and confidence in these markers accumulate. The final gauge of the usefulness of these techniques will lie in their ability to influence treatment decisions and to bring drugs to patients more quickly. The advances with sunitinib in refractory GIST serve as a model for how functional imaging can facilitate drug development. Among available biomarkers, imaging is unique in that it applies to all stages of drug development, starting from preclinical selection of drugs to clinical selection of drug dosing and target populations. Increasing awareness of this potential should lead to more widespread use. Incorporation of functional imaging end points in all stages of drug development should be encouraged. With increasing familiarity will come increasing confidence, and these techniques are likely to be accepted by researchers, governing bodies, and clinical oncologists. Although much progress has already been made, much more is needed.

We have one of the most technologically advanced healthcare systems in the world in which all patients are entitled to be treated with the latest standard of care and diagnostic tools available. One question that has been raised is whether we have "overshot" the level of care needed by the majority of our citizens. New technology comes with a steep price. Can the U.S health-care system continue to absorb the costs of new drugs, novel imaging modalities, new surgery, and radiation techniques? For example, the cost for an eight-week treatment for colon cancer has jumped from $63 for 5-fluorouracil (5-FU) with leucovorin, to $9497 with irinotecan, $11,889 with the approval of oxaliplatin with 5-FU and irinotecan, to $21,399 with bevacizumab with 5-FU/leucovorin/irinotecan, to now $30,790 for cetuximab with irinotecan (May 2004 average wholesale price). Is a 10% temporary improvement in response rate worth $17,000/month as is the case for cetuximab? Is the improvement in median survival of

4.4 months justifying the additional $4400/month by adding bevacizumab? If all 56,000 American patients with advanced colon cancer received these latest agents, the national health cost would increase by a staggering $1.2 billion (Schrag, 2004). The questions raised are difficult to address for an individual, but for society, the answer is no.

What about imaging? One of the fastest growing healthcare expenses is the use of diagnostic imaging. It is estimated that imaging accounted for ~ $75 billion in the United States alone for the year 2000. The 2005 projected costs of diagnostic imaging have jumped to a staggering $100 billion. Out of this, ~ $16 billion was felt to be unnecessary (IMV Medical Information, 2005) and in part due to defensive medicine and the inappropriate use of more expensive radiologic techniques such as CT, MRI, or PET. Doctors want to offer the latest technologies, and patients demand the best imaging. From a strict marketing standpoint, it is the profitable high-end (demanding) consumers who drive this innovation, which overshoots the needs of the routine consumer (Christensen et al., 2000). For example, if a patient receiving palliative chemotherapy has obvious regression of his lung metastasis on a chest X-ray, is a CT scan really necessary? Does it add information that will influence management? Moreover, PET scans are frequently overused to stage patients with obvious metastasis on CT scan and inappropriately used to follow response after chemotherapy. As we adopt newer functional imaging as biomarkers of benefits, we will need to ask ourselves whether the additional costs are justified in the context of the treatment being performed. On the other hand, if a functional imaging technique is adopted as a valid biomarker of tumor response, due to the high costs of these new targeted therapies, it could be justified to use functional imaging to predict early on whether a particular drug is not working, thus giving us a reason to stop the ineffective agent early on, resulting in a net cost reduction for all.

In conclusion, imaging will continue to play a large role in the current and future drug development paradigm. With the current wealth of new agents being developed, appropriate imaging will be important to assess which combinations will be most effective against the tumor, as well as potentially least harmful for the host. Given the high costs of drug development, demanding patients, and regulating agencies, long gone are the days of arbitrarily combining agents in hopes of an improved response. We must now prove at least additive benefit biologically (proof of mechanism), pharmacodynamically (proof of activity), and clinically (proof of benefit). Although functional and molecular imaging will always be important in drug development, we must be cautious in adopting these new tools in clinical practice until they are validated, and then consider them only when they will contribute further to management of patients over what standard imaging can provide. Each new advance brings us one step closer to finding the cure for cancer. With refinements in imaging equipment, techniques, and probes, the possibilities are enormous.

References

Abrams, J.S., Mooney, M., Goldberg, J., Adler, J., Ansher, S., and Smith, M. 2005. Bringing new agents to market: navigating the regulatory requirements for investigators. *AACR Education Book 12*:211–216.

Anderson, H.L., Yap, J.T., Miller, M.P., Robbins, A., Jones, T., and Price, P.M. 2003. Assessment of pharmacodynamic vascular response in a Phase I trial of combretastatin A4 phosphate. *J. Clin. Oncol. 21*:2823–2830.

Chabner, B.A., and Roberts, T.G. 2005. Chemotherapy and the war on cancer. *Nat. Rev. Cancer 5*:65–72.

Christensen, C.M., Bohmer, R., and Kenacy, J. 2000. Will disruptive innovations cure health care? *Harvard Business Review 6*:102–112.

Demetri, G.D., George, S., Heinrich, M.C., Flethcer J.A., Fletcher, C.D.M., Desai, J., Cohen, D.P., Scigalla, P., Cherrington, J.M., and van den Abbeele, A. 2003. Clinical activity and tolerability of the multi-targeted tyrosine kinase inhibitor SU11248 in patients with malignant gastrointestinal stromal tumors refractory to imatinib mesylate. *Proc. Am. Soc. Clin. Oncol.*, abstract 3273.

Demetri, G.D., von Mehren, M., Blanke, C.D., Van den Abbeele, A., Eisenberg, B., Roberts, P.J., Heinrich, M.C., Tuveson, D.A., Singer, S., Janicek, M., Fletcher, J.A., Silverman, S.G., Silberman, S.L., Capdeville, R., Kiese, B., Peng, B., Dimitrijevic, S., Druker, B.J., Corless, C., Fletcher, C.D.M., and Joensuu, H. 2002. Efficacy and safety of imatinib mesylate in advanced gastrointestinal stromal tumors. *N. Engl. J. Med. 347*:472–480.

Dimasi, J.A., Hansen, R.W., and Grabowski, H.G. 2003. The price of innovation: new estimates of drug development costs. *J. Health Econ. 22*:151–185.

Ellis, L.M. 2003. Antiangiogenic therapy: more promise and, yet again, more questions. *J. Clin. Oncol. 21*:3897–3899.

Evelhoch, J.L., LoRusso, P.M., He, Z., DelProposto, Z., Polin, L., Corbett, T.H., Langmuir, P., Wheeler, C., Stone, A., Leadbetter, J., Ryan, A.J., Blakey, D.C., and Waterton, J.C. 2004. Magnetic resonance imaging measurements of the response of murine and human tumors to the vascular-targeting agent ZD6126. *Clin. Cancer Res. 10*:3650–3657.

Floyd, E., and McShane, T. 2004. Development and use of biomarkers in oncology drug development. *Toxicol. Pathol. 32*:106–115.

Galbraith, S.M., Maxwell, R.J., Lodge, M.A., Tozer, G.M., Wilson, J., Taylor, N.J., Stirling, J.J., Sena, L., Padhani, A.R., and Rustin, G.J.S. 2003. Combretastatin A4 phosphate has tumor antivascular activity in rat and man as demonstrated by dynamic magnetic resonance imaging. *J. Clin. Oncol. 21*:2831–2842.

Galbraith, S.M., Rustin, G.J.S., Lodge, M.A., Taylor, N.J., Stirling, J.J., Jameson, M., Thompson, P., Hough, D., Gumbrell, L., and Padhani, A.R. 2002. Effects of 5,6-dimethylxanthenone-4-acetic acid on human tumor microcirculation assessed by dynamic contrast-enhanced magnetic resonance imaging. *J. Clin. Oncol. 20*:3826–3840.

Herbst, R.S., Mullani, N.A., Davis, D.W., Hess, K.R., McConkey, D.J., Charnsangavej, C., O'Reilly, M.S., Kim, H., Baker, C., Roach, J., Ellis, L.M., Rashid, A., Pluda, J., Bucana, C., Madden, T., Tran, H.T., and Abbruzzese, J.L. 2002. Development of biologic markers of response and assessment of antiangiogenic activity in a clinical trial of human recombinant endostatin. *J. Clin. Oncol. 20*:3804–3814.

Jayson, G.C., Zweit, J., Jackson, A., Mulatero, C., Julyan, P., Ranson, M., Broughton, L., Wagstaff, J., Hakannson, L., Groenewegen, G., Bailey, J., Smith, N., Hastings, D., Lawrance, J., Haroon, H., Ward, T., McGown, A.T., Tang, M., Levitt, D., Marreaud, S., Lehmann, F.F., Herold, M., and Zwierzina, H. 2002. Molecular imaging and biological evaluation of HuMV833 anti-VEGF antibody: implications for trial design of antiangiogenic antibodies. *J. Natl. Cancer Inst. 94*:1484–1493.

Juweid, M.E., and Cheson, B.D. 2006. Positron-emission tomography and assessment of cancer therapy. *N. Engl. J. Med. 354*:496–507.

Leach, M.O., Brindle, K.M., Evelhoch, J.L., Griffiths, J.R., Horsman, M.R., Jackson, A., Jayson, G.C., Judson, I.R., Knopp, M.V., Maxwell, R.J., McIntyre, D., Padhani, A.R., Price, P., Rathbone, R., Rustin, G.J., Tofts, P.S., Tozer, G.M., Vennart, W., Waterton, J.C., Williams, S.R., and Workman, P. 2005. The assessment of antiangiogenic and antivascular therapies in early-stage clinical trials using magnetic resonance imaging: issues and recommendations. *Brit. J. Cancer 92*:1599–1610.

Liu, G., Rugo, H.S., Wilding, G., McShane, T.M., Evelhoch, J.L., Ng, C., Jackson, E., Kelcz, F., Yeh, B.M., Lee, F.T., Charnsangavej, C., Park, J.W., Ashton, E.A, Steinfeldt, H.M., Pithavala, Y.K., Reich, S.D., and Herbst, R.S. 2005. Dynamic contrast-enhanced magnetic resonance imaging as a pharmacodynamic measure of response after acute dosing of AG-013736, an oral angiogenesis inhibitor, in patients with advanced solid tumors: results from a Phase I study. *J. Clin. Oncol. 23*:5464–5473.

Ludwig, J.A., and Weinstein, J.N. 2005. Biomarkers in cancer staging, prognosis and treatment selection. *Nat. Rev. 5*:845–856.

Miller, A.B., Hoogstraten, B., Staquet, M., and Winkler, A. 1981. Reporting results of cancer treatment. *Cancer 47*:207–214.

Morgan, B., Thomas, A.L., Drevs, J., Hennig, J., Buchert, M., Jivan, A., Horsfield, M.A., Mross, K., Ball, H.A., Lee, L., Mietlowski, W., Fuxius, S., Unger, C., O'Byrne, K., Henry, A., Cherryman, G.R., Laurent, D., Dugan, M., Marme, D., and Steward, W.P. 2003. Dynamic contrast-enhanced magnetic resonance imaging as a biomarker for the pharmacological response of PTK787/ZK 222584, an inhibitor of the vascular endothelial growth factor receptor tyrosine kinases, in patients with advanced colorectal cancer and liver metastases: results from two Phase I studies. *J. Clin. Oncol. 21*:3955–3964.

Park, J.W., Kerbel, R.S., Kelloff, G.J., Barrett, J.C., Chabner, B.A., Parkinson, D.R., Peck, J., Ruddon, R.W., Sigman, C.C., and Slamon, D.J. 2004. Rationale for biomarkers and surrogate endpoints in mechanism-driven oncology drug development. *Clin. Cancer Res. 10*:3885–3896.

Parulekar, W.R., and Eisenhauer, E.A. 2004. Phase I trial design for solid tumor studies of targeted, non-cytotoxic agents: theory and practice. *J. Natl. Cancer Inst. 96*:990–997.

Roberts, C., Issa, B., Stone, A., Jackson, A., Waterton, J.C., and Parker, G.J.M. 2006. Comparative study into the robustness of compartmental modeling and model-free analysis in DCE-MRI studies. *J. Magn. Reson. Imaging 23*:554–563.

Roberts, T.G., Lynch, T.J., and Chabner, B.A. 2003. The Phase III trial in the era of targeted therapy: unraveling the "Go or No Go" decision. *J. Clin. Oncol. 21*:3683–3695.

Schilsky, R.L. 2002. Endpoints in cancer clinical trials and the drug approval process. *Clin. Cancer Res. 8*:935–938.

Schrag, D. 2004. The price tag on progress—chemotherapy for colorectal cancer. *N. Engl. J. Med. 351*:317–319.

Stevenson, J.P., Rosen, M., Sun, W., Gallagher, M., Haller, D.G., Vaughn, D., Giantonio, B., Zimmer, R., Petros, W.P., Stratford, M., Chaplin, D., Young, S.L., Schnall, M., and O'Dwyer, P.J. 2003. Phase I trial of the antivascular agent combretastatin A4 phosphate on a 5-day schedule to patients with cancer: magnetic resonance imaging evidence for altered tumor blood flow. *J. Clin. Oncol. 21*:4428–4438.

Stroobants, S., Goeminne, J., Seegers, M., Dimitrijevic, S., Dupont, P., Nuyts, J., Martens, M., van den Borne, B., Cole, P., Sciot, R., Dumez, H., Silberman, S., Mortelmans, L., and van Oosterom, A. 2003. [18]FDG-positron emission tomography for the early prediction of response in advanced soft tissue sarcoma treated with imatinib mesylate (Glivec®). *Eur. J. Cancer 39*:2012–2020.

Therasse, P. 2002. Measuring the clinical response. What does it mean? *Eur. J. Cancer 38*:1817–1823.

Therasse, P., Arbuck, S.G., Eisenhauer, E.A., Wanders, J., Kaplan, R.S., Rubinstein, L., Verweij, J., Van Glabbeke, M., van Oosterom, A.T., Christian, M.C., and Gwyther, S.G. 2000. New guidelines to evaluate the response to treatment in solid tumors. *J. Natl. Cancer Inst. 92*:205–216.

Thomas, J.P., Arzoomanian, R.Z., Alberti, D., Marnocha, R., Lee, F., Friedl, A., Tutsch, K., Dresen, A., Geiger, P., Pluda, J., Fogler, W., Schiller, J.H., and Wilding, G. 2003. Phase I pharmacokinetic and pharmacodynamic study of recombinant human endostatin in patients with advanced solid tumors. *J. Clin. Oncol. 21*:223–231.

Weber, W.A., Ziegler, S.I., Thodtman, R., Hanauske, A.R., and Schwaiger, M. 1999. Reproducibility of metabolic measurements in malignant tumors using FDG PET. *J. Nucl. Med. 40*:1771–1777.

Young, H., Baum, R., Cremerius, U., Herholz, K., Hoekstra, O., Lammertsma, A.A., Pruim, J., and Price, P. 1999. Measurement of clinical and subclinical tumor response using [18F]-fluorodeoxyglucose and positron emission tomography: review and 1999 EORTC recommendations. *Eur. J. Cancer 35*:1773–1782.

Zia, M.I., Siu, L.L., Pond, G.R., and Chen, E.X. 2005. Comparison of outcomes of Phase II studies and subsequent randomized control studies using identical chemotherapeutic regimens. *J. Clin. Oncol. 23*:6982–6991.

4

Characterization of Multiple Aspects of Tumor Physiology by Multitracer Positron Emission Tomography

Dan J. Kadrmas, Thomas C. Rust, and John M. Hoffman

Introduction

Noninvasive medical imaging procedures play a central and increasingly important role in cancer diagnosis, staging, re-staging, assessment of prognosis, treatment planning, therapy monitoring, and evaluation for recurrence. Anatomic imaging modalities such as magnetic resonance imaging (MRI) and X-ray computed tomography (CT) provide high-resolution images of body structures and are capable of depicting many cancerous lesions. Although these images are of excellent quality, they provide limited metabolic or physiologic information. The technology of medicine and biology has progressed to the point where *functional, metabolic*, and *molecular* information about malignant disease can now be utilized to improve patient care—leading to the emergent field of molecular imaging, where noninvasive imaging is used to measure functional and metabolic/molecular processes on a cellular and molecular level. The dominant modality for imaging tumor physiology *in vivo* is positron emission tomography (PET) (Gambhir, 2002). In PET, a pharmaceutical or compound that (ideally) traces a specific molecular function or pathway is labeled with a positron-emitting radioisotope. The resulting radiotracer is administered in very small amounts, usually intravenously, and the distribution of the tracer is imaged. The resulting images reflect the metabolic/molecular or functional processes that the tracer is designed to target or assess. In combined PET/CT imaging, this functional information is precisely fused and localized with high-resolution CT images, providing co-registered structure and function.

The vast majority of clinical PET experience to date has been with ^{18}F-fluorodeoxyglucose (FDG), which is a marker for hexokinase activity (the rate-limiting step in glucose metabolism). Indeed, in the context of cancer imaging, PET has often been used interchangeably with FDG PET, and care should be taken to distinguish between tracer-specific issues and those of the modality as a whole. FDG PET is discussed extensively in other chapters of this volume. Since most cancerous cells exhibit markedly increased FDG uptake as compared to normal cells, FDG PET is a fairly general-use tool for cancer imaging. FDG PET is routinely used for evaluating indeterminate pulmonary nodules, staging, detecting distant metastases through whole-body imaging, and evaluating recurrent or residual disease following therapy. Though a powerful agent, FDG has several limitations: FDG uptake is not specific to neoplastic disease, and the normal accumulation of FDG is complex and variable; inflammatory responses can lead to false-positive findings; certain malignancies such as prostate cancer are not particularly FDG avid, leading to low sensitivity for FDG PET; and glucose metabolism is only one factor of interest regarding cancer assessment and characterization.

Current clinical PET and PET/CT tumor imaging is focused on *detection* tasks, such as determining the presence or absence of malignancy and detecting metastases to evaluate the extent of local, regional, and distant spread of disease. These mainstream tasks form the backbone of PET tumor imaging; however, the true value of the modality lies in its ability to image, with very high measurement sensitivity, any of a number of radiotracers specifically targeting the underlying functional, metabolic, molecular, and physiologic processes of malignant disease. Literally hundreds of positron-emitting radiotracers have been investigated, and tracers can be conceived for imaging virtually any metabolic, molecular, or physiologic target-of-interest.

Thus, while detection tasks form the current mainstream of clinical PET usage, the modality is particularly well suited to *characterizing* the molecular status of disease sites *in vivo*. Moreover, since different PET tracers assess different aspects of tumor function (Fig.1), the complementary use of multiple PET tracers can provide greater insight into disease status. Such information may potentially offer improved methods for evaluating the grade and extent of disease, making an individualized prognosis and characterization of the malignancy, selecting of the most effective therapy (both guiding choice of therapeutic regimen and image-guided localization of therapy), monitoring tumor response to therapy, and evaluating residual/recurrent disease. The field of PET tumor characterization for these applications is in its infancy, with most clinical investigations utilizing only a single tracer, and a vast array of new tracers and multitracer imaging schemes will be studied in the coming decades. This chapter provides a brief overview of the most important imaging targets and PET tracers under investiga-

tion by a number of research groups, a summary of evidence demonstrating the complementary value of using multiple PET tracers for characterizing malignant tumors, and a discussion of the technical hurdles for imaging multiple PET tracers in a clinical setting.

PET Tracers and Imaging Targets

Positron-emitting tracers have been developed for imaging many cellular and molecular targets, including glucose metabolism, blood flow, hypoxia, cellular proliferation, protein synthesis, lipid biosynthesis, membrane transport of proteins, hormone receptors, tumor receptors, angiogenesis, apoptosis, and gene expression; and the list continues to grow rapidly. Each PET tracer consists of a molecule, substrate, or drug designed to image a specific molecular or physiologic target, labeled with an appropriate positron-emitting radioisotope. The most commonly used PET radioisotopes are fluorine-18 ($T_{1/2}$ = 110 min), carbon-11 ($T_{1/2}$ = 20 min), oxygen-15 ($T_{1/2}$ = 122 sec), and nitrogen-13 ($T_{1/2}$ = 10 min), though many other radioisotopes have also been studied, including gallium-68 ($T_{1/2}$ = 68 min), rubidium-82 ($T_{1/2}$ = 75 sec), iodine-124 ($T_{1/2}$ = 4.2 days), copper-64 ($T_{1/2}$ = 12.7 hr), copper-62 ($T_{1/2}$ = 9.7 min), and others. Each radioisotope has its own means of production (e.g., cyclotron, generator, other), handling, and safety requirements, and each also has different imaging characteristics in terms of spatial resolution and radiation dosimetry. The following provides an overview of the foremost cancer imaging targets and leading PET tracers under investigation for imaging each target.

Glucose Metabolism

Glucose metabolism can be imaged using ^{11}C-glucose or ^{18}F-fluoro-2-deoxy-D-glucose (FDG). ^{11}C-glucose is chemically identical to endogenous glucose, with a natural carbon atom replaced with the positron-emitting radioisotope ^{11}C. As such, this tracer enters the full citric acid cycle,

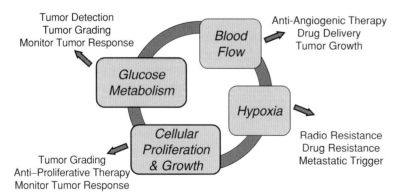

Figure 1 A number of different physiologic and metabolic/molecular factors must be measured to fully characterize malignant tumors *in vivo*, each of which has different implications for individualized patient management. Various PET tracers have been developed for imaging each of these factors and, when used in combination, provide complementary information about tumor status.

and imaging is complicated by the presence of circulating labeled metabolites. FDG, on the other hand, employs a tracer-trapping mechanism that greatly simplifies image interpretation. FDG is typically administered by bolus intravenous injection and is delivered throughout the body via the blood. Glucose transport proteins govern cellular uptake of FDG, and within the cell it is phosphorylated by hexokinase to FDG-6-phosphate. Hexokinase is the rate-limiting enzyme in glucose metabolism. Unlike natural glucose, the presence of the fluorine atom blocks further catabolism in most tissues, and FDG-6-phosphate is metabolically trapped in the cell. FDG is the most commonly used PET tracer, with numerous applications in oncology, cardiology, neurology, and inflammation imaging. Most tumors exhibit increased expression of glucose transport proteins and increased hexokinase activity. Thus, FDG is avidly taken up in many types of tumors, making it a fairly general-use tracer for cancer imaging, though false positives from inflammatory processes can also occur. The increased FDG uptake seen in inflammation is typically felt to be secondary to the utilization of FDG by the increased white blood cells present in an inflammatory process. An extensive review of FDG PET imaging can be found in Gambhir *et al.* (2001).

Blood Flow and Perfusion

In vivo measurement of tumor blood flow can provide important insight into the physiologic status of tumor sites, has implications for tumor grade and the delivery of chemotherapeutic agents, and is increasingly important for measuring tumor response to certain therapies, especially anti-angiogenic and antivascular therapies. Methods of imaging tumor blood flow are reviewed in Anderson and Price (2002) and Choyke *et al.* (2002). The most widely used and validated PET blood flow tracer is ^{15}O-water, which is freely diffusible and not affected by cellular uptake mechanisms or metabolic trapping. The short half-life of ^{15}O ($T_{1/2} = 122\,sec$) makes rapid repeat imaging feasible. However, widespread use of ^{15}O tracers is limited by the need for an on-site cyclotron and facilities to deliver the tracer quickly to the scanning suite. Imaging with ^{15}O-water is technically challenging and best performed by experienced research groups.

Several longer-lived tracers have been investigated, which are rapidly taken up and trapped in tissues in proportion to blood flow and perfusion, such as ^{13}N-ammonia, ^{82}Rb-chloride, and copper-labeled perfusion tracers such as ^{62}Cu-pyruvaldehyde-bis-N^4-methyl-thiosemicarbazone (PTSM) and ^{62}Cu-ethylglyoxal bis-thiosemicarbazone (ETS). The first two, ^{13}N-ammonia and ^{82}Rb-chloride, find frequent use for imaging myocardial perfusion, but concerns about their mechanisms for tissue extraction and trapping limit the usefulness of these tracers for imaging tumor blood flow. The copper-labeled blood flow tracers show more promise for assessing tumor blood flow, and may become a viable option

for imaging centers without on-site cyclotrons since ^{62}Cu can be produced by a portable generator. Additional development and evaluation of these tracers for measuring tumor blood flow are warranted.

Hypoxia

PET imaging of oxygen status and hypoxia has become established in recent years as a practical and effective tool for oncologic and other applications (Ballinger, 2001; Lewis and Welch, 2001). Hypoxia can lead to radioresistance, resistance to many chemotherapeutic drugs; has implications for drug delivery issues; and causes phenotypical changes resulting in more malignant and metastatic tumor behaviors. The leading radiotracers include nitroimidazole derivatives, such as ^{18}F-fluoromisonidazole (FMISO), and select copper complexes, such as Cu-diacetyl-bis-N^4-methylthiosemicarbazone (ATSM). Hypoxia selective compounds are generally retained in viable cells by a redox trapping mechanism, which proceeds at a faster rate under hypoxic conditions and slower under normoxic conditions. This leads to prolonged retention of these tracers in hypoxic cells.

The earliest PET tracer of hypoxia to be developed was FMISO, and it remains the most widely studied (Rasey *et al.*, 1986; Koh *et al.*, 1992; Casciari *et al.*, 1995). A number of papers have shown FMISO to provide valuable images of tumor hypoxia for treatment planning. The relatively slow washout of FMISO from normoxic tissues and limited contrast for hypoxic tissues prompted the development of more hydrophilic tracers such as ^{18}F-fluoroerythro-nitroimidazole (FETNIM) (Yang *et al.*, 1995; Grönroos *et al.*, 2001). These may potentially provide higher contrast images of tumor hypoxia with shorter time delays between injection and imaging. Another PET tracer under development for imaging tumor hypoxia is ^{62}Cu-diacetyl-bis-N^4-methylthiosemi-carbazone (ATSM), which has higher uptake in hypoxic tissues and faster clearance from normoxic tissues as compared to the nitroimidazoles. ATSM may provide high-contrast hypoxia imaging in as little as 15 min post-injection, though concerns about flow-dependent uptake exist that are not yet fully resolved.

Cellular Proliferation

Cellular proliferation can be measured effectively using tracers involved in cell division and deoxyribonucleic acid (DNA) synthesis. Measurement of proliferation with PET can provide information complementary to FDG for oncology applications, and it has increased the ability to detect certain cancers, monitor response to therapy, and evaluate prognosis (Kubota, 2001; Shields, 2003). Thymidine and other molecules incorporated in DNA have received the most interest as imaging agents. PET imaging of radiolabeled ^{11}C-thymidine has been established through numerous studies, but the images are complicated by circulating labeled metabolites. This led to the development of thymidine analogs such as ^{18}F-fluorothymidine (FLT). FLT remains virtually unchanged during *in vivo* administration and thus simplifies the kinetic analysis required for PET imaging. FLT is transported into cells by a carrier-mediated mechanism and simple diffusion, where it is phosphorylated by thymidine kinase and trapped. Retention of FLT within the cell primarily measures thymidine kinase activity, which is known to increase 5–10 fold during cell division. FLT PET is receiving significant attention for imaging many tumor types, especially lung tumors, and much needed comparisons with FDG are currently underway. In addition to FLT, other proliferation tracers are also under development, including 1-(2'-deoxy-2'-fluoro-ß-D-arabinofurano-syl)thy-mine (FMAU) and 1-(2'-deoxy-2'-fluoro-ß-D-arabinofuranosyl)-5-bromouracil (FBAU). Further work is required to determine the efficacy and potential roles of these for oncologic imaging.

Other Growth-Related Tracers

In addition to cellular proliferation, a number of other imaging targets related to tumor growth have been identified, including imaging of protein and lipid synthesis, and amino acid transport (Herholz *et al.*, 1998; Jager *et al.*, 2001; Narayanan *et al.*, 2002). Amino acids are the building blocks of protein, and several amino acid tracers have been developed. The most frequently studied amino acid tracer is ^{11}C-methyl-methionine (MET). MET is used primarily to image brain tumors, where FDG can be ineffective due to high background in normal brain tissue. MET and other amino acid tracers are useful for tumor detection, grading, and delineation of tumor margins, and for evaluating the effects of therapy. Another growth-related tracer is ^{11}C-acetate, which is a free fatty acid that enters into the tricarboxylic acid (TCA or Krebs) cycle after being converted to acetyl-coA. Acetate is thought to act as a precursor of amino acid or lipid synthesis in tumors, and it has been found useful for imaging prostate, hepatocellular, meningioma, glioma, nasopharyngeal, lymphoma, colon, ovarian, and renal cell cancers. ^{11}C-choline and ^{18}F-fluorocholine are other tracers of lipid synthesis found to have promise for several tumor imaging applications and are currently under investigation.

Other Tracers

Numerous other PET tracers have received significant interest for cancer imaging, for example:

- Sodium fluoride labeled with ^{18}F-fluorine is a bone-imaging agent that has been used for many years to image primary and metastatic tumors (Hawkins *et al.*, 1992).
- ^{18}F-fluoroestradiol (FES) is an estrogen hormone receptor agent that has been found effective in predicting response to hormone therapy in breast cancer (Mintun *et al.*, 1988).

- ^{18}F-Fluoro-deoxy-phenylalanine (FDOPA) has been found to be specifically useful for imaging melanoma since it is a substrate for melanin synthesis, and it is also a general indicator of large neutral amino acid transport with potential applications in neuroendocrine, pancreatic, medullary thyroid, and gastrointestinal cancers with elevated amino acid uptake or serotonin expression (Dimitrakopoulou-Strauss *et al.*, 2001; Graham, 2001; Hoegerle *et al.*, 2001).
- Annexin V is a protein marker for apoptosis, programmed cell death, that has been labeled using ^{18}F and [124]I for PET imaging (Keen *et al.*, 2005; Yagle *et al.*, 2005).
- PET imaging of gene expression has been developed in recent years, for example, using ^{18}F-fluorogancyclovir or ^{18}F-fluoropenciclovir along with the herpes simplex virus type-1 thymidine kinase reporter gene.
- PET is also a powerful modality for imaging radiolabeled peptides, and positron-emitting tags that can often be employed to study the pharmacokinetics and biodistribution of new therapeutic agents.

Complementary Value of Imaging Multiple Tracers

As can be seen from the brief overview just presented, a large number of PET tracers have been developed or are under investigation for a wide range of cancer imaging applications. Many published scientific articles have discussed the potential importance of different PET tracers for both clinical and basic science investigations (Roelcke *et al.*, 1995; Mankoff *et al.*, 2000; Kubota, 2001; Inoue *et al.*, 2002; Rajendran and Krohn, 2005). These papers point toward an expanding role for PET in characterizing tumor biology and providing individualized clinical management of cancer patients. A number of studies have utilized multiple tracers for evaluating tumor growth and response to therapy. The following summary includes example papers where different tracers were recognized as having complementary value.

Monitoring Response to Radiotherapy and Predicting Recurrence

Kubota *et al.* (1991) performed a study to test the feasibility of radiotherapy monitoring using multiple tracers. Five different tracers were studied using multitracer autoradiography techniques in a rat tumor model: FDG, ^{18}F-fluorouridine (RNA and thymidine synthesis), ^{14}C-methionine, ^{3}H-thymidine, and ^{67}Ga-citrate. This work demonstrated that different aspects of tumor physiology, as measured by these tracers, responded differently to different levels of irradiation, and also that the temporal patterns of response differed for the different tracers. For a highly effective treatment dose, FDG showed a gradual and constant decrease in uptake over 6 days following treatment. For both thymidine and methionine, a rapid 50% decrease in uptake was observed on the first day after treatment. ^{67}Ga-citrate showed a slight increase in uptake on the first day followed by a rapid decrease. FDG and ^{67}Ga-citrate showed the largest overall changes in tissue uptake, indicating that they may be valuable for monitoring response to therapy. Thymidine and methionine showed more rapid changes in uptake and were more sensitive to the difference between fully effective versus partially effective treatment, suggesting that they may be more sensitive for early detection of response and predicting recurrence. An accompanying editorial (Sasaki, 1991) suggested that successful image-guided selection of a therapeutic strategy and monitoring its effect requires combined measurement of tumor perfusion, metabolism, receptor distribution, and drug uptake.

More recently, Kubota *et al.* (1999) evaluated combined imaging of hypoxia (FMISO), glucose metabolism (^{14}C-2-deoxyglucose, 2DG) and proliferation (MET) in the same rat tumor model. They reported:

> Combined use of these tracers might provide better information on tumor characteristics. The ratio of FMISO uptake to 2DG (FDG) uptake may reflect the proportion of hypoxic tissue in the tumor, the hypoxic fraction. This fraction has been used in the field of radiation biology as an important index to predict radiosensitivity. On the other hand, the ratio of MET uptake to 2DG (FDG) uptake may correspond to the percentage of proliferative tissue, the growth fraction. This is also an important parameter with which to describe the growth kinetics of tumor tissue. Further studies correlating tumor uptake of FMISO and FDG or MET to radiotherapeutic effects are warranted. (p. 756)

Detection and Grading of Non-Hodgkin's Lymphoma

Leskinen-Kallio *et al.* (1991) performed PET scans with FDG and MET scans four hours apart on the same day in patients with non-Hodgkin's Lymphoma. MET was more effective in detecting lymphomas of all grades, while FDG was inconsistent in detecting intermediate and low-grade disease. However, FDG was better for grading high-grade lymphomas while MET was ineffective for this task. Using both tracers provided complementary value for early detection (MET) and grading (FDG) in this study. Grading is particularly important for non-Hodgkin's Lymphoma since low-grade disease typically has a slow clinical progression over several years while high-grade lymphomas may be fatal within a few weeks.

Detection and Localization of Bone Metastases

In 1998 Hoegerle *et al.* investigated dual-tracer summed Na[18]F-fluoride and FDG imaging for detection and staging of a wide variety of cancers with potential bone metasta-

ses. Whole-body imaging using this combination of tracers was considered as a potential alternative to using co-registered anatomical images from CT or MRI for the purposes of tumor localization. Their results suggested that summed images of these two tracers could provide better sensitivity and localization than FDG alone. One caveat of the summed dual-tracer approach is that it could potentially lead to false-negative findings, particularly in bone lesions with little or no reactive bone formation, in which case a combination of low Na[18]F-fluoride and high FDG uptake could result in similar activity as compared to surrounding bone. As a potential alternative, they suggested acquiring separate images of one tracer followed by a second injection of the other tracer and then later acquisition of summed images.

"Metabolic Flare" Response in Breast Cancer

Multitracer PET studies have also been performed to characterize a "metabolic flare" response in breast cancer patients treated with tamoxifen, an antiestrogen hormone therapy agent (Dehdashti *et al.*, 1999; Mortimer *et al.*, 2001). Serial PET scans were performed with FDG and FES (estrogen receptor agent) before and 7–10 days after treatment. High uptake of FES prior to treatment was a good predictor of response to therapy, and an increase in uptake of FDG after treatment was effective for showing a positive response to therapy. All patients showed decreased FES uptake after treatment due to the blockade of estrogen receptors, and responders showed a somewhat greater decrease in FES uptake as compared to nonresponders. Serial PET with FES and FDG before and after tamoxifen therapy accurately predicted response within 10 days after the start of therapy, in contrast to the several weeks often required to make this assessment by standard anatomical imaging techniques and clinical evaluation. The authors conclude that the information provided by PET will allow for optimal selection of the most appropriate systemic therapy in individual patients with advanced breast cancer.

Predicting and Monitoring Response to Chemotherapy in Breast Cancer

Several studies have used combined PET imaging of blood flow (^{15}O-water) and glucose metabolism (FDG) to predict and measure response to neoadjuvant chemotherapy in breast cancer patients (Mankoff *et al.*, 2002, 2003; Zasadny *et al.*, 2003). The rationale for this approach is that some tracers and systemic chemotherapy agents may not be delivered adequately to tumors with low blood flow. Furthermore, underperfused tumors may become hypoxic and undergo a transformation to more aggressive and therapy-resistant phenotypes (Vaupel and Hockel, 2000). Pretherapy measures of blood flow alone were not a good predictor of response to therapy, but there was a strong association between glucose metabolism and response. The ratio of low glucose metabolism to high blood flow was found to be the best predictor of a positive response to treatment and also predicted longer disease-free survival (Mankoff *et al.*, 2002). During the course of therapy, responders showed only a slightly greater reduction in glucose metabolism as compared to nonresponders. Meanwhile, changes in blood flow showed a much greater difference between responders and nonresponders, with nonresponders showing an average increase of about 50% in blood flow and responders showing an average reduction of approximately 10% (Mankoff *et al.*, 2003). The ratio of glucose metabolism to blood flow decreased for all tumors after therapy, falling to values approaching that of a normal breast in more responsive tumors (Tseng *et al.*, 2004). Overall, combined measurement of both blood flow and glucose metabolism provided more insight into breast tumor biology than either alone.

Melanoma Detection

Dimitrakopoulou-Strauss *et al.* (2001) performed multitracer PET studies with FDOPA (melanin synthesis), FDG, and ^{15}O-water in patients undergoing treatment for melanoma. The sensitivity of PET for detecting viable tumors was higher when using FDG and FDOPA in combination (95%) as compared to either tracer alone (86% for FDG; 64% for FDOPA). Another interesting finding of this work was that the pharmacokinetic data from all three tracers were not strongly correlated, indicating that each of these tracers provided different information about tumor biology. An accompanying editorial highlighted the potential of multitracer PET:

> FDG PET is an effective but imperfect tool that takes advantage of a common defect in tumor metabolism: inefficient and elevated glucose metabolism. However, this metabolic defect is apparently not present in all tumors. We need to identify other tracers that can probe alternative metabolic pathways and minimize the false-negative findings that are a significant problem with FDG imaging. These tracers may also reduce the false-positivity problems with FDG caused by uptake in normal and inflamed tissues. (Graham, 2001, p. 258)

Detection of Hepatocellular Carcinoma (HCC) and Liver Tumors

In 2003, Ho *et al.* performed a study to evaluate the usefulness of ^{11}C-acetate as a complementary tracer to FDG in the detection of hepatocellular carcinoma (HCC) and other liver tumors. HCC is known to exhibit similar or reduced glucose metabolism compared to normal liver and therefore may escape detection with FDG PET. A strong complementary relationship was found between ^{11}C-acetate and FDG for detection of liver tumors. The overall sensitivity for detecting HCC with ^{11}C-acetate PET was 87.3% as compared to 47.3%

using FDG. Vascular hepatic metastases and extrahepatic metastases showed greater FDG avidity and were detected in greater numbers using FDG, while one brain metastasis was detected using ^{11}C-acetate but not with FDG. Another interesting observation was that ^{11}C-acetate was fairly specific for HCC tumors and was negative for detection of non-HCC liver tumors, such as hemangioma, cholangiocarcinoma, and metastases from colon, breast, and lung tumors. Thus, using FDG and ^{11}C-acetate together may provide complementary information for evaluating liver tumors of unknown origin.

Detection and Characterization of Lung Cancers

Higashi *et al.* (2004) studied FDG PET, ^{11}C-acetate PET, and ^{99}Tc-sestamibi SPECT for detection and characterization of lung cancers in 23 patients. They observed that FDG PET had the highest sensitivity for detecting tumors, followed by ^{11}C-acetate, followed by ^{99}Tc-sestamibi. FDG also correlated well with the degree of cellular differentiation, aggressiveness (pleural involvement, vascular invasion, lymphatic permeation, nodal involvement), and recurrence, whereas the other tracers did not. However, ^{11}C-acetate and ^{99}Tc-sestamibi showed high uptake in slow-growing bronchioloalveolar carcinomas, whereas FDG failed to identify these lesions. These results suggest that multiple PET tracers may play important complementary roles in the detection of certain lung tumors.

Halter *et al.* (2004) studied the role of FDG and FLT PET for staging bronchial carcinomas in 28 patients. For primary lung tumor detection, FDG was found to be more sensitive than FLT (95% vs. 86%), while FLT showed higher specificity (100% vs. 71%). For detecting lymph node metastases, FDG was much more sensitive than FLT (86% vs. 57%). The overall conclusion was that FDG PET played the most important role in detection, while FLT could potentially play a secondary role by identifying cases where false-positive FDG results occur due to an associated inflammatory processes.

Hypoxia and Metabolism for Tumor Characterization and Treatment Selection

Rajendran *et al.* (2004) investigated the relationship between regional glucose metabolism (FDG) and hypoxia (FMISO) in a variety of human tumors using PET. Wide variations in tumor glucose metabolism and hypoxia were observed, including all four of the possible combinations: (1) low glucose metabolism, low hypoxia; (2) low glucose metabolism, high hypoxia; (3) high glucose metabolism, low hypoxia; and (4) high glucose metabolism, high hypoxia. These variations were observed in different cancer types and tumor sizes, and were considered to reflect ubiquitous genetic responses to hypoxic stress. The complementary information provided by FDG and FMISO was considered to be important in the clinical characterization of tumor biology and selection of effective treatments. The accompanying editorial (Larson, 2004) explains that the capability of PET to explore multiple facets of the phenotype of human cancers is opening new doors for the *in vivo* study of the biochemistry of human tumors.

Brain Tumors

Perhaps the best example of using multiple PET tracers in oncology is in the study of gliomas, which are a class of tumors that includes about 40% of all primary brain tumors and about 80% of malignant brain tumors. Since the 1980s, a large number of patient studies have been performed to investigate a variety of different PET tracers for imaging gliomas. In many of these studies, blood flow, blood volume, oxygen extraction, and oxygen metabolism were measured together using sequential administration of several ^{15}O-labeled tracers (Frackowiak *et al.*, 1980). In addition, glucose metabolism (FDG), protein synthesis (MET), proliferation (^{11}C-thymidine, FLT), and hypoxia (FMISO) have also been frequently studied in various combinations (Roelcke *et al.*, 1995; Narayanan *et al.*, 2002; Jacobs *et al.*, 2005; Van Laere *et al.*, 2005; and others). Overall, these studies suggest that PET imaging with multiple tracers can provide complementary information for detection, differential diagnosis, grading, prognosis, planning radiotherapy and chemotherapy treatments, measuring response to therapy, and detecting recurrence.

Tumor Blood Flow and Hypoxia

The relationship between tumor blood flow and hypoxia is complex and variable, and imaging both may provide valuable complementary information for characterizing tumor perfusion status and managing treatment. Several researchers have studied the relationship between the uptake of blood flow and hypoxia tracers in tumors. In 1993, Moore *et al.* and Groshar *et al.* studied the correlation between SPECT perfusion tracers of blood flow (HMPAO, ^{99m}Tc-hexamethylpropyleneamine oxime) and hypoxia (IAZA, ^{123}I-iodoazaomycine arabinoside) in a variety of tumors. A wide range of uptake patterns were observed, and hypoxia in most tumor types was associated with low flow, suggesting a complex relationship between impaired tissue perfusion and the presence of viable hypoxic cells. In 1999, Lewis *et al.* compared the uptake of PTSM and ATSM *in vitro*, using autoradiography in a tumor-bearing murine model. *In vitro*, PTSM showed uptake completely independent of oxygen concentration, while ATSM uptake was inversely related to the pO_2 of the culture media. The autoradiography results showed uniform uptake of PTSM throughout the tumors, with heterogeneous uptake of ATSM and hypoxic fractions of 15 to 45%.

Lehtiö *et al.* (2001) performed PET imaging with ^{15}O-water, FDG, and ^{18}F-FETNIM (hypoxia) in patients with untreated head and neck carcinomas. In this study, tumors with high regional uptake of ^{18}F-FETNIM also tended to have high average blood flow. Several explanations were offered to account for this phenomenon: (1) the uptake of ^{18}F-FETNIM in tissue is governed by blood flow, (2) the presence of hypoxia enhances angiogenesis leading to high average blood flow on the macroscopic level, and (3) regions with high apparent flow may remain severely hypoxic due to a low oxygen extraction ratio.

In 2003, Lehtio *et al.* further examined the relationship between ^{18}F-FETNIM (hypoxia) distribution and ^{15}O-water (blood flow) using compartment model-based simulations over the range of hypoxia levels observed in patient data. Tissue blood flow was observed to have a notable effect on detection of hypoxia, with hypoxia tracer distribution being more sensitive to changes in oxygen concentration in high-flow regions than in low-flow regions. High blood flow was considered to enhance not only the uptake of ^{18}F-FETNIM into hypoxic cells but also the washout of the tracer from surrounding normoxic cells. These studies illustrate the complex relationship between tumor blood flow and hypoxia, and support the need for additional research to understand how they are interrelated. The results of pretherapy imaging for predicting the outcome of patients treated with radiotherapy and surgery were then evaluated (Lehtio *et al.*, 2004). The results indicated that it is possible to attain prognostic information by imaging perfusion and hypoxia using PET. Large variations in the measured PET parameters were observed both between individual patients and within the tumors, which depicted the heterogeneity of tumors. These studies illustrate the complex relationship between tumor blood flow and hypoxia, and support the need for additional research to understand how they are interrelated.

Technical Challenges for Imaging Multiple Tracers

It is clear that imaging multiple PET tracers can provide significantly improved characterization of tumor status *in vivo* and may offer improved treatment selection and monitoring. Why, then, are multiple PET tracers not widely used? The answer lies in the technical and logistical challenges of imaging multiple PET tracers, and is further complicated by the plethora of tracer combinations and imaging scenarios that will require extensive clinically directed research to test and validate. Furthermore, the current technology for PET is limited to imaging only a single tracer per scanning session, and multiple scanning sessions are currently required to image multiple tracers; however, new technologies are being developed to enable imaging of certain tracer combinations in a single scanning session as discussed in the final section of this chapter.

Tracer Interference Issues

The biggest limitation for performing multitracer PET imaging is the issue of tracer interference—all PET tracers emit positrons that annihilate to produce antiparallel 511 keV photons, and the coincident photon pairs produced by one tracer are indistinguishable from those produced by another. In physics jargon, there is no explicit information in the PET measurement that allows one to differentiate the signals for each tracer. As such, the present technology permits only two options for imaging multiple PET tracers: (1) wait for extended periods, usually > 7 half-lives, between scans for each tracer; or (2) in the limited cases where the activity from the first tracer has stabilized and is fixed (except for radioactive decay), acquire a "background" scan before injecting the second tracer and utilize background subtraction techniques to obtain a corrected image of the second tracer. In either case, unless ultra-short half-life tracers such as ^{15}O-water are used, multiple scanning sessions are required. This leads to extensive use of the imaging facilities (i.e., low throughput) and image co-registration issues. In addition, if PET/CT scans are performed, multiple CT scans should not in general be acquired due to radiation dosimetry concerns (see below). In any case, multiple sequential scans with different tracers, either on the same day or different days, are necessary to obtain untainted images of each tracer, placing a significant burden on both the imaging facilities and the patient's schedule. This has been the biggest factor limiting the use of multiple PET tracers for imaging cancer patients.

Logistics

When scans with multiple PET tracers are contemplated, a number of logistical issues arise that can be much more problematic than those encountered for routine single-tracer imaging. First of all, production and delivery issues for each tracer need to be resolved. For sites with an on-site cyclotron, which generally operates in the early morning to produce the day's supply of FDG, production of secondary "research" tracers is often restricted to afternoons on a limited basis with corresponding staffing issues. To exacerbate the situation, many such research tracers are labeled with short half-life radioisotopes, requiring coordination of the cyclotron run with the tracer injection and scanning times. The use of generator-produced tracers, e.g., ^{82}Rb or ^{62}Cu-labeled, greatly simplifies the logistics of tracer availability; however, such generators are generally quite expensive and may be limited in availability to only certain days according to institutional practices.

Additional logistical issues arise in coordinating the timing of tracer injection versus imaging. Some tracers, such as FMISO, benefit from a long delay ($\geq$ 2–3 hours) between tracer administration and imaging in order to permit the tracer to fully distribute and attain high contrast in the target tissues. Other tracers, such as ^{15}O-water, require immediate injection and dynamic imaging for a timeframe of only a few minutes. Careful planning of imaging protocols and coordination between tracer production personnel and imaging staff is necessary for successful efforts at multitracer PET imaging.

Cost of Multiple Tracers

At most sites, tracers other than FDG are available on a special-order or research basis only, and are not produced on a regular basis. As such, the cost for each dose may be much higher than that for a dose of FDG. Until the clinical value of using research PET tracers is well established and the demand increases correspondingly, the cost of using multiple PET tracers will remain much higher than that of FDG alone. Still, as demand rises, the per dose costs of these newer tracers should fall accordingly, and the cost savings associated with improved image-guided patient management (if realized) may potentially greatly outweigh the additional costs associated with multiple tracers.

Dosimetry Limitations

Each PET tracer administered will bring additional radiation exposure to the patient (as well as to the technologist), and care should be taken to ensure that safe radiation practices are maintained. Here, the situation for multitracer PET is less worrisome than one might initially suspect. The limits set by the Food and Drug Administration (FDA) for application of radiation in human subjects (21 CFR 361.1) for *research studies with no immediate diagnostic benefit* are:

21 CFR 361.1 Limits

Single dose	3 rems
Annual and total dose commitment	5 rems
Other organs:	
Single dose	5 rems
Annual and total dose commitment	15 rems

With typical injected doses, most PET tracers give whole-body absorbed doses on the order of 0.1–0.3 rad, with somewhat higher doses to individual target organs depending on the tracer. In contrast, the CT portion of a typical whole-body PET/CT scan imparts closer to 1.0 rad whole-body dose. In general, a multitracer PET/CT scan with 3–4 tracers still remains within the dose limits for research scans with no immediate benefit. When considering that the most likely clinical applications of multitracer PET will be in patients with known disease for image-guide treatment purposes, the risks associated with these low levels of radiation exposure will be heavily outweighed by the potential clinical benefits to the patient.

Multitracer Image Analysis and Interpretation

Finally, the use of each additional PET tracer brings corresponding demands on image processing, data analysis, and image interpretation. These increased demands are complex and multifold. First, many PET tracers benefit from dynamic imaging techniques, resulting in much more complicated imaging protocols requiring significant expertise for data analysis and processing. Second, proper co-registration of the images for each tracer is needed, a process that is semiautomated at best and also requires significant expertise. In general, only highly advanced technologists or even medical physicists will have the skills necessary for such data management. Third, the greatly increased volume of data provided by the multitracer images will require a corresponding increase in reading expertise by the interpreting physician, including specific training in the normal uptake patterns, features, and limitations of *each* tracer. Overall, a highly trained and experienced "imaging team" is required for efficacious use of multitracer PET tumor imaging. This requirement will likely remain the case for many years until specific multitracer imaging protocols become routine and commonplace in the field.

The Future: Rapid Multitracer Positron Emission Tomography

The objective of characterizing multiple aspects of tumor physiology by multitracer PET imaging would be much more appealing if all the imaging could be completed in a single, rapid scanning session. This would increase scanner throughput for such studies, greatly simplify scheduling and staffing issues, and offer much improved patient convenience and compliance. It would also bring benefits in terms of the imaging itself. It would ensure accurate co-registration of the images for each tracer, eliminate any penchant for acquiring additional CT scans for each tracer (thereby minimizing CT dose concerns), and ensure that the multitracer images provide a true "snapshot" of tumor status at a single point in time. This last benefit has important implications for treatment monitoring, where scans may be taken a matter of days into therapy and compared with a pretreatment baseline scan. For this application, concurrent or near simultaneous imaging of each tracer would be needed to provide a robust and reproducible measure of tumor status for detecting metabolic/functional changes that occur in response to therapy.

As discussed earlier, simultaneous or near-simultaneous imaging of multiple PET tracers is impeded by a considerable technological challenge: all PET tracers give rise

to indistinguishable coincident 511 keV photons, and no explicit information is present in the signal that allows the detector to determine which events arose from which tracers. This differs from single photon emission computed tomography (SPECT) imaging, where different tracers may emit gamma rays of different energies, and energy discrimination can be employed to separate the imaging signals for each tracer. Using current technology, a PET scan acquired with multiple tracers presents an image *summed* over all tracers, and the information from each tracer is confounded by that from the other tracers. Note, however, that we carefully say that there is no *explicit* information in the PET measurement identifying which tracer gave rise to which event. Using dynamic imaging techniques, we can exploit differences in tracer distribution kinetics and radioactive decay in some cases to predict the fractional contribution and spatial distribution of each tracer to a multitracer data set. Using *a priori* information about expected tracer kinetic behaviors, known isotopic half-lives, and employing staggered injection times, we can recover clinically important measures for multiple tracers. Figure 2 presents a brief overview of previous work in this area, along with a discussion of the present status of the field, future expectations, and limitations of the approach.

Previous Work on Rapid Multitracer PET

In 1982, Huang *et al.* demonstrated that multiple PET tracers with static distributions (i.e., at equilibrium) could be imaged dynamically and individual tracer images recovered based on differences in tracer half-lives. This study used ^{18}F ($T_{1/2} = 110$ min), ^{13}N ($T_{1/2} = 9.97$ min), ^{64}Cu ($T_{1/2} = 12.7$ hr), and ^{68}Ga ($T_{1/2} = 68.3$ min) in a plastic and water phantom, and it established the basic principle on which rapid multitracer PET strategies could be built. Limitations in the performance capabilities of PET tomographs and limited experience with PET tracer kinetic analysis methods at the time precluded further work on rapid multitracer PET for a number years.

Then, in 1998 Koeppe *et al.* developed a methodology for temporally overlapping dual-tracer PET studies using a combined compartment-modeling method to obtain separate pharmacokinetic information about two different tracers injected a short time apart during a dynamic PET scan. The work was motivated by the desire to study multiple neurotransmitter-neuroreceptor systems in the same subject's brain during a short time period and under similar pharmacologic conditions, using the tracers ^{11}C-flumazenil, ^{11}C-dihydrotetrabenazine, and N-^{11}C-methyl-piperidinyl-propionate. The combined compartmental-modeling approach was evaluated for several tracer pairings using simulated dual-tracer time activity curves in a digital brain phantom. Model parameters for tracers injected only 10 to 20 min apart were estimated nearly as accurately as in

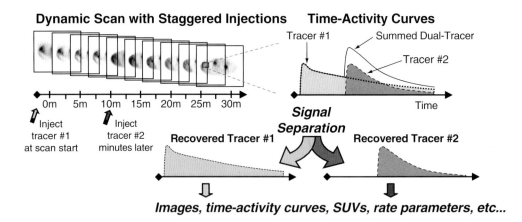

Figure 2 In rapid multitracer PET imaging, a dynamic scan is acquired while multiple PET tracers are injected at staggered intervals. The multitracer time-activity curve for each region of interest or voxel is then processed, using *a priori* knowledge of each tracer's radioactive half-life, injection time, and expected kinetic behaviors, in order to recover separate time-activity curves for each tracer. These can then be analyzed—as with conventional single-tracer PET—to provide measures such as SUVs and rate parameter estimates, and they can also be re-formed into images of each tracer. Current research is involved in developing signal separation algorithms and evaluating the accuracy and limitation of the approach.

standard single-tracer studies. These results demonstrated the feasibility of rapid dual-tracer PET imaging and showed that the accuracy of kinetic parameter estimates is dependent on the choice of tracers, injection order, injection timing, the kinetic parameter(s) of interest, and the kinetics in different brain regions. The most significant advantages in comparison to performing two independent scans were identified as reducing total scan time by 1.5 to 2 hr, obtaining neuropharmacologic measures over nearly the same time interval, and simplifying interventional protocols.

Koeppe *et al.* (2001) later extended their work to include more simulations and a pilot study in healthy volunteers. Sophisticated arterial blood sampling techniques were used, and the kinetic rate parameters for each tracer were estimated using a parallel compartmental model configuration. Results demonstrated that voxel-by-voxel estimation of parameters from multiple tracers was possible with good precision and little bias other than those from partial volume effects. The primary limiting factor was an increase in statistical uncertainty (noise) in the parameter estimates when using the dual-tracer approach as compared to conventional single-tracer imaging.

More recently, Ikoma *et al.* (2002) presented an abstract that paralleled Koeppe's work using ^{18}F-FDG ($T_{1/2} = 110$ min) and ^{11}C-flumazenil ($T_{1/2} = 20.3$ min). A parallel dual-tracer compartmental model was used, and their results were consistent with those of Koeppe. Converse *et al.* (2004) also investigated PET measurement of regional cerebral blood flow using ^{17}F-fluoromethane (inhaled, $T_{1/2} = 64.5$ sec) in the presence of a neurochemical tracer, ^{18}F-fallypride. The objective of this work was to demonstrate proof of principle

for measuring rapidly changing blood flow patterns while also measuring the neuroreceptor status over a longer timescale. Their results demonstrated the feasibility of obtaining reproducible blood flow measurements in the presence of a longer-lived tracer.

Current Status and Research

These previous efforts established the proof of principle for imaging multiple PET tracers using a dynamic imaging protocol with rapid staggered injections, prompting our group to systematically investigate and develop rapid multitracer imaging techniques for PET tumor imaging. Kadrmas and Rust (2005) presented an engineering paper studying the information content available in multitracer PET signals for recovering separate images of each tracer. This extensive simulation study included four tracers, ^{18}F-FDG ($T_{1/2} = 110$ min), ^{11}C-acetate ($T_{1/2} = 20.3$ min), and ^{62}Cu-PTSM, and ^{62}Cu-ATSM ($T_{1/2} = 9.7$ min). Dual- and triple-tracer combinations were studied with injection delays ranging from 0 min (simultaneous) to 1 hr. Information content for separating individual tracer signals was analyzed using principal component analysis (PCA) techniques, and parallel multitracer compartment-modeling methods were also studied as a more readily available means of recovering separated measures for each tracer. The bias and noise properties of the rapid multitracer methods were evaluated and compared to those for conventional single-tracer methods.

The results of that work characterized the trade-off between total imaging time (i.e., injection delay timing) and accuracy, demonstrating that accuracy of the multitracer method improves rapidly with increasing injection delays from 0 to 10 min, with a 10 min delay generally providing good accuracy with a fairly short overall imaging time. The noise increase associated with multitracer imaging was also quantified and found to be a modest increase relative to the overall time savings of the method. Analysis of quantitative imaging measures for multitracer vs. single-tracer methods was somewhat more complicated, with variable results depending on the particular imaging measure (e.g., kinetic rate parameter, net uptake parameter, or SUV) and tracer under consideration.

This work was continued with a second simulation study optimizing the acquisition protocol for rapid dual-tracer imaging of tumor hypoxia using ^{62}Cu-PTSM and ^{62}Cu-ATSM (Rust and Kadrmas, 2006). These generator-produced copper-labeled tracers were chosen to simplify tracer production and delivery issues, and also because PTSM and ATSM are particularly well suited for rapid dual-tracer imaging—the two tracers are chemically very similar with closely related uptake mechanisms, primarily differing in their redox potentials, which cause PTSM (blood flow) to be retained in all cells whereas ATSM (hypoxia) is selectively retained in hypoxic cells. This work confirmed that a single dynamic scan with 10 min delay between injections of the tracers provides a near-optimal protocol for rapid imaging of these tracers. This work also confirmed that the kinetic parameters k_1 and k_{net} (net-uptake) were accurately recovered from the rapid dual-tracer data, whereas secondary rate parameters (e.g., k_2, k_3) suffered from higher noise levels and were not robustly measured.

More recently, we have moved on to evaluating rapid multitracer PET imaging protocols in physiologic models that test these new technologies under situations that are more readily applicable to clinical imaging scenarios. The biggest challenge to testing new multitracer imaging technologies is the need for a gold standard. Since the prior development of each individual PET tracer includes extensive investigation of uptake and retention mechanisms, multitracer technologies can be evaluated by asking the question: Can multitracer PET provide the same information about each tracer as separate, single-tracer imaging? In other words, the technology of rapid multitracer PET can be evaluated using conventional single-tracer imaging as the gold standard. On the other hand, the efficacy of multitracer imaging *for particular clinical tasks* is a much broader question that will require specific clinical trials for each tracer combination and imaging application under consideration.

In order to use separate single-tracer images as a gold standard for testing rapid multitracer PET techniques, a physiologic model that permits both multitracer and repeat imaging with single tracers (after > 7 half-lives decay) is required. Such imaging experiments are not generally feasible in human subjects due to the very long (> 12 hr) experimental protocols and radiation safety issues associated with repeat

injections of multiple tracers. We have initiated an institutionally approved protocol to image canines with spontaneously occurring tumors for evaluating rapid multitracer PET tumor imaging. Dogs with preexisting tumors that are scheduled for euthanasia are recruited from regional animal shelters and veterinarians. This provides a large animal tumor model, with body habitus sufficiently large to reasonably approximate physical imaging characteristics on clinical PET scanners, which can be sedated, immobilized, and imaged repeatedly over a period of many hours as necessary to acquire both single- and multitracer scans of each tracer.

Initial results with this large animal model for dual- and triple-tracer tumor imaging with ^{18}F-FDG (glucose metabolism), ^{62}Cu-PTSM (blood flow), and ^{62}Cu-ATSM (hypoxia) were presented at the 53rd Annual Meeting of the Society of Nuclear Medicine in June 2006. The experimental imaging results largely concurred with the simulation studies previously discussed, confirming that clinically important measures of tumor glucose metabolism, blood flow, and oxygen status can be obtained from a single, rapid multitracer PET scan with a total imaging time of about one hour:

- ^{18}F-FDG: SUV R = 0.999 k_i R = 0.99
- ^{62}Cu-PTSM: SUV R = 0.96 k_1 R = 0.97
- ^{62}Cu-ATSM   SUV R = 0.94 k_1 R = 0.97

Here, SUV is the standardized uptake value, k_1 is the wash-in rate constant, k_i is the net-uptake constant for FDG (closely related to the metabolic rate of glucose metabolism), and R is Pearson's correlation coefficient comparing estimates from rapid triple-tracer imaging to those from conventional single-tracer imaging. The rapid multitracer methods have also been extended to rest-stress myocardial perfusion imaging, which has been initially tested in a human subject population (Rust *et al.*, 2006). Work on developing and evaluating new multitracer PET technologies is ongoing, with initial clinical research trials on the near horizon.

Limitations and Future Directions

While this work shows the high potential for rapid multitracer PET as a new tool for characterizing multiple aspects of tumor physiology *in vivo*, rapid multitracer PET technologies are in their infancy and significant additional research is required before routine clinical use can be considered. In terms of the technology itself, specific imaging protocols and data analysis methods need to be developed for each particular tracer combination being considered. While there is mounting evidence that short half-life/fast kinetic tracers can be reliably imaged in conjunction with a single, longer half-life/slow kinetic tracer, it is currently unclear how well the approach will perform for imaging two longer-lived tracers in conjunction. In addition, the current methods use parallel multitracer compartment modeling techniques to separate the images for each tracer, and these models require measurement of arterial input functions. While there is preliminary evidence that approximations of the input functions may be sufficient for multitracer image separation, much additional work is needed in this area. Similarly, the present methods have been evaluated on a region of interest (ROI) basis only, and improved algorithms may be necessary for robust multitracer *parametric imaging*.

The signal-separation strategies employed to recover separate images of each tracer require dynamic imaging during the injection and distribution phase of each tracer. As such, multitracer image separation can only be accomplished for the single-bed position where the dynamic imaging was performed. While this may not be a significant limitation for many tumor-characterization scenarios where the tumor site and volume of interest are known beforehand, it is a complicating factor for imaging spatially separated tumor sites. In any case, static whole-body images of long-lived tracers such as FDG can still be acquired after the dynamic multitracer scan as desired.

Looking beyond the technological status of rapid multitracer PET, an even broader area of research awaits: investigating which tracer combinations, optimized by tumor type, provide clinically useful information for image-guided selection of more effective therapies, and likewise for monitoring the early (preclinical) tumor response to therapy. In short, the advent of rapid multitracer PET technologies combined with the large number of PET tracers available literally opens the floodgates to a vast array of potential imaging applications for personalized, image-guided management of cancer.

References

Anderson, H., and Price, P. 2002. Clinical measurement of blood flow in tumors using positron emission tomography: a review. *Nucl. Med. Commun. 23*:131–138.

Ballinger, J.R. 2001. Imaging hypoxia in tumors. *Semin. Nucl. Med. 31*:321–329.

Casciari, J.J., Graham, M.M., and Rasey, J.S. 1995. A modeling approach for quantifying tumor hypoxia with [F-18]fluoromisonidazole PET time-activity data. *Med. Phys. 22*:1127–1139.

Choyke, P.L., Knopp, M.V., and Libutti, S.K. 2002. Special techniques for imaging blood flow to tumors. *Cancer J. 8*:109–118.

Converse, A.K., Barnhart, T.E., Dabbs, K.A., DeJesus, O.T., Larson, J.A., Nickles, R.J., Schneider, M.L., and Roberts, A.D. 2004. PET measurement of rCBF in the presence of a neurochemical tracer. *J. Neurosci. Methods 132*:199–208.

Dehdashti, F., Flanagan, F.L., Mortimer, J.E., Katzenellenbogen, J.A., Welch, M.J., and Siegel, B.A. 1999. Positron emission tomographic assessment of "metabolic flare" to predict response of metastatic breast cancer to antiestrogen therapy. *Eur. J. Nucl. Med. 26*:51–56.

Dimitrakopoulou-Strauss, A., Strauss, L.G., and Burger, C. 2001. Quantitative PET studies in pretreated melanoma patients: a comparison of 6-[18F]fluoro-L-dopa with 18F-FDG and (15)O-water using compartment and noncompartment analysis. *J. Nucl. Med. 42*:248–256.

Frackowiak, R.S., Lenzi, G.L., Jones, T., and Heather, J.D. 1980. Quantitative measurement of regional cerebral blood flow and oxygen metabolism in man using 15O and positron emission tomography: theory, procedure, and normal values. *J. Comput. Assist. Tomogr. 4*:727–736.

Gambhir, S.S. 2002. Molecular imaging of cancer with positron emission tomography. *Nat. Rev. Cancer 2*:683–693.

Gambhir, S.S., Czernin, J., Schwimmer, J., Silverman, D.H., Coleman, R.E., and Phelps, M.E. 2001. A tabulated summary of the FDG PET literature. *J. Nucl. Med. 42*:1S–93S.

Graham, M.M. 2001. Combined 18F-FDG-FDOPA tumor imaging for assessing response to therapy. *J. Nucl. Med. 42*:257–258.

Grönroos, T., Eskola, O., Lehtio, K., Minn, H., Marjamaki, P., Bergman, J., Haaparanta, M., Forsback, S., and Solin, O. 2001. Pharmacokinetics of [18F]FETNIM: a potential marker for PET. *J. Nucl. Med. 42*:1397–1404.

Groshar, D., McEwan, A.J., Parliament, M.B., Urtasun, R.C., Golberg, L.E., Hoskinson, M., Mercer, J.R., Mannan, R.H., Wiebe, L.I., and Chapman, J.D. 1993. Imaging tumor hypoxia and tumor perfusion. *J. Nucl. Med. 34*:885–888.

Halter, G., Buck, A.K., Schirrmeister, H., Wurziger, I., Liewald, F., Glatting, G., Neumaier, B., Sunder-Plassmann, L., Reske, S.N., and Hetzel, M. 2004. [18F] 3-deoxy-3′-fluorothymidine positron emission tomography: alternative or diagnostic adjunct to 2-[18f]-fluoro-2-deoxy-D-glucose positron emission tomography in the workup of suspicious central focal lesions? *J. Thorac. Cardiovasc. Surg. 127*:1093–1099.

Hawkins, R.A., Choi, Y., Huang, S.C., Hoh, C.K., Dahlbom, M., Schiepers, C., Satyamurthy, N., Barrio, J.R., and Phelps, M.E. 1992. Evaluation of the skeletal kinetics of fluorine-18-fluoride ion with PET. *J. Nucl. Med. 33*:633–642.

Herholz, K., Holzer, T., Bauer, B., Schroder, R., Voges, J., Ernestus, R.I., Mendoza, G., Weber-Luxenburger, G., Lottgen, J., Thiel, A., Wienhard, K., and Heiss, W.D. 1998. 11C-methionine PET for differential diagnosis of low-grade gliomas. *Neurology 50*:1316–1322.

Higashi, K., Ueda, Y., Matsunari, I., Kodama, Y., Ikeda, R., Miura, K., Taki, S., Higuchi, T., Tonami, H., and Yamamoto, I. 2004. 11C-acetate PET imaging of lung cancer: comparison with 18F-FDG PET and 99mTc-MIBI SPET. *Eur. J. Nucl. Med. Mol. Imag. 31*:13–21.

Ho, C.L., Yu, S.C., and Yeung, D.W. 2003. 11C-acetate PET imaging in hepatocellular carcinoma and other liver masses. *J. Nucl. Med. 44*:213–221.

Hoegerle, S., Altehoefer, C., Ghanem, N., Koehler, G., Waller, C.F., Scheruebl, H., Moser, E., and Nitzsche, E. 2001. Whole-body 18F dopa PET for detection of gastrointestinal carcinoid tumors. *Radiology 220*:373–380.

Hoegerle, S., Juengling, F., Otte, A., Altehoefer, C., Moser, E.A., and Nitzsche, E.U. 1998. Combined FDG and [F-18]fluoride whole-body PET: a feasible two-in-one approach to cancer imaging? *Radiology 209*:253–258.

Huang, S.C., Carson, R.E., Hoffman, E.J., Kuhl, D.E., and Phelps, M.E. 1982. An investigation of a double-tracer technique for positron computerized tomography. *J. Nucl. Med. 23*:816–822.

Ikoma, Y., Toyama, H., Uemura, K., and Uchiyama, A. (2002). *Evaluation of the reliability in kinetic analysis for dual tracer injection of FDG and flumazenil PET study*. 2001 IEEE Nuclear Science Symposium Conference Record, Piscataway, NJ, USA, IEEE.

Inoue, T., Oriuchi, N., Tomiyoshi, K., and Endo, K. 2002. A shifting landscape: what will be next FDG in PET oncology? *Ann. Nucl. Med. 16*:1–9.

Jacobs, A.H., Thomas, A., Kracht, L.W., Li, H., Dittmar, C., Garlip, G., Galldiks, N., Klein, J.C., Sobesky, J., Hilker, R., Vollmar, S., Herholz, K., Wienhard, K., and Heiss, W.D. 2005. 18F-fluoro-L-thymidine and 11C-methylmethionine as markers of increased transport and proliferation in brain tumors. *J. Nucl. Med. 46*:1948–1958.

Jager, P.L., Vaalburg, W., Pruim, J., de Vries, E.G., Langen, K.J., and Piers, D.A. 2001. Radiolabeled amino acids: basic aspects and clinical applications in oncology. *J. Nucl. Med. 42*:432–445.

Kadrmas, D.J., and Rust, T.C. 2005. Feasibility of rapid multitracer PET tumor imaging. *IEEE Trans. Nucl. Sci. 52*:1341–1347.

Keen, H.G., Dekker, B.A., Disley, L., Hastings, D., Lyons, S., Reader, A.J., Ottewell, P., Watson, A., and Zweit, J. 2005. Imaging apoptosis *in vivo* using 124I-annexin V and PET. *Nucl. Med. Biol. 32*:395–402.

Koeppe, R.A., Ficaro, E.P., Raffel, D.M., Minoshima, S., and Kilbourn, M.R. (1998). Temporally overlapping dual-tracer PET studies. In: *Quantitative Functional Brain Imaging with Positron Emission Tomography*, R.E. Carson, M.E. Daube-Witherspoon, and P. Herscovitch (Eds.). San Diego, CA: Academic Press, 359–366.

Koeppe, R.A., Raffel, D.M., Snyder, S.E., Ficaro, E.P., Kilbourn, M.R., and Kuhl, D.E. 2001. Dual-[11C]tracer single-acquisition positron emission tomography studies. *J. Cereb. Blood Flow Metab. 21*:1480–1492.

Koh, W.J., Rasey, J.S., Evans, M.L., Grierson, J.R., Lewellen, T.K., Graham, M.M., Krohn, K.A., and Griffin, T.W. 1992. Imaging of hypoxia in human tumors with [F-18]fluoromisonidazole. *Int. J. Radiat. Oncol. Biol. Phys. 22*:199–212.

Kubota, K. 2001. From tumor biology to clinical PET: a review of positron emission tomography (PET) in oncology. *Ann. Nucl. Med. 15*: 471–486.

Kubota, K., Ishiwata, K., Kubota, R., Yamada, S., Tada, M., Sato, T., and Ido, T. 1991. Tracer feasibility for monitoring tumor radiotherapy: a quadruple tracer study with fluorine-18-fluorodeoxyglucose or fluorine-18-fluorodeoxyuridine, L-[methyl-14C]methionine, [6-3H]thymidine, and gallium-67. *J. Nucl. Med. 32*:2118–2123.

Kubota, K., Tada, M., Yamada, S., Hori, K., Saito, S., Iwata, R., Sato, K., Fukuda, H., and Ido, T. 1999. Comparison of the distribution of fluorine-18 fluoromisonidazole, deoxyglucose and methionine in tumour tissue. *Eur J. Nucl. Med. 26*:750–757.

Larson, S.M. 2004. Positron emission tomography-based molecular imaging in human cancer: exploring the link between hypoxia and accelerated glucose metabolism. *Clin. Cancer Res. 10*:2203–2204.

Lehtio, K., Eskola, O., Viljanen, T., Oikonen, V., Gronroos, T., Sillanmaki, L., Grenman, R., and Minn, H. 2004. Imaging perfusion and hypoxia with PET to predict radiotherapy response in head-and-neck cancer. *Int. J. Rad. Oncol. Biol. Phys. 59*:971–982.

Lehtio, K., Oikonen, V., Nyman, S., Gronroos, T., Roivainen, A., Eskola, O., and Minn, H. 2003. Quantifying tumour hypoxia with fluorine-18 fluoroerythronitroimidazole ([18F]FETNIM) and PET using the tumour to plasma ratio. *Eur. J. Nucl. Med. Mol. Imag. 30*:101–108.

Leskinen-Kallio, S., Ruotsalainen, U., Nagren, K., Teras, M., and Joensuu, H. 1991. Uptake of carbon-11-methionine and fluorodeoxyglucose in non-Hodgkin's Lymphoma: a PET study. *J. Nucl. Med. 32*: 1211–1218.

Lewis, J.S., McCarthy, D.W., McCarthy, T.J., Fujibayashi, Y., and Welch, M.J. 1999. Evaluation of 64Cu-ATSM in vitro and *in vivo* in a hypoxic tumor model. *J. Nucl. Med. 40*:177–183.

Lewis, J.S., and Welch, M.J. 2001. PET imaging of hypoxia. *Q. J. Nucl. Med. 45*:183–188.

Mankoff, D.A., Dehdashti, F., and Shields, A.F. 2000. Characterizing tumors using metabolic imaging: PET imaging of cellular proliferation and steroid receptors. *Neoplasia 2*:71–88.

Mankoff, D.A., Dunnwald, L.K., Gralow, J.R., Ellis, G.K., Charlop, A., Lawton, T.J., Schubert, E.K., Tseng, J., and Livingston, R.B. 2002. Blood flow and metabolism in locally advanced breast cancer: relationship to response to therapy. *J. Nucl. Med. 43*:500–509.

Mankoff, D.A., Dunnwald, L.K., Gralow, J.R., Ellis, G.K., Schubert, E.K., Tseng, J., Lawton, T.J., Linden, H.M., and Livingston, R.B. 2003. Changes in blood flow and metabolism in locally advanced breast cancer treated with neoadjuvant chemotherapy. *J. Nucl. Med. 44*: 1806–1814.

Mintun, M.A., Welch, M.J., Siegel, B.A., Mathias, C.J., Brodack, J.W., McGuire, A.H., and Katzenellenbogen, J.A. 1988. Breast cancer: PET imaging of estrogen receptors. *Radiology 169*:45–48.

Moore, R.B., Chapman, J.D., Mercer, J.R., Mannan, R.H., Wiebe, L.I., McEwan, A.J., and McPhee, M.S. 1993. Measurement of PDT-induced hypoxia in Dunning prostate tumors by iodine-123-iodoazomycin arabinoside. *J. Nucl. Med. 34*:405–411.

Mortimer, J.E., Dehdashti, F., Siegel, B.A., Trinkaus, K., Katzenellenbogen, J.A., and Welch, M.J. 2001. Metabolic flare: indicator of hormone responsiveness in advanced breast cancer. *J. Clin. Oncol. 19*:2797–2803.

Narayanan, T.K., Said, S., Mukherjee, J., Christian, B., Satter, M., Dunigan, K., Shi, B., Jacobs, M., Bernstein, T., Padma, M., and Mantil, J. 2002. A comparative study on the uptake and incorporation of radiolabeled methionine, choline and fluorodeoxyglucose in human astrocytoma. *Mol. Imag. Biol. 4*:147–156.

Rajendran, J.G., and Krohn, K.A. 2005. Imaging hypoxia and angiogenesis in tumors. *Radiol. Clin. North Am. 43*:169–187.

Rajendran, J.G., Mankoff, D.A., O'Sullivan, F., Peterson, L.M., Schwartz, D.L., Conrad, E.U., Spence, A.M., Muzi, M., Farwell, D.G., and Krohn, K.A. 2004. Hypoxia and glucose metabolism in malignant tumors: evaluation by [18F]fluoromisonidazole and [18F]fluorodeoxyglucose positron emission tomography imaging. *Clin. Cancer Res. 10*:2245–2252.

Rasey, J.S., Hoffman, J.M., Spence, A.M., and Krohn, K.A. 1986. Hypoxia mediated binding of misonidazole in non-malignant tissue. *Int. J. Radiat. Oncol. Biol. Phys. 12*:1255–1258.

Roelcke, U., Radu, E.W., von Ammon, K., Hausmann, O., Maguire, R.P., and Leenders, K.L. 1995. Alteration of blood-brain barrier in human brain tumors: comparison of [18F]fluorodeoxyglucose, [11C]methionine and rubidium-82 using PET. *J. Neurol. Sci. 132*:20–27.

Rust, T.C., DiBella, E.V.R., McGann, C.J., Christian, P.E., Hoffman, J.M., and Kadrmas, D.J. 2006. Rapid dual-injection single-scan 13N-ammonia PET for quantification of rest and stress myocardial blood flows. *Phys. Med. Biol. 51*:5347–5362.

Rust, T.C., and Kadrmas, D.J. 2006. Rapid dual-tracer PTSM+ATSM PET imaging of tumour blood flow and hypoxia: a simulation study. *Phys. Med. Biol. 51*:61–75.

Sasaki, Y. 1991. Monitoring tumor radiotherapy. *J. Nucl. Med. 32*:2124–2125.

Shields, A.F. 2003. PET imaging with 18F-FLT and thymidine analogs: promise and pitfalls. *J. Nucl. Med. 44*:1432–1434.

Tseng, J., Dunnwald, L.K., Schubert, E.K., Link, J.M., Minoshima, S., Muzi, M., and Mankoff, D.A. 2004. 18F-FDG kinetics in locally advanced breast cancer: correlation with tumor blood flow and changes in response to neoadjuvant chemotherapy. *J. Nucl. Med. 45*:1829–1837.

Van Laere, K., Ceyssens, S., Van Calenbergh, F., de Groot, T., Menten, J., Flamen, P., Bormans, G., and Mortelmans, L. 2005. Direct comparison of 18F-FDG and 11C-methionine PET in suspected recurrence of glioma: sensitivity, inter-observer variability and prognostic value. *Eur. J. Nucl. Med. Mol. Imag. 32*:39–51.

Vaupel, P., and Hockel, M. 2000. Blood supply, oxygenation status and metabolic micromilieu of breast cancers: characterization and therapeutic relevance. *Int. J. Oncol. 17*:869–879.

Yagle, K.J., Eary, J.F., Tait, J.F., Grierson, J.R., Link, J.M., Lewellen, B., Gibson, D.F., and Krohn, K.A. 2005. Evaluation of 18F-annexin V as a PET imaging agent in an animal model of apoptosis. *J. Nucl. Med. 46*:658–666.

Yang, D.J., Wallace, S., Cherif, A., Li, C., Gretzer, M.B., Kim, E.E., and Podoloff, D.A. 1995. Development of F-18-labeled fluoroerythronitroimidazole as a PET agent for imaging tumor hypoxia. *Radiology 194*:795–800.

Zasadny, K.R., Tatsumi, M., and Wahl, R.L. 2003. FDG metabolism and uptake versus blood flow in women with untreated primary breast cancers. *Eur. J. Nucl. Med. Mol. Imag. 30*:274–280.

5

Whole-Body Magnetic Resonance Imaging in Patients with Metastases

Thomas C. Lauenstein

Introduction

The term *staging* refers to examinations involving patients with known (and mostly malignant) disease. The capacity to use diagnostic imaging for detection of primary malignancy and metastases is essential for therapeutic management of most cancer patients. This is particularly true for cancer entities, such as breast cancer, lung cancer, and malignant melanoma, which often metastasize to different organ systems, including liver, lungs, brain, adrenal glands, lymph nodes, and bones. Therapeutic strategies often depend on the extent of disease and on whether distant organ systems have been affected. Not long ago, patients had to undergo several different examinations for whole-body staging, including positron emission tomography (PET), computed tomography (CT), magnetic resonance tomography (MRI), X-ray examinations, and ultrasound. However, this has often been a time-consuming process harboring inconvenience for the patient. In addition to excessive time, cost concerns are also a crucial factor. Thus, it is highly attractive to implement a single imaging modality for the simultaneous depiction of different organ systems (ideally of the entire body).

During the past decade, PET/CT machines have been developed that facilitate subsequent data acquisition of different anatomical regions. Current practice often utilizes PET/CT for assessing patients suspected of having metastases and for following patients during chemotherapy to monitor tumor response. Strengths of PET/CT include obtaining even decreased tumor metabolism during chemotherapy, which is presumed as an early marker of tumor response. Limitations, however, include lack of specificity for different tumor types, false-positive activity related to inflammation or granulation-fibrosis, and certain benign tumors (Delbeke *et al.*, 2001). A further drawback of PET/CT is the ionizing radiation exposure to the patient, with an additional ~ 10–15 mSv dose from the CT component and a total dose approaching 30 mSv for the combined PET/CT (Brix *et al.*, 2005). The lifetime attributable risk for lethal cancer induction for this dose has been recently estimated to be as high as 1 per 1000 for the general population, but rises up to 1 per 100 in subjects under 20 years of age (Martin *et al.*, 2006; NAS, 2005). The PET/CT dose may be of particularly concern in younger patients, or in patients who will receive multiple studies, as is routine, for instance, in breast cancer patients who receive chemotherapy, particularly if the objective is to affect long-term disease free interval or cure in these treated patients.

A strong motivation for continued development of MRI applications in tumor assessment is the achievement of higher diagnostic accuracy relative to CT and partially also to PET/CT. This is mainly due to the considerable soft tissue contrast obtained with the MRI. Thus, detection and characterization of tumor lesions is most accurate in most organ systems, including the brain (Valk *et al.*, 1987), liver (Hawighorst *et al.*, 1999; Ward *et al.*, 2005), and other abdominal and pelvic organs (Miller *et al.*, 2006; Renken *et al.*, 2005). Furthermore, MRI has been shown to be sensitive for the detection of metastatic osseous lesions (Eustace *et al.*, 1997; Walker *et al.*, 2000), and more recently shown to be able to detect even small pulmonary nodules (Schaefer *et al.*, 2006; Schroeder *et al.*, 2005). Magnetic resonance imaging also avoids exposure to ionizing radiation, and intravenous MR exogenous contrast agents are not associated with the same risk of nephrotoxicity as exists for iodinated CT contrast agents.

Methodology of Whole-Body Magnetic Resonance Imaging

One major disadvantage of a whole-body MRI approach in the past was related to the need to reposition patients in the bore of the magnet. In addition, different surface coils often were required to allow for an optimal depiction of each anatomical region. Different strategies have been explored to overcome these limitations. One initial approach was based on the implementation of a sliding table platform enabling data selection of different anatomical regions in rapid succession (Lauenstein *et al.*, 2002a). Spine coils (which are integrated in the patient table) are used for signal reception in combination with an anteriorly positioned torso phased-array coil. The latter coil remains in the isocenter of the magnet, while the patient is sliding underneath it. This concept of a rolling table platform could be successfully employed for staging purposes of malignant tumors (Lauenstein et al., 2002a, 2002b, 2004) and whole-body MR-angiography (Goyen *et al.*, 2004). Most recent technological developments provide MRI systems with multiple input channels and automatic table movement. Specialized surface coils (e.g., phased-array and peripheral MR-angio coils, head and neck coils) can be used during the same examination. This technique allows for the acquisition of high-resolution images of different anatomical regions without the need of coil repositioning. The scanner table is automatically moved to the anatomical region in question. Hence, a total scan range of > 200 cm in the *z*-axis can be obtained (Fig. 1). Feasibility of this novel MR system for whole-body imaging was proven in an initial study for the assessment of metastatic disease (Schlemmer *et al.*, 2005).

Beyond the development in the hardware sector, improvements in imaging acquisition techniques have also been

substantial for the implementation of whole-body MRI. First, whole-body MRI concepts were based on the acquisition of fast echoplanar imaging (EPI). This imaging technique provided only limited spatial resolution, and diagnostic accuracy was only fair (Horvath *et al.*, 1999). One of the most important innovations is the use of fat-suppressed three-dimensional (3D) gradient-echo (GRE) sequences. This sequence type enables dynamic imaging of different organ systems after the intravenous administration of gadolinium. Thus, the basis of most whole-body MRI protocols is represented by gadolinium-enhanced T1w 3D GRE images of all different organ systems. Similarly, T2w single-shot

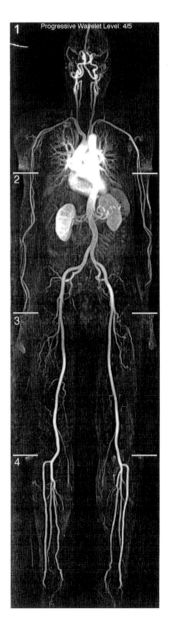

Figure 1 This image depicts how high-resolution images of various anatomical regions can be acquired without repositioning the coil. A total scan range of > 200 cm in the *z*-axis can be obtained.

fast spin echo (SSFSE) should be included in a whole-body protocol providing fast, high-resolution, and motion-insensitive images. Further data acquisition should be tailored to the individual need of the patient. Thus, it is preferable to include additional acquisition of other sequences, including short tau inversion recovery (STIR) for the assessment of the skeletal system and the pelvis, or fluid attenuation inversion recovery (FLAIR) for the evaluation of the brain. Moreover, the implementation of parallel acquisition techniques (PAT) is helpful for whole-body MRI. This imaging technique allows data acquisition with either decreased acquisition time or increased spatial resolution. The combined effect of sequence advances and hardware improvement has allowed whole-body MRI to be performed within a time range of 20 min, while maintaining diagnostic image quality.

Clinical Results of Whole-Body MRI for Tumor Staging

Depiction of Osseous Metastases

One of the first whole-body MRI strategies aimed to depict skeletal metastases in patients with malignant tumors. In an initial study, 28 patients were enrolled (Lauenstein et al., 2002a). Primary tumors included thyroid carcinoma, breast cancer, lung cancer, ovarian cancer, and testicular cancer. Patients were examined after being placed on a rolling table platform (BodySURF, System for Unlimited Rolling Field-of-view, MR-Innovation, Essen, Germany). The exam was structured into five steps extending from the head to the upper half of the tibia and fibula. For all five steps, three different MR sequences were collected in the coronal plane: T1 GRE in breath hold, Half Fourier Acquisition Single Shot Turbo Spin Echo (HASTE) with fat-suppression in breath hold, and Short Tau Inversion Recovery (STIR) were collected during quiet respiration. In addition, the spine was scanned with sagittal T1 GRE and HASTE sequences. After completing data acquisition at one station, the rolling table platform was moved manually to the next station. As a standard of reference, skeletal radionuclide scintigraphy was performed using a planar one-phase technique.

For image interpretation, the skeletal system was divided into 11 regions: head, sternum, clavicle, scapula, humerus, ribs, upper spine (cervical and thoracic), lower spine (lumbar and sacrum), pelvis, femur, and patella/tibia. The evaluation of scintigraphy and MRI was performed on a per-patient as well as per-region basis. If the reading of whole-body MR examination revealed metastases not seen by scintigraphy and the diagnosis was deemed of therapeutic relevance, a dedicated contrast-enhanced MR examination of this region was performed to resolve the discrepancy. Whole-body MR scanning was eventually performed on 26 patients because two patients could not be examined due to claustrophobia.

Scintigraphy detected bone metastases in 16 of 26 patients and in 60 of the 286 analyzed regions. Prospective analysis of all MR imaging data detected bone metastases in the same 16 patients as radionuclide scinitigraphy, resulting in a patient-based sensitivity of 100%. Regional assessment revealed 7 false-negative MR readings in the ribs ($n = 4$), head ($n = 2$), and scapula ($n = 1$). Thus, 53 of 60 regions with bone metastases were correctly identified by MRI, resulting in a region-based sensitivity of 88.3%. In addition, 28 regions in which scintigraphy had not detected bone metastases were considered positive for bone metastases. These metastatic lesions were located mainly in the spine and pelvis.

Similar findings were observed in another study enrolling 17 patients with biopsy-proven breast cancer and suspected metastases (Walker et al., 2000). Patients underwent both whole-body MRI and bone scintigraphy. For whole-body MRI a body coil was used, and a turboSTIR sequence was collected. Imaging of the entire body was performed by four overlapping coronal acquisitions and an average scan time of 20 min. Bone metastases were identified at both modalities (MRI/scintigraphy) in 11 of the 17 patients. Discrepancy between both techniques was found in 2 patients. One patient had a focal concentration of radiotracer on bone scintigraphy, which was rated suspicious for metastatic disease, which was not found to be abnormal on whole-body MRI. A clinical follow-up of 18 months revealed no evidence of metastasis. Thus, this finding was considered a false-positive scintigraphy. Another patient had marrow signal changes on MRI that were worrisome for metastatic disease. Scintigraphy, however, did not reveal any abnormality. In this patient a biopsy sample confirmed the presence of a bone metastasis. Thus, scintigraphy was false negative in this case.

The advantages of whole-body MRI over scintigraphy were confirmed by another study (Ghanem et al., 2006). A total of 129 tumor patients were examined with whole-body MRI using coronal TIRM sequences for different anatomical regions. Similarly to the previous study, skeletal scintigraphy served as the standard of reference: In 81% of all patients the whole-body MRI and skeletal scintigraphy findings were concordant: in 56 patients, both imaging modalities were negative as for the depiction of skeletal metastases, while in 49 patients whole-body MRI and skeletal scintigraphy revealed metastatic disease. However, whole-body MRI demonstrated more extensive disease in 22 of the 49 patients. In 24 patients, the imaging findings were discordant. In 15 cases, skeletal scintigraphy was negative, whereas whole-body MRI revealed skeletal metastases. In 9 cases skeletal scintigraphy was positive, whereas whole-body MRI failed to detect these metastases. Authors concluded that whole-body MRI is more accurate than skeletal scintigraphy with respect to the detection of skeletal metastases and the extent of metastastic disease.

Staging of Parenchymal Metastases

The range of diagnostic capabilities for whole-body MRI should not be limited to the assessment of a single organ system. Rather, imaging should be performed to detect metastases in all different organ systems. The implementation of 3D-GRE sequences with nearly isotropic resolution and gadolinium enhancement has broadened the possibilities for whole-body MRI. Data acquisition is performed under breath-hold conditions, ensuring consistent image quality. An initial trial including 8 patients with malignant tumors showed the feasibility of contrast-enhanced T1w 3D GRE sequences for whole-body imaging (Lauenstein *et al.*, 2002b). A good correlation with standard staging examinations including CT and bone scintigraphy was observed. In particular, multiphase dynamic liver imaging allowed for an accurate detection and characterization of hepatic mass lesions. Similarly, all other abdominal organs, including the pancreas, adrenal glands, and kidneys were visualized by MRI with a high level of diagnostic accuracy. Cerebral and bone metastases were also well depicted as enhancing focal lesions. In this preliminary study, only image quality of the lungs proved to be slightly inferior to CT scanning. However, all pulmonary metastases except a single small lesion were correctly detected. These results are confirmed by other authors, indicating that lesions larger than 5 mm in size can be adequately depicted by MRI (Vogt *et al.*, 2004). Furthermore, all skeletal and cerebral metastases were correctly depicted.

In a follow-up study, a larger patient cohort encompassing 51 patients with known malignant tumors was examined (Lauenstein *et al.*, 2004). Primary malignant tumors included breast cancer, lung cancer, and testicular cancer, all of which can metastasize to different organ systems, including brain, lungs, liver, lymph nodes, and bones. Dedicated CT and MRI scans as well as nuclear scintigraphy served as the standard of reference. The basis for whole-body MRI was formed by gadolinium-enhanced 3D-GRE of the entire body. Furthermore, supplemental data of the thorax and abdomen were acquired with fat-suppressed T2-weighted single-shot echo-train spin echo. Mean in-room time for whole-body MRI was nearly 15 min, including the time for patient and coil positioning and the acquisition of all MR data sets. In 42 of 51 patients metastatic disease was found by means of the reference scans. These findings were confirmed by whole-body MRI. However, in one patient with a single hepatic metastasis, which was subsequently proven by histology, only whole-body MRI was able to visualize this lesion. As far as an analysis on a lesion basis was concerned, there were apparent differences in the sensitivity of metastases detection. Overall, more liver metastases were shown on MRI than on CT. Some lung lesions < 6 mm in size that were detected by CT could not be identified by whole-body MRI. The impact of depicting smaller pulmonary nodules is still controversial because some of these lesions are of benign origin. Many patients with these small benign lesions have to undergo serial follow-up CT, with the attendant risks of repeat radiation exposure.

Concerning the depiction of skeletal metastases, a higher total number of bone metastases were found by MRI compared to skeletal scintigraphy. Similar to the findings of previous studies using whole-body MRI in conjunction with STIR sequences, there were regional advantages and disadvantages in osseous metastases detection. Magnetic resonance imaging showed more accurate detection of bone metastases in the spine and pelvis, whereas some metastases in the ribs could not be visualized. In addition, a high accuracy for the detection of metastases in other organ systems was found. All cerebral metastases as well as metastases in the adrenal glands were also detected by whole-body MRI. Lymph node metastases were considered present in 15 patients on whole-body MRI, and all findings were confirmed by correlating CT scans.

A more extensive whole-body protocol was recently described (Schlemmer *et al.*, 2005); 63 patients with known metastatic disease and malignant tumors, including mainly multiple myeloma, lymphoma, malignant melanoma, colon cancer, and breast cancer, were examined. Dedicated CT scans served as a standard of reference. In addition to the acquisition of contrast-enhanced T1w data from the entire body, the whole-body MRI protocol included STIR sequences for the assessment of the skeletal system and the pelvis and a FLAIR sequence for the evaluation of the brain. Mean in-room time for the entire examination amounted to ~60 min. Compared with CT, more metastases were detected by MRI in 11 of 63 patients, especially in liver, brain, lymph nodes, and the skeletal system. Therapeutic strategies had to be changed in 6 patients due to these findings. The authors concluded that whole-body MRI is feasible in clinical routine ensuring the evaluation of individual tumor spread and total tumor burden. A similar protocol was used by the same group to evaluate the impact of whole-body MRI on treatment decisions in patients with malignant melanoma (Muller-Horvat *et al.*, 2006). They compared whole-body magnetic resonance MRI and whole-body CT to detect distant metastases; 41 patients with known malignant melanoma were examined. By means of both methods, a total number of 775 metastases were found. While a total number of 730 metastatic lesions were depicted by MRI, only 522 metastases were detected on CT images. There were apparent differences regarding the diagnostic accuracy to depict metastatic disease, depending on the organ systems in question. Whole-body MRI was more accurate for the depiction of metastases in the brain, liver, spleen, and bones. However, more pulmonary lesions were seen on whole-body CT scans. Overall, therapeutic strategies were modified due to the whole-body MRI results in 24% of the patients.

Whole-Body MRI vs. PET/CT

FDG-PET/CT has been developed to provide a clinically available method for assessing tumor spread in patients with different malignancies. The FDG-PET modality detects tissues that have upregulated glucose metabolism such as malignant cells. Strengths of FDG-PET have included the capacity to scan the whole body and to be able to show decreased tumor metabolism during chemotherapy, presumed an early marker of tumor responsiveness. Limitations include lack of specificity for different tumor types, false-positive activity related to inflammation or granulation-fibrosis, and certain benign tumors. In order to overcome the problem of localization, PET/CT machines have been developed, and FDG-PET images today are viewed in conjunction with structural images from CT.

Preliminary data are available in the current literature comparing the outcome of MRI and FDG-PET/CT. These findings suggest that MRI yields higher sensitivity and specificity in certain organ systems, including detection of tumor lesions in the skeletal system as well as in parenchymal organs, whereas FDG-PET/CT shows advantages for diagnosing lymph node metastases. The accuracy of screening for bone metastases was assessed in a trial encompassing 30 patients with different oncological diseases (Schmidt *et al.*, 2007), using clinical follow-up findings as a measure of malignancy. A total of 102 malignant and 25 benign bone lesions were discovered. While 96 lesions were correctly identified by MRI, only 79 were identified by FDG-PET/CT. Furthermore, cut-off size for the detection of bone metastases was only 2 mm for MRI but 5 mm for FDG-PET/CT.

Another trial aimed to determine the staging accuracies of FDG-PET/CT and whole-body MRI in patients with different malignant diseases (Antoch *et al.*, 2003). In a prospective setting, 98 patients with various oncological diseases underwent FDG-PET/CT and whole-body MRI for tumor staging. All patients were monitored by follow-up examinations for an average of 9 months. Diagnostic accuracies of both imaging modalities were compared as for correct TNM classification of primary tumor and tumor spread. Whole-body MRI was more sensitive and specific in the detection of hepatic and skeletal lesions, whereas the extent of primary tumors and lymph nodes metastases was more reliably staged with PET/CT. Results of PET/CT were especially reliable in patients with primary lung cancer, proving the utility of this modality in this patient group.

The impact of whole-body MRI and FDG-PET/CT was also assessed in a relatively heterogeneous patient cohort with different malignant tumors (Schmidt *et al.*, 2005). As for the previously described studies, MRI was found to be more sensitive for the depiction of bone and liver metastases. Surprisingly, even lung metastases were depicted to a higher degree (albeit not statistically significant) by MRI compared to FDG-PET/CT. However, this study also showed that FDG-PET/CT had better sensitivity (98%) and specificity (83%) for lymph node metastases as compared to MRI sensitivity (80%) and specificity (75%).

In summary, whole-body MRI has been evolved as an accurate means for the detection of disease throughout the entire body. Technical advances including remote movement of the imaging table, the use of specialized surface coils, and high image quality T1w 3D GRE sequences, have rendered whole-body screening with MRI a viable method. Clinical results underline the usefulness of whole-body MRI as an accurate alternative to conventional multimodality evaluation for staging purposes. However, whole-body MR imaging is not intended to replace dedicated MR or CT examinations, which provide more detailed evaluation of individual organ systems.

References

Antoch, G., Vogt, F.M., Freudenberg, L.S., Nazaradeh, F., Goehde, S.C., Barkhausen, J., Dahmen, G., Bockisch, A., Debatin, J.F., and Ruehm, S.G. 2003. Whole-body dual-modality PET/CT and whole-body MRI for tumor staging in oncology. *JAMA 290*:3199–3206.

Brix, G., Lechel, U., Glatting, G., Ziegler, S.I., Munzing, W., Muller, S.P., and Beyer, T. 2005, Radiation exposure of patients undergoing whole-body dual-modality 18F-FDG PET/CT examinations. *J. Nucl. Med. 46*:608–613.

Delbeke, D., and Martin, W.H. 2001. Positron emission tomography imaging in oncology. *Radiol. Clin. North Am. 39*:883–917.

Eustace, S., Tello, R., DeCarvalho, V., Carey, J., Wroblicka, J.T., Melhem, E.R., and Yucel, E.K. 1997. A comparison of whole-body turboSTIR MR imaging and planar 99mTc-methylene diphosphonate scintigraphy in the examination of patients with suspected skeletal metastases. *AJR Am. J. Roentgenol. 169*:1655–1661.

Ghanem, N., Altehoefer, C., Kelly, T., Lohrmann, C., Winterer, J., Schafer, O., Bley, T.A., Moser, E., and Langer, M. 2006. Whole-body MRI in comparison to skeletal scintigraphy in detection of skeletal metastases in patients with solid tumors. *In Vivo 20*:173–182.

Goyen, M., Goehde, S.C., Herborn, C.U., Hunold, P., Vogt, F.M., Gizewski, E.R., Lauenstein, T.C., Ajaj, W., Forsting, M., Debatin, J.F., and Ruehm, S.G. 2004. MR-based full-body preventative cardiovascular and tumor imaging: technique and preliminary experience. *Eur. Radiol. 14*:783–791.

Hawighorst, H., Schoenberg, S.O., Knopp, M.V., Essig, M., Miltner, P., and van Kaick, G. 1999. Hepatic lesions: morphologic and functional characterization with multiphase breath-hold 3D gadolinium-enhanced MR angiography—initial results. *Radiology 210*:89–96.

Horvath, L.J., Burtness, B.A., McCarthy, S., and Johnson, K.M. 1999. Total-body echo-planar MR imaging in the staging of breast cancer: comparison with conventional methods—early experience. *Radiology 211*:119–128.

Lauenstein, T.C., Freudenberg, L.S., Goehde, S.C., Ruehm, S.G., Goyen, M., Bosk, S., Debatin, J.F., and Barkhausen, J. 2002a. Whole-body MRI using a rolling table platform for the detection of bone metastases. *Eur. Radiol. 12*:2091–2099.

Lauenstein, T.C., Goehde, S.C., Herborn, C.U., Treder, W., Ruehm, S.G., Debatin, J.F., and Barkhausen, J. 2002b. Three-dimensional volumetric interpolated breath-hold MR imaging for whole-body tumor staging in less than 15 minutes: a feasibility study. *AJR Am. J. Roentgenol. 179*:445–449.

Lauenstein, T.C., Goehde, S.C., Herborn, C.U., Goyen, M., Oberhoff, C., Debatin, J.F., Ruehm, S.G., and Barkhausen, J. 2004. Whole-body MR imaging: evaluation of patients for metastases. *Radiology 233*:139–148.

Martin, D.R., and Semelka, R.C. 2006. Health effects of ionising radiation from diagnostic CT. *Lancet 367*:1712–1714.

Miller, F.H., Rini, N.J., and Keppke, A.L. 2006. MRI of adenocarcinoma of the pancreas. *AJR Am. J. Roentgenol. 187*:W365–W374.

Muller-Horvat, C., Radny, P., Eigentler, T.K., Schafer, J., Pfannenberg, C., Horger, M., Khorchidi, S., Nagele, T., Garbe, C., Claussen, C.D., and Schlemmer, H.P. 2006. Prospective comparison of the impact on treatment decisions of whole-body magnetic resonance imaging and computed tomography in patients with metastatic malignant melanoma. *Eur. J. Cancer 42*:342–350.

National Academy of Sciences/Washington D.C. 2005. *Biological Effects of Ionizing Radiation (BEIR) VII.*, National Academies Press.

Renken, N.S., and Krestin, G.P. 2005. Magnetic resonance imaging of the kidney. *Semin. Ultrasound CT MR 26*:153–161.

Schaefer, J.F., Schneider, V., Vollmar, J., Wehrmann, M., Aebert, H., Friedel, G., Vonthein, R., Schick, F., and Claussen, C.D. 2006. Solitary pulmonary nodules: association between signal characteristics in dynamic contrast enhanced MRI and tumor angiogenesis. *Lung Cancer 53*:39–49.

Schlemmer, H.P., Schafer, J., Pfannenberg, C., Radny, P., Korchidi, S., Muller-Horvat, C., Nagele, T., Tomaschko, K., Fenchel, M., and Claussen, C.D. 2005. Fast whole-body assessment of metastatic disease using a novel magnetic resonance imaging system: initial experiences. *Invest. Radiol. 40*:64–71.

Schmidt, G.P., Baur-Melnyk, A., Herzog, P., Schmid, R., Tiling, R., Schmidt, M., Reiser, M.F., and Schoenberg, S.O. 2005. High-resolution whole-body magnetic resonance image tumor staging with the use of parallel imaging versus dual-modality positron emission tomography-computed tomography: experience on a 32-channel system. *Invest. Radiol. 40*:743–753.

Schmidt, G.P., Schoenberg, S.O., Schmid, R., Stahl, R., Tiling, R., Becker, C.R., Reiser, M.F., and Baur-Melnyk, A. 2007. Screening for bone metastases: whole-body MRI using a 32-channel system versus dual-modality PET-CT. *Eur. Radiol. 17*:939–949.

Schroeder, T., Ruehm, S.G., Debatin, J.F., Ladd, M.E., Barkhausen, J., and Goehde, S.C. 2005. Detection of pulmonary nodules using a 2D HASTE MR sequence: comparison with MDCT. *AJR Am. J. Roentgenol. 185*:979–984.

Valk, J., De Slegte, R.G., Crezee, F.C., Hazenberg, G.J., and Thjaha, S.I. 1987. Gadolinium-DTPA in magnetic resonance imaging of the brain. *Neurosurg. Rev. 10*:87–92.

Vogt, F.M., Herborn, C.U., Hunold, P., Lauenstein, T.C., Schroder, T., Debatin, J.F., and Barkhausen, J. 2004. HASTE MRI versus chest radiography in the detection of pulmonary nodules: comparison with MDCT. *AJR Am. J. Roentgenol. 183*:71–78.

Walker, R., Kessar, P., Blanchard, R., Dimasi, M., Harper, K., DeCarvalho, V., Yucel, E.K., Patriquin, L., and Eustace, S. 2000. Turbo STIR magnetic resonance imaging as a whole-body screening tool for metastases in patients with breast carcinoma: preliminary clinical experience. *J. Magn. Reson. Imaging 11*:343–350.

Ward, J., Robinson, P.J., Guthrie, J.A., Downing, S., Wilson, D., Lodge, J.P., Prasad, K.R., Toogood, G.J., and Wyatt, J.I. 2005. Liver metastases in candidates for hepatic resection: comparison of helical CT and gadolinium- and SPIO-enhanced MR imaging. *Radiology 237*:170–180.

6

Whole-Body Imaging in Oncology: Positron Emission Tomography/ Computed Tomography (PET/CT)

A. Bockisch, L. Freudenberg, G. Antoch, and S. Rosenbaum

Introduction

Positron emission tomography (PET) has a long history of use. In the beginning, more than 30 years ago, it was developed mainly as a research tool focused on neurology. During the last two decades, PET devices have become available on a routine basis and have become established in diagnostic procedures of multiple oncological diseases. Presently, a large number of positron-emitting radiotracers are available, which are suitable for PET imaging. However, only a small fraction is more frequently used in oncology: [^{11}C]Choline, a precursor of the biosynthesis of phosphatidylcholine, is used for staging prostate cancer (Schoder et al., 2004). [^{11}C]Methionin allows a more unspecific visualization of the protein synthesis and is well established as a metabolic marker in brain tumors (Jacobs et al., 2002). Other highly specific tracers such as ^{68}Ga-DOTATOC, relying on the density of free somatostatin receptors, are used in neuroendocrine tumors (Hofmann et al., 2001). [^{124}I]I$^+$, another highly specific tracer, is applied for imaging differentiated thyroid cancer (Freudenberg et al., 2004).

By far the most common PET radiotracer is fluorine-18-2-fluoro-2-deoxy-D-glucose (FDG), which unspecifically images and quantifies the glucose turnover. As shown for the first time in the 1920s by Warburg et al. (1924), the glucose metabolism frequently is significantly increased in malignoma. Metabolic imaging using FDG-PET has been shown to be substantially more sensitive and specific in the detection and characterization of several tumor entities (Gambhir et al., 2001). Several studies compared the accuracy of anatomic imaging (CT, MRI) and FDG-PET, showing significant differences with respect to sensitivity and specificity, especially in non-small lung cancer, lymphoma, thyroid cancer, sarcoma, gastrointestinal stromal tumors, melanoma, mesothelioma, colorectal carcinoma, head and neck tumors, and others (Gambhir et al., 2001). Based on 419 studies, including 18,402 PET examinations, Gambhir et al. (2001) described an average sensitivity and specificity of FDG-PET in staging and re-staging of several malignancies of 84% and 88%, respectively. In 30% of the patients, FDG-PET yielded in a different staging, subsequently resulting in a change of the treatment plans.

As all tissues have FDG turnover, there is some anatomic information in the FDG-PET images. However, this anatomic information is limited and frequently renders localization of a lesion and its potential infiltration into adjacent organs difficult. Thus, for maximal diagnostic benefit, functional data sets should be read in conjunction with morphologic images. Image fusion and side-by-side image evaluation of morphologic and functional data sets have been proposed (Wahl et al., 1993).

Technical Considerations

Several attempts have been made to effect image co-registration and fusion of separately acquired functional images using PET with morphology-based images acquired using CT or MRI. Either internal markers such as lung boundaries and kidneys or artificial, external markers have been used. The first method is less precise but allows using complete, independently acquired images. At present, different methods of software-based retrospective image fusion of dedicated PET and CT are applied. Co-registration errors have been best evaluated for the brain, with reported values of 1.2 mm to 6 mm. Comparatively few studies of extracerebral fusion have been published. Recent studies demonstrated an average mean error of 13 mm in plane and up to 11 mm in a z-axis direction for abdomen and thorax (Nömayr et al., 2005). The major problem of software fusion compared to hardware fusion with PET/CT is the different positioning (bending and twisting of the spine, twisting of the neck, angulation of the head, breathing pattern, or internally different bowel or bladder filling), especially with the increasing time interval between the two examinations. Lind et al. demonstrated that the quality of software-based image co-registration is essentially independent from the tracer used (Lind et al., 2004). This limitation may be overcome by collecting functional and morphologic data in one examination. Combined PET/CT devices offer a hardware solution to this problem, permitting sequential acquisition in a single scanning session. Thus, the availability of dual-modality PET/CT tomographs provides the technical basis for intrinsically aligned functional and morphologic data sets (Beyer et al., 2002). The patient rests on the bed between examinations; consequently, anatomical changes due to patient movement are minimized by the principle of investigation and the quality of fusion is optimized. Combined PET/CT today represents the best intrinsic co-registration of multimodality imaging (Pietrzyk, 2005).

As the basic idea of PET/CT is to overcome the lack or the uncertainty of anatomic or morphologic information, CT images need to be acquired in a quality that at least allows identification of morphologic structures. Consequently, CT should be acquired in the highest possible quality, meaning the routine use of oral and intravenous contrast agents (Kuehl et al., 2005). This requirement is stressed by the fact that PET/CT examinations are often used as one of the last imaging modalities in clinical routine. Therefore, no uncertainties should remain after the investigation.

The rigid combination of PET and CT promises high-quality image co-registration and improves the logistics and efficacy of PET. Using the CT data for attenuation and scatter correction shortens the duration of the investigation by approximately 30%, making PET investigation more cost effective (von Schulthess, 2000), and reduces the time of suffering for sick patients who have problems lying motionless for such a long period. Consequently, motion artifacts are also reduced and less pronounced. In addition, eliminating the rod sources of conventional PET saves maintenance costs and permits a wider opening of the tunnel, which is favorable for imaging patients in the same position as during external beam radiation treatment. In addition, the wider opening reduces claustrophobia.

Using the CT images as low-noise transmission scans also allows calculation of attenuation and scatter-corrected images with improved image quality. However, this method of attenuation correction bares some kinds of artifacts that have to be considered.

The transformation of attenuation coefficients at X-ray energies to those at 511 keV works well for soft tissues, bone, and air, but is insufficient for dense CT contrast agents, such as iodine or barium and for metal implants, such as dental fillings or prostheses. Furthermore, today's CT reconstruction algorithms lead to streak artifacts in the presence of metal implants, which are propagated into the PET image through the attenuation correction. On occasion, focally increased concentrations of high-density intravenous or oral contrast agents are seen on CT, which result in artificial tracer uptake patterns on the corrected PET images of PET/CT studies (Fig. 1). Also, metal implants may cause artificial focal uptake in corrected PET images. These foci may be misleading in the diagnosis, particularly in the presence of true lesions. It is therefore advisable to reconstruct "uncorrected" emission images without attenuation correction in addition.

Local misregistration between the CT and the PET in integrated PET/CT and the use of CT contrast media may bias the PET tracer distribution following CT-based attenuation correction. Consequently, protocol requirements for PET/CT with diagnostic CT include alternative contrast application schemes to handle CT contrast agents appropriately (Bockisch et al., 2004). Many CT IV-contrast protocol modifications are described in the literature (Beyer et al., 2005a) to avoid focal artifacts from intravenous bolus injection. Beyond the use of negative oral contrast agents instead of positive contrast agents has been proposed (Antoch et al., 2004b) for PET/CT imaging. As a result, overestimation of attenuation coefficients from high-Z materials can be avoided.

Other sources of artifacts have to be considered. When using CT for attenuation correction, the underlying algorithm requires that the emission and transmission images be acquired from the same object. A misregistration between emission and transmission investigation (e.g., due to breathing, bladder filling, or moving) necessarily results in artifacts, the most prominent being the breathing artifact.

The requirement of perfect co-registration is best approximated employing the PET/CT compared to retrospective image fusion as the patient is not moved physically between PET and CT acquisition. Nevertheless, patients should be

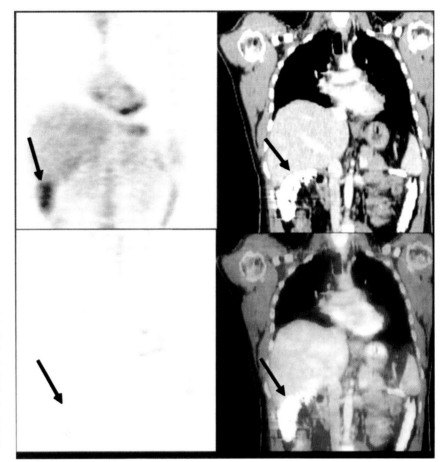

Figure 1 [18F]FDG-PET/CT of a patient with GIST; top-left side: PET, top-right side: CT, bottom-left side: uncorrected emission image without CT-based attenuation correction, bottom-left side fusion image. In the right upper abdomen, an artificial FDG accumulation is seen (arrow), implicating vital tumor tissue. CT shows positive bowel contrast within the corresponding area. No pathologic lesion is seen in the uncorrected PET image. Consequently, the uptake in the corrected PET is artificial due to overestimation of attenuation coefficients from the positive oral contrast.

supported with adequate positioning aids (e.g., knee, head and neck, and arm supports) to prevent involuntary motion during the whole examination, which may lead to local misalignment (Beyer *et al.*, 2004). Image misalignment in the thorax and abdomen due to different breathing patterns during PET and CT acquisition has been described as a source of potential artifacts in emission images after CT-based attenuation correction. Goerres *et al.* have compared different CT acquisition protocols in PET/CT imaging and have shown that image alignment in the thorax was most accurate if the CT was acquired in normal expiration breath hold, with PET acquired as usual in tidal breathing (Goerres *et al.*, 2002). This protocol, however, is limited to PET/CT tomographs with very fast CT components or CT protocols that use large table feeds per rotation, as normal expiration over the entire imaging range may not be feasible, especially when scanning uncooperative or sick patients. An alternative, limited breath-hold protocol has been suggested with breath hold in normal expiration only for the time that the CT takes to cover the lower lung and liver, which is of shorter duration. Instructing the patient before the PET/CT examinations on the breath-hold command is essential in avoiding serious respiration artifacts (Beyer *et al.*, 2004).

Future developments in hardware and software solutions of PET/CT indicate that further improvements will take place. Commercial scanners that are now available allow up to 64 slices to be simultaneously acquired in less than 0.5 sec. The reduced acquisition time of CT allows breath hold during the whole-body acquisition in normal expiration. In the context of PET/CT, the artifactual effects of respiratory motion may be minimized, and improvement of the sensitivity of detection for small lesions located particularly in the lower parts of lungs or in the liver may be achieved (Beyer *et al.*, 2005b). Finally, with respect to PET, modern scanners based on improved detector material have been proposed, acquiring a whole-body scan significantly faster than the 30 min needed today. Implementation of respiration-gated PET acquisition will lead to further improvement of co-registration, especially in the thorax and upper abdomen and significantly enhancing treatment accuracy.

Clinical Considerations

FDG is the dominant PET tracer in clinical oncology today. FDG-PET alone has been proven to be superior to CT or MRI in many malignant diseases (Gambhir *et al.*, 2001; Reske *et al.*, 2001). PET findings may be misclassified when physiologic variants of FDG accumulation are present that cannot easily be distinguished from pathology, especially in situations with changed anatomy, for example, after surgery (Rosenbaum *et al.*, 2005). PET/CT promises to resolve diagnostic problems such as ambiguous anatomic assignment of PET findings in normal and especially altered anatomy. It may offer synergetic effects of PET and CT in equivocal PET and/or CT findings. In the following we will outline the present clinical state and the expected developments of the near future.

Combined PET/CT devices have been commercially available since 2001. This technology has now spread worldwide, and as demonstrated by a huge amount of published data it has been the subject of intense clinical and scientific interest. With only a few malignant tumors not accumulating the labeled glucose tracer FDG, applications of PET/CT affect the whole field of medical and surgical oncology (see Reske, 2001). Of main interest in cancer therapy are diagnosis, staging, therapy planning, and follow-up. Another important question is the initial prognosis and the early prognosis with respect to therapy response.

Two recent studies (Antoch *et al.*, 2004c; Buell *et al.*, 2004) evaluated the accuracy of PET/CT in oncological patients with different malignancies. Their results are of interest with respect to NSCLC since patients with lung cancer represent the largest patient cohort within both patient populations. Antoch *et al.* (2004) evaluated FDG-PET/CT for tumor staging in 260 patients with solid tumors and concluded that FDG-PET/CT is able to detect significantly more lesions than FDG-PET and CT. Based on a change in the TNM stage, they reported a change in patient management in 6% of patients with FDG-PET/CT compared with FDG-PET and CT evaluated side by side. Buell *et al.* (2004) evaluated side-by-side analysis of CT and conventional FDG-PET in 733 patients with respect to patient groups that may benefit the most from the integrated PET/CT scanners. They showed that side-by-side reading of FDG-PET and CT failed to yield conclusive data with regard to lesion characterization in only 7.4% of patients. Thus, FDG-PET/CT might have been helpful in these cases.

PET imaging in the primary work-up of tumor suspicion is a relatively infrequent indication; this is in contrast to the other above-mentioned applications. Exceptions are patients with cancer of unknown primary (CUP) and cancer suspected by paraneoplastic syndrome. In ~ 2–10% of all newly diagnosed biopsy-confirmed malignancies, the site of origin is not identified by routine clinical work-up, and they are categorized as CUP. Although the prognosis of these patients is generally unfavorable with an average survival of only a few months, the detection of the occult primary is important to allow appropriate therapy planning. FDG-PET has been shown to be the most efficient method capable of localiz-ing unknown primary tumors. Detection rates of about 80% (Gambhir *et al.*, 2001) have been described in the literature. FDG-PET has been shown to be a useful technique in detecting small tumors in patients with paraneoplastic syndrome (Rees *et al.*, 2001; Frings *et al.*, 2005). However, the inability to localize foci of increased activity of FDG-PET can be challenging in respect to diagnosis, biopsy verification, and subsequent treatment planning. These problems can be overcome by PET/CT allowing an optimized therapy planning (Freudenberg *et al.*, 2005). Exact anatomic localization for further therapy planning and biopsy, for example, is also improved by PET/CT.

Initiation of a stage-adapted therapy is known to improve patient survival for a variety of malignant tumors. In staging applications, precise knowledge of the anatomic correlation of the PET finding with morphology is required (e.g., lymph node vs. organ involvement in lymphoma) or in lung cancer the exact identification of involved locoregional lymph nodes determines the stage. In the setting of cancer staging, combined PET/CT has been shown to be superior to other imaging modalities such as PET, PET and CT side by side, and MRI in most tumor types (Antoch *et al.*, 2003a, 2004a; Freudenberg *et al.*, 2004b).

FDG-PET allows depiction of malignant lymph node involvement in normal-sized lymph nodes (Fig. 2). These findings are as important as the differentiation of enlarged lymph nodes into malignant and non-malignant by the help of functional imaging with PET being precisely co-registered with the morphologic CT image. As the CT diagnosis predominantly relies on size, PET uses different functional abnormalities of the tumors. Synthesis of structural and metabolic information improves the accuracy of staging and the detection of recurrent disease and has the realistic potential to change patient management. PET/CT has some advantages over PET that may influence the clinical routine, one of these advantages being higher accuracy in anatomically localizing focal areas of abnormal tracer uptake and defining tumor extent (Antoch *et al.*, 2004c).

Clinical relevance of improved lesion detection by PET/CT has been described for several tumor entities yielding a change in the tumor–node–metastasis system stage. Beyond it, FDG-PET/CT will lead to a change in patient management in some of these patients. As an example, it is generally concluded that dual-modality FDG-PET/CT represents the most efficient and accurate approach to NSCLC staging, with a profound effect on therapy and, hence, on patient prognosis (Cerfolio *et al.*, 2004; Lardinois *et al.*, 2003; Aquino *et al.*, 2003; Antoch *et al.*, 2003a; Shim *et al.*, 2005). Antoch *et al.* observed that PET/CT findings led to a change in tumor stage in 26% of the patients compared to PET data alone, resulting in a change of treatment plans in 15%. Cerfolio *et al.*, Lardinois *et al.*, and Aquino *et al.* also found that tumor staging was significantly more accurate with integrated PET-CT than with PET alone.

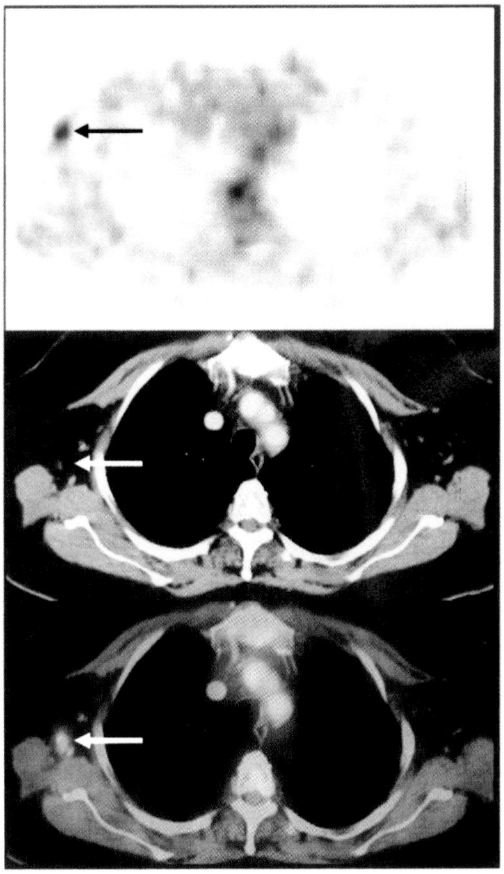

Applying FDG-PET/CT for staging reasons, we find that the results provide additional prognostic information. The incremental staging information and prognostic risk stratification of PET/CT significantly influence treatment strategies. By allowing patients with a poor prognosis to be converted from futile curative therapy, the use of PET avoids waste morbidity and saves the costs associated with that unhelpful treatment. Apart from diagnostic imaging, PET/CT is suitable for optimal planning of image-guided minimally invasive treatments such as radiofrequency ablation (RFA) of primary liver malignancies and secondary liver malignancies by providing the extent of vital tumor tissue and its underlying anatomical structure (Fig. 3). Based on PET/CT images, guided biopsy is possible, which is of importance within lesions consisting of vital tumor tissue and necrosis (Veit *et al.*, 2006).

PET/CT offers the radiation oncologist the possibility to include functional information into the target outlining (Fig. 4). For the treatment of patients with NSCLC, the use of FDG-PET images has been shown to modify the shape and volume of radiation fields in 22 to 62% of cases, mainly due to a better nodal staging and distinction of atelectasis from tumor. It also significantly reduced the interobserver and intraobserver variability (Bachaud *et al.*, 2005). In PET/CT examinations used for treatment planning of radiotherapy, the positioning of the patient is of utmost importance. The normal examination table should be replaced by a dedicated table for radiotherapy purposes, enabling additional fixation with radiotherapy masks or positioning aids.

PET/CT has an important role in re-staging after surgery and radio- or chemotherapy, as morphologic as well as functional changes may result. Scarring and necrotic

Figure 2 [18F]FDG-PET/CT, patient with breast cancer: top: PET, middle: CT, bottom: fusion image. PET unambiguously shows a pathologic lesion in the right axilla. The corresponding CT shows a non-enlarged lymph node, which would wrongly be classified as non-malignant if CT had been carried out alone.

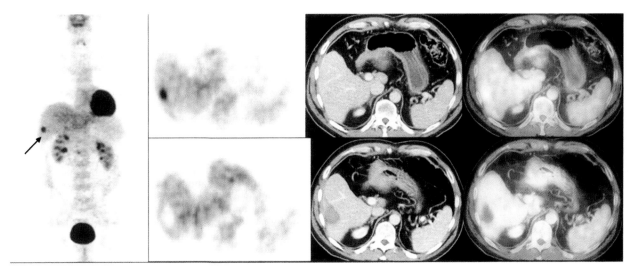

Figure 3 Left side: [18F]FDG-PET, projection image, patient with a single hepatic metastasis after colorectal carcinoma. Radiofrequency ablation (RFA) is planned for therapy. Top-left side: PET/CT (axial slices) is applied for planning RFA and to define the extent of the tumor, as well as after RFA to control the success of the minimally invasive treatment (bottom-left side).

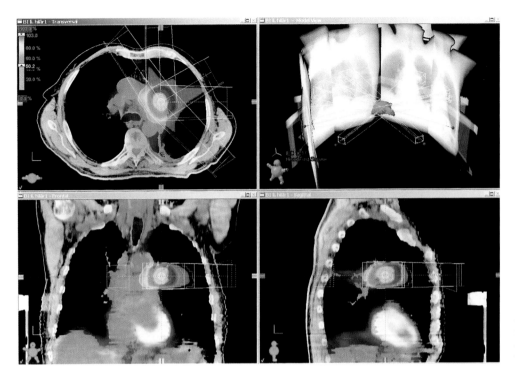

Figure 4 Patient with bronchial carcinoma after one radiotherapy. FDG-PET data are used to optimize the target volume for the following boost treatment.

masses have to be distinguished from residual vital tumor or recurrence. Anatomical imaging methods use the criterion of tumor shrinkage in order to define a good therapy response. Reduction in size, however, may not be the best indicator of response to therapy, since fibrotic tissue secondary to therapy may give the same image as a non- or partially responding mass. Metabolic imaging such as FDG-PET is a more accurate method for differentiating tumor from scar

tissue (Fig. 5). PET is superior to CT when the time interval between the beginning of therapy and re-staging for verifying therapy response is short, as changes in function precede morphologic changes. Focal FDG uptake after therapy is a relatively specific sign of viable tumor tissue and is associated with a poor prognosis. Knowledge of the shape and size of the structure-of-interest, which is readily available from the CT data, is necessary to perform a recovery

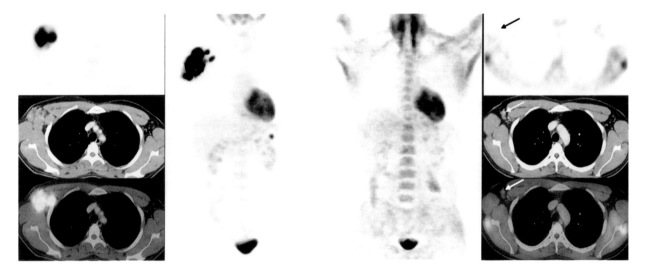

Figure 5 Prior to chemotherapy, FDG-PET/CT of a patient with lymphoma shows vital lymphoma in the right axilla and the left upper abdomen (left side axial slices and projection image) and after chemotherapy (right side axial slices and projection image). Four weeks after chemotherapy CT still shows pathologic enlarged lymph nodes in the axilla, but no pathologic glucose utilization can be seen (right-side axial slices and projection image (see arrow)). Consequently, the enlarged lymph nodes are nonvital remnants that do not require further therapy.

correction for accurate quantitation in small tumors. Furthermore, in longitudinal studies, PET/CT permits the unambiguous identification of marker lesions and provides more reliable information about response or progression of the disease (Antoch *et al.*, 2004a).

Apart from FDG, other radiotracers are available and clinically applied. Although they are used considerably less frequently today, these tracers are often promising. For example, [^{124}I]Iodine is a highly specific PET tracer used for imaging differentiated thyroid carcinoma, and ^{68}Ga-DOTATOC is a radiolabeled peptide used for somatostatin receptor scintigraphy. Less specific and quite widely established are [^{11}C]choline, a precursor of the biosynthesis of phosphatidylcholine used for staging prostate cancer, and [^{11}C]methionin, a well-established marker in brain tumor diagnosis. The more specific the tracer, the more selective will be the tissue uptake or receptor binding;, consequently, the higher the tumor-to-background ratio, the fewer the anatomical information will be within the PET image. The evaluation of tracer distribution in the body without knowing its morphological background limits image interpretation. In highly specific radiopharmaceuticals, such as, for example, [^{124}I]KI in thyroid cancer imaging, the complete lack of background information cannot be overcome by experience. Similarly, retrospective image fusion is likely to fail. This may seriously impair the diagnostic usefulness of these tracers. Anatomic information provided by PET/CT is essential to ensure the clinical application especially of high specific imaging agents (Freudenberg *et al.*, 2004) (Fig. 6). The spread of PET/CT, combined with the reliable anatomic information transferred from the CT to the PET investigation, will support the development and use of more specific tracers. A number of novel tracers are expected to be introduced into the clinical routine, which all require the precise identification of the anatomical structure underlying the functional abnormality (e.g., on atherosclerosis, angiogenesis, and hypoxia).

In conclusion, integrated PET/CT has been shown to be more accurate than PET and CT in staging in many malignancies. However, the benefits of anatomic-metabolic imaging using PET/CT can be fully exploited only if optimized acquisition protocols are implemented.

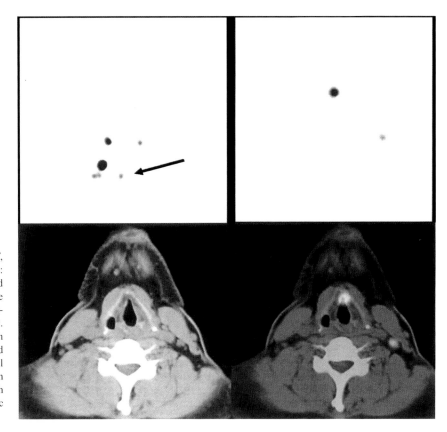

Figure 6 ^{124}Iodine PET/CT. Top-left side: PET, projection image of head and neck, top-right side: PET, axial slice of the finding, which is marked with an arrow in the projection image. Due to the high specificity of the tracer, no anatomical background can be recognized within the PET image. For further therapy planning, the exact lesion localization has to be known, which is achieved by PET/CT; bottom-left side: corresponding axial CT slice, bottom-right side: corresponding fusion image, showing iodine positive left cervical lymph node and a pretracheal lesion without morphologic correlative.

References

Antoch, G., Kanja, J., Bauer, S., Kuehl, H., Renzing-Koehler, K., Schuette, J., Bockisch, A., Debatin, J.F., and Freudenberg, L.S. 2004a. Comparison of PET, CT, and dual-modality PET/CT imaging for monitoring of imatinib (STI571) therapy in patients with gastrointestinal stromal tumors. *J. Nucl. Med. 45*:357–365.

Antoch, G., Kuehl, H., Kanja, J., Lauenstein, T.C., Schneemann, H., Hauth, E., Jentzen, W., Beyer, T., Goehde, S.C., and Debatin, J.F. 2004b. Dual-modality PET/CT scanning with negative oral contrast agent to avoid artifacts: introduction and evaluation. *Radiology 230*:879–885.

Antoch, G., Saoudi, N., Kuehl, H., Dahmen, G., Mueller, S.P., Beyer, T., Bockisch, A., Debatin, J.F., and Freudenberg, L.S. 2004c. Accuracy of whole-body dual-modality fluorine-18-2-fluoro-2-deoxy-D-glucose positron emission tomography and computed tomography (FDG-PET/CT) for tumor staging in solid tumors: comparison with CT and PET. *J. Clin. Oncol. 22*:4357–4368.

Antoch, G., Stattaus, J., Nemat, A.T., Marnitz, S., Beyer, T., Kuehl, H., Bockisch, A., Debatin, J.F., and Freudenberg, L.S. 2003a. Non-small cell lung cancer: dual-modality PET/CT in preoperative staging. *Radiology 229*:526–533.

Antoch, G., Vogt, F.M., Freudenberg, L.S., Nazaradeh, F., Goehde, S.C., Barkhausen, J., Dahmen, G., Bockisch, A., Debatin, J.F., and Ruehm, S.G. 2003b. Whole-body dual-modality PET/CT and whole-body MRI for tumor staging in oncology. *JAMA 290*:3199–3206.

Aquino, S.L., Asmuth, J.C., Alpert, N.M., Halpern, E.F., and Fischman, A.J. 2003. Improved radiologic staging of lung cancer with 2-[18F]-fluoro-2-deoxy-D-glucose-positron emission tomography and computed tomography registration. *J. Comput. Assist. Tomogr. 27*:479–484.

Bachaud, J.M., Marre, D., Dygai, I., Caselles, O., Hamelin, D., Begue, M., Laprie, A., Zerdoud, S., Gancel, M., and Courbon, F. 2005. The impact of 18F-fluorodeoxyglucose positron emission tomography on the 3D conformal radiotherapy planning in patients with non-small cell lung cancer. *Cancer Radiother. 9*:602–609.

Beyer, T., Antoch, G., Bockisch A., and Stattaus, J. 2005a. Optimized intravenous contrast administration for diagnostic whole-body 18F-FDG PET/CT. *J. Nucl. Med. 46*:429–435.

Beyer, T., Rosenbaum, S., Veit, P., Stattaus, J., Muller, S.P., Difilippo, F.P., Schoder, H., Mawlawi, O., Roberts, F., Bockisch, A., and Kuhl, H. 2005b. Respiration artifacts in whole-body (18)F-FDG PET/CT studies with combined PET/CT tomographs employing spiral CT technology with 1 to 16 detector rows. *Eur. J. Nucl. Med. Mol. Imaging 32*:1429–1439.

Beyer, T., Antoch, G., Muller, S., Egelhof, T., Freudenberg, L,S., Debatin, J., and Bockisch, A. 2004. Acquisition protocol considerations for combined PET/CT imaging. *J. Nucl. Med. 45* (Suppl 1):25–35.

Beyer, T., Townsend, D.W, and Blodgett, T.M. 2002. Dual-modality PET/CT tomography for clinical oncology. *Q. J. Nucl. Med. 46*:24–34.

Bockisch, A., Beyer, T., Antoch, G., Freudenberg, L.S., Kuhl, H., Debatin, J.F., and Muller, S.P. 2004. Positron emission tomography/computed tomography–imaging protocols, artifacts, and pitfalls. *Mol. Imaging Biol. 6*:188–199.

Buell, U., Wieres, F.J., Schneider, W., and Reinartz, P. 2004. 18FDG-PET in 733 consecutive patients with or without side-by-side CT evaluation: analysis of 921 lesions. *Nuklearmedizin 43*:210–216.

Cerfolio, R.J., Ojha, B., Bryant, A.S., Raghuveer, V., Mountz, J.M., and Bartolucci, A.A. 2004. The accuracy of integrated PET-CT compared with dedicated PET alone for the staging of patients with nonsmall cell lung cancer. *Ann. Thorac. Surg. 78*:1017–1023.

Freudenberg, L.S., Antoch, G., Jentzen, W., Pink, R., Knust, J., Gorges, R., Muller, S.P., Bockisch, A., Debatin, J.F., and Brandau, W. 2004a. Value of (124)I-PET/CT in staging of patients with differentiated thyroid cancer. *Eur. Radiol. 14*:2092–2098.

Freudenberg, L.S., Antoch, G., Schutt, P., Beyer, T., Jentzen, W., Muller, S.P., Gorges, R., Nowrousian, M.R., Bockisch, A., and Debatin, J.F. 2004b. FDG-PET/CT in re-staging of patients with lymphoma. *Eur. J. Nucl. Med. Mol. Imaging 31*:325–329.

Freudenberg, L.S., Fischer, M., Antoch, G., Jentzen, W., Gutzeit, A., Rosenbaum, S.J., Bockisch, A., and Egelhof, T. 2005. Dual modality of 18F-fluorodeoxyglucose-positron emission tomography/computed tomography in patients with cervical carcinoma of unknown primary. *Med. Princ. Pract. 14*:155–160.

Frings, M., Antoch, G., Knorn, P., Freudenberg, L., Bier, U., Timmann, D., and Maschke, M. 2005. Strategies in detection of the primary tumour in anti-Yo associated paraneoplastic cerebellar degeneration. *J. Neurol. 252*:197–201.

Gambhir, S.S., Czernin, J., Schwimmer, J., Silverman, D.H., Coleman, R.E., and Phelps, M.E. 2001. A tabulated summary of the FDG PET literature. *J. Nucl. Med. 42*:1–93.

Goerres, G.W., Kamel, E., Heidelberg, TN., Schwitter, MR., Burger, C., and von Schulthess, G.K. 2002. PET-CT image co-registration in the thorax: influence of respiration. *Eur. J. Nucl. Med. 29*:351–360.

Hofmann, M., Maecke, H., Borner, R., Weckesser, E., Schoffski, P., Oei, L., Schumacher, J., Henze, M., Heppeler, A., Meyer, J., and Knapp, H. 2001. Biokinetics and imaging with the somatostatin receptor PET radioligand (68)Ga-DOTATOC: preliminary data. *Eur. J. Nucl. Med. 28*:1751–1757.

Jacobs, A.H, Dittmar, C., Winkeler, A., Garlip, G., and Heiss, W.D. 2002. Molecular imaging of gliomas. *Mol. Imag. 1*:309–335.

Kuehl, H., and Antoch, G. 2005. How much CT do we need for PEt/CT? A radiologist's perspective. *Nuklearmedizin 44* (Suppl. 1):24–31.

Lardinois, D., Weder, W., Hany, T.F., Kamel, E.M., Korom, S., Seifert, B., von Schulthess, G.K., and Steinert, H.C. 2003. Staging of non-small-cell lung cancer with integrated positron-emission tomography and computed tomography. *N. Engl. J. Med. 19*:2500–2507.

Lind, T., Jentzen, W., Freudenberg, L., and Bockisch, A. 2004. Genauigkeit der Lokalisation von Tumoren mit Hilfe der retrospektiven Koregistrierung von PET und CT: Ein Vergleich mit PET/CT. *Nuklearmedizin 43*:A22.

Nömayr, A., Römer, W., Hothorn, T., Pfahlberg, A., Hornegger, J., Bautz, W., and Kuwert, T. 2005. Anatomical accuracy of lesion localization. *Nuklearmedizin 4*:149–155.

Pietrzyk, U. 2005. Does PET/CT render software registration obsolete? *Nuklearmedizin 44* (Suppl. 1):13–17.

Rees, J.H., Hain, S.F., Johnson, M.R., Hughes, R.A., Costa, D.C., Ell, P.J., Keir, G., and Rudge, P. 2001. The role of [18F]fluoro-2-deoxyglucose-PET scanning in the diagnosis of paraneoplastic neurological disorders. *Brain 124*:2223–2231.

Reske, S.N., and Kotzerke, J. 2001. FDG-PET for clinical use. Results of the 3rd German Interdisciplinary Consensus Conference, "Onko-PET III," July 21 and September 19, 2000. *Eur. J. Nucl. Med. 28*:1707–1723.

Rosenbaum, S.J., Lind, T., Antoch, G., and Bockisch, A. 2005. False-positive FDG PET uptake—the role of PET/CT. *Eur. Radiol. 17*:1–12.

Schoder, H., and Larson, S.M. 2004. Positron emission tomography for prostate, bladder, and renal cancer. *Semin. Nucl. Med. 34*:274–292.

Shim, S.S., Lee, K.S., Kim, B.T., Chung, M.J., Lee, E.J., Han, J., Veit, P., Antoch, G., Stergar, H., Bockisch, A., Forsting, M., and Kuehl, H. 2006. Detection of residual tumor after radiofrequency ablation of liver metastasis with dual-modality PET/CT: initial results. *Eur. Radiol. 16*:80–87.

Veit, P., Kuehle, C., Beyer, T., Kuehl, H., Bockisch, A., and Antoch, G. 2006. Accuracy of combined PET/CT in image-guided intervention of liver lesions: an *ex vivo* study. *World J. Gastroenterol. 12*:2388–2393.

von Schulthess, G.K. 2000. Cost considerations regarding an integrated CT-PET system. *Eur. Radiol. 10* (Suppl. 3):377–380.

Wahl, R.L., Quint, L.E., Cieslak, R.D., Aisen, A.M., Koeppe, R.A., and Meyer, C.R. 1993. "Anatometabolic" tumor imaging: fusion of FDG PET with CT or MRI to localize foci of increased activity. *J. Nucl. Med. 34*:1190–1197.

Warburg, O., Posener, K., and Negelein, E. 1924. Uber den Stoffwechsel der Carcinomzelle. *Biochem. Zeitschrift. 152*:309–335.

7

Whole-Body Cancer Imaging: Simple Image Fusion with Positron Emission Tomography/ Computed Tomography

Yuji Nakamoto

Introduction

Before positron emission tomography/computed tomography (PET/CT) scanners were developed, multimodal registration was performed using software on a workstation. Because both PET and CT images are digital and tomographic, it was possible to simply merge the two data sets. However, due to the image quality or software limitation, the complicated and time-consuming procedure of fusing the images did not always provide any clinically relevant merit. With the progress of computer hardware and software, as well as PET and CT devices themselves, image fusion has been established as a promising technique that can often affect therapeutic strategy, even when it is a software-based approach. This chapter discusses one of the software-based fusion methods for evaluating cancer patients.

Hardware and Software Fusion

Software-based fusion was initially applied to brain tumors at the end of the 1980s; the application of image fusion of molecular and morphological information for lesions in the body was discussed in the early 1990s; and Beyer *et al.* (2000) and his colleagues developed a prototype of an inline PET-CT system at the end of the 1990s. Subsequently, PET/CT devices have been installed in many institutes, where thousands of clinical studies are currently performed (Schoder *et al.*, 2003). Image fusion can now be obtained not only for a region, but also for the whole body.

The advantages of PET/CT are as follows: it is easy to know the anatomical localization of the tracer uptake, resulting in fewer false-positive findings by avoiding the misinterpretation of physiological uptake as pathological. Equivocal findings on CT or PET can be identified as pathological findings on fused images with more confidence, contributing to higher sensitivity, and more appropriate diagnoses based on fusion imaging can lead to more appropriate treatment. In addition, the short time required for the examination yields higher patient throughput. Among these advantages, all but the last are derived from fusion imaging. Therefore, the advantage of a PET/CT device is as follows: fused images offering many advantages can be obtained easily and in a short time using an integrated PET/CT scanner.

169

Although an increasing number of institutes have installed this device, not every institute can afford it due to economic concerns. In contrast to hardware fusion such as PET/CT, software-based fusion is more cost-effective. Recently, there has been dramatic progress in computers and software. We can currently produce fused images with minimal effort, as compared with the old system. Kim *et al.* (2005) reported that PET/CT hardware fusion was superior to software fusion and that software-based fusion was not considered an alternative due to its high rate of misregistration. However, the scanning protocol of CT, including respiratory phase during the scanning, could have been suboptimal. This is considered a problem of image acquisition rather than the software-based approach. In addition, in spite of the disadvantages of the software-based approach, they demonstrated comparable diagnostic outcomes between PET/CT and software-based fusion. In other words, as long as misregistration does not damage diagnostic accuracy, perfect registration is not always necessary in clinical settings. The advantages and disadvantages of each method are shown in Table 1.

There are mainly two types of image registration algorithms: feature-based and volume-based algorithms. In the feature-based algorithm, image registration is performed using anatomic landmarks, organ surfaces, or other fiducial markers, whereas statistical voxel dependency of the image data sets is used in the volume-based algorithm, such as the mutual information method. There is another classification of image registration: rigid and nonrigid. In rigid registration, which is also known as linear registration, images are three-dimensionally translated, rotated, or scaled without deforming them. On the other hand, in nonrigid or nonlinear registration, images can be deformed to match in nonrigid fusion. Because PET images are obtained during tidal breathing, they are susceptible to respiratory motion or peristalsis. For this reason, the two image data sets do not always match each other with only rigid registration, and image warping in nonlinear registration often provides better fused images. However, there is no evidence that deformed images reflect the true distribution of the tracer in nonrigid registration and may adversely affect image interpretation. Further investigations are required to confirm whether it has no effect.

Table 1   Advantages and Limitations of Methods

	Advantages	Disadvantages
Hardware-based fusion (PET/CT, SPECT/CT, etc.)	Excellent fused images Shorter examination time Higher patient throughput	Expensive Possibly more radiation exposure
Software-based fusion	Cost effective Easy multimodal access	Troublesome More misregistration

Fusion Technique for Cancer Imaging

As mentioned earlier, the success of PET/CT can be attributed to the development of multidetector-row CT (MDCT), which enables the scanning of the whole body in a single scanning. Therefore, if we had separate state-of-the-art MDCT and dedicated PET devices, it would be possible to obtain fairly good fused images, which may not have perfect registration, but could be helpful enough for clinical interpretation, resulting in higher diagnostic accuracy and yielding a clinical impact. In order to minimize misregistration, we started to use a fixation device for both scanning methods (Nakamoto *et al.*, 2005): rigid fusion on a pixel-to-pixel basis. Most fused images were tolerable for image interpretation without problematic manual intervention, and they often had significant clinical impact (Fig. 1). Our established method has been designed as a cost-effective and clinically acceptable approach in clinical settings.

Scanning Protocol

Positron emission tomography scan pretreatment does not differ from conventional scanning. After fasting for at least 4 hr, patients received ^{18}F-FDG while monitoring the plasma glucose level. At 50 min post-injection, patients were urged to void. They were then positioned in a 200 × 60 × 5 cm large vacuum cushion (ESFORM, Engineering System, Matsumoto, Japan), which has been widely used for the reproducible positioning of the patients in radiation therapy on the bed of a PET scanner with their arms up over their head. When air is drawn from the cushion, it becomes a rigid cradle having the shape of the patient's torso. After positioning the patient, a median line is marked on the skin from the navel to the sternum, bilateral horizontal lines, and a transverse line indicating the start of scanning on the upper thigh. External fiducial markers are not used in this procedure.

After positioning the patient in this way, data acquisition using a static emission scan is performed in 3-D mode with 2 to 3 min of acquisition in each bed position, covering from the upper thigh to the skull base. A conventional transmission scan using ^{68}Ge/^{68}Ga rod sources is then performed over the same area for 2 min per bed position. Attenuation-corrected images are made using an iterative reconstruction algorithm. After completion of the PET scan, the patient is urged to void again to get a consistent bladder shape and to reduce radiation exposure. After moving to a CT room with the fixation device, the patient is repositioned using the same molded vacuum cushion, referring to the median and bilateral surface lines marked before PET scanning. The technical parameters used for CT scanning are as follows: 120 kV peak energy, 200 to 450 mA tube electric current with automated radiation exposure control, helical pitch of 5.5 (high-speed mode), 3 mm collimation, and 5 mm reconstruction thickness.

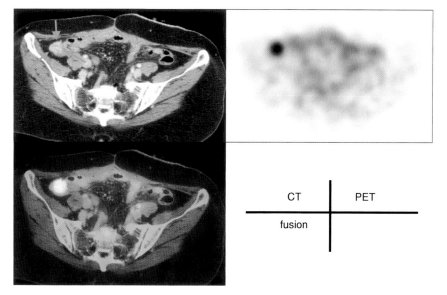

Figure 1 A representative case in which our fusion technique was applied. The patient is a 52-year-old female who had undergone surgery for rectal cancer. PET and CT scans were ordered for re-staging. There is a focal intense uptake in the right side in the pelvis, indicating a peritoneal implant. This lesion had been missed on CT. It seems difficult to differentiate a tumor from bowel only on the corresponding CT image (arrows).

During the 20 to 30 sec scan, the patient is requested to perform shallow breathing. The scanning time depends on the number of detectors. In our system, it takes ~ 30 sec because our CT scanner has four detectors. If the patient can hold the breath, the CT scan is performed during the end-expiratory phase with breath holding. Unless the use of intravenous contrast is a contraindication, contrast-enhanced CT is acquired in the venous phase—that is, 80 to 90 sec after the administration of 100 ml iohexol or iopamidol, containing 300 mg iodide per 1 ml solution at an injection rate of 2 ml/sec. Oral contrast for CT scanning is not used, but it may be preferable when available.

Image Processing

Both CT and PET data sets are transferred to a SUN workstation (ULTRA60; SUN Microsystems, Mountain View, California). Positron emission tomography images, enlarged by multiplying a zooming factor to fit the field-of-view of the CT images (50 cm), are interpolated and resliced using a matrix size of 512 × 512 and a 5 mm interval using a software package (Dr. View, Asahikasei-Joho Systems, Tokyo, Japan). We initially used this UNIX-based system, but the current LINUX version works on a personal computer. The slice showing the lower margin of the urinary bladder is then determined in both the CT and modified PET images. The PET images are shifted cranio-caudally to match the CT images. Lastly, the two sets of images are merged on a pixel-to-pixel basis for the whole body. The computing time is ~ 5 minutes per patient, although this depends on the central processing unit and computer memory.

In this protocol, CT is basically performed for diagnostic purpose, depicting morphological details, not for attenuation correction. Therefore, this technique might be characterized as PET-supported CT rather than CT-supported PET. There are some advantages of our technique. It is simple and needs only a small amount of extra time (~ 3 min) for positioning for each examination. The fusion software is commercially available, and no specific algorithm for fusion is necessary. Compared with a combined PET/CT scanner, it is cost effective, and it may be applied in institutes where stand-alone CT and PET scanners are ready to use, only by preparing a fixation device and software. Because patients do not need CT scanning twice for a diagnostic CT scan and PET/CT scan, redundant radiation exposure can be avoided, although irradiation by an external source for the transmission scan is inevitable.

This technique also has some disadvantages. Since repositioning is necessary, this method has a greater chance of misregistration for pathological or physiological uptake. As has been demonstrated in PET/CT studies, the average displacement between CT and PET is < 1 cm when we use the PET/CT device for fusion (Cohade *et al.*, 2003; Nakamoto *et al.*, 2003). On the other hand, the average displacement of pulmonary nodules was ~ 12 mm using this fusion method, although this misregistration does not necessarily influence the diagnostic accuracy. Misregistration tended to be more remarkable in patients who are severely ill and have catheters, including a central venous line. Surgery for rectal cancer often changes the shape of the bladder. External markers would be necessary in such cases instead of referring to the lower edge of the bladder in the fusion process as an internal marker. Furthermore, for patients with stiff and painful shoulders, holding their arms up during the scanning would be painful. Because the gantry of the PET device is generally smaller than that of a CT scanner, scanning the neck area with the arms up would be difficult. Moreover, radiation exposure of medical staff from patients may be problematic. We scan in this order because it is easy to reposition the patients before CT scan, because the gantry of the PET device is smaller than that of CT. However, in order to avoid unnecessary radiation exposure for the medical staff, the order should be reversed.

While CT scanning should be performed in the end-expiratory phase to get the best registration of the diaphragm (Goerres *et al.*, 2002), we adopted free breathing because breath holding for about 30 seconds was painful for some elderly patients, and it has been reported that free breathing can be used during CT in PET/CT scanning (Goerres *et al.*, 2003). Consequently, compared with conventional diagnostic CT images obtained during the end-inspiratory phase, our CT images used for fusion are a little noisy and blurred due to respiratory movement. Nonetheless, in most cases, the image quality in this study is high enough to allow proper evaluation of whether pulmonary nodules are present in the lung field, indicating pulmonary metastasis. The results would also be adequate for use in disease staging or re-staging, even though it may be difficult to accurately evaluate diffuse pulmonary disease.

In this method, CT was performed during the venous phase. The intrapelvic region must be read carefully in patients with suspected colorectal cancer in terms of the presence or absence of lymph node swelling. To more easily evaluate metastases to the iliac nodes, we began CT scanning 90 sec after injection of the intravenous contrast. However, this timing may be suboptimal for evaluation of the liver. We need further evaluation to identify a more optimal administration rate of contrast material and timing of CT scan by considering the primary tumor and expected distant metastases.

It remains unknown whether our method can really achieve better diagnostic accuracy or affect the therapeutic strategy. According to our preliminary results regarding suspected recurrent colorectal cancer, interpreting fused images provided more accurate diagnoses, as compared with interpreting CT alone, PET alone, or CT and PET side by side (Nakamoto *et al.*, 2007). It should be investigated whether it is also applicable to other malignancies.

Advanced Fusion with Advanced Software

As shown in Table 2, additional software has been developed to obtain fused images easily (Slomka *et al.*, 2003), and inexpensive or even free software is currently available. In addition, picture archiving and communication systems

Table 2 Imaging Software with Fusion Function

Name	Vendor	Type of Fusion Algorithm
Aquarius Workstation	TeraRecon	Rigid
BodyGuide	Advanced Biologic Corp.	Nonrigid
Dr. View/Linux	Asahikasei-Joho system	Rigid
Fusion 7D	Mirada solutions	Nonrigid
OsiriX	Free soft	Rigid
Virtual Place	Aze	Rigid

(PACS) have been widely distributed, and the interpretation of images displayed on a workstation has been performed in many institutes. A fusion software should also be prepared together with the PACS system, which would contribute to CT or PET interpretation at institutes without a PET/CT device. Therefore, fusion imaging is possible in routine clinical use. When CT images are obtained during the inspiratory phase, two image data sets are merged with more misregistration. If both CT and PET are scheduled, especially for staging and re-staging, CT scanning should be performed in the expiratory phase or under shallow breathing. If we need to evaluate the lung field more accurately, additional CT scanning of the lung field in the end-inspiratory phase with breath holding would be ideal.

Software fusion is not limited to PET-CT fusion (Forster *et al.*, 2003), and especially for the head and neck or in gynecology, image fusion between PET and MR might be useful. Because these areas are hardly affected by respiratory motion, image fusion is easy, with little misregistration (Fig. 2). In addition, SPECT-CT or SPECT-MR fusion is also available using software. Most software has the capability of

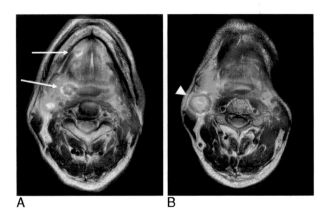

A   B

Figure 2 A case of PET-MR fusion. A 62-year-old man had surgery for left maxillary cancer and radiation therapy. PET images, which were ordered for restaging, revealed three focal uptakes in the right cervical region. PET and MR images were fused using software. One corresponded to submandibular lymph node metastasis (B: arrowhead), and two indicated the right sublingual gland and right palatine tonsil (A: arrows). Physiological uptake in the left sublingual gland or palatine tonsil may be reduced by irradiation.

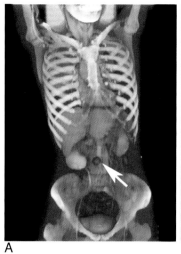
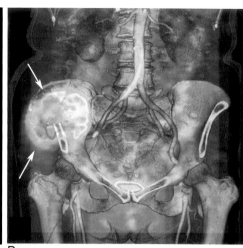

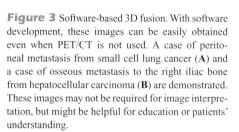

Figure 3 Software-based 3D fusion. With software development, these images can be easily obtained even when PET/CT is not used. A case of peritoneal metastasis from small cell lung cancer (**A**) and a case of osseous metastasis to the right iliac bone from hepatocellular carcinoma (**B**) are demonstrated. These images may not be required for image interpretation, but might be helpful for education or patients' understanding.   A   B

various volume-rendering techniques, which can yield three-dimensional fusion (Fig. 3). This kind of image is not always necessary for image interpretation, but it might be useful for navigation before a medical procedure or education for medical students or residents. It may also help patients to understand when they are not familiar with conventional tomographic CT or PET images.

In summary, image fusion between morphological and metabolic information can yield higher diagnostic accuracy and yield more confidence of a clinical impact. When an inline PET/CT system is available, it should be used properly. Otherwise, a software-based approach may be worth considering, and for this purpose, connectivity, compatibility, and cooperation between departments would be indispensable (Slomka, 2004). In addition, we have to familiarize ourselves with the morphological and metabolic information provided by the images in order to acquire synergistic benefits, whichever radiology or nuclear medicine is our speciality.

References

Beyer, T., Townsend, D.W., Brun, T., Kinahan, P.E., Charron, M., Roddy, R., Jerin, J., Young, J., Byars, L., and Nutt, R. 2000. A combined scanner for clinical oncology. *J. Nucl. Med. 41*:1369–1379.

Cohade, C., Osman, M., Marshall, L.T., and Wahl, R.L. 2003. PET-CT: accuracy of PET and CT spatial registration of lung lesions. *Eur. J. Nucl. Med. Mol. Imaging 30*:721–726.

Forster, G.J., Laumann, C., Nickel, O., Kann, P., Rieker, O., and Bartenstein, P. 2003. SPET/CT image co-registration in the abdomen with a simple and cost-effective tool. *Eur. J. Nucl. Med. Mol. Imaging 30*:32–39.

Goerres, G.W., Kamel, E., Heidelberg, T.N., Schwitter, M.R., Burger, C., and von Schulthess, G.K. 2002. PET-CT image co-registration in the thorax: influence of respiration. *Eur. J. Nucl. Med. Mol. Imaging 29*:351–360.

Goerres, G.W., Burger, C., Schwitter, M.R., Heidelberg, T.N., Seifert, B., and von Schulthess, G.K. 2003. PET/CT of the abdomen: optimizing the patient breathing pattern. *Eur. Radiol. 13*:734–739.

Kim, J.H., Czernin, J., Allen-Auerbach, M.S., Halpern, B.S., Fueger, B.J., Hecht, J.R., Ratib, O., Phelps, M.E., and Weber, W.A. 2005. Comparison between 18F-FDG PET, in-line PET/CT, and software fusion for restaging of recurrent colorectal cancer. *J. Nucl. Med. 46*:587–595.

Nakamoto, Y., Tatsumi, M., Cohade, C., Osman, M., Marshall, L.T., and Wahl, R.L. 2003. Accuracy of image fusion of normal upper abdominal organs visualized with PET/CT. *Eur. J. Nucl. Med. Mol. Imaging 30*:597–602.

Nakamoto, Y., Sakamoto, S., Okada, T., Matsumoto, K., Minota, E., Kawashima, H., and Senda, M. 2005. Accuracy of image fusion using a fixation device for whole body cancer imaging. *AJR. Am. J. Roentgenol. 184*:1960–1966.

Nakamoto, Y., Sakamoto, S., Okada, T., Senda, M., Higashi, T., Saga, T., and Togashi, K. 2007. Clinical value of manual fusion of PET and CT images in patients with suspected recurrent colorectal cancer. *Am. J. Roentgenol. 188*:257–267.

Schoder, H., Erdi, Y.E., Larson, S.M., and Yeung, H.W. 2003. PET/CT: a new imaging technology in nuclear medicine. *Eur. J. Nucl. Med. Mol. Imaging 30*:1419–1437.

Slomka, P.J., Dey, D., Przetak, C., Aladl, U.E., and Baum, R.P. 2003. Automated 3-dimensional registration of stand-alone (18)F-FDG whole-body PET with CT. *J. Nucl. Med. 44*:1156–1167.

Slomka, P.J. 2004. Software approach to merging molecular with anatomic information. *J. Nucl. Med. 45*:36S–45S.

8

Whole-Body Tumor Imaging: O-[¹¹C]Methyl-L-Tyrosine/Positron Emission Tomography

Kiichi Ishiwata, Kuzuo Kubota, Tadashi Nariai, and Ren Iwata

Introduction

2-Deoxy-2-[¹⁸F]fluoro-D-glucose (FDG) is the radiopharmaceutical of choice for the diagnosis of tumors by positron emission tomography (PET). Whole-body imaging with FDG-PET is routinely used to diagnose cancer; however, it has several limitations (Kubota, 2001). Because of high glucose metabolism in the normal brain, brain tumors are sometimes visualized as cold spots, or the invasive regions of tumors are poorly delineated. FDG is also taken up to some extent by inflamed tissues, and by normal organs under physiological conditions. Furthermore, the excretion of FDG through the urinary tract can make it difficult to identify tumors in the lower abdominal region. In contrast to FDG, radiolabeled amino acids such as L-[methyl-¹¹C]methionine (MET) are taken up into normal brain tissue at much lower levels, which enables imaging of the majority of low- and high-grade brain tumors. The uptake of amino acid tracers by inflamed tissues is also low. Presently, MET has been applied for diagnosing tumors in the chest region as well as the brain, but not in the abdominal region where the natural amino acids are taken up at high levels in organs such as the pancreas and liver, as confirmed by whole-body imag-

ing (Kubota, 2001). On the other hand, the artificial amino acid O-[¹⁸F]fluoroethyl-L-tyrosine was accumulated at very low levels in the human pancreas and liver but excreted from the kidneys to the bladder through the urinary tract (Wester et al., 1999). This finding could be characteristically common to artificial amino acid tracers that reflect amino acid transport.

This chapter describes the development of O-[¹¹C]methyl-L-tyrosine (OMT) and its first clinical application to whole-body imaging as well as brain tumor imaging. Artificial amino acids labeled with ¹⁸F ($t_{1/2}$ = 109.8 min) have the potential advantage that a single production is sufficient for several patients, or alternatively to be delivered to satellite PET-centers, if the tracers can be prepared with high radiochemical yields. The use of amino acids labeled with ¹¹C ($t_{1/2}$ = 20.4 min) is restricted to a few subjects in PET-centers with an on-site cyclotron; however, it has a potential advantage for patients. Multiple tracers can be administered to the individuals on the same day for a differential diagnosis with OMT-PET followed by FDG-PET. The use of ¹¹C-labeled tracers usually results in decreased radiation absorbed doses compared with the use of ¹⁸F-tracers that have longer half-lives.

Development of *O*-[^{11}C]Methyl-L-Tyrosine

Radiosynthesis

Initially, OMT was prepared with a high radiochemical yield by the methylation of L-tyrosine with [^{11}C]methyl triflate followed by purification with high-performance liquid chromatography (HPLC) (Iwata *et al.*, 2002). Later, a simple automated method using solid phase extraction without HPLC purification was developed for routine clinical use (Ishikawa *et al.*, 2005).

Tumor Imaging Potential Evaluated in a Rat Model

The evaluation of OMT was performed in rats bearing AH109A hepatoma (Ishiwata *et al.*, 2004, 2005). The uptake of OMT by the AH109A gradually increased for 60 min postinjection and was greater than in any normal tissues except for the pancreas after 15 min. However, the tumor-to-tissue uptake ratio for OMT was not as high as that for FDG. Metabolically, OMT was stable, suggesting that it is useful for imaging the transport of amino acids in tumors. In AH109A-bearing rats with the turpentine oil-induced inflammation, the inflammation-to-AH109A uptake ratio was smaller for OMT than for [^{3}H]deoxyglucose, an analog of FDG, suggesting that with OMT it is possible to distinguish between tumorous and inflamed tissues.

Dynamic Whole-Body Imaging of Normal Monkeys

We performed dynamic whole-body imaging in monkeys for 92 min post-injection to confirm the applicability of OMT-PET to the diagnosis of tumors in the whole body (Ishiwata *et al.*, 2005). Positron emission tomography showed low uptake of OMT in all normal organs except for the urinary tract and bladder, and the radioactivity remained distributed throughout the body after 20 min. These findings suggested that whole-body imaging could be done within 60 min, an appropriate scan period for the ^{11}C-tracers, which was confirmed in normal human subjects.

Radiation Dosimetry and Acute Toxicity

The acceptability of OMT for clinical use was examined (Ishiwata *et al.*, 2005). The radiation-absorbed dose of OMT was low (4.54 μSv/MBq for the whole body). No acute toxicity was found in rats at up to 2.41 mg/kg, which is 55,000-times of the postulated dose in humans. No mutagenicity in the Ames test was observed at a dose range of 0.0763-5000 μg/plate.

Whole-Body Tumor Imaging Using OMT Compared with FDG

FDG-PET is the standard for imaging in oncology. To test the possibility of whole-body tumor imaging using a new tracer, we have compared OMT-PET with FDG-PET and considered the characteristics of OMT-PET.

Subjects and Methods

Seventeen patients (13 males, 4 females, mean age 69, range 46–89) with various types of cancers or suspected of having cancer with a total of 24 lesions were examined using OMT-PET. Sixteen patients also received FDG-PET within a week. One patient suspected of having cerebral hemorrhage from a brain tumor was examined only with OMT-PET. The PET images were visually evaluated by experienced nuclear medicine physicians, and diagnostic reports were prepared. The final diagnosis for each lesion, determined by surgery, biopsy, or clinical examination after a follow-up of at least 6 months was compared to that based on the PET reports, and diagnostic efficacy was evaluated. The final diagnosis was: brain tumor, brain abscess, cerebral hemorrhage (no tumor found), lung cancer, lung infection, esophageal cancer, gastric cancer, gallbladder cancer, cholecystitis, pancreatic cancer, pancreatitis, colon cancer, and malignant lymphoma.

After fasting 4 hr or more, 740 MBq of OMT were intravenously injected into subjects, and 10 to 15 min later, whole-body imaging was performed with PET or PET/CT. FDG-PET was also performed 1 hr after the injection of 370 MBq of FDG within a week. Eight patients were studied using a dedicated PET scanner (Headtome IV, Shimadzu, Kyoto, Japan). Nine patients were studied using a combined PET and 16-row mutlidetector CT (Biograph sansation 16, Siemens, Malvern, Pennsylvania). All PET images were reconstructed by iterative reconstruction with an ordered-subset expectation maximization algorithm. Image interpretation was performed using dedicated workstations for each PET system. A quantitative evaluation of the lesion uptake of each tracer using a standardized uptake value (SUV), (tissue activity/ml tissue)/(injected radioisotope activity)/(g body weight) was performed.

Results and Discussion

Diagnostic accuracy for all lesions was calculated as follows: sensitivity of OMT 75% (12/16) and FDG 94% (15/16); specificity of OMT 75% (6/8) and FDG 43% (3/7); and accuracy of OMT 75% (18/24) and FDG 78% (18/23).

Chronic xantomatous cholecystitis showed a ring-like uptake with FDG but no significant uptake with OMT. Tumor-to-background ratios (T/B ratios) of lung cancer and brain tumor were ~ 2.0. T/B ratios of pancreatic cancer and colon

OMT-PET

Diagnostic	Malignant	Benign	Total
Positive	12	2	14
Negative	4	6	10
Total	16	8	24

FDG-PET

Diagnostic	Malignant	Benign	Total
Positive	15	4	19
Negative	1	3	4
Total	16	7	23

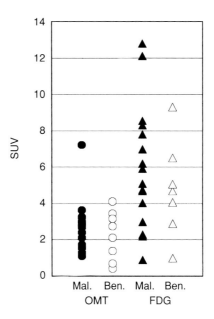

Figure 1 Distribution of the SUV of malignant and benign lesions (inflammation) obtained with OMT and FDG. No significant differences were observed between malignant and benign lesions using OMT or FDG.

cancer were ~ 1.5. Malignant lymphoma was clearly detected with OMT, but the SUV was lower than that obtained with FDG. Mean SUV values of malignant and benign lesions with OMT-PET and FDG-PET were as follows: OMT malignant 2.26 ± 1.44 ($n = 16$), OMT benign 2.25 ± 1.33 ($n = 8$), FDG malignant 5.98 ± 3.38 ($n = 16$), FDG benign 4.79 ± 2.64 ($n = 7$). There was no significant difference between malignant and benign tumors with FDG or OMT. The distribution of the SUVs is shown in Figure 1.

The uptake of OMT in the liver and pancreas was mild, but urinary excretion was observed soon after the injection. Normal uptake was lower in the brain than that in the liver and slightly higher than that in the muscle. Kidney and urine in the bladder showed the highest levels of activity. Typical images of OMT and FDG are shown in Figure 2. The results can be summarized as follows:

1. Cancerous tissue tended to take up less OMT than FDG.

2. Inflamed tissue also tended to take up less OMT than FDG.

3. In some tumors, such as esophageal cancer and gallbladder cancer, the use of OMT would avoid the false-positive results caused by the uptake of FDG in inflamed areas.

Essential amino acids labeled with ^{11}C, such as MET and L-[carboxyl-^{11}C]tyrosine, are known to accumulate in the pancreas, liver, and salivary glands. This seems to be related to the function of these organs, that is, the secretion of digestive fluids, enzymes, and plasma proteins. MET has been used for protein synthesis and transmethylation pathway in part in the liver and pancreas, and radioactivity was excreted into the duodenum after the injection (Kubota, 2001). However, most of the artificial analogues of amino acids have shown a mild uptake in the pancreas, usually lower than that in the liver. This may be explained by an absence of metabolic incorporation into proteins or other macromolecules.

In animal models, OMT has been demonstrated to be a nonmetabolized amino acid analogue, whose accumulation in tissue is regulated by amino acid transporters (Ishiwata *et al.*, 2004). In human subjects, the lower uptake in the pancreas and liver, and the lack of intestinal excretion of radioactivity even 50 min after injection, can be explained by the nonmetabolic nature of OMT. The extensive urinary excretion of OMT soon after its injection may also be related to this and, as in the case of FDG, may hinder the detection of tumors in the pelvis.

Macrophages and granulocytes consume glucose for their immune reactions. In addition to the increased metabolism of glucose in the cells responsible for immune reactions, glucose metabolism by proliferating fibroblasts and a newly formed vasculature consisting of young granulation tissue would explain the marked uptake of FDG in inflamed tissue (Kubota, 2001). In contrast to high glucose metabolism, protein synthesis by granulocytes or macrophages has been reported to be reduced, and experimental inflammation resulted in a lower uptake of amino acids than with FDG (Jager *et al.*, 2001). OMT as a tracer of amino acid transport seems to accumulate less in inflamed tissue than does FDG, as observed in the experimental model of inflammation (Ishiwata *et al.*, 2005). This is a preliminary clinical study for the types of cancers suited to this tracer. We have included a wide variety of malignant and benign lesions. This may be reflected by the very scattered distribution of SUVs for both FDG and OMT. Also, the mean SUV data for inflammation did not show any significant differences from that for tumors, despite the fact that several patients

OMT   FDG

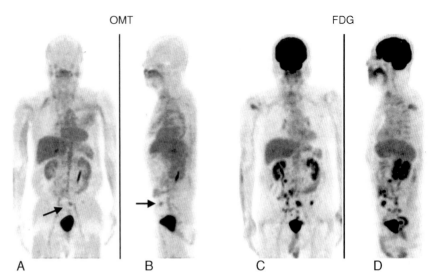

Figure 2 Maximum intensity projected (MIP) images of whole-body PET using OMT (A: frontal view; and B: lateral view) and FDG (C: frontal view; and D: lateral view). A 79-year-old man with a history of surgery for colon cancer was referred for a PET examination. FDG-PET showed multiple focal lesions in the abdomen, indicative of peritoneal and para-aortic lymph node metastasis. Surgery confirmed the metastasis. OMT-PET showed the largest of the peritoneal metastatic nodules (arrows); however, other nodules showed less uptake.

A   B   C   D

were true negative with OMT and false positive with FDG. In conclusion, OMT-PET has the potential to improve the specificity of cancer diagnosis by reducing the rate of false positives caused by inflammation.

Brain Tumor Imaging Using OMT Compared with MET

Positron-labeled amino acids have been identified as a suitable imaging probe to evaluate the pathophysiology of brain tumors using PET. As they are taken up in the normal brain far less extensively than FDG, it can delineate active brain tumor, whichever benign or malignant, with good contrast to the surrounding brain. Among the various amino acid tracers (Jager *et al.*, 2001), MET is used in most clinical studies of brain tumors because of its simple and efficient labeling procedure. Many previous clinical reports, including ours (Nariai *et al.*, 2005), suggest that MET-PET is an excellent imaging method for localizing and characterizing brain tumors. To use OMT for that purpose, the benefits of amino acid probes in brain tumor imaging as exemplified in MET-PET should be preserved.

Subjects and Methods

Fifteen pairwise scans for 13 patients (8 males, 5 females, mean age 53.5, range 28–76) with brain tumors were performed. The final pathological diagnosis of these patients was glioblastoma (4), anaplastic astrocytoma (3), anaplastic oligodendroglioma (1), oligodendroglioma (3), oligoastrocytoma (1), and metastatic tumor (1). On the day of the examination, several patients underwent routine MET-PET. One or two patients who showed an increase in the uptake of MET into cancerous regions were asked to participate in the present comparative study. After enough time had passed for the

radioactivity to decay, OMT-PET scan was performed. In the selection process patients with a nontumorous pathology and radiation necrosis were excluded.

Measurements were made of the equilibrated radioactivity 20 min after the injection of MET or OMT (250 MBq) using a PET scanner (Headtome V, Shimadzu, Kyoto, Japan). The transmission data were acquired with a rotating germanium-68 rod source for attenuation correction. To obtain regional data from exactly the same location used in the MET and OMT studies, two PET images in each patient were co-registered using an automated image registration program, and regions of interest (ROIs) were manually placed over the tumor area on a maximum of four axial images. The regional uptake of each tracer was expressed as an SUV, and the uptake into the tumor was expressed as a ratio of the SUV for the tumor to that for the contralateral normal brain (T/N ratio).

Results and Discussion

In Figure 3, representative PET axial images indicating the uptake of OMT and MET into gliomas of various grades, metastatic tumors, and normal tissue are displayed side-by-side. The images of tumors (Figs. 3A, B, C, and D) obtained with OMT-PET and MET-PET were almost identical in all subjects. Moreover, the uptake of both tracers increased as the malignancy of the tumors increased. We concluded that the ability of the two probes is identical in delineating and characterizing various brain tumors. A major difference between the OMT and MET images was noted in the glandular organs in the skull base area. As shown in Figures 3E and F, the salivary gland and pituitary gland took up more MET than did the surrounding tissues but did not accumulate OMT.

MET passes through the blood-brain barrier (BBB) and tumor plasma membrane via neutral amino acid transporters

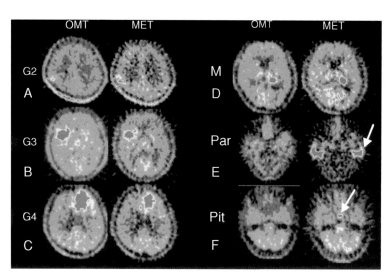

Figure 3 Representative PET images of tumor pathology and normal structure obtained with OMT and MET. Images of the same individual were co-registered using an image registration program, and axial slices with the same anatomical configuration are displayed side by side. The same color scales to express SUV were used for OMT and MET in each individual. (**A**) WHO grade 2 glioma (oligodendroglioma). (**B**) WHO grade 3 glioma (anaplastic astrocytoma). (**C**) WHO grade 4 glioma (glioblastoma). (**D**) A metastatic brain tumor (mammalian carcinoma) after gamma knife treatment that is still active. (**E**) Parotid glands (indicated as an arrow). (**F**) A normal pituitary gland (indicated as an arrow).

and is used mainly for protein synthesis. The accumulation of this probe in active tumors may reflect both increased capillary transport and increased protein synthesis by tumor cells. Increased uptake of MET in the salivary gland or pituitary gland outside the BBB may represent the vigorous use of amino acids for the synthesis of digestive enzymes and peptide hormones in these organs. On the other hand, OMT, an artificial amino acid, is also transported by neutral amino acid transporters but is not utilized for protein synthesis. It may be trapped in the amino acid pool in tumor cells reflecting the rate at which amino acids are transported. Previous reports suggested that the rate of transport of an amino acid probe reflects the malignancy of the tumor. Therefore, OMT-PET should have similar value to MET-PET for brain tumor imaging.

In the cases of the salivary and endocrinology glands outside the BBB, it is quite logical that OMT is washed away rapidly and not accumulated. The difference between OMT and MET in the rate of accumulation in the skull base organs should be as observed in whole-body imaging in the pancreas and liver, where OMT did not accumulate. This difference in behavior from MET may make OMT a better diagnostic probe for tumors on the face and skull base tumors.

In conclusion, OMT-PET may be as useful in characterizing and delineating brain tumors as MET-PET. A major difference between these two probes was in the rate at which they accumulated in the salivary glands and pituitary gland. OMT accumulated to a far lesser extent than MET. This may make it a superior imaging probe to MET in the diagnosis of tumors of the face and skull base area.

Conclusion

OMT was prepared in high radiochemical yield by a simple automated method suitable for routine clinical use.

When compared with FDG-PET, OMT-PET had smaller ratios of the uptake in tumor to that in background tissues, but may have the potential to improve the specificity of cancer diagnosis by reducing the rate of false positives caused by inflammation. For brain tumor imaging, OMT-PET had similar value to MET-PET, but may be superior in diagnosing tumors on the face and skull base area.

References

Ishikawa, Y., Iwata, R., Furumoto, S., Pascali, C., Bogni, A., Kubota, K., and Ishiwata, K. 2005. Simple automated preparation of O-[11C]methyl-L-tyrosine for routine clinical use. *Appl. Radiat. Isot. 63*:55–61.

Ishiwata, K., Kawamura, K., Wang, W.F., Furumoto, S., Kubota, K., Pascali, C., Bogni, A., and Iwata, R. 2004. Evaluation of O-[11C]methyl-L-tyrosine and O-[18F]fluoromethyl-L-tyrosine as tumor imaging tracers by PET. *Nucl. Med. Biol. 31*:191–198.

Ishiwata, K., Tsukada, H., Kubota, K., Nariai, T., Harada, N., Kawamura, K., Kimura, Y., Oda, K., Iwata, R., and Ishii, K. 2005. Preclinical and clinical evaluation of O-[11C]methyl-L-tyrosine for tumor imaging by positron emission tomography. *Nucl. Med. Biol. 32*:253–262.

Iwata, R., Furumoto, S., Pascali, C., Bogni, A., and Ishiwata, K. 2002. Radiosynthesis of O-[11C]methyl-L-tyrosine and O-[18F]fluoromethyl-L-tyrosine as potential PET tracers for imaging amino acid transport. *J. Label. Compds. Radiopharm. 46*:555–566.

Jager, P.L., Vaalburg, W., Prium, J., de Vries, E.G.E., Langen, K.J., and Piers, D.A. 2001. Radiolabeled amino acids: basic aspects and clinical applications in oncology. *J. Nucl. Med. 42*:432–445.

Kubota, K. 2001. From tumor biology to clinical PET: a review of positron emission tomography (PET) in oncology. *Ann. Nucl. Med. 15*:471–486.

Nariai, T., Tanaka, Y., Wakimoto, H., Aoyagi, M., Tamaki, M., Ishiwata, K., Senda, M., Ishii, K., Hirakawa, K., and Ohno, K. 2005. Usefulness of L-[methyl-11C]methionine-positron emission tomography as a biological monitoring tool in the treatment of glioma. *J. Neurosurg. 103*:498–507.

Wester, H.J., Herz, M., Weber, W., Heiss, P., Senekowitsch-Schmidtke, R., Schwaiger, M., and Stocklin, G. 1999. Synthesis and radiopharmacology of O-(2-[18F]fluoroethyl)-L-tyrosine for tumor imaging. *J. Nucl. Med. 40*:205–212.

9

Tumor Proliferation: 2-[^{11}C]-Thymidine Positron Emission Tomography

Paula Wells and Pat Price

Introduction

[^{18}F]-labeled fluorodeoxyglucose (^{18}F-FDG) positron emission tomography (PET) is a recognized diagnostic tool for cancer, but the potential uses of PET in oncology are far reaching and extend beyond the imaging of glucose metabolism for diagnosis. The development of alternative PET probes specific for tumor proliferation would provide useful pharmacodynamic tools to assess treatment response and assist early validation of novel anticancer agents. [^{11}C]-labeled-thymidine, the first radiotracer used for noninvasive imaging of tumor proliferation, is one of the most appropriate contenders for this role as its uptake is directly related to DNA synthesis and correlates with proliferation in human tumors. Although the historical assessment of [^{11}C]-thymidine PET has not been clear-cut, it has been demonstrated in humans as a specific measure of tumor proliferation that is a more sensitive discriminator of early clinical tumor response when compared with ^{18}F-FDG.

As a vital component for DNA synthesis, thymidine is essential for cell proliferation, and is therefore also a key molecule for measuring tumor proliferation and an important target for cancer therapy. Historically, thymidine and its analogs have been used with a variety of techniques to mea-

sure cell proliferation. More recently, this methodology has been applied to the development of positron-emitting tracers that can provide a measure of cell proliferation *in vivo* using PET. Significant advances have occurred in anticancer treatment during the last decade, with increasing emphasis on drug development aimed at novel cellular targets identified by advances in molecular biology, but these advances have only translated into modest benefit for patients. While the identification of new therapeutic targets is important, the development of more accurate and relevant methods of measuring response to treatment is also vital, especially for the early assessment of new agents. It is in the latter areas that functional imaging techniques may provide a unique insight into the effects of anticancer therapy. It is increasingly recognized that conventional radiological methods of assessing response, that is, measuring changes in tumor size with computed tomography (CT) or magnetic resonance imaging (MRI), are likely to be less applicable to the monitoring of new agents that may be cytostatic rather than cytotoxic. Furthermore, assessment based solely on change in volume occurring over several weeks cannot take account of the early changes in biological processes that may provide potentially more important prognostic information. The direct observation of tumor biology, molecular pharmacology, and the pharmacodynamic effects of treatment *in vivo* provided by functional imaging techniques such as PET may be used to develop new treatment paradigms based on more tumor-specific end points, allowing greater individualization of therapy.

Because of its relatively long half-life and hence wide availability, [^{18}F]-labeled-fluorodeoxyglucose (^{18}F-FDG) is the predominant tracer being investigated as a method of measuring cancer treatment response (Young *et al.*, 1999; Price, 2000; Brock *et al.*, 2000).^{18}F-FDG uptake reflects glucose metabolism and is used primarily in the diagnosis and staging of cancer. ^{18}F-FDG is taken up into tumor cells by glucose transporter-1 (glut-1) receptors, and uptake reflects high levels of glut-1, hexokinase 1, and cell number (Bos *et al.*, 2002; Higashi *et al.*, 1993; Smith, 1998). However, it is not a direct marker of proliferation, although correlations with histological proliferation indices have been shown (Jacob *et al.*, 2001; Folpe *et al.*, 2000). Importantly, the utilization of glucose also occurs by other cell types, such as macrophages (Kubota *et al.*, 1992), whose presence in tissues confounds the interpretation of FDG-PET images. There is also evidence that cancer treatment-induced changes in DNA cell proliferation are more pronounced than changes in glucose metabolism (Barthel *et al.*, 2003; Shields *et al.*, 1998), further supporting the need for a direct marker to image and measure cell proliferation. In contrast, radiolabeled thymidine is incorporated into DNA, and its uptake is a direct measure of cell proliferation rate. Uptake of 2-[^{11}C]-thymidine is related to DNA synthesis (Vander Borght *et al.*, 1991b) and, in comparison with ^{18}F-FDG, has been shown to be a more sensitive discriminator of early clinical response in small cell lung cancer and sarcoma (Shields *et al.*, 1998).

The search for a reliable PET marker of proliferation has therefore centered on thymidine and its analogs, but no standard has emerged to date. ^{18}F-labeled 3′-deoxy-3′-fluorothymidine (FLT) is currently the lead agent in the field because it is labeled with the longer-lived ^{18}F isotope (^{18}F has a half-life of 110 min, compared with a half-life of 20 min for ^{11}C and 2 min for ^{15}O). It is also largely resistant to metabolic degradation, but as it undergoes glucouronidation in the liver, its use is potentially limited for imaging liver tumors (Shields, 2003). Nonetheless, it is not incorporated into DNA and is not a direct measure of cell proliferation, although its uptake in tumors does correlate with histological measurements of proliferation (Buck *et al.*, 2003; Francis *et al.*, 2003). The intracellular retention of FLT occurs following phosphorylation by thymidine kinase 1 (TK1), and thus FLT uptake is a measure of TK1 activity which is only linked with cell proliferation and may be subject to poor cell-cycle checkpoint regulation in tumor cells. Another probe under investigation is ^{18}F-labeled 1-(2′-de-oxy-2′-fluoro-β-D-arabinofuranosyl)-thymidine (^{18}F-FMAU), which is incorporated into DNA and is also resistant to degradation. The liver retains high levels of ^{18}F-FMAU, again making the probe unsuitable for imaging cancers in the liver, but its slow clearance into the bladder makes it a good probe for imaging tumors in the pelvis (Shields, 2003). A recent cell-line study compared the three tracers and showed that thymidine was better than FLT and FMAU at tracking changes in proliferation. A comparison of proliferating versus quiescent cells showed up to 20-fold changes in thymidine uptake compared with a < 10-fold increase in FLT and a < 4-fold increase in FMAU (Schwartz *et al.*, 2003). In cell lines with a strong TK1 dependence for proliferation, only thymidine and FLT could detect changes in proliferation, and thymidine was better than FLT. Thus, thymidine is a more specific marker of proliferation compared to its analogs, but the short half-life of its ^{11}C radiolabel and its rapid metabolism *in vivo* have hindered its development. The following sections briefly describe [^{11}C]-thymidine-PET methodology, summarize its historical development and current research status, and discuss the need for its continued development alongside alternative proliferation probes such as ^{18}F-FLT and ^{18}F-FMAU.

[^{11}C]-Thymidine Positron Tomography Methodology

Positron emission tomography scanning is dependent on the detection of gamma rays (photons) emitted from a positron-emitting radioisotope. Positrons are emitted from proton-rich unstable isotopes such as ^{18}F or ^{11}C, which are made in a cyclotron. These short-lived radioactive isotopes are then chemically linked to a probe molecule (e.g., a drug, water, or a metabolite) to form a labeled PET tracer, which is injected intravenously into a patient. Not all tracer molecules are easy to label, but compounds containing N-, S-, or O-methyl (or ethyl) groups, proteins, and antibodies are readily radiolabeled, and some molecules may be labeled at different positions (e.g., thymidine may be labeled with ^{11}C at the methyl position or at the 2-carbonyl group). Single positrons emitted from the tracer are annihilated after combination with an electron, resulting in the simultaneous release of two photons emitted at 180° to each other. The emitted photons are coincidentally detected by scintillation detectors within the PET scanner, enabling dynamic, three-dimensional localization of the tracers' distribution within the patients' body.

Following dynamic acquisition of data, computerized tomographic images are reconstructed, and regions of interest (ROIs) are drawn following alignment of anatomical structures using other imaging techniques, such as CT. Multiple ROIs can be drawn in a number of tissues to allow parallel analysis of the distribution of a tracer in both tumor and normal tissues. Positron emission tomography can quantify the tissue concentration of a tracer with sensitivity in the range of $10^{-11} - 10^{-12}$ mol/l, and measure changes in tissue levels with time. However, in order to accurately calculate the distribution of a tracer molecule within the patient's body dynamically, many influential factors must be taken into account. These include the rate of tracer uptake by tumor or normal tissue, dispersion rate, the existence of unlabeled endogenous tracer molecule, and, importantly, the biochemistry and metabolism of the tracer within the body. Consideration of these factors has led to the development of various methodologies, parameters, and kinetic models for interpreting PET data. For example, a semiquantitative objective way of measuring tumor-tracer uptake involves the determination of the standardized uptake value (SUV). This is the simplest PET parameter, which has been widely used in the measurement of ^{18}F-FDG uptake in tumors and in studies to examine the value of tumor imaging for treatment response (Young *et al.*, 1999). It is a measure of tracer uptake in tissue at a specific time and is usually normalized against injected activity and body weight or surface area (Graham *et al.*, 2000). To account for radiolabeled metabolites produced by tracer catabolism, which may be indistinguishable from the parent in blood and tissues and interfere with the measurement of tracer kinetics, validated methods are required to measure the presence of labeled metabolites. Biochemical breakdown and/or subsequent reuptake and elimination of radiolabeled tracer must also be monitored. The subsequent application of complex kinetic models (reviewed elsewhere; see Schmidt *et al.*, 2002), which are designed to take into account all of the relevant confounding factors together, allows further analysis of PET imaging data.

When using thymidine as a tracer molecule, several specific factors related to its normal biochemistry and catabolism must be considered. Thymidine is phosphorylated by thymidine kinase in a series of reversible reactions to produce thymidine nucleotides (dTMP $\rightarrow$ dTDP $\rightarrow$ dTTP), which are subsequently incorporated into DNA. Catabolism of thymidine occurs via the action of thymidine phosphorylase (TP) to produce thymine (Fig. 1), which is subsequently broken down in the liver to β-aminoisobutyric acid (BAIB). This acid is then further catabolized, releasing CO_2 and NH_4^+ in the process, to succinyl CoA, which enters the citric acid cycle. It can be appreciated from Figure 1 that when using thymidine as a tracer molecule, the fate of the ^{11}C label is dependent on its initial position: thymidine labeled in the methyl position will result in labeled succinyl CoA, whereas thymidine labeled in the 2-carbonyl position results in labeled CO_2. Endogenously, pyrimidine nucleotides, and hence thymidine, may also be synthesized either by *de novo* or *salvage* pathways. *De novo* synthesis occurs under strict regulatory control via the production of uridine monophosphate (UMP), the precursor of all the pyrimidine mononucleotides. *Salvage* production of thymidine and thymidine nucleotides occurs as thymine and may be reconverted back into thymidine via the respective action of TP and TK. Thus, in order to effectively interpret [^{11}C]-thymidine PET images, it is important to account for the initial position of the ^{11}C label, the metabolic fate of labeled thymidine break-down products in blood and tissue, and the contribution of unlabeled endogenous thymidine.

Historical Development of Thymidine Positron Emission Tomography

Early studies utilized thymidine labeled in the methyl position: the early imaging of tumor-bearing animals following intravenous injection of [^{11}C]-methyl-thymidine was reported in 1978 (Crawford *et al.*, 1978). Concurrent early validation studies using [^{3}H]-methyl-thymidine demonstrated high tumor to tissue uptake independent of perfusion, and retention of labeled thymidine by proliferating tissues, supporting its use as a specific tracer of proliferation for tumor imaging (Larson *et al.*, 1980, 1981; Shields *et al.*, 1984). In 1988, the first use of [^{11}C]-methyl-thymidine PET in patients with non-Hodgkin's Lymphoma was reported by a research group from the University of Louvain in Belgium (Martiat *et al.*, 1988). During the 1980s, further validation and feasibility studies investigated the metabolism of radiolabeled thymidine and focused on the need for specific methodologies and kinetic models required to adequately interpret thymidine PET images. However, by the end of the 1980s, it was recognized that the presence of methyl-labeled metabolites would hamper the interpretation of PET images. It was suggested that thymidine labeled in the 2-C position would simplify image interpretation because of its rapid degradation and elimination as ^{11}CO$_2$ (Shields *et al.*, 1990), and research into thymidine labeled in the 2-C position was subsequently favored.

During the early 1990s Vander Borght *et al.* (1991b) at the University of Louvain described a method for the production of 2-[^{11}C]-thymidine. They demonstrated the probe's ability to measure proliferation *in vivo* (Vander Borght *et al.*, 1990, 1991b) and to image tumors in humans (Vander Borght *et al.*, 1994). Toward the end of the 1990s, studies concentrated on the development of kinetic modeling approaches to enable metabolite-corrected estimates of the incorporation of 2-[^{11}C]-thymidine into tissues (Mankoff *et al.*, 1998, 1999; Shields *et al.*, 1996; Gunn *et al.*, 2000b). This work paved the way for an increase in the number of studies in cancer patients and work showing the feasibility of using 2-[^{11}C]-thymidine PET in the clinical setting to measure response to therapy (Wells *et al.*, 2002a; Eary *et al.*, 1999; Shields *et al.*, 1998), tumor proliferation (Wells *et al.*, 2002c), and thymidine salvage kinetics (Wells *et al.*, 2003).

Validation Studies

Validation studies demonstrated the potential use of labeled thymidine as a specific PET tracer for imaging proliferation, and provided the necessary data required for the construction of kinetic models needed to adequately interpret

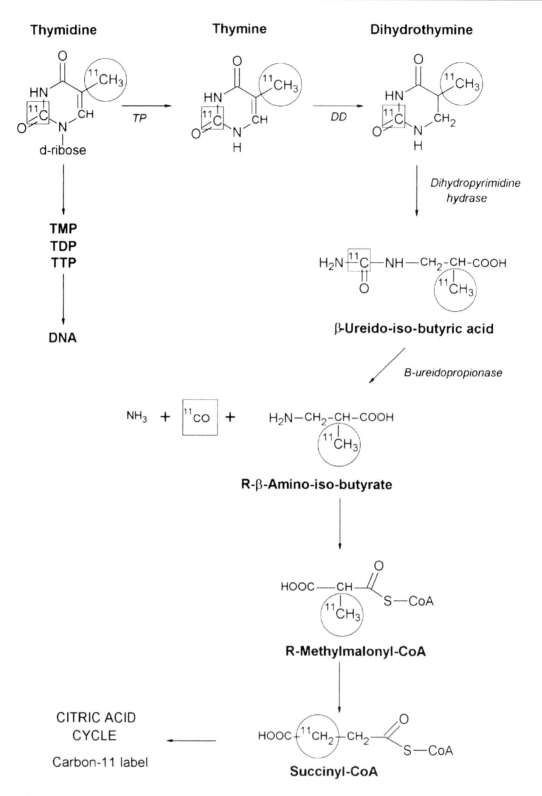

Figure 1 Thymidine metabolic pathways. The square for the 2-carbonyl group and the circle for the methyl group highlight the fate of the carbon label. Reproduced with permission from: P. Wells et al. 2004. Measuring tumor pharmacodynamic response using PET proliferation probes: the case for 2-[11C]-thymidine. Biochemica et Biophysica Acta *1705*:91–102.

thymidine PET images. When human tumor cell lines were labeled *in vitro* with [^{3}H]-methyl-thymidine, between 18% and 100% of the exogenously supplied thymidine was taken up and incorporated into DNA (Taheri *et al.*, 1982). Subsequent *in vivo* studies in mice employing ^{11}C, ^{14}C, and ^{3}H methyl-thymidine showed that the majority of the activity was in DNA, with a small amount in metabolites one hour after injection (Shields *et al.*, 1990). However, for dogs, whose metabolism more closely resembles that of humans, the opposite situation was observed with the majority of the activity in metabolites (20% thymine and 57% in other metabolites) rather than DNA. Only 33 to 49% ^{11}C activity was associated with DNA for spleen and tumor tissue at 60 min post-injection, and significant interanimal variation was noted. Together, these data confirmed that individual high-performance liquid chromatography (HPLC) analyses of blood samples would be necessary to obtain accurate input functions in humans.

A research group in Seattle implemented a four-compartment model developed by Cleaver (1967) that utilized plasma measurements of unlabeled and labeled thymidine and its metabolites obtained using HPLC, as well as determining tracer levels in tissues (measured using the PET regional time-activity curve) and the specific activity of intracellular thymidine nucleotide pools. The relative use of exogenous and endogenously synthesized thymidine and reutilization of thymidine from dying cells also had to be considered. Shields *et al.* (1987) demonstrated that exogenous radiolabeled thymidine accounted for 45% activity for a variety of cells and tissues, and that when the relative utilization of the two synthetic pathways for thymidine was manipulated by varying the concentration of exogenous radiolabeled thymidine, it was independent of the tissue, tumor, or species studied. This finding is important as it demonstrates that the endogenous pathway is not an independent variable, but is predictable from the exogenous thymidine concentration and can be ignored, resulting in a simplification of Cleaver's four-compartment model to a three-compartment model. The Seattle group also found little or no local reutilization of radiolabeled thymidine in tissues, thus, further simplifying the use of ^{11}C-labeled thymidine as an imaging agent for measuring tissue proliferation (Quackenbush *et al.*, 1988).

[^{11}C]-Methyl-Thymidine

Subsequent studies investigated [^{11}C]-methyl-thymidine metabolism and the influence of labeled metabolites on the interpretation of tissue data. The University of Louvain group first reported clinical PET imaging of non-Hodgkin's Lymphoma patients using [^{11}C]-methyl-thymidine: a high-uptake ratio of tumor to muscle was shown, and the uptake increased with increasing tumor grade, indicating that [^{11}C]-methyl-thymidine PET would be a useful method to noninvasively measure tumor proliferation *in vivo*, but a low tumor-to-intestine uptake ratio suggested that PET imaging using this tracer would be restricted to areas outside of the abdomen (Martiat *et al.*, 1988). At first, it was assumed that [^{11}C]-methyl-thymidine was not metabolized in the blood, but this assumption was subsequently found to be incorrect (Shields *et al.*, 1990). In rats, [^{11}C]-methyl-thymidine PET was not able to discriminate regenerating from nonregenerating livers *in vivo* due to the accumulation of radiolabeled metabolites (Vander Borght *et al.*, 1990). Studies in patients with head and neck cancer showed high tracer accumulation in tissues where both blood flow and metabolites were likely to influence the resulting PET images and the rapid clearance and appearance of metabolites in blood (Goethals *et al.*, 1995; van Eijkeren *et al.*, 1992). Thus, the accumulation of labeled thymidine metabolites was found to contribute to the PET signal, and also varied between tissues. A subsequent study in rats showed that despite rapid metabolism of [^{11}C]-methyl-thymidine, the majority of the ^{11}C activity was incorporated into DNA (Goethals *et al.*, 1999), a finding in keeping with the earlier studies carried out in mice. Together, the results of these studies indicated the potential usefulness of this tracer to image cell proliferation *in vivo*, but demonstrated that further studies and the application of kinetic models would be needed to account for the contribution of specific degradation products to PET images and allow the calculation of cell proliferation parameters.

2-[^{11}C]-Thymidine

As previously outlined, the rationale behind the development of 2-[^{11}C]-thymidine as a PET tracer was that its main labeled metabolite, CO_2, would be eliminated rather than accumulate in tissues. An initial validation investigation by (Vander Borght *et al.*, 1990) in partially hepatectomized rats demonstrated that, unlike ^{11}C-methyl-thymidine, 2-C-labeled thymidine discriminated regenerating from nonregenerating livers. Furthermore, tracer activity measured in extracted DNA correlated with levels of radioactivity measured in liver tissue, showing that 2-C-labeled thymidine was incorporated into DNA. The same group then developed a reproducible method for the production of 2-[^{11}C]-thymidine (Vander Borght *et al.*, 1991a) and performed subsequent dynamic PET studies, again using the rat liver regeneration model (Vander Borght *et al.*, 1991b). A twofold higher uptake was seen in regenerating compared with nonregenerating livers, which increased to sixfold at 2 hr, and again a good correlation between whole tissue and DNA radioactivity was also observed, indicating uptake of the tracer into the DNA of proliferating cells. Thus, these authors demonstrated that 2-[^{11}C]-thymidine PET could measure cell proliferation *in vivo*, and they paved the way for human studies to begin.

Validation of 2-[¹¹C]-Thymidine Positron Emission Tomography in Patients

The first clinical studies with 2-[¹¹C]-thymidine were also carried out by Vander Borght *et al.* (1994) in patients with brain tumors. The semiquantitative parameter SUV was used as a measure of thymidine uptake, and an increase was noted in 80% of the tumors compared with surrounding structures. 2-[¹¹C]-thymidine was also better at imaging recurrent tumors than ¹⁸F-FDG. Although the study demonstrated the diagnostic potential of imaging with 2-[¹¹C]-thymidine, there was no correlation between uptake of the tracer and tumor grade. This differed from the previously described study in patients with non-Hodgkin's Lymphoma where the uptake of ¹¹C-methyl-thymidine was analyzed using a three-compartment model (Martiat *et al.*, 1988). The lack of correlation between thymidine uptake and grade in the study by Vander Borght *et al.* (1994) might reflect tumor heterogeneity and the small number of low-grade tumors in the series of patients studied. The nonmodeled parameter (SUV) used to determine thymidine uptake is also likely to have influenced this result, as the variable delivery and retention of thymidine and its subsequent metabolism were not accounted for. When given intravenously, thymidine is rapidly cleared from the circulation, and in most organs only the immediate initial distribution correlates with perfusion (Shields *et al.*, 1984). However, as thymidine transports poorly across the BBB, the initial uptake in the brain reflects the number of blood vessels, which is highest in gray matter and variable in tumor and tumor blood flow. The subsequent transport of thymidine across the BBB is a prerequisite for its accumulation in tumor. Once inside the cell, the rate-limiting step to thymidine accumulation is phosphorylation of the molecule prior to incorporation into DNA. The rapid metabolism of the tracer must also be considered (Shields *et al.*, 1996). Thus, as several processes influence the delivery (number of blood vessels, blood flow, thymidine transport rate) and retention (tissue permeability, accumulation of metabolites) of 2-[¹¹C]-thymidine, its resulting PET images need to be interpreted using kinetic/mathematical models that account for these factors.

Development and Application of Kinetic Models

Although it was originally thought that the ¹¹CO$_2$ metabolite could be disregarded as it was believed to be eliminated from the lungs, subsequent animal studies demonstrated that ¹¹CO$_2$ does accumulate in tissues. Following the injection of ¹¹CO$_2$ in dogs, 58% of the total injected label was excreted through the lungs as ¹¹CO$_2$ over a 60-min period, with the rest accumulating in tissues (Shields *et al.*, 1992). Analysis of blood radioactivity in the clinical study (Vander Borght *et al.*, 1994) and in a later study by Shields *et al.* (1996) in 14 cancer patients both reported a plateau of ~ 65% of the total ¹¹C injected in blood CO$_2$ 11 min following 2-[¹¹C]-thymidine administration: the earlier study also indicated that after 17 min, ¹¹CO$_2$ or labeled bicarbonate (H¹¹CO$_3$) accounted for most of the radioactivity observed in normal brain tissue. Thus, the radioactively labeled biochemical breakdown product of 2-[¹¹C]-thymidine, ¹¹CO$_2$, and its subsequent reuptake from blood and retention in tissues, does contribute to 2-¹¹C-thymidine PET signals and influence image interpretation. In order to address this issue, methods have been developed for measuring labeled metabolites of 2-¹¹C-thymidine in blood (Shields *et al.*, 1996; Conti *et al.*, 1994), exhaled air (Gunn *et al.*, 2000a), and tissues (Gunn *et al.*, 2000b), and modeling the data.

Different kinetic modeling approaches have been used, both compartmental (Wells *et al.*, 2002a) and spectral analyses (Wells *et al.*, 2002c). As previously outlined, to describe the incorporation of thymidine into DNA, initially a four-compartment model was developed (Cleaver, 1967), but validation studies showed this could be reduced to three compartments: plasma thymidine, intracellular thymidine, and phosphorylated thymidine. This model assumes that most of the thymidine taken up by cells incorporates into DNA or is degraded, there is no reutilization of labeled metabolites for DNA synthesis, and exogenous and endogenous thymidine behave in the same way. By assuming that labeled thymidine binds irreversibly once incorporated into DNA and that reversible uptake of a tracer occurs in the tissue compartment prior to this event, tissue thymidine and thymidine nucleotides are modeled as a single compartment with reversible transport. This simplifies the model, allowing the description of thymidine incorporation into DNA as a flux constant (Mankoff *et al.*, 1998). The ratio of total label in intracellular small molecules relative to the incubating medium provides an estimate of the virtual volume of distribution of thymidine (V_{TdR}). V_{TdR} is defined as the ratio of the concentration of thymidine in tissue relative to the blood in units of micromoles per ml. Tissue is composed of an intracellular and extracellular space, and for a reliable estimate of V_{TdR} to be made, the concentration of extracellular thymidine should be similar to that of the blood.

As well as DNA uptake of thymidine, the metabolic fate of thymidine and the presence of labeled breakdown products in tissues, such as ¹¹CO$_2$ and a variety of molecules that can incorporate labeled carbon from this source, must also be accounted for in the design of valid models. Although tissues generate small amounts of thymine and other metabolites, most of the metabolites are blood borne because of the degradation of thymidine by organs such as the liver or by platelets. There are limited data on the transport and biodistribution of thymine, dihydrothymine, and BAIB *in vivo* (Covey *et al.*, 1983), but because they account for only a small fraction of the label for most tissues, they are usually considered together in the correction of data. Studies suggest that these compounds do not bind to tissue except in organs involved with degradation (Cleaver, 1967). A five-compartment model that describes the kinetics of thymidine and its metabolites (Fig. 2) has been validated by the Seattle group to take account of these complex processes (Wells *et al.*, 2002a, 2002b).

Kinetic Analysis of 2-[^{11}C]-Thymidine Positron Emission Tomography Images

Sequential $^{11}CO_2$ and 2-[^{11}C]-thymidine PET scans were carried out in four patients with malignant brain tumors to demonstrate the feasibility of modeling both tracers simultaneously (Eary *et al.*, 1999). Kinetic analysis using compartmental modeling was able to remove the confounding influence of $^{11}CO_2$, the principal metabolite, and to estimate the incorporation of thymidine into DNA. Comparison of model estimates of 2-[^{11}C]-thymidine transport versus 2-[^{11}C]-thymidine flux was able to distinguish increased uptake based solely on BBB disruption from that associated with increased cellular proliferation (Eary *et al.*, 1999). Kinetic analysis was also used in a study of 20 patients with malignant brain tumors who underwent sequential $^{11}CO_2$ and 2-[^{11}C]-thymidine PET scans. When compartmental modeling was employed (Wells *et al.*, 2002a), thymidine flux into the tumors was shown to increase with tumor grade (Wells *et al.*, 2002b).

Spectral analysis has also been investigated for the modeling of 2-[^{11}C]-thymidine PET data. In comparison with compartmental modeling, spectral analysis has no *a priori* assumptions of the number of compartments involved in the fit of data. By using metabolite-corrected plasma input function and tissue time-activity curves, the tissue impulse response function (IRF) parameter can be calculated for the delivery (IRF$_{1\,min}$) and uptake (IRF$_{60\,min}$) of thymidine by a tissue. This can then be used to derive the fractional retention of thymidine (FRT), which is calculated as IRF$_{60\,min}$/IRF$_{1\,min}$ (Wells *et al.*, 2002c, 2003). By using this methodology, the *in vivo* spectral-analysis-derived 2-[^{11}C]-thymidine PET data were shown to relate to the *ex vivo* MIB1 histological index of proliferation in human tumors (Wells *et al.*, 2002c). Seventeen patients with advanced intra-abdominal malignancies were scanned, and thymidine incorporation was measured as FRT. This was then compared with expression of the proliferation marker Ki-67, which was determined histologically from biopsies of the imaged tumors using the specific monoclonal antibody MIB1. A statistically significant correlation was obtained between the MIB1 index and FRT, but no correlation was seen with nonmodeled 2-[^{11}C]-thymidine PET parameters. The study showed that the 2-[^{11}C]-thymidine parameter FRT measured *in situ* reflects proliferation measured *ex vivo*, and the work demonstrated the potential of the technique for the early assessment of response to cancer treatment.

Pharmacodynamic Studies

Comparison of 2-[^{11}C]-Thymidine with FDG-PET and Magnetic Resonance Imaging

Shields *et al.* (1998) undertook preliminary studies to investigate the ability of 2-[^{11}C]-thymidine-PET to measure tumor response to therapy early after the initiation of treatment. 2-[^{11}C]-thymidine and ^{18}F-FDG studies were performed in six cancer patients. The study showed that both tumor proliferation and metabolism decreased after successful chemotherapy, but the effects were more pronounced for the 2-[^{11}C]-thymidine scans: tumors responding to chemotherapy had low thymidine uptake but retained relatively high glucose metabolic activity. In particular, in one patient with small cell lung cancer, a fall in 2-[^{11}C]-thymidine incorporation was seen two weeks after administration of effective salvage chemotherapy following failure of first-line treatment, where a minimal decline in thymidine incorporation was seen.

In another study by the Seattle group, 13 patients with malignant brain tumors were investigated (Eary *et al.*, 1999). In approximately half of the cases the 2-[^{11}C]-thymidine scans were qualitatively different from the other ^{18}F-FDG scans, and there was some suggestion that thymidine images

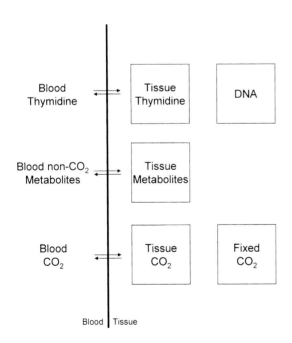

Figure 2 Five-compartment model for thymidine kinetics in blood and tissue. Reproduced with permission from J.M. Wells *et al.* 2002. Kinetic analysis of 2-[11C]thymidine PET imaging studies of malignant brain tumors: compartmental model investigation and mathematical analysis. *Molecular Imaging* 1:151–159.

demonstrated the presence of viable tumor where FDG images could not. Tumor 2-[^{11}C]-thymidine uptake appeared to be more accurately related to tumor control (two patients) and recurrence (two patients), but no consistent pattern emerged.

A further study in 20 patients with brain tumors obtained data using a five-compartment model and a dual-scanning approach. The work showed that the rate of thymidine transport into tumors was higher for MRI contrast-enhancing tumors and increased with tumor grade. On average, the transport of thymidine into tumors was lower after treatment in high-grade tumors. The model used was also able to distinguish between increased thymidine transport due to BBB breakdown and increased tracer retention associated with tumor cell proliferation (Wells et al., 2002a).

2-[^{11}C]-Thymidine PET to Detect Antitumor Activity in Clinical Drug Trials

In a pilot study, tumor 2-[^{11}C]-thymidine PET data were obtained for a group of patients enrolled in a Phase I clinical study of midostaurin (Propper et al., 2001). Midostaurin is a protein kinase C (PKC) inhibitor that has great promise as an anticancer agent: it has been shown to inhibit the proliferation of the tumor cell line in vitro, has activity toward xenografted tumor models, acts synergistically with conventional cytotoxic agents, is able to inhibit P-glycoprotein-mediated efflux activity and can reverse multidrug resistance in vitro and in vivo, and high levels of its target, PKC, have been found in various tumors (Fabbro et al., 2000). As midostau-

rin is administered orally and lacks the toxicity associated with conventional chemotherapeutic agents, pharmacodynamic measures are required to optimize drug dosing and scheduling.

Thirty-two patients with advanced solid tumors were administered with 2-[^{11}C]-thymidine and scanned before and after the first course of midostaurin therapy (Propper et al., 2001). The area under the tissue time-activity curve (Jacob et al.) was calculated pre- and post-treatment and compared with the differences in AUC for seven control patients who received no treatment between scans. In all the study patients, there was a midostaurin-induced reduction in AUC with a mean change of $-10 \pm 9\%$, compared with $1 \pm 5\%$ for the control group, which was statistically significant (Table 1). There were no significant changes in normal tissue AUC for either the control or treated group. As AUC does not allow for the accumulation of labeled metabolites, we do not consider it to be the most appropriate parameter for measuring thymidine incorporation; therefore, these findings must be interpreted with caution. However, with this caveat in mind, the pilot study showed the feasibility of obtaining repeat 2-[^{11}C]-thymidine PET scans in early-phase clinical trials of novel agents.

Discussion and Summary

[^{11}C]-thymidine was the first radiotracer for noninvasive imaging of tumor proliferation. But the short half-life of ^{11}C and its rapid metabolism in vivo have inhibited its widespread

Table 1   2-[^{11}C]Thymidine PET Feasibility Study for Measuring Pharmacodynamic Response in a Phase I Trial

Arm	Tumor AUC[a]			Normal Tissue[b] AUC		
	Scan1[c]	Scan2	Diff[d]	Scan1	Scan2	Diff
Control	12.29	12.32	0.2	6.74	5.94	−12.0
	7.83	7.80	−0.4	7.52	7.20	−4.0
	5.12	5.04	−1.6	1.94[e]	1.69	−13.0
	10.02	9.50	−5.0	7.28	6.76	−7.0
	14.83	15.04	1.4	6.74	6.33	−6.0
	5.97	6.58	10.0	6.87	6.74	−2.0
	7.19	7.20	0.01	7.24	7.38	2.0
Treated	8.90	7.66	−14.0	4.48[f]	4.52	0.9
	8.14	7.75	−5.0	2.14[e]	2.31	8.0
	7.13	7.06	−1.0	13.44	7.38	−45.0
	12.85	10.13	−21.0	6.35	5.14	−19.0

Treated patients received the protein kinase C inhibitor midostaurin. [a]AUC = area under the curve. [b]The normal tissue scanned was spleen except where indicated. [c]Paired scans were taken either one (control) or six (treated) weeks apart. [d]Diff = difference between the AUC values for the paired scans in percent. [e]Lung. [f]Bone marrow. Reproduced with permission from: D.J. Propper, et al. (2001). Phase I and pharmacokinetic study of PKC412, an inhibitor of protein kinase C. J. Clin. Oncol. 19:1485–1492.

clinical use. The main argument against the continued development of 2-[¹¹C]-thymidine PET is that short-lived isotopes like ¹¹C require a combined on-site cyclotron, sterile radiolabeling, and PET scanning facility. The result has been a drive toward finding thymidine analogs readily labeled with the longer-lived ¹⁸F isotope, such as ¹⁸F-FLT or ¹⁸F-FMAU, although studies have shown that these tracers are not as specific for cell proliferation (Schwartz et al., 2003) and, unlike thymidine are either unsuitable or limited for use in the liver (Shields, 2003; Wells et al., 2002c, 2003).

However, [¹¹C]-thymidine PET scanning of patients enrolled in early-phase clinical trials has been shown to be feasible, and it can also be argued that a PET proliferation probe with a specific purpose, for example, as a tool for pharmacodynamic studies, does not need to be as widely available as a diagnostic imaging probe. This is certainly the case for the very short-lived tracer $H_2^{15}O$, which has very limited availability but is considered the PET gold standard used specifically to assess tumor blood flow. The development of a wide range of PET tracers and early-phase pharmacodynamic studies is therefore likely to be carried out in larger cancer centers with on-site cyclotrons. Alternatively, the cyclotron/PET scanning facility does not necessarily need to be located at the Phase I study site. For example, the Phase I and pharmacokinetic study of midostaurin described previously involved 2-[¹¹C]-thymidine scanning of patients in a PET unit, which was ~ 60 miles away from the clinical Phase I center (Propper et al., 2001).

The introduction of in vivo pharmacodynamic studies into Phase I clinical trials will potentially increase the speed and efficiency of introducing new antitumor agents into clinical practice. Recent years have seen considerable growth in the number and type of anticancer agents developed. Many agents show promising early activity only to fail in randomized Phase III trials. The high rate of attrition is costly for the pharmaceutical industry, and biological proof of activity in early-phase trials is required. This is particularly important for novel targeted therapies. It is envisaged that a PET proliferation probe would have potentially wide applications in drug development. For example, drugs designed as antiproliferative, TK inhibitors and agents targeting the epidermal growth factor receptor (EGFR: which is involved in the control of cell proliferation) would all benefit from early proof-of-principle assessment. Such a probe would be useful as a tool not only for increasing our understanding of the mechanism of action of drugs in vivo, but also for the early assessment of their biological effects in humans.

It is clear that continued work is required to validate the use of ¹¹C-thymidine-PET in cancer patients. More studies are required to confirm the relationship found between a histological measure of proliferation and PET measurements of thymidine retention in tissues. These studies should decide the best modeling approach for the data and whether the collection of data can be simplified (e.g., fewer time points in dynamic scans, use of population-derived input function scales using a single time point, or use of image-derived input functions). In addition, studies are required to investigate whether the accuracy of the data collection can be increased (e.g., methods for reducing signal-to-noise ratio) and to further validate the dual thymidine and CO_2 scanning approach. Additional thought also needs to be given to alternative ways of administering radiolabeled thymidine. With the introduction of high-sensitivity 3D tomography, steady-state administration could be investigated as a method of simplifying the collection and analysis of data, and of correcting the presence of labeled metabolites. Other validation studies are required to examine the value of thymidine-PET in measuring pharmacodynamic response in cancer patients. These studies need to compare thymidine with FDG and other proliferation probes, and should be carried out in different tumor sites to evaluate site-specific differences in the accuracy of PET proliferation probes.

FDG-PET is increasingly accepted as a diagnostic tool for cancer, but PET has far greater potential than restricted application to the imaging of glucose metabolism. The development of a gold standard, proliferation-specific PET probe is required in oncology, specifically to assist the pharmacodynamic evaluation of new anticancer agents and reduce the attrition from early clinical evaluation to regulatory approval. Research to date has validated the use of [¹¹C]-thymidine as a key contender for this role, although its short half-life and rapid metabolism have led a drive away from the validation of thymidine probes toward thymidine analogs radiolabeled with ¹⁸F. However, the better specificity of [¹¹C]-thymidine as a marker of cell proliferation should be the rationale for its continued development, validation, and application as a key PET probe in oncology imaging.

References

Barthel, H., Cleij, M.C., Collingridge, D.R., Hutchinson, O.C., Osman, S., He, Q., Luthra, S.K., Brady, F., Price, P.M., and Abogaye, E.O. 2003. 3′-deoxy-3′-[18F]fluorothymidine as a new marker for monitoring tumor response to antiproliferative therapy in vivo with positron emission tomography. *Cancer Res. 63*:3791–3798.

Bos, R., Vander Hoeven, J.J., Vander Wall, E., Vander Groep, P., Van Diest, P.J., Comans, E.F., Joshi, U., Semenza, G.L., Hoekstra, O.S., Lammertsma, A.A., and Molthoff, C.F. 2002. Biologic correlates of (18)fluorodeoxyglucose uptake in human breast cancer measured by positron emission tomography. *J. Clin. Oncol. 20*:379–387.

Brock, C.S., Young, H., O′Reilly, S.M., Matthews, J., Osman, S., Evans, H., Newlands, E.S., and Price, P.M. 2000. Early evaluation of tumour metabolic response using [18F]fluorodeoxyglucose and positron emission tomography: a pilot study following the phase II chemotherapy schedule for temozolomide in recurrent high-grade gliomas. *Br. J. Cancer 82*:608–615.

Buck, A.K., Halter, G., Schirrmeister, H., Kotzerke, J., Wurziger, I., Glatting, G., Mattfeldt, T., Neumaier, B., Reske, S.N., and Hetzel, M. 2003. Imaging proliferation in lung tumors with PET: 18F-FLT versus 18F-FDG. *J. Nucl.Med. 44*:1426–1431.

Cleaver, J.E. 1967. Thymidine metabolism and cell kinetics. *Frontiers Boil.* 6:43–100.

Conti, P.S., Hilton, J., Wong, D.F., Alauddin, M.M., Dannals, R.F., Ravert, H.T., Wilson, A.A., and Anderson, J.H. 1994. High performance liquid chromatography of carbon-11 labeled thymidine and its major catabolites for clinical PET studies. *Nucl. Med. Bio.* 21:1045–1051.

Covey, J.M., and Straw, J.A. 1983. Nonlinear pharmacokinetics of thymidine, thymine, and fluorouracil and their kinetic interactions in normal dogs. *Cancer Res.* 43:4587–4595.

Crawford, E.J., Christman, D., Atkins, H., Friedkin, M., and Wolf, A.P. 1978. Scintigraphy with positron-emitting compounds.—I. Carbon-11 labeled thymidine and thymidylate. *Int. J. Nucl. Med. Biol.* 5:61–69.

Eary, J.F., Mankoff, D.A., Spence, A.M., Berger, M.S., Olshen, A., Link, J.M., O'Sullivan, F., and Krohn, K.A. 1999. 2-[C-11]thymidine imaging of malignant brain tumors. *Cancer Res.* 59:615–621.

Fabbro, D., Ruetz, S., Bodis, S., Pruschy, M., Csermak, K., Man, A., Camoichiaro, P., Wood, J., O'Reilly, T., and Meyer, T. 2000. PKC412—a protein kinase inhibitor with a broad therapeutic potential. *Anticancer Drug Des.* 15:17–28.

Folpe, A.L., Lyles, R.H., Sprouse, J.T., Conrad, E.U., 3rd, and Eary, J.F. 2000. (F-18) fluorodeoxyglucose positron emission tomography as a predictor of pathologic grade and other prognostic variables in bone and soft tissue sarcoma. *Clin. Cancer Res.* 6:1279–1287.

Francis, D.L., Freeman, A., Visvikis, D., Costa, D.C., Luthra, S.K., Novelli, M., Taylor, I., and Ell, P.J. 2003. *In vivo* imaging of cellular proliferation in colorectal cancer using positron emission tomography. *Gut* 52:1602–1606.

Goethals, P., Van Eijkeren, M., Lodewyck, W., and Dams, R. 1995. Measurement of [methyl-carbon-11]thymidine and its metabolites in head and neck tumors. *J. Nucl. Med.* 36:880–882.

Goethals P., Van Eijkeren, M., and Lemahieu, I. 1999. *In vivo* distribution and identification of 11C-activity after injection of [methyl-11C]thymidine in Wistar rats. *J. Nucl. Med.* 40:491–496.

Graham, M.M., Peterson, L.M., and Hayward, R.M. 2000. Comparison of simplified quantitative analyses of FDG uptake. *Nucl. Med. Biol.* 27:647–655.

Gunn, R.N., Ranicar, A., Yap, J.T., Wells, P., Osman, S., Jones, T., and Cunningham, V.J. 2000a. On-line measurement of exhaled [11C]CO2 during PET. *J. Nucl. Med.* 41:605–611.

Gunn, R.N., Yap, J.T., Wells, P., Osman, S., Price, P., Jones, T., and Cunningham, V.J. 2000b. A general method to correct PET data for tissue metabolites using a dual-scan approach. *J. Nucl. Med.* 41:706–711.

Higashi, K., Clavo, A.C., and Wahl, R.L. 1993. Does FDG uptake measure proliferative activity of human cancer cells? *In vitro* comparison with DNA flow cytometry and tritiated thymidine uptake. *J. Nucl. Med.* 34:414–419.

Jacob, R., Welkoborsky, H.J., Mann, W.J., Jauch, M., and Amedee, R. 2001. [Fluorine-18]fluorodeoxyglucose positron emission tomography, DNA ploidy and growth fraction in squamous-cell carcinomas of the head and neck. *ORL J. Otorhinolaryngol Relat. Spec.* 63:307–313.

Kubota, R., Yamada, S., Kubota, K., Ishiwata, K., Tamahashi, N., and Ido, T. 1992. Intratumoral distribution of fluorine-18-fluorodeoxyglucose *in vivo*: high accumulation in macrophages and granulation tissues studied by microautoradiography. *J. Nucl. Med.* 33:1972–1980.

Larson, S.M., Grunbaum, Z., and Rasey, J.S. 1980. Positron imaging feasibility studies: selective tumor concentration of 3H-thymidine, 3H-uridine, and 14C-2-deoxyglucose. *Radiology 134*:771–773.

Larson, S.M., Weiden, P.L., Grunbaum, Z., Rasey, J.S., Kaplan, H.G., Graham, M.M., Harp, G.D., Sale, G.E., and Williams, D.L. 1981. Positron imaging feasibility studies. I: characteristics of [3H]thymidine uptake in rodent and canine neoplasms: concise communication. *J. Nucl. Med.* 22:869–874.

Mankoff, D.A., Shields, A.F., Graham, M.M., Link, J.M., Eary, J.F., and Krohn, K.A. 1998. Kinetic analysis of 2-[carbon-11]thymidine PET imaging studies: compartmental model and mathematical analysis. *J. Nucl. Med.* 39:1043–1055.

Mankoff, D.A., Shields, A.F., Link, J.M., Graham, M.M., Muzi, M., Peterson, L.M., Eary, J.F., and Krohn, K.A. 1999. Kinetic analysis of 2-[11C]thymidine PET imaging studies: validation studies. *J. Nucl. Med.* 40:614–624.

Martiat, P., Ferrant, A., Labar, D., Cogneau, M., Bol, A., Michel, C., Michaux, J.L., and Sokal, G. 1988. *In vivo* measurement of carbon-11 thymidine uptake in non-Hodgkin's Lymphoma using positron emission tomography. *J. Nucl. Med.* 29:1633–1637.

Price, P. 2000. Changes in 18F-FDG uptake measured by PET as a pharmacodynamic end-point in anticancer therapy. *Br. J. Cancer 83*:281–283.

Propper, D.J., McDonald, A.C., Man, A., Thavasu, P., Balkwill, F., Braybrooke, J.P., Caponigro, F., Graf, P., Dutreix, C., Blackie, R., Kaye, S.B., Ganesan, T.S., Talbot, D.C., Harris, A.L., and Twelves, C. 2001. Phase I and pharmacokinetic study of PKC412, an inhibitor of protein kinase C. *J. Clin. Oncol.* 19:1485–1492.

Quackenbush, R.C., and Shields, A.F. 1988. Local re-utilization of thymidine in normal mouse tissues as measured with iododeoxyuridine. *Cell Tissue Kinet.* 21:381–387.

Schmidt, K.C., and Turkheimer, F.E. 2002. Kinetic modeling in positron emission tomography. *Q. J. Nucl. Med.* 46:70–85.

Schwartz, J.L., Tamura, Y., Jordan, R., Grierson, J.R., and Krohn, K.A. 2003. Monitoring tumor cell proliferation by targeting DNA synthetic processes with thymidine and thymidine analogs. *J. Nucl. Med.* 44:2027–2032.

Shields, A.F., Larson, S.M., Grunbaum, Z., and Graham, M.M. 1984. Short-term thymidine uptake in normal and neoplastic tissues: studies for PET. *J. Nucl. Med.* 25:759–764.

Shields, A.F., Coonrod, D.V., Quackenbush, R.C., and Crowley, J.J. 1987. Cellular sources of thymidine nucleotides: studies for PET. *J. Nucl. Med.* 28:1435–1440.

Shields, A.F., Lim, K., Grierson, J., Link, J. and Krohn, K.A. 1990. Utilization of labeled thymidine in DNA synthesis: studies for PET. *J. Nucl. Med.* 31:337–342.

Shields, A.F., Graham, M.M., Kozawa, S.M., Kozell, L.B., Link, J.M., Swenson, E.R., Spence, A.M., Bassingthwaighte, J.B., and Krohn, K.A. 1992. Contribution of labeled carbon dioxide to PET imaging of carbon-11-labeled compounds. *J. Nucl. Med.* 33:581–584.

Shields, A.F., Mankoff, D., Graham, M.M., Zheng, M., Kozawa, S.M., Link, J.M., and Krohn, K.A. 1996. Analysis of 2-carbon-11-thymidine blood metabolites in PET imaging. *J. Nucl. Med.* 37:290–296.

Shields, A.F., Mankoff, D.A., Link, J.M., Graham, M.M., Eary, J.F., Kozawa, S.M., Zheng, M., Lewellen, B., Lewellen, T.K., Grierson, J.R., and Krohn, K.A. 1998. Carbon-11-thymidine and FDG to measure therapy response. *J. Nucl. Med.* 39:1757–1762.

Shields, A.F. 2003. PET imaging with 18F-FLT and thymidine analogs: promise and pitfalls. *J. Nucl. Med.* 44:1432–1434.

Smith, T.A. 1998. FDG uptake, tumour characteristics and response to therapy: a review. *Nucl. Med. Commun.* 19:97–105.

Taheri, M.R., Wickremasinghe, R.G., and Hoffbrand, A.V. 1982. Functional compartmentation of DNA precursors in human leukaemoblastoid cell lines. *Br. J. Haematol.* 52:401–409.

Van Eijkeren, M.E., De Schryver, A., Goethals, P., Poupeye, E., Schelstraete, K., Lemahieu, I., and De Potter, C.R. 1992. Measurement of short-term 11C-thymidine activity in human head and neck tumours using positron emission tomography (PET). *Acta. Oncol.* 31:539–543.

Vander Borght, T.M., Lambotte, L.E., Pauwels, S.A., and Dive, C.C. 1990. Uptake of thymidine labeled on carbon 2: a potential index of liver regeneration by positron emission tomography. *Hepatology, 12*:113–118.

Vander Borght, T., Labar, D., Pauwels, S., and Lamnotte, L. 1991a. Production of [2-11C]thymidine for quantification of cellular proliferation with PET. *Int. J. Rad. Appl. Instrum. [A]* 42:103–104.

Vander Borght, T., Lambotte, L., Pauwels, S., Labar, D., Beckers, C., and Dive, C. 1991b. Noninvasive measurement of liver regeneration with positron emission tomography and [2-11C]thymidine. *Gastroenterology 101*:794–799.

Vander Borght, T., Pauwels, S., Lambotte, L., Labar, D., De Maeght, S., Stroobandt, G., and Laterre, C. 1994. Brain tumor imaging with PET and 2-[carbon-11]thymidine. *J. Nucl. Med.* *35*:974–982.

Wells, J.M., Mankoff, D.A., Eary, J.F., Spence, A.M., Muzi, M., O'Sullivan, F., Vernon, C.B., Link, J.M., and Krohn, K.A. 2002a. Kinetic analysis of 2-[11C]thymidine PET imaging studies of malignant brain tumors: preliminary patient results. *Mol. Imaging* *1*:145–150.

Wells, J.M., Mankoff, D.A., Muzi, M., O'Sullivan, F., Eary, J.F., Spence, A.M., and Krohn, K.A. 2002b. Kinetic analysis of 2-[11C]thymidine PET imaging studies of malignant brain tumors: compartmental model investigation and mathematical analysis. *Mol. Imaging* 1:151–159.

Wells, P., Gunn, R.N., Alison, M., Steel, C., Golding, M., Ranicar, A.S., Brady, F., Osman, S., Jones, T., and Price, P. 2002c. Assessment of prolif-

eration *in vivo* using 2-[(11)C]thymidine positron emission tomography in advanced intra-abdominal malignancies. *Cancer Res.* *62*:5698–5702.

Wells, P., Aboagye, E., Gunn, R.N., Osman, S., Boddy, A.V., Taylor, G.A., Rafi, I., Hughes, A.N., Calvert, A.H., Price, P.M., and Newell, D.R. 2003. 2-[11C]thymidine positron emission tomography as an indicator of thymidylate synthase inhibition in patients treated with AG337. *J. Natl. Cancer Inst.* *95*:675–682.

Young, H., Baum, R., Cremerius, U., Herholz, K., Hoekstra, O., Lammertsma, A.A., Pruim, J., and Price, P. 1999. Measurement of clinical and subclinical tumour response using [18F]-fluorodeoxyglucose and positron emission tomography: review and 1999 EORTC recommendations. European Organization for Research and Treatment of Cancer (EORTC) PET Study Group. *Eur. J. Cancer 35*:1773–1782.

^{18}F-Fluorodeoxyglucose Positron Emission Tomography in Oncology: Advantages and Limitations

Tarik Belhocine and Albert Driedger

Introduction

In today's oncology practice, ^{18}F-fluorodeoxyglucose positron emission tomography (^{18}FDG PET) has become the cornerstone for the management of many patients suffering from cancer (Maisey, 2002). Unlike morphological imaging techniques such as ultrasonography (US), computed tomography (CT), or magnetic resonance imaging (MRI), ^{18}FDG PET provides a functional image of the underlying changes of glucose metabolism in normal and abnormal tissues (Jerusalem *et al.*, 2003). Because most malignancies exhibit increased glucose metabolism, whole-body ^{18}FDG PET reflects a certain degree of tumor aggressiveness in terms of glucose tracer avidity and disease extent (Pauwels *et al.*, 1998). Not surprisingly, this form of metabolic imaging is now recognized as a procedure of choice for the purpose of staging, re-staging, and monitoring responses to treatment in various types of cancers (Gambhir *et al.*, 2001). In the present chapter, the advantages and limitations of ^{18}FDG PET in the assessment of cancer are synthesized on the basis of current knowledge.

Mechanisms of ^{18}FDG Uptake

Increased glucose metabolism has long been known to be a characteristic of malignant cells (Warburg, 1930). This biochemical feature is genetically upregulated via proliferation oncogenes such as c-fos, c-myc, c-jun, and jun-B (Mukarami *et al.*, 1992). Glucose tropism in various malignancies relies on overexpression of glucose transporters (GLUTs), such as GLUT-1, GLUT-3, and GLUT-5, and key enzymes of the glycolytic pathway, such as hexokinase, pyruvate kinase, and phosphofructokinase. ^{18}F-fluorodeoxyglucose (^{18}FDG) as a radiolabeled glucose analog follows the course of natural glucose in the body (Gatenby *et al.*, 2003). Hence, ^{18}FDG is internalized into normal and abnormal tissues via facilitative energy-independent GLUTs. Unlike the natural glucose, however, ^{18}FDG is trapped intracellularly because the second enzyme of the glycolytic pathway (glucose-6-phosphate isomerase) cannot act on the oxygen atom in $-C2$ position, which was replaced by a fluorine atom. In addition, the action of the reverse enzyme (glucose-6-phosphatase) is nearly negligible (Gallagher *et al.*, 1978). Figures 1 and 2 summarize the biochemical mechanisms underlying the ^{18}FDG uptake.

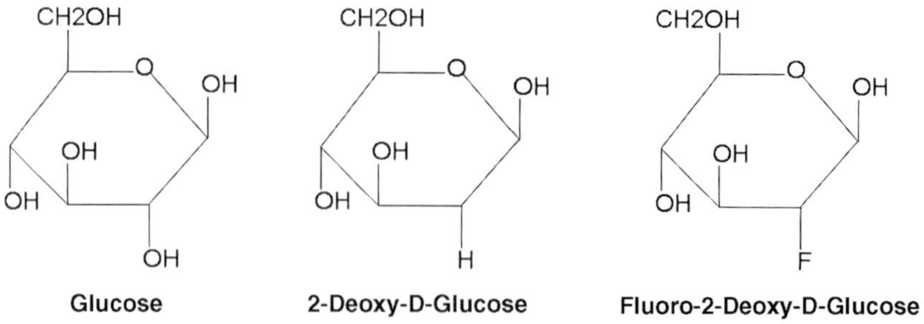

Figure 1 Synthesis of ^{18}F-fluorodeoxyglucose. Glucose, 2-deoxy-D-glucose (DG), and fluoro-2-deoxy-D-glucose (FDG) share a common chemical structure. DG derives from the original glucose molecule by substitution of the hydroxyl group in $-C2$ position with a hydrogen atom. FDG derives from DG by substitution of the hydrogen atom in $-C2$ position with a fluorine atom. ^{18}F-labeled FDG is most commonly cyclotron-produced through a nucleophilic substitution method as described by Hamacher *et al.* (1986).

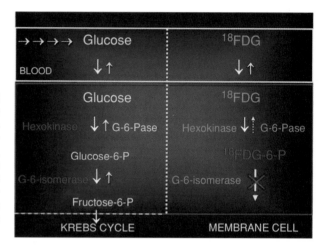

Figure 2 Mechanisms of ^{18}FDG uptake into tumor cells. Like the natural glucose molecule, ^{18}F-fluorodeoxyglucose (^{18}FDG) is avidly taken up into tumor cells via facilitative glucose transporters (GLUTs) and phosphorylated by hexokinase. Unlike glucose-6-phosphate, ^{18}FDG-6-phosphate is trapped in the tumor cell. ^{18}FDG-6-phosphate cannot be targeted by glucose-6-phosphate isomerase, an enzyme that requires the presence of an atom of oxygen on carbon 2 ($-C2$) to be active. As the activity of the reverse enzyme (glucose-6-phosphatase) is negligible, ^{18}FDG-6-phosphate bearing a negative charge accumulates in tumor cells without further significant degradation. Therefore, the tissue concentration of ^{18}FDG tracer is ultimately an indicator of the glycolytic activity related to the endogenous glucose.

^{18}FDG PET Uptake Patterns

Physiological ^{18}FDG Uptake

In normal subjects, the ^{18}FDG tracer is avidly taken up by the brain and is predominantly excreted by the urinary system through the kidneys, the ureters, and the bladder (Kato *et al.*, 1999). As a rule, the glucose tracer is slightly taken up by the liver, the spleen, the colon, and, to a lesser extent, by the salivary glands, the stomach, and the bone marrow; young subjects may also present with ^{18}FDG uptake in a normal thymus (Shreve *et al.*, 1999). In menstruating and ovulating women, physiological endometrial and ovarian ^{18}FDG uptake may be observed; similarly, ^{18}FDG uptake may be seen in lactating breasts (Lerman *et al.*, 2004; Hicks *et al.*, 2001). In nonfasting patients, increased ^{18}FDG uptake is seen in the heart; inconstantly, myocardial uptake may also be detected in long-fasting patients (Kaneta *et al.*, 2006).

Not infrequently, marked vascular ^{18}FDG uptake (e.g., aorta, iliac arteries, and femoral arteries) is observed, particularly in older patients who present with advanced vascular disease and/or atherosclerosis (Yun *et al.*, 2001). Pronounced ^{18}FDG uptake may occur in some patients with localized muscle contraction, especially in the head and neck musculature (Jackson *et al.*, 2006); under hyperinsulinic conditions,

diffuse skeletal muscle uptake is usually noted. Similarly, increased ^{18}FDG uptake has been well documented in metabolically active brown adipose tissues, particularly in young subjects and/or female patients (Hany *et al.*, 2002).

Pathological ^{18}FDG Uptake

In oncology patients, the tumor-to-background ratio (T/B) within the lungs, pleura, mediastinum, liver, spleen, skeleton, peritoneum, digestive system, and uterus is most often sufficient to allow adequate delineation of ^{18}FDG-avid tumors (Strauss *et al.*, 1991). In patients with high serum glucose levels, however, T/B may be suboptimal because of a possible competition between the ^{18}FDG tracer (as glucose analog) and endogenous glucose (Lindholm *et al.*, 1993). The sensitivity of this form of metabolic imaging is based primarily on the degree of tracer accumulation at the tumor site independent of its structural characteristics (Heinicke *et al.*, 2005). So far, the performances of ^{18}FDG PET may vary from one tumor type or subtype to another (Hoffman *et al.*, 2006). As a marker of tumor viability, the intensity of ^{18}FDG uptake usually reflects the tumor aggressiveness (Spaepen *et al.*, 2003). The intensity of glucose tracer uptake is also related to the tumor grade and degree of differentiation. Overall, ^{18}FDG uptake appears to be a marker of high-grade and/or poorly differentiated tumors, which means that ¹⁸FDG-avid cancers likely present with a certain degree of aggressiveness, thereby expressing an inherent metastatic tendency (Feine *et al.*, 1995). As such, ¹⁸FDG PET has been used as a prognostic index prior to any therapy, and also to assess the tumor chemosensitivity after one or several courses of treatment (Cascini *et al.*, 2006). Table 1 summarizes key parameters influencing the ¹⁸FDG uptake into tumor tissues.

Advantages of ¹⁸FDG PET

In most developed countries, ¹⁸FDG PET has become the imaging procedure of choice in oncology (Maisey, 2002). This relies on many technical and clinical advantages, as follows:

1. ¹⁸FDG PET is not just a scintigraphic technique; it represents the best example of *molecular imaging*, also called metabolic imaging (Wagner, 2004; Alavi *et al.*, 2004). This allows the evaluation of biochemical tumor changes, which may take place early in the malignant process as well as in the course of tumor response to treatment (Phelps, 2000). Thus, the introduction of ¹⁸FDG PET in clinical oncology has led to reconsideration of conventional Response Evaluation Criteria in Solid Tumors (RECIST) by adding metabolic PET criteria to morphologic CT criteria (Young *et al.*, 1999).

2. ¹⁸FDG PET relies on the *coincidental detection* of two annihilation photons, which significantly improves the spatial resolution and the sensitivity compared to conventional single photon emission tomography (SPECT) (Ter-Pogossian *et al.*, 1975).

3. ¹⁸FDG PET is a *flexible* imaging technique that may be readily performed in any clinical environment (private clinic, public hospital, mobile car) when the conditions related to radiopharmaceutical production and distribution are properly managed (Preusche *et al.*, 1999). In addition, the short ¹⁸F-fluorine half-life (T1/2 = 109.08 min) alleviates the need for drastic radioprotection measures, especially in case of contamination.

Table 1   Parameters Related to ¹⁸FDG Uptake into Tumor Tissues

¹⁸FDG activity injected
Serum glucose levels
GLUT expression[a]
Hexokinase expression[b]
Tumor perfusion
Tumor viability
Tumor hypoxia

Abbreviations
[a]Glucose transporter, especially GLUT-1 and GLUT-3.
[b]Hexokinase types I and II.

4. ¹⁸FDG PET is a *safe and noninvasive* imaging procedure, which allows the performance of a highly sophisticated examination with a minimal inconvenience for the patient (e.g., intravenous injection).

5. ¹⁸FDG PET is a *whole-body* imaging that enables, in a single session, the exploration of anatomic regions that are not routinely explored with CT or MRI. Hence, metabolic imaging may detect clinically or radiologically unsuspected lesions (Alberini *et al.*, 2003).

6. ¹⁸FDG PET yields a quantifiable index of tumor metabolism (Hallett, 2005), which may be obtained by means of complex kinetic models (absolute quantification) or, more practically, in relative terms by computerized semiquantitative indices such as the standardized uptake value (SUV) body weight; the SUV is a unitless score expressing the ¹⁸FDG concentration (MBq/L) within a tumor volume per injected activity (MBq) corrected by the patient's body weight (Kg). In addition to scatter correction, a transmission scan is required for attenuation correction of emission data (Meikle *et al.*, 1995). With ¹⁸FDG PET alone, the transmission is based on a rotating radioactive source such as ¹³⁷Cs (cesium), or ⁶⁸Ge (germanium) (Benard *et al.*, 1999). In the course of treatment, the calculation of sequential SUVs (e.g., delta changes pretherapy-to-posttherapy) may be particularly helpful for monitoring tumor responsiveness (Young *et al.*, 1999). The SUV score may eventually have a diagnostic value for differentiating benignity from malignancy, especially in a dual-time evaluation (e.g., early versus delayed ¹⁸FDG PET) (Hustinx *et al.*, 1999; Kumar *et al.*, 2005). Recent data have also pointed out the prognostic importance derived from SUV for prediction of outcomes (Vansteenkiste *et al.*, 1999).

7. ¹⁸FDG PET is a *highly accurate* imaging technology for detection of metabolically active tumors (see Fig. 3). Compelling data from the literature including comparative prospective and retrospective studies as well as meta-analyses have shown the superiority of ¹⁸FDG PET to morphological studies (US/CT/MRI), particularly in terms of sensitivity, and at a lesser degree by extent, in terms of specificity (Gambhir *et al.*, 2001).

8. ¹⁸FDG PET is not only an accurate diagnostic imaging procedure, but it also brings unique prognostic information. In recent years, increasing data have highlighted the importance of ¹⁸FDG tumor uptake in terms of survival; this holds true in the setting of primary staging as well as in the course of treatment (Grigsby *et al.*, 2004).

9. ¹⁸FDG PET is a valuable *research tool* in clinical and preclinical research (Phelps, 2000). In human subjects, metabolic imaging is nowadays incorporated in many research protocols dedicated to evaluating new chemotherapy drugs and/or radiation therapy sequences (Fox *et al.*, 2002). Micro-PET is also used in animal models to assess specific aspects of tumor metabolism or newly designed drugs. Table 2 summarizes the advantages of ¹⁸FDG PET in oncology.

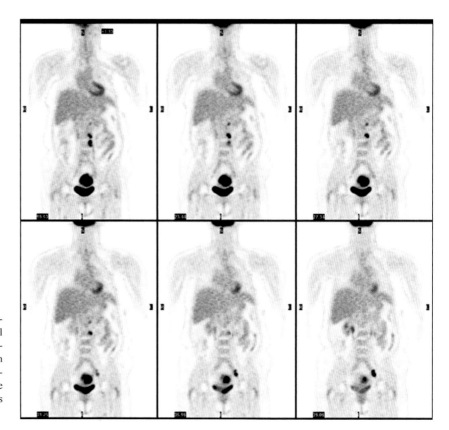

Figure 3 Initial staging with [18]FDG PET. A 59-year-old woman with a newly diagnosed endometrial cancer was referred for pretreatment staging. Whole-body [18]FDG PET showed intense tracer uptake within the primary tumor (SUV = 21.32) by SUV -bw. In addition, metabolic imaging detected multiple lymph node metastases along the left iliac and left para-aortic chains (St. Joseph's Hospital, London, Canada).

Limitations of [18]FDG PET

Despite the well-documented advantages provided by [18]FDG PET in clinical oncology and research, a number of limitations have to be noted, as follows:

1. [18]FDG PET is a high-end and costly technology that requires reliable devices, appropriate infrastructures for the [18]FDG production (e.g., linear accelerator, cyclotron), and its efficient distribution (Ter-Pogossian *et al.*, 1998). As a consequence, this imaging technique is not universally available, particularly not in developing countries.

Table 2   Advantages of [18]FDG PET in Oncology

Metabolic imaging[a]
Noninvasive procedure
Flexible technique
Whole-body assessment
Qualitative and quantitative information
High diagnostic performances
Unique prognostic information

[a][18]FDG PET is a molecular imaging.

2. [18]FDG is not a tumor-specific tracer. Besides cancer cells, inflammatory and infectious processes may exhibit increased glucose metabolism and hence, increased [18]FDG uptake (Spaepen *et al.*, 2003). Of note, macrophages, lymphocytes, neutrophil granulocytes, and fibroblasts may exhibit increased [18]FDG uptake as intensely as tumor cells, especially when the inflammation or the infection is active (Kubota *et al.*, 1992). As a consequence, such nontumoral [18]FDG uptake patterns may compromise the specificity of [18]FDG PET in oncology patients, particularly after radiation therapy or recent surgery (e.g., inflammatory changes) or after immunotherapy or chemotherapy (e.g., increased susceptibility to infection) (see Fig. 4). Recent studies suggest that serial SUVs obtained within hours of [18]FDG injection will separate malignancy from infection when the distinction must be made (Hustinx *et al.*, 1999). Table 3 summarizes the causes of false-positive results and false-negative results in [18]FDG PET imaging.

3. [18]FDG PET is limited for detection of abnormal uptakes to regions of the body with a high physiological background. Therefore, the sensitivity of metabolic imaging is most often suboptimal for detection of [18]FDG-avid metastases within the brain and the urinary tract (Larcos *et al.*, 1996).

4. [18]FDG PET lacks anatomic details for precisely localizing tumor sites. As a rule, a correlation between [18]FDG

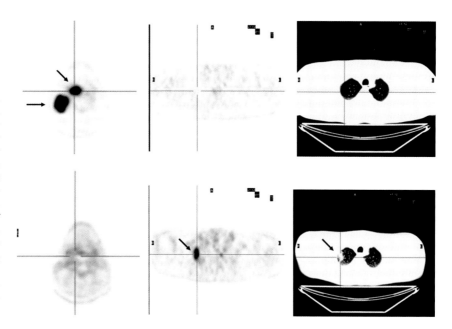

Figure 4 Post-radiation inflammatory changes. A 58-year-old man with a squamous cell carcinoma of the base of the tongue was explored by 18FDG PET. Pretreatment staging showed intense tracer uptake within the primary tumor (SUV = 8.39) by SUV-bw; an ipsilateral 18FDG-avid nodal mass was also detected (SUV = 7.80) by SUV-bw. The patient was treated by chemotherapy and radiation therapy including the right lung apex. Post-treatment evaluation performed two months after completion of chemoradiation therapy showed complete metabolic response in previously described lesions. A new 18FDG-avid focus was detected in the right lung apex, which was also seen on the co-registered CT. This uptake pattern was consistent with inflammatory changes secondary to a recent radiation treatment (St. Joseph's Hospital, London, Canada).

PET findings and CT or MRI data is recommended (Rinne et al., 1998).

5. 18FDG PET alone may be limited for differentiating between physiological and pathological uptakes (see Fig. 5); examples include focal digestive activity versus peritoneal implants, ureter stasis versus lymph node, supraclavicular muscle or brown adipose tissue uptake patterns versus lymph nodes (Cohade et al., 2003). Similarly, within the gynecological sphere, benign or physiological uptakes such as ovarian functional cysts and menstruation may be falsely

interpreted as tumors without clinical and radiological confrontation (Lerman et al., 2004).

6. 18FDG PET most often has poor sensitivity in low-grade malignancies (e.g., low-grade lymphoma), in well-differentiated cancers (e.g., carcinoid tumors), as well as in tumors with low metabolic activity (e.g., renal cell carcinoma with a low GLUT-1 activity) (Hoffmann et al., 2006).

7. 18FDG PET may be inaccurate within the first two weeks after chemotherapy; a false-negative pattern is related

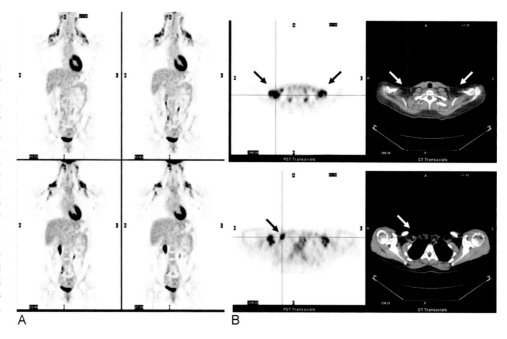

Figure 5 Physiological and pathological uptake patterns with 18FDG PET. A patient previously treated for a differentiated thyroid cancer presented with elevated thyroglobulin levels and normal post-therapy 131I scan. Whole-body 18FDG PET/CT scan was performed to detect a recurrence. On PET images alone, multiple 18FDG-avid foci were seen bilaterally and symmetrically in the neck (**A**). Correlation with the co-registered CT precisely localized these foci in metabolically active brown adipose tissue (**B**—Top). On the other hand, an asymmetrical 18FDG-avid focus was detected in the right supraclavicular region. Fused PET/CT image precisely localized this focus in a lymph node metastasis (**B**—Bottom) (St. Joseph's Hospital, London, Canada).

A   B to a temporary metabolic shutdown. As a rule, a minimal time interval of 2–3 weeks is recommended for monitoring chemosensitivity with metabolic imaging (Cremerius *et al.*, 1995).

8. [18]FDG PET most often has poor sensitivity for detecting small tumor sites that escape the spatial resolution of current PET devices (~ 4–6 mm). As a rule, [18]FDG PET has been shown to miss millimetric lymph node metastases, which may be otherwise detected by the sentinel lymph node technique (e.g., malignant melanoma, breast cancer, head and neck cancer) (Belhocine *et al.*, 2006a).

9. [18]FDG PET acquisition remains time consuming (~ 1 hr) when a radioactive source (e.g., ^{137}Cs, [68]Ge) is used for the purpose of attenuation correction. In this situation, the transmission scan duration reduces the patient's throughput considerably (Cohade *et al.*, 2003). Table 3 summarizes the limitations of [18]FDG PET in oncology, and Table 4 details potential causes of misinterpretation with [18]FDG PET.

Clinical Indications

The clinical added-value of whole-body [18]FDG PET has been widely documented in various types of cancers (Jerusalem *et al.*, 2003). Current oncological indications for the use of whole-body [18]FDG PET cover a large spectrum of known or suspected malignancies. Metabolic imaging is well recognized today for the evaluation of solitary pulmonary nodules, the initial staging of newly diagnosed malignancies, the detection of clinically or radiologically suspected recur-

Table 3 Limitations of [18]FDG PET in Oncology

Tracer synthesis
Tracer distribution
Costly technique
Nonuniversally available
Suboptimal specificity
Lack of anatomic landmarks
Time-consuming

rences, and the evaluation of tumor response in the course of treatment (Belhocine *et al.*, 2006b). [18]FDG PET also proved to be useful for the detection of unknown primary tumor and the assessment of masses ill-characterized on CT or MRI. Table 5 enumerates clinical indications currently reimbursed by Medicare in the United States.

In conclusion, the introduction of [18]FDG PET to the clinical setting has significantly changed the approach to management of oncology patients from diagnosis to treatment. In particular, [18]FDG PET offers the advantage of a noninvasive and highly sensitive imaging technique allowing the assessment of the entire body in a single session. This is critical for accurate staging of disease, treatment decision making, appropriate monitoring of tumor response, and early detection of recurrence. Owing to its limited spatial resolution and the lack of anatomic precision, [18]FDG PET remains complementary to other imaging techniques such as sentinel node detection and anatomical imaging. Multimodality hybrid imaging such as PET-CT or PET-MRI with hardware or software image fusion has overcome some of

Table 4 [18]FDG PET in Oncology: Potential Causes of Misinterpretation

Causes of False-Positive Findings	Causes of False-Negative Findings
Physiological Uptakes	Low GLUT expression (e.g., renal cell carcinoma)
—Bowel activity	Small lesions (e.g., lung micrometastase)
—Ureter stasis	High background (e.g., brain metastases)
—Brown adipose tissue	Hyperglycemia (e.g., diabetics)
—Degenerative spine disease	Metabolic shutdown post-chemotherapy
—Muscle contraction	Low-grade malignancies (e.g., low-grade lymphoma)
—Atherosclerosis (e.g., mediastinal vessels)	Well-differentiated tumors (e.g., typical carcinoid tumors)
—Endometrial and ovarian hot spots (e.g., menstruation and ovulation phases)	
Pathological Uptakes	
—Infection (e.g., tuberculosis, aspergillosis, pneumonia)	Lobular breast cancer
—Inflammatory diseases (e.g., sarcoidosis, granulomatosis, asbestosis)	Mucinous colon cancer
—Benign or premalignant diseases (e.g., colonic polyps, ovarian functional cyst, Paget's disease, esophagitis, gastritis, thyroiditis, pituitary adenoma)	Typical MALT lymphoma
	Signet cell gastric cancer
	Bronchoalveolar lung cancer (e.g., BAC with no aggressive features)
Intervention-Related Uptakes	
—After recent surgery or biopsy (inflammation)	Prostate cancer
—After radiation therapy or chemotherapy (e.g., pneumonitis, flare phenomenon)	

Table 5   ¹⁸FDG PET Indications Recognized by U.S. Medicare in Oncology

Clinical Indications	Comments
—Non-small cell lung cancer	Diagnosis–Staging–Re-staging
—Small cell lung cancer	Clinical trial
—Solitary lung nodule	Metabolic characterization of inconclusive nodule on CT scan
—Colon cancer	Diagnosis–Staging–Re-staging
—Malignant melanoma	Diagnosis–Staging–Re-staging
—Lymphoma	Diagnosis–Staging–Re-staging
—Breast cancer	Staging–Re-staging–Treatment monitoring
—Head and neck cancer	Diagnosis–Staging–Re-staging
—Esophageal cancer	Diagnosis–Staging–Re-staging
—Pancreatic cancer	Clinical trial
—Ovarian cancer	Clinical trial
—Cervical cancer	Staging as adjunct to conventional—Clinical trial
—Testicular cancer	Clinical trial
—Thyroid cancer	Staging—Elevated Tg with negative 1–131 whole-body scan[a]
—Brain cancer	Clinical trial
—Soft tissue sarcoma	Clinical trial
—All other cancers	Clinical trial

*18FDG PET indications covered by U.S. Medicare as "Coverage with Evidence Development" since January 28, 2005 include brain cancer, pancreatic cancer, ovarian cancer, small-cell lung cancer, testicular cancer, soft tissue sarcoma, re-staging or monitoring of cervical cancer, and all other cancers not listed in the table. Of note, the initial staging of cervical cancer is a covered indication in newly diagnosed and locally advanced disease with a negative CT/MRI for extra-pelvic metastases.

the aforementioned technical limitations. The development of new PET tracers is also critical to improve the specificity of metabolic imaging.

Acknowledgments

My thanks are offered to all my previous and current colleagues from different institutions in Belgium and Canada who shared their valuable experience in the field of ¹⁸FDG PET imaging, particularly Pr. Rigo and Pr. Hustinx (University Hospital Liège), Dr. Vandevivere (Middelheim Hospital in Antwerp), Pr. Flamen (Jules Bordet Institute in Brussels), and Dr. Urbain (London Health Sciences Center, Canada).

References

Alavi, A., Kung, J.W., and Zhuang, H. 2004. Implications of PET based molecular imaging on the current and future practice of medicine. *Semin. Nucl. Med. 34*:56–69.

Alberini, J-L., Belhocine, T., Hustinx, R., Daenen, F., and Rigo, P. 2003. Whole-body positron emission tomography using fluorodeoxyglucose in patients with metastases of unknown primary tumours (CUP syndromes). *Nucl. Med. Commun. 24*:1081–1086.

Belhocine, T.Z., Scott, A.M., Even-Sapir, E., Urbain, J-L., and Essner, R. 2006a. Role of nuclear medicine in the management of cutaneous malignant melanoma. *J. Nucl. Med. 47*:957–967.

Belhocine, T., Spaepen, K., Dusart, M., Castaigne, C., Muylle, K., Bourgeois, P., Bourgeois, D., Dierckx, L., and Flamen, P. 2006b. ¹⁸FDG PET in oncology: the best and the worst (Review). *Int. J. Oncol. 28*:1249–1261.

Benard, F., Smith, R.J., Hustinx, R., Karp, J.S., and Alavi, A. 1999. Clinical evaluation of processing techniques for attenuation correction with ¹³⁷Cs in whole-body PET imaging. *J. Nucl. Med. 40*:1257–1263.

Cascini, G.L., Avallone, A., Delrio, P., Guida, C., Tatangelo, F., Marone, P., Aloj, L., De Martinis, F., Comella, P., Parisi, V., and Lastoria, S. 2006. 18F-FDG PET is an early predictor of pathologic tumor response to pre-operative radiochemotherapy in locally advanced rectal cancer. *J. Nucl. Med. 47*:1241–1248.

Cohade, C., Osman, M., Pannu, H.K., and Wahl, R.L. 2003. Uptake in supraclavicular area fat ("USA-Fat"): description on 18F-FDG PET/CT. *J. Nucl. Med. 44*:170–176.

Cremerius, U., Effert, P.J., Adam, G., et al. 1998. FDG PET for detection and therapy control of metastatic germ cell tumor. *J. Nucl. Med. 39*:815–822.

Feine, U., Lietzenmayer, R., Hanke, J.P., Wohrle, H., and Muller-Schauenburg, W. 1995. 18FDG whole-body PET in differentiating thyroid carcinoma. Flipflop in uptake patterns of 18FDG and 131I. *Nuklearlmedizin 34*:127–134.

Fowler, J.S., and Ido, T. 2002. Initial and subsequent approach for the synthesis of ¹⁸FDG. *Sem. Nucl. Med. 32*:6–12.

Fox, E., Curt, G.A., and Balis, F.M. 2002. Clinical trial design for target-based therapy. *Oncologist. 7*:401–409.

Gallagher, B.M., Fowler, J.S., Gutterson, N.I., MacGregor, R.R., Wan, C.N., and Wolf, A.P. 1978. Metabolic trapping as a principle of oradiopharmaceutical design: some factors responsible for the biodistribution of [18F] 2-deoxy-2-fluoro-D-glucose. *J. Nucl. Med. 19*:1154–1161.

Gambhir, S.S., Czernin, J., Schwimmer, J., et al. 2001. A tabulated summary of the FDG PET literature. *J. Nucl. Med. 42*:1S–93S.

Gatenby, R.A., and Gawlinski, E.T. 2003. The glycolytic phenotype in carcinogenesis and tumor invasion. *Cancer. Res. 63*:3847–3854.

Grigsby, P.W., Siegel, B.A., Dehdashti, F., Rader, J., and Zoberi, I. 2004. Posttherapy [18F] Fluorodeoxyglucose positron emission tomography in carcinoma of the cervix: response and outcome. *J. Clin. Oncol. 22*:2167–2171.

Hallett, W.A. 2005. Quantification in clinical fluorodeoxyglucose positron emission tomography. *Nucl. Med. Commun. 25*:647–650. (Review.)

Hamacher, K., Coenen, H.H., and Stocklin, G. 1986. Efficient stereospecific synthesis of no-carrier-added 2-18F-fluoro-2-deoxy-D-glucose using aminopolyether supported nucleophilic substitution. *J. Nucl. Med. 27*:235–238.

Hany, T.F., Gharehpagagh, E., and Kamel, E.M. 2002. Brown adipose tissue: a factor to consider in symmetrical tracer uptake in the neck and upper chest region. *Eur. J. Nucl. Med. Mol. Imaging. 29*:1393–1398.

Hatanaka, M. Transport of sugars in tumor cell membranes. 1974. *Biochem. Biophys. Acta. 355*:77–104.

Heinicke, T., Wardelmann, E., Sauerbruch, T., *et al.* 2005. Very early detection of response to imatinib mesylate therapy of gastroinstestinal stromal tumours using 18fluoro-deoxyglucose-positron emission tomography. *Anticancer. Res. 25*:4591–4594.

Hicks, R.J., Binns, D., and Stabin, M.G. 2001. Pattern of uptake and excretion of (18)F-FDG in the lactating breast. *J. Nucl. Med. 42*:1238–1242.

Hoffmann, M., Wohrer, S., Becherer, A., Chott, A., Streubel, B., Kletter, K., and Raderer, M. 2006. ^{18}F-Fluoro-deoxy-glucose positron emission tomography in lymphoma of mucosa-associated lymphoid tissue: histology makes the difference. *Ann. Oncol. 17*:1761–1765.

Hustinx, R., Smith, R.J., Benard, F., *et al.* 1999. Dual time point fluorine-18 fluorodeoxyglucose positron emission tomography: a potential method to differentiate malignancy from inflammation and normal tissue in the head and neck. *Eur. J. Nucl. Med. 26*:1345–1348.

Jackson, R.S., Schlarman, T.C., Hubble, W.L., and Osman, M.M. 2006. Prevalence and patterns of physiologic muscle uptake detected with whole-body 18F-FDG PET. *J. Nucl. Med. Technol. 34*:29–33.

Jerusalem, G., Hustinx, R., Beguin, Y., and Fillet, G. 2003. PET scan imaging in oncology. *Eur. J. Cancer 39*:1525–1534.

Jerusalem, G., Beguin, Y., Najjar, F., *et al.* 2001. Positron emission tomography (PET) with 18F-fluorodeoxyglucose (18F-FDG) for the staging of low-grade non-Hodgkin's Lymphoma (NHL). *Ann. Oncol. 12*: 825–830.

Kaneta, T., Hakamatsuka, T., Takanami, K., *et al.* 2006. Evaluation of the relationship between physiological FDG uptake in the heart and age, blood glucose level, fasting period, and hospitalization. *Ann. Nucl. Med. 20*:203–208.

Kato, F., Tsukamoto, E., Suginami, Y., *et al.* 1999. Visualization of normal organs in whole-body FDG-PET imaging. *Kaku. Igaku. 36*:971–977.

Kubota, R., Yamada, S., Kubota, K., Ishiwata, K., Tamahashi, N., and Ido, T. 1992. Intratumoral distribution of fluorine-18-fluorodeoxyglucose *in vivo*: high accumulation in macrophages and granulation tissues studied by microautoradiography. *J. Nucl. Med. 33*:1972–1980.

Kumar, R., Loving, V.A., Chauhan, A., Zhuang, H., Mitchell, S., and Alavi, A. 2005. Potential of dual time-point imaging to improve breast cancer diagnosis with (18)F-FDG PET. *J. Nucl. Med. 46*:1819–1824.

Larcos, G., and Maisey, M.N. 1996. FDG-PET screening for cerebral metastases in patients with suspected malignancy. *Nucl. Med. Commun. 17*:197–198.

Lerman, H., Metser, U., Grisaru, D., *et al.* 2004. Normal and abnormal ^{18}F-FDG endometrial and ovarian uptake in pre- and postmenopausal patients: assessment by PET/CT. *J. Nucl. Med. 45*:266–271.

Lindholm, P., Minn, H., and Leskinen-Kallio, S. 1993. Influence of the blood glucose concentration on FDG uptake in cancer—a PET study. *J. Nucl. Med. 34*:1–6.

Maisey, M.N. 2002. Overview of clinical PET. *Br. J. Radiol. 75*:S1–S5.

Meikle, S.R., Bailey, D.L., Hooper, P.K., Eberl, S., Hutton, B.F., Jones, W.F., Fulton, R.R., and Fulham, M.J. 1995. Simultaneous emission and transmission measurements for attenuation correction in whole-body PET. *J. Nucl. Med. 36*:1680–1688.

Mukarami, T., Nishiyama, T., Shirotani, T., *et al.* 1992. Type 1 glucose transporter from the mouse which are responsive to serum, growth factors, and oncogenes. *J. Biol. Chem. 267*:9300–9306.

Pauwels, E.K.J., Ribeiro, M.J., Stoot, J.H.M.B., McCready, V.R., Bourguigon, M., and Mazière, B. 1998. FDG accumulation and tumor biology. *Nuclear. Med. Biol. 25*:317–322.

Phelps, M.E. 2000. Inaugural article: positron emission tomography provides molecular imaging of biological processes. *Proc. Natl. Acad. Sci. U.S.A. 97*:9226–9233.

Preusche, S., Fuchtner, F., Steinbach, J., Zessin, J., Krug, H., and Neumann, W. 1999. Long-distance transport of radionuclides between PET cyclotron and PET radiochemistry. *Appl. Radiat. Isot. 51*:625–630.

Rinne, D., Baum, R.P., Hor, G., and Kaufman, R. 1998. Primary staging and follow-up of high risk melanoma patients with whole-body 18F-fluorodeoxyglucose positron emission tomography: results of a prospective study of 100 patients. *Cancer 82*:1664–1671.

Shreve, P.D., Anzai, Y., and Wahl, R.L. 1999. Pifalls in oncologic diagnosis with FDG PET imaging: physiologic and benign variants. *Radiographics 19*:61–77; quiz 150–151.

Spaepen, K., Stroobants, S., Dupont, P., *et al.* 2003. [(18)F]FDG PET monitoring of tumour response to chemotherapy: does (18F)FDG uptake correlate with the viable tumour cell fraction? *Eur. J. Nucl. Med. Mol. Imag. 30*:682–688.

Strauss, L.G., and Conti, P.S. 1991. The applications of PET in clinical oncology. *J. Nucl. Med. 32*:801–820.

Ter-Pogossian, M.M., Phelps, M.E., Hoffman, E.J., and Mullani, N.A. 1975. A positron-emission transaxial tomograph for nuclear imaging (PETT). *Radiology 114*:89–98.

Ter-Pogossian, M.M., and Wagner, H.N. 1998. A new look at the cyclotron for making short-lived isotopes. 1966-classical article-. *Sem. Nucl. Med. 28*:202–212.

Vansteenkiste, J.F., Stroobants, S.G., Dupont, P.J., *et al.* 1999. Prognostic importance of the standardized uptake value on (18)F-fluoro-2-deoxyglucose-positron emission tomography scan in non-small-cell lung cancer: an analysis of 125 cases. Leuven Lung Cancer Group. *J. Clin. Oncol. 17*:3201–3206.

Wagner, H.N., Jr. 1991. Positron emission tomography at the turn of the century: a perspective. *Semin. Nucl. Med. 22*:285–288.

Warburg, O. 1930. *The Metabolism of Tumors*. London: Constable Press.

Young, H., Baum, R., Cremerius, U., *et al.* 1999. Measurement of clinical and subclinical tumour response using [18F]-fluorodeoxyglucose and positron emission tomography: review and 1999 EORTC recommendations. European Organization for Research and Treatment of Cancer (EORTC) PET Study Group. *Eur. J. Cancer 35*:1773–1782.

Yun M., Yeh, D., Araujo, Li, Jang, S., Newberg, A., and Alavi, A. 2001. F-18 FDG uptake in the large arteries: a new observation. *Clin. Nucl. Med. 26*:314–319.

11

Positron Emission Tomography Imaging of Tumor Hypoxia and Angiogenesis: Imaging Biology and Guiding Therapy

Joseph G. Rajendran and K.A. Krohn

Introduction

Integration of form and function is rapidly changing the paradigm for noninvasive diagnostic imaging, treatment planning, and monitoring response to therapy in cancer. This fusion overcomes many of the limitations of these individual imaging modalities (Herschman, 2003; Peters *et al.*, and McKay, 2001; Wahl, 2003). The phenomenal growth seen in PET imaging instrumentation—more typically integration with anatomic imaging modalities such as PET/CT—have been responsible for the rapid changes that have taken place in the field of molecular medicine. This is coupled with the availability of an expanding array of molecular probes. Together, they are providing an important bridge between the laboratory and bedside (Gambhir, 2002; Maclean *et al.*, 2003; Pomper, 2005). Patient management will benefit as the attending clinician is presented with more complete and more integrated information about the morphology as well as functional elements of the tumor's metabolism, proliferation, and death, as well its microenvironment.

The microenvironment of a tumor is constantly evolving and is largely dictated by abnormal vasculature and metabolism due to cellular proliferation. These characteristics are tumor and host specific, with differences sufficient to separate tumor from normal tissue. Hypoxia is a state of reduced oxygenation in tissue and is the most widely studied of all the microenvironmental changes. Oxygen is an essential metabolic substrate because of its critical role as the terminal electron acceptor in metabolic respiration, with levels of oxygen in tissue ranging through a continuum between normal levels (*euoxia* or *normoxia*) and total lack of oxygen (*anoxia*) without necessarily showing a clear demarcation between them. The tissue oxygen levels, commonly reported as a pressure, Po_2, can reach as low as < 5 mm Hg, with many cells surviving and adapting to these circumstances.

Although the terms *ischemia* and *hypoxia* are frequently used interchangeably, they are not the same pathophysiologically. Focal regions of hypoxia develop in many solid tumors (typically in the center) as they grow and as a direct consequence of unregulated cellular growth, resulting in a greater demand on oxygen for energy metabolism. This process is compounded by high interstitial pressure in already inefficient vascularization (Bhujwalla *et al.*, 2001). Thomlinson and Gray (1955), in explaining the mechanistic aspects of hypoxia, showed that a distance greater than 200 microns from a capillary would compromise cell viability and survival.

201

Hypoxia-Induced Changes in Tumor Behavior

Regardless of the level of perfusion or status of the vasculature in a tumor, hypoxia induces changes that reflect homeostatic attempts to maintain adequate oxygenation by increasing O_2 extraction from blood and by inducing cells to adapt by developing more aggressive survival traits through expression of new proteins. Aggressive tumors often have high microvessel density but paradoxically can show greater hypoxia (Kourkourakis et al., 2000). As a consequence of increased glycolysis seen in most hypoxic cells, lactate accumulates in cells. This will eventually lead to a dampening of glycolytic activity, even in the presence of hypoxia, a mechanism that would reduce the specificity of [F18]Fluorodeoxyglucose (FDG) as a surrogate marker for hypoxia (Rajendran et al., 2004).

A number of hypoxia-related genes have been found to be responsible for the genomic changes, and several downstream transcription factors have been identified (Hockel et al., 2001a). These include expression of endothelial cytokines such as vascular endothelial growth factor (VEGF), signaling molecules such as IL-1, TNF-alpha, and TGF-beta, and selection of cells with mutant p53 expression (Dachs and Tozer, 2000). For example, hypoxic cells do not readily undergo death by apoptosis (Hockel et al., 1999) or arrest in G1 phase of the cell cycle in response to sublethal DNA damage (Guillemin and Krasnoq, 1997). Increased glucose transporter (GLUT) activity is responsible for much of the increased glucose uptake associated with hypoxia, which can be as high as twofold temporarily (Wellmann et al., 2004).

Hypoxia-Inducible Factor (HIF)

The seminal mechanism for cellular oxygen sensing appears to be mediated by a heme-protein that uses O_2 as a substrate to catalyze hydroxylation of proline in a segment of HIF1α. This leads to rapid degradation of HIF1α under normoxic conditions (Ivan et al., 2001). However, in the absence of O_2, HIF1α accumulates and forms a heterodimer with HIF1β that is transported to the nucleus, resulting in activation of "hypoxia-responsive" genes, and a cascade of genetic and metabolic activities (Huang et al., 1996). Stabilization of HIF1α has been shown to occur early in the process of tumor development (Bos et al., 2001). Measurement of overexpressed HIF1α in tissues by immunohistochemical (IHC) staining has been suggested and used as an indirect measure of hypoxia (Marxsen et al., 2001), but the value of IHC is dampened because of the heterogeneous expression of hypoxia response within a tumor that can result in sampling errors.

Angiogenesis

Angiogenesis is the formation of new blood vessels and is also an important attribute in a number of physiological processes vital for sustaining cancer cells and promoting tumor growth (Hanahan and Weinberg, 2000). It is critical for delivering nutrients for tumor growth and in providing energy to support invasion and metastatic spread. In simple terms, angiogenesis is a failure of the balance between pro-angiogenic and anti-angiogenic signals. Tumors switch to angiogenesis under a variety of stress signals that result in tumor growth and metastases and, as a general rule, do not grow beyond a size of 1–2 mm without forming new blood vessels (Folkman, 1971). However, the network of blood vessels formed within a tumor can show significant functional deficiencies compared to normal vasculature (e.g., leakiness), and these distinctions can be exploited for imaging. In fact, the angiogenesis trigger in a tumor leads to the formation of new vessels, with capillary endothelial cell characteristics that are not found in normal tissues, and are thus attractive targets themselves.

The emergence of angiogenesis as an important target for cancer therapy has prompted a great deal of new research to understand this molecular process and how it can be manipulated with drugs. Gene expression profiling has identified several proteins that are selectively expressed by new tumor endothelial cells, including a large class of integrins, such as $\alpha_v \beta_3$ and $\alpha_v \beta_5$, providing the potential for specific targeting of therapy (Zhang et al., 2006). This has coincided with the development of molecular imaging methods that provide the potential to detect the angiogenic phenotype and to monitor treatment. Prognosis has been found to be poor when there is a paucity in angiogenesis, perhaps due to hypoxia, or when there is profound angiogenesis, probably because of increased metastatic potential (Koukourakis et al., 2000). Is this a cause-and-effect relationship of two important biological parameters or the result of the tumor genotype? Only additional long-term studies will provide the answer. While angiogenesis is a frequent consequence of hypoxia, some tumors develop extensive angiogenesis without the presence of hypoxia and vice versa, and cannot always establish a cause-and-effect relationship (West et al., 2001).

Von Hippel-Lindau syndrome is a typical example of de novo angiogenesis, where patients develop spontaneous renal tumors as a result of overexpression of HIF1α, producing multiple angiomata due to widespread angiogenesis in the absence of hypoxia. Even in the presence of aggressive angiogenesis, observed blood perfusion rates can be paradoxically lower. Perfusion in a tumor is the result of several biophysical parameters, which might cause a reduced perfusion secondary to tumor growth (Jain et al., 1998). Unfortunately, neither perfusion nor vascular permeability can provide an adequate measure of angiogenesis in the tumor, requiring the whole tumor mass to be studied to address the issue of widespread heterogeneity.

Tumor Hypoxia and Clinical Outcome: New Approach to an Old Problem

The negative influence of hypoxia on response to radiation therapy has long been recognized, with the understanding that oxygen is necessary for "fixing" in the sense of making permanent the radiation-induced cytotoxic products in tissues. In its absence, the free radicals formed by ionizing radiation recombine without producing the anticipated cellular damage (Hall, 2000). In hypoxic conditions, response to radiation is dampened for conventional radiation types and dose schemes. Even though the use of other types of radiation with a low oxygen enhancement ratio (OER) (such as fast neutrons) have been tried in the clinic to address this problem, issues related to the availability and or toxicity limit their clinical role. Clinical and preclinical experience indicates that it can take three times as much photon radiation dose to cause the same cytotoxic effect in hypoxic cells as compared to normoxic cells (Evans and Koch, 2003), although there are potential constraints in escalating the dose to this level for routine clinical use.

Apart from the issues relating hypoxia to radioresistance, we now understand that under hypoxic conditions the viable cells become aggressive, resulting in poor overall outcome due to increased metastatic potential (Hockel et al., 1999). In patients with head and neck cancer, we found the negative effect of hypoxia (based on FMISO PET imaging) on the overall survival (Rajendran et al., 2006). Hypoxia has also been found to promote resistance to a number of chemotherapeutic agents by a variety of related but independent mechanisms.

Many cancer treatment schemes that were introduced to circumvent the cure-limiting consequences of hypoxia have had less than encouraging results (Moulder and Rockwell, 1987). Most importantly, they all suffered from the lack of ability to select patients with significant tumor hypoxia who would have benefited from these types of treatments. Hypoxic cells have always remained as attractive targets for recently introduced hypoxia-activated prodrugs (Brown, 2000) that are less toxic and more effective than their early counterparts such as mitomycin C. These agents are shown to have synergistic toxicity when used with radiation and chemotherapy while exhibiting direct cytotoxic effects. While focal hypoxia within a tumor can be tackled with boost radiation using intensity-modulated radiation therapy (IMRT) (Chao et al., 2001; Rajendran et al., 2003), more diffuse hypoxia will benefit from systemic use of hypoxic cell toxins/sensitizers. Hypoxia imaging with specific tracers is likely to be an efficient tool for selecting patients who might benefit from hypoxia-directed treatment (Rischin et al., 2001). Selecting appropriate patients for a hypoxia-directed therapy will result in the greatest benefit for the individual patient and will reduce unnecessary toxicity to patients who will not benefit from hypoxia-directed cytotoxins.

The Importance of Identifying Hypoxia in Tumors

The negative association of hypoxia to treatment response and clinical outcome strongly implies that evaluating hypoxia will help in identifying tumors with a high hypoxic fraction in order to implement hypoxia-directed treatments and avoiding treatments that are oxygen-dependent. Most commonly used clinico-pathological parameters such as tumor size, grade, and extent of necrosis or blood hemoglobin status, which have historically been used to infer the presence of tumor hypoxia, have not proven to be strong indicators of prognosis. Identification of tumor hypoxia seems prudent in instituting treatments targeting hypoxia, which are capable of overcoming its cure limiting effects.

Methods to Evaluate Tumor Hypoxia

Tumor oxygenation has been evaluated directly by several methods, and tumor hypoxia was found to predict patient outcome in cancers of the uterine cervix (Hockel, 1991), lung (Koh et al., 1995), head and neck (Rajendran et al., 2006), and glioma (Muzi, 2003). As expected, most of these studies have shown significant heterogeneity in hypoxia within a tumor, between tumors, and between patients with similar tumor types.

Currently available assays for tumor hypoxia can be largely categorized as *in vivo* (invasive and noninvasive) or *ex vivo* (invasive biopsy) (Hockel et al., 2001b). To be clinically useful, an assay must distinguish normoxic regions from the regions that are hypoxic at a level relevant to cancer, Po_2 in the 5 mm Hg range. Because of the heterogeneity in hypoxia, regional levels of hypoxia should be measured for individual tumors in patients. It is important for hypoxia-directed imaging and treatment to target chronic hypoxia, as well as acute hypoxia (Rasey et al., 2000), and to directly reflect intracellular Po_2 rather than blood flow or some consequence of O_2 on subsequent biochemistry. The observed temporal heterogeneity in tissue Po_2 suggests that a secondary effect, such as intracellular redox status of thiols, will not be as relevant to cancer treatment outcome as the intracellular partial pressure of O_2. Other desirable characteristics for an ideal clinical hypoxia assay include (1) simple and noninvasive methodology, (2) lack of toxicity, (3) rapid and easy performance with consistency between laboratories, and (4) ability to quantify without the need for substantial calibration of the detection instrumentation. In addition, location of the tumor in a patient should not be a limiting factor for the assay. Lastly, due to spatial heterogeneity in the distribution of hypoxia, the assay must provide a locoregional evaluation of the tumor. Imaging in general and PET in particular have the potential to satisfy all of these requirements to be used in the clinical evaluation of hypoxia.

Polarographic Electrode Measurements of Tissue Oxygenation

Early experience evaluating oxygenation of tumors was based largely on the pioneering work done by direct measurement of O_2 levels using very fine polarographic oxygen electrodes. This assay, simply because it can be calibrated in units of mm Hg, has been referred to as a "gold standard." It is a useful gold standard in terms of attaching a number that would be comparable from laboratory to laboratory on the regional partial pressure of O_2 at the tip of the electrode. However, there are a number of drawbacks, including lack of ability to provide a complete map of a tumor, need for accessible tumor location, closer entry points, presence of blood, and blood vessels in the path. The assay is also technically challenging to perform, and there may be interlaboratory variations in the calibration of the electrodes, which might compromise patient compliance (Vaupel et al., 2001). The electrode studies have, however, been useful in teaching us that the distribution of Po_2 follows a continuum, which means that in individual tumors the imaging contrast between normoxic and hypoxic tissue will be modest—a quantitative difference more than a qualitative difference. Imaging methods for hypoxia provide a complete anatomic as well as functional map of relative oxygenation level in the primary tumor as well as regional metastases with good spatial resolution.

Evaluating Angiogenesis

Angiogenesis can be evaluated by both direct and indirect methods. Direct methods were started with largely fluorescent techniques such as intravital fluorescent video microscopy, and fluorophore coupled of fibronectin, or quenched Near Infra Red (NIR) fluorochromes to matrix metalloproteinase 2 (MMP 2) substrates, MR imaging (Bhujwalla et al., 2001), and color Doppler vascularity index (Chen et al., 2002). The simplicity of dynamic contrast-enhanced (DCE) MRI has led to fairly widespread use of this technique to measure perfusion (Stevenson et al., 2003). It provides a signal that effectively integrates vascular blood flow, blood volume, and vascular permeability, all of which are important features of the angiogenesis phenotype.

Noninvasive imaging of the $\alpha_v\beta_3$ integrins, which are abundant on vascular endothelium, has been attempted by investigators using different modalities such as MR (Sipkins et al., 1998), ultrasound (Leong-Poi et al., 2003), and PET (Beer et al., 2005), and using endostatins (Barthel, 2002). The $\alpha_v\beta_3$ integrin is a transmembrane cell-adhesion receptor that leads to tumor cells binding to extracellular matrix proteins. The receptor is highly expressed on activated endothelial cells but only weakly in mature endothelium, so that imaging receptor density measures new vasculature and not well-established capillaries. This has led to $\alpha_v\beta_3$ integrin being evaluated as a target for tumor-specific therapy of neoangiogenesis in the tumor. The arginine-glycine-aspartic acid (RGD) tripeptide recognizes the $\alpha_v\beta_3$ receptor, although it cross-reacts with other integrins. A labeled RGD-containing glycopeptide shows great promise as an imaging agent and has also been suggested as a potential therapeutic agent (Ogawa et al., 2003).

Blood flow has been used as a surrogate for angiogenesis. Methods to quantify blood flow in tumors range from PET methods to CT or MR. However, imaging and or quantifying angiogenesis itself would provide a different kind of information on the burden of neovascularity in the biological characterization of the tumor, not only for prognosis but also for therapeutic interventions.

Positron Emission Tomography (PET) in Hypoxia Imaging

Hypoxia imaging presents the special challenge of making a positive image out of low levels of O_2 visualizing an "entity" that is not present. Chemists have developed two different imaging agents to address this problem: bioreductive alkylating agents that are O_2 sensitive and metal chelates that are sensitive to the intracellular redox state that develops as a consequence of hypoxia.

Nitroimidazole Compounds

Misonidazole, an azomycin-based hypoxic cell radio sensitizer, introduced in clinical radiation oncology nearly three decades ago, binds covalently to intracellular molecules at levels that are inversely proportional to intracellular oxygen concentration below ~ 10 mm Hg. It is a lipophilic 2-nitroimidazole derivative whose uptake in hypoxic cells is dependent on the sequential reduction of the nitro group on the imidazole ring; electrons from mitochondrial electron transport are added one at a time to the electron-affinic NO_2 group. This sequence produces the radical anion with 1 e^-, the hydroxylamine with the second e^- and the totally reduced amine, $-NH_2$, after six electrons are added. This mechanism requires that the cell be alive in order to provide the electron that initiates the bioreduction step. In the absence of electron transport, the tracer is not reduced or accumulated. The one-electron reduction product is an unstable radical anion that will either give up its extra electron to O_2 or pick up a second electron. In the presence of O_2, the nitroimidazole simply goes through a futile reduction cycle and is returned to its initial state. In the absence of an alternative electron acceptor, the nitroimidazole continues to accumulate electrons to form the hydroxylamine alkylating agent and become trapped within the viable but O_2-deficient cell (Fig. 1). This unique biochemical mechanism leads to a tracer whose uptake is inversely related to the oxygen tension within the cell. If cells are reoxygenated and then exposed to a new batch of the tracer, it will not be accumulated.

[F-18] Fluoromisonidazole (FMISO) is an imaging agent derived from misonidazole, one of the earliest radiosensitizers used in clinical radiation therapy. It has a high "hypoxia-specific factor" (HSF) 20–50 (Rasey et al., 1989). Pro-drug imaging agents such as FMISO are activated by bioreduction in hypoxic tissue, but the process is inhibited by the presence of oxygen in tissues. The result is a positive image of the absence of O_2. FMISO is a highly stable and robust radio-pharmaceutical that can be used to quantify tissue hypoxia using PET technology (Grierson et al., 1989). Its easy synthesis and optimal safety profile are responsible for its ready acceptance in the clinic. After extensive clinical validation, FMISO remains the most commonly used agent for hypoxia PET imaging. Its biodistribution and dosimetry characteristics are ideal for PET imaging. The partition coefficient of FMISO is 0.41, similar to that of the blood flow agent anti-pyrine, so that initially after injection, the tissue distribution reflects blood flow, but after ~ 1 hr the distribution reflects its partition coefficient. It is homogeneously distributed with no normal tissue specificity (Martin et al., 1992).

Narrow distribution of pixel uptake values (mean T:B ≈ 1.0) after ~ 90 min has led to a simple analysis of FMISO-PET images by scaling the pixel uptake to plasma concentration. The mean value for this ratio in all tissues is close to unity, and almost all normoxic pixels have a value of < 1.2. The magnitude of the intermediate radical anion product parallels nitroreductase levels, which vary only slightly between normoxic tissues, so this factor does not affect the imaging analysis of fractional hypoxic volume. The optimum time for imaging appears to be between 90 and 120 min and can be adjusted to fit the clinic schedule so that to the patient or the imaging technologist the procedure is very similar to that of a bone scan. While the tumor:background ratio image does not show high contrast, this does not compromise image interpretation. Hypoxia images can be interpreted in several ways, both qualitatively or quantitatively.

Qualitative interpretations have been used with a scoring system to grade the uptake in a tumor compared to adjacent normal tissue (Rischin et al., 2001). After extensive validation studies, we have preferred a simple but accurate quantitation method using a venous blood sample drawn during the imaging sequence to calculate a tissue:blood ratio (Fig. 2). Other studies have used tumor-to-muscle ratio for this purpose (Yeh et al., 1996).

Fractional hypoxic volume (FHV), defined as the proportion of pixels within the imaged tumor volume having a ratio above some cut-off value, is an extrapolation from radiobiology (Rasey et al., 1996), but this requires accurate delineation of tumor margins to define the denominator. It is not the same as radiobiological hypoxic function as determined from analysis of cell survival curves. We prefer the tumor hypoxic volume (HV) parameter, which is the total number of pixels with a T:B ≥ 1.2 expressed in ml and is a measure of the extent of tissue hypoxia within a tumor, without the need for stringent demarcation of the tumor boundaries. This simple analysis is also unaffected by perfusion but only requires the viability of the hypoxic cell as defined by active electron transport. Mathematical models have been investigated for more detailed analysis of FMISO uptake but are probably too complicated for routine clinical imaging.

A typical FMISO-PET scanning protocol uses an intra-venous administration of a dose of 3.7 MBq (0.1 mCi)/kg, which results in an effective total body dose equivalent of 0.0126 mGy/MBq. Scanning begins after 90–120 min and lasts for 20 min, with blood sampling midway during the scan. A transmission scan is used for attenuation correction of emission data. Typically, one axial field-of-view (AFOV) of 15-centimeter cranio-caudal dimension centered over the tumor region is acquired. An FDG scan of the same region is routinely obtained for these patients, with care taken to reposition the patients between images.

Other Azomycin Imaging Agents

In order to improve image contrast, some scientists have developed alternative azomycin radiopharmaceuticals for

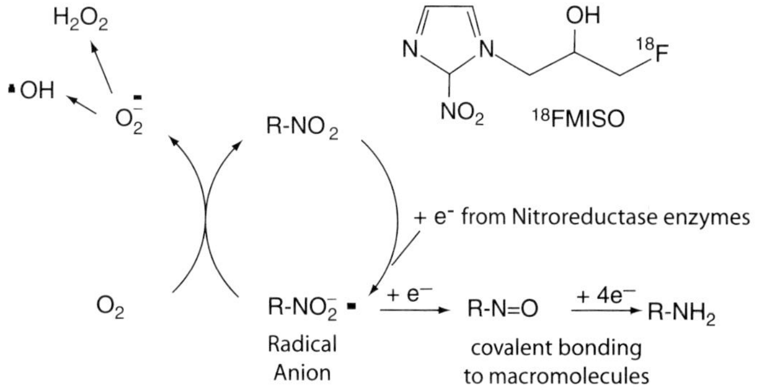

Figure 1 Structure of misonidazole showing the mechanism of action in the presence and absence of oxygen.

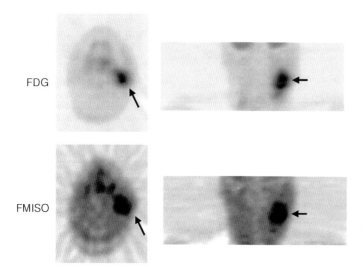

Figure 2 Corresponding FDG (top) and FMISO (bottom) images in transaxial (left) and coronal (right) of a patient with cancer of the tongue with metastatic lymph node in the left neck (arrow). The FDG SUV_{max} was 25.4, and FMISO tissue:blood $_{max}$ was 1.62.

hypoxia imaging by attempting to manipulate the rate of blood clearance (Chapman *et al.*, 2001). EF − 1 was initially developed because of the availability of an antibody stain to verify the distribution in tissue samples (Kachur *et al.*, 1999). Fluoroerythronitroimidazole (FETNIM) was developed as a more hydrophilic derivative of misonidazole that might have more rapid plasma clearance, and this could be an imaging advantage. Fluoroetanidazole has binding characteristics similar to FMISO but has been reported to have less retention in liver and fewer metabolites in animals. However, the advantages were not sufficient to carry these derivatives to wide clinical testing. Hypoxia imaging compounds based on single photon emission computerized tomography (SPECT) have been introduced with the hope of taking this technology to gamma camera imaging (Wiebe and Stypinski, 1996). Because direct halogenation of the imidazole ring does not lead to a stable radiopharmaceutical, the general approach has been to place sugar residues between the nitroimidazole and the radioiodine to stabilize the molecule to *in vivo* decomposition. The resulting images have higher contrast when imaging is typically initiated 1.5 to 2 hr after injection. However, a simple ratio analysis to infer hypoxia, as used for FMISO images, is not valid.

The success with radioiodinated azamycin arabinosides (IAZA) led to attempts to develop technetium derivatives of 2-nitroimidazole. The practical advantages of a Tc-99m label are well known in the nuclear medicine community and include ready availability at low cost, convenient half-life for hypoxia measurements, and versatile chemistry. A number of BMS compounds involving a nitroimidazole group were developed: BMS181321, HL91, and BMS194796, the last-named compound having less lipophilicity (Rumsey *et al.*, 1995). The HL91 molecule, TcBnAO, does not include a nitroimidazole; the Tc-ligand coordination chemistry is directly reduced and retained in hypoxic environments (Siim *et al.*, 2000). The resulting lack of specificity

and the need for a much higher level of hypoxia raised concerns for routine clinical applications (Zhang *et al.*, 1998).

Single photon emission computerized tomography (SPECT) radiopharmaceuticals include both the iodinated compounds (e.g., [123I] IAZA) and technetium-based agents. These radiopharmaceuticals, in contrast to PET agents, suffer from lower image contrast and less potential for quantification (Nunn *et al.*, 1995). Furthermore, the absence of a gold standard for hypoxia evaluation complicates validation of all hypoxia markers, including FMISO. Thus, treatment outcome studies are urgently needed to provide convincing evidence for the clinical value of hypoxia imaging.

The altered redox environment associated with hypoxia has led to another class of radiopharmaceuticals for imaging hypoxia. Copper bis(thiosemicarbazones) are a class of molecules evaluated as freely diffusible but retained blood flow tracers. The ^{64}Cu-labeled acetyl derivative of pyruvaldehyde bis [N4-methylthiosemicarbazonato] copper (II) complex, Cu-ATSM, has the potential advantage of a longer half-life for practical clinical use (Dehdashti *et al.*, 2003), although the mechanism of retention is less well validated than that of FMISO. Fujibayashi *et al.* (1997) showed that the intracellular retention mechanism was related to the copper reduction chemistry, Cu^{++} to Cu^{+}, which has a redox potential of −297 mV for Cu-ATSM. Several biological systems have comparable redox potentials: −315 mV for NADH and −230 mV for glutathione.

Cu-ATSM has rapid washout from normoxic areas. Copper agents are very useful for identifying regions of tissue that have higher levels of reducing agents such as NADH as a consequence of hypoxia. There is ample evidence in the literature that the concentration of NADH is increased under extended hypoxic conditions. This mechanism is distinct from that for the nitroimidazoles in that the copper agents reflect a consequence of hypoxia rather than the actual Po_2. This mechanistic difference might dampen the role of

Cu-ATSM for measuring a prompt reoxygenation response because the increased levels of NADH will persist longer. Diffusion of NADH-related reducing equivalents might make Cu-ATSM less reflective of the spatial heterogeneity of hypoxia. However, the same characteristics make the Cu agents preferable for imaging chronic hypoxia where levels of NADH can increase by severalfold. Several PET radionuclides of copper can be used for imaging (Ballinger, 2001).

With its noninvasive and less operator-dependent nature and the ability to image the entire tumor and lymphatic drainage areas in a snap-shot fashion, PET imaging will easily become the dominant method for the clinical evaluation of tumor hypoxia. The main advantage of PET is its ability to accurately quantify tissue uptake of the hypoxia tracer, independent of anatomic location of the tumor. Expanding availability of PET scanners (and now PET/CT scanners), as well as easy access to ^{18}F-labeled hypoxia tracers in the community, will bring this procedure within reach of community nuclear medicine centers. The utility of hypoxia imaging is twofold: (1) the level of pretherapy hypoxia is an important prognostic parameter and (2) change in hypoxic volume with treatment will provide a better understanding of treatment response and a target for radiation boost.

Hypoxia imaging can be combined with other indicators of tissue hemodynamics and oxygenation, such as perfusion imaging, using [^{15}O]water, and tissue markers of proteomic response to hypoxia, such as vascular density and HIF1α expression using immunocytochemistry as well as angiogenesis imaging, all complementing one another to characterize individual tumors and patients. The greatest advantage of PET/CT imaging will be the improved accuracy in localizing hypoxia and making it possible to incorporate these images into radiation treatment planning systems to safely plan and deliver a hypoxia-directed radiotherapy boost using intensity-modulated radiation therapy (IMRT) within the framework of radiobiological rationale.

Summary

Tumor hypoxia, one of the great challenges facing cancer management, can now be easily evaluated, quantified, and targeted for therapy because of recent advances in the fields of imaging, treatment planning, and delivery. Oncologists can be provided with relevant quantitative information on the tumor microenvironment, along with other biological profiles of the tumor, to effectively plan appropriate therapy that can overcome the cure-limiting effects of hypoxia by providing an objective means for treatment selection and planning. The limited quantitative potential of SPECT and MRI will be a factor in their widespread clinical use. In contrast, clinical hypoxia imaging using FMISO and Cu-ATSM are in advanced stages of clinical experience, to be studied in cooperative multicenter trials in order to validate their roles in addressing the problem of hypoxia in cancer patients. Technological advances in radiation treatment planning, such as IMRT (intensity-modulated radiation therapy) or IGRT (image-guided radiotherapy) provide us with the ability to individualize radiation delivery and target volume coverage (Alber *et al.*, 2003). With the incorporation of regional biological information such as hypoxia and proliferating vasculature in treatment planning, imaging can create a biological profile of the tumor to direct therapy (Ling *et al.*, 2000). Presence of widespread hypoxia in the tumor can be effectively targeted with a systemic hypoxic cell cytotoxin such as tirapazamine (Covens *et al.*, 2006). Information gained from angiogenesis imaging will provide additional information about the hypoxia–angiogenesis connection and complement the efforts in developing anti-angiogenesis therapy or hypoxia-targeted drugs for tumor and patient and tumor-specific treatment. Optimal characterization of therapeutic targets is essential for the development and clinical evaluation of novel drugs targeting angiogenesis and hypoxia (Hammond *et al.*, 2003). Hypoxia imaging provides information that is different from that of FDG-PET and should play a pivotal role in oncologic imaging in the very near future.

Among all the hypoxia imaging radiopharmaceuticals, Cu-ATSM images show the best contrast early after injection, but these images are confounded by blood flow. In addition, their mechanism of localization appears to be one step removed from the intracellular O$_2$ concentration. The FMISO images show less contrast than those of Cu-ATSM because of its lipophilicity and slower clearance. The criticism that FMISO is inadequate because of its clearance characteristics is negated because its uptake after 2 hr is the purest reflection of regional Po$_2$ at the time of radiopharmaceutical administration. The imaging community should make a more convincing case for clinical hypoxia imaging in characterizing tumor hypoxia for effective targeting of hypoxia. Similarly, addition of angiogenesis imaging provides complementary information that can be used to further characterize tumors and individualize the treatment approaches for the patient.

Acknowledgments

We thank Lanell Peterson and Holly Pike for their help in preparing this manuscript.

References

Alber, M., Paulsen, F., Eschmann, S.M., and Machulla, H.J. 2003. On biologically conformal boost dose optimization. *Phys. Med. Biol. 48*: N31–N35.

Ballinger, J.R. 2001. Imaging hypoxia in tumors. *Semin. Nucl. Med. 31*:321–329.

Barthel, H. 2002. Endostatin imaging to help understanding of antiangiogenic drugs. *Lancet Oncol. 3*:520.

Beer, A.J., Haubner, R., Goebel, M., Luderschmidt, S., Spilker, M.E., Wester, H.J., Weber, W.A., and Schwaiger, M. 2005. Biodistribution and pharmacokinetics of the alphavbeta3-selective tracer 18F-galacto-RGD in cancer patients. *J. Nucl. Med. 46*:1333–1341.

Bhujwalla, Z.M., Artemov, D., Aboagye, E., Ackerstaff, E., Gillies, R.J., Natarajan, K., and Solaiyappan, M. 2001. The physiological environment in cancer vascularization, invasion and metastasis. *Novartis Found. Symp. 240*:23–38; discussion 38–45, 152–153.

Bos, R., Zhong, H., Hanrahan, C.F., Mommers, E.C., Semenza, G.L., Pinedo, H.M., Abeloff, M.D., Simons, J.W., van Diest, P.J., and van der Wall, E. 2001. Levels of hypoxia-inducible factor-1 alpha during breast carcinogenesis. *J. Natl. Cancer Inst. 93*:309–314.

Brown, J.M. 2000. Exploiting the hypoxic cancer cell: mechanisms and therapeutic strategies. *Mol. Med. Today 6*:157–162.

Chao, K.S., Bosch, W.R., Mutic, S., Lewis, J.S., Dehdashti, F., Mintun, M.A., Dempsey, J.F., Perez, C.A., Purdy, J.A., and Welch, M.J. 2001. A novel approach to overcome hypoxic tumor resistance: Cu-ATSM-guided intensity-modulated radiation therapy. *Int. J. Radiat. Oncol. Biol. Phys. 49*:1171–1182.

Chapman, J.D., Schneider, R.F., Urbain, J.L., and Hanks, G.E. 2001. Single-photon emission computed tomography and positron-emission tomography assays for tissue oxygenation. *Semin. Radiat. Oncol. 11*:47–57.

Chen, C.N., Cheng, Y.M., Lin, M.T., Hsieh, F.J., Lee, P.H., and Chang, K.J. 2002. Association of color Doppler vascularity index and microvessel density with survival in patients with gastric cancer. *Ann. Surg. 235*:512–518.

Covens, A., Blessing, J., Bender, D., Mannel, R., and Morgan, M. 2006. A Phase II evaluation of tirapazamine plus cisplatin in the treatment of recurrent platinum-sensitive ovarian or primary peritoneal cancer: a gynecologic oncology group study. *Gynecol. Oncol. 100*:586–590.

Dachs, G.U., and Tozer, G.M. 2000. Hypoxia modulated gene expression: angiogenesis, metastasis and therapeutic exploitation. *Eur. J. Cancer 36*:1649–1660.

Dehdashti, F., Mintun, M.A., Lewis, J.S., Bradley, J., Govindan, R., Laforest, R., Welch, M.J., and Siegel, B.A. 2003. *In vivo* assessment of tumor hypoxia in lung cancer with 60Cu-ATSM. *Eur. J. Nucl. Med. Mol. Imaging 30*:844–850.

Evans, S.M., and Koch, C.J. 2003. Prognostic significance of tumor oxygenation in humans. *Cancer Lett. 195*:1–16.

Folkman, J. 1971. Tumor angiogenesis: therapeutic implications. *N. Engl. J. Med. 285*:1182–1186.

Fujibayashi, Y., Taniuchi, H., Yonekura, Y., Ohtani, H., Konishi, J., and Yokoyama, A. 1997. Copper-62-ATSM: a new hypoxia imaging agent with high membrane permeability and low redox potential. *J. Nucl. Med. 38*:1155–1160.

Gambhir, S.S. 2002. Molecular imaging of cancer with positron emission tomography. *Nat. Rev. Cancer 2*:683–693.

Grierson, J.R., Link, J.M., Mathis, C.A., Rasey, J.S., and Krohn, K.A. 1989. Radiosynthesis of fluorine-18 fluoromisonidazole. *J. Nucl. Med. 30*:343–350.

Guillemin, K., and Krasnoq, M.A. 1997. The hypoxic response: huffing and HIFing. *Cell 89*:9–12.

Hall, E.J. 2000. *Radiobiology for the Radiologist*. Philadelphia: Lippincott Williams & Wilkins.

Hammond, L.A., Denis, L., Salman, U., Jerabek, P., Thomas, C.R., Jr., and Kuhn, J.G. 2003. Positron emission tomography (PET): expanding the horizons of oncology drug development. *Invest: New Drugs 21*:309–340.

Hanahan, D., and Weinberg, R.A. 2000. The hallmarks of cancer. *Cell 100*:57–70.

Herschman, H.R. 2003. Molecular imaging: looking at problems, seeing solutions. *Science 302*:605–608.

Hockel, M., Schlenger, K., Hockel, S., and Vaupel, P. 1999. Hypoxic cervical cancers with low apoptotic index are highly aggressive. *Cancer Res. 59*:4525–4528.

Hockel, M., Schlenger, K., Knoop, C., and Vaupel, P. 1991. Oxygenation of carcinomas of the uterine cervix: evaluation by computerized O2 tension measurements. *Cancer Res. 51*:6098–6102.

Hockel, M., and Vaupel, P. 2001a. Biological consequences of tumor hypoxia. *Semin. Oncol. 28*:36–41.

Hockel, M., and Vaupel, P. 2001b. Tumor hypoxia: definitions and current clinical, biologic, and molecular aspects. *J. Natl. Cancer Inst. 93*:266–276.

Huang, L.E., Arany, Z., Livingston, D.M., and Bunn, H.F. 1996. Activation of hypoxia-inducible transcription factor depends primarily upon redox-sensitive stabilization of its alpha subunit. *J. Biol. Chem. 271*:32253–32259.

Ivan, M., Kondo, K., Yang, H., Kim, W., Valiando, J., Ohh, M., Salic, A., Asara, J.M., Lane, W.S., and Kaelin, W.G., Jr. 2001. HIFalpha targeted for VHL-mediated destruction by proline hydroxylation: implications for O2 sensing. *Science 292*:464–468.

Jain, R.K., Safabakhsh, N., Sckell, A., Chen, Y., Jiang, P., Benjamin, L., Yuan, F., and Keshet, E. 1998. Endothelial cell death, angiogenesis, and microvascular function after castration in an androgen-dependent tumor: role of vascular endothelial growth factor. *Proc. Natl. Acad. Sci. USA 95*:10820–10825.

Kachur, A.V., Dolbier, W.R., Jr., Evans, S.M., Shiue, C.Y., Shiue, G.G., Skov, K.A., Baird, I.R., James, B.R., Li, A.R., Roche, A., and Koch, C.J. 1999. Synthesis of new hypoxia markers EF1 and [18F]-EF1. *Appl. Radiat. Isot. 51*:643–650.

Koh, W.J., Bergman, K.S., Rasey, J.S., Peterson, L.M., Evans, M.L., Graham, M.M., Grierson, J.R., Lindsley, K.L., Lewellen, T.K., Krohn, K.A., and Griffin, T.W. 1995. Evaluation of oxygenation status during fractionated radiotherapy in human nonsmall cell lung cancers using [F-18]fluoromisonidazole positron emission tomography. *Int. J. Radiat. Oncol. Biol. Phys. 33*:391–398.

Koukourakis, M.I., Giatromanolaki, A., Sivridis, E., and Fezoulidis, I. 2000. Cancer vascularization: implications in radiotherapy? *Int. J. Radiat. Oncol. Biol. Phys. 48*:545–553.

Leong-Poi, H., Christiansen, J.P., Klibanov, A.L., Kaul, S., and Lindner, J.R. 2003. Noninvasive assessment of angiogenesis by contrast ultrasound imaging with microbubbles targeted to alpha-V integrins. *J. Am. Coll. Cardiol. 41*:430–431.

Ling, C.C., Humm, J., Larson, S., Amols, H., Fuks, Z., Leibel, S., and Koutcher, J.A. 2000. Towards multidimensional radiotherapy (MD-CRT): biological imaging and biological conformality. *Int. J. Radiat. Oncol. Biol. Phys. 47*:551–560.

Maclean, D., Northrop, J.P., Padgett, H.C., and Walsh, J.C. 2003. Drugs and probes: the symbiotic relationship between pharmaceutical discovery and imaging science. *Mol. Imaging Biol. 5*:304–311.

Martin, G.V., Caldwell, J.H., Graham, M.M., Grierson, J.R., Kroll, K., Cowan, M.J., Lewellen, T.K., Rasey, J.S., Casciari, J.J., and Krohn, K.A. 1992. Noninvasive detection of hypoxic myocardium using fluorine-18-fluoromisonidazole and positron emission tomography. *J. Nucl. Med. 33*:2202–2208.

Marxsen, J.H., Schmitt, O., Metzen, E., Jelkmann, W., and Hellwig-Burgel, T. 2001. Vascular endothelial growth factor gene expression in the human breast cancer cell line MX-1 is controlled by O2 availability *in vitro* and *in vivo*. *Ann. Anat. 183*:243–249.

Moulder, J.E., and Rockwell, S. 1987. Tumor hypoxia: its impact on cancer therapy. *Cancer Metast. Rev. 5*:313–341.

Muzi, M., Spence, A.M., Rajendran, J.G., Grierson, J.R., and Krohn, K.A. 2003. Glioma patients assessed with FMISO and FDG: two tracers provide different information. *J. Nucl. Med. 44*:878.

Nunn, A., Linder, K., and Strauss, H.W. 1995. Nitroimidazoles and imaging hypoxia. *Eur. J. Nucl. Med. 22*:265–280.

Ogawa, M., Hatano, K., Oishi, S., Kawasumi, Y., Fujii, N., Kawaguchi, M., Doi, R., Imamura, M., Yamamoto, M., Ajito, K., Mukai, T., Saji, H., and Ito, K. 2003. Direct electrophilic radiofluorination of a cyclic RGD peptide for *in vivo* alpha(v)beta3 integrin related tumor imaging. *Nucl. Med. Biol. 30*:1–9.

Peters, L., and McKay, M. 2001. Predictive assays: will they ever have a role in the clinic? *Int. J. Radiat. Oncol. Biol. Phys. 49*:501–504.

Pomper, M.G. 2005. Translational molecular imaging for cancer. *Cancer Imaging 5 (Suppl)*:S16–S26.

Rajendran, J.G., O'Sullivan, F., Peterson, L.M., Schwartz, D.L., Conrad, E.U., Spence, A.M., Muzi, M., Farwell, D.G., and Krohn, K. 2004. Hypoxia and glucose metabolism in malignant tumors: evaluation by FMISO and FDG PET imaging. *Clin. Cancer. Res. 10*:2245–2252.

Rajendran, J.G., M. J., Schwartz, D.L., Kinahan, P.E., Cheng, P., Hummel, S.M., Lewellen, B., Philips, M., and Krohn, K.A. 2003. Imaging with F-18 FMISO-PET permits hypoxia directed radiotherapy dose escalation for head and neck cancer. *J. Nucl. Med. 44*:415.

Rajendran, J.G., Schwartz, D.L., O'Sullivan, J., Peterson, L.M., Ng, P., Scarnhorst, J., Grierrson, J.R., and Krohn, K.A. 2006. Tumor hypoxia imaging with [F-18] FMISO PET in head and neck cancer: value of pre-therapy FMISO uptake in predicting survival. *Clin. Cancer Res. 12*:5435–5441.

Rasey, J.S., Casciari, J.J., Hofstrand, P.D., Muzi, M., Graham, M.M., and Chin, L.K. 2000. Determining hypoxic fraction in a rat glioma by uptake of radiolabeled fluoromisonidazole. *Radiat. Res. 153*:84–92.

Rasey, J.S., Koh, W.J., Evans, M.L., Peterson, L.M., Lewellen, T.K., Graham, M.M., and Krohn, K.A. 1996. Quantifying regional hypoxia in human tumors with positron emission tomography of [18F]fluoromisonidazole: a pretherapy study of 37 patients. *Int. J. Radiat. Oncol. Biol. Phys. 36*:417–428.

Rasey, J.S., Koh, W.J., Grierson, J.R., Grunbaum, Z., and Krohn, K.A. 1989. Radiolabelled fluoromisonidazole as an imaging agent for tumor hypoxia. *Int. J. Radiat. Oncol. Biol. Phys. 17*:985–991.

Rischin, D., Peters, L., Hicks, R., Hughes, P., Fisher, R., Hart, R., Sexton, M., D'Costa, I., and von Roemeling, R. 2001. Phase I trial of concurrent tirapazamine, cisplatin, and radiotherapy in patients with advanced head and neck cancer. *J. Clin. Oncol. 19*:535–542.

Rumsey, W.L., Kuczynski, B., Patel, B., Bauer, A., Narra, R.K., Eaton, S.M., Nunn, A.D., and Strauss, H.W. 1995. SPECT imaging of ischemic myocardium using a technetium-99m-nitroimidazole ligand. *J. Nucl. Med. 36*:1445–1450.

Siim, B.G., Laux, W.T., Rutland, M.D., Palmer, B.N., and Wilson, W.R. 2000. Scintigraphic imaging of the hypoxia marker (99m)technetium-labeled 2,2′-(1,4-diaminobutane)bis(2-methyl-3-butanone) dioxime (99mTc-labeled HL-91; prognox): noninvasive detection of tumor response to the antivascular agent 5,6-dimethylxanthenone-4-acetic acid. *Cancer Res. 60*:4582–4588.

Sipkins, D.A., Cheresh, D.A., Kazemi, M.R., Nevin, L.M., Bednarski, M.D., and Li, K.C. 1998. Detection of tumor angiogenesis *in vivo* by alpha Vbeta3-targeted magnetic resonance imaging. *Nat. Med. 4*:623–626.

Stevenson, J.P., Rosen, M., Sun, W., Gallagher, M., Haller, D.G., Vaughn, D., Giantonio, B., Zimmer, R., Petros, W.P., Stratford, M., Chaplin, D., Young, S.L., Schnall, M., and O'Dwyer, P.J. 2003. Phase I trial of the antivascular agent combretastatin A4 phosphate on a 5-day schedule to patients with cancer: magnetic resonance imaging evidence for altered tumor blood flow. *J. Clin. Oncol. 21*:4428–4438.

Thomlinson, R.H., and Gray, L.H. 1955. The histological structure of some human lung cancers and the possible implications for radiotherapy. *Br. J. Cancer 9*:537–549.

Vaupel, P., Kelleher, D.K., and Hockel, M. 2001. Oxygen status of malignant tumors: pathogenesis of hypoxia and significance for tumor therapy. *Semin. Oncol. 28*:29–35.

Wahl, R.L. 2003. Anatomolecular imaging with 2-deoxy-2-[18F]fluoro-D-glucose: bench to outpatient center. *Mol. Imaging Biol. 5*:49–56.

Wellmann, S., Guschmann, M., Griethe, W., Eckert, C., von Stackelberg, A., Lottaz, C., Moderegger, E., Einsiedel, H.G., Eckardt, K.U., Henze, G., Seeger, K., and Stackelberg, A. 2004. Activation of the HIF pathway in childhood ALL, prognostic implications of VEGF. *Leukemia 18*:926–933.

West, C.M., Cooper, R.A., Loncaster, J.A., Wilks, D.P., and Bromley, M. 2001. Tumor vascularity: a histological measure of angiogenesis and hypoxia. *Cancer Res. 61*:2907–2910.

Wiebe, L.I., and Stypinski, D. 1996. Pharmacokinetics of SPECT radiopharmaceuticals for imaging hypoxic tissues. *Q. J. Nucl. Med. 40*:270–284.

Yeh, S.H., Liu, R.S., Wu, L.C., Yang, D.J., Yen, S.H., Chang, C.W., Yu, T.W., Chou, K.L., and Chen, K.Y. 1996. Fluorine-18 fluoromisonidazole tumour to muscle retention ratio for the detection of hypoxia in nasopharyngeal carcinoma. *Eur. J. Nucl. Med. 23*:1378–1383.

Zhang, X., Melo, T., Ballinger, J.R., and Rauth, A.M. 1998. Studies of 99mTc-BnAO (HL-91): a non-nitroaromatic compound for hypoxic cell detection. *Int. J. Radiat. Oncol. Biol. Phys. 42*:737–740.

Zhang, X., Xiong, Z., Wu, Y., Cai, W., Tseng, J.R., Gambhir, S.S., and Chen, X. 2006. Quantitative PET imaging of tumor integrin {alpha}v{beta}3 expression with 18F-FRGD2. *J. Nucl. Med. 47*:113–121.

12

Noninvasive Determination of Angiogenesis: Molecular Targets and Tracer Development

Roland Haubner

Introduction

Angiogenesis-Related Disorders

Formation of blood vessels is an important process not only in the developing embryo but also in vascular remodeling in the adult. In early development, this process is referred to as vasculogenesis and is characterized by *in situ* differentiation of endothelial progenitor cells (e.g., angioblasts) into endothelial cells that assemble into a vascular labyrinth (Carmeliet and Jain, 2000). In contrast, angiogenesis is the process that results in the formation of new vessels by the sprouting of existing vessels into an avascular tissue. Angiogenesis is involved in numerous biological processes, such as embryogenesis, tissue remodeling, female reproductive cycle, and wound healing. Also, numerous disorders are characterized by either an excess or an insufficient number of blood vessels. The best known disorders are rheumatoid arthritis (Storgard *et al.*, 1999), psoriasis (Creamer *et al.*, 2002), restenosis (Bishop *et al.*, 2001), diabetic retinopathy (Chavakis *et al.*, 2002), and tumor growth (Folkman, 2002). There are a variety of other inflammatory, allergic, infectious, traumatic, metabolic, and hormonal disorders, which are characterized by upregulated vessel growth (Carmeliet, 2003). Thus, the field of angiogenesis research has evolved to become one of the most rapidly growing biomedical disciplines. The interest in basic angiogenesis research is sparked by the translational therapeutic potential aimed at developing anti-angiogenesis drugs as novel therapeutics for tumors and a number of nononcological diseases.

Under certain pathological conditions, dysfunction of this highly regulated process results in aberrant angiogenesis (Carmeliet, 2005). An understanding of this imbalance is required to develop therapeutic strategies. Most of the current knowledge of the mechanisms results from studying tumor-induced angiogenesis. Tumors larger than 1–2 mm in diameter induce formation of new blood vessels to overcome tumor dormancy (Ranieri and Gasparini, 2001). Becoming an angiogenic phenotype, the balance between pro- and anti-angiogenic factors is upset, contributing to the uncontrolled growth of the tumor. However, angiogenesis is required not only to guarantee sufficient nutrient supply but also to enable tumor cells to migrate into the surrounding tissue and to form metastases (Folkman, 1995). Although the processes inducing this "angiogenic switch" are not completely understood, it is likely that tumor-suppressor mutation, oncogene activation, and hypoxia play important roles in tumor-induced angiogenesis.

Uncontrolled angiogenesis is also involved in diabetic retinopathy. As a result of retinal ischemia, the pathologic proliferation of blood vessels is a major cause of blindness in diabetic patients (Lee *et al.*, 1998). Again, hypoxia seems to be a trigger. It is found that especially hypoxic portions of the retina release angiogenic factors that stimulate neovascularization. Abnormal ocular angiogenesis may ultimately cause severe vitreous cavity bleeding, retinal detachment, and glaucoma leading to blindness.

Rheumatoid arthritis is a chronic inflammatory condition that involves all elements of the immune response (Szekanecz *et al.*, 2005). Its etiology is complex and centers on the development of autoantibodies and immune complexes. The multistage pathogenesis involves cytokines, rheumatoid factors, and angiogenesis. New vessel formation is crucial for leukocyte extravasation during inflammatory synovitis. In analogy to tumor-induced angiogenesis, the outcome of neovascularization in the rheumatoid arthritis synovium is highly dependent on the balance or imbalance between angiogenic mediators and inhibitors. For example serum level of VEGF, TNF-α, and TGF-β are increased in rheumatoid arthritis patients. Several attempts have been made to therapeutically interfere with the cellular and molecular mechanisms under-

lying rheumatoid arthritis-associated neovascularization. One of the most promising strategies is based on TNF-α-neutralizing molecules (Feldmann *et al.*, 2005).

Psoriasis is a chronic inflammatory disease of the skin that is characterized by well-demarcated, symmetrical erythematous plaques most commonly found on trunk, elbows, knees, and scalp. Although there is evidence indicating that psoriasis is primarily lymphocyte driven, the prominence of dermal microvascular expansion in lesional skin suggests that psoriasis is also angiogenesis-dependent (Creamer *et al.*, 2002).

Molecular Background

Angiogenesis is a multistep process that is regulated by a balance between pro- and anti-angiogenic factors (Ellis *et al.*, 2002; Kuwano *et al.*, 2001) (Fig. 1). The angiogenic switch is often triggered by an insufficient nutrient supply resulting in

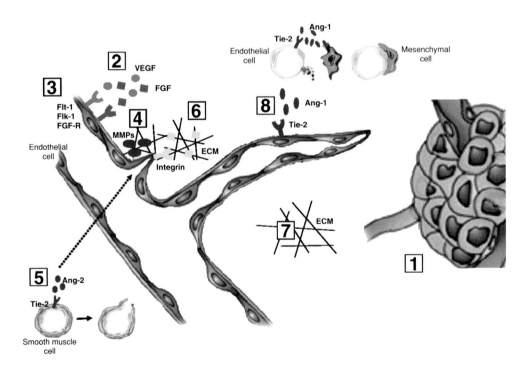

Figure 1 Schematic presentation of the key steps in tumor-induced angiogenesis. The activation of quiescent endothelial cells (**2**) can be triggered by hypoxia (**1**), inducing the expression of hypoxia response genes, such as vascular endothelial growth factor (VEGF) (**2**). However, other stimuli such as metabolic stress, inflammatory response, and genetic mutations can also activate these processes. Further angiogenesis-regulating factors are locally secreted (**2**). These include basic and acid fibroblast growth factor (bFGF, aFGF) and platelet-derived endothelial cell growth factor (PDGF). After activation, the endothelial cells express growth factor receptors (**3**) and excrete proteolytic enzymes (**4**), such as matrix metalloproteinases (MMPs) to degrade the extracellular matrix surrounding the vessels. Tie-2 is upregulated, which is involved in the capillary destabilization (**5**). Activated endothelial cells express cell-adhesion molecules like the αvβ3 integrin (**6**), which allow interaction with and migration through the extracellular matrix (ECM) during vessel formation. Finally, ECM proteins such as tenascin and collagens are produced to provide new basement membrane components (**7**). Capillary organization and stabilization are mediated by interaction of Tie-2 receptor tyrosine kinase with angiopoietin-1 (Ang-1) (**8**). The newly built endothelial cells reorganize by forming tight junctions. These new tubes connect with the microcirculation, resulting in an operational new vasculature.

hypoxic cells (Carmeliet and Jain, 2000). Activation is carried out by binding of the hypoxia-inducible factor to the hypoxia response element, which subsequently turns on expression of vascular endothelial growth factor (VEGF), a key player in the growth and maturation of vessels. Additional regulators of VEGF expression are glucose concentration, pH, and several oncogenes (Bikfalvi and Bicknell, 2002). However, other stimuli such as genetic mutations, mechanical and metabolic stress, and immune/inflammatory response can also activate production of angiogenic factors. A variety of regulating factors (e.g., transforming growth factor β [TGF-β], platelet-derived endothelial cell growth factor [PDGF], and basic and acid fibroblast growth factor [bFGF, aFGF]) are involved in these processes, and are locally secreted by numerous cells such as endothelial cells, stromal cells, and cancer cells, but can also emanate from blood and the extracellular matrix (Hagedorn and Bikfalvi, 2000; Kuwano et al., 2001).

After activation, the endothelial cells excrete proteolytic enzymes, such as matrix metalloproteinases (MMPs) and serine proteases, to degrade the basement membrane and the extracellular matrix (ECM) surrounding the vessels, allowing migration of endothelial cells in the basement membrane (Rundhaug, 2005). In the last few years, it has become clear that MMPs contribute more to angiogenesis than simply degrading ECM components. On the one hand, matrix metalloproteinases have a pro-angiogenic role by, for example, releasing matrix-bound pro-angiogenic factors. On the other hand, they can also play an anti-angiogenic role, by, for example, cleaving matrix components into anti-angiogenic factors (for details, see Rundhaug, 2005). The disruption of this balance contributes to the outcome of the angiogenic switch.

Integrins, which mediate cell-matrix interactions, are one receptor class playing a key role during migration of the endothelial cells in the basement membrane (Eliceiri and Cheresh, 2000). In addition, these receptors are not only involved in endothelial cell adhesion but are also important in the regulation of endothelial cell growth, survival, and differentiation during the angiogenic process. It has been demonstrated that monoclonal antibodies as well as low-molecular-weight reagents that recognize the integrins αvβ3 and αvβ5 block angiogenesis in murine tumor models and in retinal angiogenesis (Brooks et al., 1994, 1995; Hammes et al., 1996). However, based on several knock-out experiments, there is evidence that αvβ3 and αvβ5 are anti-angiogenic or negative regulators of angiogenesis rather than pro-angiogenic (Hynes, 2002). It is conceivable that these integrins could play both positive and negative roles in different phases of angiogenesis. In contrast, the integrin α5β1 and its ligand, fibronectin, are clearly pro-angiogenic. Genetic ablation of either integrin leads to embryonic lethality with major vascular defects (Yang et al., 1993) and antibodies or peptides blocking their interactions inhibit angiogenesis (Kim et al., 2000).

In addition, extracellular matrix proteins such as laminin, tenascin, or collagen-type IV are produced to provide new ECM components. Mesenchymal cells release angiopoietin-1, which interacts with Tie-2 receptor tyrosine kinase mediating capillary organization and stabilization (Yancopoulos et al., 2000). The newly built endothelial cells reorganize by forming tight junctions with each other, leading to tube formation. These new tubes connect with the microcirculation, resulting in an operational new vasculature.

Possible Targets for Imaging Angiogenesis

This multistep process offers several targets for therapeutic interventions (Hagedorn and Bikfalvi, 2000). Thus, great efforts are being made to develop anti-angiogenic drugs. Most of the development is focused on four major groups: (1) growth receptor antagonists for inhibition of endothelial cell activation, (2) inhibition of the degradation of the extracellular matrix by metalloproteinases (MMP) inhibitors, (3) adhesion antagonists, and (4) antagonists blocking endothelial cell function (e.g., angiostatin).

A variety of low-molecular-weight compounds blocking the function of different growth factor receptors have been developed (Rosen, 2002). Some examples are SU 5416 (Mendel et al., 2000), a potent ATP-mimetic VEGF-R2 inhibitor, SU 6668 (Hoekman, 2001), which is active against VEGF-, FGF-, and PDGF-receptor tyrosine kinase, or PTK 787 (Wood et al., 2000), which blocks VEGF-receptor kinase activity. Another class of compounds has been designed to inhibit MMP activity by binding to the substrate-cleavage site and/or the catalytic site of these enzymes. Several of these compounds such as Marimastat® (Quirt et al., 2002), Bay 129566 (Heath and Grochow, 2000), and CGS 27023A (Levitt et al., 2001) have already been studied in clinical trials. The adhesion antagonists focus on the inhibition of αvβ3-mediated cell/matrix-interaction. It is assumed that αvβ3-antagonists such as EMD 121974 (Mitjans et al., 2000) and Vitaxin™ (Patel et al., 2001) induce apoptosis by blocking these interactions. However, other models for endothelial apoptosis suggest a direct activation of caspase-3 by RGD-peptides or induction of apoptosis by direct activation of caspase-8 via unligated integrins (Hynes, 2002).

Another approach is focused on the application of endogenous angiogenesis inhibitors such as Angiostatin™, a 38 kDa fragment of plasminogen, which might inhibit ATP synthase, and Endostatin™ a 20 kDa fragment of the C-terminus of collagen XVIII (Folkman, 2002; Hajitou et al., 2002). Both proteins showed anti-angiogenic effects in preclinical studies and are now in clinical trials.

Based on knowledge of the molecular processes and data from drug development approaches, several potential targets for the design of radiolabeled compounds for monitoring of angiogenesis are available. Presently, most of the work is concentrated on the development of radiolabeled αvβ3-antagonists and MMP inhibitors. Another approach (Demartis *et al.*, 2001; Tarli *et al.*, 1999) focuses on a single-chain Fv antibody fragment that selectively binds to a particular fibronectin isoform containing the ED-B domain, which is important in vascular proliferation.

Tracer for Imaging VEGF or the VEGF Receptor

Vascular endothelial growth factor (VEGF) is a central cytokine in the angiogenic process and mediates the development of new vasculature during embryogenesis, neovascularization, and tumorigenesis. There are isoforms that are freely diffusible, including $VEGF_{165}$, $VEGF_{145}$, and $VEGF_{121}$ but also isoforms that remain cell associated, such as $VEGF_{206}$ and $VEGF_{189}$ (Cross and Claesson-Welsh, 2001). The major isoform found in tumors is $VEGF_{165}$. This diffusible form can associate with cells via a heparin-binding domain (Neufeld *et al.*, 1996). Three VEGF receptors, named VEGFR-1 (or flt-1), VEGFR-2 (orKDR/flk-1), and VEGFR-3, are known. The first two are found on vascular endothelial cells, whereas the third is expressed on lymphatic endothelial cells (Cross and Claesson-Welsh, 2001). Vascular endothelial growth factor binding not only activates endothelial cell proliferation but also stimulates an increase in vascular permeability, allowing the diffusion of proteins involved in the development of a fibrin matrix, facilitating the invasion of stromal cells into the tumor tissue (Poon *et al.*, 2001). Both VEGF and VEGF receptors are used as targets to develop tracers for monitoring angiogenesis. Despite the availability of a variety of low-molecular-weight antagonists, currently tracer development is focused on radiolabeled VEGF or radiolabeled antibodies against VEGF.

Collingridge *et al.* (2002) developed a [124]I-iodine-labeled monoclonal antibody (VG76e) that recognizes the 121, 165, and 189 isoforms of human VEGF. They investigated different labeling strategies, including direct labeling via the IodoGen method ([*I]-VG76e) and indirect labeling via the Bolton-Hunter reagent ([*I]-SHPP-VG76e) or m-N-succiniimidyl iodobenzoic acid ([*I]-SIB-VG76e), according to Zalutsky and colleagues (Vaidyanathan *et al.*, 1993). Great differences in binding affinities and immunoreactivity have been found for the antibodies labeled via different strategies, with the best results obtained for [*I]-SHPP-VG76e. In contrast, for the direct-labeled [*I]-VG76e, loss of immunoreactivity has been observed. Biodistribution and PET imaging studies using either the [125]I- or [124]I-labeled [*I]-SHPP-VG76e showed a slow and time-dependent activity accumulation in the tumor tissue, reaching peak levels not before 24 hr after tracer injection. At this time, with the exception of blood and urine, most of the normal tissue showed lower activity

concentration than the tumor. Further studies in patients are planned to evaluate the potential of this tracer.

Another approach uses a system that is based on an adapter/docking tag set. This system uses the interactions between two fragments of the ribonuclease I known as HuS and Hu-tag (Blankenberg *et al.*, 2004). The Hu-tag was fused to DNA coding for the $VEGF_{121}$ isoform. The HuS was conjugated with HYNIC, labeled with [99m]Tc. Together they form a radiolabeled protein complex between Hu-tagged $VEGF_{121}$ and the ^{99m}Tc-HuS. Such an approach can prevent loss of targeting activity, which may occur by direct labeling of proteins. Indeed, they found a marked decreased ability of the HYNIC-VEGF to stimulate the VEGFR-2 compared to native VEGF or HuS/Hu-VEGF. The authors emphasize that they can image tumor vasculature even in very small tumors. However, more detailed studies need to be carried out to confirm these preliminary results.

In contrast, Li *et al.* (2001) carried out direct labeling of $VEGF_{165}$ and $VEGF_{121}$ with ^{123}I-iodine and found, based on a variety of *in vitro* binding studies, that labeling has no influence on the functional properties of both proteins. For the $VEGF_{165}$ these data are confirmed by Cornelissen *et al.* (2005). In addition, Li *et al.* (2003) found that [^{123}I]$VEGF_{165}$ binds to a higher number of different tumor cell types compared to [^{123}I]$VEGF_{121}$. Thus, they studied [^{123}I]$VEGF_{165}$ uptake in 18 patients with gastrointestinal tumors (Fig. 2). An overall VEGF receptor sensitivity of 58% was obtained, varying from 78% for primary pancreatic cancers to 33% for lung metastasis. However, no detailed analysis of tumor tissue has been carried out to identify correlation of tracer uptake with receptor expression or vessel density. In an additional study, safety and radiation dosimetry were investigated (Li *et al.*, 2004). The data from 9 patients with pancreatic carcinoma showed favorable dosimetry, with highest absorbed organ dose in thyroid, indicating some de-iodination of the tracer.

Radiolabeled Antibody Fragment against the ED-B Domain of Fibronectin

Fibronectin, a polymorphic matrix protein, exists in several isoforms, depending on alternative splicing patterns in different regions (e.g., III CS, ED-A, ED-B) of the primary transcript (Hynes, 1985). These isoforms are involved in a variety of processes such as wound healing, cell migration, and oncogenic transformation. It has been shown that a particular isoform containing the ED-B domain, a sequence of 91 amino acids that is highly conserved in mice, rats, and humans, is important in vascular proliferation, and is widely expressed in fetal and neoplastic tissue but shows a highly restricted distribution in normal adult tissue (Castellani *et al.*, 2000). It has been demonstrated that fluorescence-labeled anti-ED-B single-chain Fv antibody fragments selectively accumulate around blood vessels in the tumor tissue in a murine tumor model (Neri *et al.*, 1997). Based on these

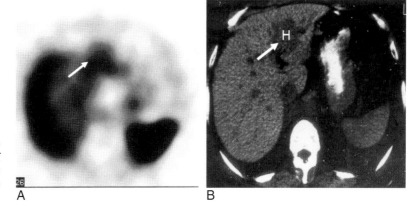

Figure 2 VEGF receptor scintigraphy. **(A)** Transverse slice of a SPECT study performed 1.5 hr after injection of [^{123}I]VEGF$_{165}$. **(B)** The pancreatic adenocarcinoma in the corresponding transverse slice of a CT scan. Arrows indicate location of the tumor. (from Li *et al.*, 2004)

A   B

results, a radioiodinated anti-ED-B antibody fragment with affinities in the picomolar range has been synthesized. The radiolabeled single-chain fragment scFv(L19) selectively binds to the ED-B domain and showed high accumulation in different animal/tumor models (e.g., F9 murine teratocarcinoma: tumor/blood ratio = 12; 24 hr p.i.) (Tarli *et al.*, 1999). In addition, immunohistochemistry and microautoradiography demonstrated selective accumulation in tumor vessels (Fig. 3A), whereas no activity accumulation was found in vessels of other organs.

An initial clinical study, using a ^{123}I-labeled dimeric single-chain fragment L19(scFv)$_2$, included 20 patients with lung, colorectal, or brain cancer (Santimaria *et al.*, 2003). In 16 of 20 patients, different levels of tracer accumulation were found either in the primary tumor or metastases. Based on the slower kinetic of antibodies and antibody fragments compared to small peptides, imaging was carried out not earlier than 6 hr after tracer injection. These data indicate that radiolabeled antibody fragments against the ED-B domain of fibronectin are potential new tracers for noninvasive angiogenesis monitoring (Fig. 3). Moreover, further modification of this fragment resulting in a trimethyl-stannyl benzoate bifunctional derivative allows labeling with ^{211}At and offers a new approach for endoradiotherapy (Demartis *et al.*, 2001). Different formats of the antibody have been tested to identify the best-suited radioimmunoconjugate (Berndorff *et al.*, 2005; Borsi *et al.*, 2002), including the single-chain fragment scFv(L19) (~ 50 kDa), the "small immunoprotein"

Figure 3 Scintigraphic detection of the ED-B domain of fibronectin. **(A)** Immunohistochemistry of a tissue section from a liver metastasis from a colon carcinoma using an anti-ED-B antibody (red) showed strong positive staining. **(B)** Localization of [^{123}I]L19(scFv)$_2$ in a patient with lung adenocarcinoma. SPECT images, obtained 6 hr after tracer injection, showing the transaxial, sagittal, and coronal projection of the thorax area, were matched to the CT scan of the same region. (from Santimaria *et al.*, 2003)

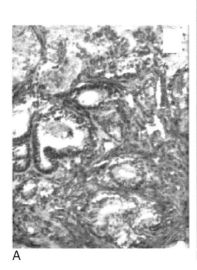

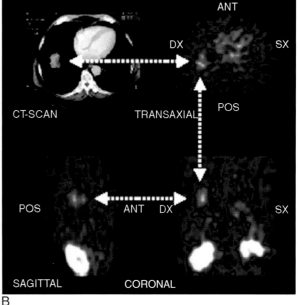

A   B

L19-SIP (~ 80 kDa), and the complete human IgG1 L19-IgG1 (~ 150 kDa). The fastest clearance but also the lowest stability were found for scFv(L19). The most favorable therapeutic index in a murine tumor model was found for the ^{131}I-labeleld L19-SIP, resulting in significant tumor growth delay and prolonged survival after a single injection. These data indicate that ED-B fibronectin-targeted radioimmunotherapy could be a new approach to treat solid tumors.

Radiolabeled MMP Inhibitors

Matrix metalloproteinases are zinc endopeptidases capable of degrading proteins of the extracellular matrix (Curran and Murray, 2000). The MMP family consists of more than 18 different members, which are divided into five classes (Hidalgo and Eckhardt, 2001). MMP activity is controlled by a balance between proenzyme synthesis and expression of endogenous MMP inhibitors, for example, tissue inhibitors of metalloproteases (TIMPs) (Gomez et al., 1997). An increased proenzyme production results in degradation of basement membrane and extracelluar matrix preparing the structural requirements for endothelial cell migration and subsequent vessel formation (Foda and Zucker, 2001). The gelatinases MMP-2 and MMP-9 are most consistently detected in malignant tissue (Nguyen et al., 2001). Their overexpression correlates with tumor aggressiveness and metastatic potential. Due to their important role in tumor-induced angiogenesis and tumor metastasis, MMPs are potential targets for therapeutic interventions (Matter, 2001; Vihinen and Kahari, 2002). Thus, great efforts are being made to develop synthetic MMP inhibitors. Numerous peptides, peptidomimetic and nonpeptidic inhibitors are described, which are in preclinical or already in clinical studies.

The disulfide bridged decapeptide with the sequence CTTHWGFTLC, found using phage display libraries, selectively inhibits MMP-2 and MMP-9 (Koivunen et al., 1999). In addition, this peptide suppresses migration of tumor and endothelial cells in vitro, and, when presented on phages, it mediates homing of these phages in the tumor vasculature. Based on these results, the radioiodinated [*I]yCTTHWGFTLC was synthesized and evaluated as a tracer to determine MMP-2/MMP-9 activity (Kuhnast et al., 2004). It was demonstrated that the modified peptide has similar inhibitory capacities for MMP-2, as found for the parent peptide, and that the tracer was not degraded by activated MMP-2 and MMP-9. However, in vivo the tracer revealed low metabolic stability and high lipophilicity, resulting in moderate tumor accumulation. Altogether, these results indicate that further improvements concerning metabolic stability as well as pharmacokinetic behavior are needed to make this compound suitable for imaging angiogenesis.

As already mentioned, owing to MMP's important role during tumor-induced angiogenesis and tumor metastasis, they are potential targets for therapeutic interventions. Thus,

numerous peptidomimetic and nonpeptidic inhibitors are currently being investigated, some of which are already in initial clinical trials.

Starting from either D-methionine, D-tryptophan, or D-valine scaffold different ^{18}F-labeled MMP-2 inhibitors have been synthesized and tested in vitro (Furumoto et al., 2002). For example, the valine-containing compound revealed an inhibitory activity against MMP-2 with an IC_{50} value of 1.9 μM. Based on another N-sulfonylamino acid derivative, a ^{11}C-labeled analog was synthesized, which showed strong inhibitory effectiveness for the gelatinases MMP-2 and MMP-9 (Kuhnast et al., 2003). A broad-range MMP inhibitor belonging to the N-sulfonylamino acid family was used as an additional lead structure for the synthesis of different [11]C- and ^{18}F-labeled derivatives (Fei et al., 2002; Zheng et al., 2002, 2003). Because initial [11]C- and ^{18}F-analogs labeled at the phenyl group are accessible only in low radiochemical yields (Fei et al., 2002), further radiolabeling was carried out at the hydroxamic acid function (Zheng et al., 2002). Some of the resulting compounds have comparable inhibitory effectiveness on MMP-1, as found for the parent compound CGS 27023A in vitro. Recently radiolabeled biphenylsulfonamide MMP inhibitors have been developed (Fei et al., 2003). Although this class of compounds was prepared from L-valine, the inhibitory effectiveness on MMP-13 for this class of compounds was found to be high. Oltenfreiter et al. (2004) labeled hydroxamic and carboxylic acid containing MMP inhibitors based on a valine or a tryptophan scaffold via an electrophilic aromatic substitution with ^{123}I-iodine. Again this compound showed high inhibition capacities on gelatinases.

In contrast to the promising in vitro data, the results of the in vivo evaluations carried out with some of these derivatives are not very promising. Some tracer biodistribution data in normal mice indicate favorable pharmacokinetics (Kuhnast et al., 2003; Oltenfreiter et al., 2004) and metabolic stability (Kuhnast et al., 2003). However, the biodistribution studies as well as micro-PET images carried out using tumor models found low tracer accumulation in the corresponding tumors. For example, for the ^{18}F-labeled D-valine-based tracer, tumor/muscle ratios were ~ 1 and tumor/blood ratios were 0.6–0.7, which were related to nonspecific binding (Zheng et al., 2003). The same group (Zheng et al., 2004) studied [11C]CGS 25966 and [11C]MSMA, and none of these tracers allowed visualization of the tumor using two different murine tumor models and a dedicated PET scanner. Oltenfreiter et al. (2005) also concluded that the investigated radioiodinated carboxylic and hydroxamic MMP inhibitor tracers do not appear suitable as tumor-imaging agents (Fig. 4). Thus, further preclinical evaluation studies have to be carried out to demonstrate and to assess the potential of radiolabeled MMP inhibitors to monitor angiogenesis. Especially with respect to their general value and the often discussed limitations of radiolabeled enzyme inhibitors for in vivo imaging

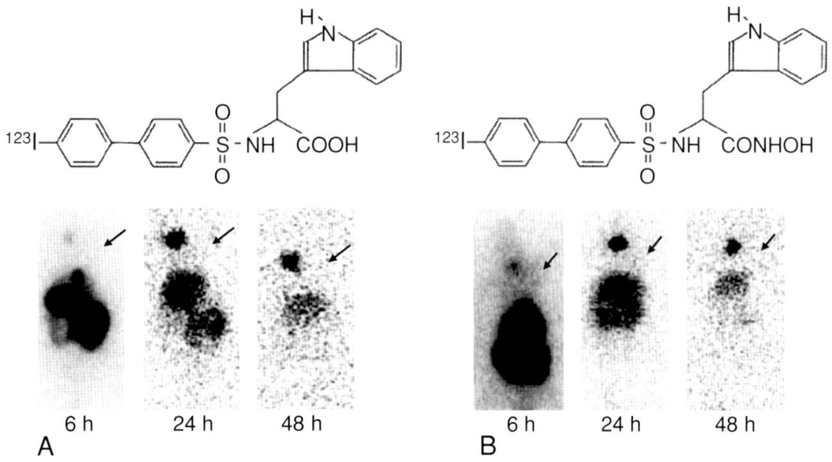

Figure 4 Imaging of MMP expression. Planar gamma camera images of A549 non-small cell lung carcinoma bearing nude mice (tumor localization is indicated by arrows) 6, 24, and 48 hr after intravenous tracer injection. Images showed almost no increased activity accumulation in the tumor compared with the background. **(A)** 2-(4′-[^{123}I]iodo-biphenyl-4-sulfonylamino)-3-(1H-indol-3-yl)-propionic acid. **(B)** 2-(4′-[^{123}I]iodo-biphenyl-4-sulfonylamino)-3-(1H-indol-3-yl)-propionamid. (from Oltenfreiter *et al.*, 2005)

Radiolabeled Integrin Antagonists

As already mentioned, the $\alpha v \beta 3$ integrin is a receptor playing an important role in mediating the migration of endothelial cells through the basement membrane during blood vessel formation. In addition, this receptor is involved in a diversity of other pathological dysfunctions, including tumor metastasis, restenosis, osteoporosis, and inflammatory processes, making it an interesting target for drug development.

Integrins are heterodimeric transmembrane glycoproteins consisting of an α- and a β-subunit. Ruoslahti and Pierschbacher (1987) found that the amino acid sequence arginine-glycine-aspartic acid (RGD, amino acid single letter code) is an important binding epitope found in several extracellular matrix proteins. Based on these findings, linear as well as cyclic peptides, including the RGD-sequence, have been developed. Kessler and coworkers (Aumailley *et al.*, 1991) synthesized the pentapeptide cyclo(-Arg-Gly-Asp-DPhe-Val-), which showed high affinity and selectivity for the $\alpha v \beta 3$ integrin. This structure was the basis of further developments of a wide range of different peptidic and nonpeptidic $\alpha v \beta 3$ antagonists.

In addition, cyclo(-Arg-Gly-Asp-DPhe-Val-) was used as lead structure for the development of radiotracers for the noninvasive determination of the $\alpha v \beta 3$ integrin status using nuclear medicine tracer techniques (Haubner and Wester, 2004). For the first evaluation of this approach, the radioiodinated peptides 3-[*I]Iodo-DTyr^4-cyclo(-Arg-Gly-Asp-DTyr-Val-) and 3-[*I]Iodo-Tyr^5-cyclo(-Arg-Gly-Asp-DPhe-Tyr-) have been synthesized (Haubner *et al.*, 1999). Both compounds showed comparable affinity and selectivity as the lead structure *in vitro* and receptor-specific accumulation in the tumor *in vivo*. However, the predominantly hepatobiliary elimination resulted in high-activity concentration in liver and intestine. Thus, several strategies to improve the pharmacokinetics of radiohalogenated peptides have been studied; they include conjugation with sugar moieties and polyethylene glycol.

The glycosylation approach (Haubner *et al.*, 2001a, 2001b) is based on the introduction of sugar amino acids (sugar derivatives with an amino and a carboxylate function). In a murine tumor model, the resulting glycopeptides [*I]Gluco-RGD (Haubner *et al.*, 2001a) and [^{18}F]Galacto-RGD (Haubner *et al.*, 2001b, 2004b) showed a clearly reduced activity concentration in liver and an increased activity uptake and retention in the tumor compared to the first-generation peptides. At the moment, [^{18}F]Galacto-RGD is evaluated in a first clinical trial demonstrating rapid predominant renal excretion and high metabolic stability, resulting in good tumor/background ratios and, thus, in high-quality images (Beer *et al.*, 2005; Haubner *et al.*, 2005). Moreover, this initial study indicates that tracer accumulation correlates with $\alpha v \beta 3$ expression on blood vessels in the tumor lesions (Fig. 5). In addition, great inter- as well as intraindividual variances in tracer accumulation are found, indicating great differences in receptor expression and demonstrating the importance of these techniques for planning and controlling corresponding anti-$\alpha v \beta 3$-directed therapies.

The technology of poly(ethlyene glycol) conjugation (PEGylation) is known to improve many properties of peptides and proteins (Harris and Chess, 2003). In many cases, it is used to prolong median circulation times and half-lives of polypeptides by shifting the elimination pathway from renal to hepatobiliary excretion. Since renal filtration is dependent on both the molecular mass and the volume occupied, this effect strongly depends on the molecular weight of the PEG moiety. In a first study, Chen *et al.* (2004c) attached a 2 kDa PEG moiety to the ε-amino function of cyclo(-Arg-Gly-

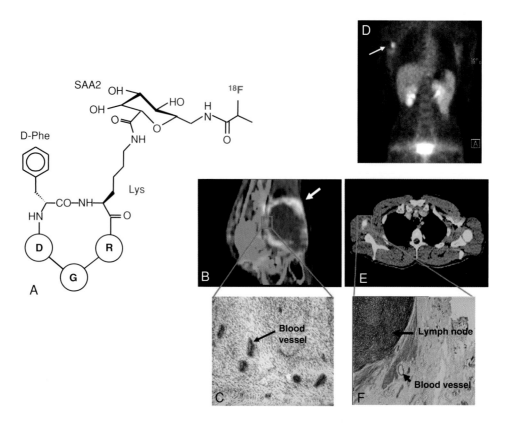

Figure 5 Noninvasive determination of the αvβ3 integrin expression. (**A**) Structure of [¹⁸F]Galacto-RGD. (**B**) Image fusion of a sagittal section of the PET-scan with the corresponding CT scan of a patient with a soft tissue sarcoma dorsal of the right knee joint. Highest tracer accumulation 170 min p.i. was found at the apical-dorsal aspect of the tumor (arrow). (**C**) Immunohistochemical staining of a peripheral tumor section using an anti-αvβ3 monoclonal antibody demonstrated intense staining predominantly of tumor vasculature. (**D**) Coronal image section of a patient with malignant melanoma and a solitary lymph node metastasis in the right axilla (arrow) 60 min after injection of [¹⁸F]Galacto-RGD. (**E**) Image fusion of an axial section of the PET-scan with the corresponding CT-scan. (**F**) Immunohistochemistry of the lymph node metastasis using an anti−αvβ3 monoclonal antibody showed intense staining predominantly of tumor cells but also of surrounding blood vessels. (from Haubner *et al.*, 2005)

Asp-ᴅTyr-Lys-) and compared the ¹²⁵I-labeled PEGylated derivative (¹²⁵I-RGD-PEG) with the radioiodinated cyclo (-Arg-Gly-Asp-ᴅTyr-Lys-) (¹²⁵I-RGD). The PEGylated derivative showed more rapid blood clearance, decreased activity concentration in the kidneys, and slightly increased activity retention in the tumor. However, tumor uptake for ¹²⁵I-RGD was higher as found for ¹²⁵I-RGD-PEG for all time points. Moreover, as explained earlier, an increased activity retention in liver and intestine was found. In addition, the effect of PEGylation was studied by comparing ⁶⁴Cu-DOTA-RGD and ⁶⁴Cu-DOTA-PEG-RGD (PEG, MW = 3.4 kDa) (Chen *et al.*, 2004a). As discussed below later in this chapter, ⁶⁴Cu-DOTA-RGD showed significant liver uptake. Thus, in this case, PEGylation reduced activity concentration in liver and small intestine and resulted in faster blood clearance, while neither the tumor uptake nor retention was affected. Altogether, these studies revealed very different effects of PEGylation on the pharmacokinetics and tumor uptake of RGD-peptides, which seems to strongly depend on the nature of the lead structure.

As already indicated, in parallel to the radiohalogenated peptides a variety of radiometallated tracers have been developed. They include peptides labeled with ¹¹¹In-indium, ⁹⁹ᵐTc-technitium, ⁶⁴Cu-copper, ⁹⁰Y-yttrium, and ¹⁸⁸Re-rhenium for diagnostic as well as potential endoradiotherapeutic purposes. Most of them are based on cyclo(-Arg-Gly-Asp-ᴅPhe/Tyr-Lys-), which is conjugated via the ε-amino function of the lysine with different chelator systems. Van Hagen *et al.* (2000) synthesized a DTPA conjugated RGD-peptide and demonstrated αvβ3 selective binding on the blood vessels of human tumor tissue sections using receptor autoradiography and immunohistochemistry. For [⁹⁹ᵐTc]DKCK-RGD, the tetrapeptide sequence H-Asp-Lys-Cys-Lys-OH was used as the chelating system (Haubner *et al.*, 2004a). Gamma-camera images 4 hr p.i. showed a clearly contrasting tumor but also high-activity concentration in the kidneys. Thus, further optimization concerning metabolic stability and pharmacokinetic behavior seems to be recommended. A DOTA conjugated RGD-peptide was labeled with ⁶⁴Cu-copper (Chen *et al.*, 2004d). This tracer showed lower tumor uptake and retention in a murine orthotopic human breast cancer model compared with the radioiodinated cyclo (-Arg-Gly-Asp-DTyr-Lys-) and unfavorable activity retention in liver and kidneys. The activity concentration in the liver could be due to transchelation of ^{64}Cu from DOTA to super-oxide dismutase and the persistent localization of the final metabolite ^{64}Cu-DOTA-Lys-OH in this tissue. Tumor/blood and tumor/muscle ratios of ~ 7–8 allowed acquisition of clear tumor/background contrast images 1 hr p.i. using a small-animal scanner. However, the highest activity concentration was found in liver, intestine, and bladder, indicating that further optimization of the tracer is needed. An approach using PEGylated RGD-peptides, resulting in decreased activity concentration in liver and small intestine, has already been discussed above (Chen *et al.*, 2004a).

RGD-4C ((Cys^2-Cys^{10},Cys^4-Cys^8)H-Ala-Cys-Asp-Cys-Arg-Gly-Asp-Cys-Phe-Cys-Gly-OH) (Assa-Munt *et al.*, 2001), an $\alpha v \beta 3$-binding disulfide-bridged undecapeptide, resulting from a phage display library, has also been used as a lead structure. A shortened derivative of RGD-4C ((Cys^1-Cys^9,Cys^3-Cys^7)H-Cys-Asp-Cys-Arg-Gly-Asp-Cys-Phe-Cys-OH) was coupled with HYNIC and labeled with ^{99m}Tc (Su *et al.*, 2002, 2003). In two murine tumor models, only marginal tumor uptake was found, which can be explained by the modest association constant of this modified ^{99m}Tc-labeled RGD-4C for $\alpha v \beta 3$ (7×10^6 M^{-1}). Thus, either the conjugation with HYNIC or the deletion of the terminal amino acids and/or the labeling with ^{99m}Tc-technetium impairs the affinity for the $\alpha v \beta 3$ integrin, resulting in a peptide that appears unsuitable for *in vivo* imaging of $\alpha v \beta 3$ expression. Further studies, including structure activity investigations and *in vivo* evaluations, have to demonstrate whether other radiolabeled RGD-4C derivatives will allow imaging of $\alpha v \beta 3$ expression. However, at the moment, radiolabeled derivatives of cyclo(-Arg-Gly-Asp-DPhe-Val-) seem to be superior.

Besides monomeric RGD peptides, multimeric compounds presenting more than one RGD site have also been introduced. The most obvious advantage of this concept is that multimeric tracer should show higher tracer uptake at the target site due to an increased apparent ligand concentration. Janssen *et al.* (2002a, 2002b) introduced a dimeric RGD peptide by conjugating cyclo(-RGDfK) via a glutamic acid linker. For radiolabeling, DOTA or HYNIC was coupled to the linker. The dimeric ^{99m}Tc-HYNIC-E-[c(RGDfK)]$_2$ showed a tenfold higher affinity for the $\alpha v \beta 3$ integrin as the monomeric ^{99m}Tc-HYNIC-c(RGDfK). Moreover, activity retention in the tumor was improved compared with the monomeric compound. However, activity retention was also high in kidneys.

The groups of Wester and Kessler (Poethko *et al.*, 2004a, 2004b; Thumshirn *et al.*, 2003) carried out a systematic study on the influence of multimerization on receptor affinity and tumor uptake. They synthesized a series of monomeric,

dimeric, tetrameric, and octameric RGD peptides. In these compounds, c(RGDfE) was conjugated via PEG linker and lysine moieties, which are used as branching units. Labeling has been carried out via a chemoselective oxime formation based on the amino-oxo function at the peptide site and an ^{18}F-labeled aldehyde. They found an increasing binding affinity in the series monomer, dimer, tetramer, and octamer. Initial PET images resulting from a clinical scanner confirm these findings. The image of mice with the $\alpha v \beta 3$ positive melanoma on the right flank and an $\alpha v \beta 3$ negative melanoma on the left flank showed an increasing activity accumulation only in the receptor positive tumor in the series monomer, dimer, and tetramer. Moreover, PET studies comparing a tetrameric structure containing four c(RGDfE) peptides with a tetrameric compound containing only one c(RGDfE) and three c(RaDFE) peptides (which do not bind to the $\alpha v \beta 3$ integrin) showed for the pseudo-monomeric tetramer a-three-fold lower activity accumulation in the tumor of a murine tumor model as for the real tetramer. This indicated that the higher uptake in the tumor is due to multimerization and is not based on other structural effects.

In another study, a dimeric cyclic RGD peptide E[c(RGDyK)]$_2$ was labeled by conjugating a prosthetic 4-[^{18}F]fluorobenzoyl moiety to the glutamate (Chen *et al.*, 2004e; Zhang *et al.*, 2006). The dimeric RGD peptide demonstrated significantly higher tumor uptake and prolonged tumor retention in comparison with a monomeric RGD peptide analog [^{18}F]FB-c(RGDyK). Moreover, the dimeric RGD peptide showed predominant renal excretion, whereas the monomeric analog was excreted primarily through the biliary route. Thus, the authors conclude that the synergistic effect of polyvalency and improved pharmacokinetics may be responsible for the superior imaging characteristics of [^{18}F]FB-E[c(RGDyK)]$_2$. Similar effects have been found for dimeric ^{64}Cu-labeled analogs (Chen *et al.*, 2004b). Moreover, the comparison with the tetrameric [^{64}Cu]DOTA-E{E[c(RGDfK)]$_2$}$_2$ (Wu *et al.*, 2005) showed significantly higher integrin-binding affinity for the tetramer than the corresponding monomeric and dimeric RGD analogs, most likely due to a polyvalence effect. Again tumor uptake was rapid and high, and the tumor washout was slow.

Summary and Conclusion

There is a keen interest in the development of methods that allow noninvasive monitoring of molecular processes involved in angiogenesis. One promising approach is based on nuclear medicine tracer techniques. Thus, several radio-labeled compounds have been developed and are currently being studied in both pre- and clinical settings. The different approaches focus on the noninvasive determination of the expression of VEGF and the VEGF receptor, the ED-B domain of fibronectin, matrix metalloproteinases, or the αvβ3 integrin. All of these proteins are involved in different steps of the angiogenesis process.

A radiolabeled antibody against VEGF, as well as radiolabeled VEGF itself, has been studied. For [^{123}I]VEGF$_{165}$ a preliminary study in 18 patients with gastrointestinal tumors has been carried out and resulted in an overall sensitivity of 58%. However, further studies correlating the signal with VEGF receptor expression have to be carried out to demonstrate the potential of this strategy.

Another approach introduced a radiolabeled antibody against the ED-B domain of a fibronectin isoform widely expressed on neoplastic tissue. The ^{123}I-labeled fragment was studied in 20 patients. In 16 patients different levels of tracer accumulation have been found. Immunohistochemical staining of different tumor tissue using an antibody against the ED-B domain has shown that, in general, the protein is expressed in the tumor vasculature. But it still has to be demonstrated that the obtained signal correlates with the protein expression and that it supplies information about the angiogenic process in the corresponding patients. Anyway, a preclinical study with a ^{131}I-labeled analog indicates that fibronectin ED-B domain-targeted radioimmunotherapy may be a new approach to treat tumors.

A peptidic and variety of different nonpeptidic MMP inhibitors have been studied for use in noninvasive determination of MMP activity. In contrast to the promising in vitro data, corresponding in vivo evaluation of some of those derivatives could not assess the potential of this class of tracer to monitor angiogenesis.

Most work has been carried out to develop tracer for monitoring αvβ3 integrin expression. As the most common lead structure, the αv-selective cyclo(-Arg-Gly-Asp-ᴅPhe-Val-) was used. Different groups demonstrated that introduction of poly(ethylene glycol), and especially carbohydrates, improved pharmacokinetic properties. Moreover, it has been shown that tracer containing two to eight RGD moieties in one compound resulted in an improved binding affinity in vitro and in an increased and prolonged uptake in αvβ3-positive tumors in murine tumor models. Moreover, preclinical as well as clinical studies, carried out mainly with [^{18}F]Galacto-RGD, strongly indicated that tracer uptake correlates with αvβ3 integrin expression. The disadvantage concerning the monitoring of tumor-induced angiogenesis is that this receptor can be expressed on activated endothelial cells as well as on tumor cells. Thus, for oncological settings it will be problematic to clearly correlate the resulting signal with neovascularization, but nevertheless αvβ3 imaging will give helpful information for planning and controlling corresponding αvβ3 targeted therapies. For other pathological processes, the signal will originate exclusively from the activated endothelial cells and, consequently may provide information on the angiogenic process noninvasively.

Altogether, great efforts are made to develop tracer for monitoring angiogenesis. At the moment, the most promising approach is based on the noninvasive determination of the αvβ3 expression, where the most intensive biological evaluation has been carried out. However, for all approaches further pre- and clinical studies have to follow, to allow final prediction about the potential of the different approaches in monitoring angiogenesis.

References

Assa-Munt, N., Jia, X., Laakkonen, P., and Ruoslahti, E. 2001. Solution structures and integrin binding activities of an RGD peptide with two isomers. Biochemistry 40:2373–2378.

Aumailley, M., Gurrath, M., Muller, G., Calvete, J., Timpl, R., and Kessler, H. 1991. Arg-Gly-Asp constrained within cyclic pentapeptides. Strong and selective inhibitors of cell adhesion to vitronectin and laminin fragment P1. FEBS Lett. 291:50–54.

Beer, A.J., Haubner, R., Goebel, M., Luderschmidt, S., Spilker, M.E., Wester, H.J., Weber, W.A., and Schwaiger, M. 2005. Biodistribution and pharmacokinetics of the αvβ3-selective tracer ^{18}F-galacto-RGD in cancer patients. J. Nucl. Med. 46:1333–1341.

Berndorff, D., Borkowski, S., Sieger, S., Rother, A., Friebe, M., Viti, F., Hilger, C.S., Cyr, J.E., and Dinkelborg, L.M. 2005. Radioimmunotherapy of solid tumors by targeting extra domain B fibronectin: identification of the best-suited radioimmunoconjugate. Clin. Cancer Res. 11:7053s–7063s.

Bikfalvi, A., and Bicknell, R. 2002. Recent advances in angiogenesis, antiangiogenesis and vascular targeting. Trends Pharmacol. Sci. 23:576–582.

Bishop, G.G., McPherson, J.A., Sanders, J.M., Hesselbacher, S.E., Feldman, M.J., McNamara, C.A., Gimple, L.W., Powers, E.R., Mousa, S.A., and Sarembock, I.J. 2001. Selective αvβ3-receptor blockade reduces macrophage infiltration and restenosis after balloon angioplasty in the atherosclerotic rabbit. Circulation 103:1906–1911.

Blankenberg, F.G., Mandl, S., Cao, Y.A., O'Connell-Rodwell, C., Contag, C., Mari, C., Gaynutdinov, T.I., Vanderheyden, J.L., Backer, M.V., and Backer, J.M. 2004. Tumor imaging using a standardized radiolabeled adapter protein docked to vascular endothelial growth factor. J. Nucl. Med. 45:1373–1380.

Borsi, L., Balza, E., Bestagno, M., Castellani, P., Carnemolla, B., Biro, A., Leprini, A., Sepulveda, J., Burrone, O., Neri, D., and Zardi, L. 2002. Selective targeting of tumoral vasculature: comparison of different formats of an antibody (L19) to the ED-B domain of fibronectin. Int. J. Cancer. 102:75–85.

Brooks, P.C., Montgomery, A.M., Rosenfeld, M., Reisfeld, R.A., Hu, T., Klier, G., and Cheresh, D.A. 1994. Integrin αvβ3 antagonists promote tumor regression by inducing apoptosis of angiogenic blood vessels. Cell 79:1157–1164.

Brooks, P.C., Stromblad, S., Klemke, R., Visscher, D., Sarkar, F.H., and Cheresh, D.A. 1995. Antiintegrin αvβ3 blocks human breast cancer growth and angiogenesis in human skin. J. Clin. Invest. 96:1815–1822.

Carmeliet, P. 2003. Angiogenesis in health and disease. Nat. Med. 9:653–660.

Carmeliet, P. 2005. Angiogenesis in life, disease and medicine. Nature 438:932–936.

Carmeliet, P., and Jain, R.K. 2000. Angiogenesis in cancer and other diseases. Nature 407:249–257.

Castellani, P., Dorcaratto, A., Pau, A., Nicola, M., Siri, A., Gasparetto, B., Zardi, L., and Viale, G. 2000. The angiogenesis marker ED-B+ fibronectin isoform in intracranial meningiomas. Acta Neurochir. 142:277–282.

Chavakis, E., Riecke, B., Lin, J., Linn, T., Bretzel, R.G., Preissner, K.T., Brownlee, M., and Hammes, H.P. 2002. Kinetics of integrin expression in the mouse model of proliferative retinopathy and success of secondary intervention with cyclic RGD peptides. Diabetologia 45:262–267.

Chen, X., Hou, Y., Tohme, M., Park, R., Khankaldyyan, V., Gonzales-Gomez, I., Bading, J.R., Laug, W.E., and Conti, P.S. 2004a. Pegylated Arg-Gly-Asp peptide: ^{64}Cu labeling and PET imaging of brain tumor $\alpha v\beta 3$-integrin expression. *J. Nucl. Med. 45*:1776–1783.

Chen, X., Liu, S., Hou, Y., Tohme, M., Park, R., Bading, J.R., and Conti, P.S. 2004b. MicroPET imaging of breast cancer αv-integrin expression with ^{64}Cu-labeled dimeric RGD peptides. *Mol. Imaging Biol. 6*:350–359.

Chen, X., Park, R., Shahinian, A.H., Bading, J.R., and Conti, P.S. 2004c. Pharmacokinetics and tumor retention of ^{125}I-labeled RGD peptide are improved by PEGylation. *Nucl. Med. Biol. 31*:11–19.

Chen, X., Park, R., Tohme, M., Shahinian, A.H., Bading, J.R., and Conti, P.S. 2004d. MicroPET and autoradiographic imaging of breast cancer αv-integrin expression using ^{18}F- and ^{64}Cu-labeled RGD peptide. *Bioconjug. Chem. 15*:41–49.

Chen, X., Tohme, M., Park, R., Hou, Y., Bading, J.R., and Conti, P.S. 2004e. Micro-PET imaging of $\alpha v\beta 3$-integrin expression with ^{18}F-labeled dimeric RGD peptide. *Mol. Imag. 3*:96–104.

Collingridge, D.R., Carroll, V.A., Glaser, M., Aboagye, E.O., Osman, S., Hutchinson, O.C., Barthel, H., Luthra, S.K., Brady, F., Bicknell, R., Price, P., and Harris, A.L. 2002. The development of [^{124}I]iodinated-VG76e: a novel tracer for imaging vascular endothelial growth factor *in vivo* using positron emission tomography. *Cancer Res. 62*:5912–5919.

Cornelissen, B., Oltenfreiter, R., Kersemans, V., Staelens, L., Frankenne, F., Foidart, J.M., and Slegers, G. 2005. *In vitro* and *in vivo* evaluation of [^{123}I]-VEGF165 as a potential tumor marker. *Nucl. Med. Biol. 32*:431–436.

Creamer, D., Sullivan, D., Bicknell, R., and Barker, J. 2002. Angiogenesis in psoriasis. *Angiogenesis 5*:231–236.

Cross, M.J., and Claesson-Welsh, L. 2001. FGF and VEGF function in angiogenesis: signalling pathways, biological responses and therapeutic inhibition. *Trends Pharmacol. Sci. 22*:201–207.

Curran, S., and Murray, G.I. 2000. Matrix metalloproteinases: molecular aspects of their roles in tumor invasion and metastasis. *Eur. J. Cancer 36*:1621–1630.

Demartis, S., Tarli, L., Borsi, L., Zardi, L., and Neri, D. 2001. Selective targeting of tumor neovasculature by a radiohalogenated human antibody fragment specific for the ED-B domain of fibronectin. *Eur. J. Nucl. Med. 28*:534–539.

Eliceiri, B.P., and Cheresh, D.A. 2000. Role of αv integrins during angiogenesis. *Cancer J. Sci. Am. 6*:S245–249.

Ellis, L.M., Liu, W., Fan, F., Jung, Y.D., Reinmuth, N., Stoeltzing, O., Takeda, A., Akagi, M., Parikh, A.A., and Ahmad, S. 2002. Synopsis of angiogenesis inhibitors in oncology. *Oncology 16*:14–22.

Fei, X., Zheng, Q.H., Hutchins, G.D., Liu, X., Stone, K.L., Carlson, K.A., Mock, B.H., Winkle, W.L., Glick-Wilson, B.E., Miller, K.D., Fife, R.S., Sledge, G.W., Sun, H.B., and Carr, R.E. 2002. Synthesis of MMP inhibitor radiotracers [^{11}C]methyl-CGS 27023A and its analogs, new potential PET breast cancer imaging agents. *J. Label. Compd. Radiopharm. 45*:449–470.

Fei, X., Zheng, Q.H., Liu, X., Wang, J.Q., Sun, H.B., Mock, B.H., Stone, K.L., Miller, K.D., Sledge, G.W., and Hutchins, G.D. 2003. Synthesis of radiolabeled biphenylsulfonamide matrix metalloproteinase inhibitors as new potential PET cancer imaging agents. *Bioorg. Med. Chem. Lett. 13*:2217–2222.

Feldmann, M., Brennan, F.M., Foxwell, B.M., Taylor, P.C., Williams, R.O., and Maini, R.N. 2005. Anti-TNF therapy: where have we got to in 2005? *J. Autoimmun. 25*:26–28.

Foda, H.D., and Zucker, S. 2001. Matrix metalloproteinases in cancer invasion, metastasis and angiogenesis. *Drug Discov. Today 6*:478–482.

Folkman, J. 1995. Angiogenesis in cancer, vascular, rheumatoid and other disease. *Nat. Med. 1*:27–31.

Folkman, J. 2002. Role of angiogenesis in tumor growth and metastasis. *Semin. Oncol. 29*:15–18.

Furumoto, S., Iwata, R., and Ido, T. 2002. Design and synthesis of fluorine-18 labeled matrix metalloproteinase inhibitors for cancer imaging. *J. Label. Compd. Radiopharm. 45*:975–986.

Gomez, D.E., Alonso, D.F., Yoshiji, H., and Thorgeirsson, U.P. 1997. Tissue inhibitors of metalloproteinases: structure, regulation and biological functions. *Eur. J. Cell Biol. 74*:111–122.

Hagedorn, M., and Bikfalvi, A. 2000. Target molecules for anti-angiogenic therapy: from basic research to clinical trials. *Crit. Rev. Oncol. Hematol. 34*:89–110.

Hajitou, A., Grignet, C., Devy, L., Berndt, S., Blacher, S., Deroanne, C.F., Bajou, K., Fong, T., Chiang, Y., Foidart, J.M., and Noel, A. 2002. The antitumoral effect of endostatin and angiostatin is associated with a down-regulation of vascular endothelial growth factor expression in tumor cells. *Faseb J. 16*:1802–1804.

Hammes, H.P., Brownlee, M., Jonczyk, A., Sutter, A., and Preissner, K.T. 1996. Subcutaneous injection of a cyclic peptide antagonist of vitronectin receptor-type integrins inhibits retinal neovascularization. *Nat. Med. 2*:529–533.

Harris, J.M., and Chess, R.B. 2003. Effect of pegylation on pharmaceuticals. *Nat. Rev. Drug Discov. 2*:214–221.

Haubner, R., Bruchertseifer, F., Bock, M., Kessler, H., Schwaiger, M., and Wester, H.J. 2004a. Synthesis and biological evaluation of a ^{99m}Tc-labeled cyclic RGD peptide for imaging the $\alpha v\beta 3$ expression. *Nuklearmedizin 43*:26–32.

Haubner, R., Kuhnast, B., Mang, C., Weber, W.A., Kessler, H., Wester, H.J., and Schwaiger, M. 2004b. [^{18}F]Galacto-RGD: synthesis, radiolabeling, metabolic stability, and radiation dose estimates. *Bioconjug. Chem. 15*:61–69.

Haubner, R., Weber, W.A., Beer, A.J., Vabuliene, E., Reim, D., Sarbia, M., Becker, K.F., Goebel, M., Hein, R., Wester, H.J., Kessler, H., and Schwaiger, M. 2005. Noninvasive visualization of the activated $\alpha v\beta 3$ integrin in cancer patients by positron emission tomography and [^{18}F]Galacto-RGD. *PLoS Med. 2*:e70.

Haubner, R., and Wester, H.J. 2004. Radiolabeled tracers for imaging of tumor angiogenesis and evaluation of anti-angiogenic therapies. *Curr. Pharm. Des. 10*:1439–1455.

Haubner, R., Wester, H.J., Burkhart, F., Senekowitsch-Schmidtke, R., Weber, W., Goodman, S.L., Kessler, H., and Schwaiger, M. 2001a. Glycosylated RGD-containing peptides: tracer for tumor targeting and angiogenesis imaging with improved biokinetics. *J. Nucl. Med. 42*:326–336.

Haubner, R., Wester, H.J., Reuning, U., Senekowitsch-Schmidtke, R., Diefenbach, B., Kessler, H., Stocklin, G., and Schwaiger, M. 1999. Radiolabeled $\alpha v\beta 3$ integrin antagonists: a new class of tracers for tumor targeting. *J. Nucl. Med. 40*:1061–1071.

Haubner, R., Wester, H.J., Weber, W.A., Mang, C., Ziegler, S.I., Goodman, S.L., Senekowitsch-Schmidtke, R., Kessler, H., and Schwaiger, M. 2001b. Noninvasive imaging of $\alpha v\beta 3$ integrin expression using ^{18}F-labeled RGD-containing glycopeptide and positron emission tomography. *Cancer Res. 61*:1781–1785.

Heath, E.I., and Grochow, L.B. 2000. Clinical potential of matrix metalloprotease inhibitors in cancer therapy. *Drugs 59*:1043–1055.

Hidalgo, M., and Eckhardt, S.G. 2001. Development of matrix metalloproteinase inhibitors in cancer therapy. *J. Natl. Cancer Inst. 93*:178–193.

Hoekman, K. 2001. SU6668, a multitargeted angiogenesis inhibitor. *Cancer J. 7*:S134–138.

Hynes, R. 1985. Molecular biology of fibronectin. *Annu. Rev. Cell Biol. 1*:67–90.

Hynes, R.O. 2002. A reevaluation of integrins as regulators of angiogenesis. *Nat. Med. 8*:918–921.

Janssen, M.L., Oyen, W.J., Dijkgraaf, I., Massuger, L.F., Frielink, C., Edwards, D.S., Rajopadhye, M., Boonstra, H., Corstens, F.H., and Boerman, O.C. 2002a. Tumor targeting with radiolabeled $\alpha v\beta 3$ integrin binding peptides in a nude mouse model. *Cancer Res. 62*:6146–6151.

Janssen, M.L.H., Oyen, W.J.G., Massuger, L.F.A.G., Frielink, C., Dijkgraaf, I., Edwards, D.S., Rajopadhye, W.J., Corstens, F.H.M., and Boerman, O.C. 2002b. Comparison of a monomeric and dimeric radiolabeled RGD-peptide for tumor imaging. *Cancer Biother. Radiopharm.* 17: 641–646.

Kim, S., Bell, K., Mousa, S.A., and Varner, J.A. 2000. Regulation of angiogenesis in vivo by ligation of integrin α5β1 with the central cell-binding domain of fibronectin. *Am. J. Pathol.* 156:1345–1362.

Koivunen, E., Arap, W., Valtanen, H., Rainisalo, A., Medina, O.P., Heikkila, P., Kantor, C., Gahmberg, C.G., Salo, T., Konttinen, Y.T., Sorsa, T., Ruoslahti, E., and Pasqualini, R. 1999. Tumor targeting with a selective gelatinase inhibitor. *Nat. Biotechnol.* 17:768–774.

Kuhnast, B., Bodenstein, C., Haubner, R., Wester, H.J., Senekowitsch-Schmidtke, R., Schwaiger, M., and Weber, W.A. 2004. Targeting of gelatinase activity with a radiolabeled cyclic HWGF peptide. *Nucl. Med. Biol.* 31:337–344.

Kuhnast, B., Bodenstein, C., Wester, H.J., and Weber, W.A. 2003. Carbon-11 labeling of an N-sulfonylamino acid derivative: a potential tracer for MMP-2 and MMP-9 imaging. *J. Label. Compd. Radiopharm.* 46:1093–1103.

Kuwano, M., Fukushi, J., Okamoto, M., Nishie, A., Goto, H., Ishibashi, T., and Ono, M. 2001. Angiogenesis factors. *Intern. Med.* 40:565–572.

Lee, P., Wang, C.C., and Adamis, A.P. 1998. Ocular neovascularization: an epidemiologic review. *Surv. Ophthalmol.* 43:245–269.

Levitt, N.C., Eskens, F.A., O'Byrne, K.J., Propper, D.J., Denis, L.J., Owen, S.J., Choi, L., Foekens, J.A., Wilner, S., Wood, J.M., Nakajima, M., Talbot, D.C., Steward, W.P., Harris, A.L., and Verweij, J. 2001. Phase I and pharmacological study of the oral matrix metalloproteinase inhibitor, MMI270 (CGS27023A), in patients with advanced solid cancer. *Clin. Cancer Res.* 7:1912–1922.

Li, S., Peck-Radosavljevic, M., Kienast, O., Preitfellner, J., Hamilton, G., Kurtaran, A., Pirich, C., Angelberger, P., and Dudczak, R. 2003. Imaging gastrointestinal tumors using vascular endothelial growth factor-165 (VEGF165) receptor scintigraphy. *Ann. Oncol.* 14:1274–1277.

Li, S., Peck-Radosavljevic, M., Kienast, O., Preitfellner, J., Havlik, E., Schima, W., Traub-Weidinger, T., Graf, S., Beheshti, M., Schmid, M., Angelberger, P., and Dudczak, R. 2004. Iodine-123-vascular endothelial growth factor-165 (^{123}I-VEGF165). Biodistribution, safety and radiation dosimetry in patients with pancreatic carcinoma. *Q. J. Nucl. Med. Mol. Imaging* 48:198–206.

Li, S., Peck-Radosavljevic, M., Koller, E., Koller, F., Kaserer, K., Kreil, A., Kapiotis, S., Hamwi, A., Weich, H.A., Valent, P., Angelberger, P., Dudczak, R., and Virgolini, I. 2001. Characterization of ^{123}I-vascular endothelial growth factor-binding sites expressed on human tumor cells: possible implication for tumor scintigraphy. *Int. J. Cancer* 91:789–796.

Matter, A. 2001. Tumor angiogenesis as a therapeutic target. *Drug Discov. Today* 6:1005–1024.

Mendel, D.B., Laird, A.D., Smolich, B.D., Blake, R.A., Liang, C., Hannah, A.L., Shaheen, R.M., Ellis, L.M., Weitman, S., Shawver, L.K., and Cherrington, J.M. 2000. Development of SU5416, a selective small molecule inhibitor of VEGF receptor tyrosine kinase activity, as an anti-angiogenesis agent. *Anticancer Drug Des.* 15:29–41.

Mitjans, F., Meyer, T., Fittschen, C., Goodman, S., Jonczyk, A., Marshall, J.F., Reyes, G., and Piulats, J. 2000. *In vivo* therapy of malignant melanoma by means of antagonists of alphav integrins. *Int. J. Cancer* 87:716–723.

Neri, D., Carnemolla, B., Nissim, A., Leprini, A., Querze, G., Balza, E., Pini, A., Tarli, L., Halin, C., Neri, P., Zardi, L., and Winter, G. 1997. Targeting by affinity-matured recombinant antibody fragments of an angiogenesis associated fibronectin isoform. *Nat. Biotechnol.* 15:1271–1275.

Neufeld, G., Cohen, T., Gitay-Goren, H., Poltorak, Z., Tessler, S., Sharon, R., Gengrinovitch, S., and Levi, B.Z. 1996. Similarities and differences between the vascular endothelial growth factor (VEGF) splice variants. *Cancer Metastasis Rev.* 15:153–158.

Nguyen, M., Arkell, J., and Jackson, C.J. 2001. Human endothelial gelatinases and angiogenesis. *Int. J. Biochem. Cell Biol.* 33:960–970.

Ogawa, M., Hatano, K., Oishi, S., Kawasumi, Y., Fujii, N., Kawaguchi, M., Doi, R., Imamura, M., Yamamoto, M., Ajito, K., Mukai, T., Saji, H., and Ito, K. 2003. Direct electrophilic radiofluorination of a cyclic RGD peptide for in vivo αvβ3 integrin related tumor imaging. *Nucl. Med. Biol.* 30:1–9.

Oltenfreiter, R., Staelens, L., Labied, S., Kersemans, V., Frankenne, F., Noel, A., Van de Wiele, C., and Slegers, G. 2005. Tryptophane-based biphenylsulfonamide matrix metalloproteinase inhibitors as tumor imaging agents. *Cancer Biother. Radiopharm.* 20:639–647.

Oltenfreiter, R., Staelens, L., Lejeune, A., Dumont, F., Frankenne, F., Foidart, J.M., and Slegers, G. 2004. New radioiodinated carboxylic and hydroxamic matrix metalloproteinase inhibitor tracers as potential tumor imaging agents. *Nucl. Med. Biol.* 31:459–468.

Patel, S.R., Jenkins, J., Papadopolous, N., Burgess, M.A., Plager, C., Gutterman, J., and Benjamin, R.S. 2001. Pilot study of vitaxin—an angiogenesis inhibitor—in patients with advanced leiomyosarcomas. *Cancer* 92:1347–1348.

Poethko, T., Schottelius, M., Thumshirn, G., Hersel, U., Herz, M., Henriksen, G., Kessler, H., Schwaiger, M., and Wester, H.J. 2004a. Two-step methodology for high-yield routine radiohalogenation of peptides: ^{18}F-labeled RGD and octreotide analogs. *J. Nucl. Med.* 45:892–902.

Poethko, T., Schottelius, M., Thumshirn, G., Herz, M., Haubner, R., Henriksen, G., Kessler, H., Schwaiger, M., and Wester, H.J. 2004b. Chemoselective pre-conjugate radiohalogenation of unprotected mono- and multimeric peptides via oxime formation. *Radiochimica Acta* 92:317–327.

Poon, R.T., Fan, S.T., and Wong, J. 2001. Clinical implications of circulating angiogenic factors in cancer patients. *J. Clin. Oncol.* 19:1207–1225.

Quirt, I., Bodurth, A., Lohmann, R., Rusthoven, J., Belanger, K., Young, V., Wainman, N., Stewar, W., and Eisenhauer, E. 2002. Phase II study of marimastat (BB-2516) in malignant melanoma: a clinical and tumor biopsy study of the National Cancer Institute of Canada Clinical Trials Group. *Invest. New Drugs* 20:431–437.

Ranieri, G., and Gasparini, G. 2001. Angiogenesis and angiogenesis inhibitors: a new potential anticancer therapeutic strategy. *Curr. Drug. Targets Immune. Endocr. Metabol. Disord.* 1:241–253.

Rosen, L.S. 2002. Inhibitors of the vascular endothelial growth factor receptor. *Hematol. Oncol. Clin. North. Am.* 16:1173–1187.

Rundhaug, J.E. 2005. Matrix metalloproteinases and angiogenesis. *J. Cell Mol. Med.* 9:267–285.

Ruoslahti, E., and Pierschbacher, M.D. 1987. New perspectives in cell adhesion: RGD and integrins. *Science* 238:491–497.

Santimaria, M., Moscatelli, G., Viale, G.L., Giovannoni, L., Neri, G., Viti, F., Leprini, A., Borsi, L., Castellani, P., Zardi, L., Neri, D., and Riva, P. 2003. Immunoscintigraphic detection of the ED-B domain of fibronectin, a marker of angiogenesis, in patients with cancer. *Clin. Cancer Res.* 9:571–579.

Storgard, C.M., Stupack, D.G., Jonczyk, A., Goodman, S.L., Fox, R.I., and Cheresh, D.A. 1999. Decreased angiogenesis and arthritic disease in rabbits treated with an αvβ3 antagonist. *J. Clin. Invest.* 103:47–54.

Su, Z.F., He, J., Rusckowski, M., and Hnatowich, D.J. 2003. *In vitro* cell studies of technetium-99 m labeled RGD-HYNIC peptide, a comparison of tricine and EDDA as co-ligands. *Nucl. Med. Biol.* 30:141–149.

Su, Z.F., Liu, G., Gupta, S., Zhu, Z., Rusckowski, M., and Hnatowich, D.J. 2002. *In vitro* and *in vivo* evaluation of a technetium-99m-labeled cyclic RGD peptide as a specific marker of αvβ3 integrin for tumor imaging. *Bioconjug. Chem.* 13:561–570.

Szekanecz, Z., Gaspar, L., and Koch, A.E. 2005. Angiogenesis in rheumatoid arthritis. *Front. Biosci.* 10:1739–1753.

Tarli, L., Balza, E., Viti, F., Borsi, L., Castellani, P., Berndorff, D., Dinkelborg, L., Neri, D., and Zardi, L. 1999. A high-affinity human antibody that targets tumoral blood vessels. *Blood* 94:192–198.

Thumshirn, G., Hersel, U., Goodman, S.L., and Kessler, H. 2003. Multi-meric cyclic RGD peptides as potential tools for tumor targeting: solid-phase peptide synthesis and chemoselective oxime ligation. *Chemistry* 9:2717–2725.

Vaidyanathan, G., Affleck, D.J., and Zalutsky, M.R. 1993. Radioiodination of proteins using N-succinimidyl 4-hydroxy-3-iodobenzoate. *Bioconjug. Chem. 4*:78–84.

van Hagen, P.M., Breeman, W.A., Bernard, H.F., Schaar, M., Mooij, C.M., Srinivasan, A., Schmidt, M.A., Krenning, E.P., and de Jong, M. 2000. Evaluation of a radiolabeled cyclic DTPA-RGD analogue for tumor imaging and radionuclide therapy. *Int. J. Cancer 90*:186–198.

Vihinen, P., and Kahari, K.M. 2002. Matrix metalloproteinases in cancer: prognostic markers and therapeutic targets. *Int. J. Cancer 99*: 157–166.

Wood, J.M., Bold, G., Buchdunger, E., Cozens, R., Ferrari, S., Frei, J., Hofmann, F., Mestan, J., Mett, H., O'Reilly, T., Persohn, E., Rosel, J., Schnell, C., Stover, D., Theuer, A., Towbin, H., Wenger, F., Woods-Cook, K., Menrad, A., Siemeister, G., Schirner, M., Thierauch, K.H., Schneider, M.R., Drevs, J., Martiny-Baron, G., and Totzke, F. 2000. PTK787/ZK 222584, a novel and potent inhibitor of vascular endothelial growth factor receptor tyrosine kinases, impairs vascular endothelial growth factor-induced responses and tumor growth after oral administration. *Cancer Res. 60*:2178–2189.

Wu, Y., Zhang, X., Xiong, Z., Cheng, Z., Fisher, D.R., Liu, S., Gambhir, S.S., and Chen, X. 2005. microPET imaging of glioma integrin $\alpha v \beta 3$ expression using ^{64}Cu-labeled tetrameric RGD peptide. *J. Nucl. Med. 46*:1707–1718.

Yancopoulos, G.D., Davis, S., Gale, N.W., Rudge, J.S., Wiegand, S.J., and Holash, J. 2000. Vascular-specific growth factors and blood vessel formation. *Nature 407*:242–248.

Yang, J.T., Rayburn, H., and Hynes, R.O. 1993. Embryonic mesodermal defects in alpha 5 integrin-deficient mice. *Development 119*:1093–1105.

Zhang, X., Xiong, Z., Wu, Y., Cai, W., Tseng, J.R., Gambhir, S.S., and Chen, X. 2006. Quantitative PET imaging of tumor integrin $\alpha v \beta 3$ expression with ^{18}F-FRGD2. *J. Nucl. Med. 47*:113–121.

Zheng, Q.H., Fei, X., DeGrado, T.R., Wang, J.Q., Lee Stone, K., Martinez, T.D., Gay, D.J., Baity, W.L., Mock, B.H., Glick-Wilson, B.E., Sullivan, M.L., Miller, K.D., Sledge, G.W., and Hutchins, G.D. 2003. Synthesis, biodistribution and micro-PET imaging of a potential cancer biomarker carbon-11 labeled MMP inhibitor (2R)-2-[[4-(6-fluorohex-1-ynyl)phen-yl]sulfonylamino]-3-methylbutyric acid [^{11}C]methyl ester. *Nucl. Med. Biol. 30*:753–760.

Zheng, Q.H., Fei, X., Liu, X., Wang, J.Q., Bin Sun, H., Mock, B.H., Lee Stone, K., Martinez, T.D., Miller, K.D., Sledge, G.W., and Hutchins, G.D. 2002. Synthesis and preliminary biological evaluation of MMP inhibitor radiotracers [^{11}C]methyl-halo-CGS 27023A analogs, new potential PET breast cancer imaging agents. *Nucl. Med. Biol. 29*:761–770.

Zheng, Q.H., Fei, X., Liu, X., Wang, J.Q., Stone, K.L., Martinez, T.D., Gay, D.J., Baity, W.L., Miller, K.D., Sledge, G.W., and Hutchins, G.D. 2004. Comparative studies of potential cancer biomarkers carbon-11 labeled MMP inhibitors (S)-2-(4'-[^{11}C]methoxybiphenyl-4-sulfonyl-amino)-3-methylbutyric acid and N-hydroxy-(R)-2-[[(4'-[^{11}C]methoxy-phenyl)sulfonyl]benzylamino]-3-methylbutanamide. *Nucl. Med. Biol. 31*:77–85.

13

Gross Tumor Volume and Clinical Target Volume: Anatomical Computed Tomography and Functional FDG-PET

Ernesto Brianzoni, Gloria Rossi, and Alfredo Proietti

Introduction

In 1993 the International Commission on Radiation Units and Measurements (ICRU) Publication (no. 50) gave precise indications in order to define a common language and establish similar models of behavior for all radiotherapy centers. These guidelines especially regarded the aims of therapy, the volume definition, and the quantity of the dose. It is fundamental to define the aims of the therapy in order to decide which levels of dosage should be delivered, which volumes have to be treated, and how accurate we have to be.

We distinguished three categories of therapy:

- Radical treatment for malignancies: In these cases the aim of the therapy is to reduce the number of malignant cells to a level that allows permanent local tumor control. We have to irradiate the evident tumor portion and a surrounding area where there is a certain probability of tumor development and where there would not be any clinically evident malignant cells. These two portions are often treated with different dose levels. When

the tumor is surgically removed, it is opportune to irradiate the remaining tissue that could be affected but in a subclinical stage.

- Palliative treatment: The aim of palliative radiotherapy is to reduce the symptoms of the disease when it is impossible to control the tumor locally. The irradiated volume can also partially contain the tumor volume or not.
- Nonmalignant disease therapy.

Prescribing a radiation dose delivery involves not only the determination of the Gy quantity to administer, but also the exact tumor volume definition and the volume that should be protected, with a respective tolerated dose level (organs at risk). These are radiotherapy limitations that must be evaluated in advance.

For the definition of volume, Figure 1 shows the criteria to be used to determine the zones and the consequent dose levels (ICRU 50, 1993):

The GTV is the gross tumor volume, that is, the evident tumor.

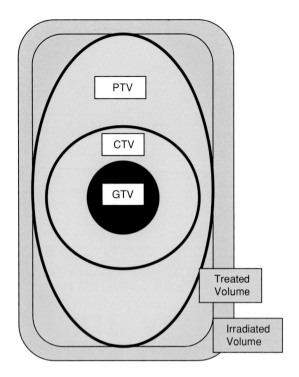

Figure 1 Definition of the volumes in radiotherapy planning in accordance with ICRU Publication no. 50 (1993).

The CTV is the clinical target volume, that is, the area surrounding the tumor that could have subclinical suspect disease. For example, regional lymph nodes, NO (according to the TNM-classification [International Union Against Cancer, 2004]), is considered to need treatment. The CTV is a clinical concept.

The PTV is the planning target volume, that is, the volume inclusive of GTV, CTV, and a margin that takes into account a possible variation in shape, size, and position relative to the treatment beams and organ motion. As we can see in Figure 1, the variations might not be homogeneous in the three directions. The PTV, as a geometrical concept, ensures the prescribed dose in the CTV.

The Treated Volume is the volume that receives a dose important for cure or palliation.

The Irradiated Volume is the volume that receives a dose important for normal tissue tolerance.

In accordance with the ICRU, the dose prescription must be set to an ICRU reference point, so that:

● It will be clinically evident and representative of the PTV dose.
● It will be clearly definable and not ambiguous.
● The dose inside will be accurately determined.
● The region in which it is located will not be a high dose gradient.

These requirements are satisfied when the reference point is located in the center or in the PTV central zone and on the

beam axis, or near it. If this is impossible, however, it necessarily has to be inside the PTV, where the dose is significant, and, therefore, where it is expected to have the maximal tumor cell concentration.

It is hoped that the distribution of the effectively delivered dose will be as homogeneous as possible inside the PTV. It is necessary to evaluate the level of homogeneity registered near the reference point dose, as well as the minimum and maximum value inside the PTV. For a more accurate evaluation, other indicators, such as the mean dose value with standard deviation or dose-volume histogram, can be used. Generally, a variance of ±5% with respect to the prescribed dose can be considered acceptable. In radiotherapy several imaging modalities, such as computed tomography (CT), ultrasound (US), and magnetic resonance imaging (MRI), can be used. In addition to these methods, in recent years positron emission tomography (PET) has become popular but has not completely replaced the previous methods. Rather, PET has complemented them and added a new facet of information that has changed targeting measuring the biological target volume (BTV) (Ling *et al.*, 2000). When a baseline PET scan shows that a tumor has high tracer avidity, then this modality has a high rate of accuracy in staging, targeting, and determining recurrent carcinomas, as well as in evaluating the biological effects of radiotherapy. In particular, PET/CT scanning allows the definition of the boundaries of the tumor with a precise mapping and tends to change ~ 17–70% of treatment plans for cancer patients (Messa *et al.*, 2006).

The final objective of radiation oncology is to ensure that no tumor survives to a high-dose concentration delivery. But the problem is how substantial a dose is necessary? Which volumes are to be considered? How do we define the marginal volumes? The dose depends on the tumor type and on its biology, and the area depends on the best available imaging methods.

The attempt to obtain the best image is the actual goal of the radiation oncologist, who exploits intense narrow multiangle beam delivery and computed optimization plans to track targets and minimize side effects. The PET imaging can help the oncologist in achieving this goal, because PET functional imaging is characterized by *in vivo* physiology, can differentiate between susceptibility and resistance to a therapy within a tumor, and with corresponding anatomical imaging (CT) can define tumor area more accurately. Finally, whole-body ^{18}F-FDG PET has been proven to be a very effective imaging modality for the staging of many malignant tumors, in particular lung cancer, malignant melanoma, lymphoma, colorectal cancer, and head and neck tumors.

Radioprotection of the Patient

The radioprotection of the patient is a relatively recently recognized problem in comparison with protecting the public and workers. It has been developed in a different way because the validity of some principles generally adopted in radio-protection never applies to medical application. In this situation the cost-benefit analysis can be on the same level or all to the advantage of the latter.

All kinds of radiotherapy submit the patient to a certain risk, and an effort to completely eliminate this risk can lead to therapeutic failure and death: a treatment can be harmful when a dose is too high because of excessive diffusion in the surrounding normal tissue at or because of an insufficient dose. If the dose is too low to sterilize, the tumor can select resistant cells, and if it is shared out in too small a volume the tumor can grow. In ICRP 26 and ICRP 60 we find three fundamental radioprotection principles: (1) justification, (2) optimization, and (3) dose limitation. The first principle establishes that every treatment has to be made only after an accurate evaluation of the benefit deriving from it. The second principle, optimization, involves enhancing of the whole process, from the dosimetric study to the treatment plan, from the execution of the single-therapy setting to periodical check without neglecting an adequate quality control protocol on the main and minor devices. The third principle is probably the most difficult to apply in radiotherapy. While for people working in this environment the aim of radioprotection is to avoid irradiation, in radiotherapy the objective is to obtain the best balance between the need to irradiate the disease with a lethal dose and the need to obtain the minimum risk of side effects (this is the ALARA principle, as low as reasonably achievable). The PET/CT images for radiotherapy planning contributes to the therapy optimization operating within the parameters of the ALARA principle.

Method

As explained earlier regarding dose optimization and correct image visualization, we have developed a method that uses PET/CT imaging to define and improve radiotherapy planning. The aim of the PET/CT registration is to establish an exact point-to-point correspondence between the voxels of the different modalities, making a direct comparison possible. There are three different ways to consider fusion: (1) visual, (2) semi-hardware, and (3) complete.

The *visual* fusion is a separate visualization on different monitor images from CT images and PET images; later, the operator makes a sort of imaginary fusion (virtual). In the *semi-hardware* fusion, images are acquired in a sequential way during the same examination by hybrid scanner (as in our case) where the transmitted and emitted data are required at intervals as long as necessary to transfer the pallet from the CT position to the PET position. The final images are fused by an operating system that uses CT data for both attenuation correction in the PET images and for anatomic lesion definition and localization.

In an ideal way, real co-registration would occur only if emitted and transmitted data were acquired at the same time and instantaneously, so as to prevent respiratory and involuntary movement artifacts (*complete*). In the semi-hardware co-registration, we allow an anatomical-functional fusion that could be used in nuclear medicine (NM) practice to find and localize lesions, and also with some care in radiotherapy planning (RTP) for the optimization of the target volume definition. In fact, treatment planning is organized in the radiotherapy unit through devices (accelerators) that have mechanical and technical characteristics differing from those of NM devices (scanners). To avoid this inconvenience, it is sufficient during the NM examination to use the same equipment as used in the RTP. In order to limit variations in position, immobilization of the patient for both the scan and subsequent therapy is performed using a flat table and an immobilization device (Fig. 2), which are customized for each patient (using conforming body casts, thermoplastic face masks, head holders, and Belly Boards). The correct positioning of the patient on the mechanical devices is necessary to avoid trivial mistakes that could lead to enormous GTV miscalculation. To accomplish this goal, we use a centering laser both in PET/CT acquisition and in radiotherapy planning. Using a laser in transverse plane at a level corresponding to the bulk of the tumor, three markers are placed to establish a reference slice within the CT data. Within this slice, a reference point called a pseudo-isocenter focused on the tumor is established. From this reference point, the precise target is identified, and this point is shifted to a "true" isocenter. We use a laser system mounted on the PET room, which is identical to the one used in the accelerator room, so as to have the same geometrical configuration without needing to adjust the value.

Eighty-four patients (60 males and 24 females) submitted to RT were included in our study; 64 patients were affected by lung cancer (41 NSCLC, 23 SCLC), 10 by head and neck high-grade non-Hodgkin's Lymphoma (Nhl), 5 by head and neck carcinoma, 3 by paraaortic lymph nodes from ovarian carcinoma, and 2 by mammary lymph nodes. The patient age range was 36 to 81 years; the mean age was 61.9 years. PET/CT examination was performed in the heterogeneous group of patients with different aims for RT after a PET/CT confirmation study: preoperative (6 cases), curative after chemotherapy (45 cases), adjuvant after surgery (21 cases), radical (6 cases), and relapsed (6 cases). The purpose was simulation for RT planning, according to the expectation that RT would be the most likely therapeutic option. All the patients included in this study have active lesions in PET imaging.

For patients who submitted to simulation, for examination and treatment, we used a linear accelerator of 15 MV. Next they were submitted to PET examination in the same position initially assumed for RT immobilization. The simulation scan is very important because it serves as a template for the delivery of radiation throughout the course of treatment.

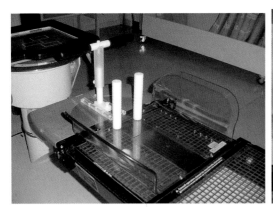 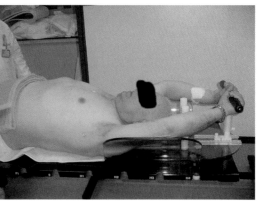

Figure 2 Immobilization device Wing-Board and RT pallet.

Because the patient will be expected to assume this same position before receiving each of the 25 to 40 apportioned doses over the course of 4 to 6 weeks, the precise, rapid reproducibility of this position is fundamental to ensure the correct delivery of the prescribed dose.

The PET/CT protocol requires patient fasting for 6 hr before the examination. The patient is first subjected to complete anamnesis, and serum glucose levels are measured before ^{18}F-FDG administration to verify an acceptable value (the cut-off is 140 mg/dl); then they are injected with a solution of ^{18}F-FDG in a dose of 5.18 MBq/Kg, relaxing for an hour drinking water before the examination. We acquire a scout image first to select the area involved, and then we perform a spiral CT examination with a dual-slice scanner. In the gantry PET, the 3D emissive acquisition with beds 16 cm long and time of 3 min/bed begins. A flat tabletop insert on the PET/CT scanner was utilized to achieve the same position obtained in the radiation treatment room. Immobilization of 43/64 patients with lung cancer was performed with a comfortable device for supporting the patient's arms overhead (Med-Tec extended (Wing-Board), while 21/64 patients with a Vac-Lok cushion were similarly treated with arms overhead. The isocenter was chosen for each patient and marked on the skin surface with external localization wires. Fifteen patients with head and neck Nhl and carcinoma were subjected to immobilization with a thermoplastic mask system. For the other pathologies the immobilization devices were the Belly Board and Vac-Lok cushion. The treatment position was supine, with arms up for lung cancer and thorax lesions and down for head and neck cases. Using the simulator lasers, patients were aligned and marked to define the coordinate system to be used for the treatment planning with external markers. In patients submitted to RT, proper patient alignment was obtained and then repeated in the radiation treatment room by using external lasers in every session.

Taking into account the imaging modalities, PET and CT were performed with the same technical equipment, the integrated LSO PET/CT scanner. Computed tomography

scan acquisitions were performed on a spiral CT dual slice, with a slice thickness of 4 mm and a pitch of 1. Images were acquired using a matrix of 512 × 512 pixels and a pixel size of ~ 1 mm and reconstructed for treatment planning system workstations with a thickness of 3.4 mm. The same thickness was used for PET images. These data were acquired using a matrix of 128 × 128 pixels, with a slice thickness of 3.4 mm. The final imaging resolution for clinical practice is ~ 6.5 mm. Positron emission tomography (PET) scans were performed ~ 45 – 60 min after the intravenous administration of FDG in the dose previously defined. Computed tomography data are used by software to evaluate the attenuation correction of the emission images. The PET images were reconstructed by the iterative method OSEM (Ordered Subset EM) (2 iterations, 8 subsets) with a Gaussian filter of 5 mm.

An important question regards the image fusion. Intensity-based registration, requiring a strict correlation between pixels in one image and the corresponding pixels in the second image, achieved a very strong correlation in integrated images from the same equipment. Therefore, the co-registration of PET and CT data obtained with the integrated PET/CT scanner could improve the diagnostic accuracy of image interpretation (Lardinois et al., 2003). Moreover, a strong interchange was required between radiation oncologist and nuclear medicine specialist for proper image analysis and interpretation.

Our method used to define volume in the PET images is achieved by dual approach. We have considered a certain number of patients with the same disease characteristics for whom we have a histological report. We took into account all the axial sections in the PET images. We used different thresholds (20%, 30%, 40%, 50%, 60%, and 70%), and we delimited the areas visualized with these values. Then we made a "volumization" by multiplying the sum of all areas in every threshold value for the slice thickness, thereby obtaining the volume. This value was then compared with the histological volume, and from this we chose the best threshold to use. In the majority of cases, the result was 40%. After this approach, we compared the volume calculated in this way to a value obtained with a mathematical approach to its definition in the image, from which we used a Laplacian filter with a gradient to select the border line. Then we decided the area of the single slice apart from the visualization threshold. In this case, too, the best comparison was with a 40% threshold.

Discussion

Of the 84 patients selected for this study, 75 were included in the evaluation of the influence of PET on RT volume. The remaining nine were not included because information provided by PET led to modification of the stage and of the management strategy from radical RT to palliative therapy. In 40 of the aforementioned 75 cases (53%), the PET information did not significantly change the GTV or CTV delineated on CT images, whereas in the other 35 appreciable differences were observed. In 16/35 cases, the target volume was decreased by addition of the PET information to the CT data, leading to a reduction in the treated volumes and, consequently, a lower risk of radiation toxicity. In these cases, we considered the smaller volume on the PET image to represent the treatment volume. In 6/16 patients, there was a decrease in GTV because of clear differentiation between tumor tissue and peritumoral but nonneoplastic atelectasis. In 10/16 the target volume decreased owing to exclusion of a peripheral area of atelectasis.

Similarly, some parenchymal areas of atelectasis, highly suspected to be tumor localizations on the basis of CT, showed no metabolic activity on FDG-PET images. Accordingly, it can be concluded that a substantial reduction in the size of radiation portals may be obtained when PET is used for treatment planning in patients with lesion-associated atelectasis (Nestle *et al.*, 1999). In the other 19/35 cases, the target volume was increased. In 10/19 patients lymph node involvement that was neither obvious nor suspected on CT images alone was well demonstrated by FDG-PET studies. This finding underlines the effectiveness of PET in combination with CT in assessing the extent of locoregional lymph node involvement in many neoplastic conditions. There was one clear example of an increase in CTV owing to PET: CT images showed primary lung cancer in the left upper lobe (Fig. 3A), but no evidence of mediastinal lymph node involvement. Positron emission tomography images revealed a pathological level of FDG uptake not only in the left upper lobe (Fig. 3B), but also in the subcarinal region, indicating metastatic lymph node extension (Fig. 3C). Three-dimensional conformal treatment planning was performed, choosing the volume based on FDG uptake, which was larger than the CT-based CTV (Fig. 3D). In this case, the PET data reduced the likelihood of geographic misses and improved the likelihood of achieving local tumor control.

In 9/19 cases, GTV was increased on the basis of comparison between PET images and CT data, illustrating the better definition of GTV that resulted from the addition of PET to CT (Giraud *et al.*, 2002).

In the case of one patient, an area of high metabolic activity was observed on PET beyond the tumor volume as assessed on CT, where the area of atelectasis was judged to be wider. Positron emission tomography led to inclusion of the area in question in the target volume, which was accordingly better delineated. Three-dimensional conformal treatment planning, commonly using CT to accurately delineate the target lesion volume and normal surrounding tissues, has been able to precisely conform the dose distribution to CTV.

Ling (Ling *et al.*, 2000) summarized imaging advances that have potential application in radiation oncology and emphasized the need to adequately identify various target volumes as defined by ICRU Report No. 50 and ICRU Report No. 62. They proposed the new concept of a biological target volume (BTV), which can be derived from biological images that will substantially improve target delineation, treatment planning, and RT delivery, incorporating both physical and biological aspects for a multidimensional conformal therapy.

Many methods have been published regarding image fusion and registration from different modalities, and they were reviewed in a summary publication (Perez *et al.*, 2002). With the co-registration method, it was possible to obtain a good correlation between the images (Rosenman, 2001), but this correlation was very strong in integrated images from the same equipment, first performed in the study of Lardinois (2003). Although some reports of RT planning using the integrated PET/CT suggest a significant improvement in image co-registration, some problems in PET and CT information acquisition remain to be solved (Lardinois *et al.*, 2003). Three-dimensional conformal RT decision making has opted to treat only gross disease and to eliminate the elective nodal irradiation due to PET/CT imaging; in this way it is possible to reduce the irradiation of normal tissues, thus keeping toxicity within acceptable levels. We already have seen that an identical setup between two different imaging modalities is fundamental to being able to compare the resulting images. In relevant literature (Toloza *et al.*, 2003), we found that mediastinal nodal involvement was more sensitive with FDG-PET (84%) than CT (57%) and also more specific (89% versus 82%); so that by PET findings we can decide whether or not a lymph node was considered pathological, while by CT we can localize the lesions exactly. Many studies have been performed for testing the combined imaging modality PET/CT, which resulted in better RT volume definition (Messa *et al.*, 2006).

Some authors have performed their studies using a visual method of fusion (virtual). Kiffer *et al.* (1998), performing

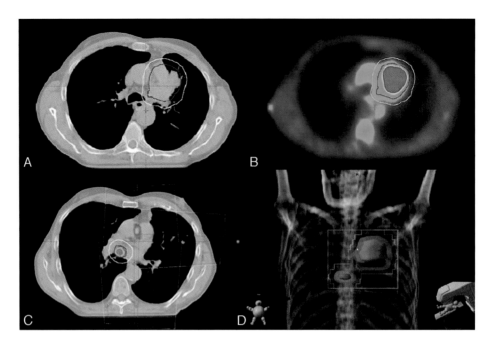

Figure 3 (**A**) CT image showing primary lung cancer in the left upper lobe. The red line defines the GTV, and the yellow line defines the CTV. (**B**) Positron emission tomography reveals pathological FDG uptake (purple and green area) in the left upper lobe at the same level as the CT image in A. (**C**) The fusion image documents that FDG uptake is also present in the subcarinal region, indicating metastatic lymph node extension not visible on CT. The red line defines the GTV, and the yellow line defines the CTV. In this image a part of the treatment field of radiotherapy planning is seen (yellow wedges). (**D**) 3D conformal treatment planning was performed, choosing the volume based on FDG uptake, which encompassed lymph node disease. This figure clearly reveals the increase in GTV (red volume) and the consequent increase in CTV (yellow volume) due to inclusion of lymph nodes in the subcarinal region

PET/CT on 15 patients, noted a CTV modification with PET scanning in 4 cases (27%), with an increase in target volume definition in all 4 cases. A similar increase in CTV delineation for RT treatment planning was performed by Giraud *et al.* (2001), analyzing fusion in co-registration images through CT and PET in 12 patients. They observed an increased CTV in 5/12 cases (41%). Positron emission tomography could change the shape and dimension of GTV and CTV in a significant number of patients, and these variations were strongly influenced by lymph node staging. Similarly, Munley *et al.* (1999), in a retrospective study, evaluated 35 lung cancer patients delineating pre-irradiation target volume with standard CT only or in addition to PET scanning and CT/PET imaging co-registration, used to perform RT planning. Their study resulted in an increased modification in CTV definition in 12 cases (34%) because of lymph node staging.

Nestle *et al.* (1999), have demonstrated that, in cases where atelectasis was present, use of a PET scanner might facilitate a reduction in field sizes. In 34 patients studied, they observed CTV changes in 12 cases, with RT volume decreased in 9/12 cases for atelectasis, excluding areas not involved on PET images. FDG-PET imaging can help to distinguish between tumor and atelectasis, making use of CT data: we can in fact reduce the field size in radiotherapy planning. Another advantage of PET in the RTP decisions is to distinguish between tumor tissue and nonneoplastic areas: a focus of inflammatory area near the tumor, also suspected as local extension on CT images, could be assessed by PET because of little or no metabolic activity.

Mah *et al.* (2002) analyzed 30 patients with NSCLC on CT scans who were treated with RT and underwent CT simulation and FDG-PET scanning in the treatment position by means of co-registration. In 7/30 cases (23%), PET information changed the therapy from radical to palliative, whereas in 5/23 remaining patients (22%) FDG-PET scan data more easily permitted an increased target volume definition than using CT scan data alone. Other authors used an image fusion by software using CT and PET devices separately.

Vanuytsel *et al.* (2000), comparing CT and PET-CT in volumetric studies for defining tumor extension in patients with NSCLC, considered for curative RT, observed that the combination of PET-CT significantly improved the accuracy in the assessment of lymph node staging. In 73 patients studied, the CT defined volume was identical to the PET-CT defined volume in 28 cases, leaving 45 patients (62%) in whom the additional acquisition of PET data changed treatment volumes. In 16/73 patients (22%), the PET-CT defined volume was larger than the only CT defined volume, while in 29/73 cases (40%) was smaller. Therefore, the combined use of a CT scan and FDG-PET images instead of CT scan alone improves GTV delineation leading to a substantial reduction in the irradiated lung volume in selected patients.

MacManus *et al.* (2002) evaluated the impact of FDG-PET staging in radical RT of nonsurgically treatable NSCLC. In 102 patients who received definitive RT after PET scanning, there was a significant increase in the target volume in 22 cases because of the inclusion of structures previously considered uninvolved by the tumor, whereas in 16 patients there was a significant decrease in the target volume because of the exclusion of areas of lung consolidation with low FDG uptake, or because uninvolved nodes were not treated. They observed a consistent variation in RT target volume in 38/102 (37%) patients and reported that 30% of patients with locally advanced NSCLC became ineligible for curative RT because of the metastases that FDG-PET demonstrated.

Erdi *et al.* (2002), performing both CT simulation and PET scanning in the RT treatment position in 11 patients, noted that the incorporation of PET data improved definition of the primary lesion by including positive lymph nodes into the CTV, because PET scanning had higher sensitivity than CT in detecting mediastinal metastases in the NSCLC. In 7/11 cases, they observed an increase in target volume (average increase of 19%) to incorporate lymph nodal metastases. In the other 4 patients, the target volume was smaller (average decrease of 18%); the reduction of CTV in 2 of these patients was due to excluding peritumoral atelectasis and trimming the target volume to avoid delivering higher radiation doses to the nearby spinal cord or heart. Finally some authors use a hybrid PET/CT system (semi-hardware fusion).

Bradley *et al.* (2004a, 2004b), in a prospective trial, evaluated 26 patients with NSCLC before RT. Computed tomography simulation was followed by ^{18}F-FDG-PET using the same immobilization device. Comparing the target volume contours outlined with CT alone and PET-CT co-registered images, they observed that PET significantly altered the target volume for 3D-CRT in 14/24 eligible patients (58%). Positron emission tomography permitted the separation of tumor focus from atelectasis in 3 cases, while detection of unsuspected nodal involvement was obtained by FDG-PET in 10/24 (42%) patients. Bradley's data and the reported literature (Perez *et al.*, 2003), suggested that radiation targeting with fused FDG-PET and CT images resulted in alterations of RT planning in over 50% of patients by comparison with CT targeting only.

Our last work (Brianzoni *et al.*, 2005), showing better delineation of GTV and CTV with PET/CT fusion in 24/55 (44%) of eligible patients, confirmed the literature review. This suggested that biological targeting with PET could change the RT volume significantly in about 50% of cases,

in the range between 30% and 60% of patients (Bradley *et al.*, 2004a). At present it is impossible to have a complete co-registration method as described previously. The results of these reports suggest that FDG-PET is a highly sensitive imaging modality that could better visualize tumor extension and radiation field definition, biologically characterizing and accurately delineating the target volume to optimize RT planning. Two important problems need to be solved: (1) the delineation of GTV edges on PET images (Paulino and Johnstone, 2004), and (2) both the tumor motion secondary to respiratory movements for RT in thoracic lesions and organ movement. We will discuss the subject in more detail later.

Problems and Their Solutions

In PET imaging, the registration inaccuracies related to several artifacts are more present in PET than in CT, and they have great importance. The most common sources of errors are: (1) partial volume effects, (2) patient motion, (3) image resolution, and (4) window display level. We have made no efforts to attempt to correct the PET data for partial-volume effects. The main problem we encounter when we use different imaging modalities to obtain a single image to work with involves the match precision. We can obtain it by using reference markers, but it would be impossible to avoid registration problems linked to involuntary movements such as respiratory, cardiac, and peristalsis that also involve the markers. Moreover, the CT examination is shorter than the whole-body PET scan, which takes ~ 20 min in a standard person. So, in this case it is impossible to compare two images acquired in such a different way. This problem is evident in lung cancer when the lesions are in the lower lobes. In order to exploit the great potential of PET/CT imaging in RT planning, it is fundamental to eliminate or at least to minimize inaccuracies caused by patient respiration. Errors introduced as a result of respiration include an artificial enlargement of the active lesion, well beyond the effect of partial volume, and lesion misplacement. The only possible solution is to use a respiratory gating in which the PET data acquisition could be triggered to register data only during certain parts of the respiratory cycle, thereby minimizing respiratory artifacts (Nehmeh *et al.*, 2002) with a great loss of data.

In fact, some have tried to minimize the errors asking patients to hold their breath for a short time when exhaling during the chest CT examination. This represents a compromise for CT because smaller lesions are better seen with a breath hold during maximal lung expansion, but asking the patient to hold his or her breath after exhaling is more practical for planning and subsequent therapy. It is also easier for the patient to perform (Bujenovic, 2004). We avoid all types of breath-holding because the available data indicate that a good image can be obtained under normal breathing (Visvikis *et al.*, 2003). Another technique is the use of dynamic imaging to obtain organ movement models in association with reconstruction algorithms without affecting PET performance (Pevsner *et al.*, 2006). Moreover, we used patient-specific immobilization to minimize this kind of problem. There is another solution—that is, shortening acquisition time with a new scanner, such as PET Time of Flight (TOF).

Positron emission tomography TOF is a recurrent idea in the development of nuclear imaging. It has not been developed because of the difficulty in finding an ideal crystal, fast and bright. This scanner type would be the fifth generation of PET, and its basic principle is based on measurement of the actual time difference between detection of two coincident gamma rays originating from the same annihilation process and using it to reduce noise, improve image quality, make shorter imaging times, and make a lower dose delivery. We also take into account the fact that two different imaging modalities are being used. Thus, to have a more accurate utilization of PET volumes in RT planning we have to check the relationship between the coordinates of the PET/CT images and of the RT. We solve this problem by using an intensity-based registration plus a laser positioning of three reference markers on the patient's body.

In radiotherapy patients, we can often find atelectasia or necrosis near the tumor environment, and this leads to a problematic approach in defining lesion volume and size. In both cases, CT images help us to define and reduce the problems, even if it is sometimes necessary to make a personalized interpretation of the images considered. If the question is localized near the tumor, usually we consider all the area and put it inside the GTV. Computed tomography images have set windows and centers, which are optimized for displaying various tissue densities, and these values are known by default. It is not true in the case of PET images. On PET it is very difficult to establish the margins of the tumor for the contouring physician.

The main problem is to establish *a priori* the best threshold for visualization of the lesion. This can obviously depend on the tumor type and position because changing the window levels may change the interpretation of lesion margin. We can overestimate or underestimate the target margin, and so administer an overdose or an underdose to the patient. For example, in pulmonary carcinomas, PET/CT is one of the principal methods of visualization of the lesion that makes quantifying its volume possible. The result is closely connected with the imaging method because obviously the uptake is modified according to the imaging threshold. The literature reports work conducted on establishing the imaging threshold for use in representing the target volume, with values ranging from 40 to 50% (Erdi *et al.*, 1997). The major difficulty associated with standardizing the calculation is, therefore, to identify the uptake threshold that is nearest to the clinical reality and that allows a precise volumetric calculation and target definition.

Our solution has been to use the 40% threshold and this decision is also due to the results of our study regarding this subject in which we considered different thresholds for the pulmonary lesions and found which one better correlates with real lesions. In the volume definition we now use a visual technique that could be improved and is faster by use of a mathematical algorithm that automatically selects the volume involved on the functional image, taking into account atelectasia or necrosis.

Another question we need to deal with is the choice of the radiopharmaceutical used. The most widespread choice is undoubtedly ^{18}F-FDG. In our center we usually consider primarily ^{18}F-FDG for the majority of tumors (lung and head and neck). Our aim is to obtain good images that can be used to plan a radiotherapy treatment and from which we can see functionality and find lesions. Another goal of radiotherapy is to identify the presence or absence of tumor hypoxia, an important and common condition that affects the tumor microenvironment as a resistance factor. So, in this case probably the most promising choices for PET radiopharmaceuticals in the radiotherapy planning imaging are ^{18}F-FASA, ^{18}F-MISO, and Cu-ATSM; these last two were recently compared in a study (O'Donoghue *et al.*, 2005). In addition, we can find other oncological radiopharmaceuticals for PET imaging with different characteristics: for visualizing nonpathological areas connected with soft tissue infections, for evaluating different tumor aspects (comparing different lesion uptakes with different radiotracers), or for the proliferation of cells by entering the salvage pathway of DNA synthesis, for the tumor response, for the measurement of thymidine-kinase 1 activity, hypoxia (Rajendran *et al.*, 2006), and angiogenesis (Haubner, 2006).

Once all the data have been acquired, they are sent to the radiation treatment software: in this phase, it is fundamental that manufacturers of this software validate the Digital Imaging and Communications in Medicine (DICOM) compatibility of every CT or PET scanner before data are accepted. In our case we compare the DICOM compatibility of every software and license we use, and we ensure the correct data transfer through the intranet with a complex quality control on the net. After the transfer, data are fused in the RTP system because prefused CT-PET images will not be accepted. We use a standard automated program that uses intensity-based registration.

The PET scanners of the last decades have always been limited regarding spatial resolution, which is always $\geq 6\,mm$. This obviously does not allow the definition of small lesions, particularly in anatomically complex zones (thorax and abdomen).

We must consider that all detectors surround the patient, and that all acquired data contribute to reconstructing an image of the *in vivo* radioisotope distribution. The events to be considered are only the "true coincidences," but they are not the only ones. Two alternative erroneous coincident events could be detected; scattered events and random events. A system's intrinsic spatial resolution can be optimized only if the scanner has sufficient sensitivity or a higher sensitivity that leads to a good resolution and so to a better signal-to-noise ratio. And, consequently, to a better disease visualization as with the new high-resolution PET scanner. On the other hand, minimizing the random and scattered events can lead to improvement in the *in vivo* quantitative accuracy, as with the PET TOF system. It is therefore fundamental that a quality control system will be set up that will help avoid every malfunction or erroneous data interpretations.

Another possible future development is linked to the PET/MRI fusion imaging: MRI provides high spatial resolution and very good soft tissue contrast, better than that provided by the CT. Co-registering PET and MRI can lead to some excellent anatomical information for the *in vivo* functional process. A serious problem to solve is that the PET photomultiplier tube cannot operate under a magnetic field, so it is necessary to engineer a system with optical fibers to drive the light outside the magnetic field.

Expected Improvement

Positron emission tomography allows differentiation between tumor and peritumoral atelectasis and changing treatment volumes. It is very useful in assessing lymphnodal status or can confirm CT data for better delineation of GTV and CTV, showing the superiority of combined modality PET/CT versus CT alone in RT volume definition and optimizing the treatment with respect to the ALARA principle.

The possibility of PET/CT use introduces another concept, the biological target volume. With BTV it is possible have nonuniform dose delivery to smaller volumes inside the GTV (Rajendran *et al.*, 2006). Moreover, we can study hypoxia, and so we can characterize the tumor and its microenvironment and plan individualized treatment. It is possible to use PET/CT images for intensity-modulated radiation therapy (IMRT) planning with ^{18}F-FDG or the other radiotracers cited before.

Intensity-modulated radiotherapy planning is an advanced mode of high-precision radiotherapy that utilizes computer-controlled X-ray accelerators to deliver precise radiation doses to a malignant tumor or specific areas within the tumor. The radiation dose is designed to conform to the 3D shape of the tumor by modulating or controlling the intensity of the radiation beam to focus a higher radiation dose on the tumor in correspondence to higher PET radiopharmaceutical uptake, while minimizing radiation exposure to surrounding normal tissues. Moreover, with a single PET/CT scan, we can obtain diagnostic information and a therapeutic application.

References

Bradley, J.D., Perez, C.A., Dehdashti, F., and Siegel, B.A. 2004a. Implementing biologic target volumes in radiation treatment planning for non-small cell lung cancer. *J. Nucl. Med. 45* (Suppl.) S96–S101.

Bradley, J., Thorstad, W.L., Mutic, S., Miller, T.R., Dehdashti, F., Siegel, B.A., Bosch, W., and Bertrand, R.J. 2004b. Impact of FDG-PET on radiation therapy volume delineation in non-small cell lung cancer. *Int. J. Radiat. Oncol. Biol. Phys. 59*:78–85.

Brianzoni, E., Rossi, G., Ancidei, S., Berbellini, A., Capoccetti, F., Cidda, C., D'Avenia, P., Fattori, S., Montini, G.C., Valentini, G., and Proietti, A. 2005. Radiotherapy planning: PET/CT scanner performances in the definition of gross tumor volume and clinical target volume. *Eur. J. Nucl. Med. Mol. Imag. 32*:1392–1399. Erratum in: *Eur. J. Nucl. Med. Mol. Imag. 32*:1491. Algranati, Carlo [added].

Bujenovic, S. 2004. The role of positron emission tomography in radiation treatment planning. *Semin. Nucl. Med. 34*:293–299. (Review.)

Erdi, Y.E., Mawlawi, O., Larson, S.M., Imbriaco, M., Yeung, H., Finn, R., and Humm, J.L. 1997. Segmentation of lung lesion volume by adaptive positron emission tomography image thresholding. *Cancer 15. 80*:2505–2509.

Erdi, Y.E., Rosenzweig, K., Erdi, A.K., Macapinlac, H.A., Hu, Y.C., Braban, L.E., Humm, J.L., Squire, O.D., Chui, C.S., Larson, S.M., and Yorke, E.D. 2002. Radiotherapy treatment planning for patients with non-small cell lung cancer using positron emission tomography (PET). *Radiother. Oncol. 62*:51–60.

Giraud, P., Grahek, D., Montravers, F., Carette, M.F., Deniaud-Alexandre, E., Julia, F., Rosenwald, J.C., Cosset, J.M., Talbot, J.N., Housset, M., and Touboul, E. 2001. CT and 18F-deoxyglucose (FDG) image fusion for optimization of conformal radiotherapy of lung cancers. *Int. J. Radiat. Oncol. Biol. Phys. 49*:1249–1257.

Giraud, P., Elles, S., Helfre, S., De Rycke, Y., Servois, V., Carette, M.F., Alzieu, C., Bondiau, P.Y., Dubray, B., Touboul, E., Housset, M., Rosenwald, J.C., and Cosset, J.M. 2002. Conformal radiotherapy for lung cancer: different delineation of the gross tumor volume (GTV) by radiologists and radiation oncologists. *Radiother. Oncol. 62*:27–36.

Haubner, R. 2006. Alpha (v)beta (3)-integrin imaging: a new approach to characterise angiogenesis? *Eur. J. Nucl. Med. Mol. Imag. 33* (Suppl.) 13:54–63.

Kiffer, J.D., Berlangieri, S.U., Scott, A.M., Quong, G., Feigen, M., Schumer, W., Clarke, C.P., Knight, S.R., and Daniel, F.J. 1998. The contribution of 18F-fluorodeoxyglucose positron emission tomographic imaging to radiotherapy planning in lung cancer. *Lung Cancer 19*:167–177.

International Union Against Cancer. 2004. TNM Classification of Malignant Tumors, 5th edition, Wittekind, C., Greene, F.L., and Hutter, R.V. P. (Eds). Berlin, Heidelberg, New York: Springer-Verlag, p. 166.

Lardinois, D., Weder, W., Hany, T.F., Kamel, E.M., Korom, S., Seifert, B., von Schulthess, G.K., and Steinert, H.C. 2003. Staging of non-small-cell lung cancer with integrated positron-emission tomography and computed tomography. *N. Engl. J. Med. 348*:2500–2507.

Ling, C.C., Humm, J., Larson, S., Amols, H., Fuks, Z., Leibel, S., and Koutcher, J.A. 2000. Towards multidimensional radiotherapy (MD-CRT): biological imaging and biological conformality. *Int. J. Radiat. Oncol. Biol. Phys. 47*:551–560.

Mac Manus, M.P., Hicks, R.J., Ball, D.L., Kalff, V., Matthews, J.P., Salminen, E., Khaw, P., Wirth, A., Rischin, D., and McKenzie, A. 2001. F-18 fluorodeoxyglucose positron emission tomography staging in radical radiotherapy candidates with non-small cell lung carcinoma: powerful correlation with survival and high impact on treatment. *Cancer 92*:886–895.

Mah, K., Caldwell, C.B., Ung, Y.C., Danjoux, C.E., Balogh, J.M., Ganguli, S.N., Ehrlich, L.E., and Tirona, R. 2002. The impact of ^{18}FDG-PET on target and critical organs in CT-based treatment planning or patients with poorly defined non-small-cell lung carcinoma: a prospective study. *Int. J. Radiat. Oncol. Biol. Phys. 52*:339–350.

Messa, C., Di Muzio, N., Picchio, M., Gilardi, M.C., Bettinardi, V., and Fazio, F. 2006. PET/CT and radiotherapy. *Q. J. Nucl. Med. Mol. Imag. 50*:4–14.

Munley, M.T., Marks, L.B., Scarfone, C., Sibley, G.S., Patz, E.F., Jr., Turkington, T.G., Jaszczak, R.J., Gilland, D.R., Anscher, M.S., and Coleman, R.E. 1999. Multimodality nuclear medicine imaging in radiation treatment planning for lung cancer: challenges and prospects. *Lung Cancer. 23*:105–114.

Nehmeh, S.A., Erdi, Y.E., Ling, C.C., Rosenzweig, K.E., Schoder, H., Larson, S.M., Macapinlac, H.A., Squire, O.D., and Humm, J.L. 2002. Effect of respiratory gating on quantifying PET images of lung cancer. *J. Nucl. Med. 43*:876–881.

Nestle, U., Walter, K., Schmidt, S., Licht, N., Nieder, C., Motaref, B., Hellwig, D., Niewald, M., Ukena, D., Kirsch, C.M., Sybrecht, G.W., and Schnabel, K. 1999. ^{18}F-deoxyglucose positron emission tomography (FDG-PET) for the planning of radiotherapy in lung cancer: high impact in patients with atelectasis. *Int. J. Radiat. Oncol. Biol. Phys. 44*:593–597.

O'Donoghue, J.A., Zanzonico, P., Pugachev, A., Wen, B., Smith-Jones, P., Cai, S., Burnazi, E., Finn, R.D., Burgman, P., Ruan, S., Lewis, J.S., Welch, M.J., Ling, C.C., and Humm, J.L. 2005. Assessment of regional tumor hypoxia using 18F-fluoromisonidazole and 64Cu(II)-diacetyl-bis(N4-methylthiosemicarbazone) positron emission tomography: comparative study featuring microPET imaging, Po2 probe measurement, autoradiography, and fluorescent microscopy in the R3327-AT and FaDu rat tumor models. *Int. J. Radiat. Oncol. Biol. Phys. 61*:1493–1502.

Paulino, A.C., and Johnstone, P.A.S. 2004. FDG-PET in radiotherapy treatment planning: Pandora's box? *Int. J. Radiat. Oncol. Biol. Phys. 59*:4–5.

Perez, C.A., Bradley, J., Chao, C.K., Grigsby, P.W., Mutic, S., and Malyapa, R. 2002. Functional imaging in treatment planning in radiation therapy: a review. *Rays 27*:157–173.

Pevsner, A., Davis, B., Joshi, S., Hertanto, A., Mechalakos, J., Yorke, E., Rosenzweig, K., Nehmeh, S., Erdi, Y.E., Humm, J.L., Larson, S., Ling, C.C., and Mageras, G.S. 2006. Evaluation of an automated deformable image matching method for quantifying lung motion in respiration-correlated CT images. *Med. Phys. 33*:369–376.

Rajendran, J.G., Hendrickson, K.R., Spence, A.M., Muzi, M., Krohn, K.A., and Mankoff, D.A. 2006. Hypoxia imaging-directed radiation treatment planning. *Eur. J. Nucl. Med. Mol. Imag. 33* (Suppl.) 13:44–53.

Rosenman, J. 2001 Incorporating functional imaging information into radiation treatments. *Semin. Radiat. Oncol. 11*:83–92.

Toloza, E.M., Harpole, L., and McCrory, D.C. 2003. Noninvasive staging of non-small cell lung cancer: a review of the current evidence. *Chest 123*:137S–146S.

Vanuytsel, L.J., Vansteenkiste, J.F., Stroobants, S.G., De Leyn, P.R., De Wever, W., Verbeken, E.K., Gatti, G.G., Huyskens, D.P., and Kutcher, G.J. 2000. The impact of 18F-fluoro-2-deoxy-D-glucose positron emission tomography (FDG-PET) lymph node staging on the radiation treatment volumes in patients with non-small cell lung cancer. *Radiother. Oncol. 55*:317–324.

Visvikis, D., Costa, D.C., Croasdale, I., Lonn, A.H., Bomanji, J., Gacinovic, S., and Ell, P.J. 2003. CT-based attenuation correction in the calculation of semi-quantitative indices of [18F]FDG uptake in PET. *Eur. J. Nucl. Med. Mol. Imag. 30*:344–353.

14

Post-Treatment Changes in Tumor Microenvironment: Dynamic Contrast-Enhanced and Diffusion-Weighted Magnetic Resonance Imaging

Benedicte F. Jordan, Jean-Philippe Galons, and Robert J. Gillies

Introduction

The development of new anticancer therapies and the optimal implementation of currently available treatments are limited in part by the lack of information regarding the metabolism and pathophysiology of individual tumors. Early indicators of treatment response that could also provide information on the spatial heterogeneity of response would be of significant benefit for both experimental and clinical trials. There is now increasing awareness of the need to obtain evidence of drug activity through the use of surrogate markers of response during early clinical trials.

One promising method for noninvasively assessing tumor physiology and metabolism is magnetic resonance imaging (MRI). This chapter presents the potential of dynamic contrast-enhanced MRI (DCE-MRI) and diffusion-weighted MRI (DW-MRI) to monitor post-treatment changes in the tumor microenvironment in both the preclinical and clinical settings. DCE-MRI is widely used in the diagnosis and staging of cancer and is emerging as a promising method for monitoring tumor response to treatment. It has been used experimentally to monitor the effectiveness of a variety of treatments, including chemotherapy, radiotherapy, hormonal manipulation, and novel therapeutic approaches, such as anti-angiogenic drugs. Experimental evidence has also placed diffusion MRI in a new perspective for clinical oncology because apparent diffusion coefficient of water (ADCw) has been shown to be a novel indicator of tumor response to therapy. Diffusion-weighted MRI can detect tumor response to chemotherapy quantitatively, sensitively, and early in the treatment regimen. While DCE-MRI provides information regarding tumor vasculature, ADCw has been shown to be sensitive to cellular volume fractions (cellularity). Because they image different markers of response, DCE- and DW-MRI may show differences in amplitude and timing of response. Hence, these techniques are complementary and could be combined in experimental studies.

Dynamic contrast-enhanced magnetic resonance imaging is able to characterize microvasculature, which provides information regarding tumor microvessel structure and function. Consequently, it has been employed for tumor characterization, staging, and therapy monitoring. Characterization of tumor vasculature by DCE-MRI involves acquisition of a series of T1-weighted images before, during, and after bolus IV injection of a contrast agent. The change in signal with time reflects the exchange of contrast agent between the intravascular space (IVS) and extravascular-extracellular space (EES). Exchange kinetics depend on the blood flow, vessel permeability, vessel surface area, fractional volumes of IVS and EES, and the blood concentration of the contrast agent as a function of time (i.e., the arterial or venous input functions). The tumor (and blood) contrast agent concentrations can be inferred from the magnitudes of the signal changes, and these can be used to extract values for parameters of the underlying vascular physiology (*vide infra*). Generally, treatment-induced changes in these parameters reflect changes in blood flow and/or the permeability-surface area product (PSP). Acquisition pulse sequences can be designed that are sensitive to perfusion and blood volume (primarily T2* methods) and/or permeability and EES (primarily T1 methods).

A distinction is made between diffusible and blood-pool tracers because they behave differently and yield different information (Daldrup *et al.*, 1998; Padhani *et al.*, 2001). Diffusible tracers range from freely diffusible tracers, such as ^2H_2O, and can often include small-molecular-weight contrast agents, such as chelates of gadolinium. Extraction fractions (i.e., the ratio of extravascular to intravascular concentrations during the first pass) for these agents vary from 0.5 to 1.0, depending on the agent and the vasculature. Extraction fractions are lower in tight endothelial such as brain microvessels and higher in leaky vessels such as those undergoing active remodeling (e.g., in tumors). In addition, contrast agents affect the spins of blood water, which in turn can diffuse into the interstitium and into cells. Blood-pool tracers are usually larger molecules and hence diffuse into the interstitium much more slowly, if at all. They are also cleared more slowly, yielding flatter vascular input functions. Slower kinetics allow for higher dynamic range in quantification of vascular leakage and acquisition of much higher-resolution images, which can be important in pathodiagnosis.

Contrast Media

An appropriate tracer for monitoring flow-limited perfusion is water, because the net capillary permeability to water is assumed to be much higher than its flow. Deuterium-labeled water is MR-detectable, with little toxicity to the host. Accordingly, deuterated water has been used as a tracer to evaluate both average and localized tumor perfusion by means of ^2H-MR spectroscopy (^2H-MRS) and imaging. The determination of permeability-dominated perfusion requires a tracer that permeates through capillaries at a rate slower than its flow. Gadolinium-based chelates, such as di-N-methylglucamine-gadoliniumdiethylenetriamine pentaacetic acid (GdDTPA), have been widely used in clinics to investigate permeability-dominated perfusion in various tumor types and diseases (Brasch *et al.*, 2000; Knopp *et al.*, 2001; Padhani *et al.*, 2001; Preda *et al.*, 2006). A detailed overview of contrast agents for MRI is provided by A. Jasanoff in this volume.

Contrast agents (CA) diffuse from the blood into the extracellular space of tissues at a rate determined by the permeability of the capillaries and their surface area. T1 relaxation time shortening caused by the contrast medium leads to enhancement in T1-weighted imaging sequences. The early phase of contrast enhancement (first-pass) includes the arrival of CA and lasts many cardiac cycles. In this phase, the increased signal seen on T1-weighted images arises from both the vascular and interstitial compartments. In tumors, 12 to 45% of the CA can leak into the EES during the first pass (Daldrup *et al.*, 1998). Contrast medium also begins to diffuse into tissue compartments further removed from the vasculature including areas of necrosis and fibrosis. Over a period typically lasting several minutes to half an hour, the contrast agent diffuses back into the vasculature from which it is excreted by the kidneys (usually) or by the liver.

Extracellular contrast agents can be divided in three groups: (1) low-molecular-weight agents (< 1000 Da) that rapidly diffuse in the EES and are in widespread clinical use; (2) large molecular agents (> 30,000 Da) designed for prolonged intravascular retention, which are also called macromolecular contrast media (MMCM) or blood-pool agents, and are in early-to-late clinical testing; and (3) experimental targeted agents intended to accumulate at sites of concentrated neoangiogenesis. Additional groups under development are the superparamagnetic compounds, which are either small particles of iron oxides (SPIO; coated diameter > 50 nm) or ultra small (USPIO) (coated diameter 10–30 nm). All these different agents increase the capabilities of DCE-MRI by utilizing their various enhancement properties to assess differences in vascular permeability. Finally, tissue-specific agents of various molecular size have been developed, such as lymph node-specific agents, those specific for atherosclerotic plaques, and those that accumulate in the cells of the reticuloendothelial system (RES) (Artemov *et al.*, 2004). Also, nanoparticles can be targeted to receptors by monoclonal antibodies covalently bound or attached via biotin-avidin linkers, respectively (Artemov *et al.*, 2004), and these are generally limited to endothelial epitopes. Integrin $\alpha v \beta 3$ receptors were successfully imaged in the neovasculature of rabbit tumors and bFGF-induced cornea. Also, avidin/biotin pretargeting has been used for *in vivo* MR imaging of HER-

2/neu receptors, using two-step labeling with biotinylated MAb and GdDTPA-labeled avidin (Artemov *et al.*, 2004). Technical aspects of DCE-MRI are described in the present volume by A. Jackson.

Acquisition of T1 Dynamic Contrast-Enhanced Data

DCE-MRI can be performed on most clinical MRI systems with a field strength superior to 1.0 Tesla. Due to their superior T1-contrast and shorter acquisition times, gradient-echo sequences are generally preferred over spin-echo pulse sequences. T1-weighted gradient-echo saturation recovery/inversion recovery snapshot sequences (e.g., turboFLASH) or echo-planar sequences are typically used (Padhani and Husband, 2001; Knopp *et al.*, 2001). Each of these techniques enables the tissue T1 relaxation time to be estimated, and thus allows quantification of contrast medium concentration. After baseline acquisition, a slow bolus injection of 0.1 ml/kg gadolinium chelate is usually injected in 40 to 60 sec. The choice of sequence and parameters used is dependent on the intrinsic advantages and disadvantages of the sequences, taking into account T1 sensitivity, anatomical coverage, acquisition times, susceptibility to artifacts arising from magnetic field inhomogeneities, and accuracy for quantification. Critical for this application is that the MRI sequence should have a nearly linear relation between contrast concentration and signal intensity. In fact, exact linearity is never perfectly achieved in MRI but can only be approximated with gradient-echo images using low flip angles and low doses of gadolinium chelates. The classical trade-off in DCE-MRI is to find a compromise between spatial and temporal resolution: the temporal resolution needs to be sufficiently fast to detect several imaging points during the initial passage of the contrast agent through the targeted tissue. Also, very important is the acquisition of baseline images to reliably quantify contrast enhancement.

Analysis of T1 Dynamic Contrast-Enhanced Data

Low Molecular Contrast Medium

Practically, a series of T1-weighted images is acquired starting before a short (bolus) injection and is continued as uptake by the tissue and usually washout from the tissue are observed (Padhani and Husband, 2001; Knopp *et al.*, 2001). Consequently, DCE-MRI studies produce time-series images that enable pixel-by-pixel analysis of contrast kinetics within a tumor. These "time-signal" curves can be analyzed with descriptive "heuristic" tools, such as onset time, initial slope, time to peak, rate of washout, or maximum intensity time ratio (semi-quantitative parameters). The uptake integral

or initial area under the signal intensity curve or contrast medium concentration (IAUGC) curve has also been studied. These methods are valuable and easy to apply; however, they provide no insight into the underlying physiology. Moreover, they are highly dependent on the imaging protocol and scanner. Finally, the only semiquantitative nature of these approaches does not truly permit across-patient analysis. Signal enhancement of healthy tissue may serve as a reference, but a more direct reference is to measure concentration time curves of the contrast agent in the feeding vessels, via, for example, the arterial input function (AIF). Therefore, many models have been developed to analyze quantitatively DCE kinetic data. Fast MRI routines and the development and application of tracer kinetic modeling techniques now allow a fuller understanding of the physiological basis of observations noted in DCE-MRI examinations. Quantitative techniques use pharmacokinetic modeling techniques that are usually applied to changes in tissue contrast agent concentrations. Signal intensity changes observed during dynamic acquisition are used to estimate contrast agent concentration *in vivo*. Concentration-time curves are then mathematically fitted by using one of a number of recognized pharmacokinetic models, and quantitative kinetic parameters are derived. The choice of the pharmacokinetic model depends on physicochemical and pharmacological properties of the tracer and the applied MR method for the detection of tracer concentration changes in the volume of interest.

Tofts (1999) unified all the different parameters used in those models by proposing a standardization of quantities that determine the dynamic behavior of diffusible contrast agents. With better quantification methodology and MR instrumentation, the estimation of each parameter is now approaching the "true" (absolute) values underlying pathophysiologic processes that are being measured. Although we can continue to improve the calculations of the "true" values, they will ultimately be limited by the complexity of the underlying pathophysiology and the variations of techniques. However, even with very primitive methodologies and quantification, there is preliminary evidence that tracer kinetic modeling can be a powerful tool in the management of cancer.

Most methods of analyzing dynamic contrast-enhanced T1-weighted data acquired with low molecular contrast medium have used a compartmental analysis to obtain some combination of the three principal parameters: the transfer constant K^{trans} in min^{-1} (volume transfer constant between blood plasma and EES), the rate constant K_{ep} in min^{-1} (rate constant between blood plasma and EES), and the volume of extravascular extracellular space (EES) per unit volume of tissue space, V_e (no unit) (Tofts *et al.*, 1999). The transfer constant and the EES relate to the fundamental physiology, whereas the rate constant is the ratio of the transfer constant to the EES: $K_{ep} = K^{trans}/V_e$. The rate constant can be derived from the shape of the tracer concentration versus time data, whereas the transfer constant and EES require access to absolute values of tracer concentration. The transfer constant K^{trans} has several physiologic interpretations, depending on the balance between capillary permeability and blood flow in the tissue of interest. In high-permeability situations (where flux across the endothelium is flow limited), a common situation in tumors, the transfer constant is equal to the blood plasma flow per unit volume of tissue. In the other limiting case of low permeability, where tracer flux is permeability limited, the transfer constant is equal to the permeability surface area product between blood plasma and the EES, per unit volume of tissue. Because low-molecular-weight contrast media do not cross cell membranes, the volume of distribution is effectively the EES (V_e). The main kinetic models are the flow-limited (Kety) model (high permeability), the permeability surface (PS) limited model (low permeability), the mixed flow and PS limited model, the clearance model, and the generalized kinetic model, all of which have been reviewed in Tofts (1999). Alternatively, without an input function, the area under the curve (IAUGC as an alternative semiquantitative end point) can be used to yield an ad hoc solution that is robust. However, IAUGC does not have a simple relation to tissue perfusion and permeability.

Limitations reside in the fact that the model chosen may not exactly reflect the data obtained, and each model makes a number of assumptions that may not be valid for every tissue or tumor type. First, it is assumed that tracer in the EES has arrived directly from a nearby capillary. Models are invalid in nonperfused tumor regions because tracer uptake in these regions is due to diffusion processes from distant perfused microvessels. Second, the different compartments contain the well-mixed tracer in a uniform concentration throughout the compartment. The high interstitial fluid pressure that exists in solid tumors may be a major cause for a heterogeneous distribution of macromolecules because it leads to radially outward convection that opposes the inward diffusion. Third, the increase in T1 relaxation rate is proportional to the concentration of the tracer. Assumptions for the measurement of tissue contrast agent concentration also lead to errors. Reliable methods for measuring arterial input function for routine DCE-MRI studies are currently emerging (Rijpkema et al., 2001). It has been suggested that classical models lead to systematic overestimation of K^{trans} in tumors. Nonetheless, if contrast agent concentration can be measured accurately and the type, volume, and method of administration of contrast agent are consistent, then it is possible to directly compare pharmacokinetic parameters obtained on different subjects, and it is important to note that quantitative kinetic parameters can provide insights into underlying tissue pathophysiologic processes that semiquantitative descriptors cannot.

Macromolecular Contrast Medium

Albumin-Gd-DTPA has a distribution volume of 0.05 l/kg (which closely approximates the body's relative blood volume

indicating its vascular distribution) and a plasma half-life of 3 hr in rats, which produces nearly constant enhancement of normal, nonleaky tissues for 30 min or longer after injection. The T1 relaxivity (R1) of albumin-(Gd-DTPA)n is substantially higher compared with low molecular gadolinium chelates. The R1 of albumin-(Gd-DTPA)n is $14.8 \, \text{mM}^{-1} \, \text{s}^{-1}$ relative to gadolinium concentration. For comparison, the R1 value of Gd-DTPA is $4.9 \, \text{mM}^{-1} \, \text{s}^{-1}$. Thus, by binding it to human albumin, the molar relaxivity of each Gd-DTPA chelate is ~ 3-fold increased (Preda et al., 2006).

Pharmacokinetic models have been developed to relate the initial fast and slow phase of the MMCM uptake to vascular volume and permeability surface area product. Extravasation of the Gd-BSA macromolecular contrast agent is often assumed to be described by a permeability-limited two-compartment model with unidirectional transport of contrast agent on the timescale of the study (Bhujwalla et al., 2003). Signal enhancement in the DCE-MRI data is converted to Gd-BSA concentration using the relaxivity measured in vitro at 37°C assuming a linear relationship between Gd concentration and relaxation rate enhancement. The Gd-BSA versus time data is fitted to a straight line for each pixel, to obtain a slope (related to vascular permeability) and y-axis intercept (related to the vascular volume). Thus, the slope of $\Delta(1/T1)$ ratios versus time in each pixel is used to compute PSP, and the intercept of the line at zero time is used to compute vascular volume.

Dynamic Contrast-Enhanced–MRI in Experimental Oncology

DCE-MRI provides a powerful tool for the rapid evaluation of the acute pharmacodynamic effect of a variety of treatments such as chemotherapy, hormonal manipulation, radiotherapy, and novel therapeutic approaches (antivascular agents, immunotherapy), most notably in the case of mechanisms that affect tumor perfusion. Evidence is mounting that DCE-MRI measurements correlate with immunohistochemical surrogates of tumor angiogenesis. Many excellent articles reviewing preclinical studies have been published (Knopp et al., 2001; Padhani et al., 2005).

Our group recently investigated changes in the tumor microenvironment in response to inhibition of HIF-1α using *PX-12* and *PX-478* (Jordan et al., 2005a, 2005b). Albumin-Gd-DTPA was used to determine vascular permeability and volume fraction in HT-29 xenografts. *PX-12* caused a rapid 63% decrease in the average tumor blood vessel permeability within 2 hr of administration. The decrease lasted 24 hr and had returned to pretreatment values by 48 hr. The changes in vascular permeability were not accompanied by alterations in average tumor vascular volume fraction. There was a decrease in tumor and tumor-derived VEGF in plasma at 24 hr after treatment with *PX-12*, but not at earlier time points. However, tumor redox active Trx-1 showed a rapid decline within 2 hr following *PX-12* administration that was maintained for 24 hr. The rapid decrease in tumor vascular permeability caused by *PX-12* administration coincided with a decrease in tumor redox active Trx-1 and preceded a decrease in VEGF.

PX-478 induced a dramatic reduction in tumor blood vessel permeability within 2 hr after treatment after a single dose of 125 mg/kg, which persisted until 24 hr post-treatment and had returned to control values by 48 hr. Although some individual changes (positive or negative) in tumor vascular volume fraction were sometimes observed, the mean change between groups was not statistically significant. Hence, we conclude that the mechanism underlying the change in PSP is due to alterations in permeability, with little or no change in surface area, because surface area changes will also be reflected in the vascular volume estimation. In comparison, the anti-VEGF antibody, Avastin®, reduced both the permeability and vascular volume. Importantly, *PX-478* had no effect on the perfusion behavior of a drug-resistant tumor system, A-549. The time course for the decrease in HIF-1a and VEGF was different from the changes in PSP measured by DCE-MRI. The differences between these responses are unknown but may also indicate that the effect of *PX-478* on hemodynamics is not mediated through VEGF (i.e., permeability factors other than VEGF might be involved in the response to *PX-478*). However, it also remains possible that the hemodynamics is affected by local concentrations or threshold values of VEGF, and these cannot yet be measured. The current findings suggest that DCE-MRI may also be useful in assessing the response to inhibition of HIF-1, although we have to keep in mind that this study was performed with a large molecular contrast agent that is not available in the clinical setting. We suggest, however, that DCE-MRI may also be useful clinically for screening and preselecting patients for therapy with anti–HIF-1.

Dynamic Contrast-Enhanced–MRI in Clinical Oncology

Because DCE-MRI is noninvasive, the tumor can be monitored longitudinally over a period of time to study the changes in tumor vascularity occurring during growth and alterations induced by various kinds of therapy. Initial results in the clinic using the low-molecular-weight contrast agent Gd-DTPA indicate that DCE-MRI is useful for both diagnosis and prognosis (review by Padhani). Moreover, DCE-MRI can serve as a pharmacodynamic indicator of biological activity for antivascular cancer drugs by helping to define the biologically active dose. Because DCE-MRI is used for the selection of antivascular drugs that advance into efficacy trials, there is a crucial need for standardization, in terms

of both techniques and data interpretation in the clinic. The following paragraphs describe some typical studies showing the relevance of the use of DCE-MRI in monitoring tumor response to therapy (it is not aimed at being an exhaustive review of all the works performed in the field of DCE-MRI).

Monitoring the Effects of Radiation Therapy

The prognostic value for tumor radiosensitivity and long-term tumor control was assessed with DCE-MRI in patients with advanced cervical cancer (Mayr *et al.*, 2000). Interestingly, the quantity of low-enhancement regions significantly predicted subsequent tumor recurrence. The group of DeVries (Hein *et al.*, 2003) observed microcirculatory changes during chemoirradiation in patients with cT3 rectal carcinoma. Comparison of perfusion index values and radiation dose showed a significant increase in the first and second weeks of treatment, thereby suggesting that DCE-MRI offers the potential for individual optimization of therapeutic procedures. De Lussanet *et al.* (2005) evaluated radiation therapy-related microvascular changes in locally advanced rectal cancer with DCE-MRI. Tumor Kps was 77% lower in the RT-treated group than in the control group, and histogram analyses showed that RT reduced both magnitude and intratumor heterogeneity of Kps.

Monitoring the Effects of Chemotherapy

The use of fast dynamic contrast-enhanced sequences for identifying residual tumor before surgery was illustrated by van der Woude *et al.* (1995). They followed 21 patients treated with neoadjuvant chemotherapy followed by surgery. Late and gradually enhancing or nonenhancing areas corresponded histopathologically to regions of chemotherapy-induced necrosis, mucomyxoid degeneration, or fibrosis, while viable tumor areas showed early enhancement with rapid washout of contrast agent. Similar results were observed in locally advanced breast cancer. For example, Hayes *et al.* (2002) analyzed K^{trans} histograms before and after one course of chemotherapy (mitoxantrone + méthotrexate, epirubicin + cisplatin + 5-fluorouracil, or cyclophosphamide + doxorubicin). The absolute change in the K^{trans} values correlated negatively with the pretreatment values, particularly for responding patients. Greater changes were observed in the upper extremes of the K^{trans} histogram than in the median values after one course of treatment. Those examples and many other published works suggest that decreasing enhancement rates, flattening of the signal intensity time course, and reduced degree of enhancement seem to be the hallmarks of early tumor response to chemotherapy.

Monitoring the Effects of Antivascular Therapy

Combretastatin A4 phosphate was evaluated in human tumors (escalating doses from 5 to 114 mg/m^2) in terms of blood flow and vascular permeability in tumor and normal tissue. Rat tumor K^{trans} was reduced by 64% 6 hr after treatment with CA4P (Galbraith *et al.*, 2003). Significant reductions were seen in tumor K^{trans} in 6 of 16 patients treated at > or = 52 mg/m^2, with a significant group mean reduction of 37% and 29% at 4 and 24 hr, respectively, after treatment. No reduction was seen in muscle K^{trans} or in kidney AUC in group analysis of the clinical data. Using semiquantitative analysis, Dowlati *et al.* (2002) observed a significant decline in gradient peak tumor blood flow by DCE-MRI in 6 of 7 patients treated at 60 mg/m^2.

The pharmacodynamic effects of PTK/ZK (PTK787/ ZK 222584, an orally active inhibitor of VEGF) were evaluated by assessing changes in contrast-enhancement parameters of metastatic liver lesions in patients with advanced colorectal cancer treated in two ongoing, dose-escalating Phase I studies (Morgan *et al.*, 2003). They found that patients with a best response of stable disease had a significantly greater reduction in Ki at both day 2 and at the end of cycle 1 compared with progressors. They showed that it may be possible to subsequently predict anti-angiogenic drug efficacy in patients who have colorectal cancer on the basis of the degree of change on DCE-MRI.

Both Galbraith *et al.* (2003) and Morgan *et al.* (2003) reported a strong inverse correlation between a decrease in transfer constant and plasma levels of CA4P and PTK/ZK. Such information can lead to the selection of the dose of drug to be used in combination with other therapies for trials with efficacy end points.

HuMV833 is a humanized version of a mouse monoclonal anti-VEGF antibody (MV833) that has antitumor activity against a number of human tumor xenografts (Jayson *et al.*, 2002). It has been tested in 20 patients with progressive solid tumors at 0.3, 1, 3, or 10 mg/kg. Permeability was strongly heterogeneous between and within patients and between and within individual tumors. All tumors showed a reduction in k(fp) 48 hr after the first treatment. Another antibody, bevacizumab (Avastin®), a recombinant humanized monoclonal antibody to VEGF, was administered to patients with locally advanced breast cancer (Wedam *et al.*, 2006). Cycle 1 (15 mg/ kg on day 1) was followed by six cycles of bevacizumab with doxorubicin (50 mg/m^2) and docetaxel (75 mg/m^2) every 3 weeks. DCE-MRI was performed at baseline and after cycles 1, 4, and 7. A median decrease of 34.4% in the inflow transfer rate constant, 15.0% in the backflow extravascular-extracellular rate constant, and 14.3% in extravascular-extracellular volume fraction were observed.

Limitations

Experience has demonstrated some limitations, such as nonspecificity and inconsistent predictive value of therapy response. There are a number of areas for improvement that will allow a fair assessment of the role of DCE-MRI. The different clinical approaches make it difficult to make meaningful comparisons between techniques, tissue types, and data obtained from different imaging centers.

A major source of variability in the DCE-MRI literature relates to the method of contrast administration. The dose and method of administration of contrast agent affect modeling procedures and clinical results. Typically, contrast agents are given as a bolus or an infusion. Recent work has suggested that short injection times are optimal for fast DCE-MRI imaging techniques, especially when evaluating lesions with high microvessel permeability for ECF contrast agents. Conversely, slower infusion methods may be better when the temporal resolution of the study is longer (Padhani *et al.*, 2005).

The presence of motion can invalidate functional vascular parameter estimates, particularly for pixel-by-pixel analyses. Methods for overcoming or minimizing these effects include the application of navigator techniques or imaging in the nonaxial plane and subsequently registering the dynamic data before kinetic analysis.

Tumor heterogeneity poses considerable difficulties within and among patients, which largely has not been taken into account when incorporating imaging strategies into early-phase clinical trials. User-defined whole tumor regions of interest (ROIs) yield graphic outputs with a good signal-to-noise ratio, but lack spatial resolution, are prone to partial volume averaging errors, and result in overly reduced data. Feature extraction has several advantages, including the appreciation of the heterogeneity of enhancement and obviating selective user-defined ROIs. Histogram and principal components analyses have been used to quantify the heterogeneity of tumors for comparative and longitudinal studies and to monitor the effects of treatment.

Conclusions and Perspectives

DCE-MRI has evolved from an experimental technique to a clinically feasible adjunct procedure that can be integrated into a standard morphologic imaging protocol. It does provide unique noninvasive functional information on the properties of tumors related to microcirculation (distribution volume, permeability, and perfusion). This information can improve diagnostic characterization, follow-up of therapy, and tumor staging; and it provides tools to facilitate advanced molecular imaging.

All the studies described here show that successful treatment results in a decrease in the rate of enhancement along with a decreased amplitude and a slower washout, and that poor response can result in persistent abnormal enhancement, however judged (semiquantitatively or quantitatively). However, the changes on DCE-MRI may be nonpredictive because the therapy may induce physiologic changes in the tumor without affecting overall patient survival. Nonetheless, there is still growing evidence that DCE-MRI could have an important role to play in the management of many cancer patients. However, progress is hindered by the large variations in the methods of acquisition and analysis of DCE-MR images. Furthermore, a number of pharmacokinetic models are available, using different simplifications of the underlying physiology.

Better reproducibility is essential to realize the full potential of DCE-MRI. There are two sources of variance: experimental and biological. Experimental variance should be reduced with consensus on acquisition methodologies. Technical improvements that could be implanted to substantially improve the performance of DCE-MRI include parallel imaging, motion robustness (e.g., navigator echoes), better registration algorithms, pulse sequences providing greater coverage, and quantitative pulse sequences. A consensus report on the acquisition and analysis of DCE-MRI data has been generated by a consortium of U.S. and European researchers (Evelhoch *et al.*, 2005). It is also possible that experimental variability will be reduced with improved image quality and thus, there is a need to explore DCE-MRI in the clinic at 3T or higher fields. Biological variability may be reduced by improved understanding of the biology underlying contrast transfer between blood and extravascular space, but ultimately may be limited by the biology of the tumor, the biology of the response, and the chemistry of the contrast agent. As noted above, larger molecular weight agents appear to have greater reproducibility in animals.

In addition, there is a need to evaluate the relationship of DCE-MRI measurements to clinical response on a larger scale (both pretreatment and early after treatment), because reduction of tumor vessel permeability may not be coupled to improved outcome. More important, there should be an evaluation of the potential for DCE-MRI to predict tumor response to specific classes of drugs, an approach known as Theranostics. Finally, the use of DCE to monitor or predict normal tissue toxicity is also worthy of investigation.

Diffusion Magnetic Resonance Imaging

For the last ten years **diffusion MRI** has been under active investigation as a biomarker of antitumor therapeutic efficacy. Early indicators of treatment response that could also provide information on the spatial heterogeneity of response would be of significant benefit for both experimental and clinical trials. There is a crucial need for using noninvasive imaging to facilitate the evaluation of the responsiveness

of experimental tumors in preclinical therapeutic studies. Because molecular and cellular changes precede macroscopic changes in tumor size, it would be ideal to have an assay that could quantify these changes in both clinical cancer therapeutics and preclinical drug trials.

Apparent diffusion is distinct from molecular diffusion because the molecular displacement of water in tissues is inhibited by membrane barriers. Diffusion-weighted imaging has become a major contrast for tissue assessment by MRI (Bammer, 2003; Norris, 2001). Demonstration of the remarkable sensitivity of water diffusion to ischemia in the brain initiated a new field within MRI, which prompted clinical interest in this novel MRI contrast. The potentials of diffusion MRI and MRS for oncology recently emerged and are still under development.

Diffusion MRI pulse sequences incorporate two additional magnetic field gradients that make the intensity of the MR signal dependent on the mobility of the signal source, that is, water molecules (Bammer, 2003). The first of these two gradient pulses imparts a phase shift to each water molecule proportional to its initial location. The second gradient pulse will remove this phase shift if the water molecule remains at its original location. Any molecular movement between first and second pulses will lead to incomplete rephasing and signal attenuation. The amount of signal loss is a direct reflection of water mobility, that is, the greater signal loss implies greater molecular mobility.

Signal attenuation resulting from the application of rectangular gradients is given by the Stejskal-Tanner equation (1965):

$$\frac{S}{S_0} = e^{-\gamma^2 G^2 \delta^2 \left(\Delta - \frac{\delta}{3}\right) D} \tag{1}$$

where γ is the gyromagnetic ratio of given nucleus, D is the diffusion coefficient of water, G is the strength of the gradient pulse, δ is the duration of the gradient pulse, and Δ is the separation of the gradient pulse. The term $\gamma^2 G^2 \delta^2 (\Delta - \delta/3)$ is the diffusion-weighting factor or *b-value*.

Practically, a series of diffusion-weighted images at different b-values can be used to calculate an apparent diffusion coefficient for water (ADC) by fitting the signal decay (pixel per pixel) to Equation (1) (Fig. 1). In media without diffusion barriers, the calculated ADC is identical to the physical diffusion coefficient of water, D (ca. 3.2×10^{-5} cm^2 s^{-1} at 37°). In biological tissues where the MR signal originates from multicompartments, the exact physical description underlying ADC values is far more complex (Norris, 2001). Nevertheless, enough data are in hand to indicate that ADC values are dominated by the presence of diffusion barriers (restriction effects) and that they can also be influenced by the presence of flow. Phenomenologically, flow effects can be reduced if only b-values > 50 sec/mm^{-2} are used to calculate the ADC, as most contributions of flow to the diffusion signal are eliminated by that point. Above 50 sec/mm^{-2}, the ADC is thought to be dominated by the presence of diffusion

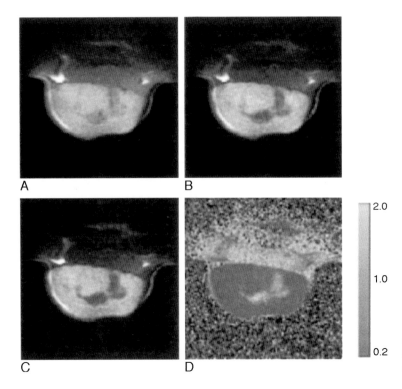

Figure 1 Diffusion images. DWI obtained from a 12-days-old MCF7 tumor at different b-values (**A**) b = 0.027 × 10^9 s/m^2. (**B**) b = 0.249 × 10^9 s/m^2. (**C**) b = 0.442 × 10^9 s/m^2. (**D**) ADC map calculated from the images shown in A through C.

barriers in both the intra- and extracellular space. The physical diffusion coefficients of intra- and extracellular water are not known with certainty. Nevertheless, because water is "trapped" (on the NMR timescale) inside of the cells, the apparent diffusion of water within the cells is lower than that in the extracellular space. Hence, the measured ADC is sensitive to cell volume. An important aspect of diffusion MRI is that the b-value is a function of both the gradient strength, G, and the evolution time, Δ. In the high G/short Δ regime most often encountered clinically, water diffusion can be parsed into two distinct components, which are most sensitive to discriminating necrotic from nonnecrotic tissues. In the weak G/long Δ regime, most often encountered clinically, different diffusion components coalesce into a single exponential, which is most sensitive to the tortuosity of the system.

Treatment of tumors may result in damage and/or killing of cells, thus altering the integrity of cell membranes or size of cells, thereby increasing the fractional volume of the interstitial space due. These changes have been shown to increase the diffusion of water in the damaged tumor tissue (Kauppinen, 2002; Moffat *et al.*, 2004; Ross *et al.*, 2003). Successful anticancer therapies are correlated to early increases in tumor ADC in both animals and humans. This is likely a consequence of reductions in cell volume, which are a general response to effective chemotherapy. Such predictions have been borne out by diffusion measurements in perfused cells and in *in vivo* systems wherein cell volume was

accurately correlated with ADC. These findings have placed diffusion MRI in a new perspective for clinical oncology.

In anisotropic systems, the measured ADC depends on the directionality of the diffusion gradients. Hence, diffusion in many biological systems is anisotropic. Such distributions can be characterized with diffusion tensor imaging (DTI), wherein diffusion coefficients are measured along nondegenerate axes to characterize the diffusion tensor. Signal attenuation in a diffusion experiment is proportional to the product of the diffusion tensor with the field gradient vectors. Using a combination of diffusion weighting along the z-, x-, and y-gradient, one can determine the orientation-independent diffusion in the form of the trace of the diffusion tensor (D_{av}). The resulting D_{av} indicates the volume and time-averaged diffusivity in the tissue. Most available evidence suggests that diffusion in tumors is isotropic, even in neuronal lesions, although diffusion in the normal surrounding tissues can acquire some anisotropic features, presumably from cell crowding.

Diffusion-Weighted MRI Methods

The greatest challenge in the implementation of diffusion imaging is to acquire quantitative diffusion-weighted images in the presence of physiological motion that are free from artifacts (Bammer, 2003). The greatest technical difficulty is thus to overcome the effects of macroscopic motion, while retaining the sensitivity to the microscopic motion. To create diffusion-weighted contrast, DWI pulse sequences must be sensitive to molecular motion on the order of several micrometers and consequently are also sensitive to bulk tissue motion. Even small (submillimeter) displacements of the tumor during the diffusion-encoding phase will cause large phase changes in the resultant echo signal. Because bulk motion on this level is likely to be different during each echo acquisition, each echo will be perturbed differently from one excitation to the next. For this reason, patient motion during the diffusion-sensitizing period produces phase errors that manifest as ghosting.

The net result of bulk motion in the presence of the diffusion-encoding gradients is an unpredictable zero order phase term and a net shift of the recorded signal away from the center of the k-space. In general, these shifts are different for each phase-encoding step, but if more than one echo per excitation are recorded (e.g., with interleaved EPI) all echoes that belong to that particular interleaf are affected by the same amount of k-space shift.

Removing the conventional phase encoding is an option to overcome motion-induced phase artifacts. This can be accomplished either by means of line-scan diffusion imaging or by applying k-space trajectories, such as used for radial or spiral imaging techniques, which are less vulnerable to motion. The main issue with line-scan diffusion methods is that they are limited in spatial resolution and SNR. Also, the widespread use of spiral scanning has been limited by the lack of time-varying gradient-waveform capabilities and the lack of appropriate image reconstruction resources. Another very promising method to minimize ghosting artifacts is to use an additional non–phase-encoded echo immediately prior to or after the imaging echo. This additional echo is termed *navigator echo*. The main intention behind the navigator echo correction method is that both echoes are diffusion-weighted and contain the phase terms from bulk motion, but only the imaging echo contains the additional phase encoding to form the image (Bammer, 2003). Despite all these readout strategies, the most common form of data acquisition is still a single-shot readout, in particular single-shot echo planar imaging (SSEPI) because the acquired phase error due to bulk motion is equal in each phase-encoding step and therefore does not affect the image reconstruction. Nevertheless, SSEPI methods are inherently limited in spatial resolution and are extremely sensitive to changes in magnetic susceptibility.

There is now renewed interest in RAD (radial acquisition of Fourier data) methods due to their insensitivity to motion and flow and novel properties for rapid data acquisition (Seifert et al., 2000; Trouard et al., 1999). Two attributes largely explain the insensitivity of RAD methods to motion in diffusion-weighted (DW) MRI (Trouard et al., 1999). First, the large phase errors associated with motion during the diffusion weighting can be removed in the image reconstruction process by employing a magnitude-only

FBPR algorithm. This also removes the effects of Fourier data shifts when they are in the direction of the readout gradient. Second, the residual artifacts in RAD images are manifested as radial blurring or streaking originating from the region of motion. This is in contrast to the ghosting Cartesian MRI, where artifacts are constrained to lie in the phase-encode direction, with intensity that can be completely displaced from the original site of the motion.

Diffusion MRI in Experimental Oncology

Numerous works illustrate the ability of tumor ACDw to detect early changes after treatments such as chemotherapy, radiation therapy, photodynamic therapy, and gene therapy in experimental tumors (reviewed in Kauppinnen, 2002). A key common finding in the follow-up of different therapies with DW imaging is that tumor volume as determined from T1 or T2-weighted or contrast agent-enhanced MRI starts to reduce upon cytotoxic drug treatment only days after diffusion MRI shows positive treatment response. Hence, diffusion MRI has high potential as an early and quantitative biomarker of response in experimental oncology where novel therapies for solid malignant tumors are being investigated.

An extensive discussion of the modeling for water diffusion *in vivo* has been published by Norris *et al.* (2001), and the translation of these models into oncology is addressed by Kauppinen (2002). Substantial MRI data from different tumor types as reviewed tend to suggest that the density of viable cells might be the key factor affecting the water apparent diffusion coefficient in tumors. The high ADC in responding tumors following cytotoxic drug treatment is likely due to increased ECS and reduced cellularity, that is, fraction of intracellular space and liberation of water from cells.

The first important application of DW-MRI was the assessment of ischemic injury, primarily in brain stroke. The ADC decreases profoundly and rapidly following ischemic injury, and this is accompanied by changes in the cell morphology. Hence, given the rapid cell-based alterations that can occur in ADC, the fact that anticancer therapies are cell based, and that DW-MRI provides the high contrast, it was logical to predict that the ADC would be altered by successful cytotoxic therapies.

A major remaining question in this area of research concerns the mechanism(s) of cell death responsible for changes in the ADC. Apparent diffusion coefficients increase in response to chemo-, radio-, and gene therapies. Many of these therapies work through induction of apoptosis or programmed cell death. Could DWI discriminate between necrosis and apoptosis? In first analysis, apoptosis and necrosis have the same net effect on the ADC measured at low b-value as they both correspond to a decrease in the intracellular volume fraction either through shrinkage (apoptosis) or disruption (necrosis). A potential discriminating parameter is the size of the intracellular space and the value of intracellular diffusion in apoptotic cells. Characterization of these parameters would require more sophisticated measurement of diffusion properties within the treated tumor, including the measurement of diffusion at very short diffusion time and the analysis of restriction in the intracellular space.

For example, our group investigated the combination chemotherapy response of human breast cancer tumor xenografts sensitive or resistant to paclitaxel, an inhibitor of microtubule depolymerization, by monitoring changes in the ADC (Galons *et al.*, 1999) (Fig. 1). Paclitaxel-treated animals were injected intraperitoneally with a single dose (27 mg/kg) immediately after the first MRI experiment and given subsequent booster injections (18 mg/kg) every other day. Diffusion-weighted images were obtained by using a diffusion-weighted stimulated echo pulse sequence at three different b-values. We measured ADCs in three orthogonal directions and calculated the trace of the ADC, a parameter independent of orientation. Our results indicated a clear, substantial, and early increase in the ADC after successful therapy in drug-sensitive tumors, while no change could be observed in the ADC in p-glycoprotein positive resistant tumors. Similarly, paclitaxel arrested growth in all MCF7/S tumors and had no effect on the tumors from MCF7/D40 cells. These changes in the ADC were apparent 2 days after commencement of chemotherapy, with no significant changes in tumor volumes. The higher values observed after treatment of the drug-sensitive tumors were consistent with a decrease in the intracellular water after paclitaxel-induced apoptosis.

We further characterized the utility of DW-MRI to predict the response of prostate cancer xenografts to docetaxel, a drug that belongs to the taxoid family, in the preclinical setting (Jennings *et al.*, 2002). The LnCaP cell line (derived from a lymph node metastasis of a human prostatic adenocarcinoma) was implanted in SCID mice that were treated with doses between 0 and 60 mg/kg, delivered in three fractions of 0.5, 0.25, and 0.25 total dose on days 0, 4, and 6, respectively. Apparent diffusion coefficient maps were generated by fitting the signal intensity to a single monoexponential decay over a low b-value range (b max 800 sec/mm²). Mice were imaged on day 0, 2, and 4. The data showed that tumor volumes and secreted prostate-specific antigen (PSA) both responded strongly to docetaxel in a dose-responsive manner. Concomitantly, ADC values increased significantly after 2 days of treatment even at the lowest doses (10 mg/kg) (Fig. 2). The change in ADC was shown to be an earlier indicator of response than tumor volume or serum PSA level.

We recently investigated the efficacy of inhibition of the HIF-1α pathway using diffusion-weighted MRI on HT-29 (a tumorigenic nonmetastatic human colon carcinoma cell line) tumor-bearing SCID mice (Jordan *et al.*, 2005a). Clinically, HIF-1α overexpression has been shown to be a marker of highly aggressive diseases and has been associated with poor prognosis and treatment failure in a number of cancers, including breast, ovarian, cervical, oligodendroglioma, esophageal, and oropharyngeal cancers. HIF-1α presence correlates with tumor grade as well as vascularity. PX-478 (S-2-amino-3-[4V-N,N,-bis(2-chloroethyl)amino]-phenyl

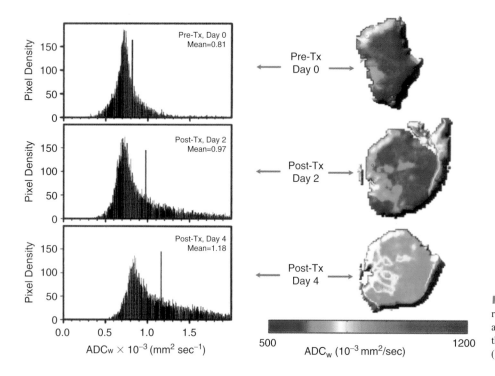

Figure 2 ADC analyses. Images on the right show ADC maps from LnCaP tumors at days 0, 2, and 4 relative to docetaxel therapy. These are converted to histograms (left) for statistical analyses.

propionic acid N-oxide dihydrochloride) is a novel agent soon to enter clinical testing that suppresses both constitutive and hypoxia-induced levels of HIF-1α in cancer cells. The inhibition of tumor growth by PX-478 is positively associated with HIF-1α levels in a variety of different human tumor xenografts in SCID mice. Diffusion-weighted images were obtained at three b-values (25, 500, and 950 sec/mm²), with a time resolution of 13 min for a complete data set. As in the previous study, images were reconstructed using a filtered backprojection algorithm of magnitude data to minimize motion artifacts. Imaging was performed before treatment and at 2, 12, 24, 36, and 48 hr after injection of a single dose of 125 mg/kg IP. At early time points (2 and 12 hr), ADC values were not significantly different between control and treated groups. A substantial increase in mean relative tumor ADC and a right shift in ADC histograms of tumors were observed for the treated groups at 24 and 36 hr post-treatment (94.5 ± 4.8%, $p = 0.005$, and 38.4 ± 4.9%, $p = 0.01$, respectively), before returning to pretreatment mean ADC values by 48 hr post-treatment. The increase in tumor ADC was correlated with a decrease in vessel permeability consistent with cell death and modification of the intracellular to extracellular water populations ratio (Fig. 3).

Diffusion MRI in Clinical Oncology

Largely because of the strong preclinical findings, DW-MRI monitoring of therapy is being investigated in a clinical setting. Hardware limitations and specific absorption rate (SAR) in clinical scanners preclude clinical diffusion measurements from generating the full dynamic range of data

that is available preclinically. Nonetheless, a number of clinical DW-MRI studies have already demonstrated its potential to noninvasively image anticancer therapy responses. Also, recent studies have begun to carry out these measurements in organs other than the brain, which is technically more demanding due to motion. Here are some examples illustrating the change in tumor ADC following therapy in the clinical setting.

Effect of Radiation Therapy on Tumor Apparent Diffusion Coefficient

The group of Chenevert demonstrated that ionizing radiation can sensitize breast carcinoma cells to tumor necrosis factor-related apoptosis-inducing ligand (TRAIL)-induced apoptosis (Chinnaiyan *et al.*, 2000). Increased water mobility was observed in combined TRAIL- and radiation-treated tumors but not in tumors treated with TRAIL or radiation alone. Histological analysis confirmed the loss of cellularity and increased numbers of apoptotic cells in TRAIL- and radiation-treated tumors.

In brain cancers, Mardor *et al.* (2003) have studied the feasibility of using DW-MRI at 0.5T for radiation response monitoring in early malignant brain lesions. They also evaluated the additional information obtained from high b-value DWI, which is more sensitive to low-mobility water molecules (such as intracellular or bound water), in increasing the sensitivity to response. With high DWI, all responding lesions showed increase in the diffusion parameter, and all nonresponding lesions showed no change or decrease. The changes in the diffusion parameters measured one week after initiating treatment were correlated with later tumor

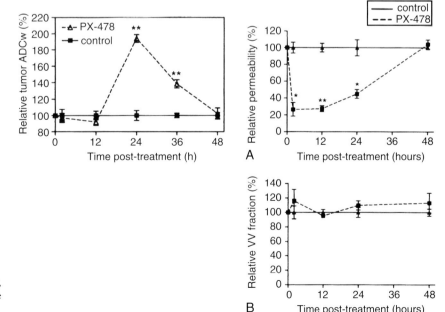

Figure 3 Left, apparent diffusion coefficient, and right, permeability (**A**) and vascular volume fraction (**B**) in response to *PX-478*.

response or no response. They further used high diffusion-weighted MRI in pretreatment prediction of brain tumor response to radiotherapy. They observed that ADC and R_D (a diffusion index reflecting tissue viability) correlated significantly with tumor recurrence, implying that tumors with low pretreatment diffusion values (indicating high viability) responded better to radiotherapy than tumors with high diffusion values (indicating necrosis).

Effect of Chemotherapy on Tumor Apparent Diffusion Coefficient

Mardor *et al.* (2001) have monitored the effects of intratumoral convection-enhanced drug delivery (CEDD) in three brain tumor patients treated with Taxol. Clear changes in the images and the water diffusion parameters were observed shortly after the initiation of treatment. Initially, a bright area corresponding to decreased diffusion appeared, followed by the appearance of a dark area of increased diffusion within the bright area. The time to appearance of the dark area varied among the patients, suggesting different response rates. Again, the ADC changes were correlated with the onset of necrosis due to the treatment.

Hein *et al.* (2003) have monitored the response of primary carcinoma of the rectum to preoperative chemoradiation by measuring tumor ADC. Nine patients undergoing preoperative combined chemoradiation for clinical stage T3 carcinoma were analyzed. Comparison of mean ADC and cumulative radiation dose showed a significant *decrease* of mean ADC at the second, third, and fourth weeks of treatment. These investigators concluded that cytotoxic edema and fibrosis were responsible for this decrease in ADC. They further showed a correlation between pretreatment perfusion indices and ADC with therapy outcome after chemoradiation. Mean tumor water ADC values before and after chemotherapy and chemoradiation in 14 patients with locally advanced rectal cancer have also been evaluated by Dzik-Jurasz *et al.* (2002). Similar to other studies in other cancers, they found a strong negative correlation between mean pretreatment tumor water ADC and percentage size change of tumors after chemotherapy and chemoradiation. However, they also observed a decrease in ADC following therapy, which is consistent with Hein's observations in the same cancers but is apparently discrepant with other studies in other cancers, which usually show an increase in ADC in responding patients. The authors associate the drop in ADC with a sloughing of dying parts of the lesions into the lumen of the rectum. Hence, the domains of the lesion that remained were not responding and were apparently healthy. This is consistent with the observations of Kremser *et al.* (2003), who also monitored changes in rectal carcinoma ADC following chemoradiation. In these studies, a significant increase in the ADC was observed during the first week of therapy in respondeers, followed by a steady decrease. In the nonresponder group, no initial increase of ADC values

was observed after the first week of therapy, and ADC values were significantly lower in the nonresponder group during the remaining duration of therapy.

Our group recently tested the hypothesis that changes in water mobility will quantitatively presage tumor responses in patients with metastatic liver lesions from breast cancer (Theilmann *et al.*, 2004). A total of 13 patients with metastatic breast cancer and 60 measurable liver lesions were monitored by diffusion MRI after initiation of new courses of chemotherapy (taxane, vinorelbine, capecitabine, paclitaxel, and trastuzumab). Diffusion-weighted SSEPI images were obtained through the entire liver. Diffusion weighting was applied in the superior/inferior direction with b = 0, 150, 300, 450 sec/ mm^2. Magnetic resonance images were obtained prior to, and at 4, 11, and 39 days following, the initiation of therapy for determination of volumes and ADC values. The data indicate that diffusion MRI can predict response by 4 or 11 days after commencement of therapy, depending on the analytic method. The highest concordance was observed in tumor lesions that were < 8 cm^3 in volume at presentation. These results suggest that diffusion MRI can be useful in predicting the response of liver metastases to effective chemotherapy.

We reviewed here the major findings showing that both T1 DCE-MRI and diffusion-weighted imaging are able to monitor tumor response to therapy, clinically and preclinically. Some studies have also suggested the potential of the techniques to *predict* tumor response. This point is still currently under investigation and would be of particular interest in screening and preselecting patients for a particular therapy. As illustrated in the present report, DCE and diffusion MRI reflect different markers of tumor response and are complementary methods. There is a high interest in combining the two techniques in future studies. In consequence, the combination of these modalities is likely to have a major impact in drug development and in clinical assessment of tumor treatment. A future challenge for imaging methods is to differentiate between cancer recurrence and necrosis/apoptosis, a very significant issue for clinical decision making. To this end both DCE and diffusion MRI have also shown great potential.

References

Artemov, D., Bhujwalla, Z.M., and Bulte, J.W. 2004. Magnetic resonance imaging of cell surface receptors using targeted contrast agents. *Curr. Pharm. Biotechnol.* 5:485–494.

Bammer, R. 2003. Basic principles of diffusion-weighted imaging. *Eur. J. Radiol.* 45:169–184.

Bhujwalla, Z.M., Artemov, D., Natarajan, K., Solaiyappan, M., Kollars, P., and Kristjansen, P.E. 2003. Reduction of vascular and permeable regions in solid tumors detected by macromolecular contrast magnetic resonance imaging after treatment with antiangiogenic agent TNP-470. *Clin. Cancer Res.* 9:355–362.

Brasch, R.C., Li, K.C., Husband, J.E., Keogan, M.T., Neeman, M., Padhani, A.R., Shames, D., and Turetschek, K. 2000. *In vivo* monitoring of tumor angiogenesis with MR imaging. *Acad. Radiol.* 7:812–823.

Chinnaiyan, A.M., Prasad, U., Shankar, S., Hamstra, D.A., Shanaiah, M., Chenevert, T.L., Ross, B.D., and Rehemtulla, A. 2000. Combined effect of tumor necrosis factor-related apoptosis-inducing ligand and ionizing radiation in breast cancer therapy. *Proc. Natl. Acad. Sci. U.S.A* 97:1754–1759.

Daldrup, H., Shames, D.M., Wendland, M., Okuhata, Y., Link, T.M., Rosenau, W., Lu, Y., and Brasch, R.C. 1998. Correlation of dynamic contrast-enhanced MR imaging with histologic tumor grade: comparison of macromolecular and small-molecular contrast media. *AJR Am. J. Roentgenol.* 171:941–949.

de Lussanet, Q.G., Backes, W.H., Griffioen, A.W., Padhani, A.R., Baeten, C.I., van Baardwijk, A., Lambin, P., Beets, G.L., van Engelshoven, J.M., and Beets-Tan, R.G. 2005. Dynamic contrast-enhanced magnetic resonance imaging of radiation therapy-induced microcirculation changes in rectal cancer. *Int. J. Radiat. Oncol. Biol. Phys.* 63: 1309–1315.

Dowlati, A., Robertson, K., Cooney, M., Petros, W.P., Stratford, M., Jesberger, J., Rafie, N., Overmoyer, B., Makkar, V., Stambler, B., Taylor, A., Waas, J., Lewin, J.S., McCrae, K.R., and Remick, S.C. 2002. A phase I pharmacokinetic and translational study of the novel vascular targeting agent combretastatin a-4 phosphate on a single-dose intravenous schedule in patients with advanced cancer. *Cancer Res.* 62:3408–3416.

Dzik-Jurasz, A., Domenig, C., George, M., Wolber, J., Padhani, A., Brown, G., and Doran, S. 2002. Diffusion MRI for prediction of response of rectal cancer to chemoradiation. *Lancet* 360:307–308.

Evelhoch, J., Garwood, M., Vigneron, D., Knopp, M., Sullivan, D., Menkens, A., Clarke, L., and Liu, G. 2005. Expanding the use of magnetic resonance in the assessment of tumor response to therapy: workshop report. *Cancer Res.* 65:7041–7044.

Galbraith, S.M., Maxwell, R.J., Lodge, M.A., Tozer, G.M., Wilson, J., Taylor, N.J., Stirling, J.J., Sena, L., Padhani, A.R., and Rustin, G.J. 2003. Combretastatin A4 phosphate has tumor antivascular activity in rat and man as demonstrated by dynamic magnetic resonance imaging. *J. Clin. Oncol.* 21:2831–2842.

Galons, J.P., Altbach, M.I., Paine-Murrieta, G.D., Taylor, C.W., and Gillies, R.J. 1999. Early increases in breast tumor xenograft water mobility in response to paclitaxel therapy detected by non-invasive diffusion magnetic resonance imaging. *Neoplasia* 1:113–117.

Hayes, C., Padhani, A.R., and Leach, M.O. 2002. Assessing changes in tumour vascular function using dynamic contrast-enhanced magnetic resonance imaging. *NMR Biomed.* 15:154–163.

Hein, P.A., Kremser, C., Judmaier, W., Griebel, J., Pfeiffer, K.P., Kreczy, A., Hug, E.B., Lukas, P., and DeVries, A.F. 2003. Diffusion-weighted magnetic resonance imaging for monitoring diffusion changes in rectal carcinoma during combined, preoperative chemoradiation: preliminary results of a prospective study. *Eur. J. Radiol.* 45:214–222.

Jayson, G.C., Zweit, J., Jackson, A., Mulatero, C., Julyan, P., Ranson, M., Broughton, L., Wagstaff, J., Hakannson, L., Groenewegen, G., Bailey, J., Smith, N., Hastings, D., Lawrance, J., Haroon, H., Ward, T., McGown, A.T., Tang, M., Levitt, D., Marreaud, S., Lehmann, F.F., Herold, M., and Zwierzina, H. 2002. Molecular imaging and biological evaluation of HuMV833 anti-VEGF antibody: implications for trial design of antiangiogenic antibodies. *J. Natl. Cancer Inst.* 94:1484–1493.

Jennings, D., Hatton, B.N., Guo, J., Galons, J.P., Trouard, T.P., Raghunand, N., Marshall, J., and Gillies, R.J. 2002. Early response of prostate carcinoma xenografts to docetaxel chemotherapy monitored with diffusion MRI. *Neoplasia* 4:255–262.

Jordan, B.F., Runquist, M., Raghunand, N., Baker, A., Williams, R., Kirkpatrick, L., Powis, G., and Gillies, R.J. 2005a. Dynamic contrast-enhanced and diffusion MRI show rapid and dramatic changes in tumor microenvironment in response to inhibition of HIF-1alpha using PX-478. *Neoplasia* 7:475–485.

Jordan, B.F., Runquist, M., Raghunand, N., Gillies, R.J., Tate, W.R., Powis, G., and Baker, A.F. 2005b. The thioredoxin-1 inhibitor 1-methylpropyl 2-imidazolyl disulfide (PX-12) decreases vascular permeability in tumor xenografts monitored by dynamic contrast enhanced magnetic resonance imaging. *Clin. Cancer Res.* 11:529–536.

Kauppinen, R.A. 2002. Monitoring cytotoxic tumour treatment response by diffusion magnetic resonance imaging and proton spectroscopy. *NMR Biomed.* 15:6–17.

Knopp, M.V., Giesel, F.L., Marcos, H., Tengg-Kobligk, H., and Choyke, P. 2001. Dynamic contrast-enhanced magnetic resonance imaging in oncology. *Top. Magn. Reson. Imaging* 12:301–308.

Kremser, C., Judmaier, W., Hein, P., Griebel, J., Lukas, P., and de Vries, A. 2003. Preliminary results on the influence of chemoradiation on apparent diffusion coefficients of primary rectal carcinoma measured by magnetic resonance imaging. *Strahlenther. Onkol.* 179:641–649.

Mardor, Y., Pfeffer, R., Spiegelmann, R., Roth, Y., Maier, S.E., Nissim, O., Berger, R., Glicksman, A., Baram, J., Orenstein, A., Cohen, J.S., and Tichler, T. 2003. Early detection of response to radiation therapy in patients with brain malignancies using conventional and high b-value diffusion-weighted magnetic resonance imaging. *J. Clin. Oncol.* 21:1094–1100.

Mardor, Y., Roth, Y., Lidar, Z., Jonas, T., Pfeffer, R., Maier, S.E., Faibel, M., Nass, D., Hadani, M., Orenstein, A., Cohen, J.S., and Ram, Z. 2001. Monitoring response to convection-enhanced taxol delivery in brain tumor patients using diffusion-weighted magnetic resonance imaging. *Cancer Res.* 61:4971–4973.

Mayr, N.A., Yuh, W.T., Arnholt, J.C., Ehrhardt, J.C., Sorosky, J.I., Magnotta, V.A., Berbaum, K.S., Zhen, W., Paulino, A.C., Oberley, L.W., Sood, A.K., and Buatti, J.M. 2000. Pixel analysis of MR perfusion imaging in predicting radiation therapy outcome in cervical cancer. *J. Magn. Reson. Imag.* 12:1027–1033.

Moffat, B.A., Hall, D.E., Stojanovska, J., McConville, P.J., Moody, J.B., Chenevert, T.L., Rehemtulla, A., and Ross, B.D. 2004. Diffusion imaging for evaluation of tumor therapies in preclinical animal models. *MAGMA.* 17:249–259.

Morgan, B., Thomas, A.L., Drevs, J., Hennig, J., Buchert, M., Jivan, A., Horsfield, M.A., Mross, K., Ball, H.A., Lee, L., Mietlowski, W., Fuxuis, S., Unger, C., O'Byrne, K., Henry, A., Cherryman, G.R., Laurent, D., Dugan, M., Marme, D., and Steward, W.P. 2003. Dynamic contrast-enhanced magnetic resonance imaging as a biomarker for the pharmacological response of PTK787/ZK 222584, an inhibitor of the vascular endothelial growth factor receptor tyrosine kinases, in patients with advanced colorectal cancer and liver metastases: results from two phase I studies. *J. Clin. Oncol.* 21:3955–3964.

Norris, D.G. 2001. The effects of microscopic tissue parameters on the diffusion weighted magnetic resonance imaging experiment. *NMR Biomed.* 14:77–93.

Padhani, A.R., and Husband, J.E. 2001. Dynamic contrast-enhanced MRI studies in oncology with an emphasis on quantification, validation and human studies. *Clin. Radiol.* 56:607–620.

Padhani, A.R., and Leach, M.O. 2005. Antivascular cancer treatments: functional assessments by dynamic contrast-enhanced magnetic resonance imaging. *Abdom. Imaging* 30:324–341.

Preda, A., van Vliet, M., Krestin, G.P., Brasch, R.C., and van Dijke, C.F. 2006. Magnetic resonance macromolecular agents for monitoring tumor microvessels and angiogenesis inhibition. *Invest. Radiol.* 41:325–331.

Rijpkema, M., Kaanders, J.H., Joosten, F.B., van der Kogel, A.J., and Heerschap, A. 2001. Method for quantitative mapping of dynamic MRI contrast agent uptake in human tumors. *J. Magn. Reson. Imag.* 14:457–463.

Ross, B.D., Moffat, B.A., Lawrence, T.S., Mukherji, S.K., Gebarski, S.S., Quint, D.J., Johnson, T.D., Junck, L., Robertson, P.L., Muraszko, K.M., Dong, Q., Meyer, C.R., Bland, P.H., McConville, P., Geng, H., Rehemtulla, A., and Chenevert, T.L. 2003. Evaluation of cancer therapy using diffusion magnetic resonance imaging. *Mol. Cancer Ther.* 2:581–587.

Seifert, M.H., Jakob, P.M., Jellus, V., Haase, A., and Hillenbrand, C. 2000. High-resolution diffusion imaging using a radial turbo-spin-echo sequence: implementation, eddy current compensation, and self-navigation. *J. Magn. Reson. 144*:243–254.

Stejskal, E.O., and Tanner, J.E. 1965. Use of spin echo in pulsed magnetic field gradient to study anistropic, restricted diffusion and flow. *J. Chem. Phys. 43*:3579–3603.

Theilmann, R.J., Borders, R., Trouard, T.P., Xia, G., Outwater, E., Ranger-Moore, J., Gillies, R.J., and Stopeck, A. 2004. Changes in water mobility measured by diffusion MRI predict response of metastatic breast cancer to chemotherapy. *Neoplasia 6*:831–837.

Tofts, P.S., Brix, G., Buckley, D.L., Evelhoch, J.L., Henderson, E., Knopp, M.V., Larsson, H.B., Lee, T.Y., Mayr, N.A., Parker, G.J., Port, R.E., Taylor, J., and Weisskoff, R.M. 1999. Estimating kinetic parameters from dynamic contrast-enhanced T(1)-weighted MRI of a diffusable tracer: standardized quantities and symbols. *J. Magn. Reson. Imag. 10*:223–232.

Trouard, T.P., Theilmann, R.J., Altbach, M.I., and Gmitro, A.F. 1999. High-resolution diffusion imaging with DIFRAD-FSE (diffusion-weighted radial acquisition of data with fast spin-echo) MRI. *Magn. Reson. Med. 42*:11–18.

van der Woude, H.J., Bloem, J.L., Verstraete, K.L., Taminiau, A.H., Nooy, M.A., and Hogendoorn, P.C. 1995. Osteosarcoma and Ewing's sarcoma after neoadjuvant chemotherapy: value of dynamic MR imaging in detecting viable tumor before surgery. *AJR Am. J. Roentgenol. 165*: 593–598.

Wedam, S.B., Low, J.A., Yang, S.X., Chow, C.K., Choyke, P., Danforth, D., Hewitt, S.M., Berman, A., Steinberg, S.M., Liewehr, D.J., Plehn, J., Doshi, A., Thomasson, D., McCarthy, N., Koeppen, H., Sherman, M., Zujewski, J., Camphausen, K., Chen, H., and Swain, S.M. 2006. Antiangiogenic and antitumor effects of bevacizumab in patients with inflammatory and locally advanced breast cancer. *J. Clin. Oncol. 24*:769–777.

15

In Vivo Molecular Imaging in Oncology: Principles of Reporter Gene Expression Imaging

Tarik F. Massoud

Introduction

It would have been unthinkable some decades ago to envision the extent to which progress would be made in observations of living subjects, as afforded by modern-day imaging techniques. Molecular imaging is the latest addition in this astounding imaging evolution, bringing *in vivo* observations to a new and more meaningful dimension. Its novelty lies in the fact that unlike traditional means of imaging patients or living experimental animals that rely on nonspecific macroscopic physical, physiological, or metabolic changes to differentiate pathological from normal tissues, molecular imaging seeks to shed new light on both structure and function by creating images that directly or indirectly reflect specific cellular and molecular events (e.g., gene expression) that can reveal pathways and mechanisms responsible for disease within the context of physiologically authentic and intact living subject environments (Massoud and Gambhir, 2003).

This change in emphasis from a nonspecific to a more specific imaging approach represents a significant paradigm shift in radiology. The impact of this shift in philosophy means that imaging can now provide the potential for (1) understanding a patient's abnormal biology in a quick,

noninvasive manner, and with less labor than is achievable by conventional pathology or clinical chemistry-based assays, (2) earlier detection and characterization of disease and its pathogenesis, and (3) assessment of therapeutic effectiveness at a molecular level, long before phenotypic change. Many of the attributes of this new imaging discipline are already being exploited in the laboratory, where molecular imaging techniques are currently used in research animals to develop and validate these novel imaging strategies, with a view to future extrapolation to the clinical setting. Experimental molecular imaging techniques are also laying a strong foundation that will ultimately transform the understanding of integrative mammalian biology. A more comprehensive discussion of factors contributing to the emergence of molecular imaging, the particular advantages of these approaches, and the general goals potentially achievable in biomedical research and clinical practice by adopting molecular imaging strategies have been reviewed recently (Weissleder and Mahmood, 2001; Massoud and Gambhir, 2003).

Many integral components and subdisciplines in the make-up of molecular imaging (e.g., basic molecular cell biology, chemistry, pharmacology, medical therapeutics, medical physics, bioengineering and biomathematics, and bioinformatics) are presently contributing to the intensive exploration in laboratory research surrounding this new field, particularly through the use and refinement of experimental animal models (Cherry and Gambhir, 2001; Chatziioannou, 2002; Contag and Bachmann, 2002; Massoud and Gambhir, 2003). One of the molecular imaging subdisciplines least familiar to imaging specialists, and arguably one that holds great future promise in oncologic imaging, is that of reporter gene expression imaging (Gambhir *et al.*, 1999; Blasberg, 2002). This chapter describes the basic principles and recent technological developments in reporter gene expression imaging in living subjects. The fact that current applications of these new techniques are mostly limited to experimental small-animal models should not diminish their relevance or interest to clinical oncologists and radiologists. Knowledge of the fundamentals of reporter gene expression imaging is essential for at least two reasons: (1) these novel imaging methods would constitute the same techniques potentially translatable into future clinical practice and applicable to future molecular imaging of cancer patients, and (2) these novel analytical research techniques, adapted from standard *in vitro* assays used in laboratory biological research, are likely to be used with increasing frequency within academic research centers by a new breed of clinician-scientists, who, through their research endeavors, will continue building the foundations for future improved molecular imaging in clinical practice.

Reporter Gene Expression Imaging: A Subfield of Molecular Imaging

Although the term *imaging* may be clearly defined as the creation of a visual representation of the measurable property of a person, object, or phenomenon, confusion exists regarding the term *molecular imaging*. This is not surprising because this term is borrowed from molecular biology, which itself is "an elusive term whose definition depends on who is doing the defining" (Weaver, 1999). Molecular biology can be defined very broadly as *the attempt to understand biological phenomena in molecular terms*. Unfortunately, this definition makes molecular biology difficult to distinguish from biochemistry (Weaver, 1999). The corollary of this is the use of the term *molecular imaging* in a broad sense as it applies to the targeting of any molecule in a specific manner to obtain images. In this sense, *molecular imaging* may be applied to almost the entire field of nuclear medicine imaging, where specific molecules are tagged with radionuclides for imaging their distribution *in vivo*. Accordingly, the use of ^{131}I approximately 40 years ago for assessment and imaging of thyroid function in recurrent thyroid cancer would constitute one of the earliest applications of molecular imaging. Another example of this generic use of the term applies to magnetic resonance spectroscopy (MRS)

where characteristic imaging spectra are obtained from small volumes of tissue subjected to magnetic resonance, depending on their chemical or molecular composition (Castillo *et al.*, 1996).

A more restrictive but useful definition of molecular biology is *the study of gene structure and function at the molecular level* (Weaver, 1999). A gene may be defined as a locus of co-transcribed DNA exons that ultimately results in the production of a peptide or protein. Genes are hereditary units controlling identifiable traits of an organism. Rigorous exploration is taking place in the biological sciences to determine the patterns of gene expression that encode normal biological processes. There is also a growing belief that diseases result from alterations in normal regulation of gene expression that transition cells to phenotypes of disease. These alterations in gene expression can result from interactions with the environment, hereditary deficits, developmental errors, and the aging process (Phelps, 2000). Molecular imaging of gene expression is the process by which a gene product, made via the two steps of transcription and translation, can be visualized, quantified, and located in intact living subjects. The achievement of molecular imaging of gene expression with the use of particular genes, termed *imaging reporter genes*, forms the basis of reporter gene expression imaging in living subjects. Previously, to obtain anything akin to this information had been nearly impossible (aside from whole-body imaging of small transparent animals) other than by *in vitro* or cell-culture methods.

A glossary of molecular imaging terminology was published recently (Wagenaar *et al.*, 2001) to facilitate an understanding of the molecular and cell biology concepts at the heart of reporter gene expression imaging and other molecular imaging strategies. Further information can be found in several previously published review articles (Gambhir *et al.*, 1999; Weissleder and Mahmood, 2001; Blasberg and Gelovani-Tjuvajev, 2002; Massoud and Gambhir, 2003), and at the Web site www.mi-central.org, which serves as a useful Internet resource for a wide variety of molecular imaging information.

Principles of Reporter Gene Expression Imaging

A dictionary might define a reporter as one who broadcasts news or carries a message. This colloquial meaning of the word is quite apt when characterizing reporter systems in molecular biology and imaging. Reporter molecules broadcast their presence by producing a signal that can be measured in the laboratory by bench top or cell-culture techniques, or with imaging instrumentation in the case of molecular imaging. More precisely, a reporter gene is one with a readily measurable phenotype that can be distinguished easily from a background of endogenous proteins

(Alam and Cook, 1990). Molecular and cell biologists might typically use reporter genes (DNA that codes for reporter protein molecules) to determine how the expression of other genes of interest is regulated under various conditions. Thus, reporter genes are used to study: (1) promoter/enhancer elements involved in gene expression (promoters are short stretches of DNA that signal RNA polymerase to begin transcription of a gene, and enhancers are DNA binding sites for protein factors that boost gene transcription), (2) inducible promoters to look at the induction (the gradual or complete switching on or off) of gene expression, and (3) endogenous gene expression through the use of transgenes containing endogenous promoters fused to the reporter (Gambhir, 2000). In all these cases, the expression of a gene of interest can be studied if it is linked to the expression of a reporter gene (the transcription of which can be tracked), for example, by their sharing of the same promoter/enhancer elements. Researchers always look for reporter systems that are sensitive, convenient to use, and with assays that yield rapid, quantitative, and reproducible results with a wide dynamic range under a variety of conditions (Gambhir *et al.*, 1999; Naylor, 1999).

Customary methods in biomedical research to monitor reporter gene expression include: (1) tissue biopsy or gross pathological observation, with or without histochemical or immunohistochemical staining for reporter gene proteins, (2) *in situ* hybridization with probes targeted at reporter gene messenger RNA, and (3) blood sampling when the reporter gene product is a secretable protein (e.g., alkaline phosphatase) (Gambhir *et al.*, 1999). These conventional methods to detect reporter proteins are hindered by their inability to noninvasively determine the location, magnitude, and extent of gene expression in a living subject. To image gene expression in living subjects, it is possible to target either genes externally transferred into cells of organ systems (transgenes) or endogenous genes. Most current applications of reporter gene imaging are of the former variety, and this will be stressed in the examples provided in this chapter. The expression of endogenous genes can also be imaged indirectly if a promoter that is endogenous to the cell drives the reporter gene. Thus, whenever the endogenous gene is upregulated, so is the reporter gene (Doubrovin *et al.*, 2001; Green *et al.*, 2002).

There are two different strategies for interrogating the myriad biological processes that could be targeted for molecular imaging. The first strategy is a direct one that uses *de novo* synthesis of unique molecular probes targeted to a specific molecular marker(s)/target(s), such as a receptor, a transporter, or an enzyme. For reasons outlined previously (Massoud and Gambhir, 2003), the development and validation of these specific imaging agents are time consuming and require significant effort. The second general strategy to image specific molecular and cellular events is an indirect one, and imaging reporter systems can be grouped under this approach. This strategy entails the use of a pre-targeting

molecule (a reporter gene under the control of one of many possible promoters) that is subsequently activated (to yield a reporter protein) upon occurrence of a specific molecular event (promoter switch-on and reporter gene expression). Following this, a molecular probe (the reporter probe) specific for the activated pre-targeting molecule (reporter protein) is used to image its activation (Fig. 1). This approach provides a generalizable system that may be used to image *many* different biological processes with the same reporter probe and different pre-targeting molecules (on account of the diversity of possible promoters that can form part of these pre-targeting molecules). This is an attractive means to indirectly visualize transcriptional and post-transcriptional regulation of gene expression, protein–protein interactions, or trafficking of proteins or cells in living subjects. The downside, however, is the necessity to introduce one or more foreign proteins/genes into a cell, and the delivery of the reporter gene may be a limitation of this strategy in living subjects. Conceptually, the latter is less of an issue in the context of gene therapy approaches where a therapeutic gene needs to be delivered in any case, or for molecular imaging of transgenic animals expressing the reporter gene already as part of their construct. When adopting this strategy, it is important to determine how accurately the reporter protein reproduces regulation and function of the corresponding endogenous pathway, thus proving that the reporter does not perturb the underlying biological process being examined.

Accordingly, an imaging reporter gene driven by a promoter of choice *must first be introduced into the cells of interest*. This is a common feature for all delivery vectors in a reporter gene-imaging paradigm; that is, a complementary DNA expression cassette (an imaging cassette) containing the reporter gene of interest must be used. The promoter can be constitutive, that is, switched on all the time, or inducible; it can also be cell-specific (endogenous) or foreign to the cell (e.g., promoters of viral origin). If the imaging reporter gene is transcribed, an enzyme or receptor product is made, capable of trapping or interacting with an imaging reporter probe, which may be a substrate for an enzyme or a ligand for a receptor. The trapping/interaction with the probe leads to an imaging signal, be it from a radioisotope, a photochemical reaction, or a magnetic resonance metal cation, depending on the exact nature of the probe itself (see below). Unlike most conventional reporter gene laboratory methods (e.g., chloramphenicol acetyl transferase, LacZ/β-galactosidase, alkaline phosphatase, Bla/β-lactamase, etc. [Spergel *et al.*, 2001]), reporter gene molecular imaging techniques offer the possibility of monitoring the location, magnitude, and persistence of reporter gene expression in intact living animals or humans.

The ideal imaging reporter gene/probe would have the following characteristics (Gambhir, 2000): (1) To prevent an immune response, the reporter gene should be present in mammalian cells but not expressed; (2) specific reporter

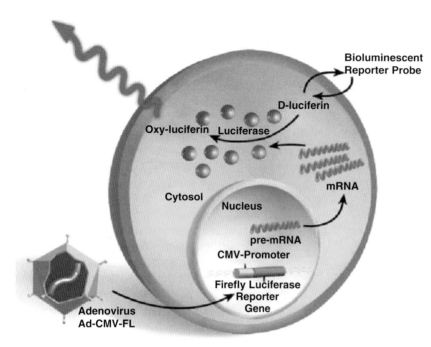

Figure 1 Schematic diagram of the principle of reporter gene imaging using the enzyme Firefly luciferase. Once the cell is transduced with a viral vector containing the imaging gene cassette, a promoter of choice drives the transcription of the imaging reporter gene (*Fluc*). If the promoter leads to transcription of *Fluc*, then translation of the imaging reporter gene mRNA leads to a protein product (the enzyme Firefly luciferase) that can interact with the imaging reporter probe (D-Luciferin). This interaction is a chemiluminescent reaction that catalyzes the transformation of the substrate D-Luciferin into oxyluciferin in a process dependent on ATP, Mg^{++}, and O_2, leading to the emission of light, which can be detected using low-light sensing instruments.

probe should accumulate only where the reporter gene is expressed; (3) no reporter probe should accumulate when the reporter gene is not expressed; (4) the product of the reporter gene should also be nonimmunogenic; (5) the reporter probe should be stable *in vivo* and not be metabolized before reaching its target; (6) the reporter probe should rapidly clear from the circulation and not interfere with detection of a specific signal; (7) the reporter probe or its metabolites should not be cytotoxic; (8) the size of the reporter gene and its driving promoter should be small enough to fit into a delivery vehicle (plasmids, viruses), except for transgenic applications; (9) natural biological barriers must not prevent the reporter probe from reaching its destination; and (10) the image signal should correlate well with levels of reporter gene mRNA and protein *in vivo*. No single imaging reporter gene/probe system currently meets all these criteria. Therefore, the development of multiple systems provides a choice based on the application of interest. The availability of multiple reporter gene/reporter probes also allows monitoring of the expression of more than one reporter gene in the same living animal.

Categories of Reporter Gene Expression Imaging Systems

A broad classification of imaging reporter systems consists of those in which the gene product is intracellular or is associated with the cell membrane (reviewed by Gross and Piwnica-Worms, 2005). Examples of the former include thymidine kinase, green fluorescent protein, the luciferases, xanthine phosphoribotransferase, cytosine deaminase, and tyrosinase. Examples of reporter proteins on or in the cell surface include the dopamine-2 receptor, the receptors for somatostatin or transferrin, and the sodium iodide symporter. The major advantages of intracellular protein expression are the relatively uncomplicated expression strategy and the likely lack of recognition of the expression product by the immune system. The relative theoretical disadvantage is the presence of potentially unfavorable kinetics, requiring the need for the substrate to penetrate into a cell. The major advantages of surface-expressed receptors and acceptors are favorable kinetics (sometimes avoiding the need for the tracer to penetrate into a cell) and the fact that synthetic reporters can be engineered to recognize already approved imaging drugs. What follows are brief descriptions of some PET-, SPECT-, and MRI-based reporter systems, and separate emphasis on optical-based reporter systems.

The herpes simplex virus type-1 thymidine kinase (HSV1-*tk*) enzyme phosphorylates a wide range of nucleoside analogs, allowing selective antiherpetic and viral vector-based gene therapies. This enzyme also forms the basis of a well-studied isotope-based imaging reporter gene/reporter probe system adapted for PET imaging, and including, for example, the reporter probe 9-(4-[^{18}F]-fluoro-3-hydroxymethylbutyl)-guanine (^{18}F-FHBG) or ^{18}F-fluoropenciclovir (^{18}F-FPCV) (Iyer *et al.*, 2001). Saito *et al.* (1982, 1984) first proposed that the HSV1-*tk* gene might be used as a marker gene for the early detection of herpes encephalitis. This reporter system was subsequently developed in 1996 using ^{131}I-labeled 2'fluoro-2'-deoxy-1-beta-D-arabinofuranosyl-5-iodo-uracil (FIAU) for SPECT imaging (Tjuvajev *et al.*, 1996). Two main categories of substrates—uracil nucleoside derivatives labeled with radioactive iodine (e.g., FIAU) (Tjuvajev *et al.*, 1995), and acycloguanosine derivatives labeled with radioactive ^{18}F-Fluorine (e.g., ^{18}F-FPCV, ^{18}F-FHBG)—have been investigated in the last few years as reporter probes for imaging HSV1-*tk* reporter gene expression (Namavari *et al.*, 2000). These radiolabeled reporter probes are transported into cells, and are trapped as a result of phosphorylation by HSV1-tk. When used in nonpharmacological tracer doses, these substrates can serve as PET or SPECT targeted reporter probes by their accumulation in only the cells expressing the HSV1-*tk* gene. More recently, a mutant version of this gene, HSV1-*sr39tk*, was derived using site-directed mutagenesis to obtain an enzyme more effective at phosphorylating ganciclovir (and also less efficient at phosphorylating thymidine), with consequent gain in imaging signal (Gambhir *et al.*, 2000).

The Dopamine-2 receptor (*D2R*) reporter gene has also been validated for PET imaging of reporter gene expression while using ^{18}F-fluoroethylspiperone (FESP) as the reporter probe ligand (MacLaren *et al.*, 1999). More recently, a mutant D2R that uncouples signal transduction while maintaining affinity for FESP has also been reported (Liang *et al.*, 2001).

Two general types of reporter systems are applicable to MRI-based molecular imaging, and have been reviewed by Louie *et al.* (2002). One imaging system relies on molecular probes that are sensitive to the activity of β-galactosidase, the product of the classic marker gene *LacZ*. The synthesis of a molecular probe in which gadolinium is protected by a carbohydrate "cap" that is β-galactosidase-cleavable would result in a probe with variable water access. This would provide a molecular probe of variable relaxivity because the interaction between water protons and paramagnetic metal centers of probes results in signal enhancement on T1-weighted images. If an external physiological process regulates water access, then the probe would be a reporter of the physiological process itself. Using the *Xenopus* embryo, Louie *et al.* (2000) have demonstrated the ability of these probes and MRI to detect gene expression in living subjects. Unfortunately, current enzyme-cleavable probes do not freely cross cell membranes (thus requiring direct intracellular injection), and the kinetics of cleavage are quite slow. However, these probes are useful for specific applications in tissues that are amenable to direct injection, (e.g., in developmental biology research).

An alternative to this conditional reporter probe is to couple MRI probes to targeting moieties. Weissleder *et al.* (2000) have highlighted the use of the transferrin receptor as a potential intracellular transporter of iron-oxide nanoparticles. The transferrin receptor is found in most cells and is part of the iron regulatory system. The receptor binds to transferrin, an iron-carrying protein, and transports it into the cell. Normal expression of the receptor is under feedback regulation to prevent excessive cellular iron uptake. However, cells can be engineered to overexpress transferrin and therefore accumulate monocrystalline iron-oxide nanoparticles intracellulary. This increased iron content results in differential MRI signal from these cells depicted on gradient-echo images, which are particularly sensitive to the presence of paramagnetic ions. Additional studies are required to further assess this system, including measurement of the effect of overexpressing the receptor on normal cellular function, and how well normal systems tolerate increased levels of freely circulating and intracellular iron. Another variation on this theme entails the use of the tyrosinase reporter gene leading to a greater cellular production of melanin and subsequent trapping of heavy metals by melanin binding, thus changing cell relaxivity and enhancing the MRI signal (Enochs *et al.*, 1997; Weissleder *et al.*, 1997). A recent evaluation of this reporter system has revealed the feasibility of its regulated expression when placed under the control of regulated promoter elements (Alfke *et al.*, 2003).

Principles of Optical Reporter Gene Imaging in Living Subjects

Many optical-imaging techniques have already been developed for *in vitro* and *ex vivo* applications in molecular and cellular biology. An extension of this concept toward noninvasive *in vivo* reporter gene expression imaging with light photons represents an interesting avenue for extracting relevant biological information from living subjects. Progress in optical molecular imaging strategies has been derived from the recent development of targeted bioluminescence probes, near-infrared fluorochromes, activatable near-infrared fluorochromes, and red-shifted fluorescent proteins (Weissleder, 2001).

A relatively recent addition to the list of reporter gene expression imaging techniques described above is bioluminescence imaging, a noninvasive optical-imaging modality that allows sensitive and quantitative detection of bioluminescence reporter genes in intact living small research animals (Contag and Bachmann, 2002; Massoud and Gambhir, 2003). Bioluminescence refers to the enzymatic generation of visible light by living organisms. In this chapter, particular emphasis is placed on the topic of bioluminescence imaging because it is perhaps the molecular imaging modality least familiar to clinical oncologists and radiologists, and yet, there has been a recent veritable explosion in the assortment and extent of its experimental applications in research laboratories. The main advantage of optical bioluminescence imaging is that it can be used to detect very low levels of signal because the light emitted is virtually background-free.

Although not precisely characterized to date, the sensitivity of bioluminescence imaging is thought to be in the 10^{-15} to 10^{-17} mole/l range, the highest for any available molecular imaging modality. (Sensitivity of PET is $\sim 10^{-11}$–10^{-12} mole/l, and that of MRI $\sim 10^{-3}$–10^{-5} mole/l [Massoud and Gambhir, 2003].) It is quick and easy to perform, and it allows relatively inexpensive and rapid testing of biological hypotheses and proofs of principle in living experimental models. It is also uniquely suited for high-throughput imaging because of its ease of operation, short acquisition times (typically 10–60 sec), and the possibility of simultaneous measurement of several anesthetized living mice. Bioluminescence imaging is well suited for use with small-animal models, is relatively easily accessible to researchers in their laboratory setting, and offers particular flexibility in experimental investigations of molecular mechanisms of disease. Despite many technological advances in this field, the clinical uses of this imaging modality are likely to be limited owing to inherent limitations of photon scatter and absorption in living tissues. Nevertheless, of particular relevance to clinicians is the fact that many of the current applications of bioluminescence imaging would likely provide the theoretical background and experimental feasibility necessary for potential extrapolation and translation into future clinical practice using other more clinically applicable modalities for molecular imaging of patients.

The light emission in bioluminescence follows a chemiluminescent reaction that can take place under physiological conditions within living cells when adenosine triphosphate (ATP) is required, or it can be extracellular (e.g., Renilla luciferase; see below) when the reaction is independent of ATP. The most commonly used bioluminescence reporter gene for research purposes has been the luciferase from the North American Firefly (*Photinus pyralis*; *Fluc*). Luciferase genes have also been cloned from a variety of other organisms, including corals (*Tenilla*), jellyfish (*Aequorea*), sea pansy (*Renilla, Rluc*), several bacterial species (*Vibrio fischeri, Vibrio harveyi*), and dinoflagellates (*Gonyaulax*) (Hastings, 1996). Several of these genes, including *Fluc*, have been modified for optimal expression in mammalian cells, and these have been used for many years in bioassays for ATP quantification and to study gene expression in transfected cells in culture. Firefly luciferase (61 kDa) catalyzes the transformation of its substrate D-Luciferin into oxyluciferin in a process dependent on ATP, Mg^{++}, and O$_2$, leading to the emission of light that can be detected using low-light sensing instruments, including standard luminometers. These biochemical assays are typically conducted on cell lysates, although there are several reports of live cell assays that use *Fluc*, reviewed by Edinger *et al.* (2002).

Some luciferins require the presence of a cofactor to undergo oxidation, such as FMNH$_2^+$, Ca^{2+}, or ATP. Complexes that contain a luciferase, a luciferin, and generally requiring O$_2$ are also called photoproteins. Although the most common luciferin–luciferase system used in molecular imaging is that derived from the Firefly *Photinus*, the sea pansy *Renilla* luciferase, which uses a different substrate (coelenterazine), and is not ATP- or Mg^{++}-dependent, has also been validated recently for applications in living subjects (Bhaumik and Gambhir, 2002). *Renilla* luciferase enzyme (36 kDa) is capable of generating a flash of blue light (460–490 nm, peak emission at 482 nm) upon reaction with its substrate. The synthetic humanized *Renilla* luciferase gene (*hRluc*) is a systematically redesigned *Renilla* luciferase gene, encoding the same 311-residue protein as wild-type Renilla luciferase, but yielding only codon changes for higher expression in mammalian cells. Both colorimetric (e.g., rhodamine red) and fluorescent (e.g., GFP) reporter proteins require an external source of light for excitation and emit light at a different wavelength for detection thus making them more susceptible to background noise (autofluorescence). In contrast, the bioluminescence luciferase enzymes and substrate systems described above have several characteristics that make them useful reporter proteins. Firstly, Firefly luciferase does not need external light excitation and self-emits light from green to yellow wavelengths (560–610 nm, peak emission at 562 nm) in the presence of D-Luciferin, ATP, magnesium, and oxygen. Second, the fast rate of enzyme turnover ($T_{1/2} = 3$ hr) in the presence of substrate D-Luciferin allows for real-time measurements because the enzyme does not accumulate intracellularly to the extent of other reporters. Third, the relationship between the enzyme concentration and peak height of emitted light *in vitro* is linear up to 7–8 orders of magnitude. Therefore, these properties potentially allow for sensitive noninvasive imaging of *Fluc* (and *Rluc*) reporter gene expression in living subjects.

Broadening the use of Firefly luciferase as a bioluminescence reporter from biochemical and cell-culture assays to living subjects was reliant upon the development of low-light imaging systems (see below) and two other crucial observations (Edinger *et al.*, 2002). The first observation was the demonstration that D-Luciferin would seem to circulate within minutes throughout many body compartments (also readily crossing the blood-brain barrier) after intravenous or intraperitoneal administration and rapidly enters many cells (Contag *et al.*, 1997). Studies are currently underway to accurately quantify the uptake kinetics and biodistribution of the substrate D-Luciferin (as well as coelenterazine). The second discovery was that the level and spectrum of emitted light from *Fluc* expressing mammalian cells is adequate to penetrate tissues of small research animals, such as mice and rats, and can be detected externally with low-light imaging cameras (Contag *et al.*, 1995).

Several factors governing interaction of emitted light with tissues deserve particular consideration. The absorption coefficient of light depends on its wavelength (more light is absorbed as the wavelength decreases below 600 nm) and on results from absorbers such as hemoglobin (the main absorber), lipids, and water. Since the emission spectrum of

Firefly luciferase is very broad, the lower end of the spectrum is absorbed to a greater extent within tissues, resulting in relatively more red-shifted light emitted from the surface, particularly when the source of light is in a deep location. The blue spectrum emitted from *Renilla* luciferase is absorbed to an even greater extent than that of Firefly luciferase, but this is counteracted by the much greater initial quantum yield from *Renilla* luciferase. Recently, Bhaumik *et al.* (2004) have found the measurable signal from C6 cells transfected with *hRluc* to be 30- to 40-fold higher than that from C6 cells transfected with *Fluc*, when implanted subcutaneously in the same mouse. The difference in light emission in cell culture is even greater at 120-fold. For deeper tissues (e.g., the lungs) the measurable light when using higher doses of coelenterazine is also higher for cells transfected with *hRluc*, even after absorption by deeper tissues. Additional studies are still needed to directly compare Firefly luciferase and synthetic Renilla luciferase in living subjects.

The signal intensity of measurable light is further determined to a large extent by attenuation of light owing to the effects of scattering. Scattering results from changes in the refractive index at cell membranes and organelles. The signal intensity from a depth of 1 cm is attenuated by a factor of $\sim 10^{-2}$ for wavelengths at ~ 650 nm (Rice *et al.*, 2001). This scatter results in the relatively poor spatial resolution of bioluminescence imaging when compared to other modalities that rely on more penetrating electromagnetic radiation to generate images (e.g., PET, SPECT, CT). The spatial resolution of bioluminescence images is depth-dependent, being slightly worse or equal to the depth of the object; that is, an object 3–5 mm deep has an ~ 3–5 mm spatial resolution.

In fluorescence imaging, an excitation light of one wavelength (in the visible light range of 395–600 nm) illuminates the living subject, and a charge-coupled device (CCD) camera (usually a less sensitive version than the cooled CCD required in bioluminescence detection, for technical reasons discussed by Golden and Ligler (2002)) collects an emission light of shifted wavelength. Cells tagged with fluorescently labeled antibodies or those in which expression of the green fluorescent protein (*GFP*) reporter gene (or its variants [Lippincott-Schwartz *et al.*, 2001; Remington, 2002]) is introduced can be followed by this technique. GFP is a protein from the jellyfish *Aequorea victoria* that has become very popular over the last decade as a reporter in fixed and cultured cells and tissues. Wild-type GFP emits green (509 nm) light when excited by violet (395 nm) light. The variant EGFP has a shifted excitation spectrum to longer wavelengths and has increased (35-fold) brightness. Between 1000 and 10,000 fluorescently labeled cells in the peritoneal cavity of a mouse can be imaged on its external surface (Kaneko *et al.*, 2001). It may be necessary to surgically expose internal organs prior to their imaging (Bouvet *et al.*, 2002; Yang *et al.*, 2002), although this is true of bioluminescence imaging as well. The two main advantages of fluorescence imaging

is that it can be used as a reporter in both live and fixed cells/tissues and no substrate is required for its visualization (Spergel *et al.*, 2001). This simple reflectance-type of fluorescence imaging has been used extensively in studies of feasibility and development of these approaches (Kamiyama *et al.*, 2002; Li *et al.*, 2002). However, these systems are not quantitative, and the image information is surface-weighted (anything closer to the surface will appear brighter compared with deeper structures) (Weissleder, 2001). Direct comparisons of bioluminescence and fluorescence imaging have not been published to date, although these are currently underway in our laboratory. One clear difference between the two modalities is the observation of significantly more background signal due to autofluorescence of tissues in fluorescence imaging as compared to bioluminescence imaging.

In contrast to fluorescence imaging in the visible light range, the use of the near-infrared (NIR) spectrum in the 700–900 nm range maximizes tissue penetration and minimizes autofluorescence from nontarget tissue (Weissleder, 2002). This is because hemoglobin and water, the major absorbers of visible and infrared light, respectively, have their lowest absorption coefficients in the NIR region. A number of NIR fluorochromes have recently become available (Lin *et al.*, 2002) that can be coupled to affinity molecules (peptides, antibodies) or that are activatable. This type of NIR fluorescence reflectance imaging is still limited to targets that are fairly near the illuminated surface.

A newer approach to fluorescence imaging of deeper structures employs fluorescence-mediated tomography (Ntziachristos *et al.*, 2002; Ntziachristos and Weissleder, 2002). The subject is exposed to continuous wave or pulsed light from different sources, and detectors are arranged in a spatially defined order in an imaging chamber to capture the emitted light. Mathematical processing of this information results in a reconstructed tomographic image. Resulting images have a resolution of 1–2 mm, and the fluorochrome detection threshold is in the nanomolar range. Recent attempts at constructing a CCD-based scanner for tomography of fluorescent NIR probes have also yielded encouraging results. Prototype instruments attain better than 3 mm resolution, have linear detection within more than two orders of magnitude of fluorochrome concentration, and can detect fluorescent objects at femtomolar quantities in small-animal-like geometries (Ntziachristos and Weissleder, 2002). Fluorescence-mediated tomography is still in its infancy, requiring extensive mathematical validation prior to practical implementation.

Instrumentation and Techniques for Bioluminescence Imaging

It is apparent from the preceding discussion that in spite of knowing precisely the exogenous or endogenous gene or gene product targeted for imaging, reporter gene expression imaging in living subjects presents more theoretical and practical challenges than *in vitro* or cell culture detection. This is primarily because of the need for molecular probes to be biocompatible, the presence of additional delivery barriers in a living subject, and the necessity for developing special *in vivo* amplification strategies. Also needed are imaging systems with high spatial/temporal resolution and sensitivity suitable for small laboratory animals and, ideally, systems that can ultimately be translated to the human patient. A more detailed discussion of all the general requirements for performing molecular imaging in living subjects can be found elsewhere (Massoud and Gambhir, 2003).

Considerable efforts have been directed in recent years toward the development of noninvasive high-resolution imaging technologies for imaging living small animals (Massoud and Gambhir, 2003). As such, there has been a great need to adapt clinical imaging methods for noninvasive assays of biochemical processes. The various existing imaging technologies differ in five main aspects: spatial and temporal resolution, depth penetration, energy expended for image generation (ionizing or nonionizing, depending on which component of the electromagnetic radiation spectrum is exploited for image generation), availability of injectable/biocompatible molecular probes, and the respective detection threshold of probes for a given technology. Planar imaging (e.g., in bioluminescence imaging) is generally fast, the data sets generated are small, and imaging can be done in high-throughput fashion at the expense of internal resolution. Tomographic imaging is usually quantitative and capable of displaying internal anatomic structures and/or functional information, but generally requires longer acquisition time and higher energy expenditure. Volumetric image acquisition results in the highest spatial information content, although it can generate very large data sets. The general characteristics of several molecular imaging techniques used for reporter gene expression imaging (e.g., PET, SPECT, MRI) are well known to radiological specialists and have been described in detail and compared elsewhere (Massoud and Gambhir, 2003). Fluorescence imaging is also comprehensively described in several review articles (Weissleder and Mahmood, 2001). Here, the technical aspects of bioluminescence imaging are elaborated upon more fully, because these concepts are likely to be novel to most clinical imaging specialists and oncologists.

A fundamental issue in bioluminescence imaging of living subjects is how to detect light emitted from the subject. In this regard, several technical advances for imaging very low levels of visible light have now emerged, allowing the use of highly sensitive detectors in living subjects, and not simply restricted to cell cultures and small transparent animals. CCD detectors are made of silicon crystals sliced into thin sheets for fabrication into integrated circuits using similar technologies to those used in making computer silicon chips.

For a detailed overview of CCD technology, refer to Spibey *et al.* (2001). One of the properties of silicon-based detectors is their high sensitivity to light, allowing them to detect light in the visible to near-infrared range. When light photons at wavelengths between 400 and 1000 nm strike a CCD pixel with energy of 2–3 eV, the CCD camera can convert these light photons into electrons. A CCD contains semiconductors that are connected so that the output of one serves as the input of the next. In this way, an electrical charge pattern, corresponding to the intensity of incoming photons, is read out of the CCD into an output register and amplifier at the edge of the CCD for digitization. Older intensified CCD cameras had much lower sensitivities than newer generation cooled CCD cameras. The reason for this is that thermal noise, termed *dark current*, from thermal energy within the silicon lattice of a CCD chip results in constant release of electrons. Thermal noise is dramatically reduced if the chip is cooled; dark current falls by a factor of 10 for every 20°C decrease in temperature (Spibey *et al.*, 2001). For bioluminescence imaging, CCD cameras are usually mounted in a light-tight specimen chamber and are attached to a cryogenic refrigeration unit for camera cooling to −120°C to −150°C. A camera controller, linked to a computer system is used for data acquisition and analysis.

Bioluminescence imaging of living subjects requires that the gene encoding the bioluminescence reporter protein be transferred to cells or tissues of interest, which can be accomplished using one of three gene transfer methods: *ex vivo*, *in vivo*, or as part of a transgenic construct. When cells transfected *ex vivo*, and transiently or stably expressing the bioluminescence reporter gene, are injected into the research animal, the light emitted from the gene-marked cells can be monitored externally. To generate such an image, the animals are anesthetized and placed in a light-tight chamber equipped with the CCD camera. A gray-scale reference image (digital photograph) is acquired under weak illumination, and then in complete darkness the photons emitted from within the body of the animal are detected externally using a range of integration times from 1 sec to several minutes. The data are transferred to a computer equipped with image acquisition, overlay, and analysis software for quantification. A bioluminescence image is most often shown as a color image representing light intensity (usually from blue for least intense to red for most intense) that is superimposed on the gray-scale photographic image in order to display the anatomical origin of photon emission. Usually a region of interest is manually selected over an area of signal intensity, and the maximum or average intensity is recorded as photons/sec/cm^2/steradian (steradian is a unit of solid angle). Whenever the exposure conditions (including time, f/stop, height of sample shelf, binning ratio, and time after injection with optical substrate) are kept identical, the measurements are highly reproducible (to within 6%).

Future Outlook

Many developments in reporter gene expression imaging are anticipated during the next decade. Significant conceptual and technological advances will most likely be seen across the five main general requirements for imaging mentioned earlier: knowledge of molecular targets, availability of molecular probes, overcoming of delivery barriers, development of amplification strategies, and availability of appropriate instrumentation. The merger of molecular biology and medical imaging is facilitating rapid growth of this new field by providing methods to monitor an ever increasing number of cellular/molecular events adapted from conventional molecular assays, including reporter gene assays. The current frenetic pace of advancements in biotechnology and functional genomics (Subramanian *et al.*, 2001) is resulting in parallel progress in molecular imaging innovations and applications.

The growth in knowledge of available cellular/molecular targets is also resulting in the development of newer molecular imaging probes. Active search for better reporter systems is ongoing for all molecular imaging modalities and techniques. As an example, with regard to bioluminescence imaging, it is known that the luciferases comprise a whole family of photoproteins that use different substrates and emit light of varying wavelengths. Unfortunately, substrates for many luciferases from different organisms are not readily available, which precludes their use in biomedical research applications. Current searches are underway for naturally occurring reporters (with available substrates) that may emit more red-shifted light and, therefore, would likely result in improved light transmission through deeper body structures. Moreover, an increasing number of bioluminescence reporter genes may undergo site-directed mutagenesis for the purpose of yielding reporter proteins that are also more red-shifted and/or with codon changes for higher expression in mammalian cells. Improving the thermostability of Firefly luciferase has already been investigated using mutagenesis directed at amino acid position 354 (White *et al.*, 1996). An intriguing future possibility might entail the genetic engineering of cells or creation of transgenic animals that could make their own substrates (e.g., D-Luciferin and/or coelenterazine) without having to provide these substrates by injection, in the case of imaging in living subjects.

A new class of molecular imaging probes is being developed for imaging of cells that have available cell-surface targets for specific protein binding. Bifunctional chimeric proteins, each containing a cell-surface targeting protein fused to a bioluminescence reporter protein can be used to image cancer cells without recourse to prior expression of the reporter protein via the delivery of imaging transgenes, as in conventional reporter gene imaging. To date, this novel approach has been attempted with an anti-CEA diabody and synthetic *Renilla* luciferase fusion protein to image CEA-expressing xenografts in mice (Venisnik *et al.*, 2006). Ongoing experiments will determine the feasibility of these novel imaging approaches prior to potential future clinical applications.

Many existing reporter probes should eventually give way to newer generations of probes that are more sensitive and specific. PET assays will need to move toward generalized reporter probes where the chemistry behind radioisotope labeling remains relatively similar, but the underlying molecular structure can be easily modified to image a new molecular target. These generalizable reporter probes will facilitate the easier use of customized imaging approaches. To this aim, a greater investment in chemistry research and the development of a larger number of smart molecular imaging probes will be necessary (Massoud and Gambhir, 2003). It is also anticipated that closer ties between molecular biologists and imaging researchers will produce imaging assays that are more sensitive to low-level biological events. This need for enhancing the sensitivity of imaging will dictate to some extent future greater exploitation and use of optical imaging, which currently has the highest inherent sensitivity for target detection at limited depths. As optical technologies have changed biotechnology, they could also change imaging in living subjects by providing more sophisticated methods for imaging molecular events.

Linked to the search for better reporters is the development of better imaging instrumentation. Improved instrumentation will make use of advances in detector technology, including the exploitation of solid-state detector technology and better image reconstruction techniques. This should help to produce newer generations of cameras, likely with better resolution, sensitivity, and even higher-throughput time, which will aid substantially in the screening of mice (Kudo *et al.*, 2002). Given the inherent advantages of optical imaging, these approaches are likely to be used increasingly in experimental feasibility studies and for bridging imaging studies from small animals to larger ones and humans. Advances in fluorescence-mediated tomography are described earlier. There are also ongoing developments for construction of tomographic three-dimensional imaging systems that can accurately quantify bioluminescence in deep heterogeneous media in living subjects. Although progress is being made, these attempts are hindered currently by the complex data that have to be acquired and analyzed as a series of two-dimensional images from multiple viewing angles. These data may then used to model surface radiance of photons emitted from deep within tissues by mathematical techniques dependent on diffusion equations and partial-current boundary condition models. In addition, newer multimodality imaging systems for small animals will provide anatomical and functional image registration. Several microPET/CT scanners are in current development, as are attempts to build instruments that combine MRI or optical imaging with PET.

This chapter discusses the principles and recent technological advances in molecular imaging of reporter gene expression. This approach is emerging as a valuable tool for monitoring the expression of genes in animals and humans. Further development of more sensitive and selective reporters, combined with improvements in detection technology, will consolidate the position of reporter gene-imaging technology as a versatile method for understanding intracellular biological processes and the molecular basis of cancer.

References

Alam, J., and Cook, J.L. 1990. Reporter genes: application to the study of mammalian gene transcription. *Anal. Biochem. 188*:245–254.

Alfke, H., Stoppler, H., Nocken, F., Heverhagen, J.T., Kleb, B., Czubayko, F., and Klose, K.J. 2003. In vitro MR imaging of regulated gene expression. *Radiology 228*:488–492.

Bhaumik, S., and Gambhir, S.S. 2002. Optical imaging of Renilla luciferase reporter gene expression in living mice. *Proc. Natl. Acad. Sci. USA 99*:377–382.

Bhaumik, S., Lewis, X.Z., and Gambhir, S.S. 2004. Optical imaging of Renilla luciferase, synthetic Renilla luciferase, and Firefly luciferase reporter gene expression in living mice. *J. Biomed. Optics 9*:578–586.

Blasberg, R. 2002. Imaging gene expression and endogenous molecular processes: molecular imaging. *J. Cereb. Blood. Flow. Metab. 22*:1157–1164.

Blasberg, R.G., and Gelovani-Tjuvajev, J. 2002. *In vivo* molecular-genetic imaging. *J. Cell. Biochem. Suppl. 39*:172–183.

Bouvet, M., Wang, J., Nardin, S.R., Nassirpour, R., Yang, M., Baranov, E., Jiang, P., Moossa, A.R., and Hoffman, R.M. 2002. Real-time optical imaging of primary tumor growth and multiple metastatic events in a pancreatic cancer orthotopic model. *Cancer Res. 62*:1534–1540.

Castillo, M., Kwock, L., and Mukherji, S.K. 1996. Clinical applications of proton MR spectroscopy. *AJNR Am. J. Neuroradiol. 17*:1–15.

Chatziioannou, A.F. 2002. Molecular imaging of small animals with dedicated PET tomographs. *Eur. J. Nucl. Med. 29*:98–114.

Cherry, S.R., and Gambhir, S.S. 2001. Use of positron emission tomography in animal research. *Ilar. J. 42*:219–232.

Contag, C.H., and Bachmann, M.H. 2002. Advances in *in vivo* bioluminescence imaging of gene expression. *Annu. Rev. Biomed. Eng. 4*:235–260.

Contag, C.H., Contag, P.R., Mullins, J.I., Spilman, S.D., Stevenson, D.K., and Benaron, D.A. 1995. Photonic detection of bacterial pathogens in living hosts. *Mol. Microbiol. 18*:593–603.

Contag, C.H., Spilman, S.D., Contag, P.R., Oshiro, M., Eames, B., Dennery, P., Stevenson, D.K., and Benaron, D.A. 1997. Visualizing gene expression in living mammals using a bioluminescent reporter. *Photochem. Photobiol. 66*:523–531.

Doubrovin, M., Ponomarev, V., Beresten, T., Balatoni, J., Bornmann, W., Finn, R., Humm, J., Larson, S., Sadelain, M., Blasberg, R., and Gelovani Tjuvajev, J. 2001. Imaging transcriptional regulation of p53-dependent genes with positron emission tomography in vivo. *Proc. Natl. Acad. Sci. USA 98*:9300–9305.

Edinger, M., Cao, Y.A., Hornig, Y.S., Jenkins, D.E., Verneris, M.R., Bachmann, M.H., Negrin, R.S., and Contag, C.H. 2002. Advancing animal models of neoplasia through *in vivo* bioluminescence imaging. *Eur. J. Cancer 38*:2128–2136.

Enochs, W.S., Petherick, P., Bogdanova, A., Mohr, U., and Weissleder, R. 1997. Paramagnetic metal scavenging by melanin: MR imaging. *Radiology 204*:417–423.

Gambhir, S.S. 2000. Imaging gene expression: concepts and future outlook. In: *Diagnostic Nuclear Medicine*. Schiepers, C. (Ed.). pp. 253–272. Berlin: Springer-Verlag.

Gambhir, S.S., Barrio, J.R., Herschman, H.R., and Phelps, M.E. 1999. Assays for noninvasive imaging of reporter gene expression. *Nucl. Med. Biol. 26*:481–490.

Gambhir, S.S., Bauer, E., Black, M.E., Liang, Q., Kokoris, M.S., Barrio, J.R., Iyer, M., Namavari, M., Phelps, M.E., and Herschman, H.R. 2000. A mutant herpes simplex virus type 1 thymidine kinase reporter gene shows improved sensitivity for imaging reporter gene expression with positron emission tomography. *Proc. Natl. Acad. Sci. USA 97*:2785–2790.

Golden, J., and Ligler, F. 2002. A comparison of imaging methods for use in an array biosensor. *Biosens. Bioelectron. 17*:719–725.

Green, L.A., Yap, C.S., Nguyen, K., Barrio, J.R., Namavari, M., Satyamurthy, N., Phelps, M.E., Sandgren, E.P., Herschman, H.R., and Gambhir, S.S. 2002. Indirect monitoring of endogenous gene expression by positron emission tomography (PET) imaging of reporter gene expression in transgenic mice. *Mol. Imaging Biol. 4*:71–81.

Gross, S., and Piwnica-Worms, D., 2005. Spying on cancer: molecular imaging *in vivo* with genetically encoded reporters. *Cancer Cell 7*:5–15.

Hastings, J.W. 1996. Chemistries and colors of bioluminescent reactions: a review. *Gene 173*:5–11.

Iyer, M., Barrio, J.R., Namavari, M., Bauer, E., Satyamurthy, N., Nguyen, K., Toyokuni, T., Phelps, M.E., Herschman, H.R., and Gambhir, S.S. 2001. 8-[F-18]fluoropenciclovir: an improved reporter probe for imaging HSV1-tk reporter gene expression *in vivo* using PET. *J. Nucl. Med. 42*:96–105.

Kamiyama, M., Ichikawa, Y., Ishikawa, T., Chishima, T., Hasegawa, S., Hamaguchi, Y., Nagashima, Y., Miyagi, Y., Mitsuhashi, M., Hyndman, D., Hoffman, R.M., Ohki, S., and Shimada, H. 2002. VEGF receptor antisense therapy inhibits angiogenesis and peritoneal dissemination of human gastric cancer in nude mice. *Cancer Gene Ther. 9*:197–201.

Kaneko, K., Yano, M., Yamano, T., Tsujinaka, T., Miki, H., Akiyama, Y., Taniguchi, M., Fujiwara, Y., Doki, Y., Inoue, M., Shiozaki, H., Kaneda, Y., and Monden, M. 2001. Detection of peritoneal micrometastases of gastric carcinoma with green fluorescent protein and carcinoembryonic antigen promoter. *Cancer Res. 61*:5570–5574.

Kudo, T., Fukuchi, K., Annala, A.J., Chatziioannou, A.F., Allada, V., Dahlbom, M., Tai, Y.C., Inubushi, M., Huang, S.C., Cherry, S.R., Phelps, M.E., and Schelbert, H.R. 2002. Noninvasive measurement of myocardial activity concentrations and perfusion defect sizes in rats with a new small-animal positron emission tomograph. *Circulation 106*:118–123.

Li, X., Wang, J., An, Z., Yang, M., Baranov, E., Jiang, P., Sun, F., Moossa, A.R., and Hoffman, R.M. 2002. Optically imageable metastatic model of human breast cancer. *Clin. Exp. Metastasis 19*:347–350.

Liang, Q., Satyamurthy, N., Barrio, J.R., Toyokuni, T., Phelps, M.P., Gambhir, S.S., and Herschman, H.R. 2001. Noninvasive, quantitative imaging in living animals of a mutant dopamine D2 receptor reporter gene in which ligand binding is uncoupled from signal transduction. *Gene Ther. 8*:1490–1498.

Lin, Y., Weissleder, R., and Tung, C.H. 2002. Novel near-infrared cyanine fluorochromes: synthesis, properties, and bioconjugation. *Bioconjug. Chem. 13*:605–610.

Lippincott-Schwartz, J., Snapp, E., and Kenworthy, A. 2001. Studying protein dynamics in living cells. *Nat. Rev. Mol. Cell Biol. 2*:444–456.

Louie, A.Y., Duimstra, J.A., and Meade, T.J. 2002. Mapping gene expression by MRI. In: Toga, A.W., and Mazziotta, J.C. (Eds.), *Brain Mapping: the Methods*, pp. 819–828. San Diego, CA: Academic Press.

Louie, A.Y., Huber, M.M., Ahrens, E.T., Rothbacher, U., Moats, R., Jacobs, R.E., Fraser, S.E., and Meade, T.J. 2000. *In vivo* visualization of gene expression using magnetic resonance imaging. *Nat. Biotechnol. 18*:321–325.

MacLaren, D.C., Gambhir, S.S., Satyamurthy, N., Barrio, J.R., Sharfstein, S., Toyokuni, T., Wu, L., Berk, A.J., Cherry, S.R., Phelps, M.E., and Herschman, H.R. 1999. Repetitive, non-invasive imaging of the dopamine D2 receptor as a reporter gene in living animals. *Gene Ther.* 6:785–791.

Massoud, T.F., and Gambhir, S.S. 2003. Molecular imaging in living subjects: seeing fundamental biological processes in a new light. *Genes Dev.* 17:545–580.

Namavari, M., Barrio, J.R., Toyokuni, T., Gambir, S.S., Cherry, S.R., Herschman, H.R., Phelps, M.E., and Satyamurthy, N. 2000. Synthesis of 8-[18F] fluoroguanine derivatives: *in-vivo* probes for imaging gene expression with PET. *Nucl. Med. Biol.* 27:157–162.

Naylor, L.H. 1999. Reporter gene technology: the future looks bright. *Biochem. Pharmacol.* 58:749–757.

Ntziachristos, V., Tung, C.H., Bremer, C., and Weissleder, R. 2002. Fluorescence molecular tomography resolves protease activity *in vivo*. *Nat. Med.* 8:757–760.

Ntziachristos, V., and Weissleder, R. 2002. Charge-coupled-device based scanner for tomography of fluorescent near-infrared probes in turbid media. *Med. Phys.* 29:803–809.

Phelps, M. 2000. Inaugural article: positron emission tomography provides molecular imaging of biological processes. *Proc. Natl. Acad. Sci. USA* 97:9226–9233.

Remington, S.J. 2002. Negotiating the speed bumps to fluorescence. *Nat. Biotechnol.* 20:28–29.

Rice, B.W., Cable, M.D., and Nelson, M.B. 2001. *In vivo* imaging of light-emitting probes. *J Biomed. Opt.* 6:432–440.

Saito, Y., Price, R.W., Rottenberg, D.A., Fox, J.J., Su, T.L., Watanabe, K.A., and Philips, F.S. 1982. Quantitative autoradiographic mapping of herpes simplex virus encephalitis with a radiolabeled antiviral drug. *Science* 217:1151–1153.

Saito, Y., Rubenstein, R., Price, R.W., Fox, J.J., and Watanabe, K.A. 1984. Diagnostic imaging of herpes simplex virus encephalitis using a radio-labeled antiviral drug: autoradiographic assessment in an animal model. *Ann. Neurol.* 15:548–558.

Spergel, D.J., Kruth, U., Shimshek, D.R., Sprengel, R., and Seeburg, P.H. 2001. Using reporter genes to label selected neuronal populations in transgenic mice for gene promoter, anatomical, and physiological studies. *Prog. Neurobiol.* 63:673–686.

Spibey, C.A., Jackson, P., and Herick, K. 2001. A unique charge-coupled device/xenon arc lamp based imaging system for the accurate detection and quantitation of multicolour fluorescence. *Electrophoresis* 22: 829–836.

Subramanian, G., Adams, M.D., Venter, J.C., and Broder, S. 2001. Implications of the human genome for understanding human biology and medicine. *JAMA J. Am. Med. Assoc.* 286:2296–2307.

Tjuvajev, J.G., Finn, R., Watanabe, K., Joshi, R., Oku, T., Kennedy, J., Beattie, B., Koutcher, J., Larson, S., and Blasberg, R.G. 1996. Noninvasive imaging of herpes virus thymidine kinase gene transfer and expression: a potential method for monitoring clinical gene therapy. *Cancer Res.* 56:4087–4095.

Tjuvajev, J.G., Stockhammer, G., Desai, R., Uehara, H., Watanabe, K., Gansbacher, B., and Blasberg, R.G. 1995. Imaging the expression of transfected genes *in vivo*. *Cancer Res.* 55:6126–6132.

Venisnik, K.M., Olafsen, T., Loening, A.M., Iyer, M., Gambhir, S.S., and Wu, A.M. 2006. Bifunctional antibody-Renilla luciferase fusion protein for *in vivo* optical detection of tumors. *Protein Eng. Des. Sel.* 19:453–460.

Wagenaar, D.J., Weissleder, R., and Hengerer, A. 2001. Glossary of molecular imaging terminology. *Acad. Radiol.* 8:409–420.

Weaver, R.F. 1999. A brief history. In: Weaver, R.F. (Ed.), *Molecular Biology*, pp. 3–17. Boston: McGraw-Hill.

Weissleder, R. 2001. A clearer vision for *in vivo* imaging. *Nat. Biotechnol.* 19:316–317.

Weissleder, R. 2002. Scaling down imaging: molecular mapping of cancer in mice. *Nat. Rev. Cancer* 2:11–18.

Weissleder, R., and Mahmood, U. 2001. Molecular imaging. *Radiology* 219:316–333.

Weissleder, R., Moore, A., Mahmood, U., Bhorade, R., Benveniste, H., Chiocca, E.A., and Basilion, J.P. 2000. *In vivo* magnetic resonance imaging of transgene expression. *Nat. Med.* 6:351–355.

Weissleder, R., Simonova, M., Bogdanova, A., Bredow, S., Enochs, W.S., and Bogdanov, A., Jr. 1997. MR imaging and scintigraphy of gene expression through melanin induction. *Radiology* 204:425–429.

White, P.J., Squirrell, D.J., Arnaud, P., Lowe, C.R., and Murray, J.A. 1996. Improved thermostability of the North American firefly luciferase: saturation mutagenesis at position 354. *Biochem. J.* 319:343–350.

Yang, M., Baranov, E., Wang, J.W., Jiang, P., Wang, X., Sun, F.X., Bouvet, M., Moossa, A.R., Penman, S., and Hoffman, R.M. 2002. Direct external imaging of nascent cancer, tumor progression, angiogenesis, and metastasis on internal organs in the fluorescent orthotopic model. *Proc. Natl. Acad. Sci. USA* 99:3824–3829.

16

Medical Radiation-Induced Cancer

Hitoshi Shibuya

Introduction

Radiation is one of the most extensively researched carcinogens, and induction of carcinogenesis by low doses of radiation (1–10 Gy) has been demonstrated by the significantly higher incidence of cancers among workers who handle radioactive substances and among atomic-bomb survivors (Amemiya *et al.*, 2005). The use of diagnostic radiology and radiotherapy has been increasing worldwide. One of the unique features of radiation used in medicine is the dosage range from a few milli-Gy, for most diagnostic examinations, to many tens of Gy, for the treatment of cancer.

Although the effects of even lower doses are still somewhat unclear, there has been increasing interest in the possibility that exposure to diagnostic X-rays (doses of < 10 mGy) may involve a considerable increase in risk of cancer. Dental diagnostic X-rays performed many years ago have also been linked to increased cancer risk (Preston-Martin *et al.*, 1988, UNSCEAR, 2000). Of the 3 mSv annual global per capita effective dose estimated for the year 2000, 2.4 mSv is from the natural background and 0.5 mSv from diagnostic medical exams (UNSCEAR, 2000; Ron, 2003).

Some investigators have reported that radiation therapy for both benign and malignant disease appears to cause second cancers when substantial doses are administered to normal, healthy organs (Amemiya *et al.*, 2005). Moreover, the significant improvement in cancer treatment over the last several decades has resulted in longer survival and a growing number of high-dose-radiation-related second cancers (Arai *et al.*, 1991; Yamamoto *et al.*, 2002). Second primary cancers have been emphasized as an important radiation-induced injury among the increasing numbers of cancer patients who have been cured by radiotherapy. Because of the paradoxical aspect of ionizing radiation in both helping to cure cancer and causing it, we must provide information on radiation-induced cancer as well as the usefulness of radiation therapy to patients, relatives, and physicians in clinical practice in order to support rational decision making, particularly in relation to the risks of other treatments.

Epidemiologic investigations of people receiving medical radiation in the course of diagnosis or treatment have provided a great deal of information on the several levels of cancer risk following a broad spectrum of medical practices, and the data have been an important complement to the atomic-bomb survivor studies. The risk associated with diagnostic X-rays has been estimated by extrapolating risk estimates from populations exposed to a range of doses, such as the atomic-bomb survivors exposed to 0–4 Gy (Pierce and Preston, 2000). While most epidemiological data are compatible with linear extrapolations from exposures at high doses or higher dose rates, they cannot entirely exclude other possibilities (Ron, 1998; Brenner *et al.*, 2003). As the field of epidemiology advances, research and our understanding of the health effects of prolonged and low-dose exposure should improve.

Diagnostic Radiation Exposure

Diagnostic X-rays are the largest human-made source of radiation exposure of the general population. While radiation doses from most diagnostic examinations are low, the

Cancer Imaging: Instrumentation and Applications

collective dose is large, because millions of people of all ages receive them, and they account for ~ 15% of total annual exposure from all sources worldwide (Ron, 2003). It is often difficult to estimate cancer risk associated with diagnostic X-ray examinations by epidemiologic methods for a variety of reasons. Doses are generally low, and determining the dose to each organ is complicated because the dose record of each X-ray examination cannot usually be obtained. Most investigators have estimated the risk of radiation-induced cancer based on the assumption that small doses of radiation can cause cancers, and their estimates of the cancer risk from diagnostic radiology has ranged from 0.6 to 1.8% of all cancers (Berrington de Gonzàlez et al., 2004). Most investigators have estimated the risk of radiation-induced cancer based on the assumption that there is no threshold dose below which radiation exposure does not cause cancer. They also assumed that the individuals who received diagnostic X-rays had the same mortality rates as the general population. Another assumption is that the effect of radiation from diagnostic X-rays is the same as from atomic-bomb radiation (Pierce and Preston, 2000). If any of these assumptions is incorrect, cumulative radiation-induced risks will be lower than estimated (Ron, 1998; Brenner et al., 2003).

Organ-specific radiation doses in pediatric radiology vary with age of the patient and the dose. They are probably lower than in adults for many common radiographic examinations, but may be higher for computed tomography (CT) scans. Brenner et al. (2000) estimated the cumulative risk of cancer mortality from 600,000 annual CT examinations in children under 15 years of age, and concluded that their cumulative risk of cancer mortality from CT examinations is much higher than in adults. A few studies of tuberculosis patients who underwent multiple fluoroscopy examinations, generally as adolescents or young adults, and who received total doses of 0.5–1 Gy, have shown that the risk of breast cancer declined with age at the time of exposure, with little increase in risk occurring after menopause (Howe and McLaughlin, 1996). Similar findings have been obtained among the atomic-bomb survivors, and their risk declined with age at the time of exposure.

An earlier validation study of dental X-rays found a high incidence of salivary gland malignancies that was almost identical to their incidence among atomic-bomb survivors (Preston-Martin et al., 1998). Little (2002) compared the risk coefficients of atomic-bomb survivors to those from studies of patients exposed to diagnostic radiation and concluded that the risk was smaller among the patients than atomic-bomb survivors of similar age, sex, and length of follow-up. He suggested that the difference might not only be due to the lower dose rate, but also to variation in background cancer rates in Japan compared with most of the Western countries where the patient studies were conducted.

Therapeutic Radiation Exposure

Radiation therapy for benign diseases was relatively common from the 1930s to the 1960s, but has declined since 1970. When exposed to moderate doses of X-radiation, such as those most often used to treat benign diseases, excess cancer risks have been observed in or near the radiation field. Excess cancers of the thyroid, hypopharynx, and skin have been reported in adult patients previously irradiated for ankylosing spondylitis, tinea capitis, hemangiomas, and benign diseases of the head and neck, including tuberculous lymphadenitis (Amemiya et al., 2005). Long-term follow-up after radiation therapy for benign diseases of the head and neck has revealed excess primary cancers of the head and neck, with a shortest latency period of 7 years. Histological diagnoses of these patients were squamous cell carcinoma of the head and neck or adenocarcinoma in the thyroid (Miyahara et al., 1998; Amemiya et al., 2005).

Second primary malignancies are serious complications of high-dose radiotherapy for malignant disease. Significant improvement in cancer treatment over the past few decades has resulted in longer survival and a growing number of radiation-related second cancers. Accurate epidemiological surveys of radiation-induced cancer require a substantial number of patients surviving long after radiation therapy and careful follow-up and accurate patient registration (Arai et al., 1991; Ron, 2003). The risk of a second cancer has been shown to increase with time and radiation dose, but the latency period of second cancers differs according to organ. Many investigators have shown that the risk of cancer of the lung, rectum, and bladder starts to increase 10 years after exposure, whereas leukemia develops within 2 to 3 years after exposure, and the peak occurrence of leukemia is between 5 and 6 years after radiotherapy for cancer. The increased risk of most of the cancers induced except leukemia patients persists from several decades to the end of life (Amemiya et al., 2005). When the risk patterns of second cancers have been investigated over time after exposures, it has often been difficult to distinguish a radiation-induced second cancer from a recurrence after a much longer latency period, if the second cancer has the same pathological features as the first cancer (Amemiya et al., 2005). In addition, only a few populations have been followed for the rest of their lives (Ron, 1998).

Radiotherapy-related second primary cancers develop subsequent to most first primary cancers, if survival is long enough, but the risk of a second malignancy is particularly high following radiotherapy for childhood cancer (Jemal et al., 2002). Over 80% of Hodgkin's disease patients are treated with radiotherapy, frequently with high doses to large fields, and second cancers are a leading cause of mortality in Hodgkin's disease survivors. Children with Hodgkin's disease are of particular interest because the 5-year survival rate for childhood Hodgkin's disease is over 90%, and radiation-induced excess breast cancer has been observed in relatively young female patients in multiple studies (Clemons *et al.*, 2000; Jemal *et al.*, 2003). This age-related effect of exposure is consistent with the pattern observed in atomic-bomb survivors, but the magnitude of the excess risk was lower in the cancer patients (Little, 2002).

The risk of a second malignancy was also higher in prostate cancer patients who received radiotherapy than in a surgically treated group, and there was an increased risk of carcinoma of the bladder, rectum, lung, and sarcomas within the treatment field in the irradiated group (Brenner *et al.*, 2000). Radiotherapy for prostate carcinoma has been found to be associated with a fairly small but statistically significant increase in the risk of second solid tumors, particularly in long-term survivors. In absolute terms, the estimated risk of developing a radiation-associated second malignancy was 1 out of 290 among all prostate carcinoma patients treated with radiotherapy (Brenner *et al.*, 2000).

After radiation therapy for uterine cervix cancer, a significant excess of second cancers associated with radiation has been found in certain organs within the irradiation field, such as the rectum and bladder, but not in organs outside it. According to Arai *et al.* (1991), the incidence of late recurrence of uterine cancer in the 10-year to 20-year period after radiation therapy is 10 times the rate after surgery alone. They suspected that a fairly substantial number of radiation-induced cervical cancers of the same histological type detected after a long latency period have been counted as recurrences. They stated that if recurrences of uterine cancer occur more than 10 years after radiation therapy, they were assumed to be radiation-induced cancers, and the incidence of second cancers of the uterus would be similar to the incidence of second cancers of the rectum and bladder (Arai *et al.*, 1991).

Few studies have been done regarding the risk of radiation-induced cancers after radiotherapy for squamous cell carcinoma of head and neck (SCH) (Amemiya *et al.*, 2005). We investigated a large population of patients with stage I and II (early-stage) SCH treated by radiotherapy in a single institution and compared the results of radiation therapy in that population with the results of radiation therapy of early-stage malignant lymphoma to determine the incidence of radiation-induced cancer after radiation therapy (Amemiya *et al.*, 2005). Most of the patients were followed until death, and the incidence of radiation-induced cancer and cause of death were ascertained (Fig. 1). The 10-year survival rate of the early-stage head and neck cancer patients was 71%, and it was 61% among the malignant lymphoma patients.

The histological diagnosis of every second cancer in and near the radiation therapy field in the malignant lymphoma was different from the diagnosis of the primary lesion and squamous cell carcinomas. In the SCH patients, on the other hand, the histological diagnosis of most of the second cancers was the same as the first cancer and squamous cell carcinomas. Five radiation-induced cancers occurred in the

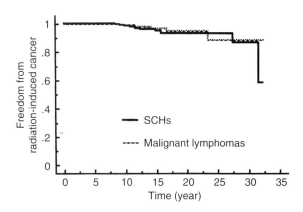

Figure 1 Freedom from induced cancer in previously irradiated patients with early-stage squamous cell carcinoma of the head and neck (SCH) and in patients with early-stage malignant lymphoma of the head and neck.

early-stage malignant lymphoma patients more than 8 years after the radiation therapy. The last regional nodal metastasis after treatment of the early-stage head and neck cancers was diagnosed at 6 years 6 months, and we defined second cancers in and around the treated area in patients with an over 8-year recurrence-free period as radiation-induced cancers. The crude incidence and the 10-year probability by actuarial life-table method of radiation-induced cancer in the malignant lymphoma population was 1.4% (5/355) and 0.8% each. The crude incidence and the 10-year probability by actuarial life-table method of second cancers in or near the irradiated field among the SCH population more than 8 years later was 1.8% (25/1358) and 1.6%, each (Fig. 2).

The incidence of induced cancer was higher in the SCH population than in the malignant lymphoma population, but the curve for freedom from radiation-induced cancer in early-stage head and neck cancer was similar to the curve for radiation-induced cancer in early-stage malignant lymphoma. Twelve of the 25 radiation-induced cancers in the SCH population were treated by surgery, and surgery was successful in 8 patients. Eight of the 25 radiation-induced cancers in the SCH population were treated by radiation, and the treatment was not successful in all 8 cases. There were another 6 post-irradiation precancerous lesions in the SCH population called pseudo-tumor occurring with a slightly lower incidence (0.22% = 6/2719) than radiation-induced (Oota *et al.*, 2003) (Fig. 3). The average radiation dose used in the treatment of SCH population was ~ 60 Gy, and ~ 50% higher than the average dose used to treat malignant lymphoma. A linear no-threshold model adequately describes the dose-response relationship for solid tumors, although at extremely high doses the risk appears to flatten out (Ron, 1998).

The differential diagnosis between radiation-induced cancer and late recurrence in the head and neck has become more complex because of the high frequency of naturally

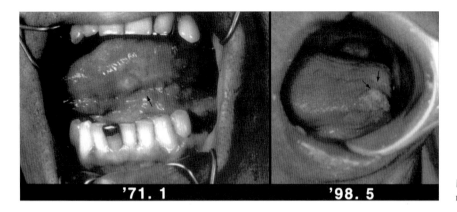

Figure 2 Second tongue cancer 27 years after radium needle treatment for tongue cancer.

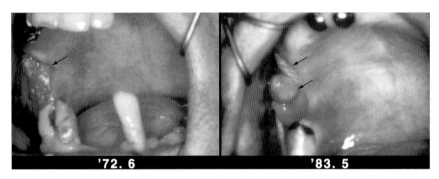

Figure 3 Post-irradiation polypoid pseudo-tumor 11 years after radiation therapy for carcinoma of the gingivo-buccal groove.

occurring multiple head and neck cancers. A study of 1609 patients with early-stage SCH treated at our hospital between 1956 and 1999 revealed an incidence of a second malignant neoplasm in the respiratory and upper digestive tracts to be 2.3% per year (Yamamoto *et al.*, 2002).

Discussion

The numerous epidemiologic studies of exposure to medical radiation and cancer incidence have been remarkably informative and have provided a complement to studies of the atomic-bomb survivors. In general, the results have been consistent with the findings in the atomic-bomb survivors—that is, that young age at the time of exposure increases the risk of radiation-related tumors at many sites and that the radiation-related tumor risks persist throughout life. On the other hand, the medical studies suggest that fractionation can diminish the excess risk at some sites, such as the lung, and that extremely high radiation doses lower risk, probably because of cell killing. Since radiation is widely used in medicine and its use appears to be increasing worldwide, there is an increasing need for additional data to estimate the long-term effects of the diagnostic and therapeutic uses of radiation.

References

Amemiya, K., Shibuya, H., Yoshimura, R., and Okada, N. 2005. The risk of radiation-induced cancer in patients with squamous cell carcinoma of the head and neck and its results of treatment. *Brit. J. Rad.* 78:1028–1033.

Arai, T., Nakano,T., Fukuhisa, K., Kasamatsu, T., Tsunemoto, R., Masubuchi, K., Yamauchi, K., Hamada, T., Fukuda, T., Noguchi, H., and Murata, M. 1991. Second cancer after radiation therapy for cancer of the uterine cervix. *Cancer 67*:398–405.

Berrington de Gonzàlez, A., and Darby, S. 2004. Risk of cancer from diagnostic X-rays' examinations for the UK and 14 other countries. *Lancet 363*:345–351.

Brenner, D.J., Curtis, R.E., Hall, E.J., and Ron, E. 2000. Second malignancies in prostate carcinoma patients after radiotherapy compared with surgery. *Cancer 88*:398–406.

Brenner, D.J., Ellisto, C.D., Hall, E.J., and Berdon, W.E. 2001. Estimated risks of radiation-induced fetal cancer from pedatric CT. *A.J.R. 176*: 289–296.

Brenner, D.J., Doll, R., Goodhead, D.T., Hall, E.J., Land, C.E., Little, J.B., Lubin, J.H., Preston, D.L., Preston, R.J., Ron, E., Sachs, R.K., Samet, K.M., Setlow, R.B., and Zaider, M. 2003. Cancer risks attributable to low doses of ionizing radiation: assessing what we really know. *Proc. Nat. Acad. Sci. USA 1000*: 13761–13766.

Clemons, M., Loijens, L., and Goss, O. 2000. Breast cancer risk following irradiation for Hodgkin's disease. *Cancer Treat. Rev. 26*:291–302.

Howe, G.R., and McLaughlin, J. 1996. Breast cancer mortality between 1950 and 1987 after exposure to fractionated moderate-dose-rate ionizing radiation in the Canadian fluoroscopy cohort study and comparison with breast cancer mortality in the atomic-bomb survivors study. *Radiat. Res. 145*:694–707.

Jemal, A., Thomas, A., Murray, T., and Thun, M. 2002. Cancer statistics, 2002. *C.A. Cancer J. Clin. 52*:23–47.

Little, M.P. 2002. Comparison of the risks of cancer incidence and mortality following radiation therapy for benign and malignant disease with the cancer risks observed in the Japanese a-bomb survivors. *Int. J. Radiat. Biol. 78*:145–163.

Miyahara, H., Sato, T., and Yoshino, K. 1998. Radiation-induced cancers of the head and neck region. *Acta Otolaryngol. Suppl. 533*:60–64.

Oota, S., Shibuya, H., Hamagaki, M., Yoshimura, R., Iwaki, H., Kojima, M., and Takagi, M. 2003. Oral pseudotumor: benign polypoid masses following radiation therapy. *Cancer 97*:1353–1357.

Pierce, D.A., and Preston, D.L. 2000. Radiarion-related cancer risks at low doses among atomic bomb survivors. *Radiat. Res. 154*:178–186.

Preston-Martin, S., Thomas, D.C., White, S.C., and Cohen, D. 1988. Prior exposure to medical and dental X-ray related to tumors of the parotid gland. *J. Natl. Cancer Inst. 80*:943–949.

Ron, E. 1998. Ionizing radiation and cancer risk: evidence from epidemiology. *Radiat. Res. 150*:530–541.

Ron, E. 2003. Cancer risks from medical radiation. *Health Phys. 85*: 47–59.

Travis, L.B., Hill, D.A., Dores, G.M., Gospodarowicz, M., van Leeuwen, F.E., Holowaty, E., Glimelius, B., Andersson, M., Wiklund, T., Lynch, C.F., Van't Veer, M.B., Glimelius, I., Storm, H., Pukkala, E., Stovall, M., Curtis, R., Boice. J.D., Jr., and Gilbert, E. 2003. Breast cancer following radiotherapy and chemotherapy among young women with Hodgkin's disease. *JAMA 290*:465–475.

United Nations Scientific Committee on the Effects of Atomic Radiation (UNSCEAR) 2000. Sources and effects of atomic radiation. Ionizing radiation. New York: United Nations; Sales publication. E. IX4.

Yamamoto, E., Shibuya, H., Yoshimura, R., and Miura, M. 2002. Site specific dependency of second primary cancer in early stage head and neck squamous cell carcinoma. *Cancer 94*:2007–2014.

III

Applications to Specific Cancers

Adrenal Lesions: Role of Computed Tomography, Magnetic Resonance Imaging, ¹⁸F-Fluorodeoxyglucose-Positron Emission Tomography, and Positron Emission Tomography/ Computed Tomography

Rakesh Kumar, Vivek Anand, and Suman Jana

Introduction

The adrenal glands were first described in 1563 by Eustachius, and they play a very important role in endocrine function to maintain life. Adrenal glands, also known as supra-renal glands (located above the kidneys), are two deep yellow-colored retroperitoneal organs. In the adult, each gland weighs ~ 4 grams. The supero-inferior length of the adrenal gland varies from 2 to 6 cm. The left adrenal gland is slightly larger than the right adrenal gland. The right adrenal gland is located in an area just superior to the right kidney, medial to the right lobe of the liver, lateral to the crus of the right hemi-diaphragm, and posterior to the inferior vena cava. The right adrenal gland is variable in shape. It may be pyramidal, or it may resemble an elongated comma lying in the crease between the liver and the crus of the diaphragm (Brunt and Moley, 2004). It may also be shaped like an inverted letter V or Y (Fig. 1A). The left adrenal gland extends along the medial border of the left kidney from the upper pole to the hilus. It lies behind the pancreas, the lesser sac, and it rests posteriorly on the diaphragm (Brunt and Moley, 2004). The left adrenal gland is also variably shaped. It may be crescentic-shaped or triangular, or it may sometimes be shaped like an inverted letter V or Y or an inverted letter L (Fig. 1B).

Each adrenal gland has two distinctively functioning portions: the outer cortex and the inner medulla. The adrenal cortex is yellow, surrounding the pale grayish inner medulla. The medulla makes up to 20% of the total weight of the adrenal

269

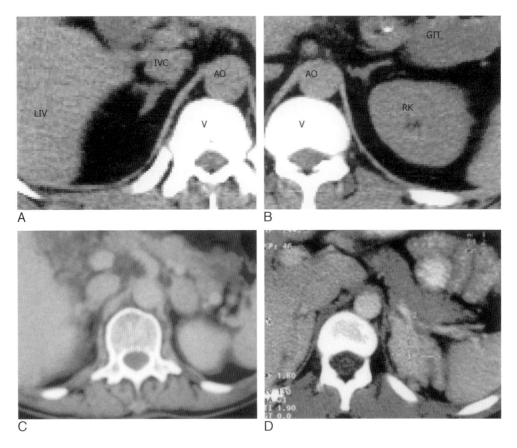

Figure 1 Bilateral normal adrenal glands: NCCT axial section of abdomen showing bilateral normal adrenal glands (**A, B**). Bilateral adrenal adenoma (**C**): CECT axial section showing moderately enhancing soft tissue mass arising from bilateral adrenals. Bilateral adrenal hyperplasia (**D**): CECT axial section showing enlarged bilateral adrenals.

gland (Brunt and Moley, 2004). It is sometimes difficult to distinguish between the two zones due to the variability of adrenal cortex thickness, which frequently differs according to the location. Although intimately related anatomically, the adrenal cortex and the adrenal medulla are quite separate internal secretory glands. The adrenal medulla contains catecholamine-producing cells, also known as chromaffin cells. The primary cathecholamines produced by the adrenal medulla include norepinephrine and epinephrine. The adrenal cortex comprises three zones—zona glomerulosa, zona fasciculata, and zona reticularis—and synthesizes three main functionally different categories of hormones (Table 1). All of the adreno-cortical hormones are derived from cholesterol and share a common structural formula. The zona fasciculate contains large, clear lipid laden cells. The extent to which the zona fasciculate is present plays an important role in the imaging characteristics of adrenal lesions.

Excess hormone production from either medulla or any zone of the cortex will lead to hormonal imbalance, which will be manifested with hormone-specific clinical signs and symptoms. In this scenario an imaging modality is used to

Table 1   Major Hormones Synthesized in Adrenal Cortex

Zone	Hormone Category	Major Hormone
Zona glomerulosa	Mineralocorticoids	Aldosterone
Zona fasciculata	Glucocorticoids	Cortisol, coticosterone
Zona reticularis	Adrenal androgens	Dehydroepiandosterone

detect and assess the nature of the adrenal lesion. On the other hand, more frequently, an adrenal lesion can be found incidentally on computed tomography (CT), magnetic resonance imaging (MRI), or ultrasonography (USG). The widespread use of high-resolution anatomic imaging modalities in patients with suspected abdominal and lower chest disease commonly leads to the detection of an unexpected adrenal mass. These adrenal masses have been called "incidentalomas" by virtue of their serendipitous detection. The next step after detection of an adrenal lesion is to determine whether or not this lesion is malignant and whether or not it is secretory

Table 2 **Imaging Modalities of Adrenal Glands**

Structural	Plain X-rays, USG, CT, and MRI
Functional	Metaiodobenzylguanidine labeled with I-131 or I-123 MIBG. I-131 Beta-iodomethyl-19-norcholesterol (NP-59), 75-Se-6-Betaselenomethyl-norcholesterol, PET, etc.
Structural and functional	PET/CT and SPECT/CT

(i.e., whether it is producing excess hormone). The secretory status of an adrenal lesion is determined through appropriate biochemical blood and/or urine tests. Appropriate screening tests should be performed when clinical signs and symptoms are present. In the absence of any specific signs and symptoms, all incidentaloma patients should be screened for subclinical Cushing's syndrome and pheocromocytoma, as these disorders could be present in ~ 15% of cases (Mantero et al., 2000). On the other hand, imaging modalities play a major role in determining the malignant nature of the adrenal mass. As the majority (85% or more) of the incidentalomas are nonsecretory, different imaging techniques are used very often to evaluate an adrenal lesion (Brunt and Moley, 2004). Determination of secretory status of an adrenal lesion is outside the scope of this discussion; therefore, the rest of the discussion focuses on the role of imaging.

The imaging techniques such as USG, CT, MRI, and positron emission tomography (PET) have played an important role in defining physiological and pathological conditions of the adrenal glands. Various imaging modalities can be broadly divided into structural, functional, and structural and functional (Table 2). Integrated information obtained from anatomic and functional imaging is essential for characterization of adrenal disease.

Computed Tomography

Currently, CT is the primary imaging modality for adrenal imaging. Widespread use of CT in clinical practice makes it an ideal noninvasive technique for evaluating adrenal gland morphology owing to its widespread availability, the speed with which examinations can be performed, its superior spatial resolution, and quantification of contrast washout patterns (Gross and Shapiror, 2005). The introduction of spiral CT and more recently multidetector-row helical CT, has allowed rapid thin (3 mm)-slice imaging of the adrenal glands during various phases of contrast enhancement.

With the widespread use of CT, an increasing fraction of clinically silent adrenal lesions not related to the primary indication for CT scanning are being reported. Similarly, an increasing number of patients with adrenals that appear benign on CT scans are being identified to harbor metastatic disease. A variety of CT characteristics may be employed in an attempt to differentiate adrenal adenomas from nonadenomas. Such characteristics include lipid content, smooth border, round or oval shape, sharp margins, maintenance of adrenal configuration, lack of calcification within or on the edge of the tumor, homogeneity of the mass, and lack of enhancement after contrast (Korobkin et al., 1996). However, none of them is individually helpful to rule out adrenal nonadenoma with great confidence.

Adrenal adenomas are usually asymptomatic, incidentally discovered, common benign tumors found in 1% of all patients undergoing abdominal CT and are found in 3% of autopsies (Dunnick et al., 1996). Computed tomography usually demonstrates a well-defined, homogeneous, low-density rounded mass with sharp margin (Fig. 1C) (Kawashima et al., 1998). The use of noncontrast-enhanced CT (NCCT) for benign adrenal mass characterization depends on the fact that adrenal adenomas contain a large number of lipid-rich cells, often resulting in Hounsfield unit (HU) values near or below zero. In general, the unenhanced scans of adrenal lesions with attenuation values up to 18 HU exhibit a sensitivity of 86% and a specificity of 88% in identifying benign adrenal adenomas. The specificity increases, approaching 100% as the HU value falls to zero. Use of delayed contrast-enhanced CT (CECT) to differentiate benign adrenal adenomas from nonadenomas has demonstrated that adrenal adenomas have lower attenuation values than that of nonadenomas on delayed CECT scans between 3 and 50 min after contrast infusion (Korobkin et al., 1998; Szolar and Kammerhuber, 1998). Some studies indicate that adrenal lesions with attenuation thresholds of less than or equal to 24 HU after contrast administration were benign adenoma. The studies showed that adenomas enhanced more than nonadenomas at 30, 60, and 90 sec after contrast administration. Moreover, the loss of contrast enhancement and the relative percentage of loss of contrast enhancement were significantly greater for adenomas than nonadenomas, when the scans were delayed for as long as 30 min after contrast infusion.

Standard CECT images of the adrenal glands are obtained ~ 60 sec after the beginning of bolus intravenous injection of contrast material. Studies suggest that at this time the attenuation values of adenomas and metastatic adrenal lesion are nearly identical. Adenomas lose enhancement more rapidly, as early as 5 min after contrast injection, so attenuation values 10–15 minutes after contrast administration can be used to differentiate adenomas from other adrenal masses (Dunnick et al., 2002). Adrenal masses with an attenuation value < 30 to 40 HU on 15 min delayed CECT are almost always adrenal adenomas (Korobkin et al., 1998). In addition to the delayed CT attenuation itself, it is also possible to calculate the percentage washout of initial enhancement: the optimal threshold for enhancement washout at 15 min is 60%, resulting in sensitivity of 88% and a specificity of 96% for the diagnosis of adenoma (Korobkin et al., 1998).

The two most commonly used methods for contrast washout evaluation are as follows. The patient is first scanned without contrast infusion, then at 70 sec and 15 min after contrast administration. The percent enhancement washout is calculated by the formula:

$$\frac{E-D}{E-U}\times 100$$

where (all values are in HU)

E is the 70-sec intravenous postcontrast enhancement value

D is the 15-min intravenous postcontrast enhancement value

U is the unenhanced value

If percent enhancement washout is > 60%, the lesion is labeled benign.

If no unenhanced values are available, the relative washout can be used. The formula for relative washout is

$$\frac{E-D}{E}\times 100$$

The adrenal lesion is benign (adenoma) if the relative washout value is greater than 40% (Korobkin, 2000).

Studies published by Dunnick *et al.* (2002) and Boland *et al.* (1998) suggest that CT is helpful in accurate diagnosis of benign lesions. CT densitometry, based on detecting the presence and amount of lipid within an adrenal mass, can be used to accurately differentiate benign adrenal lesions from metastases (Boland *et al.*, 1998). Using pooled data from multiple published studies of calculated and corresponding threshold values of unenhanced attenuation values, Boland *et al.* (1998) found that optimal sensitivity (71%) and specificity (98%) for the diagnosis of adrenal adenoma resulted from choosing a threshold attenuation value of 10 HU on NCCT. If the adrenal mass is inhomogeneous or has a density equal to or > 10 HU, the diagnosis is uncertain (a lipid-poor adenoma or a malignant lesion) and CECT scanning is done to assess the washout of initial enhancement in the lesion. Adenomas are enhanced significantly after intravenous contrast administration and show more rapid washout of the contrast than adrenal metastases.

In a recent study, Hamrahian *et al.* (2005) attempted to distinguish adrenocortical adenoma/hyperplasia from nonadenomas based on NCCT attenuation values, tumor size, and a combination of HU and tumor size. Their study included 151 adrenal lesions and supported the proposal that 10 HU in an NCCT is a safe cut-off value to differentiate adrenal adenomas/hyperplasia from nonadenomas (Fig. 2). Their data also suggest that 20 HU may be an acceptable cut-off value if the mass is 4 cm or smaller, particularly in patients without any history of malignancy. Caoili *et al.* (2002) evaluated a protocol by combining attenuation threshold values

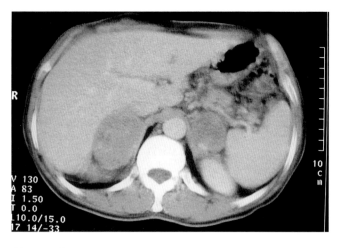

Figure 2 Bilateral adrenal metastases: CECT axial section showing moderately enhancing soft tissue mass arising from bilateral adrenals in a known case of carcinoma lung suggestive of metastases.

of 10 HU or less on NCCT and a percentage enhancement washout threshold of 60% for adrenal lipid-poor adenomas. The authors found that the sensitivity and specificity of this protocol for characterizing adrenal mass as an adenoma versus a nonadenoma were 98% and 92%, respectively. The specificity of this protocol was reported as 97% when adenomas were compared only with metastases. In a study attempting to characterize lipid-poor adrenal masses, Pena *et al.* (2000) concluded that the relative washout percentage is more accurate for the differentiation of adenomas from metastases than are the absolute attenuation values. However, the diagnosis of adrenal adenomas based on attenuation values on unenhanced or delayed CECT is often not feasible in clinical practice. Moreover, the usefulness of mean CT attenuation of adrenal masses on CECT is limited because there is too much overlap between the two groups to accurately differentiate between adrenal adenomas and nonadenomas (Allard *et al.*, 1990).

At autopsy, 27% of the oncology patients are found to have adrenal metastases. Thirty to 40% of patients with metastatic breast and lung carcinoma have adrenal metastases, whereas 50% of patients with melanomas have metastatic lesions to the adrenal glands (Macari *et al.*, 1998). CT findings demonstrate that metastases are ill defined, larger, with inhomogeneous central areas with irregular, thick enhancing rims (Fig. 2). They usually demonstrate an attenuation of > 20 HU on NCCT scans. On delayed CECT, the attenuation values are usually higher and the metastases remain enhanced more than adenomas; at 30 min, metastases show an attenuation of > 40 HU. In a recent study, Blake *et al.* (2006a) concluded that noncalcified, nonhemorrhagic adrenal lesions with precontrast attenuation of > 43 HU should be considered suspicious for malignancy.

Computed tomography has been shown to have suboptimal sensitivity for detecting adrenal metastases. Allard *et al.*

(1990) found that only 20 to 41.1% of metastatic adrenal lesions were interpreted as positive on CT scanning in patients with lung cancer undergoing autopsy. Porte *et al.* (1999) reported a series of 443 patients with operable lung cancer, 32 of whom had an adrenal mass 1 cm or more in size. Based on HU units, CT misdiagnosed 21% of adrenal adenomas as metastases and 11% of the adrenal adenomas as metastases. Sensitivity for characterizing a lesion as benign has ranged from 47% at a threshold of 2 HU to 88% at a threshold of 20 HU in a meta-analysis of 10 CT studies (Boland *et al.*, 1998). Moreover, diagnosis on the basis of attenuation measurement in unenhanced or delayed contrast-enhanced CT is often not feasible. Pagani (1984) found a 12% incidence of adrenal metastases in patients with non-small cell lung cancer and normal adrenal glands; the false-negative adrenal lesions on CT imaging were subsequently diagnosed as true positive on FDG-PET scanning. Gupta *et al.* (2001), found that a considerable difference in the efficacy of CT and FDG-PET in differentiation of benign from malignant adrenal masses in lung cancer patients (Fig. 3A, B). They found sensitivity, specificity, accuracy, positive-predictive value (PPV), and negative-predictive value (NPV) for CT imaging to be 72%, 33%, 56%, 61%, and 30%, respectively. In contrast, the sensitivity, specificity, accuracy, PPV, and NPV of PET imaging were found to be 94%, 91%, 93%, 94%, and 91%, respectively.

Magnetic Resonance Imaging

In recent years, MRI has become another imaging modality to aid the characterization of indeterminate adrenal masses (Mitchell *et al.*, 1992; Haider *et al.*, 2004). Due to increased fluid content in the lesions of adrenal cancer and metastases, it appears bright on T2-weighted MRI images. However, there is significant overlap T1- and T2-weighted MRI images of adenoma and metastases. With the introduction of higher field strength magnets (1.5T or higher), chemical shift imaging, and dynamic gadolinium-enhanced imaging, MRI has shown promising results with adrenal gland lesion characterization (Fig. 3C, D). In a review of 42 patients with lung cancer, chemical shift MRI was recommended for initial use in evaluating adrenal masses in lung cancer patients (Mitchell *et al.*, 1992; Schwartz *et al.*, 1995). The chemical shift imaging (CSI) primarily identifies protons in the body that are located either within water molecules or within lipid molecules, thus allowing separation of fat from water contributions in an image. This capability plays an essential role in adrenal imaging because certain adrenal lesions contain significant amounts of lipids. This imaging is based on the principle that the hydrogen protons in water and lipid molecules resonate at different frequencies (Israel, 2004). In this technique, when the protons of water and lipid are aligned in the same direction, they are "in-phase," and when opposite from each

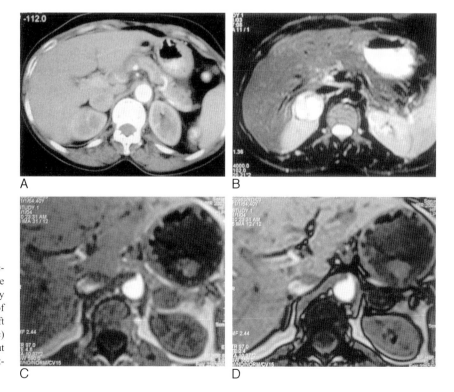

Figure 3 Pheochromocytoma: CECT axial section showing an enhancing soft tissue mass in the right suprarenal region (**A**). The mass is brightly hyperintense on T2W MR axial section suggestive of pheochromocytoma (**B**). Adenoma on chemical shift imaging: T1W acquisitions a longer TE (4.4 msec) [in-phase] (**C**) and short TE (2.2 msec at 1.5 T) [out of phase] (**D**). Left adenoma appears darker on out-phase images.

other, they are "out-of-phase." The MRI signal intensity is maximum when they are in-phase, whereas the signal intensity is reduced when they are out-of-phase. This in- and out-of-phase process is the "chemical shift" technique. Benign adenomas lose signal on out-of-phase images and appear relatively bright on in-phase images. The chemical shift change can be detected either by quantitative methods or simple visual analysis. Two ratios have been defined in CSI.

$$\text{SI Index} = \frac{1-[SI(in)-SI(opp)]}{SI(in)}$$

and

$$\text{Adrenal-to-Spleen Ratio} = \frac{SI\,adrenal\,(opp)}{SI\,spleen\,(opp)} \Big/ \frac{SI\,adrenal\,(in)}{SI\,spleen\,(in)}$$

An SI index of > 16.5% and an adrenal-to-spleen ratio of < 0.71 is suggestive of adenoma/benign adrenal lesions. For a benign adrenal lesion characterization, the reported sensitivity and specificity were 87–100% and 92–100%, respectively, whereas failure rate for diagnosis in lipid-poor adenomas has been 13 to 17% (Korobkin et al., 1995). Burt et al. (1995) conducted a prospective study to assess the efficacy of adrenal lesion characterization by MR imaging and found the false-positive rate to be 67%. Because of these limitations on CT and MR imaging, other functional adrenal imaging modalities such as F-18 FDG-PET are essential for further characterization of an adrenal lesion. PET has an established role, and study findings in literature support the role of PET in patients with extracranial cancer (Kumar et al., 2005, 2006).

Positron Emission Tomography and Positron Emission Tomography/ Computed Tomography

F-18-fluorodeoxyglucose-PET (^{18}F-FDG-PET) permits acquisition of functional information and, when fused with

CT imaging, results in accurate localization and metabolic characterization of adrenal lesions. ^{18}F-fluorodeoxyglucose is the most commonly used radiotracer for PET and PET/CT imaging. FDG is a glucose analog, which is taken up preferentially by malignant cells because of their increased glucose metabolism. Like glucose, FDG is transported into cells by means of a glucose transporter protein and begins to follow the glycolytic pathway. Once inside the cell, [18]F- FDG is phosphorylated into ^{18}F-FDG-6-phosphate (similar to glucose being converted to glucose-6-phosphate by the same enzyme). ^{18}F-FDG-6-phosphate cannot continue through glycolysis because it is not a substrate for enzyme glucose-6-phosphate isomerase. As a result, ^{18}F-FDG-6-phosphate is biochemically trapped within the cell. This process of metabolic trapping constitutes the basis of PET imaging. Such imaging makes it possible to calculate a specific uptake value, normalized to the injected dose, which is called a standardized uptake value (SUV). The SUV provides an approximate indicator that correlates with FDG metabolism (which will be proportional to the glucose metabolism). A lesion with an SUV > 2.5 is considered to have a high probability of malignancy. However, that is not always true. Standardized uptake values are calculated according to the following formula:

$$\frac{\text{Mean ROI activity (MBq/g)}}{\text{Injected dose (MBq)/Body weight (g)}}$$

where MBq = a mega-Becquerel, and g = grams.

Recently, the role of ^{18}F-FDG-PET and PET/CT in characterizing adrenal lesions has been evaluated in cancer patients (Blake et al., 2006b; Jana et al., 2006; Kumar et al., 2004). The results of these studies are encouraging and justify the use of PET for metastatic disease evaluation in these patients with a sensitivity and specificity ranging from 92 to 100% and from 80 to 100% (Table 3). In studies involving PET, Boland et al. (1995) reported a sensitivity and specificity of 100% with ^{18}F-FDG-PET in 20 patients with cancer. Erasmus et al. (1997) studied 33 adrenal lesions in 27 patients with lung cancer. Positron emission tomography findings were

Table 3 Results of Published PET Studies in Oncology Patients with Adrenal Lesions

Study	Year	Imaging Modality	Sensitivity	Specificity	Accuracy
Boland et al.	1995	PET	100%	100%	100%
Erasmus et al.	1997	PET	100%	80%	94%
Maurea et al.	1999	PET	100%	93%	96%
Yun et al.	2001	PET	100%	94%	96%
Gupta et al.	2001	PET	94%	92%	93%
Kumar et al.	2004	PET	93%	90%	92%
Jana et al	2006	PET /PET-CT	93%	96%	95%
Ur Metser et al.	2006	PET-CT	100%	98%	—
Blake et al.	2006	PET-CT	100%	94%	95%

interpreted as positive when ^{18}F-FDG uptakes were higher in the adrenal mass than the background.

Gupta *et al.* (2001) evaluated 30 patients with bronchogenic carcinoma and considered adrenal ^{18}F-FDG uptake to be abnormal when it were higher than liver uptake. Yun *et al.* (2001), Kumar *et al.* (2004), and Jana *et al.* (2006) used similar criteria and interpreted ^{18}F-FDG uptake of the adrenal glands as positive if it were equal to or greater than that of the liver. Their results indicate that if a lesion shows F18-FDG uptake less than that of the liver, or shows uptake that is significantly higher than the liver, the study can be interpreted with high confidence unless the patient has pheochromocytoma, that can be excluded by biochemical markers (Yun *et al.*, 2001).

In the largest study, Kumar *et al.* (2004) evaluated the performance of ^{18}F-FDG-PET in characterizing 113 adrenal masses in 94 patients with lung cancer. Comparing FDG uptake in adrenal lesion to background activity in liver, we found overall sensitivity of 93%, specificity of 90%, and accuracy of 92% (Fig. 4A). In our recent study involving 80 adrenal lesions in 74 patients, PET demonstrated sensitivity of 93% and specificity of 96% for detection of metastases when adrenal uptake exceeding liver uptake was considered PET positive (Jana *et al.*, 2006). A maximum SUV of 3.4

was 95% sensitive and 86% specific, while an average SUV of 3.1 was found to be 95% sensitive and 90% specific. Interestingly, we found visual interpretation as accurate as SUV interpretation. In our study, FDG/PET was most useful in the 52.5% of cancer patients with inconclusive adrenal lesions on CT (Fig. 4B).

In a recent ^{18}F-FDG-PET/CT study, Metser *et al.* (2006) concluded that in evaluation of adrenal masses with F18-FDG-PET/CT for differentiating benign from malignant adrenal masses in oncology patients, combined information from the ^{18}F-FDG-PET and unenhanced CT portions of a PET/CT study is more specific than ^{18}F-FDG-PET information alone. They evaluated 150 patients with malignancy who presented with adrenal mass; the intensity of ^{18}F-FDG uptake, expressed as standardized uptake value (SUV), was determined from receiver operating characteristic curves. An SUV cut-off value of 3.1 was used to compare malignant lesions and adenomas. They found that when malignant lesions were compared with adenomas, PET data using an SUV cut-off of 3.1 yielded a sensitivity, specificity, PPV, and NPV of 98.5%, 92%, 89.3%, and 98.9%, respectively. In another study involving ^{18}F-FDG-PET/CT, Blake *et al.* (2006b) interpreted F18-FDG uptake as positive when the maximum SUVs of the adrenal lesion exceeded hepatic

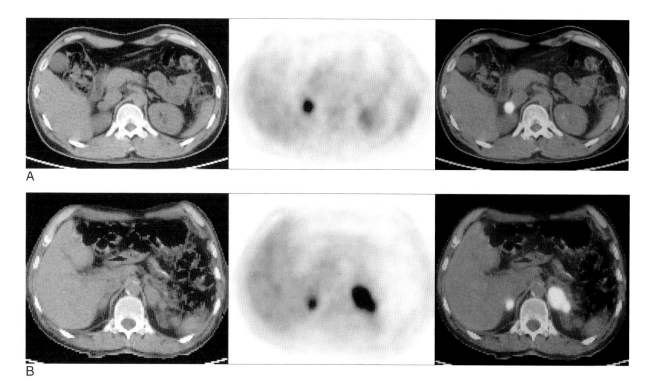

Figure 4 (**A**) Right adrenal metastasis: Axial section CT shows right adrenal mass. Intense FDG uptake (significantly more than liver) was seen in PET and PET/CT images; (**B**) bilateral adrenal metastases: Coronal and axial section CT shows left adrenal mass and doubtful right adrenal mass. Intense FDG uptake (significantly more than liver) was seen in PET and PET/CT images in bilateral adrenal masses.

maximum SUVs. In their study, sensitivity, specificity, PPV, NPV, and accuracy of ^{18}F-FDG-PET/CT in differentiating malignant from benign adrenal masses in patients with proved or suspected malignancy were found to be 100%, 93%, 81%, 100%, and 95%, respectively.

Although PET results are encouraging, several inherent problems are associated with FDG-PET imaging. These include lack of widespread availability, uptake in other abdominal structures, such as superior renal calyx (hot urine), that can obscure the adrenal gland, and limited resolution of PET, which leads to difficulty in imaging very small adrenal lesions. However, the recent addition of CT to PET has further improved the value of PET as PET/CT provides functional and structural information in the same setting. The common causes of false-positive adrenal lesions on ^{18}F-FDG-PET imaging are benign adenomas and pheochromocytomas (Yun et al., 2001; Shulkin et al., 1999). Both the benign and malignant pheochromocytomas have been shown to accumulate ^{18}F-FDG, although uptake is greater in malignant as compared to benign pheochromocytoma (Fig. 5) (Shulkin et al., 1999). The common causes of false-negative F18-FDG-PET results are small-size lesions, necrotic metastasis, and metastases from neuroendocrine tumours (Yun et al., 2001; Erasmus et al., 1998). Small metastatic lesions can be missed because of the limited resolution of ^{18}F-FDG-PET and PET/CT or the absence of sufficient tumor cells with increased glycolysis.

^{18}F-FDG-PET and PET/CT imaging has been found to be a reliable noninvasive imaging technique for differentiating benign from malignant adrenal masses. It has demonstrated a high sensitivity, specificity, and overall accuracy for detecting adrenal metastases in patients with malignancy. ^{18}F-FDG-PET imaging is likely to be useful in presurgical staging of cancer patients demonstrating adrenal lesion on CT scanning. Adrenal lesions with an FDG uptake equal to or slightly higher than that of the liver on FDG-PET should be read as indeterminate because these properties can be seen in either benign or malignant lesions. In such patients, an additional imaging study with MRI should be performed for further characterization of the lesions. Positron emission tomography and PET/CT have an additional advantage of evaluating the other parts of the body (head and neck, chest and pelvis) to stage the extent of the malignant disease.

Fine-Needle Aspiration (FNA) Biopsy

Cytology from a specimen obtained by FNA cannot distinguish a benign adrenal lesion from adrenal carcinoma. However, it can differentiate an adrenal tumor and a metastatic tumor (Brunt et al., 2004). Thus, FNA may be indicated when there is a suspicion for metastatic lesion in the adrenal gland. Adrenal biopsy is a relatively invasive procedure and is associated with a failure rate of 14–50% after the first

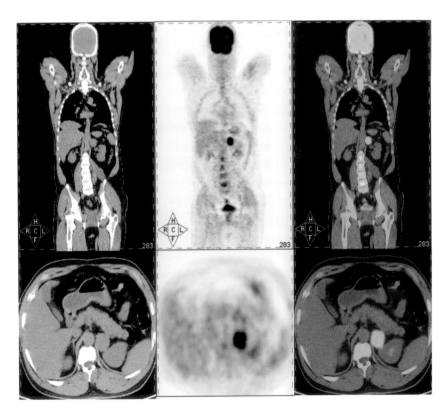

Figure 5 Pheochromocytoma: Coronal and axial section CT shows left adrenal mass. Intense FDG uptake (significantly more than liver) was seen in PET and PET/CT images in the left adrenal mass. In this case PET/CT was false positive.

attempt due to either nondiagnostic pathology or the failure to obtain adequate tissue (Benardino *et al.*, 1985; Ettinghausen and Burt, 1991; Silverman, 1993). This procedure also is associated with a reported complication rate of 8.4–11.3% (Benardino *et al.*, 1985; Mody *et al.*, 1995). The commonly reported complications are pneumothorax, pain, perinephric hemorrhage, sub-capsular and intra-hepatic hematoma and hepatic needle tract metastases depending on the approach to the adrenal gland (Benardino *et al.*, 1985; Ettinghausen, 1991; Mody *et al.*, 1995; Silverman, 1993). There are reported cases of hypotension and a drop of hematocrit requiring blood transfusion as a complication of adrenal biopsy (Benardino *et al.*, 1985). Before attempting FNA of an adrenal lesion, pheochromocytoma should always be excluded with normal values of 24-hr urinary excretion of fractionated metanephrines and catecholamines (Brunt and Moley, 2004). Therefore (due to the above limitations associated with FNA), a noninvasive imaging modality is always the first test of choice to distinguish a benign adrenal lesion from a malignant adrenal mass, and FNA is usually used at the end when noninvasive modalities could not succeed.

Summary

Adrenal lesions are more commonly detected incidentally due to the widespread use of high-resolution anatomical imaging modalities. Once an adrenal lesion is detected, the two questions that arise are (1) whether it is secretory (functioning) and (2) whether it is malignant. Hormonal assays of the blood and/or urine with or without intervention are used to determine the secretory status. On the other hand, imaging modalities such as CT, MRI, PET, or PET/CT are used to answer the second question. Noncontrast CT is the most easily available and also the most commonly used imaging modality. At the time when an adrenal lesion was detected, the patient already had a noncontrast CT.

The current literature shows that if an adrenal lesion has all the following characteristics in the noncontrast CT there is a 98–100% chance (specificity) that the lesion is benign and does not need further evaluation. The characteristics are: (1) unilateral location and less than 4 cm diameter, (2) uniform round shape with homogeneous density, smooth contour, and sharp margins, and (3) a CT attenuation value of less than 10 HU. There is also no need for further evaluation when a lesion can be identified as malignant with all the following characteristics: (1) more than 4 cm diameter, irregular shape, and inhomogeneous density, (2) tumor calcification, and (3) CT attenuation value of more than 40 HU. Therefore, if CT is conclusive, other imaging studies are not required to characterize the adrenal lesion (Boland *et al.*, 1998; Dunnick and Korobkin, 2002; Jana *et al.*, 2006; Szolar and Kammerhuber, 1998). On the other hand, a significant number (up to 50%) of lesions will be identified as indeterminate following the above criteria for a benign as well as malignant lesion (Jana *et al.*, 2006; Allard *et al.*, 1990). Another imaging modality is required in this condition to determine the nature of the adrenal lesion noninvasively. The options are contrast CT with delayed enhancement, MRI with chemical shift, and FDG-PET or PET/CT. If the patient has a known cancer outside the adrenal gland, then the next possible best test is FDG-PET or PET/CT. Positron emission tomography or PET/CT, being a whole-body imaging modality, provides not only information related to the nature of the adrenal lesion but also information related to the overall current stage (and grade) of the nonadrenal cancer, therefore, impacting the overall management of the patient's disease. The visual criteria, that is, adrenal uptake higher than liver uptake, were found to be as good as using SUV values to identify a lesion as malignant (Jana *et al.*, 2006). When FDG-PET is inconclusive (i.e., mild uptake but not conclusively higher than the liver uptake with CT findings suspicious for malignancy), either contrast CT with washout measurements (when the attenuation of the lesion lies between 25 and 40 HU on prior noncontrast CT) or MRI with chemical shift (when the attenuation of the lesion lies between 10 and 25 HU on prior noncontrast CT, i.e., enough fat present in the lesion to produce a conclusive chemical shift) is a good alternative. If it also fails to identify a lesion conclusively as malignant or benign and there is suspicion for metastatic disease, then a CT-guided FNA should be considered, provided that the correct diagnosis can significantly influence the patient's management, e.g., isolated adrenal metastases from lung cancer (otherwise respectable lung cancer) can potentially undergo adrenalectomy with increased survival (Ettinghausen and Burt, 1991). If the lesion is more than 6 cm and there is suspicion for adrenal cancer, a surgical resection of the mass is the next best step. Before any patient goes for either surgery or FNA, a subclinical pheochromocytoma should be excluded by appropriate blood and/or urine test. Finally, adrenal cysts, adrenal hemorrhage, and myelolipoma are usually easily characterized in noncontrast CT because of their distinctive imaging characteristics and do not require any further investigation.

References

Allard, P., Yankaskas, B.C., Fletcher, R.H., Parker, L.A., and Halvorsen, R.A., Jr. 1990. Sensitivity and specificity of computed tomography for the detection of adrenal metastatic lesions among 91 autopsied lung cancer patients. *Cancer 66*:457–462.

Bernardino, M.E., Walther, M.M., Phillips, V.M., Graham, S.D., Jr, Sewell, C.W., Gedgaudas-McClees, K., Baumgartner, B.R., Torres, W.E., and Erwin, B.C. 1985. CT-guided adrenal biopsy: accuracy, safety and indications. *Am. J. Roentgenol. 144*(1):67–69.

Blake, M.A., Kalra, M.K., Sweeney, A.T., Lucey, B.C., Maher, M.M., Sahani, D.V., Halpern, E.F., Mueller, P.R., Hahn, P.F., and Boland, G.W. 2006a. Distinguishing benign from malignant adrenal masses: multidetector row CT protocol with 10-minute delay. *Radiology 238*:578–585.

Blake, M.A., Slattery, J., Kalra, M.K., Halpern, E.F., Fischman, A.J., Mueller, P.R., and Boland, G.W. 2006b. Adrenal lesions: characterisation with fused PET/CT image in patients with proved or suspected malignancy—initial experience. *Radiology 238*:970–977.

Boland, G.W., Goldberg, M.A., Lee, M.J., Mayo-Smith, W.W., Dixon, J., McNicholas, M.M., and Mueller, P.R. 1995. Indeterminate adrenal mass in patients with cancer: evaluation at PET with 2-[F-18]-fluoro-2-deoxy-D-glucose. *Radiology 194*:131–134.

Boland, G.W., Lee, M.J., Gazelle, G.S., Halpern, E.F., McNicholas, M.M., and Mueller, P.R. 1998. Characterization of adrenal masses using unenhanced CT: an analysis of the CT literature. *Am. J. Roentgenol. 171*:201–204.

Brunt, L.M., and Moley, J. 2004. The pituitary and adrenal glands. In: Townsend, C.M., Beauchamp, R.D., Evers, B.M., and Mattox, K.L. (Eds.), *Sabiston Textbook of Surgery* (17th ed.). Philadelphia: W.B. Saunders, pp. 1035–1066

Burt, M., Heelan, R., Coit, D., McCormack, P.M., Bains, M.S., Martini, N., Rusch, V., and Ginsberg, R.J. 1995. Prospective evaluation of unilateral adrenal masses in patients with operable non-small cell lung cancer. Impact of magnetic resonance imaging. *J. Thorac. Cardiovasc. Surg. 109*:814–815.

Caoili, E.M., Korobkin, M., Francis, I.R., Cohan, R.H., Platt, J.F., Dunnick, N.R., and Raghupathi, K.I. 2002. Adrenal masses: characterisation with combined unenhanced and delayed enhanced CT. *Radiology 222*:629–633.

Copeland, P.M. 1983. The incidentally discovered adrenal mass. *Ann. Intern. Med. 98*:940–945.

Dunnick, N.R., and Korobkin, M. 2002. Imaging of adrenal incidentalomas: current status. *Am. J. Roentgenol. 179*:559–568.

Dunnick, N.R., Korobkin, M., and Francis, I. 1996. Adrenal radiology: distinguishing benign from malignant adrenal masses. *Am. J. Roentgenol. 167*:861–867.

Erasmus, J.J., McAdams, H.P., Patz, E.F., Jr, Coleman, R.E., Ahuja, V., and Goodman, P.C. 1998. Evaluation of primary pulmonary characinoid tumors using FDG PET. *Am. J. Roentgenol. 170*:1369–1373.

Erasmus, J.J., Patz, E.F., Jr, Mcadams, H.P., Murray, J.G., Herndon, J., Coleman, R.E., and Goodman, P.C. 1997. Evaluation of adrenal masses in patients with bronchogenic carcinoma using 18F-FDG-PET. *Am. J. Roentgenol. 168*:1357–1360.

Ettinghausen, S.E., and Burt, M.E. 1991. Prospective evaluation of unilateral adrenal masses in patients with operable non-small-cell lung cancer. *J. Clin. Oncol. 9*:1462–1466.

Falk, T.H.M., and Sandler, M.P. 1994. Classification of silent adrenal masses: time to get practical. *J. Nucl. Med. 35*:1152–1154.

Fishman, E.K., Deutch, B.M., Hartman, D.S., Goldman, S.M., Zerhouni, E.A., and Siegelman, S.S. 1987. Primary adrenocortical carcinoma: CT evaluation with clinical correlation. *Am. J. Roentgenol. 148*:531–535.

Gross, M.D., Korobkin, M., and Hussain, H. 2005. Adrenal gland imaging. In: Jameson, J.L., and DeGroot, L.J. (Eds.), *Endocrinology* (5th ed.). Philadelphia: W.B. Saunders, pp. 2425–2453.

Gross, M.D., and Shapiro, B. 1993. Clinical review 50: clinically silent adrenal masses. *J. Clin. Endocrinol. Metab. 77*:885–888.

Gupta, N.C., Geoffrey, M., Tamim, W.J., Rogers, J.S., Irisari, L., and Bishop, H.A. 2001. Clinical utility of PET-FDG imaging in differentiation of benign from malignant adrenal masses in lung cancer. *Clin. Lung Cancer 3*:59–64.

Haider, M.A., Ghai, S., Jhaveri, K., and Lockwood, G. 2004. Chemical shift MR imaging of hyper attenuating (> 10 HU) adrenal masses: does it still have a role? *Radiology 231*:711–716.

Hamrahian, A.H., Ioachimescu, A.G., Remer, E.M., Motta-Ramirez, G., Bogabathina, H., Levin, H.S., Reddy, S., Gill, I.S., Siperstein, A., and Bravo, E.L. 2005. Clinical utility of no contrast computed tomography attenuation value (Hounsfield units) to differentiate adrenal adenomas/hyperploids from non adenomas: Cleveland Clinic Experience. *J. Clin. Endocrinol. Metab. 90*:871–877.

Hussain, S., Belldegrun, A., Seltzer, S.E., Richie, J.P., Gittes, R.F., and Abrams, H.L. 1985. Differentiation of malignant from benign adrenal masses: predictive indices on computed tomography. *Am. J. Roentgenol. 144*:61–65.

Israel, G.M., Korobkin, M., Wang, C., Hecht, E.N., and Krinsky, G.A. 2004. Comparison of unenhanced CT and chemical shift MRI in evaluating lipid-rich adrenal adenomas. *AJR Am. J. Roentgenol. 183*:215–230.

Jana, S., Zhang, T., Milstein, D.M., Isasi, C.R., and Blaufox, M.D. 2006. FDG-PET and CT characterization of adrenal lesions in cancer patients. *Eur. J. Nucl. Med. and Mol. Imag. 33*:29–35.

Kawashima, A., Sandler, C.M., Fisherman, E.K., Charnsangavej, C., Yasumori, K., Honda, H., Ernst, R.D., Takahashi, N., Raval, B.K., Masuda, K., and Goldman, S.M. 1998. Spectrum of CT findings in non-malignant disease of the adrenal gland. *Radiographics 18*:393–412.

Korobkin, M. 2000. CT characterization of adrenal masses: the time has come. *Radiology 217*:629–632

Korobkin, M., Brodeur, F.J., Francis, I.R., Quint, L.E., Dunnick, N.R., and Londy, F. 1998. CT time attenuation washout curves of adrenal adenomas and non adenomas. *Am. J. Roentgenol. 170*:747–752.

Korobkin, M., Brodeur, F.J., Yutzy, G.G., Francis, I.R., Quint, L.E., Dunnick, N.R., and Kazerooni, E.A. 1996. Differentiation of adrenal adenomas from non adenomas using CT attenuation values. *Am. J. Roentgenol. 166*:531–536.

Korobkin, M., Lombardi, T.J., Aisen, A.M., Francis, I.R., Quint, L.E., Dunnick, N.R., Londy, F., Shapiro, B., Gross, M.D., and Thompson, N.W. 1995. Characterisation of adrenal masses with chemical shift and gadolinium enhanced MR imaging. *Radiology 197*:411–418.

Kumar, R., Xiu, Y., Yu, J.Q., Takalkar, A., El-Haddad, G., Potenta, S., Kung, J., Zhuang, H., and Alavi, A. 2004. F18-FDG PET in evaluation of adrenal lesions in patients with lung cancer. *J. Nucl. Med. 45*:2058–2062.

Kumar, R., Loving, V., Chauhan, A., Zhuang, H., and Alavi, A. 2005. Dual time point imaging and its potential to improve breast cancer diagnosis with F18-fluorodeoxyglucose positron emission tomography. *J. Nucl. Med. 46*:1819–1824.

Kumar, R., Yan, X., Zhuang, H., and Alavi, A. 2006. F18-fluorodeoxyglucose positron emission tomography in primary cutaneous lymphoma. *Br. J. Dermatol. 155*:357–363.

Kumar, R., Nadig, M., and Chauhan, A. 2005. Positron emission tomography: clinical application in oncology: part I. Expert Rev. *Anticancer Ther. 5*:1079–1094.

Macari, M., Rofsky, N.M., Naidich, D.P., and Megibow, A.J. 1998. Nonsmall cell lung carcinoma: usefulness of unenhanced helical CT of the adrenal glands in an unmonitored environment. *Radiology 209*:807–812.

Mantero, F., Terzolo, M., Arnaldi, G., Osella, G., Masini, A.M., Ali, A., Giovagnetti, M., Opocher, G., and Angeli, A. 2000. A survey on adrenal incidentaloma in Italy. Study group on Adrenal Tumors of the Italian Society of Endocrinology. *J. Clin. Endocrinol. Metab. 85*:637–642.

Maurea, S., Mainolfi, C., Bazzicalupo, L., Panico, M.R., Imparato, C., Alfano, B., Ziviello, M., and Salvatore, M. 1999. Imaging of adrenal tumours using FDG-PET: comparison of benign and malignant lesions. *Am. J. Roentgenol. 173*:25–29.

Mitchell, D.G., Crovello, M., Matteucci, T., Petersen, R.O., and Miettinen, M.M. 1992. Benign adrenocortical masses: diagnosis with chemical shift MR imaging. *Radiology 185*:345–351.

Mitnick, J.S., Bosniak, M.A., Megibow, A.J., and Naidich, D.P. 1983. Non functioning adrenal adenomas discovered incidentally on computed tomography. *Radiology 148*:495–499.

Mody, M.K., Kazerooni, E.A., and Korobkin, M. 1995. Percutaneous CT-guided biopsy of adrenal masses: immediate and delayed complications. *J. Comput. Assist. Tomogr. 19*(3):434–439.

Pagani, J.J. 1984. Non small cell lung carcinoma adrenal metastases: computed tomography and percutaneous needle biopsy in their diagnosis. *Cancer 52*:1058–1060.

Pena, C.S., Boland, G.W.L., Hahn, P.F., Lee, M.J., and Mueller, P.R. 2000. Characterization of indeterminate (lipid poor) adrenal masses: use of washout characteristics at contrast enhanced CT. *Radiology 217*:798–802.

Porte, H.L., Ernst, O.J., Delebecq, T., Metois, D., Lemaitre, L.G., and Wurtz, A.J. 1999. Is computed tomography guided biopsy still necessary for the diagnosis of adrenal masses in patients with respectable non-small cell lung cancer? *Eur. J. Cardiothorac. Surg. 15*:597–601.

Schwartz, L.H., Panicek, D.M., Koutcher, J.A., Brown, K.T., Getrajdman, G.I., Heelan, R.T., and Burt, M. 1995. Adrenal masses in patients with malignancy: prospective comparison of echo-planar, fast spin echo, and chemical shift MR imaging. *Radiology 197*:421–425.

Shulkin, B.L., Thompson, N.W., Shapiro, B., Francis, I.R., and Sisson, J.C. 1999. Pheochromocytomas: imaging with 2-[18F] fluoro-2-deoxy-D-glucose PET. *Radiology 212*:35–41.

Silverman, S.G., Mueller, P.R., Pinkney, L.P., Koenker, R.M., and Seltzer, S.E. 1993. Predictive value of image-guided adrenal biopsy: analysis of results of 101 biopsies. *Radiology 187*:715–718.

Stoner, H.B., Whiteley, H.J., and Emery, J.L. 1953. Effect of systemic disease on adrenal cortex of children. *J. Pathol. Bacteriol. 66*:171–183.

Szolar, D.H., and Kammerhuber, F.H. 1998. Adrenal adenomas and non adenomas: assessment of washout at delayed contrast enhanced CT. *Radiology 207*:369–375.

Metser, U., Miller, E., Lerman, H., Lievshitz, G., Avital, S., and Even -Sapir, 2006. 18F-FDG PET/CT in evaluation of adrenal masses. *J. Nucl. Med. 47*:32–37.

Yun, M., Kim, W., Alnafisi, N., Lacorte, L., Jang, S., and Alavi, A. 2001. 18F-FDG PET in characterizing adrenal lesions detected on CT or MRI. *J. Nucl. Med. 42*:1795–1799.

2

Hemangioendothelioma: Whole-Body Technetium-99m Red Blood Cell Imaging-Magnetic Resonance Imaging

Cuneyt Turkmen and Izzet Rozanes

Introduction

The term *hemangioendothelioma* describes a group of vascular neoplasm showing histologic features and clinical behavior intermediate between the benign hemangiomas and the anaplastic angiosarcomas. Hemangioendotheliomas commonly present with an enlarging mass and have been reported in the skin, soft tissue, liver, bones, lungs, heart, intestines, nervous system, retroperitoneum, and many other body sites. However it is most common in liver, soft tissue, and bone. These lesions can produce a variety of clinical symptoms depending on their location or in some cases they can be asymptomatic. Noninvasive imaging modalities used for diagnosis of hemangioendothelioma include ultrasonography (US), computed tomography (CT), magnetic resonance imaging (MRI), and scintigraphic techniques (three-phase bone scan, sulfur colloid imaging, Technetium-99m (Tc-99m) red blood cell imaging, 18F-fluorodeoxyglucose positron emission tomography, etc.). The determination of the initial test of choice usually depends on localization of the lesion, and often more than one imaging technique are needed for a prompt and reliable diagnosis. The management

of these tumors can include conservative measures in some cases and aggressive intervention in others. Several treatments of hemangioendothelioma have been attempted. Best results are surgical excision with a wide margin (Lai *et al.*, 1991). The role of adjuvant radiotherapy or chemotherapy was not well established until now (Weiss and Enzinger, 1995). Transplantation of the liver is considered in patients with liver hemangioendothelioma if all other treatment strategies fail. The prognosis of hemangioendothelioma usually is much more favorable than that of angiosarcoma; prolonged survival (5–28 years) has been reported after surgical resection or liver transplantation.

Recent advances in imaging methods and combining anatomical and functional imaging techniques provide a more accurate determination of the extent of the disease. Functional imaging modalities have an inherently low spatial resolution, but when combined with a cross-sectional anatomical imaging technique such as CT or MRI, they allow tumor function to be accurately detected. In this context, Tc-99m red blood cell imaging and MRI have emerged as two complementary imaging modalities in the diagnosis of hemangioendothelioma. This chapter will review the utility of MRI as well as other conventional imaging modalities and whole-body Tc-99m red blood cell imaging in the evaluation of hemangioendothelioma.

Histopathologic Classification

Hemangioendotheliomas that formerly included spindle cell hemangioendothelioma, endovascular papillary angioendothelioma (Dabska tumor), and epithelioid hemangioendothelioma have been defined as vascular tumors of "intermediate" malignancy. Accumulating data on clinical behavior and pathologic features of hemangioendothelioma has led to a revision of histopathological classification of these rare tumors. According to this revision, spindle cell hemangioendothelioma has been renamed spindle cell hemangioma, which is recognized as an entirely benign and nonrecurring lesion. Similarly, as many as 20 to 30% of epithelioid hemangioendotheliomas may give rise to distant metastases; hence these tumors have been redesignated as malignant. In the recent WHO-classification of soft tissue tumors, intermediate vascular tumors are subcategorized into locally aggressive and rarely metastazing subsets (Fletcher, 2006).

In the category of locally aggressive intermediate tumors, the entity of kaposiform hemangioendothelioma, which was first recognized in the early 1990s, has been introduced. This is a very rare neoplasm that affects mainly infants and children and that arises mainly in the skin, subcutis, and deep soft tissues, including the retroperitoneum. Although it seems that kaposiform hemangioendothelioma is associated with a high mortality rate, the deaths are almost always related to locally invasive effects or as a result of bleeding and consumption coagulopathy (Kasabach–Merritt syndrome). So far, no metastasizing case of kaposiform hemangioendothelioma has been reported, and it seems that the prognosis in kaposiform hemangioendothelioma is related mainly to size, anatomical site, and depth of the lesion.

In the rarely metastasizing, intermediate category, endovascular papillary angioendothelioma has been renamed papillary intralymphatic angioendothelioma. Today lesions described under the rubric Dabska tumor are seen to include not only this entity but also examples of retiform hemangioendothelioma, which occurs most often in the distal extremities of young adults and which often recurs locally (and repeatedly) but only rarely metastasizes. This category also includes composite hemangioendothelioma, which is an exceedingly uncommon vascular tumor characterized, in most cases, by a complex admixture of histologically benign, intermediate, and malignant components, most often consisting of retiform hemangioendothelioma and epithelioid hemangioendothelioma. These tumors, which are most commonly seen in the distal extremities, often recur locally but only rarely metastasize.

Clinical Presentation and Radiology of Hemangioendothelioma

Although hemangioendothelioma has no definite diagnostic features, imaging findings of hemangioendothelioma vary according to the imaging modality of choice and the localization of lesion.

Hemangioendothelioma of Bone

Epithelioid hemangioendothelioma occurs in the calvarium, spine, femur, tibia, and feet of adults during the second or third decade. Multiple lesion may be present, either in the same bone (particularly in the tibia or fibula), in adjacent bones in the same limb, or in widely separated bones. Nearby or distant soft tissues and skin may also be involved. It is more common in men than women and is found in the metaphysis or epiphysis.

On radiological examination, epithelioid hemangioendotheliomas are expansive, osteolytic, and poorly demarcated lesions. They have a distinctive "soap-bubble" matrix with a sclerotic margin. No periosteal reaction is present. Lesions with particularly ill-defined margins and loss of trabeculae are considered more aggressive. CT scan findings are noncontributory as they only reflect additional soft tissue details, but lesions do enhance with contrast media. MRI findings are also nonspecific. The radiological differential includes metastatic carcinoma, Ewing's sarcoma, telangiectatic osteosarcoma, lymphoma, fibrous dysplasia, and aneurysmal bone cyst (Murphey et al., 1995).

Hemangioendothelioma of the Liver

There are two distinct forms of hemangioendothelioma of the liver: infantile hemangioendothelioma and the epithelioid hemangioendothelioma (EHE), which occur in the adult population. Infantile hemangioendothelioma is the third most common hepatic tumor in children (representing 12% of all childhood hepatic tumors), the most common benign vascular tumor of the liver in infancy, and the most common symptomatic liver tumor during the first 6 months of life. Approximately 85% of affected patients present by 6 months of age and in ~ 45–50% of cases these patients also have cutaneous hemangiomas. The tumor has a 2:1 female predilection. The lesions may be single or multiple, and calcifications are seen at histopathologic analysis in 50% of cases. Infantile hemangioendotheliomas are usually benign, but malignant sarcomas have been reported to arise in existing hemangioendotheliomas. Most tumors continue to grow during the first year of life and then spontaneously regress, probably due to thrombosis and scar formation. At sonography, infantile hemangioendothelioma appears as a complex, mostly solid hepatic lesion with variable hypo- and hyperechoic echotexture. In cases of significant arteriovenous shunting, dilated hepatic vasculature with prominent blood flow at Doppler US is typical. If large vascular spaces are present, anechoic regions with detectable flow may be seen. The lesions are often well demarcated from the surrounding liver parenchyma.

At unenhanced CT, infantile hemangioendothelioma usually manifests as a well-defined mass that is hypoattenuating relative to the normal liver parenchyma. In ~ 16–40% of cases, the lesion is heterogeneous with central high-attenuation areas due to hemorrhage or calcifications. At contrast-enhanced CT, the enhancement pattern may resemble that of an adult giant hemangioma, with "nodular" peripheral puddling of contrast material in the early phase, subsequent peripheral pooling, and central enhancement with variable delay. In larger tumors, central enhancement is often lacking due to fibrosis, hemorrhage, or necrosis. Conversely, small lesions, which tend to be multifocal, frequently enhance completely and typically do not demonstrate hemorrhage or necrosis.

At unenhanced MR imaging, the lesions have low signal intensity on T1-weighted images and high signal intensity on T2-weighted images. In tumors with arteriovenous shunting and high blood flow, flow voids may be observed on T2-weighted images. Because of the simultaneous presence of hemorrhage, necrosis, and fibrosis, the mass often appears heterogeneous on both T1- and T2-weighted images. After intravenous administration of gadopentetate dimeglumine, the lesions usually show an enhancement pattern similar to that described at CT. In some cases, however, the lesions may show complete "rim enhancement" at dynamic gadolinium-enhanced MR imaging (as at CT), which might confuse the differential diagnosis of hepatic tumors in infants. At angiography, a dilated and elongated hepatic artery and early filling of dilated draining hepatic veins may be seen in a hemangioendothelioma with significant arteriovenous shunting. Pooling of contrast material in large vascular spaces may be present. Because of the increased vascular supply to these tumors, a striking decrease in the aortic caliber is often seen distal to the celiac artery origin. This finding is also recognizable at US, CT, and MR imaging (Roos *et al.*, 2003).

Hepatic epithelioid hemangioendothelioma is a rare tumor of vascular origin first defined as a specific entity in 1982. Clinical manifestation is variable, usually with nonspecific symptoms such as right upper quadrant pain and weight loss. Some patients present with Budd-Chiari syndrome or liver failure. Although tumor growth may be progressive and may lead to hepatic failure, metastasis, and death, the prognosis is considered more favorable than that of other liver malignancies.

At sonography, discrete nodules may be seen, or the liver may have a diffusely heterogeneous echotexture in regions of extensive diffuse involvement. Echogenicity of individual lesions is variable. Most frequently, the lesions are hypoechoic relative to adjacent hepatic parenchyma, but masses may be hyperechoic and isoechoic relative to background liver. The internal architecture of a nodule may be complex and heterogeneous. Most of the lesions are peripheral, extending to the capsular margin. Capsular retraction adjacent to the mass is seen in < 5% of patients. CT or plain X-ray may depict hepatic parenchymal calcifications. Tumor involvement can be widespread with extensive confluent masses and few traceable signs of portal or hepatic veins. After administration of IV contrast material on CT, some tumor nodules display marginal enhancement during the arterial phase. On contrast-enhanced scans, the tumor nodules may become isodense to liver parenchyma. The extent of such involvement may be better defined on unenhanced images.

Magnetic resonance imaging shows the lesions on T1-weighted images as being of low intensity relative to uninvolved liver parenchyma, with some lesions containing central areas of lower signal intensity than the remainder of the tumor. On T2-weighted images, lesions tend to be of heterogeneously increased signal. Some lesions may have a target appearance due to the presence of a central sclerotic zone and a peripheral region of cellular proliferation. Central areas of reduced signal may correspond to areas of hemorrhage, coagulation necrosis, and calcification; peripheral high signal intensity corresponds to edematous connective tissue and viable tumor. After IV contrast administration of gadopentetate dimeglumine, peripheral enhancement occurs with a thin nonenhancing rim corresponding to a narrow avascular zone between normal liver parenchyma and the nodules (Fig. 1). Ferumoxides-enhanced T1-weighted images more clearly define the extent of tumor than other images, but distinction between normal liver and tumor may be difficult on all sequences (Lyburn *et al.*, 2003). A recent report describes the termination of a hepatic or portal vein at or just within the periphery of epithelioid hemangioendothelioma in four patients. The author describes this finding as "the lollipop sign" and considers it to be a specific radiological finding (Alomari, 2006). However, in our opinion similar findings can be seen in patients with hepatocellular carcinoma where invasion and thrombosis of portal and/or hepatic veins is a very common finding.

Lung Epithelioid Hemangioendothelioma

Epithelioid hemangioendothelioma in its pulmonary form was originally described by Dail and Liebow as an "intravascular bronchioalveolar tumour"; these authors noted the tumor's remarkable propensity to invade pulmonary vessels and small airways. Since then, < 50 cases have been described in the literature worldwide. It is a tumor of borderline malignancy, which tends to follow an intermediate course between hemangioma and conventional angiosarcoma. In the typical pulmonary forms, epithelioid hemangioendothelioma presents with nonspecific symptoms, such as chest pain, cough,

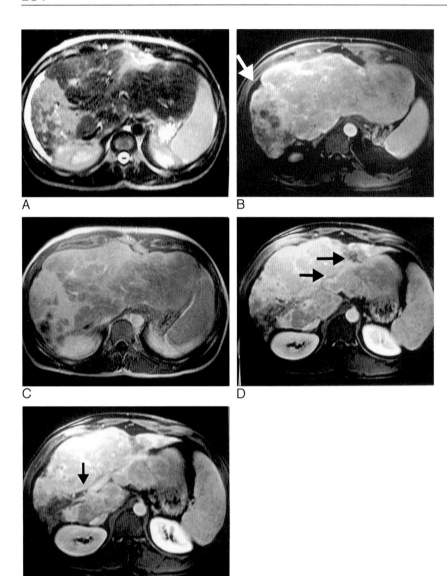

Figure 1 Forty-five-year-old male with biopsy-proven epithelioid hemangioendothelioma of the liver. (**A**) T2W axial scan of the liver. Right lobe 7 cm mass and left lobe 4 cm mass have a higher signal intensity than normal liver. (**B**) Post-GdDTPA arterial phase image of the upper liver depicting ill-defined mass in segments 7 and 8, with peripheral enhancement and capsular retraction (arrow). (**C**) Post-GdDTPA portal phase of the upper liver. Most of the mass has a higher signal than normal liver with some nonenhancing areas. (**D**) Post-GdDTPA arterial phase image of the mid-liver depicting two additional masses in the left liver lobe (arrows). (**E**) Post-GdDTPA portal phase image of the mid-liver showing right portal vein thrombosis (arrow) reminiscent of "the lollipop sign."

or sputum, or it may remain asymptomatic. It usually affects middle-aged patients, with a female predominance, although cases in children and in the elderly have been described.

Multifocal nodular densities up to 2 cm in diameter, with well- or ill-defined margins, are the most common feature of pulmonary epithelioid hemangioendothelioma on chest radiography; these are often mistaken for metastatic disease, but they show little or no growth on serial radiography. The presence of a pleural effusion or hilar or mediastinal lymphadenopathy is rare. The thoracic CT usually reveals more nodules than those in the chest radiography. In long-standing cases, extensive calcification of the nodules and insterstitial involvement can be seen (Diaz *et al.*, 2004).

Technetium-99m Red Blood Cell Imaging

The use of radioactive nuclides in the labeling of erythrocyte dates to the work of Nobel Laureate George de Hevesy, who introduced the use of phosphorus (P) 32-labeled erythrocytes for the determination of blood volume in patients. While a variety of radiolabels have been used in the past, Tc-99m has gained widespread use for imaging due to its ready availability, low cost, and ideal imaging energy. Technetium-99m-labeled autologous red blood cells are routinely used for the noninvasive evaluation of cardiac function, the localization of gastrointestinal bleeding sites, the splenic imaging, and the determination of total red blood cell mass.

Red blood cells labeled with 99mTc are also useful to constitute a suitable intravascular agent for imaging of vascular tumors.

Methodological Aspects of Tc-99m Red Blood Cell Imaging

Although it is technetium in the +7 (pertechnetate) oxidation state that crosses the intact erythrocyte membrane, only technetium that has been reduced to a lower oxidation state will firmly bind hemoglobulin. It has been shown that in red blood cells labeled with Tc-99m, the majority (87%) of radioactivity was associated with the globulin chain of the hemoglobin molecule. Standardized kit formulations using stannous pyrophosphate as a reducing agent are available. Because of the ready availability of good quality commercial kits, enabling rapid and reliable erythrocyte labeling, this technique has greatly facilitated the clinical application of RBC labeling. Several methods have been employed to label red blood cells, including *in vivo*, *in vitro*, and a combination of these methods (Callahan and Bruce, 2006). The selection of the method of labeling red blood cells with Tc-99m depends on personal preference and the clinical indication. The modified *in vivo* method had highlabeling efficiency without the added efforts and risks associated with *in vitro* and *in vivo* techniques.

In vitro labeling of erythrocytes requires a 10–15 ml sample of blood. Stannous citrate is then added to provide ~ 1.5 µg of stannous ion and additionally to help prevent coagulation of the blood sample. After 5 min of gentle agitation, the syringe is centrifuged. The supernatant that contains any excess stannous ion is then discharged. The resultant packed red blood cells are then mixed with 15 to 30 mCi (550–1110 MBq) of Tc-99m pertechnetate. After another 5 min of gentle agitation, the mixture is considered properly incubated and is reinjected into the patient for subsequent imaging. An excellent labeling efficiency (98%) can be achieved by this technique (Walton, 1998). However, the increased time, blood handling, and radiation exposure for the technologists and the need for centrifuge have precluded clinical acceptance of the *in vitro* technique. When an *in vitro* technique is used for radiolabeling autologous red blood cells, a safe policy and procedures must be in place and implemented to ensure that administration of labeled cells to the wrong patient is prevented.

The *in vivo* labeling technique, as the name describes, takes place within the bloodstream. In this method, labeling is accomplished with two consecutive intravenous injections, first of cold stannous pyrophosphate (10 to 20 µg per kg) and then of 99mTc pertechnetate. The stannous ion is allowed to circulate for 30 min, which results in maximum uptake by the red blood cell. A dose of 15 to 30 mCi (550–1110 MBq) of Tc-99m pertechnetate is then injected intravenously. The red

blood cells will be labeled over the succeeding 5 to 10 min. The labeling efficiency of this method ranges from 85 to 95%. This technique has the advantage of being the easiest to perform because it is the least labor intensive and results in the lowest radiation exposure to personnel. However, the quality of images obtained with the *in vivo* method was often suboptimal (Murphy and Port, 2003).

The modified *in vivo* technique represents a compromise between the two previous methods. Increased labeling efficiency, compared with the *in vivo* technique, is achieved by tagging the red blood cells with Tc-99m pertechnetate outside the body, whereas less labor and exposure for the technologist is achieved by *in vivo* red blood cell preparation with stannous ion. In this technique stannous pyrophosphate solution containing ~ 1 mg of stannous chloride dihydrate is injected intravenously. It is important that sufficient time is allowed for distribution and clearance of extracellular stannous ion and pyrophosphate within the intravascular pool. After 20 to 30 min, 3–5 ml of blood are withdrawn into a shielded syringe containing 15 to 30 mCi (550–1110 MBq) of Tc-99m pertechnetate and 1 ml of acid-citrate-dextrose (ACD) solution. After 10 min of incubation, the red blood cells are reinjected (Murphy and Port, 2003). Compared with the *in vitro* method, this technique is less time consuming, but the tagging efficiency of 90 to 93%, is lower (Callahan *et al.*, 1982).

It is important that the Tc-99m is firmly and quantitatively bound to the cells and that this labeling persists *in vivo* during the imaging period. Some of the free circulating pertechnetate will be taken up by the thyroid, the kidneys, and the gastric mucosa. Such a distribution pattern results in lower blood-to-background activity ratios, poor detection of vascular abnormality, and images that may be difficult or impossible to interpret. In addition, a number of drugs and solutions interfere with RBC labeling through various mechanisms. (Adalet and Cantez, 1994). The following causes have been reported to induce suboptimal red blood cell labeling: (1) injection through a line containing heparin or dextrose, (2) inadequate administration of stannous ion, (3) prior intravenous iodinated radiographic contrast media (within 24 hr), (4) excess stannous ion, (5) decreased hematocrit, (6) use of initial technetium generator elution, (7) several blood pressure and cardiac drugs (hydralazine, prazosin, methyldopa, propranolol, digoxin, and quinidine), (8) oxidation of Tc-99m with exposure to air, and (9) cytotoxic, immunosuppressive, and antibiotic medications.

Radiation Dosimetry

For the adult, the usual administered activity is 15–30 mCi (555–1110 MBq) autologous red blood cells labeled with Tc-99m using the *in vivo*, modified *in vivo*, or *in vitro* techniques. The usual administered activity in children is 0.2–0.4 mCi/kg (7–15 MBq/kg) with a minimum dose of

2–4 mCi (70–150 MBq). Tc-99m-labeled red blood cells distribute within the blood pool, with an estimated volume of distribution of ~ 4–7% of body weight. The estimated biological half-life is approximately 24–30 hr. Mean organ doses received from Tc-99m red blood cells labeled *in vivo* were calculated by the MIRD method using biodistribution data reported in the literature. The effective total body radiation doses received from Tc-99m red blood cells labeled *in vivo* were found to be 0.0085 mSv/MBq for adults and 0.025 mSv/MBq for children. The organ receiving the largest radiation dose was found to be the heart (0.023 mGy/MBq for adults and 0.062 mGy/MBq for children), followed closely by the bladder and stomach (ICRP-53, 1987). Relatively high doses are also received by the blood, spleen, and lungs. Intermediate absorbed doses are received by the thyroid and kidneys, whereas organs with small blood concentrations and the remainder of the body receive the smallest doses. The major portion of the absorbed doses delivered to the stomach and the thyroid is due to the presence of free pertechnetate (Callahan and Bruce, 2006; Ponto, 1988).

The Potential Role of Tc-99m Red Blood Cell Imaging in the Management of Hemangioendothelioma

Although the differential diagnosis between hemangioma, hemangioendothelioma, and hemangiosarcoma is based on histopathologic findings, diagnostic imaging methods are essential for locating the lesions and also useful for orienting a possible surgical approach (Lai *et al.*, 1991). In the literature, only limited numbers of cases have been reported with imaging characteristics of hemangioendothelioma so far, and initial misdiagnosis is not uncommon due to unfamiliarity of the lesions. Although this is a relatively rare condition, advances in imaging modalities should lead to a prompt diagnosis of hemangioendothelioma and early initiation of treatment, which may reduce residual tumor and sequel. It is of paramount importance to correctly identify these vascular lesions, as biopsy of these lesions may lead to uncontrolled hemorrhage and has been reported to be fatal.

Anatomic imaging studies like radiography, US, CT, or MRI are quite effective diagnostic tools for locating hemangioendotheliomas. However, unusual features of numerous atypical forms of hemangiomatous lesions make diagnosis on anatomical images particularly difficult and thus multiple imaging studies are often necessary, even in referral centers, before a definitive diagnosis can be made. Moreover, MRI is superior to CT in characterizing soft tissue lesions, but even the MRI is unable to distinguish categorically hemangiomatous lesions from hypervascular metastasis (Yoon *et al.*, 2003). In this context, evaluation of these patients with Tc-99m-labeled red blood cells and combination with the

anatomical imaging allows correct identification and accurate differentiation from other benign or malign lesions. Clinical effectiveness of Tc-99m-labeled red blood cells is based on its ability to distribute primarily within the intravascular pool of the body and to leave this compartment at a slow rate. However, because all vascular tumors are fundamentally composed of blood-filled vascular channels, it is not possible to distinguish each other based on the imaging characteristics in Tc-99m red blood cell imaging. As the classic finding of hemangiomatous lesions on Tc-99m red blood cell imaging, a characteristic discordance has been described between the perfusion image and that of the pool because of the reduced flow and increased blood pool (Camarero *et al.*, 1999). This perfusion blood-pool mismatch, not encountered in other lesions, may help in the specific diagnosis of vascular tumor (Front *et al.*, 1984). However, decreased flow is not observed in small and/or deeply situated lesions, due to limited resolution of dynamic imaging. Also, dynamic imaging requires information regarding the location of lesion(s) before imaging. On the other hand, in contrast to findings in adult patients, the increased uptake in both the early and delayed phases on scintigraphic studies with Tc-99m-labeled red blood cells was reported in cases with infantile hemangioendothelioma in liver (Keslar *et al.*, 1993; Miller *et al.*, 1987; Gianni *et al.*, 1997; Park *et al.*, 1996). Therefore, although the perfusion characteristics of these lesions can vary, an increase in delayed blood-pool activity within the lesion is typical of hemangiomatous lesions, and only rarely do other hypervascular tumors (e.g., hepatocellular carcinoma) present a similar scintigraphic pattern (Swayne *et al.*, 1991). Rabinowitz *et al.* (1984) reported four cases of hepatocellular carcinoma that demonstrated increased activity on delayed images. In contrast to this report, Kudo *et al.* (1989) found no cases demonstrating increased activity on either planar or SPECT delayed images in a large series of hepatocellular carcinoma patients. On the other hand, Miller *et al.* reported four cases with hepatic tumors other than hemangiomatous lesion that have increased red blood cell activity when compared with the surrounding liver parenchyma, but none were equal to the heart blood pool in activity. They have suggested that using the activity of heart blood pool as a cut-off allows the accurate differentiation of infantile hemangioendothelioma from other lesions that are the major differential concern in children: hepatoblastoma, metastatic neuroblastoma, nodular hyperplasia, and fibromuscular hematoma.

The greatest problem in trying to better define and analyze the clinical effectiveness of Tc-99m-labeled red blood cells in the diagnosis of hemangioendothelioma is the availability of only relatively small case numbers. Based on the experience with hemangiomatous lesions, it appears that Tc-99m-labeled red blood cell scintigraphy provides the most specific, noninvasive method for making the diagnosis of vascular tumors, although the sensitivity varies depending on the imaging protocol, lesion size, and location. The sensitivity and specificity of Tc-99m-labeled red blood cell scintigraphy are ~ 70–80% and 100%, respectively, in the diagnosis of vascular tumors (Birnbaum *et al.*, 1990; Krause *et al.*, 1993). The sensitivity of this technique is significantly improved by single photon emission computed tomography (SPECT) imaging, although its diagnostic value is limited when lesions are smaller than 1 cm or are located in topographically unfavorable sites (Ziessman *et al.*, 1991; Birnbaum *et al.*, 1990). False-negative results have been reported in cases of hemangiomatous lesions with extensive thrombosis and/or fibrosis or in lesions smaller than 1.4 cm (Brant *et al.*, 1987; Ziessman *et al.*, 1991; Rabinowitz *et al.*, 1984). Based on the available information, red blood cell activity persists in the heart and major blood vessels, making detection of the activity related to small hemangiomatous lesions adjacent to these vascular structures difficult on SPECT images. Fusion imaging, combining functional information deriving from SPECT with the anatomical details of CT or MRI, can solve this problem, allowing the precise localization of sites of increased uptake. Schillaci *et al.* (2004) reported that hybrid imaging proved to be useful in the correct characterization of liver lesions located near the heart or major intrahepatic vessels, allowing accurate anatomical assessment of sites of increased blood-pool activity on SPECT images. SPECT-CT had a significant impact on results in 33.3% of the patients with lesions defined as indeterminate on SPECT images.

Based on our reported experience with RBC imaging in hemangioendothelioma, it appears that early diagnosis of hemangioendothelioma could be possible with a whole-body imaging technique, especially localized in deep soft tissue or bone even in asymptomatic parts of the body (Turkmen *et al.*, 2006). In this context, whole-body Tc-99m-labeled red blood cell imaging has potential for detecting these lesions, while anatomical imaging techniques generally can be used on limited and symptomatic parts of the body. Furthermore, the utilization of whole-body Tc-99m-labeled red blood cell imaging also allows a relatively noninvasive method of sequential monitoring of these patients during courses of therapy (Fig. 2). Treatment of this tumor should comprise wide surgical excision. Unfortunately, however, many lesions are technically difficult to resect and are prone to recur, especially in Kaposiform because of their widely infiltrative growth. In these patients as in our case, whole-body Tc-99m-labeled red blood cell imaging is an effective tool for follow-up.

Summary

Hemangioendothelioma is a rare vascular tumor of intermediate malignancy that commonly arises in soft tissues, liver, bone, and lung, and has a clinical course between that of a benign hemangioma and a malignant angiosarcoma. Clinical manifestation is nonspecific and variable. Most lesions are hypoechoic on sonography, hypodense on CT, hypointense on T1-weighted MR imaging, and hyperintense on T2-weighted MR imaging. But unusual features of numerous atypical forms of hemangioendothelioma make diagnosis of anatomical images particularly difficult, and conventional imaging methods with low specificity are only helpful in suggesting the diagnosis. Therefore, many published cases are initially misdiagnosed. Combining anatomic information with functional imaging is a powerful diagnostic tool for improved diagnosis of hemangioendothelioma, which can be applied to a combination of whole-body Tc-99m-labeled red blood cell imaging and MRI data.

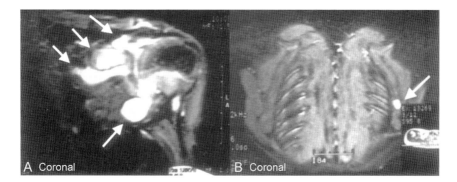

Figure 2 MRI scans of the left shoulder in patient with history of surgical resections of hemangioendothelioma located in the soft tissue of the left elbow revealed new foci localized in the soft tissue of the left shoulder and the left hemi-thorax lateral wall (**A** and **B**). Tc-99m red blood cell

(Continued)

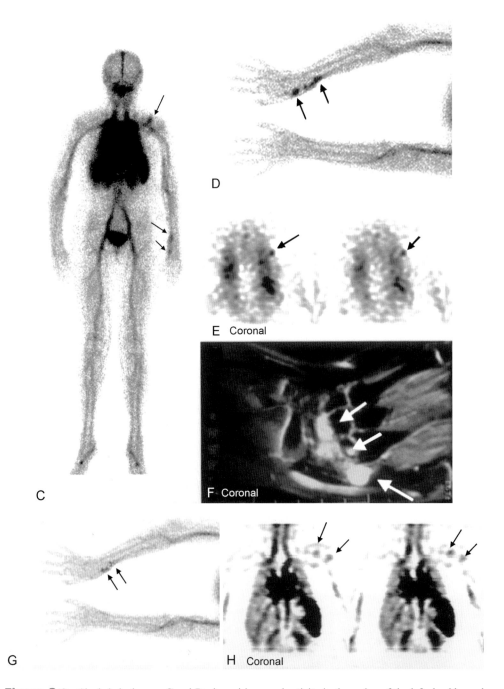

Figure 2 Cont'd whole-body scan **C** and **D**: showed increased activity in the region of the left shoulder and left wrist. After SPECT imaging, it was possible to identify more accurately the pathologic accumulation in the left hemi-thorax wall (**E**). The new foci revealed by scintigraphy in the left wrist confirmed by MRI (**F**), and according to the diagnostic imaging findings, she was reoperated on and lesions located in the left wrist and left shoulder were removed by surgical resection. Three months following the operation, Tc-99m red blood cell imaging was performed to evaluate the efficiency of surgical resection. It showed persistent increased activity in the regions of the left shoulder and left wrist (**G** and **H**). When we compared images with the first study, the size and intensity of the activities in the left shoulder and left wrist were decreased but had not disappeared.

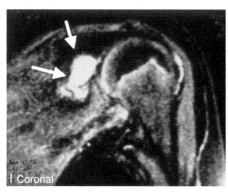
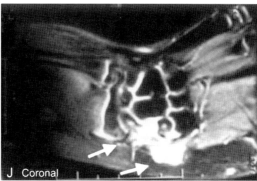

Figure 2 Cont'd: Repeated MR scans showed the lesions located in the left shoulder (**I**) and left wrist (**J**) corresponding with red blood cell imaging. (From Türkmen, C., Unal, S., Sanli, Y., and Kebudi, R. 2006. Technetium-99m red blood cell imaging of multicentric kaposiform hemangioendothelioma. *Eur. J. Nucl. Med. Mol. Imag. 33*:232–233. Copyright ©, with kind permission of Springer Science and Business Media).

References

Adalet, I., and Cantez, S. 1994. Poor-quality red blood cell labeling with Technetium-99m: case report and review of the literature. *Eur. J. Nucl. Med. 21*:173–175.

Alomari, AI. 2006. The lollipop sign: a new cross-sectional sign of hepatic epithelioid hemangioendothclioma. *Eur. J. Radiol. 59*:460–464.

Beaubien, E.R., Ball, N.J., and Storwick, G.S. 1998. Kaposiform hemangioendothelioma: a locally aggressive vascular tumor. *J. Am. Acad. Dermatol. 38*:799–802.

Birnbaum, B.A., Weinreb, J.C., Megibow, A.J., Sanger, J.J., Lubat, E., Kanamuller, H., Noz, M.E., and Bosniak, M.A. 1990. Definitive diagnosis of hepatic hemangiomas: MR imaging versus Tc-99m-labeled red blood cell SPECT. *Radiology 176*:95–101.

Brant, W.E., Floyd, J.L., Jackson, D.E., and Gilliland, J.D. 1987. The radiological evaluation of hepatic cavernous hemangioma. *JAMA 8*:2471–2474.

Callahan, R.J., and Bruce, A.D.P. 2006. Radiolabeling formed elements of blood: methods and mechanisms. In: Henkin, R.E., Boles, M.A., Dillehay, G.L., Halama, J.R., Karesh, S.M., Wagner, R.H., and Zimmer, A.M. (Eds.), *Nuclear medicine* (2nd ed). Philadelphia: Mosby-Year Book, pp. 407–412.

Callahan, R.J., Froelich, J.W., McKusick, K.A., Leppo, J., and Strauss, H.W. 1982. A modified method for the *in vivo* labeling of red blood cells with Tc-99m: concise communication. *J. Nucl. Med. 23*:315–318.

Camarero, A., Delgado, M., Lorente, R., Rayo, J.I., and Ramos, J.L. 1999. Multicentric epithelioidal hemangioendothelioma of bone: diagnostic imaging. *Clin. Nucl. Med. 24*:1002–1004.

Dail, D.H., Liebow, A.A., Gmelich, J.T., Friedman, P.J., Miyai, K., Myer, W., Patterson, S.D., and Hammar, S.P. 1983. Intravascular, bronchiolar, and alveolar tumor of the lung (IVBAT): an analysis of twenty cases of a peculiar sclerosing endothelial tumor *Cancer 51*:452–464.

Diaz, R., Segura, A., Calderero, V., Cervera, I., Aparicio, J., Jorda, M.V., and Pellin, L. 2004. Central nervous system metastases of a pulmonary epithelioid hemangioendothelioma. *Eur. Respir. J. 23*:483–486.

Fletcher, C.D. 2006. The evolving classification of soft tissue tumors: an update based on the new WHO classification. *Histopathology 48*:3–12.

Front, D., Israel, O., Groshar, D., and Weininger, J. 1984. Technetium-99m-labeled red blood cell imaging. *Semin. Nucl. Med. 14*:226–250.

Gianni, W., De, Vincentis, G., Graziano, P., Ierardi, M., Fimognari, F.L., Banci, M., Gazzaniga, P., Cacciafesta, M., Di, Tondo, U., Scopinaro, F., and Marigliano, V. 1997. Scintigraphic imaging of hepatic epithelioid hemangioendothelioma. *Digestion 58*:498–500.

ICRP-53. 1987. Radiation dose to patients from radiopharmaceuticals. A report of a Task Group of Committee 2 of the International Commission on Radiological Protection. *Ann. ICRP 18*:1–377.

Keslar, P.J., Buck, J.L., and Selby, D.M. 1993. From the archives of the AFIP. Infantile hemangioendothelioma of the liver revisited. *Radiographics 13*:657–670.

Krause, T., Hauenstein, K., Studier-Fischer, B., Schuemichen, C., and Moser, E. 1993. Improved evaluation of Technetium-99m-red blood cell SPECT in hemangioma of the liver. *J. Nucl. Med. 34*:375–380.

Kudo, M., Ikekubo, K., Yamamoto, K., Ibuki, Y., Hino, M., Tomita, S., Komori, H., Orino, A., and Todo, A. 1989. Distinction between hemangioma of the liver and hepatocellular carcinoma: value of labeled RBC-SPECT scanning. *Am. J. Roentgenol. 152*:977–983.

Lai, F.M., Allen, P.W., Yuen, P.M., and Leung, P.C. 1991. Locally metastasizing vascular tumor: spindle cell, epithelioid, or unclassified hemangioendothelioma? *Am. J. Clin. Pathol. 96*:660–663.

Lyburn, I.D., Torreggiani, W.C., Harris, A.C., Zwirewich, C.V., Buckley, A.R., Davis, J.E., Chung, S.W., Scudamore, C.H., and Ho, S.G. 2003. Hepatic epithelioid hemangioendothelioma: sonographic, CT, and MR imaging appearances *Am. J. Roentgenol. 180*:1359–1364.

Mac-Moune, Lai, F., To, K.F., Choi, P.C., Leung, P.C., Kumta, S.M., Yuen, P.P., Lam, W.Y., Cheung, A.N., and Allen, P.W. 2001. Kaposiform hemangioendothelioma: five patients with cutaneous lesion and long follow-up. *Mod. Pathol. 14*:1087–1089.

Miller, J.H. 1987. Technetium-99m-labeled red blood cells in the evaluation of hemangiomas of the liver in infants and children. *J. Nucl. Med. 28*:1412–1418.

Murphey, M.D., Fairbairn, K.J., Parman, L.M., Baxter, K.G., Parsa, M.B., and Smith, W.S. 1995. From the archives of the AFIP. Musculoskeletal angiomatous lesions: radiologic-pathologic correlation. *Radiographics 15*:893–917.

Murphy, P.B., and Port, S.C. 2003. Radionuclide evaluation of left ventricular function. In: Sandler, M.P., Coleman, E.R., Patton, J.A., Wackers, F.J. Th., and Gottschalk, A. (Eds.), *A Diagnostic Nuclear Medicine* (4th ed.). Philadelphia: Lippincott Williams & Wilkins, pp. 239–271.

Park, C.H., Hwang, H.S., Hong, J., and Pak, M.S. 1996. Giant infantile hemangioendothelioma of the liver: scintigraphic diagnosis. *Clin. Nucl. Med. 21*:293–295.

Ponto, J.A. 1988. Dosimetry of Technetium-99m red blood cells labeled *in vivo*. *Clin. Nucl. Med. 13*:342–344.

Rabinowitz, S.A., McKusick, K.A., and Straus, H.W. 1984. 99mTc red blood cell scintigraphy in evaluating focal liver lesions. *Am. J. Roentgenol. 143*:63–68.

Roos, J.E., Pfiffner, R., Stallmach, T., Stuckmann, G., Marincek, B., and Willi, U. 2003. Infantile hemangioendothelioma. *Radiographics* 23:1649–1655.

Schillaci, O., Danieli, R., Manni, C., Capoccetti, F., and Simonetti, G. 2004. Technetium-99m-labelled red blood cell imaging in the diagnosis of hepatic hemangiomas: the role of SPECT/CT with a hybrid camera. *Eur. J. Nucl. Med. Mol. Imaging. 31*:1011–1015.

Swayne, L.C., Diehl, W.L., Brown, T.D., and Hunter, N.J. 1991. False-positive hepatic blood pool scintigraphy in metastatic colon carcinoma. *Clin. Nucl. Med. 16*:630–632.

Turkmen, C., Unal, S., Sanli, Y., and Kebudi, R. 2006. Technetium-99m red blood cell imaging of multicentric kaposiform hemangioendothelioma. *Eur. J. Nucl. Med. Mol. Imaging 33*:232–233.

Walton, S. 1998. Radionuclide ventriculography. In: Murray, I.P.C., and Ell, P.J (Eds.), *Nuclear Medicine in Clinical Diagnosis and Treatment* (2nd ed.). Edinburgh: Churchill Livingstone, pp. 1319–1332.

Weiss, S.W., and Enzinger, F.M. 1995. *Soft Tissue Tumors* (3rd ed.). St. Louis: Mosby-Year Book.

Yoon, S.S., Charny, C.K., Fong, Y., Jarnagin, W.R., Schwartz, L.H., Blumgart, L.H., and DeMatteo, R.P. 2003. Diagnosis, management, and outcomes of 115 patients with hepatic hemangioma. *J. Am. Coll. Surg. 197*:392–402.

Ziessman, H.A., Silverman, P.M., Patterson, J., Harkness, B., Fahey, F.H., Zeman, R.K., and Keyes, J.W., Jr. 1991. Improved detection of small cavernous hemangiomas of the liver with high-resolution three-headed SPECT. *J. Nucl. Med. 32*:2086–2091.

3

Malignant Bone Involvement: Assessment Using Positron Emission Tomography/ Computed Tomography

Einat Even-Sapir

Introduction

Bone metastases are the most common malignant bone tumor. Skeletal involvement varies in different human malignancies, with breast cancer being the leading cause for bone metastases in women and prostate cancer in men, followed by lung cancer (Padhani and Husband, 1998). Bone is the first site of relapse in 50% of patients with breast cancer and in 80% of patients with prostate cancer (Clamp *et al.*, 2004).

The extent of tumor spread remains a principal predictor of clinical outcome and is a major determinant of treatment strategy in cancer patients. Cure by removal of the primary cancer is unlikely to be achieved in the presence of disseminated disease where adjuvant systemic therapy is indicated. This implies that rigorous detection of metastatic disease is required to ensure optimal staging and treatment (Rybak and Rosenthal, 2001; Maffioli *et al.*, 2004; Thurairaja *et al.*, 2004). In the past, treatment of bone metastases has focused on symptom control by using effective analgesics and palliative radiotherapy. However, in the last decade, with the introduction of bisphosphonate therapy, treatment of bone metastases has improved. Bisphosphonates are

pyrophosphate analogs that potently inhibit osteoclast-induced bone resorption and have proved highly effective in decreasing the incidence of skeletal-related complications (Clamp *et al.*, 2004). Many patients with bone metastases are asymptomatic, and metastases are only incidentally detected (Seregni *et al.*, 1993). Patients with metastatic disease mainly in bone tend to live longer than patients with visceral metastases. However, extended survival means that patients are more likely to develop complications as a result of bone metastases. Symptoms occur mainly when lesions increase in size with extensive bone destruction causing bone pain, hypercalcemia, or accompanying complications, which are of clinical relevance including pathologic fractures, vertebral collapse, epidural involvement, nerve root invasion, and spinal cord compression (Angtuaco *et al.*, 2004).

Various morphologic and functional imaging modalities are being used for assessment of malignant bone involvement. Imaging may be undertaken for screening in tumors, which have a high incidence of bone metastases or may be performed in symptomatic patients (Fogelman *et al.*, 2005). The purpose of imaging is to identify malignant bone involvement as early as possible, to determine the extent of the disease, to evaluate the presence of complications, to monitor response to therapy, and occasionally to guide biopsy (Padhani and Husband, 1998; Schirrmeister *et al.*, 1999; Rybak and Rosenthal, 2001; Hamaoka *et al.*, 2004).

Assessment of malignant bone involvement is a common indication for patients' referral to nuclear medicine. Various radiopharmaceuticals may be used for this goal, both single photon-emitting tracers detected by gamma cameras and positron-emitting tracers detected by positron emission tomography (PET) technology. Scintigraphic lesions often require further validation with a contemporaneous morphologic imaging modality, mainly CT. Recently, hybrid techniques composed of either SPECT or PET installed in the same gantry with CT became commercially available. Functional and anatomical data can be acquired in the same clinical setting without changing the patient positioning, with automatic generation of fused images, which combine data of both modalities (Even-Sapir, 2005).

SPECT and PET Imaging of Malignant Bone Involvement: Technological and Radiochemical Aspects

Detection of malignant bone involvement is based on either direct visualization of tumor infiltration or detection of bone reaction to the presence of malignant cells. It is, therefore, essential to understand the pathophysiology of metastatic spread to bone. Bone tissue consists of cortical, trabecular, and marrow components. Normally, the bone undergoes constant remodeling, maintaining a balance between osteoclastic (resorptive) and osteoblastic activities. Bone involvement by cancer usually occurs by hematogenous spread (Galasko, 1982; Hamaoka *et al.*, 2004). The venous system is the main pathway for transport of tumor cells to bone, which does not contain lymphatic channels (del Regato *et al.*, 1977). It is well established that the vertebral epidural and perivertebral veins play a significant role in the transport of cancer cells to the vertebral bone marrow (Yuh *et al.*, 1989). However, tumor may occasionally extend from disease in the neighboring soft tissue. The vast majority of bone metastases initiates as intramedullary lesions. Bone marrow micrometastases are viable cells with proliferative and tumorigenic potential. Therefore > 90% of bone metastases are found in the distribution of the red active marrow, which in adults is located in the axial skeleton (Kricun, 1985). The most common sites for metastatic spread in decreasing order are the vertebral column, pelvis, proximal femurs, skull, and upper extremities. In some tumor types, a predilection for specific sites is present, for example, pelvic bones in prostate and bladder cancer and peripheral long bones in lung cancer (Fogelman *et al.*, 2005). Tumor cells may destroy bone directly or produce mediators that stimulate reabsorption by osteoclasts (Roodman, 2004). As the metastatic lesion

enlarges within the marrow, the surrounding bone undergoes osteoclastic (resorptive) and osteoblastic (depositional) activity. Based on the balance between the two processes, the radiographic appearance of a bone metastasis may be lytic, sclerotic (blastic), or mixed. In general, rapidly growing aggressive tumors tend to be lytic, while sclerosis is considered to indicate slower tumor growth rate.

Sclerosis may also be a sign of repair following treatment (Padhani and Husband, 1998; Blake *et al.*, 2001). The incidence of lytic, blastic, and mixed types of bone metastases is different in various tumor types. Lytic lesions may be seen in almost all tumor types. Invariably, lytic lesions may be detected in bladder, kidney, and thyroid cancer and in multiple myeloma. Blastic lesions are frequently seen in prostate and breast cancers, occasionally in lung, stomach, pancreas, and cervix carcinomas, and infrequently in colorectal cancer (Padhani and Husband, 1998).

Detecting malignant bone involvement by the various imaging modalities either is based on direct visualization of tumor cells or reflects the secondary bone reaction to the presence of malignant cells. Among the tracers used in nuclear medicine for assessment of malignant bone involvement is ^{18}F-fluorodeoxyglucose (^{18}F-FDG), which directly accumulates in tumor cells and may therefore identify malignant bone involvement even at early stages when confined to the marrow before cortical bone reaction has occurred. In contrast, increased accumulation of ^{99m}Tc-MDP–methylene diphosphonate (the tracer used for bone scintigraphy) in bone metastases depends on the presence of secondary reactive osteoblastic changes (Blake *et al.*, 2001; Cook and Fogelman, 2001; Rohren *et al.*, 2004; Even-Sapir, 2005).

Imaging Using Single Photon-Emitting Tracers and Gamma Cameras

^{99m}Tc-MDP–methylene diphosphonate is the most commonly used bone tracer for detection of bone metastases with gamma cameras, identifying the bone reaction to the presence of malignant cells. The compound, which is an analog of pyrophosphate, is chemisorbed onto bone surface, and its uptake depends on local blood flow and osteoblastic activity. The focal accumulation of ^{99m}Tc-MDP in bone metastases is due to the increased osteoblastic reaction, commonly accompanying bone metastases. As little as 5 to 10% change in lesion to normal bone uptake ratio is required to detect bony lesions on bone scintigraphy preceding their detection on plain radiographs or CT by 2–18 months (Blake *et al.*, 2001). Based on these characteristics, bone scintigraphy (BS) with ^{99m}Tc-MDP is highly sensitive for the detection of osteoblastic-type metastases predominating in patients with prostate cancer and also seen in patients with breast or lung cancer. In the past, virtually all patients with newly diagnosed prostate, breast, or lung cancer underwent a baseline ^{99m}Tc-MDP-BS and then annual follow-up studies. This "automatic" referral of cancer patients to BS was possible through the wide availability of gamma cameras and the low cost of radio-pharmaceuticals. This approach, however, was abandoned in many places, and BS is indicated only in patients who are at high risk for bone metastases or have a clinical suspicion of malignant bone involvement. The past performance of BS in all cancer patients has, however, formed the grounds for our current knowledge on the incidence of bone metastases in the different disease stages (Smith *et al.*, 1999). Presently, the use of ^{18}F-FDG-PET whole-body imaging (which will be discussed later) in the routine imaging algorithm of various human malignancies may obviate in many patients the need to perform a separate bone scintigraphy.

The BS procedure was initiated as two-dimensional (planar) data. Later, with the introduction of single photon emission computerized tomography (SPECT) providing reconstructed data in three planes—transaxial, coronal, and sagittal—it became apparent that the latter technology improves the diagnostic accuracy of BS for detection of bone pathology. It was reported that SPECT detects 20 to 50% more lesions than planar BS and allows for a straigtforward comparison with other tomography-based techniques such as CT and MRI (Gates, 1998). The better localization of lesions by SPECT has been reported to improve the specificity of BS. In the vertebral column, for instance, different disease processes tend to involve different parts of the vertebra. Accurate localization of a scintigraphic lesion within the vertebra by SPECT has been reported to improve the specificity of ^{99m}Tc-MDP-BS, differentiating between benign and malignant sites of uptake (Even-Sapir *et al.*, 1993). However, SPECT has been limited, at least until recently, to a relatively localized skeletal region due to the fact that it considerably increased the study acquisition time. Only in the past year have novel software algorithms, which allow the performance of rapid multifield of view SPECT, become commercially available, transferring BS to the era of becoming a full tomographic procedure (Even-Sapir *et al.*, 2006).

Despite its favorable characteristics, ^{99m}Tc-MDP-BS, even when SPECT is performed, has some major limitations: it is insensitive for detection of early bone marrow involvement and is not as sensitive for detection of pure lytic metastases as it is for osteoblastic ones. It cannot accurately separate active malignant disease from the repair process as the latter is also associated with high bone turnover; therefore, it is of a limited value for monitoring response to therapy, and accumulation of ^{99m}Tc-MDP is not specific for malignancy and may be detected in other bone conditions associated with high bone turnover, including trauma, osteomyelitis, osteoporosis, metabolic bone disease, and degenerative changes. The detection of a solitary, or only a few bone lesions on BS, often indicates the need to further assess these lesions by correlating the scintigraphic abnormalities with a recent CT (Hamaoka *et al.*, 2004). Hybrid systems composed of gamma camera and CT are now commercially available. The latter systems will be discussed further in this chapter.

Imaging Using Positron-Emitting Tracers and Positron Emission Tomography

Positron emission tomography (PET) provides whole-body tomographic data and is characterized by a high-contrast resolution, and ability to perform absolute quantitation of tracer uptake (Figs. 1 and 2). Measurements of the regional skeletal kinetic parameters using compartmental modeling and nonlinear regression analysis have been reported to have a role in differentiating malignant from benign lesions as well as for monitoring response to therapy (Cook and Fogelman, 2001; Aoki *et al.*, 2001; Dimitrakopoulou-Strauss *et al.*, 2002; Rohren *et al.*, 2004). The number of PET devices has been rapidly growing, changing from being mainly a research tool into a routine modality in the imaging algorithm of oncologic patients. Positron emission tomography technology is based on the detection of a pair of annihilation photons produced when a positron (having the same mass as electrons and positively charged) is emitted from a radioisotope. Once produced, the positron gradually loses

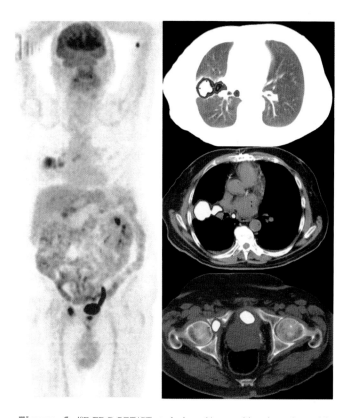

Figure 1 ^{18}F-FDG PET/CT study in a 64-year-old male patient with non-small cell lung carcinoma. On the left, a PET overview. On the right, three fused PET/CT images detecting increased ^{18}F-FDG uptake in the primary lung lesion (top image), in hilar and infracarinal-involved lymph nodes (middle image) and in a lytic bone metastasis at the right acetabulum (lower image). Tumoral lesions are marked by a red sign. Due to the presence of remote metastases, surgical removal of the primary lung cancer was denied.

kinetic and annihilates with the production of two photons, which leave the annihilation site in opposite directions and hit simultaneously two opposite detectors in the ring surrounding the body. These photons represent the distribu-

tion of radiotracer in the body. This instrumentation has improved because its development and the system resolution for clinical imaging may reach 4–5 mm (Rohren *et al.*, 2004).

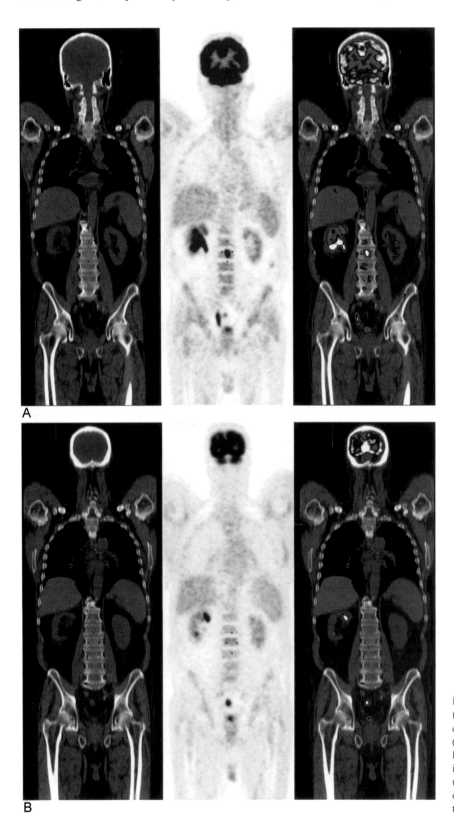

Figure 2 ^{18}F-FDG PET/CT baseline study (**A**) and follow-up study after chemotherapy (**B**) in a 56-year-old male patient with non-Hodgkin's Lymphoma. (**A**) At diagnosis, from left to right, coronal CT, PET, and fused PET/CT images illustrate early bone involvement represented as a focal site of increased uptake on the PET data with normal appearing bone on CT. (**B**) After a successful therapy, PET reverted to normal.

Two main PET tracers are clinically used for assessment of malignant bone involvement: ^{18}F-fluorodeoxyglucose (^{18}F-FDG), which is the most commonly used tracer for detection of both soft tissue and bone tumor sites, and the specific bone-seeking agent, ^{18}F-fluoride.

[18]F-Fluorodeoxyglucose (^{18}F-FDG)

As a glucose analog, [18]FDG gains entry into cells by glucose membrane transporter proteins and is overexpressed in many tumor cells. It is then trapped within tumor cells in which dephosphorylation is slow. The normal red marrow demonstrates a low-intensity [18]FDG uptake. Increased marrow uptake may suggest the presence of early bone marrow malignant involvement prior to an identifiable bone reaction, therefore, preceding the detection of early metastases by BS and CT (Fig. 2). Although ^{18}F-FDG-PET has been reported to be appropriate for detecting all types of bone metastases, there are data suggesting that ^{18}F-FDG-PET is more sensitive in detecting lytic-type metastases than in detecting sclerotic ones. It is assumed that the avidity of ^{18}F-FDG in lytic metastases reflects the high glycolitic rate and the relative hypoxia characterizing this type of metastases, while sclerotic metastases are relatively acellular, less aggressive, not prone to hypoxia, and therefore show lower or no ^{18}F-FDG avidity (Cook *et al.*, 1998; Burgman *et al.*, 2001).

Detection of bone metastases by ^{18}F-FDG-PET may be affected by therapy. Detection of both soft tissue and bone metastases with ^{18}F-FDG-PET is highly susceptible to previous chemotherapy. Performance of ^{18}F-FDG-PET soon after chemotherapy (less than two weeks apart) may result in metabolic shutdown of the tumor cells and a false-negative PET study. At different time points after radiotherapy, bone included in the radiation field may show increased, normal, or reduced ^{18}F-FDG uptake compared to the neighboring bone. Treatment with granulocyte colony stimulating factors (GCSF) may induce a diffusely increased FDG uptake in the marrow, which can mask malignant infiltration (Sugawara *et al.*, 1998; Clamp *et al.*, 2004). A recognized effect of anti-estrogen therapy, which is commonly applied in patients with breast cancer, is the "flare" reaction. This phenomenon is presumed to reflect an initial agonist effect of the drug before its antagonist effect supervenes. Clinically, it may be difficult to differentiate a "flare" reaction from disease progression in patients with bone-dominant metastatic disease (Mortimer *et al.*, 2001). Bone scintigraphy may show "new" sites that are actually responsive lytic lesions undergoing a repair process. "Flare phenomenon" can also be seen on ^{18}F-FDG-PET. Dehdashti *et al.* (1999) have reported an increase in ^{18}F-FDG uptake in responsive patients, as early as 10 days after initiation of tamoxifen treatment, compared with several weeks required to make this assessment on the basis of clinical presentation.

Though not a tumor-specific tracer, [18]FDG-PET is less hampered by nonmalignant uptake in benign bone lesions compared with BS. However, false-positive increased ^{18}F-FDG uptake may be detected in benign lesions, mainly in the presence of histiocytic or giant cells, which play a major role in the host response to injury and infection, with energy predominantly supplied by intracellular glucose metabolism. Among the benign lesions reported as showing increased [18]FDG uptake, osteoblastoma, brown tumor, aneurysmal bone cyst, sarcoidosis, recent trauma, and osteomyelitis may be found (Cook *et al.*, 1996; Aoki *et al.*, 2001).

Generally, uptake of ^{18}F-FDG is higher in malignant bone lesions than in benign lesions, but overlap does exist (Aoki *et al.*, 2001). Compartmental modeling for evaluation of the full ^{18}F-FDG kinetics may assist in differentiating malignant from benign bone lesions in special occasions (Dimitrako-poulou-Strauss *et al.*, 2002). With the use of hybrid PET/CT, the benign nature of the PET lesions may be discerned (Metser *et al.*, 2005; Even-Sapir, 2005).

[18]F-Fluoride

In contrast with [18]FDG that is valuable in detecting both soft tissue and bone abnormalities, ^{18}F-fluoride, which was first introduced by Blau *et al.* (1962), is a PET bone-seeking agent with an uptake mechanism similar to that of the single photon-emitting tracer, ^{99m}Tc-MDP. Fluoride ions exchange with hydroxyl groups in hydroxyapetite crystal bone to form fluoroapatite and are deposited at the bone surface where bone turnover is greatest. Similarly to ^{99m}Tc-MDP, accumulation of ^{18}F-fluoride uptake in bone metastases reflects increased regional blood flow and high bone turnover. ^{18}F-fluoride has better pharmacokinetic characteristics compared to those of ^{99m}Tc-MDP. The bone uptake of the former is twofold higher, and in contrast with ^{99m}Tc-MDP, it does not bind to protein. The capillary permeability of ^{18}F-fluoride is higher, and its blood clearance is faster, resulting in a better target-to-background ratio. Regional plasma clearance of ^{18}F-fluoride was reported to be 3–10 times higher in bone metastases than that in normal bone (Blake *et al.*, 2001; Cook and Fogelman, 2001).

[18]F-fluoride-PET is a highly sensitive modality for detection of bone abnormalities, taking advantage of both the high performance of PET technology and the favorable characteristics of ^{18}F-fluoride. Although, as mentioned above, the mechanism of uptake of ^{18}F-fluoride depends on bone turnover, it is very sensitive for detecting not only osteoblastic metastases but also lytic metastases, as the latter even when considered "pure lytic" do have minimal osteoblastic activity, which is enough for detection by ^{18}F-fluoride-PET. ^{18}F-fluoride-PET is therefore an optimal modality for detection of both blastic- and lytic-type bone metastases (Schirrmeister *et al.*, 1999a,b, 2001; Cook and Fogelman, 2001; Even-Sapir *et al.*, 2004, 2006).

As in the case with ^{99m}Tc-MDP, ^{18}F-fluoride is not tumor-specific and accumulates excessively in benign bone lesions. Because of its high sensitivity, ^{18}F-fluoride-PET is prone to a higher false-positive rate by detecting nonmalignant lesions, including those that are usually not detected by ^{99m}Tc-MDP-BS, such as uncomplicated small cysts (Even-Sapir et al., 2004). It is not possible to differentiate benign from malignant lesions based on the intensity of ^{18}F-fluoride uptake (Cook and Fogelman, 2001). Lesions detected on ^{18}F-fluoride-PET therefore require correlation with CT and/or MRI for further validation (Schirrmeister et al., 1999a,b). The use of novel hybrid PET/CT systems has significantly improved this limited specificity of ^{18}F-fluoride PET, as the CT part of the study allows morphologic characterization of the scintigraphic lesion and accurate separation between benign lesions and metastases.

We performed ^{18}F-fluoride-PET/CT studies in 44 cancer patients and found a statistically significant improvement in the specificity of ^{18}F-fluoride-PET/CT (97%) compared with ^{18}F-fluoride-PET alone (72%). The high sensitivity of ^{18}F-fluoride-PET was reflected by the detection of increased ^{18}F-fluoride uptake in 16 bone metastases with normal CT appearance and in 4 patients who had a false-negative BS. ^{18}F-fluoride-PET/CT was also found valuable in suggesting the cause of bone pain in symptomatic patients by detecting relevant benign bone lesions and by detecting, on the CT part of the study, a soft tissue tumor mass invading the sacral foramen (Even-Sapir et al., 2004).

Due to its higher cost and lower availability, ^{18}F-fluoride-PET is not a routine imaging modality for detecting malignant bone involvement in spite of its high sensitivity. In most countries, ^{18}F-fluoride-PET is not reimbursed by the insurance companies. The clinical added value of this modality taking into consideration the results of cost-effective analysis is yet to be determined. At present, ^{18}F-fluoride-PET and, more recently, PET/CT are reserved for patients who are at high risk for bone metastases, particularly if the more routinely used modality is ^{99m}Tc-MDP-BS or if ^{18}F-FDG-PET seems to be inaccurate or inconclusive (Langsteger et al., 2006; Even-Sapir et al., 2006).

Functional-Anatomic Hybrid Imaging: SPECT-CT and PET-CT

Novel integrated systems composed of SPECT or PET (functional) and CT (anatomic), installed in a single gantry, have been recently introduced in routine clinical practice. Data of the two modalities are acquired at the same clinical setting, without changing the patient positioning, allowing for generation of fused images on which each lesion is characterized by its tracer uptake (SPECT or PET) and morphologic appearance (CT). The CT part of hybrid imaging may range from low-dose nondiagnostic CT to full-dose multislice diagnostic CT with IV contrast injection (Keidar et al., 2003; Antoch et al., 2003).

The number of hybrid functional-anatomic systems used in clinical practice is growing fast. The relative ease by which the fused data are obtained has made it a diagnostic tool, and many experts refer to hybrid imaging as a novel imaging concept. Image quality of the PET or SPECT data may be improved using CT maps for attenuation correction. Accumulated data from many recently published reports suggest improvement in the diagnostic accuracy of PET/CT imaging compared to PET alone or even to side-by-side reading of PET and CT performed separately (Lardinois et al., 2003; Kostakoglu et al., 2004; Metser et al., 2005). The presence of bone metastases may be hampered by nearby physiologic uptake sites. For instance, it is difficult to detect skull metastases due to the high physiologic ^{18}F-FDG uptake in the adjacent brain cortex. This limitation may be overcome with SPECT/CT or PET/CT, where physiologic and pathologic sites of uptake can be differentiated based on accurate localization of the scintigraphic abnormality using the CT data as anatomic guidelines (Kostakoglu et al., 2004).

There are several SPECT and PET tracers, including ^{131}Iodine, ^{111}In-somatostatin, ^{67}Ga-citrate (SPECT tracer), and ^{18}F-FDG (a PET tracer), which may identify soft tissue and bone tumor sites (Keidar et al., 2003). SPECT/CT and PET/CT may assist in localizing the scintigraphic abnormality to the correct tissue, that is, being a soft tissue or skeletal metastasis. It was previously reported that bone lesions that showed increased ^{18}F-FDG uptake were misinterpreted as located in soft tissue, thus yielding a falsely low calculated sensitivity for ^{18}F-FDG-PET in detecting bone metastases (Nakamoto et al., 2003).

SPECT/CT and PET/CT have been found to improve the specificity of ^{99m}Tc-MDP, ^{18}F-FDG-PET, and ^{18}F-fluoride-PET, which may accumulate in access to not only in tumor sites but also in benign bone lesions. In a previous report by Metser et al. (2004), on the clinical added value of ^{18}F-FDG-PET/CT in detecting malignant bone involvement in the spine compared with ^{18}F-FDG-PET alone, the latter was incorrect in determining the level of abnormality in 15% of lesions and in determining the part of the vertebra involved in 18% lesions. The CT part of the PET/CT study was found to be valuable in identifying complications, including epidural involvement and neural foramen invasion, and was reported to occur in ~ 10% of vertebral metastases. These complications require an early diagnosis and treatment prior to the development of permanent neurological deficits (Spuentrup et al., 2001).

PET/CT can be used for radiotherapy planning. The CT information obtained from this instrument can be used for the purpose of volume planning, and the PET data can be used to better delineate the tumor margins. Ultimately, a more rational approach to radiotherapy planning is an achievable goal by PET/CT (Ell, 2006).

Monitoring Response of Bone Metastases to Therapy

Malignant bone involvement is considered unmeasurable. Determining complete or partial response can be difficult. Even when clinical complete remission has been achieved, "normalization" of bone may be delayed after the disappearance of other soft tissue sites of the disease. Moreover, bone may remain morphologically abnormal even when the disease is "burnt out." Radiotracers whose accumulation reflects high bone turnover (i.e., ^{99m}Tc-MDP and ^{18}F-fluoride) are inadequate for accurate assessment of therapy response, as both viable bone metastasis and repair process are associated with increased bone turnover and may appear similar. Moreover, a recognized effect of antihormonal therapy, which is commonly applied in patients with breast and prostate cancer, is the "flare" reaction (Mortimer *et al.*, 2001). This phenomenon is presumed to reflect an initial agonist effect of the drug before its antagonist effect. Clinically, in patients with bone-dominant metastatic disease, it may be difficult to differentiate a "flare" reaction from disease progression. Bone scintigraphy may show "new" sites that are actually responsive lytic lesions undergoing a repair process. Tracers, which detect malignant involvement by a direct visualization of the tumor tissue (such as ^{18}F-FDG), may be beneficial, as favorable response to therapy is manifested by decline in the intensity of ^{18}F-FDG uptake in the skeletal lesions. Reduction in ^{18}F-FDG uptake was reported to be in a good correlation with the clinical response and tumor markers in patients with bone-dominant disease (Stafford *et al.*, 2001).

Imaging of Bone Involvement in Common Human Malignancies

Solid Tumors

Breast Cancer

Bone is the most common site of metastases in breast cancer patients. Among patients with metastatic breast disease, bone is the first site of metastasis in 26–50% of patients and may develop in 30–85% of patients in the later course of the disease (Hamaoka *et al.*, 2004). The risk for bone involvement increases with disease stage from 0.8 to 2.6% in early stages (I and II) to 16.8 to 40.5% in advanced stages (III and IV) (Schirrmeister *et al.*, 1999b; Hamaoka *et al.*, 2004; Maffioli *et al.*, 2004). Bone scintigraphy, which is the most commonly used modality for detection of bone metastases, is indicated in patients with advanced disease or when bone involvement is clinically suspected and is no longer recommended in asymptomatic patients with early-stage cancer (Smith *et al.*, 1998; Maffioli *et al.*, 2004).^{18}F-FDG-PET has been introduced recently in the imaging algorithms of patients with breast cancer, mainly those with infiltrating ductal type (Eubank and Mankoff, 2004). This modality permits the detection of both soft tissue and skeletal sites of breast cancer (Schirrmeister *et al.*, 2001a; Wahl, 2001).

Bone metastases of breast cancer may be lytic, sclerotic, or mixed in their radiographic appearance. Osteolytic lesions predominate but 15–20% of patients have osteoblastic lesions. These data have a direct impact on the sensitivity of the

various scintigraphic techniques in detecting bone metastases, as blastic and lytic lesions may differ in their tracer avidity (Hamaoka *et al.*, 2004; Langsteger *et al.*, 2006). Cook *et al.* (1998) reported a higher detection rate of bone metastases by ^{18}F-FDG-PET compared with BS in patients with breast cancer. The superiority of ^{18}F-FDG-PET was reflected mainly in the detection of bone metastases, which are predominantly lytic with only minimal osteoblastic reaction, overlooked on BS. Nakai *et al.* (2005) in a study of 89 patients with breast cancer, studied the sensitivity of ^{18}F-FDG-PET and BS for detection of bone metastases based on their morphologic CT appearance. While significantly superior to BS in detecting lytic, mixed-type metastases and lesions with no visible cortical changes (probably reflecting early marrow involvement), ^{18}F-FDG-PET was somewhat limited in depicting blastic metastases. Similar findings were reported by Abe *et al.* (2005), who compared the diagnostic accuracy of ^{18}F-FDG-PET and BS in detecting bone metastasis in 44 breast cancer patients. ^{18}F-FDG-PET was superior to BS in the detection of osteolytic lesions, but inferior in the detection of osteoblastic lesions. False-negative lesions of bone scintigraphy were mostly bone marrow metastases that were clearly detected by ^{18}F-FDG-PET. Lonneux *et al.* (2000), in their report on 33 patients also illustrated the superiority of ^{18}F-FDG-PET in detecting bone marrow infiltration.

In a prospective study on 80 patients who presented to Memorial Sloan-Kettering Cancer Center for operative treatment of breast cancer, Port *et al.* (2006) reported conventional imaging and ^{18}F-FDG-PET to be equally sensitive in diagnosing the presence of metastatic disease in patients with high-risk, operable breast cancer, but ^{18}F-FDG-PET generated fewer false-positive results. Conventional imaging studies resulted in a higher number of findings that generated additional tests and biopsies that ultimately had negative results (17% vs. 5% for PET). Moreover, in 5% of the study patients, accounting for 50% of patients with bone metastases, ^{18}F-FDG-PET imaging identified additional sites of disease, which affected treatment decisions.

In view of the favorable results of assessing the presence of malignant bone involvement with ^{18}F-FDG-PET, several authors have raised the question of whether performance of a separate BS is still indicated in patients with breast cancer, who undergo ^{18}F-FDG-PET study. The somewhat lower sensitivity of ^{18}F-FDG-PET in detecting sclerotic-type metastases has encouraged some authors to recommend complementary use of BS and ^{18}F-FDG-PET for optimizing the detection of both sclerotic and lytic-type metastases (Eubank and Mankoff, 2004; Nakai *et al.*, 2005). The use of hybrid PET-CT imaging in a single setting now simplifies this issue. Sclerotic lesions overlooked by the PET part of the study can be clearly identified by the CT data. On this basis, the high sensitivity of ^{18}F-FDG-PET in detecting marrow and lytic lesions and the high sensitivity of CT in detecting sclerotic lesions may be complementary, similar to the complementary role of BS and ^{18}F-FDG-PET performed separately (Even-Sapir, 2005).

After successful therapy, patients with bone metastases may show response and disease stabilization. A major role of follow-up imaging techniques is to accurately monitor response to therapy separating active metastasis from bone repair. Monitoring response to anti-estrogen therapy in breast cancer patients is particularly difficult owing to the "flare" reaction characterized clinically by pain and erythema in soft tissue lesions and increased pain in bone lesions (Mortimer et al., 2001). Bone scintigraphy has a major drawback for monitoring the response of bone metastases to treatment, as detection of higher-intensity uptake or increase in the number of lesions on follow-up BS does not unequivocally represent disease progression. Paradoxically, this pattern may, in fact, indicate an early good response to therapy when pure lytic lesions that were overlooked by a baseline BS become detectable once associated with the repair process.

A potential advantage of ^{18}F-FDG-PET is in the assessment of response to therapy given the direct mechanism of ^{18}F-FDG uptake, which is related to tumor cell activity rather than to the osteoblastic reaction. Serial ^{18}F-FDG-PET studies seemed more accurate than serial BS in treatment control of patients with bone metastases (Gallowitsch et al., 2003). A change in ^{18}F-FDG uptake has been reported to be valuable in indicating "flare." The change in ^{18}F-FDG uptake may be detected as early as 10 days after initiation of treatment compared with the several weeks that are often required to make this assessment on the basis of clinical symptoms (Dehdashti et al., 1999; Stafford et al., 2001).

Prostate Cancer

Prostate cancer is the most common malignancy in men. Accurate staging of newly diagnosed prostate cancer, including the assessment of malignant bone involvement, is essential for guiding treatment. Early accurate detection or exclusion of bone metastasis is extremely important in order to allow correct selection of patients with localized disease for radical curative treatments, prevent patients who bear metastasis from undergoing unnecessary radical therapies, and, conversely, select patients who may benefit from treatment of early bone metastasis (Thurairaja et al., 2004). As the disease evolves, patients may experience biochemical progression, local recurrence, or metastatic spread. The most frequent sites of metastasis are lymph nodes and bone; 90% of patients who die of prostate cancer harbor bone metastases (Gomez et al., 2004). The extent of osseous metastatic disease from prostate cancer is an independent prognostic factor (Riguad et al., 2002).

Patients with prostate cancer are categorized at diagnosis as low-risk or high-risk patients based on clinical nomograms, which include prostate-specific-antigen (PSA) levels and Gleason score at biopsy and clinical stage (Fricke et al., 2003; Schoder and Larson, 2004). Low-risk patients

are unlikely to have metastatic bone involvement. Therefore, the routine use of BS for primary staging in all newly diagnosed prostate cancer patients is no longer recommended. This method, which is the most commonly used modality for detecting bone metastases, is now reserved for patients with high-risk cancer and in clinically or laboratory suspected disease, including elevated serum alkaline phosphatase levels, bone pain, or equivocal bone lesions on CT (Schoder and Larson, 2004; Fogelman et al., 2005).

Although bone metastases of prostate cancer are of osteoblastic type, the results of recent reports raise some doubts as to whether BS is as effective for confirming metastatic bone disease as was previously perceived (Schirrmeister et al., 1999a, 2001b). The role of ^{18}F-FDG, the most commonly used PET tracer in oncologic patients, seems to be limited in detecting metastases of prostate cancer. It has been speculated that glucose utilization of prostate tumor cells is not enhanced significantly compared to normal cells and that prostate cancer cells may have an alternative source of energy supply. A large fraction of prostate cancer possesses a relatively low metabolic rate (Schoder and Larson, 2004; Jana and Blaufox, 2006). Another disadvantage of ^{18}F-FDG is the overlap in uptake intensity in prostate cancer and in benign prostate conditions, such as hyperplasia (Oyama et al., 1999). More recent publications have suggested that [18]FDG-PET is not an unsuitable modality in selected patients with prostate cancer, particularly those with a poorly differentiated subtype (Morris et al., 2002; Fricke et al., 2003; Oyama et al., 2004). The diagnostic accuracy of ^{18}F-FDG-PET in patients with prostate cancer is still a controversial issue.

Other PET tracers, including [11]C- or ^{18}F-labeled choline, acetate, and ^{18}F-fluorodihydrotestosterone, have been suggested for assessment of both soft tissue and bone metastases in patients with prostate cancer (Schoder and Larson, 2004; Jana and Blaufox, 2006; Langsteger et al., 2006). Choline is incorporated by conversion into phosphorylcholine, which is a component of the cell membrane; because tumor cells duplicate quickly, synthesis of the cell membrane is also rapid and therefore associated with increased choline accumulation. Choline may be labeled by [18]F (half-life of 110 min) or [11]C (half-life of 20 min) (Schmid et al., 2005). Acetate uptake in tumor cells is proportional to lipid synthesis (Swinnen et al., 2003). Accumulation of labeled acetate in prostate cancer cells reflects the increased fatty acid synthesis and overexpression of the enzyme fatty acid synthase characterizing these cells (Swinnen et al., 2003). ^{18}F-fluorodihydrotestosterone is an analog of dihydrotestosterone, a ligand of the androgen receptor, which plays an important role in the proliferation of prostate cancer. Preliminary published data offer encouraging results on its clinical use in staging and re-staging of patients with prostate cancer (Larson et al., 2004).

As mentioned earlier, ^{18}F-fluoride is a highly sensitive PET tracer for detection of bone metastases. Schirrmeister et al.

(1999a,b, 2001a,b) reported the superiority of ^{18}F-fluoride-PET for detection of bone metastases over BS in patients with various human malignancies, including prostate cancer. In a recent publication by our group, BS (planar and SPECT acquisitions) and ^{18}F-fluoride PET/CT were performed on the same day in patients with high-risk prostate cancer. ^{18}F-fluoride-PET imaging, taking advantage of the better performance of PET technology combined with the better pharmacokinetic characteristics of ^{18}F-fluoride, resulted in a better sensitivity for lesion detection on both patient-based and lesion-based analysis compared with ^{99m}Tc-MDP planar and SPECT/BS. As a PET/CT hybrid system was used, the morphology of sites, which showed increased ^{18}F-fluoride uptake, was automatically correlated with the CT data, separating benign from malignant sites of uptake with high specificity. Moreover, early bone metastases were clearly detected by ^{18}F-fluoride-PET, while CT showed a falsely normal-appearing bone. In this series, detection of bone metastasis solely by ^{18}F-fluoride-PET/CT indicated initiation of androgen withdrawal and bisphosphonate therapy and warranted withholding radiotherapy in newly diagnosed patients. In advanced hormone refractory cases, such findings warranted chemotherapy. On the other hand, a negative ^{18}F-fluoride-PET/CT study, also in the presence of equivocal finding on other imaging modalities and despite adverse clinical parameters, allowed us to offer radiotherapy or radical prostatectomy with a curative intent to high-risk patients, who otherwise would be managed in a palliative approach. Although ^{18}F-fluoride-PET/CT is not yet a routine procedure, based on these findings we feel that it might be valuable to exploit its high sensitivity and specificity in selected patients with prostate cancer where the presence of bone metastasis cannot be definitely confirmed or equally excluded by other imaging modalities (Even-Sapir et al., 2006).

The monitoring response of bone metastases to therapy remains a challenge in prostate cancer. As previously mentioned, ^{99m}Tc-MDP and ^{18}F-fluoride are not useful for monitoring response to therapy, as tumor progression and bone repair may present similarly. The use of ^{18}F-FDG for monitoring the response of prostate cancer metastases to therapy is limited to those cases characterized by ^{18}F-FDG avidity (Oyama et al., 2001; Morris et al., 2002). This approach was reported beneficial, particularly in poorly differentiated tumors and in patients with androgen-independent cancer (Kurdziel et al., 2003). Other studies reported a decline in the intensity of ^{18}F-fluorodihydrotestosterone and ^{18}F-choline as indicating a favorable response to therapy. These are, however, preliminary observations that require further validation in larger series (Jana and Blaufox, 2006).

Lung Cancer

Prognosis of patients with non-small cell lung carcinoma (NSCLC) depends on the stage of the disease and the ability to completely remove the tumor. Bone metastases are diagnosed at initial presentation in 3.4–60% of patients with

NSCLC. Bone pain is usually considered an indicator of skeletal metastases. However, up to 40% of lung cancer patients with proven bone metastases are asymptomatic (Bury et al., 1998; Lardinois et al., 2003).

Before the era of ^{18}F-FDG-PET, the staging algorithm of patients with NSCLC included CT of the thorax through the liver and adrenals, CT and/or MRI of the brain, and BS. Inconclusive bony lesions identified on BS were further assessed by CT, MRI, or even biopsy (Schirrmeister et al., 2001b). Recently, ^{18}F-FDG-PET and PET-CT were reported valuable in assessing the presence of soft tissue and bone spread in patients with NSCLC, obviating the need to perform a separate BS (Lardinois et al., 2003; Rohren et al., 2004) (Fig. 1). Investigating 110 consecutive patients with NSCLC, Bury et al. (1998) reported ^{18}F-FDG-PET to be superior to BS in detecting bone metastases, with accuracy of 96% and 66% for each of the modalities, respectively. ^{18}F-FDG-PET was reported to be of higher positive-predictive value and lower false-positive rate compared with BS.

Hematological Malignancies

Lymphoma

In recent years, ^{18}F-FDG-PET has become a routine imaging modality for staging and for monitoring response to therapy in patients with lymphoma, replacing in many centers the role of ^{67}Ga scintigraphy in these patients. ^{18}F-FDG-PET may detect early marrow infiltration, and is therefore highly sensitive for assessment of early bone involvement in lymphoma (Moog et al., 1999). Lymphoma involvement is commonly marrow-based. Bone marrow involvement is found at presentation in ~ 50–80% of the patients with low-grade Non-Hodgkin Lymphoma (NHL), 25–40% of high-grade NHL, and 5–14% of Hodgkin's Disease (HD) at diagnosis, reaching 32% later in the course of the disease. Pakos et al. (2005) performed a meta-analysis of the literature on the issue of the ability of ^{18}F-FDG-PET to evaluate bone marrow infiltration in the staging of lymphoma. Thirteen studies with a total of 587 patients were enrolled. Comparing PET findings with those on bone marrow biopsy (BMB) showed that the calculated sensitivity and specificity of ^{18}F-FDG-PET were 51% and 91%, respectively. However, some of the patients in whom positive PET findings were considered false positive due to negative BMB marrow turned out to be true positive when repeat biopsy was carried out using the positive PET site to guide the optimal biopsy site. Subgroup analysis showed a sensitivity of PET in assessing marrow involvement in patients with HD and in aggressive types of NHL.

When interpreting a baseline ^{18}F-FDG-PET study prior to therapy, a pattern of heterogeneous patchy marrow activity should raise the suspicion of marrow lymphomatous involvement. A pattern of diffuse uptake, mainly in HD, is more commonly associated with reactive hematopoietic changes or myeloid hyperplasia (Carr *et al.*, 1998). As neither bone marrow biopsy nor imaging using ^{18}F-FDG-PET or MRI is completely reliable as a single technique, their complementary usage was suggested by Kostakoglu and Goldsmith (2000) for assessment of marrow involvement in lymphoma patients. After chemotherapy and/or following granulocyte colony-stimulating factors (G-CSF), assessment of activity of disease in the marrow by ^{18}F-FDG-PET after therapy (mainly chemotherapy and the administration of granulocyte colony stimulating factors—GCSF) is hampered by the resemblance between active lymphoma infiltration and reactive marrow changes and by the effect chemotherapy and GCSF have on distribution of the tracer in the marrow (Cook *et al.*, 1996; Clamp *et al.*, 2004; Kazama *et al.*, 2005). Diffusely increased splenic uptake often accompanies G-CSF stimulated marrow uptake and was therefore suggested as a "clue" for the correct diagnosis (Sugawara *et al.*, 1998).

^{18}F-FDG-PET is also more sensitive than CT alone for detecting early lymphomatous bone involvement. When performing ^{18}F-FDG-PET/CT, unexpected bone involvement may be identified by increased ^{18}F-FDG uptake with normal CT appearance when bone involvement is early, prior to identifiable bone destruction (Fig. 2). The delay in detecting lymphomatous bone involvement on CT reflects its relatively low sensitivity in assessing malignant marrow infiltration and the fact that detection of a malignant bone involvement on CT depends on the presence of considerable bone destruction (Padhani and Husband, 1998).

Primary bone involvement occurs in 3–5% of patients with non-Hodgkin's Lymphoma (NHL). Secondary bone involvement occurs in up to 25% of them. Primary bone involvement is rare in Hodgkin's disease (HD). Secondary bone involvement occurs in 5–20% of patients with HD during the course of the disease but in only 1–4% at presentation (Baar *et al.*, 1999; Guermazi *et al.*, 2001). Moog *et al.* (1999) have reported ^{18}F-FDG-PET to be more sensitive and specific than ^{99m}Tc-MDP bone scintigraphy for detection of osseous involvement of lymphoma. Lymphomatous bone involvement is the result of hematogeneous spread or direct extension from adjacent soft tissue disease. Bone involvement upstages disease to stage 4 and is indicative of an aggressive disease with a poor outcome unless it is an extension of disease from adjacent soft tissue disease. Then, bone involvement does not alter staging. It is, therefore, of clinical relevance in accurately separating the two conditions when interpreting ^{18}F-FDG-PET/CT. On the CT part of study, the radiographic features of bone lymphoma are nonspecific. Lymphoma lesions may appear on CT to be predominantly osteolytic but may also be sclerotic or mixed (Edeiken-Monroe *et al.*, 1990; Guermazi *et al.*, 2001). A valuable contribution of the CT data of PET/CT in lymphoma patients is that it allows for identification of vertebral collapse, the presence of soft tissue paravertebral masses, epidural masses, or neural foramen invasion, and complications, that may accompany vertebral disease more commonly in lymphoma patients requiring special attention and appropriate therapy (Guermazi *et al.*, 2001; Metser *et al.*, 2004).

Multiple Myeloma

Multiple myeloma (MM) is a clonal B-lymphocyte neoplasm of plasma cells accounting for 10% of hematologic malignancies. The hallmark of this malignancy is the presence of a monoclonal protein, M protein, produced by the abnormal plasma cells, in the blood and/or urine. The effect of abnormal plasma cells is that of excessive bone resorption and inhibition of bone formation (Bataille and Horoosseau, 1997; Terpos *et al.*, 2005).

In the past, the X-ray (XR) has been the primary imaging modality for detecting bone changes in MM and is included in the Durie-Salmon clinical staging criteria of MM. This imaging modality is, however, of only limited sensitivity for detection of bone involvement because ~ 50% bone destruction must be present for radiographic bone lesion to be detectable. Computerized tomography (CT) is a more sensitive tool for detecting the bone-destructive effects of MM (Avva *et al.*, 2001). Because myeloma lesions tend to be predominantly lytic, BS is considered less sensitive than XR and CT, overlooking almost half of the abnormal sites of disease identified radiographically (Woolfenden *et al.*, 1980). Scintigraphic abnormalities associated with myeloma may appear as "cold" lesions or sites of increased ^{99m}Tc-MDP uptake, mainly when fractures are present. Soft tissue uptake may be detected in association with calcification within a plasmocytoma or secondary amyloidosis (Angtuaco *et al.*, 2004).

Myelomatous marrow involvement precedes bone destruction and experience with modalities, which can identify early marrow involvement, including MRI and ^{18}F-FDG-PET, is now evolving. Magnetic resonance imaging (MRI) has been used in patients with MM for assessing of the actual tumor burden in the marrow and the presence of accompanying complications. Spinal compression fractures caused by bone destruction or by a mass may occur in 55–70% of patients with MM (Schmidt *et al.*, 2005). The image features of MM on MRI, however, may not be specific, resembling other disease processes such as reactive marrow changes or increased hematopoiesis. The use of ^{18}F-FDG-PET in patients with MM is accumulating. Durie *et al.* (2002) assessed the role of ^{18}F-FDG-PET in 66 patients with MM and monoclonal gamopathy of undetermined significance (MGUS). Their results suggested that a positive ^{18}F-FDG-PET can reliably detect active MM, while a negative study strongly supports the diagnosis of MGUS. In a series of 43 patients, Schirrmeister *et al.* (2002) reported a sensitivity of 93% for detection of osteolytic MM by ^{18}F-FDG-PET. This system has been reported to identify unexpected medullary and extramedullary sites of disease missed by XR, CT, or BS (Durie *et al.*, 2002; Schirrmeister *et al.*, 2002). Detection of extramedullary sites of disease and residual ^{18}F-FDG uptake on follow-up study after stem-cell transplantation were shown to be poor prognostic factors (Durie *et al.*, 2002). In a recent report by Nanni *et al.* (2006) on 28 patients with MM, ^{18}F-FDG-PET/CT and MRI of the spine were shown to have a complementary role. While the former modality detected more lesions, all of which were located outside the field of view of MRI, the latter modality was found to be superior to ^{18}F-FDG PET-CT in diagnosing an infiltrative pattern in the spine. The authors therefore suggested a complementary use of the two modalities in the staging of MM. In another recent report by Mahfouz *et al.* (2005), ^{18}F-FDG-PET was found valuable in detecting infection in patients with MM. Of 248 myeloma patients, 165 infections were identified in 143 patients, including musculoskeletal-related infections (i.e., discitis, osteomyelitis, septic arthritis, and cellulitis). Based on ^{18}F-FDG-PET findings, work-up and therapy were modified in 55 cases. Twenty cases of infection were silent but clinically relevant. These ^{18}F-FDG-PET findings in patients with MM may also be relevant in other immunosuppressed conditions.

In conclusion, ^{18}F-FDG, the most commonly used PET tracer, is a glucose analog that directly identifies tumor tissue characterized by high metabolic activity. It is, therefore, sensitive for detection of early bone marrow involvement prior to any identifiable bone changes. It is highly sensitive for detection of lytic-type bone metastases and somewhat less so for detection of osteoblastic metastases. The introduction of ^{18}F-FDG-PET in the imaging algorithms of various human malignancies often obviates the need to perform a separate bone scintigraphy for assessment of bone involvement. In ^{18}F-FDG-avid tumors, successful therapy is represented by a decline in the intensity of ^{18}F-FDG uptake. ^{18}F-fluoride is a bone-seeking PET tracer. Although its uptake depends, similarly to ^{99m}Tc-MDP used for bone scintigraphy, on regional blood flow and osteoblastic activity, the better spatial resolution of PET and the favorable pharmacokinetic characteristics of ^{18}F-fluoride make ^{18}F-fluoride-PET a highly sensitive modality for detecting both lytic and blastic lesions, but it is not yet a routine procedure and is therefore reserved for selected high-risk patients.

Novel hybrid systems composed of PET and CT allow for acquisition of both modalities at the same clinical setting and the generation of fused functional-anatomical images. This novel imaging technique has been found to improve the diagnostic accuracy of the scintigraphic techniques in detecting malignant bone involvement.

References

Abe, K., Sasaki, M., Kuwabara, Y., Koga, H., Baba, S., Hayashi, K., Takahashi, N., and Honda, H. 2005. Comparison of 18FDG-PET with 99mTc-HMDP scintigraphy for the detection of bone metastases in patients with breast cancer. *Ann. Nucl. Med. 19*:573–579.

Angtuaco, E.J.C., Fassas, A.B.T., Walker, R., Sethi, R.H., and Barlogie, B. 2004. Multiple myeloma: clinical review and diagnostic imaging. *Radiology 231*:11–23.

Antoch, G., Vogt, F.M., Freudenberg, L.S., Nazaradeh, F., Goehde, S.C., Barkhausen, J., Dahmen, G., Bockisch, A., Debatin, J.F., and Ruehm, S.G. 2003. Whole-body dual-modality PET/CT and whole-body MRI for tumor staging in oncology. *JAMA 290*:3199–3206.

Aoki, J., Watanabe, H., Shinozaki, T., Takagishi, K., Ishijima, H., Oya, N., Sato, N., Inoue, T., and Endo, K. 2001. FDG PET of primary benign and malignant bone tumors: standardized uptake value in 52 lesions. *Radiology 219*:774–777.

Avva, R., Vanhemert, R., Barlogie, B., Munshi, N., and Angtuaco, E.J. 2001. CT guided biopsy of focal lesions in patients with multiple myeloma may reveal new and more aggressive cytogenetic abnormalities. *Am. J. Neuro. Radiol. 22*:781–785.

Baar, J., Burkes, R.L., and Gospodarowicz, M. 1999. Primary non-Hodgkin's Lymphoma of bone. *Semin. Oncol. 26*:270–275.

Bataille, R., and Harousseau, J.L. 1997. Multiple myeloma. *N. Engl. J. Med. 336*:1657–1664.

Blake, G.M., Park-Holohan, S.J., Cook, G.J., and Fogelman, I. 2001. Quantitative studies of bone with the use of ^{18}F-fluoride and ^{99m}Tc-methylene diphosphonate. *Semin. Nucl. Med. 31*:28–49.

Blau, M., Nagler, W., and Bender, M.A. 1962. A new isotope for bone. *Scan. Nucl. Med. 3*:332–334.

Burgman, P., Odonoghue, J.A., Humm, J.L., and Ling, C.C. 2001. Hypoxia-induced increase in FDG uptake in MCF7 cells. *J. Nucl. Med. 42*:170–175.

Bury, T., Barreto, A., Daenen, F., Barthelemy, N., Ghaya, B., and Rigo, P. 1998. Fluorine-18 deoxyglucose positron emission tomography for the detection of bone metastases in patients with non-small cell lung cancer. *Eur. J. Nucl. Med. 25*:1244–1247.

Carr, R., Barrington, S.F., Madan, B., O'Doherty, M.J., Saunders, C.A.B., Jvan der Walt, J., and Timothy, A.R. 1998. Detection of lymphoma in bone marrow by whole-body positron emission tomography. *Blood 91*:3340–3346.

Clamp, A., Danson, S., Nguyen, H., Cole, D., and Clemons, M. 2004. Assessment of therapeutic response in patients with metastatic bone disease. *Lancet Oncol. 5*:607–616.

Cook, G.J., Fogelman, I., and Maisey, M.N. 1996. Normal physiological and benign pathological variants of 18-fluoro-2-deoxyglucose positron-emission tomography scanning: potential for error interpretation. *Semin. Nucl. Med. 26*:308–314.

Cook, G.J., Houston, S., Rubens, R., Maisey, M.N., and Fogelman, I. 1998. Detection of bone metastases in breast cancer by ^{18}FDG PET: differing metabolic activity in osteoblastic and osteolytic lesions. *J. Clin. Oncol. 16*:3375–3379.

Cook, G.J., and Fogelman, I. 2001. The role of positron emission tomography in skeletal disease. *Semin. Nucl. Med. 31*:50–61.

Dehdashti, F., Flanagan, F.L., and Mortimer, J.E. 1999. Positron emission tomographic assessment of "metabolic flare" to predict response of metastatic breast cancer to antiestrogen therapy. *Eur. J. Nucl. Med. 26*:51–56.

del Regato, J.A. 1977. Pathways of metastatic spread of malignant tumors. *Semin. Oncol. 4*:33–38.

Dimitrakopoulou-Strauss, A., Strauss, L.G., Heichel, T., Wu, H., Burger, C., Bernd, L., and Ewerbeck, V. 2002. The role of quantitative ^{18}F-FDG PET studies for the differentiation of malignant and benign bone lesions. *J. Nucl. Med. 43*:510–518.

Durie, B.G.M., Waxman, A.D., D'Agnolo, A., and Williams, C.M. 2002. Whole-body ^{18}F-FDG PET identifies high-risk myeloma. *J. Nucl. Med. 43*:1457–1463.

Edeiken-Monroe, B., Edeiken, J., and Kim, E.E. 1990. Radiologic concepts of lymphoma of bone. *Radiol. Clin. North. Am. 28*:841–864.

Ell, P.J. 2006. The contribution of PET/CT to improved patient management. *Br. J. Radiol. 79*:32–36.

Eubank, W.B., and Mankoff, D.A. 2004. Current and future uses of positron emission tomography in breast cancer imaging. *Semin. Nucl. Med. 34*:224–240.

Even-Sapir, E., Martin, R.H., Barnes, D.C., Pringle, C.R., Iles, S.E., and Mitchell, M.J. 1993. Role of SPECT in differentiating malignant from benign lesions in the lower thoracic and lumbar vertebrae. *Radiology 187*:193–198.

Even-Sapir, E., Metser, U., Flusser, G., Zuriel, L., Kollender, Y., Lerman, H., Lievshitz, G., Ron, I., and Mishani, E. 2004. Assessment of malignant skeletal disease: initial experience with 18F-fluoride PET/CT and comparison between 18F-fluoride PET and 18F-fluoride PET/CT. *J. Nucl. Med. 45*:272–278.

Even-Sapir, E. 2005. Imaging of malignant bone involvement by morphologic, scintigraphic, and hybrid modalities. *J. Nucl. Med. 46*:1356–1367.

Even-Sapir, E., Metser, U., Mishani, E., Lievshitz, G., Lerman, H., and Leibovitch, I. 2006. The detection of bone metastases in patients with high-risk prostate cancer: 99mTc-MDP planar bone scintigraphy, single- and multi-field-of-view SPECT, 18F-fluoride PET, and 18F-fluoride PET/CT. *J. Nucl. Med. 47*:287–297.

Fogelman, I., Cook, G., Israel, O., and Van der Wall, H. 2005. Positron emission tomography and bone metastases. *Semin. Nucl. Med. 35*:135–142.

Fricke, E., Machtens, S., Hofmann, M., van den Hoff, J., Bergh, S., Brunkhorst, T., Meyer, G.J., Karstens, J.H., Knapp, W.H., and Boerner, A.R. 2003. Positron emission tomography with 11C-acetate and 18F-FDG in prostate cancer patients. *Eur. J. Nucl. Med. Mol. Imag. 30*:607–611.

Galasko, C.S. 1982. Mechanisms of lytic and blastic metastatic disease of bone. *Clin. Orthop. 169*:20–27.

Gallowitsch, H.J., Kresnik, E., Gasser, J., Kumnig, G., Igerc, I., Mikosch, P., and Lind, P. 2003. F-18 fluorodeoxyglucose positron-emission tomography in the diagnosis of tumor recurrence and metastases in the follow-up of patients with breast carcinoma: a comparison to conventional imaging. *Invest. Radiol. 38*:250–256.

Gates, G.F. SPECT bone scanning of the spine. 1998. *Semin. Nucl. Med. 28*:78–94.

Gomez, P., Manoharan, M., Kim, S.S., and Soloway, M.S. 2004. Radionuclide bone scintigraphy in patients with biochemical recurrence after radical prostatectomy: when is it indicated? *Br. J. Urol. Int. 94*:299–302.

Guermazi, A., Brice, P., de Kerviler, E.E., Ferme, C., Hennequin, C., Meignin, V., and Frija, J. 2001. Extranodal Hodgkin disease: spectrum of disease. *Radiographics 21*:161–179.

Hamaoka, T., Madewell, J.E., Podoloff, D.A., Hortobagyi, G.N., and Ueno, N.T. 2004. Bone imaging in metastatic breast cancer. *J. Clin. Oncol. 22*:2942–2953.

Hricak, H., Schoder, H., Pucar, D., Lis, E., Eberhardt, S.C., Onyebuchi, C.N., and Scher, H.I. 2003. Advances in imaging in the postoperative patient with a rising prostate-specific antigen level. *Semin. Oncol. 30*:616–634.

Jana, S., and Blaufox, M.D. 2006. Nuclear medicine studies of the prostate, testes, and bladder. *Semin. Nucl. Med. 36*:51–72.

Kazama, T., Faria, S.C., Varavithya, V., Phongkitkarun, S., Ito, H., and Macapinlac, H.A. 2005. FDG PET in the evaluation of treatment for lymphoma: clinical usefulness and pitfalls. *Radiographics 25*:191–207.

Keidar, Z., Israel, O., and Krausz, Y. 2003. SPECT/CT in tumor imaging: technical aspects and clinical applications. *Semin. Nucl. Med. 33*:205–218.

Kostakoglu, L., and Goldsmith, S.J. 2000. Fluorine-18 fluorodeoxyglucose positron emission tomography in the staging and follow-up of lymphoma: is it time to shift gears? *Eur. J. Nucl. Med. 27*:1564–1578.

Kostakoglu, L., Hardoff, R., Mirtcheva, R., and Goldsmith, S.J. 2004. PET/CT fusion imaging in differentiating physiologic from pathologic FDG uptake. *Radiographics 24*:1411–1431.

Kotzerke, J., Volkmer, B.G., Neumaier, B., Gschwend, J.E., Hautmann, R.E., and Reske, S.N. 2002. Carbon-11 acetate positron emission tomography can detect local recurrence of prostate cancer. *Eur. J. Nucl. Med. Mol. Imag. 29*:1380–1384.

Kricun, M.E. 1985. Red-yellow marrow conversion: its effect on the location of some solitary bone lesions. *Skeletal Radiol. 14*:10–19.

Kurdziel, K.A., Figg, W.D., Carrasquillo, J.A., Huebsch, S., Whatley, M., Sellers, D., Libutti, S.K., Pluda, J.M., Dahut, W., Reed, E., and Bacharach, S.L. 2003. Using positron emission tomography 2-deoxy-2-[18F]fluoro-D-glucose, 11CO, and 15O-water for monitoring androgen independent prostate cancer. *Mol. Imaging Biol. 5*:86–93.

Langsteger, W., Heinisch, M., and Fogelman, I. 2006. The role of fluorodeoxyglucose, 18F-dihydroxyphenylalanine, 18F-choline, and 18F-fluoride in bone imaging with emphasis on prostate and breast. *Semin. Nucl. Med. 36*:73–92.

Lardinois, D., Weder, W., Hany, T.F., Kamel, E.M., Korom, S., Seifert, B., von Schulthess, G.K., and Steinert, H.C. 2003. Staging of non-small-cell lung cancer with integrated positron-emission tomography and computed tomography. *N. Engl. J. Med. 348*:2500–2507.

Larson, S.M., Morris, M., Gunther, I., Beattie, B., Humm, J.L., Akhurst, T.A., Finn, R.D., Erdi, Y., Pentlow, K., Dyke, J., Squire, O., Bornmann, W., McCarthy, T., Welchl, M., and Scher, H. 2004. Tumor localization of 16beta-(18)F-fluoro-5alpha-dihydrotestosterone versus (18)F-FDG in patients with progressive, metastatic prostate cancer. *J. Nucl. Med. 45*:366–373.

Lonneux, M., Borbath, I., Berliere, M., Kirkove, C., and Pauwels, S. 2000. The place of whole-body PET FDG for the diagnosis of distant recurrence of breast cancer. *Clin. Positron Imag. 3*:45–49.

Maffioli, L., Florimonte, L., Pagani, L., Butti, I., and Roca, I. 2004. Breast cancer: diagnostic and therapeutic options. *Eur. J. Nucl. Med. Mol. Imag. 31*(suppl 1):S143–S148.

Mahfouz, T., Miceli, M.H., Saghafifar, F., Stroud, S., Jones-Jackson, L., Walker, R., Grazziutti, M.L., Purnell, G., Fassas, A., Tricot, G., Barlogie, B., and Anaissie, E. 2005. 18F-fluorodeoxyglucose positron emission tomography contributes to the diagnosis and management of infections in patients with multiple myeloma: a study of 165 infectious episodes *J. Clin. Oncol. 23*:7857–7863.

Metser, U., Lerman, H., Blank, A., Lievshitz, G., Bokstein, F., and Even-Sapir, E. 2004. Malignant involvement of the spine: assessment by ^{18}F-fluorodeoxyglucose PET/CT. *J. Nucl. Med. 45*:279–284.

Metser, U., Golan, O., Levine, C.D., and Even-Sapir, E. 2005. Tumor lesion detection: when is integrated positron emission tomography/computed tomography more accurate than side-by-side interpretation of positron emission tomography and computed tomography? *J. Comput. Assist. Tomogr. 29*:554–559.

Moog, F., Kotzerke, J., and Reske, S.N. 1999. FDG PET can replace bone scintigraphy in primary staging of malignant lymphoma. *J. Nucl. Med. 40*:1407–1413.

Morris, M.J., Akhurst, T., Osman, I., Nunez, R, Macapinlac, H., Siedlecki, K., Verbel, D., Schwartz, L., Larson, S.M., and Scher, H.I. 2002. Fluorinated deoxyglucose positron emission tomography imaging in progressive metastatic prostate cancer. *Urology 59*:913–918.

Mortimer, J.E., Dehdashti, F., and Siegel, B.A. 2001. Metabolic flare: indicator of hormone responsiveness in advanced breast cancer. *J. Clin. Oncol. 19*:2797–2803.

Nakai, T., Okuyama, C., Kubota, T., Yamada, K., Ushijima, Y., Taniike, K., Suzuki, T., and Nishimura, T. 2005. Pitfalls of FDG-PET for the diagnosis of osteoblastic bone metastases in patients with breast cancer. *Eur. J. Nucl. Med. Mol. Imag. 32*:1253–1258.

Nakamoto, Y., Osman, M., and Wahl, R.L. 2003. Prevalence and patterns of bone metastases detected with positron emission tomography using F-18 FDG. *Clin. Nucl. Med. 28*:302–307.

Nanni, C., Zamagni, E., Farsad, M., Castelluccim P., Tosi, P., Cangini, D., Salizzoni, E., Canini, R., Cavo, M., and Fanti, S. 2006. Role of (18)F-FDG PET/CT in the assessment of bone involvement in newly diagnosed multiple myeloma: preliminary results. *Eur. J. Nucl. Med. Mol. Imag.* 2:1–7.

Oyama, N., Akino, H., Suzuki, Y., Kanamaru, H., Sadato, N., Yonekura, Y., and Okada, K. 1999. The increased accumulation of [¹⁸F]fluoro-deoxyglucose in untreated prostate cancer. *Jpn. J. Clin. Oncol.* 29:623–629.

Oyama, N., Akino, H., Suzuki, Y., Kanamaru, H., Ishida, H., Tanase, K., Sadato, N., Yonekura, Y., and Okada, K. 2001. FDG PET for evaluating the change of glucose metabolism in prostate cancer after androgen ablation. *Nucl. Med. Commun.* 22:963–969.

Oyama, N., Ponde, D.E., Dence, C., Kim, J., Tai, Y.C., and Welch, M.J. 2004. Monitoring of therapy in androgen-dependent prostate tumor model by measuring tumor proliferation. *J. Nucl. Med.* 45:519–525.

Padhani, A., and Husband, J. 1998. Bone metastases. In: Husband, J.E.S., and Reznek, R.H. (Eds.), *Imaging in Oncology*. Oxford, Isis Medical Media Ltd., pp. 765–787.

Pakos, E.E., Fotopoulos, A.D., and Ioannidis, J.P. 2005. 18F-FDG PET for evaluation of bone marrow infiltration in staging of lymphoma: a meta-analysis. *J. Nucl. Med.* 6:958–963.

Petren-Mallmin, M., Andreasson, I., Ljunggren, O., Ahlstrom, H., Bergh, J., Antoni, G., Langstrom, B., and Bergstrom, M. 1998. Skeletal metastases from breast cancer: uptake of F18-fluoride measured with positron emission tomography in correlation with CT. *Skelet. Radiol.* 27:72–76.

Port, E.R., Yeung, H., Gonen, M., Liberman, L., Caravelli, J., Borgen, P., and Larson, S. 2006. (18)F-2-fluoro-2-deoxy-D-glucose positron emission tomography scanning affects surgical management in selected patients with high-risk, operable breast carcinoma. *Ann. Surg. Oncol.* 13:677–684.

Rigaud, J., Tiguert, R., and Le Normand, L. 2002. Prognostic value of bone scan in patients with metastatic prostate cancer treated initially with androgen deprivation therapy. *J. Urol.* 168:1423–1426.

Roodman, G.D. 2004. Mechanisms of bone metastasis. *N. Engl. J. Med.* 350:1655–1664.

Rohren, E.M., Turkington, T.G., and Coleman, R.E. 2004. Clinical applications of PET in oncology. *Radiology* 231:305–332.

Rybak, L.D., and Rosenthal, D.I. 2001. Radiological imaging for the diagnosis of bone metastases. *Q. J. Nucl. Med.* 45:53–64.

Schirrmeister, H., Guhlmann, A., Elsner, K., Kotzerke, J., Glatting, G., Rentschler, M., Neumaier, B., Trager, H., Nussle, K., and Reske, S.N. 1999a. Sensitivity in detecting osseous lesions depends on anatomic localization: planar bone scintigraphy versus 18F PET. *J. Nucl. Med.* 40:1623–1629.

Schirrmeister, H., Guhlmann, A., Kotzerke, J., Santjohanser, C., Kuhn, T., Kreienberg, R., Messer, P., Nussle, K., Elsner, K., Glatting, G., Trager, H., Neumaier, B., Diederichs, C., and Reske, S.N. 1999b. Early detection and accurate description of extent of metastatic bone disease in breast cancer with fluoride ion and positron emission tomography. *J. Clin. Oncol.* 17:2381–2389.

Schirrmeister, H., Kuhn, T., Guhlmann, A., Santjohanser, C., Horster, T., Nussle, K., Koretz, K., Glatting, G., Rieber, A., Kreienberg, R., Buck, A.K., and Reske, S.N. 2001a. Fluorine-18 2-deoxy-2-fluoro-D-glucose PET in the preoperative staging of breast cancer: comparison with the standard staging procedures. *Eur. J. Nucl. Med.* 28:351–358.

Schirrmeister, H., Glatting, G., Hetzel, J., Nussle, K., Arslandemir, C., Buck, A.K., Dziuk, K., Gabelmann, A., Reske, S.N., and Hetzel, M.

2001b. Prospective evaluation of clinical value of planar bone scan, SPECT and 18F-labeled NaF PET in newly diagnosed lung cancer. *J. Nucl. Med.* 42:1800–1804.

Schirrmeister, H., Bommer, M., Buck, A.K., Muller, S., Messer, P., Bunjes, D., Dohner, H., Bergmann, L., and Reske, S.N. 2002. Initial results in the assessment of multiple myeloma using F-18 FDG PET. *Eur. J. Nucl. Med. Mol. Imag.* 29:361–366.

Schmid, D.T., John, H., Zweifel, R., Cservenyak, T., Westera, G., Goerres, G.W., von Schulthess, G.K., and Hany, T.F. 2005. Fluorocholine PET/CT in patients with prostate cancer initial experience. *Radiology* 235:623–628.

Schmidt, G.P., Schoenberg, S.O., Reiser, M.F., and Baur-Melnyk, A. 2005. Whole-body MR imaging of bone marrow. *Eur. J. Radiol.* 55:33–40.

Schoder, H., and Larson, S.M. 2004. Positron emission tomography for prostate, bladder, and renal cancer. *Semin. Nucl. Med.* 34:274–292.

Schoder, H., Herrmann, K., Gonen, M., Hricak, H., Eberhard, S., Scardino, P., Scher, H.I., and Larson, S.M. 2005. 2-[18F]fluoro-2-deoxyglucose positron emission tomography for the detection of disease in patients with prostate-specific antigen relapse after radical prostatectomy. Clin. *Cancer. Res.* 11:4761–4769.

Seregni, E., Agresti, R., Bombardieri, E., and Buraggi, G.L. 1993. Bone scintigraphy in breast cancer: a ten years follow up study. *J. Nucl. Biol. Med.* 37:57–61.

Smith, T.J., Davidson, N.E., Schapira, D.V., Grunfeld, E., Muss, H.B., Vogel, V.G. III, and Somerfield, M.R. 1998. American Society of Clinical Oncology 1998 update of recommended breast cancer surveillance guidelines. *J. Clin. Oncol.* 17:1080–1082.

Spuentrup, E., Buecker, A., Adam, G., van Vaals, J.J., and Guenther, R.W. 2001. Diffusion-weighted MR imaging for differentiation of benign fracture edema and tumor infiltration of the vertebral body. *Am. J. Roent.* 176:351–358.

Stafford, S.E., Gralow, J.R., and Schubert, E.K. 2001. Use of serial FDG-PET to measure the response of bone-dominant breast cancer to therapy. *Acad. Radiol.* 9:913–921.

Sugawara, Y., Fisher, S.J., Zasadny, K.R., Kison, P.V., Baker, L.H., and Wahl, R.L.1998. Preclinical and clinical studies of bone marrow uptake of fluorine-18-fluorodeoxyglucose with or without granulocyte colony-stimulating factor during chemotherapy. *J. Clin. Oncol.* 16:173–180.

Swinnen, J.V., Van Veldhoven, P.P., Timmermans, L., De Schrijver, E., Brusselmans, K., Vanderhoydonc, F., Van de Sande, T., Heemers, H., Heyns, W., and Verhoeven, G.J.V. 2003. Fatty acid synthase drives the synthesis of phospholipids partitioning into detergent-resistant membrane microdomains. *Biochem. Biophys. Res. Commun.* 302:898–903.

Terpos, E., Politou, M., and Rahemtulla, A. 2005. The role of markers of bone remodeling in multiple myeloma. *Blood Rev.* 19:125–142.

Thurairaja, R., McFarlane, J., Traill, Z., and Persad, R. 2004. State-of-the-art approaches to detecting early bone metastasis in prostate cancer. *Br. J. Urol. Int.* 94:268–271.

Wahl, R.L. 2001. Current status of PET in breast cancer imaging, staging, and therapy. *Semin. Roentgenol.* 36:250–260.

Woolfenden, J.M., Pitt, M.J., Durie, B.G., and Moon, T.E. 1980. Comparison of bone scintigraphy and radiography in multiple myeloma. *Radiology* 134:723–728.

Yuh, W.T., Zachar, C.K., Barloon, T.J., Sato, Y., Sickels, W.J., and Hawes, D.R. 1989. Vertebral compression fractures: distinction between benign and malignant causes with MR imaging. *Radiology* 172:215–218.

4

Bone Metastasis: Single Photon Emission Computed Tomography/ Computed Tomography

Daisuke Utsunomiya and Seiji Tomiguchi

Introduction

Nuclear medicine imaging provides excellent functional information on the region where anatomical change is present or not present. The anatomic information obtained from this technique is, however, generally quite limited. In contrast, computed tomography (CT) is an excellent anatomic imaging modality. Combination of the functional information from nuclear medicine imaging and the anatomic information from CT imaging can improve diagnostic capability and facilitate image interpretation.

The frequency with which bone metastases are detected varies considerably with the methodology used. Since the introduction of Technetium (Tc)-99m-based scan agents, bone scintigraphy has been the standard method for detecting bone metastases. Its excellent sensitivity makes it useful in screening for bone metastases. Tracer accumulates in the reactive new bone that is formed in response to the lesion. In addition, the amount of accumulation is sensitive to the level of blood flow. Thus, most metastatic lesions, especially osteoblastic lesions, show increased tracer uptake. Bone scintigraphy, however, suffers from a lack of specificity. Tracer accumulation may occur in any skeletal location with an elevated rate of bone turnover and thus may accompany trauma, infection, or arthropathy. The probability that an abnormal bone scan represents metastatic tumor is related to the number of abnormal foci. In a patient with multiple and randomly distributed foci of increased uptake and a known primary tumor, the scan suggests metastases. However, a small number of bone metastases is not rare in clinical practice. The precise anatomic localization of the tracer uptake may clarify the nature of the abnormality. Careful analysis of uptake pattern and intensity and the use of single photon emission computed tomography (SPECT) are helpful for making a correct diagnosis in some cases. However, reliable differentiation between malignant and benign uptake is often difficult because of the complex anatomy of skeletal system and lower spatial resolution of bone scintigraphy. On the other hand, CT has higher spatial resolution, but structural changes of early bone metastasis shown on CT are often subtle and difficult to assess without corresponding functional information. Combining functional and anatomic data should improve diagnostic accuracy. Obtaining functional and anatomic data on different devices, however, necessarily leads to errors in realignment because of the motion of patients, posture difference at imaging, or other effects. A robust mode for inherent registration between SPECT and high-resolution CT images is achieved by image fusion using a combined SPECT/CT system. Image fusion is an exciting area where there is the potential to positively influence patient management, particularly in the field of oncology. This chapter describes the principal and clinical applications of SPECT/CT for imaging bone metastases.

Bone Metastasis

Overview of Bone Metastasis

Bone metastases are unfortunately common and one of the most frequent causes of pain in cancer patients. They can also cause bones to break and high calcium levels in the blood (calcium is released from damaged bones). Bone metastases also cause other symptoms and complications that can lower the ability to maintain usual activities and lifestyle. Four kinds of solid tumors account for 80% of all patients with bone metastases: breast cancer and prostate, lung and renal carcinoma. The exact incidence of bone metastasis is unknown, but it is estimated that 350,000 people die with bone metastases annually in the United States (Mundy, 2002). Furthermore, once tumors metastasize to bone, they are usually difficult to cure: only 20% of patients with breast cancer are still alive five years after the discovery of bone metastasis (Coleman, 2001). Most bone metastases result from hematogenous dissemination of cancer cells. Micrometastases are present in the bone marrow in 25–75% of patients with common malignancies. The mechanism of development and growth of bone metastases is a multistep process that requires complex interactions between the metastatic cells and the tissue. During this process, several biochemical mediators are delivered, and bone resorption occurs. Besides molecular and biologic characteristics of both neoplastic and normal host cells, other factors may play a role in bone localization of malignant cells, such as the vascular ways of spreading, and the speed and amount of blood flow toward specific areas. Bone constitutes a well-defined microcompartment supplied primarily by the bloodstream. In this structure most bone marrow is found, where the particular capillary structures and the reduction of the blood speed may favor the seeding of metastatic cells. Vascular sinusoids are lined by endothelial cells, and they lack a basement membrane.

Types of Bone Metastasis

Metastases have been characterized as osteolytic or osteoblastic. This classification actually represents two extremes of a continuum in which dysregulation of the normal bone remodeling process occurs. Patients can have both osteolytic and osteoblastic metastasis. Most patients with breast cancer and renal carcinoma have predominantly osteolytic lesions. In addition, secondary formation of bone occurs in response to bone destruction. This reactive process makes it possible to detect osteolytic lesions by means of bone scintigraphy, which identifies sites of active bone formation. In contrast, the lesions in prostate cancer are predominantly osteoblastic. There is also increased bone resorption in the osteoblastic lesions of prostate cancer; thus agents that block bone resorption can decrease bone pain and the risk of pathologic fractures.

Therapy for Bone Metastasis

A close relationship exists between bone destruction and tumor growth. In a large, randomized, double-blind, placebo-controlled study of biphosphonates that block bone resorption, administration of this drug was associated with a decrease in both the incidence of bone metastasis and the death rate in patients with breast cancer who were at high risk for bone metastasis (Powles *et al.*, 2002).

Anticancer drugs and hormones are also used to control the tumor growth, reduce bone pain, and decrease the risk of skeletal fractures in patients. Anticancer agents are used to kill cancer cells throughout the body. Hormone therapy uses drugs to prevent hormones from forming or acting on cells to promote the cancer growth.

Radiation is useful in relieving pain and controlling the growth of tumor cells in the area of the bone metastasis. It may be used to prevent a fracture or as a treatment for spinal cord compression. Radiation therapy uses high-energy ionizing radiation to injure or destroy cancer cells. Typically, radiation is administered once a day in 10 treatments over a two-week period. The full effects of this treatment may take two to three weeks to occur. Side effects of radiation therapy may include skin changes in the area being treated and a temporary increase in symptoms of bone metastasis. Another type of radiation therapy, radiopharmaceutical therapy, involves injecting into a vein a beta-emitting radioactive substance such as strontium-89. This substance is attracted to areas of bone containing cancer. Providing radiation directly to the bone in this way destroys active cancer cells in the bone and can relieve symptoms. Two important side effects are decreased blood counts, with increased risk of bleeding, and rarely, leukemia.

Surgery for bone cancer is performed to prevent or to treat a bone fracture. It usually involves removing the tumor and stabilizing the bone to prevent a fracture. Metal rods, plates, screws, wires, nails, or pins may be surgically inserted to strengthen or provide structure to the bone damaged by metastasis.

Other treatments for bone metastases and their symptoms include physical therapy and drug and nondrug approaches to control pain. Many different drugs or combinations of drugs can be used to treat pain from bone metastases. The principal drug type used to treat bone metastases is the nonsteroidal anti-inflammatory agents that stop prostaglandins, which seem to be responsible for much of the bone pain. Non-drug approaches to managing pain include the use of heat and cold, relaxation techniques, and therapeutic beds or mattresses.

Technical Aspects for Single Photon Emission Computed Tomography/ Computed Tomography

Combining Single Photon Emission Computed Tomography/Computed Tomography

Combined SPECT/CT systems make use of a full diagnostic CT scanner in combination with a dual-headed gamma camera. Early work (Hasegawa et al., 1991) combined anatomical (CT) and functional (SPECT) by using a single material, high-purity germanium, as the detector for both modalities. The X-ray CT images were, in addition, used for generating attenuation correction maps to increase the accuracy of the gamma camera data. Their early work is important because, for the first time, it highlighted the possibility that a single device was capable of performing both anatomical and functional imaging. A dual-headed gamma camera system equipped with a low-power X-ray tube that rotates around the patient along with the gamma detectors was introduced in clinical use (Bocher et al., 2000). This X-ray-tube-based CT system, however, has poor performance, and the lower-resolution anatomical images may often be insufficient for image interpretation (Horger et al., 2004). In order to improve the quality of CT images, we have designed a SPECT/CT system that combines a gantry-free SPECT scanner with a high-performance multidetector row CT scanner (Fig. 1) (Utsunomiya et al., 2006). The two commercial devices are juxtaposed so that the CT imaging table can move with the patient directly into the SPECT scanner prior to CT scanning. Recently, the potential of SPECT/CT scanners has been recognized by the manufacturers of medical imaging equipment. Having the gamma camera and CT scanner on the same gantry allows straightforward fusion of the two data sets. The CT provides accurate anatomical localization of the functional information within the gamma camera scan. These combined scanners are suitable for assessing the bone lesions in cancer patients.

Technical Parameters in Bone Scintigraphy

Tc-99m-labeled polyphosphate, pyrophosphate, and diphosphonate were primarily used for bone scintigraphy. Polyphosphate and diphosphonate have slow clearance, and pyrophosphate is relatively unstable in vivo. These

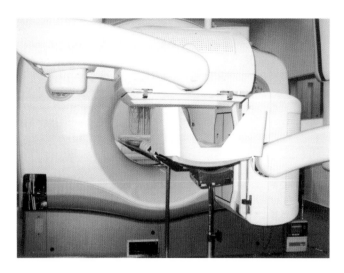

Figure 1 Photograph of the combined SPECT/CT system of Kumamoto University. SPECT and CT (MDCT) scanners are adjacent, which obviates repositioning the patient because the CT patient table extends into gantry-free SPECT system.

radiopharmaceuticals are, therefore, rarely used. Recently, Tc-99m-methylene diphosphonate (MDP) or Tc-99m-hydroxymethylene diphosphonate (HMDP) has been used for bone scintigraphy. After an intravenous injection, most of the injected dosage is localized in the skeleton. The remainder of the dose is distributed in soft tissue and plasma from which it is excreted slowly in the urine.

Whole-body planar bone imaging in the anterior and posterior positions is performed at about three hours following the injection of 555 MBq (15 mCi) of Tc-99m MDP or HMDP. Scintigraphic examinations are performed with dual-head detectors equipped with a low-energy, general-purpose, or high-resolution collimators. A magnification factor of 1.25 in a 64×64, or 128×128 matrix is used for SPECT data acquisition. Orbits of $360°$ are the norm for bone SPECT. The filtered backprojection (FBP) method has been used most commonly for SPECT image reconstruction in routine clinical practice. Iterative reconstruction (i.e., maximum-likelihood expectation-maximization [ML-EM] or ordered subsets estimation maximization [OSEM]) has been found to be more effective than classical FBP for bone SPECT because of its better ability to reconstruct low-count projection data. Attenuation correction of the radionuclide data is not routinely used in bone SPECT, although it has some efficacy in the cervical spine region. Reducing bladder activity before pelvic imaging is preferable to the many postacquisition solutions that have been proposed. On the basis of findings on planar scintigrams that show a small number of abnormal foci (four or less), SPECT and nonenhanced CT imaging are performed. SPECT scanning is a lengthy process, typically

10–15 min for one body region. Bone SPECT scanning is not appropriate for all cancer patients from the viewpoint of patient throughput and cost. SPECT scanning is not necessary for patients with no abnormal foci. Also, we suggest that SPECT scanning is not necessary for patients with multiple (five or more), randomly distributed foci of increased uptake of varying size, shape, and intensity because they are highly suggestive of bone metastases.

Technical Parameters in Computed Tomography

The following parameters are used for unenhanced CT scans: the tube voltage, 120 kV; the tube electric current, 140 mA; and 2.5 mm or less collimation for three-dimensional reconstruction. CT images are reconstructed with a standard reconstruction algorithm and a 512×512 matrix and 35–40 cm field-of-view. In assessing cervical spine, CT images are also used for photon attenuation correction. Contrast-enhanced CT scan is not routinely performed for assessing bone lesions.

Single Photon Emission Computed Tomography/Computed Tomography Image Fusion

Generally, image registration and fusion are performed using either software-based or hardware-based methods.

Software-based fusion enables the user to take two separate data sets acquired on two separate modalities at two different times and, by locating certain common features, fuse the images in space. Internal anatomical structures seen on both CT and bone SPECT images are used to determine the geometric transformation. Anatomical structures chosen as internal markers include the bones themselves, kidneys, and urinary tracts. Before the advent of combined SPECT/CT scanners, the registration could only be performed manually or using software-based methods. The manual approach takes considerable time and generally corrects for rigid misalignment only. In many instances, the labor-intensive procedure of registering images acquired on separate scanners limits the applicability of that approach. Furthermore, the skeletal system is complex and flexible, and thus fusion of SPECT and CT images on separate modalities at two different times may often lead to registration error.

Hardware-based methods include the hybrid combined scanners. Combined SPECT/CT scanners perform image registration "mechanically" by performing the two scans successively while minimizing patient movement through the use of a common couch and the appropriate "sliding" of one scan with respect to another. Although sophisticated image fusion software exists, the convenience, for both patient and physician, of imaging anatomy and function in a single scan cannot be overemphasized.

Clinical Applications for Single Photon Emission Computed Tomography/ Computed Tomography Fusion

When compared with planar bone imaging in a variety of clinical settings, SPECT can produce an increase in lesion detectability. However, differentiation between bone metastasis and benign lesion may often be difficult using bone scintigraphy alone. Correlation of SPECT and CT or magnetic resonance imaging (MRI) is necessary for determining the specific region and anatomical change of such indeterminate lesions. Fused SPECT and CT imaging is best for the purpose. A combined SPECT/CT system provides rigorous registration of functional and anatomical information.

Diagnosis on Bone Scintigraphy

Bone metastases do not affect all the bones with the same pattern and frequency, but, generally, they prefer the spine, pelvis, and proximal bones of the extremities. The distinction of benign from malignant lesions often depends on identifying the pedicle and determining whether its uptake is abnormal in association with a vertebral body lesion. Malignant lesions are more frequent when scan changes are seen in the pedicle, in the vertebral body with the extension to the pedicle, in central parts of the body, in the entire vertebra, and in cold lesions with a marginal increased uptake. The location of lesions on SPECT images provides useful information to help with differentiating between benign and malignant lesions. The determination of SPECT imaging, however, is often insufficient for the precise localization of bone lesions (e.g., facet joint vs. pedicle; femoral head vs. hip joint). Thus, bone scintigraphy often requires correlation with anatomical imaging techniques such as CT or MRI in order to increase the specificity of scintigraphic findings.

Diagnosis on Computed Tomography

CT scanning alone has a limited impact on the clinical detection of skeletal metastases. Although CT is more sensitive than conventional radiography for detecting lytic or sclerotic bone lesions, it is a cumbersome tool for screening the entire skeleton. CT can detect metastases within bone marrow before bone destruction has occurred. Tumor within the marrow causes an increase in attenuation due to fat replacement. An attenuation difference of more than 20 Hounsfield Units between right and left extremities is considered abnormal. Such findings are, however, subtle and easily overlooked.

Advantages of Single Photon Emission Computed Tomography/Computed Tomography for Differentiation of Benign and Malignant Lesions

SPECT/CT fusion provides increased diagnostic confidence in differentiating between malignant and benign bone lesions when analyzing the findings of scans performed in cancer patients. After additional review of fused scintigraphic and CT images, approximately 20% of all abnormal tracer uptake lesions are reclassified correctly as benign or malignant (Utsunomiya *et al.*, 2006). Fused images facilitate the differentiation of benign from metastatic foci that are difficult to differentiate on scintigraphic and CT images viewed side by side. In our receiver operating characteristic (ROC) analysis in which reviewers scored the degree of confidence as to whether a site of abnormal radiotracer uptake represented a bone metastasis, the areas under the ROC curve were 0.59–0.77 for scintigraphic images, 0.83–0.89 for separate data sets of scintigraphic and CT images, and 0.95–0.97 for fused images (Utsunomiya *et al.*, 2006). Results demonstrate the increased diagnostic confidence obtained with fused SPECT/CT images compared with separate data sets of scintigraphic and CT images in differentiating malignant from benign bone lesions. The information gained by SPECT and CT image fusion can be greater than the sum of their individual contributions. Regarding benign lesions, fused images are especially useful for differentiating osteoarthritis (Fig. 2). Metastatic foci that represent subtle changes and that are overlooked on two separate sets of bone scintigraphic and CT images can be detected on fused images (Fig. 3).

Clinical Indication of Fused Imaging of Bone

There is little doubt that the fusion of functional or anatomical imaging can be a considerable help in guiding cancer-patient care. At the same time, fused images may not be required for all imaging studies. Therefore, it is necessary to attempt to identify those clinical areas where image fusion is most effective in influencing patient management and outcome. The following indications are suggested: (1) a patient with a small number (four or less) of abnormal tracer uptake; (2) a patient with abnormal tracer uptake near the articulation; and (3) a patient with abnormal uptake in the rib (side-by-side visual correlation between SPECT and CT is especially difficult).

Pitfalls and Limitations

False-negative interpretations of fused images may be encountered owing to a metastatic lesion being undetectable or overlooked on bone scintigraphic or CT images. Osteolytic bone metastases sometimes show negative bone scintigraphic findings. Positron emission tomography with the glucose analog may be superior to bone scintigraphy in detecting such lesions. Also, abnormal foci near the articulations on bone scintigraphy that show subtle or no anatomical change on CT images may be misinterpreted as osteoarthritis. Positive bone scintigraphic images that show negative CT images may require intensive follow-up studies or MRI. These false-negative cases are pitfalls in image interpretation of fused SPECT/CT images.

Combined dual-modality scanners have undoubtedly simplified image registration and fusion. However, the underlying registration mode remains rigid, which cannot compensate for involuntary nonrigid motion of thoracic and abdominal organs. On bone SPECT/CT imaging, potential

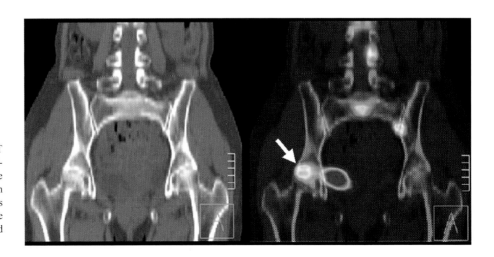

Figure 2 A case with lung cancer. CT image (left) shows no significant anatomical change. Fused image shows precise localization of abnormal tracer uptake in right hip joint (arrow). This finding was suggestive of osteoarthritis. Later bone scans and disease-free follow-up helped confirm the absence of bone metastasis.

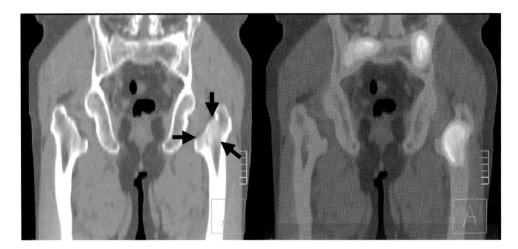

Figure 3 A case with prostate cancer. CT image shows subtle increased density of the left femur (arrows). Fused image shows abnormal tracer in the subtle osteoblastic lesion, which can be easily overlooked on CT image alone. Later bone scans and CT scans helped confirm the bone metastasis.

registration errors in the thorax are due to breathing. Because a SPECT scan is an average image over many breathing cycles and a CT scan is a breath-hold image, the fusion of SPECT with CT images would require respiratory gating of the SPECT scan. However, this is not a promising approach, owing to the substantial resulting increase in imaging time. An automated three-dimensional elastic registration algorithm to correct for nonrigid misalignment in SPECT/CT images can improve the "mechanical" registration of a combined SPECT/CT scanner (Shekhar *et al.*, 2005).

The challenges of combining functional and anatomical imaging in a single scanner are not only technical. Financial, operational, and political issues may assume varying levels of importance when attempting to introduce dual-modality imaging systems into a hospital environment. However, since combined functional-anatomical scanning is emerging as an effective cancer imaging method, such transient issues will hopefully not influence the eventual introduction of dual-modality tomographs in the clinical arena. Commercial PET/CT and SPECT/CT scanners are realities. New combined scanners such as SPECT/MR or PET/MR for human studies may follow at a later time. Ultimately, the imaging of anatomy and function separately on different scanners will be replaced by an integrated disease-management approach whereby anatomy and function will be routinely imaged and interpreted together, allowing accurate assessment and staging of malignant disease.

In conclusion, image fusion of bone SPECT and CT offers an important advantage over assessment of two separate data sets for improved anatomic localization of a suspected site of increased uptake on bone scanning. This provides increased diagnostic confidence in differentiating between malignant and benign bone lesions when analyzing the scans of cancer patients.

References

Bocher, M., Balan, A., Krausz, Y., Shrem, Y., Lonn, A., Wilk, M., and Chisin, R. 2000. Gamma camera-mounted anatomical X-ray tomography: technology, system characteristics and first images. *Eur. J. Nucl. Med. 27*:619–627.

Coleman, R.E. 2001. Metastatic bone disease: clinical features, pathophysiology and treatment strategies. *Cancer Treat Rev. 27*:165–176.

Hasegawa, B.H., Stebler, B., Rutt, B.K., Martinez, A., Gingold, E.L., Barker, C.S., Faulkner, K.G., Cann, C.E., and Boyd, D.P. 1991. A prototype high-purity germanium detector system with fast photon-counting circuitry for medical imaging. *Med. Phys. 18*:900–909.

Horger, M., Eschmann, S.M. Pfannenberg, C., Vonthein, R., Besenfelder, H., Claussen, C.D., and Bares, R. 2004. Evaluation of combined transmission and emission tomography for classification of skeletal lesions. *Am. J. Roentgenol. 183*:655–661.

Mundy, G.R. 2002. Metastasis to bone: causes, consequences and therapeutic opportunities. *Nat. Rev. Cancer. 2*:584–593.

Powles, T., Paterson, S., Kanis, J.A., McCloskey, E., Ashley, S., Tidy, K.A., Rosenqvist, K., Smith, I., Ottestad, L., Legault, S., Pajunen, M., Nevantaus, A., Mannisto, E., Suovuori, A., Atula, S., Nevalainen, J., and Pylkkanen, L. 2002. Randomized, placebo-controlled trial of clodronate in patients with primary operable breast cancer. *J. Clin. Oncol. 20*:3219–3224.

Shekhar, R., Walimbe, V., Raja, S., Zagrodsky, V., Kanvinde, M., Wu, G., and Bybel, B. 2005. Automated 3-dimensional elastic registration of whole-body PET and CT from separate or combined scanners. *J. Nucl. Med. 46*:1488–1496.

Utsunomiya, D., Shiraishi, S., Imuta, M., Tomiguchi, S., Kawanaka, K., Morishita, S., Awai, K., and Yamashita, Y. 2006. Added value of SPECT/CT fusion in assessing suspected bone metastasis: comparison with scintigraphy alone and nonfused scintigraphy and CT. *Radiology 238*:264–271.

5

Bone Cancer: Comparison of ^{18}F-Fluorodeoxyglucose-Positron Emission Tomography with Single Photon Emission Computed Tomography

Takayoshi Uematsu

Introduction

Bone metastases are the most common malignant bone tumor. Skeletal involvement occurs in 30 to 70% of all cancer patients, with breast cancer being the leading cause for bone metastases in women and prostate cancer in men, followed by lung cancer (Padhani and Husband, 1998). Early detection of bone cancer is essential for optimal therapy. The purpose of imaging is to identify bone cancers as early as possible, to determine the full extent of disease, to evaluate the presence of complications that may accompany malignant bone involvement, including pathologic fractures and spinal cord compression, to monitor response to therapy, and, occasionally, to guide biopsy if histologic confirmation is needed (Hamaoka et al., 2004; Padhani and Husband, 1998). The diagnosis and treatment of bone metastases before the development of significant neurologic and functional deficits might improve outcomes in bone cancer patients. Appropriate imaging is able to assist in the early detection of bone cancers.

Radioisotope bone scan has been the standard initial imaging method for the detection of skeletal metastases because of its great sensitivity and the ability to examine the whole skeleton in a single examination with low cost (Hamaoka et al., 2004; Padhani and Husband, 1998). Moreover, bone single photon emission computed tomography (SPECT) is superior to fluorine-18-fluorodeoxyglucose (^{18}F-FDG) positron emission tomography (PET) as a tumor-specific tracer in detecting bone metastases in breast cancer (Uematsu et al., 2005). Bone SPECT has proven superior to planar bone scan imaging in detecting various bone diseases, resulting in increased sensitivity and specificity (Savelli et al., 2001).

There is increasing interest in the use of PET tracers for the investigation of various aspects of skeletal disease, particularly for the diagnosis of bone metastases. FDG has been assessed, and early results suggest that the agent has roles to play in the clinical management of patients. Use of FDG-PET in the evaluation and management of patients with bone cancer continues to increase; however, currently FDG-PET has no established clinical role in the clinical evaluation of bone cancer. There are, however, reports that bone scan is less effective than FDG-PET in detecting bone metastases (Cook *et al.*, 1998; Moon *et al.*, 1998), while there are reports that FDG-PET has lower sensitivity for detecting breast cancer bone metastases than bone scan (Kao *et al.*, 2000; Gallowitsch *et al.*, 2003; Uematsu *et al.*, 2005). Therefore, FDG-PET has not yet found a role in the clinical evaluation of bone metastases, especially in breast cancer. Understanding the advantages and disadvantages of different isotope imaging modalities, that is, FDG-PET and bone SPECT, in detecting bone cancer will assist the clinician in patient screening and treatment planning. In this chapter, we discuss the use of FDG-PET and bone SPECT in the evaluation of bone cancer.

What Is 18F-Fluorodeoxyglucose-Positron Emission Tomography?

Positron emission tomography is an imaging technique that enables the evaluation of tissue metabolism and physiology *in vivo* with positron-emitting radionuclides. The positron is a positively charged electron that is emitted widely and is used in clinical PET oncology. FDG accumulation reflects the rate of glucose utilization in a tissue, because FDG is transported into a tissue by the same mechanisms of glucose transport and is trapped in the tissue as FDG-6-phosphate, which is a poor substrate for the further enzyme systems of glycolysis or glycogen storage. FDG-PET imaging has successfully demonstrated a high uptake of FDG into several tumor tissues *in vivo*. As more aggressive tumors may have increased rates of glycolysis in comparison with less aggressive lesions and normal tissue, metabolic evaluation with FDG-PET has been used to distinguish benign from malignant lesions and to assess tumor grades (Wahl, 2002).

The fundamental signal in PET results from the mutual annihilation of the positron and an electron. This results in the production of two annihilation photons, each having energy corresponding to the mass of an electron and a neutrino. The two photons are emitted exactly $180°$ apart with respect to the electron-positron pair. The near-simultaneous detection of a pair of annihilation photons represents one event or count in the image. Positron emission tomography devices are typically fairly expensive, in part because of the thick detector materials required to stop the energetic 511-keV photons resulting from positron annihilation. The disadvantages of PET are its high cost ($2097.22, according to the Medicare fee schedule for Harris County, Texas), its relative lack of availability, and the additional time required for scanning over that of other imaging modalities (Hamaoka *et al.*, 2004).

Use of FDG-PET in the evaluation and management of patients with bone cancer continues to increase; however,

currently FDG-PET has no established clinical role in the clinical evaluation of bone cancer. Estimates of the sensitivity of FDG-PET for detecting bone metastasis range from 62 to 100%, and specificity from 96 to 100% (Hamaoka *et al.*, 2004). FDG-PET is more sensitive for detecting osteolytic metastases but less sensitive for detecting osteoblastic metastases (Cook *et al.*, 1998; Uematsu *et al.*, 2005). For detecting purely osteolytic or marrow metastases, FDG-PET may be more sensitive than bone scan because those lesions involve little to no osteoblastic activity (Cook *et al.*, 1998; Uematsu *et al.*, 2005). Both osteolytic and osteoblastic processes are important for bone metastases, so the difference between bone scan and FDG-PET for the detection of bone tumor is likely related to the difference in the mechanism by which disease is detected by these two modalities. Bone scan detects the osteoblastic response to bone destruction by tumor cells, and FDG-PET detects the metabolic activity of the tumor cells.

FDG-PET has shown promise for monitoring the response of primary tumors and other nonosseous tumors to treatment. However, the clinical role for FDG-PET in monitoring the response of bone metastases remains undefined at this time (Hamaoka *et al.*, 2004). Chemotherapy in conjunction with granulocyte colony-stimulating factor can lead to increased FDG uptake by hyperplastic bone marrow, which can be difficult to distinguish from diffuse marrow involvement by tumors.

What Is Bone Single Photon Emission Computed Tomography?

Single photon emission computed tomography requires that molecules labeled with a radionuclide emit gamma-ray photons or high-energy X-ray photons. In contrast to PET, only a single photon is detected per event, and that photon is emitted directly from the radioactive atom. Gamma-ray photons are emitted from the nucleus as a result of the relaxation of neutrons and protons that are in an excited energy state in the nucleus. X-ray photons may result from alternate nuclear relaxation or decay processes that involve the removal of an inner shell atomic electron. When an outer shell electron fills this inner shell vacancy, X-rays may be emitted from the atom. Single photon-emitting radionuclides can be created using a nuclear reactor by bombarding reactor-generated neutrons onto high atomic number targets or as a product of the fission process itself (Levin, 2005).

Single photon emitters can also be produced using a nuclear generator, which creates short-lived positron-emitting radionuclides from the decay of a long-lived parent isotope. Single photons are ejected at the speed of light from every radioactive atom attached to the molecules of the SPECT probe distributed throughout the body of the subject. The emitted photons interact with electrons and nuclei of nearby atoms of the tissue through Compton scatter or photoelectric absorption. Unlike a beam of positrons traversing matter, energetic photons do not slow down from interactions in body tissues or external detector materials, but rather the photon beam is attenuated (Levin, 2005).

Photons that escape from the body can be used for SPECT imaging. In the most common SPECT system configuration, the subject is surrounded by one or more position-sensitive gamma-ray photon-detector panels, which typically are large scintillation detectors. Single photon emission computed tomography acquisition consists of detecting and positioning many single photons traversing the detectors and can take 20 min to an hour depending on parameters such as the collimator used, the size of the imaging subject region of interest, and the amount of activity available. Similar performance parameters such as photon sensitivity, spatial resolution, and energy resolution that characterize a PET system are also used for SPECT. The combined effects of these performance parameters dictate a SPECT system's molecular sensitivity (Levin, 2005).

Many of the instrumentation requirements for PET apply to SPECT, with a few exceptions: Because collimators are required for SPECT, the detectors are not configured in rings but rather in flat panels called heads that must rotate around the patient to view the photon activity from all angles. Only one rotating head is required for SPECT, but most systems have two heads to improve system sensitivity. Because photon energies are lower in SPECT, crystals do not have to be as thick, dense, and of a high atomic number in order to have high intrinsic detection efficiency. Most of the world's SPECT systems use NaI (Tl) scintillation crystals. Because the collimator determines the geometric efficiency and spatial resolution performance of SPECT, the detector crystal design requirements are somewhat relaxed. For example, most clinical systems use a continuous sheet of NaI (Tl) scintillation crystals rather than discrete crystal arrays. In principle, SPECT data from the distribution of a single photon emitting molecular probe are acquired and organized into 2D projections in a very similar manner to that described previously for PET (Levin, 2005).

Bone SPECT uses the same radionuclide markers as bone scanning. Bone scanning is the most commonly used means of detecting bone metastasis (Hamaoka et al., 2004; Padhani and Husband, 1998); it visualizes increases in osteoblastic activity and skeletal vascularity. A bone scan is generally considered sensitive for detecting osteoblastic bone metastases on whole-body images, which can be obtained at reasonable cost ($212, according to the Medicare fee schedule for Harris County, Texas) (Hamaoka et al., 2004). False-negative findings can occasionally result when pure osteolytic metastases are growing rapidly, when bone turnover is slow, or when the site is avascular (Cook et al., 1998). The advantage of a bone scan is not for diagnosis but rather for screening,

as it is widely available and can produce rapid whole-body images at reasonable cost.

There is no argument that bone SPECT is superior to planar bone images; its sensitivity for the diagnosis of bone metastases is 85%, and its specificity is 99% (Uematsu et al., 2005). It is particularly difficult to detect small abnormalities and evaluate the exact anatomic site of abnormalities of the thoracic vertebrae by planar bone scan because of the ribs and sternum, and the morphological complexity of the thoracic vertebrae. In planar bone scan, some solitary abnormal accumulations often cause diagnostic confusion because of their low specificity. Abnormally increased focal accumulation does not always mean metastasis, and abnormal findings are often caused by many other conditions such as osteoarthritis, compression fracture, discitis, and spondylitis. Compared with planar bone scanning, SPECT allows more accurate anatomic localization of increased uptake. Tomographic reconstructions provide a more precise display of tracer accumulation, which helps differentiate structures that would otherwise overlap on planar images.

As the anatomic location of tracer uptake is an important clue to the precise diagnosis, the specificity of SPECT is better than that of planar imaging. For bone scintigraphy, many authors have reported the benefits of bone SPECT (Savelli et al., 2001; Uematsu et al., 2005). It is known that bone SPECT increases image contrast and improves lesion detection and localization compared with planar scintigraphy. However, bone SPECT is a time-consuming procedure that might limit its routine use. In most studies that describe the utility of bone SPECT, the acquisition time ranged from 20 to 40 min, and the total protocol schedule of bone scintigraphy takes ~ 1 hr. Therefore, it is necessary to identify the clinical areas in which SPECT is most effective in influencing patient care and outcome.

Although very little information is available on the use of SPECT in routine screening, routine bone SPECT is superior to FDG-PET in detecting bone metastases in breast cancer (Uematsu et al., 2005). Our study is the first to compare bone SPECT and FDG-PET in breast cancer. The intention of our report was to pay attention to the usefulness of bone scanning, especially bone SPECT, in detecting bone metastases in breast cancer, but not other cancers, such as lung cancer. The goal was to see whether FDG-PET can replace bone scanning, including SPECT, for diagnosing bone metastases from less aggressive tumors, such as breast cancer.

The time course for the appearance of clinically detected distant metastases of breast cancer is very long. It is common for metastases to manifest 10 years or more after the initial diagnosis of breast cancer (Harris et al., 2000). During the long manifestation of bone metastases, many breast cancer patients, except the low-risk subset that never develop bone metastases, will be treated with adjuvant hormone and/or chemotherapy according to guidelines (National Comprehensive Cancer Network, 2005). Adjuvant hormone and/or chemotherapy may change purely osteolytic lesions into mixed or osteoblastic bone metastases (Rosenthal *et al.*, 1997). Breast cancer is a heterogeneous disease, and some patients, whose survival duration may be only a few months, have aggressive disease. FDG-PET may be helpful in a carefully selected subgroup of patients in advanced stages of breast cancer because the advantage of whole-body FDG-PET imaging is its ability to detect metastases in different sites and organs in a single examination. Patients with advanced stages of breast cancer who have no treatment may have osteolytic lesions with higher FDG uptake levels. However, these osteolytic lesions may be detected by conventional diagnostic imaging, and these advanced breast cancer patients may also have osteosclerotic lesions. Therefore, osteoblastic metastases with advanced breast cancer may be undetectable by FDG-PET. Bone scanning is not recommended for patients with stage 1 or 2 breast cancer because of the low return. Some studies have shown that the majority of patients are symptomatic at the diagnosis of bone metastases (American Society of Clinical Oncology, 1997).

Many breast cancer patients have more indolent disease that is responsive to hormone therapy or chemotherapy. With adjuvant hormone and/or chemotherapy, breast cancer tends to result in mixed bone metastases (Rosenthal *et al.*, 1997). On bone scanning, the false-negative rate was only 0.08% in 1267 consecutive cases of breast cancer (Coleman *et al.*, 1998). These results suggest that cases of breast cancer, especially stages 1 and 2 postoperative breast cancer, with purely osteolytic metastases only, are not common in our opinion. Our results that bone scanning is more sensitive than FDG-PET for osteosclerotic lesions, and that for osteolytic lesions FDG-PET detects more abnormalities than bone scanning, agree with previously documented findings (Cook *et al.*, 1998). Some reports indicate that FDG-PET has lower sensitivity for detecting breast cancer bone metastases than bone scanning (Kao *et al.*, 2000; Gallowitsch *et al.*, 2003). Some reports also indicate the relatively low sensitivity of FDG-PET in the detection of bone metastases (Moon *et al.*, 1998). FDG-PET currently has no established clinical role in the clinical evaluation of bone metastases from breast cancer. Bone SPECT has improved both the sensitivity and specificity of bone scanning because of the precise location of lesions on tomographic images. Routinely performed bone SPECT is practicable and cost-effective, and improves the sensitivity and specificity of bone scanning; however, it takes much longer. Whole-body bone SPECT might commonly replace whole-body planar scanning for routine examinations because technical improvements in gamma cameras will enable bone SPECT images in a short time (Kobayashi *et al.*, 2005).

FDG-PET vs. Bone SPECT for Bone Metastases in Various Human Malignancies

Breast Cancer

A higher number of false-negative FDG-PET findings of bone tumor than nonskeletal metastases in breast cancer have been reported (Moon *et al.*, 1998). There were 41 sites of recurrent or metastatic disease in 29 patients. On a patient basis, the sensitivity of FDG-PET was 93% and the specificity 79%, and on a lesion basis, the sensitivity was 85% and specificity 79%. However, the sensitivity for bone lesions was 69% vs. 96% for nonosseous lesions ($p < 0.05$). The authors concluded that the sensitivity for bone metastases appeared lower than for other organs. In support of this conclusion, Gallowitsch *et al.* (2003) conducted a retrospective analysis of 62 women with breast cancer. Of these, 38 had isotope bone scans in addition to FDG-PET. On a patient basis, no difference in sensitivity was found for either technique but the specificity was better for FDG-PET. In lesion-based analysis, however, the sensitivity for bone scanning was much higher, although the specificity was less. In the total study population, 21 patients received chemotherapy and 15 antihormonal therapy. It is not clear what relationship, if any, prior treatment had to these findings. However, adjuvant hormone and/or chemotherapy may change purely osteolytic lesions into mixed or osteoblastic bone metastases (Rosenthal *et al.*, 1997).

Cook *et al.* (1998) reported that bone scanning detected the osteoblastic response to bone destruction by tumor cells and FDG-PET detected the metabolic activity of the tumor cells. They also studied 23 patients with breast cancer with progressive bone metastases. On the basis of their pretreatment bone X-rays, each patient had his or her metastatic disease classified as lytic, sclerotic, or a mixed pattern. They found that patients with either a lytic or a mixed pattern of disease had a higher number of lesions identified on FDG-PET than on bone scan, but for the subgroup with sclerotic lesions, a lower number was seen. Furthermore, the patients in whom FDG uptake could be calculated, sclerotic metastases showed a lower uptake of FDG than lytic lesions. In addition, the survival of patients with a mixed pattern or sclerotic disease was significantly greater than those with predominantly lytic metastases. This study shows that lytic bone metastases are more FDG-sensitive than sclerotic. Clearly, lytic metastases may have a higher glycolytic rate and because of their aggressive nature with rapid growth, could outstrip their blood supply, rendering the lesion relatively hypoxic. Hypoxia has been shown in some cell lines to increase FDG uptake (Clavo *et al.*, 1995). Another factor is that sclerotic metastases are relatively acellular and therefore contain a smaller volume of viable tumor tissue within an individual lesion.

A confirmed effect of anti-estrogen therapy commonly applied in patients with breast cancer is the "flare reaction" characterized by pain and erythema in soft tissue lesions and increased pain in bone lesions (Mortimer et al., 2001). This phenomenon is presumed to reflect the initial agonist effect of the drug before its antagonist effect supervenes. Clinically, it may be difficult to differentiate the flare reaction from disease progression (Mortimer et al., 2001). Consecutive bone scan may show an increase in uptake at sites of previously detected metastases or new sites, which are actually responsive lytic lesions undergoing a repair process with increased osteoblastic activity. The initial agonist effect to therapy is also associated with increased tumor FDG uptake. A change in FDG uptake can be detected as early as 10 days after the initiation of treatment compared with the several weeks that are often required to make this assessment on the basis of clinical symptoms (Mortimer et al., 2001).

Bone SPECT is superior to FDG-PET in detecting bone metastases in breast cancer (Uematsu et al., 2005). In our opinion, bone SPECT is more advantageous than PET as a whole-body screening modality for detecting bone metastases from breast cancer because of its low cost and because purely osteolytic metastases only are not common in breast cancer. Figure 1 shows that the low sensitivity of FDG-PET in detecting osteoblastic bone metastases when compared with traditional bone scanning and bone SPECT.

Prostate Cancer

The staging of newly diagnosed prostate cancer is essential for guiding treatment (Lee et al., 2000). Patients with low-risk prostate cancer are unlikely to have metastatic disease on bone scan (Abuzallouf et al., 2004; Lee et al., 2000). Bone scanning is the most widely used method for evaluating skeletal metastases of prostate carcinoma. The role of FDG-PET seemed limited in this type of malignancy as both the soft tissue and bone metastases were reported to be FDG negative or to show only low-intensity uptake in many patients (Shreve et al., 1996). It has been speculated that the glucose use of prostate tumor cells is not enhanced significantly compared with normal cells and that prostate cancer cells may have an alternative source of energy supply (Oyen et al., 2001). On the basis of these two studies, it is concluded that FDG-PET does not perform well in the identifying skeletal metastases, even in untreated patients with prostate cancer, and in those who have received treatment; the results may be extremely poor.

Despite the relatively disappointing early reports, more recent publications suggest that FDG-PET is not an unsuitable modality for the assessment of patients with prostate cancer but needs to be used in selected groups of patients using adequate imaging techniques. PET/CT was suggested to overcome the problem of pelvic tumor sites obscured by radioactive urine (Schoder and Larson, 2004). Morris et al.

(2002) found that FDG-PET appropriately discriminated active bone tumor from scintigraphically negative lesions. Interestingly, all but one lesion seen on bone scan alone were stable on follow-up when compared with the baseline bone scan, whereas all FDG-PET lesions reflected active disease in subsequent studies. FDG-PET was used to monitor the response to treatment, and a decline in tumor glucose uptake was measured as early as 48 hr after androgen withdrawal, preceding any change in tumor volume or in PSA levels (Schoder and Larson, 2004).

Lung Cancer

Surgical resection offers the highest probability of a favorable outcome in patients with non-small cell lung cancer (NSCLC). However, the survival of patients who undergo surgery remains low, probably because of presurgical understaging. Bone metastases are diagnosed at initial presentation in 3.4 to 60% of patients with NSCLC (Even-Sapir et al., 2005). Bone pain is usually considered an indicator of bone metastases, but up to 40% of lung cancer patients with proven bone metastases are asymptomatic (Bury et al., 1998; Lardinois et al., 2003). Clinical staging at presentation has been performed by means of CT of the thorax through the liver and adrenals, CT or MRI of the brain, and bone scan for assessment of bone involvement. This staging algorithm remains the most commonly used in places where FDG-PET is not a routine staging modality of lung cancer. FDG-PET and PET/CT were recently reported to be of value in assessing the presence of soft tissue and bone spread in patients with NSCLC, obviating the need to perform a separate bone scan (Bury et al., 1998; Lardinois et al., 2003). They showed FDG-PET to be superior to bone scanning in detecting bone metastases. They reported that FDG-PET had a high positive-predictive value and a lower false-positive rate compared with a bone scan.

Lymphoma

Primary bone involvement occurs in 3 to 5% of patients with non-Hodgkin's Lymphoma, and 25% have secondary bone involvement. Primary bone involvement is rare in Hodgkin's disease (HD). Secondary bone involvement occurs in 5 to 20% of patients with HD during the course of disease but in only 1 to 4% at presentation (Even-Sapir et al., 2005). Lymphomatous bone involvement is the result of hematogenous spread or direct extension from adjacent soft tissue disease. Bone involvement upgrades the disease to stage 4 and is indicative of aggressive disease with a poor outcome. The extension of disease from adjacent disease in the soft tissue to bone, however, does not alter staging. The radiographic features of bone lymphoma are nonspecific. Lesions may often be multiple. They are predominantly osteolytic but may be sclerotic or mixed.

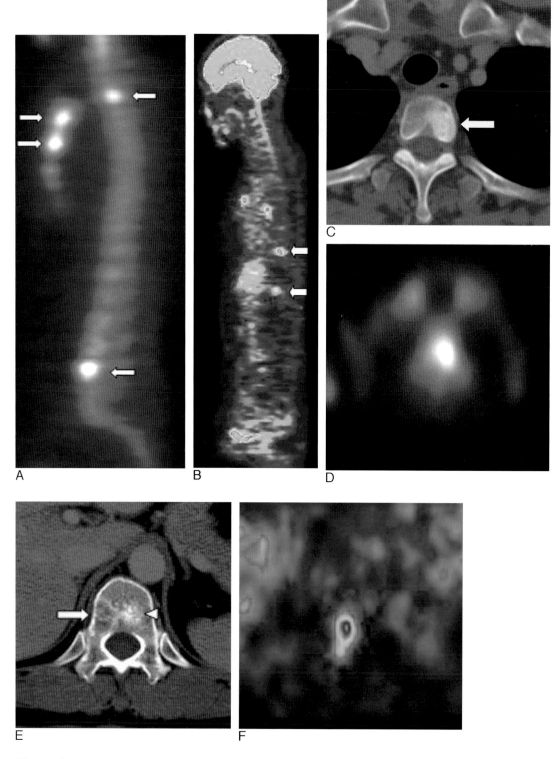

Figure 1 Multiple osteoblastic and osteolytic metastases in a 52-year-old woman who underwent lumpectomy for invasive ductal cancer in the upper inner quadrant of the left breast. **(A)** A sagittal bone scan shows abnormalities in the sternum and in the axial skeleton at T2, L4 vertebral bodies (arrows). **(B)** A sagittal FDG-PET slice shows abnormalities in the axial skeleton at T9 and T12 (arrows). **(C)** A CT axial slice through the upper thorax at T2 shows osteoblastic metastasis in the posterior part of the vertebral body (arrow). CT slices show osteophytes at L4 vertebral bodies (not shown). **(D)** An axial bone SPECT image shows the vertebral body at T2 of increased 99mTc HMDP uptake. **(E)** A CT axial slice through the upper thorax at T12 vertebral body shows osteolytic metastasis (arrow) in the posterior part of the vertebral body. A faint sclerotic deposit (arrowhead) in the same vertebral body shows no associated increase in the uptake of 99mTc HMDP and FDG. **(F)** An axial FDG-PET slice image shows the vertebral body at T12 of increased FDG.

[67]Gallium scintigraphy has been found to be a sensitive imaging modality for detecting bone involvement in lymphoma, mainly with the administration of high doses of ^{67}Ga and the use of SPECT. Both lytic and sclerotic lesions were reported to be ^{67}Ga sensitive. The lymphoma-seeking properties of ^{67}Ga rather than its bone-seeking properties are presumably the primary cause of increased ^{67}Ga uptake in lymphoma involving the bone. Israel et al. (2002) reported that ^{67}Ga SPECT was found to be both sensitive and specific for monitoring the response of bone lymphoma to therapy. Persistent increased ^{67}Ga uptake in a skeletal disease site at the end of therapy has been shown to indicate active disease, whereas a negative ^{67}Ga study suggests complete response and a favorable outcome, regardless of its appearance on follow-up CT, which may remain abnormal even when the disease is cured (Israel et al., 2002).

Lymphoma involvement is commonly marrow based. Magnetic resonance imaging is a sensitive modality for detecting marrow involvement; however, it is not a routine modality for the staging of lymphoma. In recent years, FDG-PET has been used for staging and for monitoring the response to therapy in patients with lymphoma, replacing the use of ^{67}Ga scintigraphy in many centers. FDG-PET can detect early marrow involvement, and therefore the sensitivity is superior to that of bone scanning for the assessment of early bone involvement in lymphoma (Moog et al., 1998). FDG-PET is also more sensitive than CT for detecting bone involvement. When performed by means of a hybrid PET/CT system, unexpected bone involvement can be identified by increased FDG uptake with either corresponding abnormalities on the CT data of the study or a normal CT appearance when bone involvement without bone destruction is early. The delay in detecting lymphomatous bone involvement on CT reflects its relatively low sensitivity in assessing malignant marrow involvement, and the fact that the detection of malignant bone involvement on CT depends on the presence of a considerable amount of bone destruction (Israel et al., 2002).

It has been suggested that FDG-PET could replace the blind marrow-sampling or may be used as a guide to an appropriate biopsy site (Moog et al., 1998). FDG-PET can identify patients with HD who are at high risk of marrow involvement. Assessment by FDG-PET of disease activity in the marrow after therapy is hampered by the resemblance of active lymphoma infiltration to reactive marrow changes, and by the effect of chemotherapy and granulocyte colony-stimulating factors on tracer distribution in the marrow (Cook et al., 1996).

Multiple Myeloma

Multiple myeloma (MM) is a clonal B-lymphocyte neoplasm of plasma cells. It accounts for 1% of all malignant diseases and represents 10% of hematologic malignancies (Even-Sapir et al., 2005). The hallmark of MM is the presence of a monoclonal protein (M protein) produced by abnormal plasma cells in the blood or urine. Once the diagnosis is suspected, a radiographic skeletal survey, bone marrow aspiration, and biopsy are performed (Angtuaco et al., 2004). The effects of abnormal plasma cells are excessive bone resorption and inhibition of bone formation. The clinical presentations of MM are bone pain, severe osteopenia, and skeletal fractures, including multilevel spinal cord compression fractures. In clinical practice for MM patients, imaging is complementary to measurements of biochemical markers of bone turnover.

X-ray is the primary imaging modality for detecting bone changes in MM. Computed tomography is a sensitive tool for detecting the bone-destructive effects of MM. Multiple myeloma findings that can be detected on CT include lytic lesions, expansile lesions with soft tissue masses, diffuse osteopenia, and fractures (Avva et al., 2001). Bone scan is considered less sensitive than X-ray and CT due to the presence of only minimal osteoblastic activity in most myeloma lesions, which are predominantly lytic (Woolfenden et al., 1980). Almost half of the abnormal sites of disease identified radiographically were reported to be overlooked by bone scan. Scintigraphic abnormalities associated with myeloma may appear as increased sites of ^{99m}Tc-MDP uptake, mainly in the presence of fractures, or as cold lesions. Magnetic resonance imaging has recently been used in patients with MM to assess actual tumor burden in the marrow and the presence of accompanying complications. Experience with FDG-PET in patients with MM is rapidly expanding. Previous reports have shown that FDG-PET can detect unexpected medullary and extramedullary disease sites missed by X-ray, CT, and bone scan. Schirrmeister et al. (2002) reported 93% sensitivity for the detection of osteolytic MM by FDG-PET.

Endemic Nasopharyngeal Cancer

Nonkeratinizing nasopharyngeal carcinoma (NPC), endemic in southern China, Southeast Asia, North Africa, and Alaska, is an epithelial neoplasm with WHO histologic classification of type 2 (differentiated nonkeratinizing carcinoma) or type 3 (undifferentiated carcinoma). It differs from squamous cell carcinomas of the head and neck in etiology, natural history, and response to treatment. Endemic NPC has a greater tendency for early locoregional spread, whereas its higher sensitivity to radiotherapy and chemotherapy produces a better prognosis. Overt distant metastasis has been detected in up to 11% of NPC patients at initial diagnosis, and the skeleton is the most frequent site involved in 70 to 80% of patients with distant metastases. FDG-PET is more sensitive than bone scanning for detecting bone metastasis in endemic NPC at initial staging (Liu et al., 2006).

Renal Cell Carcinoma

Renal cell carcinoma (RCC) accounts for 2% of all cancers. Initially, RCC is clinically asymptomatic. Due to delayed diagnosis, bone metastases occur in ~ 10% of patients at their first presentation. Bone scanning in RCC frequently underestimates metastatic spread due to its primarily osteolytic growth. Therefore, the necessity of performing a bone scan as part of a routine preoperative work-up or postoperative follow-up for patients with RCC has been questioned. Bone scanning has no diagnostic role in RCC patients with a high pretest probability for bone metastases due to abnormal laboratory tests, pain, or confirmed nonosseous metastases (Staudenherz *et al.*, 1998). Presently, no reports on the utility of FDG-PET in RCC bone metastases are available.

Hepatocellular Carcinoma

Extrahepatic metastases from hepatocellular carcinoma (HCC) are not uncommon. The incidence of extrahepatic HCC was reported in 37% of patients, and the frequent sites of metastases are the lung, lymph nodes, and bone. Although most extrahepatic metastases occur in patients at an advanced stage, accurately diagnosing HCC recurrence is necessary to manage the disease and decide the treatment strategy. FDG-PET is less successful in the detection of primary HCC because of variable FDG uptake in HCC. Sugiyama *et al.* (2004) reported that FDG-PET revealed two bone metastases that were not identified by a bone scan. As bone metastases from HCC are osteolytic, FDG-PET is expected to be sensitive for the detection of bone metastases from HCC.

Esophageal Cancer

The majority of patients with esophageal carcinomas have an advanced disease at the time of diagnosis. The major distant metastases of esophageal carcinomas involve the lymph nodes, liver, lungs, and bones. Kato *et al.* (2005) reported that FDG-PET revealed that three patients with false-negative findings on their bone scan had true-positive findings with FDG-PET; all of these lesions were osteolytic metastases.

Summary

It is apparent that while FDG-PET is used extensively in oncological practice, its role in the identification of bone metastases is far from clear. For breast cancer, several studies showed that FDG-PET is less sensitive than a bone scan. There is general agreement that FDG-PET has improved specificity and that there can be no argument that the two techniques have a complementary role if bone metastases are not to be missed. There is convincing evidence that for prostate cancer, FDG-PET is less sensitive than bone scanning, and this may be tumor specific, reflecting the morphology of the metastases. For lymphoma and myeloma, FDG-PET is clearly better than a bone, scan, presumably because FDG-PET can identify marrow-based disease at an early stage.

The morphology of the metastasis itself appears to be relevant. At least in breast cancer, different patterns of FDG uptake have been shown in sclerotic, lytic, or mixed lesions. It has been suggested that while there may be differences in the glycolytic rate between these types of bone metastases, sclerotic lesions have a much smaller tumor volume relative to the size of the metastases and may simply be less likely to be identified. Furthermore, the precise localization of metastasis in the skeleton may be important with regard to the extent of the metabolic response induced. Clearly, previous treatment is highly relevant. Adjuvant hormone and/or chemotherapy may change purely osteolytic lesions into mixed or osteoblastic bone metastases. In this case, a bone scan is superior to FDG-PET in detecting bone metastases.

Bone cancer is a heterogeneous disease and some patients, whose survival duration may be a few months, have aggressive disease. FDG-PET may be helpful in a carefully selected subgroup of patients in advanced stages and with aggressive bone cancer because patients with aggressive and advanced bone cancer who receive no treatment may have osteolytic lesions with higher FDG uptake levels. Bone SPECT has improved both the sensitivity and specificity of bone scanning at low cost because of the precise location of lesions on tomographic images.

Finally, understanding the advantages and disadvantages of bone scanning and FDG-PET in detecting breast bone metastases will assist the clinician in bone cancer patient screening and treatment planning. FDG-PET and bone scanning might be complementary in their ability to detect bone metastases in bone cancer. Aggressive metastatic bone tumors such as lung cancer are more lytic, and theoretically should have increased sensitivity for FDG-PET imaging. FDG-PET is an expensive imaging modality and its cost-effectiveness in diagnosing bone cancer is more difficult to ascertain. A larger study population and more outcome data are necessary to confirm the cost-effectiveness of FDG-PET in diagnosing bone cancer. On the other hand, less aggressive tumors such as breast or prostate cancer, or tumors rendered less aggressive by chemotherapy or radiation, are more likely to have sclerotic metastases and be more sensitive to detection by traditional bone scanning imaging. Routinely performed bone SPECT is practicable and cost-effective, and improves the sensitivity and specificity of bone scanning. Whole-body bone SPECT might replace whole-body planar scanning for routine examination because technical improvements in gamma cameras will enable bone SPECT images in a short time. FDG-PET is not a powerful tool for the detection of osteoblastic bone metastases. Bone scanning remains the most important investigation for the detection of osteoblastic and mixed bone cancer. Tumor biology is never simple, and recent evidence has questioned many of these traditional assumptions. However, it is very important to know the biology of each bone cancer and the morphology of each bone metastasis for a good modality choice for bone cancer diagnosis.

References

Abuzallouf, S., Dayes, I., and Lukka, H. 2004. Baseline staging of newly diagnosed prostate cancer: a summary of the literature. *J. Urol. 171*:2122–2127.

Angtuaco, E.J.C., Fassas, A.B.T., Walker, R., Sethi, R.H., and Barlogie, B. 2004. Multiple myeloma: clinical review and diagnostic imaging. *Radiology 231*:11–23.

American Society of Clinical Oncology. 1997. Recommended breast cancer surveillance guidelines. *J. Clin. Oncol. 15*:2149–2156.

Avva, R., Vanhemert, R., Barlogie, B., Munshi, N., and Angtuaco, E.J. 2001. CT-guided biopsy of focal lesions in patients with multiple myeloma may reveal new and more aggressive cytogenetic abnormalities. *Am. J. Neuroradiol. 22*:781–785.

Bury, T., Barreto, A., Daenen, F., Barthelemy, N., Ghaya, B., and Rigo, P. 1998. Fluorine-18 deoxyglucose positron emission tomography for the detection of bone metastases in patients with non-small cell lung cancer. *Eur. J. Nucl. Med. 25*:1244–1247.

Clavo, A.C., Brown, R.S., and Wahl, R.L. 1995. Fluorodeoxyglucose uptake in human cancer cell lines is increased by hypoxia. *J. Nucl. Med. 36*:1625–1632.

Coleman, R.E., Rubens, R.D., and Fogelman, I. 1988. Reappraisal of the baseline bone scan in breast cancer. *J. Nucl. Med. 29*:1045–1049.

Cook, G.J., Fogelman, I., and Maisey, M.N. 1996. Normal physiological and benign pathological variants of 18-fluoro-2-deoxyglucose positron-emission tomography scanning: potential for error interpretation. *Semin. Nucl. Med. 26*:308–314.

Cook, G.J.R., Houston, S., Rubens, R., Maisey, M.N., and Fogelman, I. 1998. Detection of bone metastases in breast cancer by ^{18}FDG PET: differing metabolic activity in osteoblastic and osteolytic lesions. *J. Clin. Oncol. 16*:3375–3379.

Even-Sapir, E. 2005. Imaging of malignant bone involvement by morphologic, scintigraphic, and hybrid modalities. *J. Nucl. Med. 46*:1356–1367.

Gallowitsch, H.J., Kresnik, E., Gasser, J., Kumnig, G., Igerc, I., Mikosch, P., and Lind, P. 2003. F-18 fluorodeoxyglucose positron-emission tomography in the diagnosis of tumor recurrence and metastases in the follow-up of patients with breast carcinoma: a comparison to conventional imaging. *Invest. Radiol. 38*:250–256.

Hamaoka, T., Madewell, J.E., Podoloff, D.A., Hortobagyi, G.N., and Ueno, N.T. 2004. Bone imaging in metastatic breast cancer. *J. Clin. Oncol. 22*:2942–2953.

Harris, J.R., Lippman, M.E., Morrow, M., and Osbone, C.K. 2000. *Disease of the Breast* (2nd ed.). Philadelphia: Lippincott Williams and Wilkins, pp. 407–423.

Israel, O., Mekel, M., Bar-Shalom, R., Epelbaum, R., Hermony, N., Haim, N., Dann, E.J., Frenkel, A., Ben-Arush, M., and Gaitini, D. 2002. Bone lymphoma: ^{67}Ga scintigraphy and CT for prediction of outcome after treatment. *J. Nucl. Med. 43*:1295–1303.

Kao, C.H., Hsieh, J.F., Tsai, S.C., Ho, Y.J., and Yen, R.F. 2000. Comparison and discrepancy of 18F-2-deoxyglucose positron emission tomography and Tc-99m MDP bone scan to detect bone metastases. *Anticancer Res. 20*:2189–2192.

Kato, H., Miyazaki, T., Nakajima, M., Takita, J., Kimura, H., Faried, A., Sohda, M., Fukai, Y., Masuda, N., Fukuchi, M., Manda, R., Ojima, H., Tsukada, K., Kuwano, H., Oriuchi, N., and Endo, K. 2005. Comparison between whole-body positron emission tomography and bone scintigraphy in evaluating bony metastases of esophageal carcinomas. *Anticancer Res. 25*:4439–4444.

Kobayashi, K., Okuyama, C., Kubota, T., Nakai, T., Ushijima, Y., and Nishimura, T. 2005. Do short-time SPECT images of bone scintigraphy improve the diagnostic value in the evaluation of solitary lesions in the thoracic spine in patients with extraskeletal malignancies? *Ann. Nucl. Med. 19*:557–566.

Lardinois, D., Weder, W., Hany, T.F., Kamel, E.M., Korom, S., Seifert, B., von Schulthess, G.K., and Steinert, H.C. Staging of non-small-cell lung cancer with integrated positron-emission tomography and computed tomography. *N. Engl. J. Med. 348*:2500–2507.

Lee, N., Fawaaz, R., Olsson, C.A., Benson, M.C., Petrylak, D.P., Schiff, P.B., Bagiella, E., Singh, A., and Ennis, R.D. 2000. Which patients with newly diagnosed prostate cancer need a radionuclide bone scan? An analysis based on 631 patients. *Int. J. Radiat. Oncol. Biol. Phys. 48*:1443–1446.

Levin, C.S. 2005. Primer on molecular imaging technology. *Eur. J. Nucl. Med. Mol. Imaging 32*:S325–S345.

Liu, F.-Y., Chang, J.T., Wang, H.-M., Liao, C.-T., Kang, C.-J., Ng, S.-K., Chan, S.-C., and Yen, T.-C. 2006. [18F] Fluorodeoxyglucose positron emission tomography is more sensitive than skeletal scintigraphy for detecting bone metastasis in endemic nasopharyngeal carcinoma at initial staging. *J. Clin. Oncol. 24*:599–604.

Moog, F., Bangrter, M., Kotzerke, J., Guhlmann, A., Frickhofen, N., and Reske, S.N. 1998. 18-F-fluorodeoxyglucose-positron emission tomography as a new approach to detect lymphomatous bone marrow. *J. Clin. Oncol. 16*:603–609.

Moon, D.H., Maddahi, J., Silverman, D.H., Glaspy, J.A., Phelps, M.E., and Hoh, C.K. 1998. Accuracy of whole body fluorine-18-FDG PET for detection of recurrent or metastatic breast carcinoma. *J. Nucl. Med. 39*:431–435.

Morris, M.J., Akhurst, T., Osman, I., Nunez, R., Macapinlac, H., Siedlecki, K., Verbel, D., Schwartz, L., Larson, S.M., and Scher, H.I. Fluorinated deoxyglucose positron emission tomography imaging in progressive metastatic prostate cancer. *Urology 59*:913–918.

Mortimer, J.E., Dehdashti, F., and Siegel, B.A. 2001. Metabolic flare: indicator of hormone responsiveness in advanced breast cancer. *J. Clin. oncol. 19*:2797–2803.

National Comprehensive Cancer Network (NCCN). Practice guidelines in oncology. Breast Cancer. Version 2.2005 (www.nccn.org).

Oyen, W.J.G., Witjes, J.A., and Corstens, F.H.M. 2001. Nuclear medicine techniques for the diagnosis and therapy of prostate carcinoma. *Eur. Urol. 40*:294–299.

Padhani, A., and Husband, J. 1998. Bone metastases. In: Husband, J.E.S., and Reznek, R.H. (Eds.), *Imaging in Oncology.* Oxford: Isis Medical Media Ltd., pp. 765–787.

Rosenthal, D.I. 1997. Radiologic diagnosis of bone metastases. *Cancer 80*:19–20.

Shreve, P.D., Grossman, H.B., Gross, M.D., and Wahl, R.L. 1996. Metastatic prostate cancer: initial finding of PET 2-deoxyglucose-[F-18]fluoro-D-glucose. *Radiology 199*:751–756.

Savelli, G., Maffioli, L., Maccauro, M., Deckere, E.D., and Bombardieri, E. 2001. Bone scintigraphy and the added value of SPECT (single photon emission tomography) in detecting skeletal lesions. *Q. J. Nucl. Med. 45*:27–37.

Schirrmeister, H., Bommer, M., Buck, A.K., Muller, S., Messer, P., Bunjes, D., Dohner, H., Bergmann, L., and Reske, S.N. 2002. Initial results in the assessment of multiple myeloma using F-18 FDG PET. *Eur. J. Nucl. Med. Mol. Imaging 29*:361–366.

Schoder, H., and Larson, S.M. 2004. Positron emission tomography for prostate, bladder, and renal cancer. *Semin. Nucl. Med. 34*:274–292.

Staudenherz, A., Steiner, B., Kainberger, F., and Leitha, T. 1998. Is there a diagnostic role for bone scanning of patients with a high pretest probability for metastatic renal cell carcinoma? *Cancer 85*:153–155.

Sugiyama, M., Sakahara, H., Torizuka, T., Kanno, T., Nakamura, F., Futatsubashi, M., and Nakamura, S. 2004. 18F-FDG PET in the detection of extrahepatic metastases from hepatocellular carcinoma. *J. Gastroenterol. 39*:961–968.

Uematsu, T., Yuen, S., Yukisawa, S., Aramaki, T., Morimoto, N., Endo, M., Furukawa, H., Uchida, Y., and Watanabe, J. 2005. Comparison of FDG PET and SPECT for detection of bone metastases in breast cancer. *Am. J. Roentgenol. 184*:1266–1273.

Wahl, R.L. 2002. *Positron Emission Tomography*. Philadelphia: Lippincott Williams and Wilkins, pp.1–65.

Woolfenden, J.M., Pitt, M.J., Durie, B.G.M., and Moon, T.E. 1980. Comparison of bone scintigraphy and radiology in multiple myeloma. *Radiology 134*:723–728.

6

Bone Metastasis in Endemic Nasopharyngeal Carcinoma: ^{18}F-Fluorodeoxyglucose-Positron Emission Tomography

Feng-Yuan Liu and Tzu-Chen Yen

Introduction

Nasopharyngeal carcinoma (NPC) occurs from the epithelial lining of the nasopharynx. Anatomically, the nasopharynx is bounded anteriorly by the nasal choanae, superiorly by the sphenoid, and posteriorly by the clivus and the first two cervical vertebrae. The initial development of NPC usually occurs at the lateral pharyngeal recess (fossa of Rosenmüller) or the ostium of the eustachian tube. NPC is rare in the United States and developed European countries (< 1/100,000 per year) but endemic in southern China, Taiwan, Southeast Asia, Middle East, Africa, Alaska, northern Canada, and Greenland (Busson *et al.*, 2004). Cantonese in Hong Kong and southern China have the highest incidence of NPC (15 to 50/100,000 per year). The World Health Organization histological classification proposed in 1978 classified NPC into three groups: type I as keratinizing squamous cell carcinoma; type II as differentiated nonkeratinizing carcinoma; and type III as undifferentiated carcinoma. Type I tumors behave more like the squamous cell carcinomas of the head and neck in other sites and are similarly associated with smoking and alcohol-drinking, while tumors of

types II and III are consistently associated with the Epstein-Barr virus (EBV). The vast majority of NPC patients in the endemic areas are of type II or III.

Because there is no significant difference in the pathogenesis and clinical behavior of types II and III tumors, they are usually collectively called nonkeratinizing NPC or undifferentiated carcinoma of the nasopharyngeal type (UCNT). Under microscope, the tumor cells appear polygonal with round or oval nuclei with distinct nucleoli. There are usually preactivational lymphoid T-cells intermingled with the tumor cells. The malignant tumor cells are immunoreactive with cytokeratin, and electron microscopy has proved that the tumor cells are of squamous origin. The EBV genome is contained in the nuclei of malignant NPC cells and can be detected in the peripheral circulation in patients with endemic or nonkeratinizing NPC. Premalignant lesions have also been shown to harbor EBV, suggesting that the infection occurs before or early in the process of carcinogenesis. The corresponding protein products of the EBV genome are associated with the highly invasive behavior of the carcinoma. In addition to the EBV, nonkeratinizing NPC is also associated with nonviral carcinogens

321

and genetic predisposition. Salted fish, salted meat, and rancid butter have been linked with the pathogenesis of NPC. Epidemiological and chromosomal studies also indicate the presence of genetic predisposition. NPC occurs more frequently in males with a male-to-female ratio of 2 to 3.5. All age groups may be involved. However, the peak incidence is among persons 40 to 60 years old. In Africa there is a minor peak between young people of 10 to 25 years old.

Diagnosis and Staging

Patients with NPC can present with symptoms ranging from epistaxis, nasal obstruction, tinnitus, cranial nerve palsy, headache, diplopia, to most frequently, neck masses (Wei and Sham, 2005). Symptoms such as anorexia and weight loss are uncommon. Because the nasopharynx is a deep-seated structure and the nasal and aural symptoms are nonspecific, a large proportion of patients with NPC are diagnosed only when the tumor has reached an advanced stage. An endoscopic examination with tumor biopsy from the nasopharynx is the standard procedure for diagnosis. If the clinical suspicion for NPC is high, cross-sectional imaging by positron emission tomography-computed tomography (PET-CT) or magnetic resonance imaging (MRI) should be undertaken even if the suspected tumor is not visible with endoscopic examination. A definitive diagnosis of NPC needs a positive biopsy taken from the tumor in the nasopharynx.

The staging system according to the American Joint Committee on Cancer and International Union Against Cancer (AJCC/UICC) in 2002 is summarized in Table 1. Magnetic resonance imaging (MRI) of the head and neck is currently the preferred imaging modality for local tumor staging (Ng et al., 1997). MRI is better than computed tomography (CT) for visualizing soft tissue structures and for tumor differentiation. MRI is also able to detect the marrow infiltration by tumor in the skull base. The PET-CT imaging of a patient with NPC is shown in Figure 1. For N-staging, both MRI and ^{18}F-fluorodeoxyglucose (FDG) positron emission tomography (PET) or PET-CT can yield complementary findings (Ng et al., 2004). There are different ways for lymphatic spreading from nasopharynx to the neck, with some routes escaping the retropharyngeal nodes (Liu et al., 2006). In our institution, only 10% of NPC patients are of N0 stage. About two out of every three patients are of stage N2 or N3. The PET imaging of an NPC patient with unilateral lymph node metastases (stage N1) is demonstrated in Figure 2.

Distant metastasis in NPC is strongly associated with the N stage (Liu et al., 2006). Because the majority of NPC patients have lymphatic spreading, it is expected that the rate of distant metastasis in NPC is higher than that in squamous cell carcinomas of the head and neck. Overt distant metastasis has been detected in up to 11% of NPC patients at initial staging by conventional studies, with the skeleton, involved

in 70 to 80% of patients with distant metastasis, as the most frequent metastatic site (Chiesa and De Paoli, 2001). In contrast, pulmonary metastasis is the most frequent in the squamous cell carcinomas of the head and neck. Considering that the most frequent sites of distant metastasis are bone, chest, and liver, whole-body skeletal scintigraphy, chest X-ray, and abdominal ultrasonography have been used for surveying distant metastasis traditionally. However, the sensitivities of these conventional examinations seem to be low (Chang et al., 2005). A significant portion of patients initially considered as M0 will develop distant metastasis shortly after the primary treatment (Caglar et al., 2003). From our clinical experience, FDG-PET seems promising for detecting distant metastasis in NPC patients. The PET imaging of an NPC patient with multiple bone metastases is shown in Figure 3.

Table 1   Staging for Nasopharyngeal Carcinoma (AJCC 2002)

Primary Tumor (T)	
TX	Primary tumor cannot be assessed
T0	No evidence of primary tumor
Tis	Carcinoma *in situ*
T1	Tumor confined to the nasopharynx
T2	Tumor extends to soft tissues of oropharynx and/or nasal cavity
	T2a without parapharyngeal extension
	T2b with parapharyngeal extension
T3	Tumor invades bony structures and/or paranasal sinuses
T4	Tumor with intracranial extension and/or involvement of cranial nerves, infratemporal fossa, hypopharynx, orbit, or masticator space
Regional lymph nodes (N)	
NX	Regional lymph nodes cannot be assessed
N0	No regional lymph node metastasis
N1	Unilateral metastasis in lymph node(s), 6 cm or less in greatest dimension, above the supraclavicular fossa
N2	Bilateral metastasis in lymph node(s), 6 cm or less in greatest dimension, above the supraclavicular fossa
N3	Metastasis in a lymph node(s) > 6 cm and/or to supra clavicular fossa
	N3a greater than 6 cm in dimension
	N3b extension to the supraclavicular fossa
Distant metastasis (M)	
MX	Distant metastasis cannot be assessed
M0	No distant metastasis
M1	Distant metastasis
Stage grouping	
Stage 0	Tis N0 M0
Stage 1	T1 N0 M0
Stage 2A	T2a N0 M0
Stage 2B	T2b N0 M0 or T0-2 N1 M0
Stage 3	T0-2 N2 M0 or T3 N0-2 M0
Stage 4A	T4 N0-2 M0
Stage 4B	Any T N3 M0
Stage 4C	Any T Any N M1

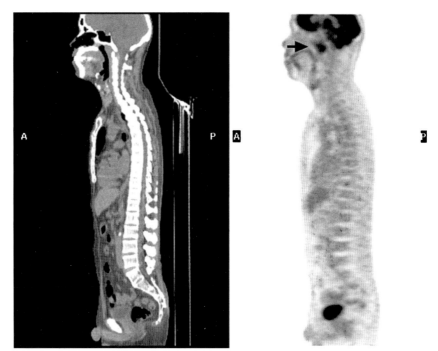

Figure 1 Sagittal images of ^{18}F-FDG PET-CT of a patient with NPC at primary staging. The PET image disclosed obviously increased FDG radioactivity at the nasopharyngeal tumor (arrow), in addition to the physiological activities at the brain and in the urinary bladder. Note also that the FDG radioactivity at the vertebral bone marrow is normal and not elevated.

A large-scaled prospective study has been conducted to address this question.

Management

Nonkeratinizing NPC has high sensitivity to radiotherapy and chemotherapy at the initial stage of treatment. This accounts for its better survival as compared to those of the squamous cell carcinomas of the head and neck in spite of its more aggressive regional and distant metastases. Radiotherapy had been the standard treatment in NPC patients for a long time. A total dose of 75 or more Gy is

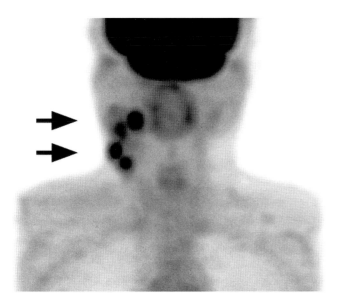

Figure 2 The anterior projection image of ^{18}F-FDG-PET of a patient with NPC indicated multiple metastatic lymphadenopathies in the right neck (arrows).

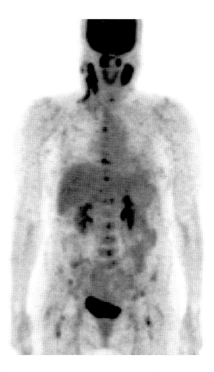

Figure 3 The anterior projection image of ^{18}F-FDG-PET of a patient with NPC indicated multiple distant metastases in the skeletal system. Note also that this patient had metastatic lymphadenopathies involving the right supraclavicular fossa and was of stage N3b.

given to the primary tumor and 65 to 70 Gy to the involved neck nodes. Because of the high incidence of occult neck node involvement, prophylactic neck radiation with a dose of 50–60 Gy is usually given. Two-dimensional techniques had been used up to the early 1990s, with a resulting 5-year overall survival of 55–60%. With newer techniques such as intensity-modulated radiation therapy (IMRT) and the concurrent use of chemotherapy, the overall survival has been increased to > 75%. IMRT can overcome some limitations of older radiotherapeutic techniques. It has achieved excellent locoregional control and decreased the salivary function impairment.

Several studies have compared the results of the use of chemotherapy in combination with radiotherapy for treating locoregional advanced NPC (Ma and Chan, 2006). Chemotherapy may decrease the chance of distant failure by eradicating micrometastases. It may enhance the effect of radiotherapy when administered concurrently, and may facilitate locoregional control by decreasing the tumor loading when administered prior to radiotherapy. The superiority of concurrent chemoradiotherapy (CCRT) over radiotherapy alone has been supported in recent meta-analyses. Prophylactic gastrostomy tubes can be placed in patients before treatment to decrease the possibility of malnutrition due to increased toxicity of CCRT, and thus decrease treatment interruptions.

For NPC patients with overt distant metastases, platinum-based combination chemotherapy has become the standard treatment. Cisplatin and infusional 5-FU can achieve a response rate of 66–76%. More intensive combinations may give a higher response rate at the cost of increased toxicities and are usually not recommended. A minority of patients with distant metastasis can achieve long-term disease-free survival after chemotherapy. Consolidation radiotherapy or CCRT for locoregional and metastatic tumor sites may be given if the tumor response for systemic chemotherapy is satisfactory. Newer treatment modalities such as targeted therapy, gene therapy, and immunotherapy are under research and development.

There is a striking difference in the sensitivity to radiotherapy and chemotherapy between the early and later courses of treatment for NPC (Faivre et al., 2004). For patients with locoregional recurrence without distant failure or for patients with sole-site distant relapse, curative-intent treatment may still be considered (Liu and Yen, 2006). However, for rerecurrent or metastatic patients who cannot achieve complete response after curative-intent treatment, the prognosis remains dismal. NPC cells may become more and more resistant to therapy after a cascade of molecular mutations and selections. Thus, early detection, accurate staging, and optimal initial treatment are the keys to improve survival of NPC patients. FDG-PET or PET-CT may be valuable in providing more accurate primary staging and in detecting patients with early relapse.

Bone Metastasis

Bone is the most common site to which NPC metastasizes. Bone consists of cortical, trabecular, and marrow components. In adults, most of the red marrow is located in axial bones and proximal femora and humeri (Roodman, 2004). At its early stage, bone metastasis starts in the bone marrow, predominantly the highly vascularized red marrow. Before cortical bone invasion becomes obvious, there are probably plenty of active tumor cells occupying the bone marrow. The bone matrix undergoes constant remodeling, which involves maintaining a dynamic balance between osteoclastic and osteoblastic activities. Bone metastasis has traditionally been characterized as osteolytic or osteoblastic, although the two processes frequently intermingle with each other. Pure osteolytic lesions develop in multiple myeloma. The myeloma cells inhibit almost all osteoblastic activity. Patients with breast cancer usually have predominantly osteolytic lesions, but variant degrees of osteoblastic activity are also present. Different lesions in the same patient also have different osteolytic and osteoblastic activities. Generally, lesions with active tumor proliferation have higher osteolytic activity, while lesions under resolution or repair have higher osteoblastic activity and may appear sclerotic. In contrast to breast cancer, patients with prostate cancer have predominantly osteoblastic lesions, although osteolytic markers are also elevated. The majority of bone metastases in NPC, like breast cancer, are predominantly osteolytic or mixed lesions.

Cook et al. (1998) studied 23 breast cancer patients with bone metastases and found that FDG-PET is superior to bone scintigraphy in the detection of osteolytic metastases. In contrast, osteoblastic metastases show lower metabolic activity and are frequently undetectable by PET. In osteoblastic metastases, there are usually fewer tumor cells and the tumor activity may be lower than that in osteolytic lesions.

For prostate cancer, FDG-PET is limited in detecting lymph node and soft tissue metastases. In the earlier studies, the ability of FDG-PET to detect bone metastases in prostate cancer seemed disappointing. Yeh et al. (1996) studied 13 prostate cancer patients with bone metastases and found that only ~ 18% of metastatic lesions were FDG-avid. Shreve et al. (1996) evaluated 34 patients and found that 65% of untreated bone metastases were FDG-avid. In a more recent and stricter study by Morris et al. (2002), FDG-PET identified 78% of bone lesions, while bone scan identified 94%. The lesions identified by FDG-PET only evolved into active lesions on bone scan thereafter, while those lesions identified by bone scan only remained stationary. It is possible that FDG-avid lesions were more active or aggressive and non-FDG-avid lesions were stable or regressive. In a recent study by Even-Sapir et al. (2006), ^{18}F-fluoride PET-CT is considered to be a more sensitive and specific modality for detecting bone metastases in prostate cancer.

Skeletal scintigraphy using Technetium-99m (^{99m}Tc)-labeled diphosphonates is the most popular method for detecting bone metastasis because of its low cost and wide availability. However, early bone metastasis, especially when the majority of tumor cells are confined in the bone marrow, is frequently missed. A significant portion of patients with advanced NPC initially considered as M0 will develop distant metastasis after treatment with a median time of < 1 year. Caglar et al. (2003) studied 171 NPC patients without evidence of distant metastasis at initial staging and found 26 (15%) patients developed bone metastasis at follow-up with a median time of 10.5 months. It is reasonable to presume that subclinical metastasis undetected by skeletal scintigraphy at initial staging was present.

In our study (Liu et al., 2006), patients with nonkeratinizing NPC before treatment were prospectively enrolled. Both FDG-PET and whole-body skeletal scintigraphy were performed at primary staging. Bone metastasis was considered to be present if there was reliable evidence identified within one year after primary diagnosis, either before or after treatment. Thirty (15%) out of 202 eligible patients were found to have bone metastasis. FDG-PET has a sensitivity of 70%, a specificity of 99%, and an accuracy of 95%, while skeletal scintigraphy has a sensitivity of 37%, a specificity of 98%, and an accuracy of 89%. FDG-PET was more sensitive than skeletal scintigraphy in the patient-based analysis ($P = 0.006$) and in the region-based analysis at the spine ($P = 0.001$). Advanced N stage was the most significant risk factor for bone metastasis ($P < 0.0001$), and the coexistence of hepatic metastasis was a prognosticator of poor survival ($P = 0.017$). It is concluded that FDG-PET is much more sensitive and accurate than skeletal scintigraphy for detecting bone metastasis in endemic NPC at initial staging, especially for lesions in the vertebral spine.

For comparing different sites of bone metastasis, the skeletal system was divided into four regions: the spine (including the whole vertebral column), the pelvis (including the iliac, ischial, and pubic bones), the thorax (including ribs and sternum), and the appendix (including extremities, scapulae, and clavicles), with the head excluded from the analysis. The spine and pelvis are the more frequently involved sites, followed by the thorax and the appendix. In addition to the vertebrae, FDG-PET is also superior to skeletal scintigraphy for lesions in the pelvic bones and extremities. This is probably related to the larger marrow space at these sites. Metastatic NPC cells probably proliferate in the marrow space first and then invade to the trabecular or cortical bones. For the thoracic cage, there seemed to be an opposite, albeit small and insignificant, inclination for skeletal scintigraphy to be more sensitive. This may be due to the smaller rib marrow space, which limits the number of proliferating tumor cells and the size of lesion. FDG-PET might not detect small lesions due to partial-volume effect and respiratory motion. In contrast, the osteoblastic reaction in the ribs seems to be easily detected by skeletal scintigraphy.

There was also a study that revealed skeletal scintigraphy to be more sensitive for lesions in the skull and thorax than that in the spine and pelvis (Schirrmeister et al., 1999).

The most significant risk factor for distant metastasis is the N stage. None of the 25 patients with stage N0 has distant metastasis, while 89% of patients with distant metastasis are of stage N3. This may lead to the assumption that tumor cells responsible for distant metastasis originate in the lymph nodes rather than in the primary tumor. Some steps of tumor transformation in the metastatic lymph node might make the tumor cell acquire the traits for distant metastasis. Further genotypic and phenotypic studies are required for validation of this assumption.

As in many other cancers, we believe that disseminated tumor cells can be present in the bone marrow in patients with locoregionally advanced NPC. However, the majority of disseminated tumor cells will not develop into persistent metastasis in bone. The key by which some cells can establish persistent metastatic foci is still unclear. Chemotherapy can possibly eliminate the majority of disseminated tumor cells and some small metastatic foci. This contributes, at least in part, to the superiority of CCRT over radiotherapy alone in the treatment of NPC. However, some metastatic foci may not be eradicated and will grow into overt lesions after CCRT. The optimal management protocols, including dosing, combination schedule, and incorporation of novel treatment, need to be further investigated for these patients with locoregionally advanced NPC. For patients with early distant metastasis detected by FDG-PET, high-dose combination chemotherapy followed by consolidation treatment for locoregional and metastatic sites can be tried.

We have also presented a case report of an NPC patient with subclinical sacral metastasis (Liu and Yen, 2006). Neither FDG-PET nor skeletal scintigraphy revealed the presence of bone metastasis at initial staging. However, sacral metastasis was detected by follow-up FDG-PET three months after CCRT and confirmed by histopathology. This patient received further chemotherapy and radiotherapy. Six cycles of cisplatin-based combination chemotherapy (cisplatin 50 mg/m^2 biweekly with oral tegafur plus uracil) were administered first. Regional radiotherapy with a total dose of 51 Gy was then delivered to the sacral area by 3D conformal radiotherapy technique concurrent with another cycle of cisplatin-based combination chemotherapy. The patient tolerated the treatment well and remains without evidence of residual or recurrent malignancy to date.

For patients with bone metastasis, concurrent hepatic metastasis was found to be a poor prognosticator of survival. This is consistent with previous studies that showed hepatic metastasis to be a poor prognosticator in NPC patients. In contrast, more favorable survivals have been demonstrated in patients with distant metastases confined to the lungs or mediastinal/hilar lymph nodes. This is quite interesting and may be related to different traits of tumor cells in different metastatic sites.

In our study, NPC patients with bone metastasis had a median survival of 20 months. The survival was not significantly better for patients with bone metastasis undetected at primary staging than for those with initially detectable bone metastasis ($P = 0.620$). This strengthens the concept that the patients with bone metastasis detected shortly after treatment actually had subclinical bone or bone marrow metastasis before treatment.

Whole-body MRI has been demonstrated to be sensitive for detecting bone marrow metastasis. PET or PET-CT utilizing ^{18}F-fluoride was also shown to be highly sensitive for malignant bone disease. Further investigations for these different modalities to detect bone or bone marrow metastasis, in addition to FDG-PET, are interesting topics. FDG-PET also has great potential in predicting and assessing treatment response, either for locoregional tumors or distant metastases.

Combined metabolic and anatomic imaging by PET-CT, with its rapidly increasing availability, is expected to have great impact in providing more accurate staging, treatment response prediction, and post-therapeutic evaluation for patients with cancers. Facilitated by this newer imaging modality, optimal treatments for NPC patients of different stages can be further pursued, with the hope that both locoregional and distant failures can be further decreased in the near future.

References

Busson, P., Keryer, C., Ooka, T., and Corbex, M. 2004. EBV-associated nasopharyngeal carcinomas: from epidemiology to virus-targeting strategies. *Trends Microbiol. 12*(8):356–360.

Caglar, M., Ceylan, E., and Ozyar, E. 2003. Frequency of skeletal metastases in nasopharyngeal carcinoma after initiation of therapy: should bone scans be used for follow-up? *Nucl. Med. Commun. 24*(12):1231–1236.

Chang, J.T., Chan, S.C., Yen, T.C., Liao, C.T., Lin, C.Y., Lin, K.J., Chen, I.H., Wang, H.M., Chang, Y.C., Chen, T.M., Kang, C.J., and Ng, S.H. 2005. Nasopharyngeal carcinoma staging by (18)F-fluorodeoxyglucose positron emission tomography. *Int. J. Radiat. Oncol. Biol. Phys. 62*(2):501–507.

Chiesa, F., and De Paoli, F. 2001. Distant metastases from nasopharyngeal cancer. *ORL J. Otorhinolaryngol. Relat. Spec. 63*(4):214–216.

Cook, G.J., Houston, S., Rubens, R., Maisey, M.N., and Fogelman, I. 1998. Detection of bone metastases in breast cancer by [18]FDG-PET: differing metabolic activity in osteoblastic and osteolytic lesions. *J. Clin. Oncol. 16*(10):3375–3379.

Even-Sapir, E., Metser, U., Mishani, E., Lievshitz, G., Lerman, H., and Leibovitch, I. 2006. The detection of bone metastases in patients with high-risk prostate cancer: ^{99m}Tc-MDP planar bone scintigraphy, single- and multi-field-of-view SPECT, ^{18}F-fluoride PET, and ^{18}F-fluoride PET/CT. *J. Nucl. Med. 47*(2):287–297.

Faivre, S., Janot, F., and Armand, J.P. 2004. Optimal management of nasopharyngeal carcinoma. *Curr. Opin. Oncol. 16*(3):231–235.

Liu, F.Y., Chang, J.T., Wang, H.M., Liao, C.T., Kang, C.J., Ng, S.H., Chan, S.C., and Yen, T.C. 2006. [^{18}F]fluorodeoxyglucose positron emission tomography is more sensitive than skeletal scintigraphy for detecting bone metastasis in endemic nasopharyngeal carcinoma at initial staging. *J. Clin. Oncol. 24*(4):599–604.

Liu, F.Y., and Yen, T.C. 2006. Nasopharyngeal carcinoma and bone metastasis. *Am. J. Oncol. Rev. 5*(5):2–4.

Liu, L.Z., Zhang, G.Y., Xie, C.M., Liu, X.W., Cui, C.Y., and Li, L. 2006. Magnetic resonance imaging of retropharyngeal lymph node metastasis in nasopharyngeal carcinoma: patterns of spread. *Int. J. Radiat. Oncol. Biol. Phys. 66*(3):721–730.

Ma, B.B.Y., and Chan, A.T.C. 2006. Systemic treatment strategies and therapeutic monitoring for advanced nasopharyngeal carcinoma. *Expert Rev. Anticancer Ther. 6*(3):383–394.

Morris, M.J., Akhurst, T., Osman, I., Nunez, R., Macapinlac, H., Siedlecki, K., Verbel, D., Schwartz, L., Larson, S.M., and Scher, H.I. 2002. Fluorinated deoxyglucose positron emission tomography imaging in progressive metastatic prostate cancer. *Urology 59*(6):913–918.

Ng, S.H., Chang, J.T., Chan, S.C., Ko, S.F., Wang, H.M., Liao, C.T., Chang, Y.C., and Yen, T.C. 2004. Nodal metastases of nasopharyngeal carcinoma: patterns of disease on MRI and FDG-PET. *Eur. J. Nucl. Med. Mol. Imaging 31*(8):1073–1080.

Ng, S.H., Chang, J.T., Ko, S.F., Yen, P.S., Wan, Y.L., Tang, L.M., and Tsai, M.H. 1997. Nasopharyngeal carcinoma: MRI and CT assessment. *Neuroradiology 39*(10):741–746.

Roodman, G.D. 2004. Mechanisms of bone metastasis. *N. Engl. J. Med. 350*(16):1655–1664.

Schirrmeister, H., Guhlmann, A., Eisner, K., Kotzerke, J., Glatting, G., Rentschler, M., Neumaier, B., Trager, H., Nussle, K., and Reske, S.N. 1999. Sensitivity in detecting osseous lesions depends on anatomic localization: planar bone scintigraphy versus 18F PET. *J. Nucl. Med. 40*:1623–1629.

Shreve, P.D., Grossman, H.B., Gross, M.D., and Wahl, R.L. 1996. Metastatic prostate cancer: initial findings of PET with 2-deoxy-2-[F-18]fluoro-D-glucose. *Radiology 199*(3):751–756.

Wei, W.I., and Sham, J.S.T. 2005. Nasopharyngeal carcinoma. *Lancet 365*(9476):2041–2054.

Yeh, S.D., Imbriaco, M., Larson, S.M., Garza, D., Zhang, J.J., Kalaigian, H., Finn, R.D., Reddy, D., Horowitz, S.M., Goldsmith, S.J., and Scher, H.I. 1996. Detection of bony metastes of androgen-independent prostate cancer by PET-FDG. *Nucl. Med. Biol. 23*(6):693–697.

7

Colorectal Polyps: Magnetic Resonance Colonography

Dirk Hartmann and Juergen F. Riemann

Colorectal Cancer Screening

Colorectal cancer (CRC) remains the second leading cause of cancer death for both women and men (Ries *et al.*, 1999) with more than 130,000 newly diagnosed cases and 50,000 deaths each year in the United States alone (Landis *et al.*, 1998). Most colon cancers develop from nonmalignant colonic adenomas or polyps over a comparatively long time period ranging between 24 and 60 months (O'Brien *et al.*, 1990). Reflecting this adenomatous pathogenesis of most colorectal cancers, polyp screening with subsequent polypectomy has been shown to constitute an effective approach for decreasing the incidence of this malignant tumor (Winawer *et al.*, 1993). Thus, colorectal screening for polyps may be considered one of the most promising preventive measures in medicine.

Most available colorectal screening modalities, including testing for occult fecal blood or double-contrast barium enema, are associated with insufficient diagnostic accuracy (Ahlquist *et al.*, 1993; Rex *et al.*, 1997). Conventional optical colonoscopy has been established as an accurate method to examine the colon, with high sensitivity and specificity regarding the detection of colorectal polyps. Despite the availability of sufficient screening options, colorectal cancer remains a considerable cause of morbidity and mortality. This discrepancy between theoretical potential and clinical reality is caused mainly in poor patient acceptance, which reflects considerable procedural pain coupled with the rigors of preparatory bowel cleansing as well as the risk of complications such as perforations and limits the acceptance of colonoscopy for colorectal cancer screening. Although various psychologic factors inhibit the acceptance of cancer screening programs in general, efforts targeting the colon have been particularly problematic. Even in countries with free access to the diagnostic measure, participation in cancer screening programs based on optical colonoscopy is suboptimal. Rex *et al.* (1997) showed that, even when offered free of charge, a huge majority of patients refused to undergo conventional colonoscopy for primary CRC screening. All these facts have motivated the development and evaluation of additional modalities to assess the large bowel, including virtual colonoscopy.

Virtual Colonoscopy

Virtual colonoscopy (VC) is based on computed tomographic (CT) or magnetic resonance imaging (MRI) three-dimensional (3D) data sets. Virtual colonoscopy is not limited to endoscopic viewing. The 3D data sets can be scrolled in a traditional two-dimensional mode on a workstation in any desired plane. This type of multiplanar reformation analysis depicts the colonic lumen and the colonic wall in relation to the surrounding abdominal morphology. Even in the presence of a stenotic tumor, the entire colon can be assessed, which often is not possible in conventional colonoscopy. Another characteristic of virtual colonoscopy is the possibility of simultaneously assessing all other abdominal organs within the displayed field-of-view. Especially in patients with colorectal cancer, the simultaneous assessment of the liver can be helpful for approving or excluding the presence of liver metastases.

Available large, prospective multicenter studies comparing computed tomographic colonography (CTC) and conventional colonoscopy have shown a wide variation in results (Pickhardt et al., 2003; Cotton et al., 2004; Rockey et al., 2005). The reasons for the variability reported in these studies include variation in the study population relative to the risk for neoplasia, variation in the techniques used to prepare the patients and perform the studies, differences in computed tomographic colonography (CTC) technology, and variability in the manner in which CTCs have been read. In the most important study using the latest techniques, the per-polyp sensitivities were 86% and 92% and per-patient sensitivities 89% and 94% for a cut-off size of 6 to 10mm, respectively, comparable to conventional colonoscopy (Pickhardt et al., 2003).

Despite promising results, the future of CT colonography as a screening method remains uncertain because potential healthy people are exposed to considerable doses of ionizing radiation. The radiation issue may even evolve into a public health concern, because screening examinations of the colon should be repeated at regular intervals (every 3–5 years). Therefore, it seems reasonable to focus on MRI for colorectal cancer screening. The technique is not associated with any radiation exposure or other harmful side effects. Furthermore, contrast agents applied in conjunction with MRI are characterized by a more favorable safety profile than CT contrast agents because they lack any nephrotoxicity and are associated with far fewer anaphylactoid reactions (Murphy et al., 1996; Prince et al., 1996).

Magnetic Resonance Colonography

Techniques

Before the examination, bowel preparation must be performed in a manner similar to that required for conventional colonoscopy, and patients should be screened for general contraindications to MRI, such as presence of metallic implants or severe claustrophobia. Hip prostheses, which are generally not considered a contraindication to MRI, may lead to strong artifacts in the region of the rectum and sigmoid colon and impede a sufficiently diagnostic image quality. Therefore, patients with hip prosthesis should not be examined.

Similar to contrast-enhanced three-dimensional MR angiography, MR colonography is based on the principles of ultrafast imaging (Luboldt et al., 2000). Because data acquisition must be performed under breath-holding conditions, the use of 1.5 T scanners equipped with strong gradient

systems is mandatory. A combination of two large flex surface coils should be used for signal reception to ensure the coverage of the entire large bowel. A sufficient distension of the large bowel loops must be accomplished. In their physiologic state, most bowel segments are collapsed and cannot be depicted properly. Bowel distension must be achieved by administrating distending media. Eventually, a high contrast between the bowel wall and the bowel lumen is important. Contrast mechanisms that allow the accurate display of the colonic wall depend strongly on the MR sequences applied and the use of intravenous and rectal contrast agents. Currently, two techniques are being evaluated for MR colonography. Based on the signal within the colonic lumen, they can be differentiated as "bright lumen" and "dark lumen" MRC.

Bright Lumen Magnetic Resonance Colonography

"Bright lumen" MRC is based on the principles of ultra-fast sequences collected after the confines of a single breath hold. After bowel cleansing in a manner similar to that required for conventional colonoscopy and after placement of a rectal enema tube, the colon is filled with the patient in a prone position using 1000 to 2000 ml of a water-based enema with paramagnetic contrast (1:100). To reduce bowel motion, the use of intravenously administered spasmolytic agents (e.g., 20 mg scopolamine or 1 mg glucagon) before the bowel filling is helpful. To ensure safe and complete bowel filling and distension, the filling process can be monitored using nonslice select sequences that provide an update every 2–3 sec. After sufficient colonic distension has been achieved, a data set of the abdomen encompassing the entire colon is collected. After the collection of a localizer sequence, two- or three-dimensional fast imaging with steady-state precession sequences is collected. Different vendor-specific names for these sequences have been introduced: TrueFISP (Siemens Medical Solutions, Erlangen, Germany), Balanced Fast Field Echo (Philips Medical Systems, Best, The Netherlands), and FIESTA (General Electric Medical Systems, Milwaukee, Wisconsin). Image features are characterized by a mixture of T1 and T2 contrast, which leads to a homogeneous bright signal of the colonic lumen. To compensate for the presence of residual air exhibiting "filling defects" similar to polyps within the colonic lumen, data sets have to be collected in both the prone and supine patient positions. On the data sets, only the colonic lumen is bright, whereas all other tissues remain low in signal intensity. The resulting contrast between the colonic lumen and surrounding structures is the basis for subsequent virtual colonographic viewing.

The detection of colorectal polyps with "bright lumen" MRC relies on the visualization of filling defects. Differential considerations for such a filling defect beyond polyps include air bubbles as well as residual fecal material. To permit differentiation, data sets are collected in both the prone and supine patient position: air and fecal material move, while polyps remain stationary.

Dark Lumen Magnetic Resonance Colonography

"Dark lumen" MRC focuses on the colonic wall. It is based on contrast between a brightly enhancing colonic wall and a homogeneously dark colonic lumen. The technique differs from "bright lumen" MRC. Instead of a gadolinium containing enema, only tap water is rectally applied, rendering low signal on heavily T1-weighted 3D gradient-echo (GRE) acquisitions. However, the administration of gases like carbon dioxide is possible. The gas is signal-less and permits delineation of the contrast-enhanced colonic wall and masses.

To obtain a bright colonic wall, it is necessary to apply paramagnetic contrast intravenously. After a first precontrast T1-weighted, three-dimensional gradient echo data set, paramagnetic contrast should be administered intravenously at a dosage of 0.2 mmol/kg. A rapid injection of normal saline should follow the paramagnetic contrast application. After a delay of 75 sec, the three-dimensional acquisition should be repeated. Because of the stable contrast enhancement of the colonic wall over a relatively long time period, the acquisition of the T1-weighted three-dimensional gradient echo sequence can be repeated. This repetition is important mainly in case of insufficient image quality (e.g., because of patient movement or technical problems). Data collection is done in a coronal plane for the three-dimensional T1-weighted sequences.

As residual air exhibits no signal in the colonic lumen, the examination needs to be performed only in the prone position. Furthermore, the "dark lumen" MRC copes with the problem of residual stool in a simple manner: if lesion enhances, it is a polyp; if it does not, it represents stool. A further advantage of "dark lumen" MRC relates to the fact that it permits direct analysis of the bowel wall. This might facilitate the evaluation of inflammatory changes in inflammatory bowel diseases. Increased contrast uptake and bowel thickening, as recorded on contrast-enhanced T1-weighted images has already been shown to correlate well with the degree of inflammation (Schreyer et al., 2006; Rottgen et al., 2006).

Data Interpretation

After finishing the MR examination, the pre- and postcontrast three-dimensional data sets should be transferred to a postprocessing workstation. At first, the contrast-enhanced three-dimensional T1-weighted images should be interpreted in the multiplanar reformation mode. This modality allows the radiologist to scroll through the data set in three orthogonal planes. Whenever a colorectal lesion is suspected, the identical part of the large bowel is to be analyzed on the corresponding native scan. By measuring signal intensities of the lesions in native and postcontrast scan, a contrast-enhancement value can be calculated. A secure differentiation between residual stool particles and real colorectal masses is possible. Colorectal masses are always strongly enhanced.

A special software tool can be used to enable the perception of the MR source data and virtual endoscopic views of the colon. MR data also should be assessed based on virtual endoscopic renderings. A virtual endoscopic fly-through improves depiction, especially of small lesions. The three-dimensional depth perception also allows the evaluation of haustral fold morphology, which enhances the observer's ability to distinguish haustral folds from colorectal masses. The virtual fly-through should be performed in an antegrade and retrograde direction, which may help to visualize both sides of haustral folds and reduce the risk of missing relevant lesions.

Fecal Tagging

Magnetic resonance colonography still requires bowel cleansing in a manner similar to conventional colonoscopy because fecal matter can mimic the appearance of colonic masses. The cleansing can be achieved with fecal tagging, a concept based on modulating the signal intensity of stool by adding contrast-modifying substances to regular meals. The signal intensity of stool is adapted to the signal properties of the rectal enema, and fecal material becomes virtually invisible. There are various theoretical approaches to fecal tagging.

A possible strategy for fecal tagging is based on rendering the colonic lumen dark by means of a rectal enema of barium sulfate and visualization of colonic polyps and other pathologies by virtue of their enhancement after the intravenous injection of paramagnetic contrast agent (Lauenstein et al., 2002). The colon is then imaged with an ultrafast, heavily T1-weighted 3D gradient-echo sequence. The darkened colonic lumen is well delineated from the bright, contrast-enhanced colonic wall. Beyond the rectal enema, the colonic lumen contains air and stool. Whereas air exhibits no signal, stool can be quite signal-rich on T1-weighted images, reflecting manganese or iron in various foods. To assimilate the signal of stool to the dark barium sulfate enema filling the colonic lumen, the stool signal must be reduced. To this end, barium sulfate can be used as the oral "fecal tagging" agent. The agent is not absorbed and mixes well with the stool. Fecal tagging with barium was used successfully in a volunteer study (Lauenstein et al., 2001). The study showed that ingestion of 200 ml of a barium sulfate-containing contrast agent with each of four low-fiber meals before the MR examination leads to a low signal of stool on T1-weighted gradient-echo images, which renders fecal material virtually indistinguishable from the administered water enema. The patient acceptance was not increased by using barium-based fecal tagging instead of bowel cleansing procedures, because the ingestion of the tagging agent was considered as unpleasant as bowel purgation (Goehde *et al.*, 2005). Today, all strategies for fecal tagging will need to be validated in larger patient cohorts before any clinical use takes place.

Diagnostic Performance of Magnetic Resonance Colonography

In contrast to computed tomographic colonography, only limited data exist comparing MR colonography and conventional colonoscopy in the detection of colorectal polyps (Table 1). In a recent trial, MR colonography with the dark lumen technique was compared with conventional colonoscopy, which served as the standard of reference (Hartmann *et al.*, 2006). One hundred patients with different clinical indications were examined prospectively. Magnetic resonance colonography was followed by subsequent conventional colonoscopy on the same time. Regarding data analysis, endoscopic and histological results were compared with MRC. In 49 patients, 107 colorectal masses were depicted by means of endoscopy. The sensitivity rate of MR colonography for adenomas on a per-polyp analysis was 100% for adenomas larger than 10mm and 84.2% for adenomas between 6 and 9mm in diameter. When using a per-patient analysis, the overall sensitivity rate for the detection of colorectal masses was 90%. There were a few false-positive results, and specificity of MR colonography amounted to 96%. In summary, MR colonography showed a high accuracy for the detection of adenomas and carcinomas larger than 5mm.

The outlined results were confirmed by other trials. In a recently published study of Ajaj *et al.* (2003), 122 subjects with suspected colorectal disease (48 polyps) underwent "dark lumen" MR-colonography followed by conventional colonoscopy. None of 30 polyps measuring ≤ 5mm identified by conventional colonoscopy were detected on MRC

images. In the 6–10mm size group, MRC correctly detected 16 of 18 documented lesions on conventional colonoscopy. In addition, two polyps ≥ 10mm and all nine colorectal carcinomas were correctly seen on MRC images.

One major issue relates to the inability of MR colonography to detect colorectal masses smaller than 5mm. Small colorectal lesions probably will become detectable by MR colonography in the future. New technical refinements, including parallel acquisition techniques, will be implemented (Steidle *et al.*, 2004; Griswold *et al.*, 2002), and spatial resolution may be increased. Flat adenomas are likely to remain elusive, however.

In another study, the diagnostic accuracy of "bright lumen" MRC was compared with the "dark lumen" technique (Lauenstein *et al.*, 2005). The detection of colorectal masses and inflammatory lesions was separately assessed for dark and bright lumen MR colonography. Image quality also was analyzed, and all patients underwent conventional colonoscopy as the standard of reference. Sensitivity of the "dark lumen" MR colonography amounted to 78.9%. There were no false-positive results. By means of the "bright lumen" MR colonography, two additional polyps could not be detected. The sensitivity rate only amounted to 68.4%. Because of the inability to distinguish residual stool particles from real colorectal masses, false-positive results were reported in 5 patients. Image quality was superior to that of "dark lumen" MR colonography because of fewer motion artifacts. "Bright lumen" MR colonography should be considered a complementary imaging modality, but the main diagnostic evaluation should be based on the "dark lumen" data.

Indications of Magnetic Resonance Colonography

There are several proven indications for MR colonography. In patients with incomplete endoscopy caused by stenoses or elongated bowel segments, virtual colonoscopy (based on either MRI or CT) has been shown to provide useful additional information (Hartmann *et al.*, 2005; Ajaj *et al.*, 2005; Gryspeerdt

Table 1   Studies Comparing MRC and Conventional Colonoscopy

Author	Year	Subjects (*n*)	Total Lesions (*n*)	Per-Polyp Sensitivity (%) 6–9mm	Per-Polyp Sensitivity (%) ≥ 10mm	Per-Patient Sensitivity (%) 6–9mm	Per-Patient Sensitivity (%) ≥ 10mm	Per-Patient Specificity (%) 6–9mm	Per-Patient Specificity (%) ≥ 10mm
Luboldt*	2000	132	189	61	96	Overall (a) 93		Overall (a) 99	
Pappalardo*	2000	70	130	96	100	Overall (a) 96		Overall (a) 93	
Ajaj**	2003	122	59 (9 carcinomas)	16/18 sensitivity: NR	11/11 sensitivity: NR	NR	NR	NR	NR
Hartmann**	2006	100	114 (7 carcinomas)	84 for adenomas	100 for adenomas	84 for adenomas	100 for adenomas	99 for adenomas	100 for adenomas

*Bright lumen MR colonography; ** dark lumen MR colonography; (a): alternate category definition; NR: not reported *et al.*, 2005; Neri *et al.*, 2002). A recent trial evaluated the impact of MR colonography in patients who had undergone incomplete colonoscopy (Hartmann *et al.*, 2005). Thirty-two patients with incomplete endoscopy for different reasons (high-grade stenosis in 26 patients, extreme patient intolerance in one patient, and technical challenges associated with an elongated colon in five patients) underwent same-day dark lumen MRC. Of the 26 patients with high-grade stenosis, 19 underwent surgery with histopathological confirmation of the initial diagnosis. Follow-up colonoscopy was carried out in 14 patients with surgically treated stenosis. In 6 out of these 14 patients, nine polyps identified at the initial MRC were confirmed and removed during a postoperative conventional colonoscopy.

There are still no evident data regarding the impact of MR colonography on colorectal cancer screening. Because most colorectal cancers develop over a period of several years from adenomatous polyps, this pathogenesis makes colorectal cancer to a large extent preventable. Detection and removal of polyps eliminate the risk of subsequent malignant degeneration. Implementations of screening programs have been shown to reduce the incidence of colorectal cancer by more than 80% (Winawer *et al.*, 1993). Magnetic reconance imaging actually includes all properties, which is necessary for a successful screening tool. The technique is not associated with any exposure to ionizing radiation and lacks any other known harmful side effects. Because of its noninvasive character, patient acceptance is not negatively impacted. Although MRI has been found to be an accurate means for the depiction of relevant colorectal masses, we must be aware that these results were based on trials performed in preselected patient cohorts. Further studies are needed to evaluate the value of MR colonography in a screening population.

Future Directions

Over the last decade, major technological advances in MRI scanners have allowed the ability to scan patients faster using thinner slices. This allows for improved quality of MR colonography examinations. Some research centers are currently evaluating alternative displays that allow viewing larger areas of the colonic surface at one time. A "virtual pathology" view bisects the colon along its longitudinal axis, opening the colon so that it may be inspected like a surgical pathologic specimen. The accuracy of these novel visualization methods needs to be determined.

Computer-aided detection (CAD) of colorectal lesions is also under investigation as a way to shorten interpretation times. Computer software that allows automated polyp detection is under development. These computer algorithms are typically based on a presumed hemispheric shape or curvature of polyps. Another area under investigation is the development of fecal and fluid tagging protocols. Because of the reluctance of some patients to undergo any form of cathartic preparations, we do believe that validation of "fecal tagging" for screening will be important to further increase compliance. However, there are several additional reasons why we believe that MRC without catharsis will not represent a singular solution. Magnetic resonance colonography should offer a same-day polypectomy for significant polyps detected at MRC. This "one-stop" service requires only a single preparation. This practice would not be possible with a "fecal tagging" approach, since patients requiring polypectomy for MRC-detected lesions would first need to undergo additional preparation prior to conventional colonoscopy. Such a "one-stop" service will only be possible with an excellent cooperation between radiologist and gastroenterologists.

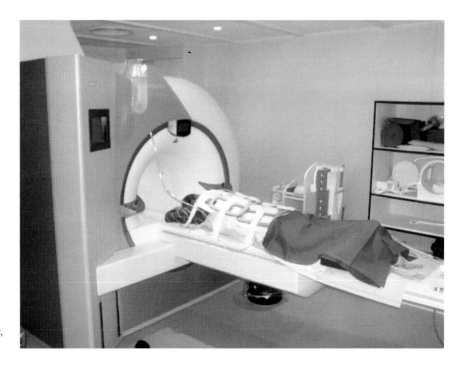

Figure 1 For filling the colon with tap water, the patient is placed in the prone position.

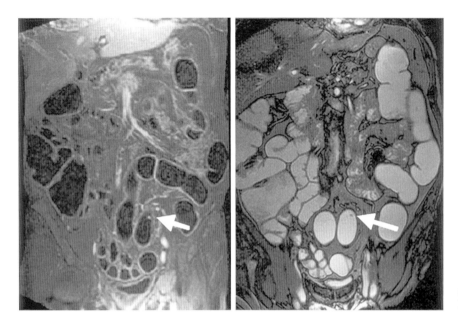

Figure 2 Small polyp in the sigmoid colon (left side: bright lumen MRC; right side: dark lumen MRC).

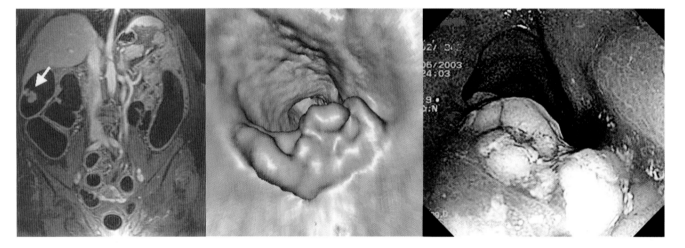

Figure 3 Large polyp in the right flexur detected using dark lumen MRC.

References

Ahlquist, D.A., Wieand, H.S., Moertel, C.G., McGill, D.B., Loprinzi, C.L., O'Connell, M.J., Mailliard, J.A., Gerstner, J.B., Pandya, K., and Ellefson, R.D. 1993. Accuracy of fecal occult blood screening for colorectal neoplasia. A prospective study using Hemoccult and HemoQuant tests. *JAMA 269*:1262–1267.

Ajaj, W., Lauenstein, T.C., Pelster, G., Holtmann, G., Ruehm, S.G., Debatin, J.F., and Goehde, S.C. 2005. MR colonography in patients with incomplete conventional colonoscopy. *Radiology 234*:452–459.

Ajaj, W., Pelster, G., Treichel, U., Vogt, F.M., Debatin, J.F., Ruehm, S.G., and Lauenstein, T.C. 2003. Dark lumen magnetic resonance colonography: comparison with conventional colonoscopy for the detection of colorectal pathology. *Gut 52*:1738–1743.

Cotton, P.B., Durkalski, V.L., Pineau, B.C., Palesch, Y.Y., Mauldin, P.D., Hoffman, B., Vining, D.J., Small, W.C., Affronti, J., Rex, D., Kopecky, K.K., Ackerman, S., Burdick, J.S., Brewington, C., Turner, M.A., Zfass, A., Wright, A.R., Iyer, R.B., Lynch, P., Sivak, M.V., and Butler, H. 2004. Computed tomographic colonography (virtual colonoscopy): a multicenter comparison with standard colonoscopy for detection of colorectal neoplasia. *JAMA 291*:1713–1719.

Goehde, S.C., Descher, E., Boekstegers, A., Lauenstein, T., Kuhle, C., Ruehm, S.G., and Ajaj, W. 2005. Dark lumen MR colonography based on fecal tagging for detection of colorectal masses: accuracy and patient acceptance. *Abd. Imag. 30*:576–583.

Griswold, M.A., Jakob, P.M., Heidemann, R.M., Nittka, M., Jellus, V., Wang, J., Kiefer, B., and Haase, A. 2002. Generalized autocalibrating partially parallel acquisitions (GRAPPA). *Magn. Reson. Med. 47*:1202–1210.

Gryspeerdt, S., Lefere, P., Herman, M., Deman, R., Rutgeerts, L., Ghillebert, G., Baert, F., Baekelandt, M., and Van Holsbeeck, B. 2005. CT colonography with fecal tagging after incomplete colonoscopy. *Eur. Radiol. 15*:1192–1202.

Hartmann, D., Bassler, B., Schilling, D., Adamek, H.E., Jakobs, R., Pfeifer, B., Eickhoff, A., Zindel, C., Riemann, J.F., and Layer, G. 2006. Colorectal polyps: detection with dark-lumen MR colonography versus conventional colonoscopy. *Radiology 238*:143–149.

Hartmann, D., Bassler, B., Schilling, D., Pfeiffer, B., Jakobs, R., Eickhoff, A., Riemann, J.F., and Layer, G. 2005. Incomplete conventional colonoscopy: magnetic resonance colonography in the evaluation of the proximal colon. *Endoscopy 37*:816–820.

Landis, S.H., Murray, T., Bolden, S., and Wingo, P.A. 1998. Cancer statistics, 1998. *CA Cancer J. Clin. 48*:6–29.

Lauenstein, T.C., Ajaj, W., Kuehle, C.A., Goehde, S.C., Schlosser, T.W., and Ruehm, S.G. 2005. Magnetic resonance colonography: comparison of contrast-enhanced three-dimensional vibe with two-dimensional FISP sequences: preliminary experience. *Invest. Radiol. 40*:89–96.

Lauenstein, T.C., Goehde, S.C., Ruehm, S.G., Holtmann, G., and Debatin, J.F. 2002. MR colonography with barium-based fecal tagging: initial clinical experience. *Radiology 223*:248–254.

Lauenstein, T.C., Holtmann, G., Schoenfelder, D., Bosk, S., Ruehm, S.G., and Debatin, J.F. 2001. MR colonography without colonic cleansing: a new strategy to improve patient acceptance. *Am. J. Roentgenol. 177*:823–827.

Luboldt, W., Bauerfeind, P., Wildermuth, S., Marincek, B., Fried, M., and Debatin, J.F. 2000. Colonic masses: detection with MR colonography. *Radiology 216*:383–388.

Murphy, K.J., Brunberg, J.A., and Cohan, R.H. 1996. Adverse reactions to gadolinium contrast media: a review of 36 cases. *Am. J. Roentgenol. 167*:847–849.

Neri, E., Giusti, P., Battolla, L., Vagli, P., Boraschi, P., Lencioni, R., Caramella, D., and Bartolozzi, C. 2002. Colorectal cancer: role of CT colonography in preoperative evaluation after incomplete colonoscopy. *Radiology 223*:615–619.

O'Brien, M.J., Winawer, S.J., Zauber, A.G., Gottlieb, L.S., Sternberg, S.S., Diaz, B., Dickersin, G.R., Ewing, S., Geller, S., Kasimian, D., *et al.* 1990. The National Polyp Study. Patient and polyp characteristics associated with high-grade dysplasia in colorectal adenomas. *Gastroenterology 98*:371–379.

Pappalardo, G., Polettini, E., Frattaroli, F.M., Casciani, E., D'Orta, C., D'Amato, M., and Gualdi, G.F. 2000. Magnetic resonance colonography versus conventional colonoscopy for the detection of colonic endoluminal lesions. *Gastroenterology 119*:300–304.

Pickhardt, P.J., Choi, J.R., Hwang, I., Butler, J.A., Puckett, M.L., Hildebrandt, H.A., Wong, R.K., Nugent, P.A., Mysliwiec, P.A., and Schindler, W.R. 2003. Computed tomographic virtual colonoscopy to screen for colorectal neoplasia in asymptomatic adults. *N. Engl. J. Med. 349*:2191–2200.

Prince, M.R., Arnoldus, C., and Frisoli, J.K. 1996. Nephrotoxicity of high-dose gadolinium compared with iodinated contrast. *J. Magn. Reson. Imaging 6*:162–166.

Rex, D.K., Rahmani, E.Y., Haseman, J.H., Lemmel, G.T., Kaster, S., and Buckley, J.S. 1997. Relative sensitivity of colonoscopy and barium enema for detection of colorectal cancer in clinical practice. *Gastroenterology 112*:17–123.

Ries, L.A.G., Eisner, M.P., Kosary, C.L., Hankey, B.F., Miller, B.A., Clegg, L., and Edwards, B.K. 1999. SEER Cancer Statistics Review, 1973–1996. Bethesda, MD: National Cancer Institute.

Rockey, D.C., Paulson, E., Niedzwiecki, D., Davis, W., Bosworth, H.B., Sanders, L., Yee, J., Henderson, J., Hatten, P., Burdick, S., Sanyal, A., Rubin, D.T., Sterling, M., Akerkar, G., Bhutani, M.S., Binmoeller, K., Garvie, J., Bini, E.J., McQuaid, K., Foster, W.L., Thompson, W.M., Dachman, A., and Halvorsen, R. 2005. Analysis of air contrast barium enema, computed tomographic colonography, and colonoscopy: prospective comparison. *Lancet 365*:305–311.

Rottgen, R., Herzog, H., Lopez-Haninnen, E., and Felix, R. 2006. Bowel wall enhancement in magnetic resonance colonography for assessing activity in Crohn's disease. *Clin. Imaging 30*:27–31.

Schreyer, A.G., Scheibl, K., Heiss, P., Feuerbach, S., Seitz, J., and Herfarth, H. 2006. MR colonography in inflammatory bowel disease. *Abdom. Imag., 31*:302–307.

Steidle, G., Schafer, J., Schlemmer, H.P., Claussen, C.D., and Schick, F. 2004. Two-dimensional parallel acquisition technique in 3D MR colonography. *Rofo. 176*:1100–1105.

Winawer, S.J., Zauber, A.G., Ho, M.N., O'Brien, M.J., Gottlieb, L.S., Sternberg, S.S., Waye, J.D., Schapiro, M., Bond, J.H., Panish, J.F., *et al.* 1993. Prevention of colorectal cancer by colonoscopic polypectomy. The National Polyp Study Workgroup. *N. Engl. J. Med. 329*: 1977–1981.

8

Early Bile Duct Carcinoma: Ultrasound, Computed Tomography, Cholangiography, and Magnetic Resonance Cholangiography

Jae Hoon Lim

Introduction

Early bile duct cancer is defined as carcinoma limited to the mucosa or fibromuscular layer of the bile duct (Mizumoto et al., 1993). With few exceptions, these tumors have no lymph node metastasis, venous invasion, perineural, or lymphatic infiltration. Radiological diagnosis of early bile duct carcinoma is important because patients with early bile duct cancer, if resected, have an excellent prognosis, the cumulative 5-year-survival rate being 83–100% (Mizumoto et al., 1993; Bhuiya et al., 1993).

Pathology of Early Bile Duct Cancer

Tumor may arise anywhere in the bile ducts, intrahepatic, hilar, or extrahepatic ducts. The tumor is within the bile ducts and presents with nodular, polypoid, cast-like appearances and varies in size from 1 to 5 cm, or larger (Lim et al., 2006). In some patients with early bile duct carcinoma, the tumor is large and extensive, involving both intrahepatic and extrahepatic ducts. This is probably because tumor cells grow and spread superficially along the bile duct mucosa and do not invade deeply into the fibromuscular layer (Iwahashi et al., 1998; Lim et al., 2003, 2004). However large, early bile duct cancer is limited to the mucosa or fibromuscular layer and does not penetrate beyond fibromuscular layer. The tumor-bearing fibromuscular layer may be thickened, varying from 1.5 to 2.0 mm. Histologically, the tumor is papillary adenocarcinoma, well-differentiated tubular adenocarcinoma, or well-differentiated papillotubular adenocarcinoma.

Sonographic Features

Sonograms will show an intraductal soft tissue mass with well-defined echogenic lines of the bile duct wall (Fig. 1) (Lim et al., 2006). On axial scans to the bile ducts, circular or curved lines of outer margins are well delineated.

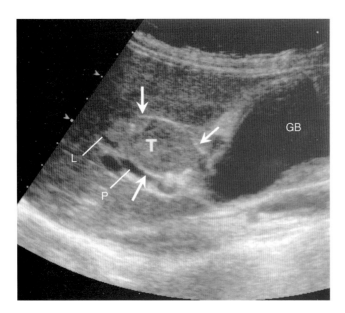

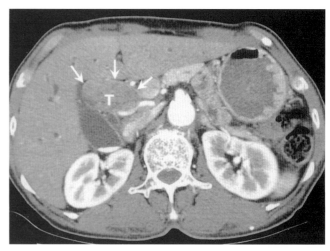

Figure 2 Early bile duct carcinoma of the extrahepatic duct. Contrast-enhanced CT scan shows intraductal mass (T) filling the entire extrahepatic duct. Note a well-preserved, thin, enhancing wall (arrows).

Figure 1 Early bile duct carcinoma of the right hepatic duct extending downward to the common hepatic duct. Sonogram of the liver shows a tumor (T) filling the right hepatic duct. Note the well-preserved thin echogenic lines (arrows) representing the wall of the intrahepatic bile duct. L = lumen of right hepatic duct, P = right branch of portal vein, GB = gallbladder.

Sonographic demonstration of the bile duct wall and its integrity are the most valuable finding for the evaluation of early bile duct carcinoma (Lim *et al.*, 2006). The bile duct wall is more echogenic than the tumor mass because of the periductal fat. Due to the fibrofatty tissue of the perimuscular layer, the intrahepatic and extrahepatic bile duct wall was delineated as clear, thin, echogenic lines on longitudinal scans and rings on axial scans.

Computed Tomography Features

Computed tomography shows an intraductal soft tissue mass with varying size. Mean attenuation is 40 HU (range, 35–45) on precontrast scan and is 100 HU (mean, 85–150) on postcontrast CT scan. The outer surfaces of the bile duct harboring masses are sharply defined without infiltration of the adjacent periductal fat (Fig. 2) (Lim *et al.*, 2006). In patients with intrahepatic and hilar cholangiocarcinoma, the outer margin of the tumor-bearing bile duct is usually not distinctly delineated due to lack of intrahepatic periductal fat or partial volume averaging. In some patients, the bile duct is enhanced as a thin tube or ring on contrast-enhanced CT images; its thickness is 0.5–1.0 mm.

On CT images, the wall of the normal extrahepatic duct is delineated as a thin ring. In patients with early bile duct carcinoma, the bile ducts harboring a tumor mass are clearly delineated as a sharply defined outer margin or as a thin, enhancing ring, sometimes more densely enhanced than the

tumor mass. The thickened fibromuscular layer of the tumor-bearing bile duct wall seems to be responsible for the sharp margin of the bile duct or encircling ring. The periductal fat is clear and not infiltrated. Even in patients whose tumor mass is large and extensive, ductal wall integrity will be preserved and there is no evidence of periductal infiltration on sonograms or CT images.

Cholangiography and Magnetic Resonance Cholangiographic Features

On cholangiograms, the size, shape, and extent of tumors are well demonstrated. The outer surfaces of tumor-bearing bile ducts are irregular due to the papillary surface of the tumor per se (Fig. 3). It is not possible to evaluate whether or not the tumor involves the outer surface of the bile ducts (Lim *et al.*, 2006). Depending on the location, the degree of bile duct patency, and technique of the endoscopist, only distal or proximal margins of the tumor are visualized. Sometimes the tumor may be too small to visualize, or the tumor may be masked by mucin. In some patients, with mucin-producing variant, there is a large amount of intraductal mucin, presenting as ovoid, elongated, or amorphous filling defects, simulating intraductal tumors (Lim *et al.*, 2004, 2006).

Bile ducts proximal to the tumor are dilated depending on the degree of obstruction by the tumors. In some patients the bile duct is completely obstructed, but in the majority, bile ducts are only partially obstructed. In some patients, the entire biliary tree was dilated markedly due to excessive mucin, even though the bile duct was not completely obstructed. The reason is that the mucin is thick and viscid and bile flow is impaired (Lim *et al.*, 2004). On MR cholangiograms, the tumor size and extent are well demonstrated.

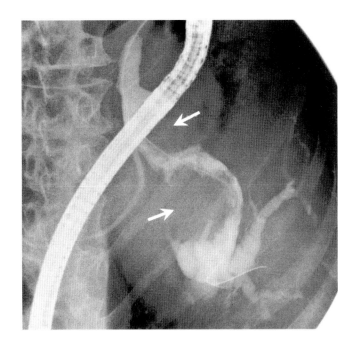

Figure 3 Early bile duct carcinoma of the extrahepatic duct. Endoscopic retrograde cholangiogram shows intraductal tumor of the extrahepatic duct (arrows). Note irregular ragged appearance representing papillary surface of the tumor.

In patients with papillary carcinoma, the papillary surface of the tumor is well depicted. The dilated biliary tree is well demonstrated in all. It is not possible to evaluate the depth of tumor invasion or periductal infiltration.

Comparison between Pathology and Imaging

On the basis of the intact bile duct wall, which has well-preserved echogenic lines of the tumor-bearing duct wall on sonograms and a clear outer margin of the bile duct without periductal fat infiltration on CT images, it is possible to make a diagnosis of early bile duct carcinoma by imaging (Lim *et al.*, 2006). However large and extensive the mass is, the bile duct wall remains intact and is visualized as smooth, well-defined echogenic lines on sonograms and as a sharply defined outer margin or as a thin enhancing ring on CT images. There is no difference in image findings between early carcinoma confined to the mucosa and that involved in the fibromuscular layer of the bile duct wall. In some patients in which the bile duct wall is enhanced, the tumor-bearing fibromuscular layer of the duct is thickened up to 2.0 mm.

However, there are limitations to the imaging diagnosis of early bile duct carcinoma. It is not always possible to visual-

ize the distal part of the common bile duct by sonography due to duodenal or colon gas. On CT images, it is difficult to determine whether the bile duct wall or periductal tissue has been infiltrated because of partial-volume averaging with adjacent organs such as the pancreas, or because of scanty fat around the bile ducts. It is difficult to determine periductal tumor infiltration in intrahepatic bile duct tumors because there is little periductal fat in the portal triads. In this regard, sonography is better for determining periductal tumor infiltration because the periductal fat can be delineated as echogenic. It is not possible to distinguish between invasion of the mucosa from invasion of the fibromuscular layer by sonography or CT. Although cholangiography and MR cholangiography allow the size, shape, and extent of a tumor to be precisely evaluated, it is not possible to determine the depth of tumor invasion in the bile duct wall. When a tumor mass is small and located at the confluence or branching area of the intrahepatic bile ducts, the mass cannot be depicted due to the complex anatomy of the bile ducts. Therefore, it is not possible to correctly stage the tumor as in two of our patients.

Recently, endoscopic sonography of the bile ducts is increasingly being used because the resolution of endoscopic ultrasound is better than transabdominal sonography. Thus, a small tumor can be detected, and the depth of tumor invasion can be better evaluated. In this regard, endoscopic biliary sonography offers an improved means for the diagnosis and staging of early bile duct carcinoma (Mukai *et al.*, 1992; Tamada *et al.*, 2001).

References

Bhuiya, M.R., Nimura, Y., Kamiya, J., Kondo, S., Nagino, M., and Hayakawa, N. 1993. Clinicopathologic factors influencing survival of patients with bile duct carcinoma: multivariate statistical analysis. *World J. Surgery 17*:653–657.

Iwahashi, N., Hayakawa, N., Yamamoto, H., Maki, A., Kawabata, Y., Murayama, A., Nimura, Y., Kamiya, J., Nagino, M., and Mori, N. 1998. Mucosal bile duct carcinoma with superficial spread. *J. Hepatob. Pancreat. Surg. 5*:221–225.

Lim, J.H. 2003. Cholangiocarcinoma: morphologic classification according to growth pattern and imaging findings. *AJR 181*:819–827.

Lim, J.H., Jang, K.T., Choi, D., Lee, W.J., and Lim, H.K. 2006. Early bile duct carcinoma: comparison of imaging features with pathologic findings. *Radiology 238*:542–548.

Lim, J.H., Yoon, K.H., Kim, S.H., Kim, H.Y., Lim, H.K., Song, S.Y., and Nam, K.J. 2004. Intraductal papillary mucinous tumor of the bile ducts. *RadioGraphics 24*:53–67.

Mizumoto, R., Ogura, Y., and Kusuda, T. 1993. Definition and diagnosis of early cancer of the biliary tract. *Hepatogastroenterology 40*:69–77.

Mukai, H., Nakajima, M., Yasuda, K., Mizuno, S., and Kawai, K. 1992. Evaluation of endoscopic ultrasonography in the preoperative staging of carcinoma of the ampulla of Vater and common bile duct. *Gastrointest. Endosc. 38*:676–683.

Tamada, K., Inui, K., and Menzel, J. 2001. Intraductal ultrasonography of the bile duct system. *Endoscopy 33*:878–885.

9

Incidental Extracolonic Lesions: Computed Tomography

Revathy B. Iyer and Chaan S. Ng

Introduction

Colorectal carcinoma (CRC) is the second most common malignant tumor in the Western world, and is a leading cause of morbidity and mortality in the United States and other industrialized countries. There were 145,000 estimated new cases in the United States in 2005, resulting in 56,000 estimated deaths (Jemal *et al.*, 2005). Most colon cancers are thought to develop directly from adenomatous polyps (Muto *et al.*, 1975). The histology of the polyp as well as the size are important in determining which are premalignant. The risk for developing invasive carcinoma in unresected polyps is 2.5% at 5 years, 8% at 10 years, and 24% at 20 years, indicating that this is a disease that has a long lead time for development, and is therefore ideally suited for early intervention and prevention.

Efforts to detect and screen for this tumor would seem to offer prospects for major impact on this malignancy. The ideal screening test for colorectal cancer should be safe, accurate, and inexpensive. Currently available screening tests include fecal occult blood testing, sigmoidoscopy/colonoscopy, air contrast barium enema, and, more recently, computed tomography (CT) colonography. Direct visualization of the colon, via colonoscopy, is generally considered to be the gold-standard modality for assessing the colon. However, it has a number of limitations, including the need for bowel cleansing, patient sedation, relative invasiveness, and

risk of bowel perforation. Air (or double) contrast barium enema has been considered the radiological gold standard. It is a fluoroscopic technique that offers indirect visualization of the colon. As with colonoscopy, it requires bowel cleansing and carries some risk of bowel perforation and, in addition, requires some degree of patient mobility and sphincter control. Both techniques are essentially luminal evaluations of the colon, that focus principally on visualization of the mucosal detail. Both techniques are unable to detect abnormalities beyond the colonic mucosa, except occasionally by inference due, for example, to extraluminal mass effect or luminal narrowing.

Advances in CT, which is intrinsically a transaxial technique, have permitted its potential utility as a means to evaluate the colon. These advances have included high spatial resolution, high-speed data acquisition, and three-dimensional (3D) reconstruction algorithms. Three-dimensional reconstruction of transaxial, isometric, source data sets enables multiplanar reconstructions and creation of surface- and volume-rendered images. It is possible with navigation software to "fly through" the colon as though viewing the colon via an endoscope—hence the term *virtual colonoscopy* or *CT colonography* (CTC).

Minimum preparation CT (MPCT) is essentially an abdomino-pelvic CT, but it utilizes prolonged administration of oral contrast medium, and typically without the administration of intravenous contrast media. It has been suggested as a means of evaluating the colon in patients who would have difficulty with colonoscopy or barium enema, such as the frail, elderly, or disabled patient. The technique does not have the high technical demands of CT colonography of high-resolution data sets and 3D reconstructions, since it does not set out to attempt to detect small colonic lesions, as does CTC. In this chapter, we review the reported studies describing extracolonic findings on CT in both CT colonography and minimal preparation CT. The techniques are quite different in their acquisition details and potential clinical application. We discuss some of the issues raised by the detection of extracolonic findings at CT and of evaluating their contribution. We also briefly discuss the practical implications and handling of specific findings.

Computed Tomography Colonography Technique

Computed tomography colonography, or virtual colonoscopy, was first described over 10 years ago by Vining *et al.* (1994). "Virtual" refers to the use of helical CT image data to reconstruct a 3D endoluminal perspective of the colon similar to that seen by the endoscopist during colonoscopy. This colonography requires rapid image acquisition during breath-holding; therefore, helical CT using a multidetector scanner that will allow rapid imaging of the abdomen and pelvis is a necessity. A workstation for coordinated evaluation of 2D and 3D reconstructions is also necessary for interpreting these studies.

Prior to the procedure, colonic cleansing similar to that used for colonoscopy or barium enema using low residue diet and laxatives is generally performed. During the procedure, a rectal tube is placed, and the colon is slowly insufflated with room air or carbon dioxide to the maximum that is tolerated by the patient. Manual insufflation may be performed with a Foley catheter attached to a rectal tube, usually requiring ~ 50 puffs of air. Semiautomatic mechanical insufflators are preferred because they allow better control of pressure and volume of gas delivered, although patients with colonic strictures may be problematic. Carbon dioxide also tends to be resorbed faster than room air, resulting in a shorter period of discomfort for the patient (Stevenson *et al.*, 1992). Slow insufflation is important in order to decrease the incidence of spasm and discomfort. Glucagon or other spasmolytics may be given. After ~ 2 liters of air or carbon dioxide is insufflated into the colon with a rectal tube, scans of the entire colon are obtained at 1–3 mm collimation in the supine and prone positions. Supine and prone scans are important to redistribute gas and fluid in the colon, so that the entire colonic wall is visualized. Typical scanning parameters utilized in multidetector (16 or 64 row) CT scanners include 1.25 mm scan thickness, 0.8 mm reconstruction interval, 120 kVp, 140 mA.

Image data are then transferred to a workstation where 2D and 3D images may be viewed. The former images should be viewed with multiple window settings, including lung and soft tissue windows, in order to optimize visualization of polyps. Overall sensitivity for polyp detection is dependent on polyp size and has ranged between 55% and 93% (Cotton *et al.*, 2004; Fenlon *et al.*, 1999; Johnson *et al.*, 2003; Pickhardt *et al.*, 2003; Yee *et al.*, 2001).

Minimal Preparation Computed Tomography Technique

Minimal preparation CT (MPCT) was originally suggested in the 1990s as a means of evaluating patients for the possibility of colonic cancer. The original concept was that MPCT was relatively noninvasive, as compared to the gold-standard techniques of colonoscopy and barium enema. The latter techniques require bowel cleansing, the introduction of a rectal tube and insufflation of air and/or barium, and a degree of patient mobility and cooperation. Colonoscopy usually requires some type of sedation, and barium enema, an antispasmodic of some kind (for example, glucagon or Buscopan). These requirements are particularly challenging for the frail, elderly, disabled or immobile, and cognitively impaired; many such patients also consider the procedures embarrassing. Minimal preparation CT simply requires the oral ingestion of positive contrast medium, typically 1–2 liters of dilute meglumine and sodium amidotrizoate (Gastrografin, Schering, Berlin, Germany) over the course of 48 hr prior to the scan. No rectal intubation or muscle relaxants are used. Patients are scanned in a conventional supine position, typically without intravenous contrast initially. Intravenous contrast is only suggested, by some centers, if there are some equivocal findings on the initial noncontrast evaluation. Computed tomography is undertaken with a conventional diagnostic scanning dose (120 kVp, 320 mA). Early studies, undertaken on nonhelical and single-slice helical CT scanners, typically utilized 10–15 mm collimation. Thinner collimations are now possible with multidetector CTs. Meta-analysis suggests an overall sensitivity of 83% (95% CI 76–89%), and specificity of 90% (85–94%) for detection of colorectal carcinomas using this technique (Koo *et al.*, 2006).

Extracolonic Findings in Computed Tomography Colonography and Minimum Preparation Computed Tomography

Both CTC and MPCT are directed principally toward detecting colonic lesions, and, because of the cross-sectional nature of CT, other organs are also visualized. Detection of extracolonic lesions is thereby a byproduct of the examination. Such findings may be previously already known. Others may be completely asymptomatic and incidental to the original purpose of the scan (hence the term *incidentaloma*), or in those in whom the evaluation is undertaken for symptomatic reasons, they may provide an explanation for the symptoms or signs. It is the latter two situations that are of particular interest in this discussion. The findings may be highly relevant to the overall evaluation of the colonic tumor, or they may be unrelated and purely incidental.

Extracolonic Findings in Computed Tomography Colonography

Extracolonic lesions are frequently seen on CT colonography studies. These may be classified to be of low, moderate, or high significance (Tables 1 and 2). Hara *et al.* (2000) first reported an overall incidence of 11% of significant extracolonic findings. Since that time, multiple other studies have also reported that extracolonic findings are not unusual in a screening population. Extracolonic findings on non contrast enhanced CT colonography have been reported in 18% to 85% of patients (as summarized in Table 3). While many of these findings tended to be benign or of no clinical significance, 7 to 23% of them have been reported to be clinically significant. Examples of insignificant incidental findings include hepatic or renal cysts and calcifications, as well as normal variants (for example, Fig. 1). These are considered to be benign and require no further work-up.

Findings of moderate importance are those that do not require immediate intervention but should be further evaluated for possible future intervention. Such intermediate lesions include gallstones, indeterminate renal lesions, adrenal lesions that are probably benign, uterine fibroids, and hiatal hernias. Lesions of major importance typically do require medical or surgical intervention, and these may include lymphadenopathy, aortic aneurysm, and solid masses in abdominal or pelvic viscera that may represent incidental malignancies. Extracolonic cancers that have been incidentally found during CT colonography studies include those of ovarian, lung, renal, hepatic, pancreatic, biliary, and bladder origin as well as lymphoma (Xiong *et al.*, 2005).

Table 1 Incidental Lesions Considered to Be of Low Significance in CT Colonography Studies

Cysts (renal, hepatic, ovary, bone)	Calcifications (vascular, prostatic,
Granulomata (hepatic, splenic,	appendix, mitral valve)
lung)	Bone island
Diverticula (colon, bladder, gastric)	Fatty liver
Pleural plaques	Degenerative joint disease
Uterine fibroids	Congenital (malrotation, urachal
Hiatal hernia	remnant, horseshoe kidney,
Lipoma	vascular anomalies, spenules, etc.)

Table 2 Incidental Lesions Considered to Be of Moderate to High Significance in CT Colonography Studies

Calculi (renal, ureteral, bladder, gallbladder)	Lymphadenopathy
	Biliary dilation
Mass/Nodule (renal, adrenal, hepatic, pancreatic, ovarian, bladder, lung)	Organ enlargement (uterus, liver, spleen, prostate)
	Ascites
Hernias (abdominal wall, inguinal, large hiatal)	Aneurysms

When intravenous contrast is not utilized, characterization of some incidentally detected lesions proves to be difficult. Hepatic and renal lesions that are not clearly cystic on noncontrast CT prove particularly difficult. Aneurysms, gallstones, hernias, and renal calcifications do not require contrast for identification or characterization (for example, Fig. 2). While most CTC studies are performed without the use of intravenous contrast enhancement, a few studies have used intravenous contrast media. These have shown an even larger number of incidental findings that may not be evident on noncontrast scans (Yee *et al.*, 2005). Spreng *et al.* (2005) reported that of all the extracolonic lesions found in their study, 71% were found on contrast-enhanced CT and 29% on nonenhanced CT. The use of intravenous contrast revealed lesions such as vascular thrombosis, which could not be diagnosed on noncontrast studies. Additional work-up for incidentally found lesions was also higher in this study, where 31% of patients who had findings on contrast-enhanced CT required additional work-up as compared to 13% of patients who had findings on noncontrast CT (Yee *et al.*, 2005). These figures concur with those of other studies that have evaluated the overall percentage of patients who have required additional

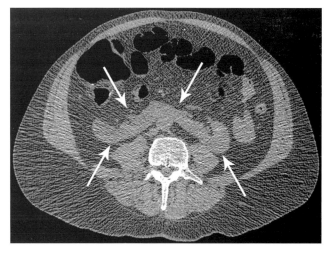

Figure 1 59-year-old male with incidental horseshoe kidney found on screening CT colonography (*arrows*).

Table 3   Extracolonic Findings on CT Colonography

Author	Ginnerup Pedersen et al.	Gluecker et al.	Pickhardt et al.	Hellstrom et al.	Rajakapsa et al.	Chin et al.	Spreng et al.	Yee et al.
Year of Publication	2003	2003	2003	2004	2004	2005	2005	2005
Population	Diagnostic	Screening	Screening	Diagnostic	Diagnostic	Screening	Diagnostic	Screening Diagnostic
Number of Patients	75	681	1233	111	250	432	102	500 (all male)
Age (Range), Years	Median 61 (33–78)	Mean 64 (41–80)	Median 57.8 (Not provided)	Median 66 (19–86)	Mean 62.5 (Not provided)	Not provided (50–69)	Mean 66 (20–91)	Mean 62.5 (30–90)
Intravenous Contrast	No	No	No	No	No	No	Yes 72/102 No 30/102	(Not provided)
Number of Patients with Extracolonic Findings (%)	49 (65%)	469 (69%)	223 (18%)	94 (85%)	83 (33%)	118 (27%)	With C: 68/72 (94%) No C: 23/30 (77%)	315 (63%)
Number of Patients with Major / Important Findings (%)	9 (12%)	88(13%)	56 (4–5%)	26 (23%)	17* (12.5%)*	32 (7%)	With C: 22/72 (31%) No C: 4/30 (13%)	45 (9%)

For a list of major/important findings requiring further work-up, see Table 2.

With C, with intravenous contrast; No C, without intravenous contrast.

Diagnostic, patients with symptoms.

*Quoted as 17 highly significant findings, out of 136 extracolonic overall findings (which were found in 83 patients). The number of patients with significant findings has not been provided.

work-up with noncontrast CT. These studies found that 12 to 14% of patients are further evaluated with imaging or other intervention (Ginnerup Pedersen *et al.*, 2003; Xiong *et al.*, 2005).

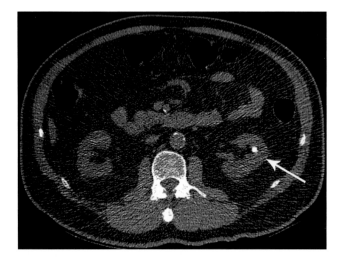

Figure 2 64-year-old man with incidental left renal calculi on screening CT colonography (*arrow*).

The population of patients being evaluated also makes a difference to the number of incidental findings that may be encountered. A low-risk screening population is different from a population that is at higher risk (Chin *et al.*, 2005). Hellstrom *et al.* (2004) found that major extracolonic findings were overrepresented in patients with malignant disease—75% as compared to 17% in those patients without malignancy. Other findings such as benign and clinically silent malignant tumors also tend to increase in elderly patients. In our review of 44 patients with colorectal cancer who presented for follow-up imaging for surveillance, CT detected significant extracolonic disease in 5 patients, or 11%. These findings included 3 extracolonic metastases, 1 new lung cancer, and 1 mesenteric desmoid tumor. A study by Yee *et al.* (2005), however, did not find a significant difference in the number of extracolonic findings in their evaluation of 500 men, when comparing those with average risk of colon cancer (who constituted 38% of the study population), versus those with high risk of colon cancer (61% of the study population). In a population over the age of ~ 50, vascular lesions such as aneurysms are also detected more frequently. Because of their age, these patients are at greater risk for aneurysms. The incidence of abdominal aortic aneurysm is 5% as reported by sonographic screening studies in patients over 50 years of age. Similar statistics are reported on CT colonography studies because the population of patients examined is of similar age (Hellstrom *et al.*, 2004).

Detection of extracolonic findings will also be influenced by the CT colonography technique. Many advocate the use of lower tube current in order to decrease the overall radiation dose, particularly in patients who are undergoing screening studies (Hara *et al.*, 1997). The use of lower tube current on the order of 70–140 mA allows excellent detail of the colonic wall because of the high contrast between gas in the colon and soft tissue of the colonic wall. However, the solid viscera are not as well evaluated at these lower tube currents. The increase in image noise resulting from very thin collimation and low tube current affects the ability to detect extracolonic abnormalities. Patient body habitus is yet another factor that contributes to image noise and ability to adequately visualize lesions in the solid viscera, such as the liver and kidneys, particularly on low-dose CT examinations. Studies using a higher tube current have reported a larger percentage of incidental extracolonic findings (Spreng *et al.*, 2005).

Costs for the work-up of incidental findings have been estimated in a few studies. They range between $28 and $34 per patient for immediate follow-up studies, such as additional imaging (Chin *et al.*, 2005; Gluecker *et al.*, 2003; Rajapaksa *et al.*, 2004; Yee *et al.*, 2005). Intangible costs include morbidity of additional studies and treatment; psychological consequences such as anxiety for the patient should also be considered. The medicolegal implications of failing to diagnose clinically important extracolonic lesions by CT colonography remain an unknown.

Extracolonic Findings in Minimum Preparation Computed Tomography

There have been comparatively limited numbers of reports detailing the extracolonic findings at MPCT. Most have been relatively anecdotal and have not attempted a systematic evaluation. Some attempt has been made to classify the findings by grade of seriousness or severity of the findings. Extracolonic findings have been reported in 16 to 32% of cases, of which 8 to 23% have been notionally considered to be of moderate to high significance or importance. The reported series are summarized in 4. One report has attempted a more rigorous evaluation, examining the potential contribution of the extracolonic findings to, for example, the staging of the CRC disease, detection of non-CRC malignancy, and, importantly, insight into the accuracy of these findings (Ng *et al.*, 2004). A possible scheme for evaluating such findings is presented in Fig. 3.

Extracolonic Findings Relevant to Staging Colorectal Cancer

Extracolonic abnormalities that are detected in the same patient in whom a (truly positive) CRC is detected may be relevant to staging the disease by, for example, demonstrating local extracolonic extension of disease, or liver or nodal metastases. The TNM staging and Dukes' classification of CRC are presented in Table 5.

Local Extent of Disease

TNM stage T3 disease may be appreciated as a mass or soft tissue stranding in the adjacent pericolic fat, or irregularity in the outer margin of the bowel wall (Horton *et al.*, 2000; Thoeni, 1997). The absence of these features does not exclude microscopic extension of disease. Unfortunately, CT cannot distinguish the layers of the bowel wall; hence, the depth of invasion into the bowel wall cannot be assessed (i.e., TNM stages T1 and T2 disease). In comparison to CT, MRI and endorectal ultrasound are better able to delineate the bowel wall layers in the rectum and can make a better contribution to such local staging. Invasion into adjacent organs can be detected, for example, muscle (abdominal or pelvic), small bowel, visceral organs, pelvic organs, and bones (TNM stage T4). However, differentiation of simple abutment of tissues and invasion can sometimes be difficult to distinguish on CT.

Nodal Metastatic Disease

Computed tomography may assist in nodal staging (TNM stage N disease). However, the only available CT criterion at present is based on nodal size. The relative sensitivity and specificity for detecting nodal metastatic disease depends on the cut-off size used: a short-axis nodal dimension of 1–1.5 cm is the typical size cut-off used, with nodes larger than this value considered suspicious for harboring metastases. However, size is an unreliable criterion because small nodes can harbor micrometastases, while large nodes can be reactive to the tumor or associated inflammatory conditions. The latter may be more common, for example, with perforated tumors. Nodal metastatic disease normally spreads in a contiguous fashion, from local pericolic nodes to mesenteric nodes, which for rectal and recto-sigmoid tumors includes the superior hemorrhoidal and inferior mesenteric territories, and for colonic tumors includes the superior mesenteric and ileo-colic mesenteric nodes. Metastases may involve peri-portal and retrocrural nodes. The sensitivity for the detection of nodal metastatic disease has been reported to be in the range of 22 to 84% (Hundt *et al.*, 1999).

Distant Metastatic Disease

Extracolonic findings may be relevant to the staging of distant metastatic disease (TNM stage M disease). Sites of metastatic disease include the liver, lung, adrenal, peritoneum, ovaries, and bone. Liver metastases appear as low-density lesions on noncontrast CT; however, this appearance is not specific because benign lesions may be similar. Foci of fine calcification may be seen in mucinous adenocarcinomas. If intravenous contrast is given, liver

Table 4   Extracolonic Findings on Minimum Preparation CT (Reproduced and Adapted with Kind Permission from Elsevier, Koo et al., 2006)

Author	Day et al.	Lipscomb et al.	Domjan et al.	Robinson et al.	Ng et al.	Kealey et al.
Year of publication	1993	1996	1998	2002	2004	2004
Population	Clinical suspicion for CRC	Clinical suspicion for CRC	Clinical suspicion for CRC	Clinical suspicion for CRC	Clinical suspicion for CRC	Clinical suspicion for CRC
No. of patients	37	55	118	195	1077	68
Age (range), years	Mean 80 (71–88)	Mean 77 (70–92)	Mean 84 (73–94)	Median 76 (47–96)	Median 80 (72–85)	Mean 81 (62–93)
Total extracolonic Findings (%)	12 (32%)*	9 (16%)*	22 (18.4%)*	54** (28%)*	261 cases (24%) 344 findings (32%)	14 (21%)*
Major Findings (%)	6/37 (16%)	9/55 (16%)	10/118 (8.4%)	37/195 (17%)	251/1077 (23)	11/68 (16%)
Minor Findings (%)	6/37 (16%)	Not stated	12/118 (10%)	17/195 (9%)	93/1077 (9%)	3/68 (4%)
Breakdown of Findings — Major	Hepatic mets (2); Ascites and obstructed ureter (1); Abdominal wall involvement (1); Gynecological mass (2)	Gastric leiomyosarcoma (1); AAA (1); Hepatic mets (2); No hepatic mets [with colon Ca] (3); Cirrhosis with portal hypertension (1); Pleural effusion (1)	Hepatic mets (2); Para-aortic lymphadenopathy (1); Ovarian masses (2); Pancreatic mass (1); AAA (3); Internal iliac	CBD obstruction with calculi (4); Cirrhosis (1); Pancreatitis (2); Cardiothoracic disease (11); AAA (4); aneurysm (1); Renal Ca (2); Bladder Ca (1); Lung Ca (2); Ovarian Ca (2); Pancreatic Ca (1); Unknown primary (2)	**With Cancer** Liver mass (22); Ascites (3); Abdo. wall mets (7); Nodal mass (4); Renal/adrenal mass (2); Bladder lesion (1); Cholangio Ca (1); Pelvic mass (2); AAA (3) — **Without Cancer** Liver mass (20); Diffuse liver abnormality (7); Ascites (15); Abdo. wall mets (9); Nodal mass (17); Splenic mass (1); Bowel inflammation (17); Gastric mass (19); Pancreatic mass (9); Renal/adrenal mass(16); Bladder lesion (8); Splenic mass (6); Pelvic mass (26); AAA (31)	Lymphoma (1); Ascites (3); Pleural effusion (1); AAA (2); Pleural plaques (1); Hydronephrosis (2); Colitis (1); Bowel obstruction (6)
Minor	Gallstones (2); Renal cyst (2); Fibroid (1); Hepatic granulomata (1)	Nil	Porcelain gallbladder (1); Gallstones (11)	Renal disease (4); Uterine leiomyoma (3); Gastric leiomyoma (3); Pancreatic atrophy (3); Splenomegaly (2); Crohn's disease (2)	Benign bowel abnormality (4); Hydro/pyonephrosis(2); Ovarian cyst (2); Thrombus (1); Lung disease (4); Others (2) — Abdo. abscess (10); Benign bowel abnormality (18); Biliary pathology (11); Hydro/pyonephrosis (7); Ovarian cyst (14); Thrombus (2); Lung disease (6); Bone disease (8); Others (2)	TB psoas abscess (1); Inguinal hernia (1); Porcelain gallbladder (1) (36 diverticulose and 1 gallstone excluded from original paper)

CRC, colorectal carcinoma; AAA, abdominal aortic aneurysm; Ca, carcinoma; CBD, common bile duct; Abdo, abdominal; mets, metastases; TB, tuberculosis

*Not stated whether on a "per finding," "per patient," or "per case" basis.

**Includes 4 patients with metastatic CRC who were excluded from the original paper.

Table 5   TNM Staging and Dukes' Classification of Colorectal Cancer

TNM classification

T-stage	T1	Invades the submucosa
	T2	Invades the muscularis propria
	T3	Invades through muscularis into subserosa, pericolic, or perirectal tissues
	T4	Invades into adjacent organs
N-stage	N0	No nodal metastases
	N1	1–3 nodal metastases
	N2	≥ 4 pericolic nodal metastases
M-stage	M0	No distant metastases
	M1	Distant metastases

Modified Dukes' classification

Dukes' Classification		TNM equivalent
A	Limited to bowel wall	T1 N0 M0
B1	Extension into serosa or mesenteric fat	T2 N0 M0
B2		T3 N0 M0
C1	Lymph node metastases	T2 N1 M0
C2		T3 N1 M0
D	Distant metastases	Any T Any N M1

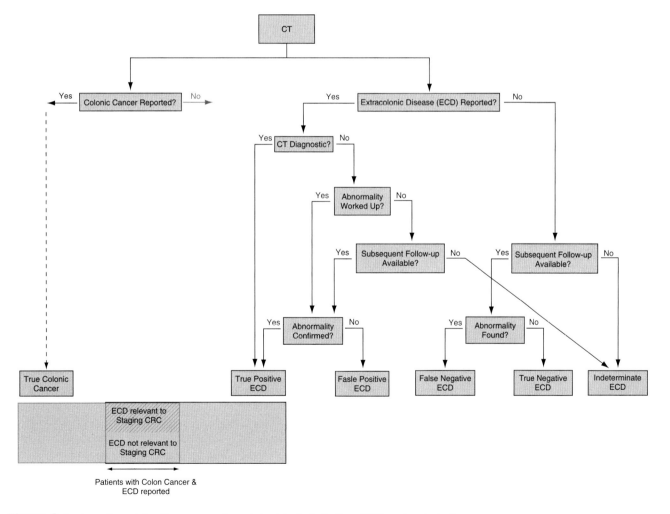

Figure 3 A scheme for evalating the accuracy of reported extracolonic findings. ECD = extracolonic disease.

metastases typically show irregular peripheral enhancement. The sensitivity of contrast-enhanced CT for the detection of liver metastases varies with lesion size but overall is ~ 60% (Horton *et al.*, 2000).

Peritoneal carcinomatosis is manifest as peritoneal nodules or implants, or as a peritoneal soft tissue mass ("cake") and/or ascites. In women, metastases may occur to the ovaries (Krukenberg tumors). Bony metastases are best viewed on CT bone windows and are typically lytic. Abdominal scans may detect metastases in the lung bases. Overall preoperative CT staging accuracy is reported to be in the range of 48 to 77% (Horton *et al.*, 2000; Hundt *et al.*, 1999). It should be noted that these figures are for contrast-enhanced rather than noncontrast CT.

Extracolonic findings incidentally detected, at the same CT examination as colonic tumors were detected, were found to be potentially important in staging the colorectal malignancy in 32 (39%) of the 83 cases identified at the same evaluation, for example, liver, nodal, and peritoneal metastases (Ng *et al.*, 2004). Other extracolonic findings in these patients were not relevant to staging the disease, for example, abdominal aortic aneurysms. Although most authors would document and consider the presence of metastatic disease on CT to be an important factor in staging, some argue that the *absence* of evidence of metastatic disease is equally important because it impacts on management (Lipscomb *et al.*, 1996).

Extracolonic Findings Unrelated to Staging of Colon Cancer

In an MPCT study of 1077 cases, 284 extracolonic findings unrelated to staging of the colonic cancer were reported in 221 cases (21%). The most common findings were abdominal aortic aneurysms, 31 cases (31/1077, 2.9%); pelvic masses, 26 cases (2.4%); and liver lesions, 20 cases (1.9%) (Ng *et al.*, 2004). Further breakdown of findings is presented in Table 4. It is important to recognize that not all these reported findings proved to be correct. Of 204 of these findings which had some form of supplementary evaluation, 44 (22%) proved to be incorrect. It is also instructive to observe that of the 284 reported findings in this group, only 124 (44%) were actively followed up or evaluated further. The value, or otherwise, of intravenous contrast media has not been evaluated in these MPCT studies. The impact of the costs of further work-up and outcomes, such as overall survival, has also not been evaluated.

Comparison of Reported Studies

Comparisons across the reported series are difficult for a number of reasons. Study populations vary, ranging from screening series involving a general population to symptomatic and/or high-risk patients, or even patients with known colonic tumors. The latter groups would be expected to have a higher yield of extracolonic lesions. The age range of the study population, which in turn may be affected by the study group, can also be expected to affect the results, since the prevalence of many lesions increases with age.

Several studies have stratified their extracolonic findings according to perceived severity or clinical importance or significance, for example, "major" versus "minor." Comparison between studies is difficult because definitions of severity vary between series. In addition, there have been differences between series in what constitutes a "reportable" finding; some series have included extracolonic findings that others have disregarded. These have usually been at the "minor" end of the scale, typically benign lesions, such as cysts or diverticular disease, where some authors have argued that further work-up of such lesions is unnecessary. This inevitably affects the overall lesion detection rate and should be borne in mind.

An important determinant of the lesion detection capabilities of CT for extracolonic, and indeed colonic, lesions relies on the specifics of the CT acquisition technique. In general, thinner collimation (better spatial resolution), higher radiation dose (higher signal to noise), and utilization of intravenous contrast media improve both lesion detection and characterization. Not only are there fundamental differences in the CT techniques between MPCT and CTC, but there are also substantial differences in the details of the scanning protocols within each of the two techniques, contributing to further variances. Interinstitutional and interobserver differences may also play a role, but have not been rigorously studied. Any improvements in lesion detection rate should be balanced against the costs of data acquisition and risks to the patient, for example, of radiation burden and adverse reactions to intravenous contrast media.

Evaluation of the Contribution of Incidental Extracolonic Findings

The detection of previously unknown extracolonic lesions would seem intuitively to be advantageous; early detection of abnormalities should in principle allow early intervention and treatment. For example, 24 (2%) previously unknown extracolonic malignancies were detected in an MPCT study of 1077 cases (Ng *et al.*, 2004). These cases included ovarian, pancreatic, renal, biliary, endometrial, and lung carcinomas, lymphoma, retroperitoneal sarcoma, and metastases from a variety of primary sources. This was in the context of detecting 83 (8%) colonic malignancies in the same study. However, studies evaluating any improvements in outcome measures, such as survival or mortality, have yet to be undertaken.

Any positive contribution of such findings should be balanced against the effect of false-positive findings. These include the unnecessary risks and costs of additional work-up, and effects on patient anxiety. There have been no studies of MPCT to evaluate the additional costs of such evaluations, although there have been some evaluations of the financial implications of such findings in CTC studies (Chin *et al.*, 2005; Gluecker *et al.*, 2003; Rajapaksa *et al.*, 2004; Yee *et al.*, 2005). Thus, in assessing the value of incidental lesion detection, careful review should be done to determine the true lesion detection rate (i.e., it is not sufficient to just report that a lesion was detected). In evaluating the contribution of such findings, there needs to be some mechanism to confirm or refute that it was correctly detected and characterized. Similarly, some means should be found to confirm truly negative status. The latter is extremely difficult to establish, and there have been no rigorous evaluations of this aspect in reported series. There would seem to be little prospect of achieving this confirmation in retrospective studies, as patients with negative findings are generally not further evaluated. In most situations, detection of such false-negative results can only be anecdotally uncovered and have not been systematically evaluated. A scheme for evaluating extracolonic lesion detection accuracy is presented in Fig. 3.

Evaluation of the accuracy of lesion detection has two main components: first, detecting the lesion (i.e., seeing the lesion); and second, characterizing the lesion (i.e., correctly diagnosing the pathological nature of the lesion). Clearly, it is a prerequisite that before attempting any form of lesion characterization the lesion needs to be detected in the first place. Lesion detection may be faulty not only in terms of reporting a spurious lesion that is in fact not present ("false positive"), but also failing to detect a lesion that is truly present ("false negative"). The characterization of lesions can also fail in false-positive and false-negative respects—for example, characterizing a lesion as a metastasis when it is in fact benign or characterizing a lesion as benign when it is in fact a metastasis. Rigorous evaluation of the true independent contribution of lesion detection also requires exclusion of lesions that are already known.

Part of the difficulty in evaluating the accuracy of extracolonic findings reported in MPCT and CTC is the relative paucity of active follow-up evaluations in these patients by clinicians. For example, only 44% of extracolonic findings in an MPCT study of 1077 cases were actively followed up (Ng *et al.*, 2004). Interestingly, this is not too dissimilar to the follow-up rate of only 18% in patients with "moderate" or "serious" findings, in a study of the use of noncontrast CT for renal stone evaluation in an Emergency Department setting (Messersmith *et al.*, 2001). In the above MPCT study of 1077 patients with symptoms and/or signs suspicious of a colonic tumor, 10% of the patients had extracolonic findings that could potentially have accounted for their presenting

symptoms (Ng *et al.*, 2004). This, however, is a function of the patient population and referral patterns, and the latter may be broadening as the contribution of the technique is becoming evident to clinicians.

Incidental findings come to light in a variety of other imaging procedures, such as abdominal and pelvic ultrasound, where one study of 1000 symptomatic patients has reported 9% significant incidental findings (Mills *et al.*, 1989) and a noncontrast CT study for renal stones in an Emergency Room setting has reported incidental findings in 45% of cases, of which approximately half were considered to be of moderate or serious concern (Messersmith *et al.*, 2001). The prevalence of incidentally detected abdominal lesions is probably increasing, largely because of the increasing use and quality of imaging (Westbrook *et al.*, 1998).

Practical Implications and Handling of Extracolonic Findings in Specific Organs

General Considerations Regarding Lesion Detection and Characterization in Computed Tomography

Lesion detection in CT is a function of morphological and contrast (density) factors. Morphological factors include detection of deformation or alteration of expected normal anatomy; that is, the lesion displays "mass effect." The conspicuity of lesions is also influenced by the contrast, or CT "density," differences between lesion and background. A lesion with similar density to its surrounding tissue is relatively inconspicuous, compared to lesions that are of higher or lower density. Lesion to background density differences in solid organs can typically be accentuated with the use of intravenous contrast enhancement; morphologic features may also be more conspicuous. Such density differences may vary with scanning time (or "scan delay") after the administration of intravenous contrast medium. The optimum delay varies with different lesions and indeed can vary with lesions of a given pathological type. Imaging during multiple time points during intravenous contrast administration, "multiphasic" scanning, can increase lesion detection sensitivity. The enhancement pattern of lesions may assist in the characterization of lesions. For example, in the context of liver lesions, simple cysts do not enhance at all, whereas hemangiomas typically show globular peripheral enhancement and metastases typically show irregular peripheral enhancement.

Other technical factors also come into play in lesion detection, and hence also in the capabilities of lesion characterization, in particular, spatial resolution and X-ray dose. In simple terms, spatial resolution increases with reducing

CT slice thickness. Conventional, nonhelical, and single-slice helical scanners, for which many older studies are based, typically used 10-mm slice thicknesses, with a range of perhaps 7–15 mm. Current multislice CT scanners, for routine scanning, use substantially thinner slice thicknesses of typically 5 mm. For CT colonography, slice thicknesses are typically 1–3 mm. A CT image requires the delivery of X-ray photons to the detector. In simple terms, the larger the number of photons, the higher the "signal to noise" and the better the object or lesion can be visualized. The price for this better visualization is an increased radiation dose, which is undesirable in general but particularly in an evaluation used in a screening context. Although small lesions can be difficult to detect and characterize, conversely, very large lesions may also present challenges—not so much in terms of detection, but in determining the site and organ of origin, which is a critical component of lesion characterization.

Liver

The overall incidence of hepatic lesions increases with age, as does the proportion of malignant lesions (Little *et al.*, 1991). Pathological entities include: (1) benign lesions, such as simple cysts, hemangiomas, focal nodular hyperplasia, and adenomas; (2) metastases; and (3) primary hepatobiliary tumors, such as hepatoma and cholangiocarcinoma. In autopsy series, benign hepatic lesions have been reported in up to 52% of the general population (Karhunen, 1986). Diffuse parenchymal abnormalities include fatty liver and cirrhosis. The latter is associated with regenerating nodules, dysplastic nodules, and hepatoma, which cannot be reliably distinguished by imaging.

Detection and Characterization of Liver Lesions

Both the detection and characterization of focal liver lesions improve with increasing lesion size. Lesions smaller than 1 to 1.5 cm cannot, in general, be characterized with much confidence; conversely, very large lesions, perhaps > 10 cm, can also be difficult to characterize accurately. A number of technical factors also influence liver lesion detection and characterization, as discussed above, including CT slice thickness, X-ray dose, and the use of intravenous contrast media. For example, simple cysts have well-defined margins, no significant wall thickness, fluid density centrally, and do not enhance with intravenous contrast media.

Some parenchymal liver disorders can be suggested on noncontrast CT, including fatty infiltration, which causes homogeneous or heterogeneous reduction in the density of the liver. Cirrhosis can be suggested if the liver is shrunken, has an irregular surface, and/or there are signs of portal hypertension, such as splenomegaly and ascites. Such morphological features, however, are relatively insensitive for the detection of cirrhosis and can only be appreciated in advanced disease.

The detection of focal liver lesions is limited when low signal-to-noise (low radiation dose) CT techniques are employed and in the absence of intravenous contrast media (noncontrast CT). Lesion characterization in the liver is also severely compromised with the lack of intravenous contrast media.

In a study of 64 patients with incidentally discovered solid hepatic lesions, in well patients, using relatively old imaging technology, the majority (75%) had benign lesions (Little *et al.*, 1991) and 25% had neoplasms, of which 17% were malignant. They found that the presence of a malignant liver lesion increased with age. An earlier study from the same institution, with 36 lesions, reported similar findings of benignity and malignancy of 81% and 19%, respectively (Little *et al.*, 1990). In the latter study, the authors reported that size or multiplicity of lesions was not helpful in making this distinction.

In a study of 1454 patients in a heterogeneous study population, using relatively old CT technology (10-mm slice thickness, and nonhelical scans) but with intravenous contrast media enhancement, small focal liver lesions measuring up to 15 mm were relatively common, being detected in 17% of cases (Jones *et al.*, 1992). When the subset of those with a known malignancy was evaluated, 51% were found to have benign lesions and 26% metastases. Interestingly, for patients with no known malignancy, and sufficient follow-up, none proved to have metastases. In a similar type of study of 2978 patients, with a known malignancy, using relatively old CT technology (10-mm slice thickness, and nonhelical scans) and with intravenous contrast media enhancement, small lesions measuring up to 10 mm were detected in 12.7% of cases. Of these, as many as 80% were considered to be benign by follow-up.

In a study of 100 patients with no history of malignancy, cirrhosis, or suspected or known liver lesion, using thin section (5 mm) CT and intravenous contrast, benign hepatic lesions were found in 33 cases (Volk *et al.*, 2001). The average size of these lesions was < 10 mm (9.4 mm, range 3–30 mm). These studies suggest that liver lesions are commonly detected by contrast-enhanced CT. The lesion detection rate is likely to be lower with the noncontrast and low-dose CT techniques typically employed in CTC and MPCT. Nevertheless, the data from contrast-enhanced studies suggest that the vast majority of these lesions can be expected to be benign. The possibility of metastatic disease, however, does increase with age and in the presence of a known malignancy. In an MPCT study of 1077 cases, focal liver lesions were reported in 42 (42/1077, 4%), of which half (21/1077, 2%) were confirmed to be malignancies. Eleven of these confirmed focal liver malignancies were relevant to staging the 83 patients with colorectal tumors concurrently detected (11/83, 13%) (Ng *et al.*, 2004).

Work-Up of Liver Lesions

Liver lesions cannot be adequately characterized with noncontrast CT. The use of IV contrast medium and multiphasic CT assists in lesion detection and characterization, but still has limitations (Green and Woodward, 2005) (see Fig. 4). Work-up of lesions incidentally detected on CT include contrast-enhanced, multiphasic, thin-section CT, MRI, and ultrasound (see Fig. 5). Where available, ultrasound can be augmented by the use of micro-bubble ultrasound contrast agents, which can increase lesion detection and characterization.

Adrenal

The prevalence of adrenal lesions in autopsy series is probably in the range of 1–8% (Barzon et al., 2003; Graham and McHenry, 1998), although figures as high as 32% have been reported (Thompson and Young, 2003). The prevalence increases with age, with ~ 0.2% in the young, 3% in those over 50 years, and 6.9% in subjects over 70 years of age (Barzon et al., 2003; Zarco-Gonzalez and Herrera, 2004). Adrenal nodules and masses may be primary or secondary tumors. Primary adrenal tumors may be functioning or nonfunctioning; functioning tumors include pheochromocytoma, aldosteronomas, and adrenocortical tumors, either benign or their malignant counterparts. Metastases are more common than primary functioning tumors. The overall risk of malignancy in the general population is low, of the order of 0.025% (Barzon et al., 1999). In subjects with known extra-adrenal malignancies, metastases are reportedly detected in 6 to 20% (Barzon et al., 2003). The frequency of metastases in adrenal incidentalomas in patients with an absence of a cancer history is reportedly in the range 0–21%, and in those with a cancer history it is substantially higher, in the range 32–73% (Kloos et al., 1995; Zarco-Gonzalez and Herrera, 2004). The

most common sites of primary tumor origin are lung, breast, renal, melanoma, stomach, colon, and lymphoma (Barzon et al., 2003; Duh, 2002). Larger lesions (> 3 cm) have a higher risk of malignancy. The incidence of benign adenomas in those without a cancer history has been reported to be in the range 36–94% (Brunt and Moley, 2001).

Detection and Characterization of Adrenal Lesions

The detection of adrenal lesions relies largely on morphological aspects of the adrenal gland, which are well appreciated against the low-density background of the retroperitoneal fat that surrounds it. Unlike the evaluation of many other visceral organs, the use of intravenous contrast medium does not add appreciably to the lesion detection ability of CT. Adrenal nodules as small as 1 cm can be well appreciated provided the CT slice thickness is thin enough, such as of the order of 5 mm or less, which is commonly employed in the types of CT scan under consideration in this chapter. The thinner the CT collimation, the smaller the nodules that can be detected.

Incidental adrenal lesions have been reported in 0.35–4.36% of patients imaged by CT, in studies typically employing older 10-mm slice thickness scanners (Barry et al., 1998; Barzon et al., 2003; Brunt and Moley, 2001; Graham and McHenry, 1998; Kloos et al., 1995). The lesion detection rate has increased over the years with advances in CT scanning technology, most notably the capability for thinner collimation images, and the detection rate now approaches that of autopsy series. In MPCT series, adrenal lesions have been reported in 0–2% of cases (Table 4 and Ng et al., 2004).

Work-Up of Adrenal Lesions

There is a substantial literature that discusses the evaluation and work-up of incidentally detected adrenal lesions

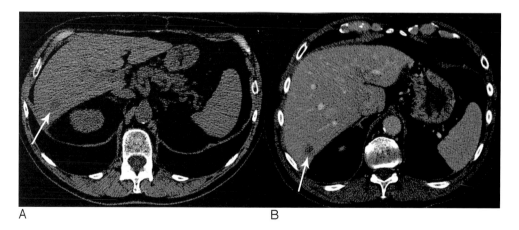

A   B

Figure 4 71 year-old male with history of colon cancer who presented for surveillance. **(A)** Noncontrast prone CT colonography image shows low-attenuation lesion in right lobe of liver (*arrow*). Note the general "grainy" appearance of the image, due to the relatively low signal to noise. **(B)** Contrast-enhanced CT shows ill-defined enhancing lesion that was biopsy-proven metastatic disease from colon primary (*arrow*). Note the better signal to noise in this diagnostic quality CT; the liver lesion is also more conspicuous with the aid of intravenous contrast medium. Irregular peripheral contrast enhancement is typical of metastatic disease.

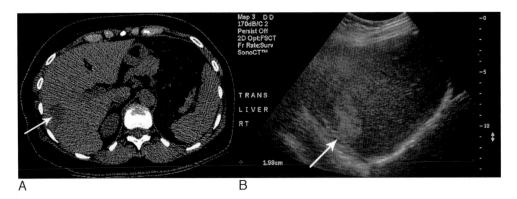

Figure 5 52-year-old woman who presented for screening CT colonography. **(A)** Noncontrast CT colonography image shows low-attenuation lesion in the right lobe of the liver (*arrow*). **(B)** Follow-up sonogram of the liver shows well-defined echogenic lesion compatible with an incidental hepatic hemangioma (*arrow*).

(Barry *et al*., 1998; Barzon *et al*., 2003; Brunt and Moley, 2001; Frilling *et al*., 2004; Graham and McHenry, 1998; Kloos *et al*., 1995; Schteingart, 2000; Thompson and Young, 2003). Algorithms include biochemical, hormonal, and metabolite assays, and/or imaging with CT, MRI, or nuclear medicine studies.

Noncontrast CT, as is typically employed in the CT studies under discussion, is fortuitously of value in characterizing adrenal lesions. For example, myelolipomas, which are benign fat-containing lesions, typically display foci of gross fat on CT, which can be identified as areas with CT density < 0 Hounsfield Units (fat has low CT density). Adenomas are relatively common benign entities. Typically, their cells are relatively rich in lipid content, which can be exploited for diagnostic purposes. Such lesions, for example, on noncontrast CT typically exhibit low density. A variety of noncontrast CT density cut-off values have been suggested to distinguish adenomas from malignant entities, each resulting in slightly different sensitivities and specificities. Commonly used cut-off values are in the range 10–15 Hounsfield Units, with lower cut-off values giving lower sensitivity, but higher specificity for the diagnosis of adenoma (Dunnick and Korobkin, 2002; Korobkin and Francis, 1997; Mayo-Smith *et al*., 2001). The relativeincreased lipid content of adenomas can also be detected by in- and out-of-phase (or "oppose" phase) MRI imaging, because the presence of lipid results in a drop of MRI signal on out-of-phase images, compared to in-phase images (Dunnick and Korobkin, 2002; Korobkin and Francis, 1997; Mayo-Smith *et al*., 2001). The use of delayed (10–15 min) intravenous contrast enhancement in CT can also assist in the diagnosis of adenoma, because adenomas "wash out" more rapidly than malignant tumors such as metastases (Dunnick and Korobkin, 2002). The lesions need to be of an adequate size for the above assessments, typically > 1 cm.

Renal

The incidence of renal cancers in autopsy series is ~ 2% (Luciani *et al*., 2000). There has been a dramatic increase in the number of incidentally detected renal tumors during the last 20 years, largely as a result of the use of CT and ultrasound. As many as 40% of renal tumors are discovered incidentally (Bretheau *et al*., 1998). An encouraging finding is that incidentally detected renal cancers have a lower stage, grade, and incidence of metastatic disease at presentation (Luciani *et al*., 2000). Incidentally detected renal cancers may be expected to improve overall prognosis, although this has not yet been conclusively demonstrated.

Detection and Characterization of Renal Lesions

Renal lesions may be solid, cystic, or a complex combination of these components. The majority of solid renal masses are renal cell carcinomas. Benign entities such as oncocytomas and other malignant tumors such as lymphoma or metastases are much rarer. Cystic lesions have a spectrum of pathological causes ranging from benign cysts to cystic renal cell carcinomas. Bosniak (1997) has derived a classification for cystic lesions based on their imaging appearances, which assists in assessing their risk of malignancy, ranging from Type I (benign simple cysts) to Type IV (frankly malignant).

Solid lesions, particularly if they are small, can be extremely difficult to detect on noncontrast CT scans because their densities are usually very similar to normal background renal parenchyma. Cystic lesions typically have densities lower than normal renal parenchyma, in the region of 0 Hounsfield Units, but when they are small they can also be difficult to detect. Characterization of renal lesions, including differentiation of solid from cystic, is also extremely difficult without the use of intravenous contrast media. This is particularly the case in the evaluation of cystic lesions, where the detection of subtle septations or solid mural nodules is extremely limited without intravenous contrast media. Lesions need to be bigger than 1–1.5 cm for a reasonable attempt at characterizing them. In MPCT series, renal lesions have been reported in 0–5% of cases (Table 4; Ng *et al.*, 2004).

Work-Up of Renal Lesions

Work-up of renal lesions is directed toward determining whether the lesion is solid or cystic, and if cystic, the degree of "complexity" (or Bosniak classification). This can be achieved by ultrasound, contrast-enhanced CT, or contrast-enhanced MRI. The role of biopsy or fine needle aspiration (FNA) is debated, but is generally considered to be limited partly because of the difficulty of accurate diagnosis on limited biopsy material, and consideration that the majority of solid renal masses are primary carcinomas. In the presence of a known malignancy, such as lymphoma or another primary tumor, pathological material, however, should be sought because treatment options may be significantly affected.

Pancreas

The most common pancreatic mass is adenocarcinoma. Such tumors located in the head of the pancreas typically present with painless jaundice, relatively early in their natural history. On the other hand, tumors in the body and tail of the pancreas tend to be relatively asymptomatic until late in their natural history, when they present with large masses. Pancreatic lesions may also be cystic, and these are most commonly due to pseudocysts (80–90%) (Green and Woodward, 2005), which in turn are most commonly secondary to a background of pancreatitis. There is a range of other solid and cystic pancreatic masses, which include serous cystadenoma, mucinous cystadenoma and cystadenocarcinoma, neuroendocrine tumors (which may be functioning or nonfunctioning), solid pseudopapillary (or papillary cystic and solid) tumors, intraductal papillary mucinous neoplasms, nonepithelial tumors, and metastases.

Detection and Characterization of Pancreatic Lesions

Pancreatic masses can be extremely difficult to detect on CT, especially when small and particularly without the aid of intravenous contrast media enhancement. The only clues to the presence of a mass on noncontrast or contrast-enhanced CT may be contour deformities, which may be extremely subtle, and/or the presence of biliary or pancreatic duct dilatation. Determining the pathological nature of pancreatic masses is also limited, even with high-resolution, thin-collimation, contrast-enhanced multiphasic CT.

The incidence of asymptomatic, incidentally detected pancreatic tumors appears to be increasing, probably because of the increase in the quantity and quality of imaging (Fitzgerald *et al.*, 2003; Sheehan *et al.*, 2000). In a series of 336 patients with a pancreatic mass, 14 (4%) patients had no symptoms and were incidental, their lesions being detected by CT undertaken for other indications (Sheehan *et al.*, 2000). In a study of 53 patients with surgically resected pancreatic tumors, 7 (13%) were asymptomatic (Fitzgerald *et al.*, 2003).

Although the majority of pancreatic masses are adenocarcinomas, it is interesting to note that among the asymptomatic, incidental lesions, these authors found a disproportionate number of relatively unusual tumors, many with more favorable diagnoses. Unfortunately, CT was found to be unreliable at distinguishing between these tumors ((Fitzgerald *et al.*, 2003; Sheehan *et al.*, 2000). In an MPCT study of 1077 cases, three (0.3%) previously unknown pancreatic carcinomas were detected (Ng *et al.*, 2004).

Work-Up of Pancreatic Lesions

Pancreatic lesions can be further evaluated by high-resolution, thin-collimation, contrast-enhanced multiphasic CT or MRI, or by endoscopic ultrasound. Imaging, however, has limitations in arriving at a pathological diagnosis. Imaging-guided percutaneous or endoscopic biopsy or FNA can be undertaken. Cystic lesions can be aspirated and be evaluated for mucin and amylase content, which can help in characterizing cystic neoplasms. Such interventions, however, are associated with all the usual risks of biopsy, and in addition bowel perforation and pancreatitis. Because of the limitations of imaging in providing a definitive diagnosis, some consider that resectable masses should proceed to surgery without intervening biopsy (Fitzgerald *et al.*, 2003).

Biliary Lesions

Gallstones are extremely common, and increase in prevalence with age. The majority are of limited clinical significance, and some reported MPCT series have not even reported on them unless considered to be associated with gallbladder inflammation (cholecystitis) or biliary obstruction (biliary colic). Computed tomography is not as sensitive as ultrasound at detecting biliary calculi. Primary malignancy of the biliary tree (cholangiocarcinoma), particularly of the extrahepatic biliary ducts, is usually small and typically very difficult to detect by CT, and especially on noncontrast CT.

Ovarian Lesions

Ovarian masses can be appreciated on CT as adnexal lesions. Such masses may be solid, cystic, or mixed solid and cystic. It is generally considered that ovarian lesions > 5 cm in diameter should be further evaluated and/or surgically treated, particularly in postmenopausal women. Physiological cysts are common in premenopausal women, but these would be expected to regress with time. Computed tomography, particularly noncontrast CT, has difficulty in evaluating the internal structure of cysts for solid components or septations, particularly if these are small; 45% of cases in one series considered to be suspicious for ovarian carcinoma proved to be incorrect on further evaluation (Ng *et al.*, 2004). Evaluation with transvaginal ultrasound is probably the most practical approach. Ovarian tumors commonly metastasize to the peritoneum, and indeed peritoneal carcinomatosis, which may be manifest as peritoneal nodules or an omental "cake," may be a presenting feature of an occult ovarian primary malignancy.

Uterine, Cervical, and Prostatic Lesions

Uterine, endometrial, and cervical malignancies cannot be reliably detected on CT, either noncontrast or contrast enhanced. These lesions are usually small, and although uterine masses are very common, they are far more likely to be benign leiomyomas (fibroids) than a malignancy, but differentiation from leiomyosarcomas cannot be reliably made. Prostatic enlargement can be subjectively appreciated on CT, but benign prostatic hypertrophy is extremely common, and CT is neither sensitive nor specific for the detection of prostatic carcinoma.

Gastric and Small Bowel Lesions

Although the CT techniques under discussion have some efficacy in detecting colonic lesions, they have very limited efficacy in detecting gastric and small bowel lesions. Apparent masses may be due to rugal folds, under distension, or peristalsis. Over half of all possible gastric lesions reported in one series were unsubstantiated on follow-up (Ng *et al.*, 2004). Gastric masses, such as leiomyomas (Ng *et al.*, 2004), and small bowel masses, such as lymphoma or those associated with Crohn's disease, can occasionally be detected on CT.

Abdominal Aortic Aneurysm and Other Vascular Abnormalities

The abdominal aorta is considered to be aneurysmal if > 3 cm in diameter (Green and Woodward, 2005). The risk of rupture progressively increases with the size of the aneurysm. Surgical intervention is generally considered appropriate for lesions > 5–5.5 cm. Abdominal aortic aneurysms increase with age and are easily detected on noncontrast CT. In reported MPCT series, their prevalence appears to be in the range of 2–3% (Table 4). Splenic and renal artery aneurysms may also be detected. Vascular occlusions can be detected with the appropriate administration of intravenous contrast media but cannot be detected on noncontrast CT. The clinical relevance of venous thromboses in the femoral or iliac veins is the risk of pulmonary emboli, and hence clinical consideration for anticoagulation.

Nodal Disease

The presence of abnormally enlarged nodes can be an indication of malignancy. Their anatomical location and distribution can offer an indication of the possible primary source of malignancy or possibly of lymphoma, and can provide staging information. Adenopathy can be detected on noncontrast CT, although sometimes differentiation from unenhanced vessels is difficult. Nodal enlargement is the only available criterion for assessing the possibility of nodal abnormality. A variety of size cut-offs have been suggested (Vinnicombe *et al.*, 1995). However, the use of size criteria has a number of limitations, including the possibility that enlarged nodes may be reactive. Biopsy or FNA is required for a tissue diagnosis.

Peritoneal and Retroperitoneal Lesions

Soft tissue masses can be detected on CT in the background of low-density peritoneal and retroperitoneal fat. Peritoneal nodules and masses are commonly due to tumor implants and may also be associated with ascites (peritoneal carcinomatosis). This can be asymptomatic in the early stages of disease. Retroperitoneal masses are rare. They may be due to pathological entities such as non-Hodgkin's Lymphoma, sarcomas, or metastases. Percutaneous biopsy of these lesions can generally be undertaken safely.

Musculoskeletal, Bony, and Soft Tissue Lesions

Focal bony lesions may be detected on CT as lucent or sclerotic abnormalities. Differentiation between benign and malignant lesions can be difficult. Hemangiomas are common benign lesions and have a characteristic typical appearance, but benign bone islands can be impossible to distinguish from other sclerotic lesions on CT.

Intrathoracic Disease

Computed tomography imaging of the abdomen includes images of the lung bases. Pulmonary nodules and masses can occasionally be detected, as can pleural lesions or effusions. These can be benign or may be related to primary or metastatic malignancies. Calcified lung nodules are commonly due to old granulomatous disease. Calcified pleural plaques are typically related to previous exposure to asbestos.

Conclusions

Extracolonic findings in CTC and MPCT are incidental to, or a byproduct of, the main purpose of these evaluations, which are undertaken principally to detect colorectal tumors. Such incidentally detected findings appear to be common, with reports in the range of 16–85% for overall findings, and with significant (moderate, serious, major, or important) findings in the range of 4–23%. Comparisons across the various reported series are difficult because the number and range of reported findings detected are inevitably affected by the nature of the study populations, patient ages, definitions of what constitutes reportable findings and classification of their seriousness, specific details of the CT techniques, and rigor of determining the accuracy of the reported findings.

Some extracolonic findings may contribute to staging the primary colonic tumor (if one is detected at the same evaluation), or early detection of other malignancies or diseases. The abnormalites detected may be associated with significant morbidity or mortality. However, the impact of such findings on costs and overall survival have yet to be determined. The limitations of the techniques, which have been primarily designed for a separate purpose, are such that they should not be used to "exclude" extracolonic lesions. The power of CT is its ability to detect abnormalities outside the colon in the course of evaluating the colon itself. The rate of incidental findings will very likely increase with the increasing use and quality of imaging techniques of all forms and with the aging population.

References

Barry, M.K., van Heerden, J.A., Farley, D.R., Grant, C.S., Thompson, G.B., and Ilstrup, D.M. 1998. Can adrenal incidentalomas be safely observed? *World J. Surg. 22*:599–603; discussion 603–604.

Barzon, L., Sonino, N., Fallo, F., Palu, G., and Boscaro, M. 2003. Prevalence and natural history of adrenal incidentalomas. *Eur. J. Endocrinol. 149*:273–285.

Barzon, L., Scaroni, C., Sonino, N., Fallo, F., Paoletta, A., and Boscaro, M. 1999. Risk factors and long-term follow-up of adrenal incidentalomas. *J. Clin. Endocrinol. Metab. 84*:520–526.

Bretheau, D., Koutani, A., Lechevallier, E., and Coulange, C. 1998. A French national epidemiologic survey on renal cell carcinoma. Oncology Committee of the Association Francaise d'Urologie. *Cancer 82*:538–544.

Brunt, L.M., and Moley, J.F. 2001. Adrenal incidentaloma. *World J. Surg. 25*:905–913.

Chin, M., Mendelson, R., Edwards, J., Foster, N., and Forbes, G. 2005. Computed tomographic colonography: prevalence, nature, and clinical significance of extracolonic findings in a community screening program. *Am. J. Gastroenterol. 100*:2771–2776.

Cotton, P.B., Durkalski, V.L., Pineau, B.C., Palesch, Y.Y., Mauldin, P.D., Hoffman, B., Vining, D.J., Small, W.C., Affronti, J., Rex, D., Kopecky, K.K., Ackerman, S., Burdick, J.S., Brewington, C., Turner, M.A., Zfass, A., Wright, A.R., Iyer, R.B., Lynch, P., Sivak, M.V., and Butler, H. 2004. Computed tomographic colonography (virtual colonoscopy): a multicenter comparison with standard colonoscopy for detection of colorectal neoplasia. *JAMA 291*:1713–1719.

Duh, Q.Y. 2002. Adrenal incidentalomas. *Br. J. Surg. 89*:1347–1349.

Dunnick, N.R., and Korobkin, M. 2002. Imaging of adrenal incidentalomas: current status. *Am. J. Roentgenol. 179*:559–568.

Fenlon, H.M., Nunes, D.P., Schroy, P.C., 3rd, Barish, M.A., Clarke, P.D., and Ferrucci, J.T. 1999. A comparison of virtual and conventional colonoscopy for the detection of colorectal polyps. *N. Engl. J. Med. 341*:1496–1503.

Fitzgerald, T.L., Smith, A.J., Ryan, M., Atri, M., Wright, F.C., Law, C.H., and Hanna, S.S. 2003. Surgical treatment of incidentally identified pancreatic masses. *Can. J. Surg. 46*:413–418.

Frilling, A., Tecklenborg, K., Weber, F., Kuhl, H., Muller, S., Stamatis, G., and Broelsch, C. 2004. Importance of adrenal incidentaloma in patients with a history of malignancy. *Surgery 136*:1289–1296.

Ginnerup Pedersen, B., Rosenkilde, M., Christiansen, T.E., and Laurberg, S. 2003. Extracolonic findings at computed tomography colonography are a challenge. *Gut 52*:1744–1747.

Gluecker, T.M., Johnson, C.D., Wilson, L.A., Maccarty, R.L., Welch, T.J., Vanness, D.J., and Ahlquist, D.A. 2003. Extracolonic findings at CT colonography: evaluation of prevalence and cost in a screening population. *Gastroenterology 124*:911–916.

Graham, D.J., and McHenry, C.R. 1998. The adrenal incidentaloma: guidelines for evaluation and recommendations for management. *Surg. Oncol. Clin. N. Am. 7*:749–764.

Green, D.E., and Woodward, P.J. 2005. The management of indeterminate incidental findings detected at abdominal CT. *Semin. Ultrasound CT MR 26*:2–13.

Hara, A.K., Johnson, C.D., MacCarty, R.L., and Welch, T.J. 2000. Incidental extracolonic findings at CT colonography. *Radiology 215*:353–357.

Hara, A.K., Johnson, C.D., Reed, J.E., Ahlquist, D.A., Nelson, H., Ehman, R.L., and Harmsen, W.S. 1997. Reducing data size and radiation dose for CT colonography. *Am. J. Roentgenol. 168*:1181–1184.

Hellstrom, M., Svensson, M.H., and Lasson, A. 2004. Extracolonic and incidental findings on CT colonography (virtual colonoscopy). *Am. J. Roentgenol. 182*:631–638.

Horton, K.M., Corl, F.M., and Fishman, E.K. 2000. CT evaluation of the colon: inflammatory disease. *Radiographics 20*:399–418.

Hundt, W., Braunschweig, R., and Reiser, M. 1999. Evaluation of spiral CT in staging of colon and rectum carcinoma. *Eur. Radiol. 9*:78–84.

Jemal, A., Murray, T., Ward, E., Samuels, A., Tiwari, R.C., Ghafoor, A., Feuer, E.J., and Thun, M.J. 2005. Cancer statistics, 2005. *CA Cancer J. Clin. 55*:10–30.

Johnson, C.D., Harmsen, W.S., Wilson, L.A., Maccarty, R.L., Welch, T.J., Ilstrup, D.M., and Ahlquist, D.A. 2003. Prospective blinded evaluation of computed tomographic colonography for screen detection of colorectal polyps. *Gastroenterology 125*:311–319.

Jones, E.C., Chezmar, J.L., Nelson, R.C., and Bernardino, M.E. 1992. The frequency and significance of small (less than or equal to 15 mm) hepatic lesions detected by CT. *Am. J. Roentgenol. 158*:535–539.

Karhunen, P.J. 1986. Benign hepatic tumours and tumour like conditions in men. *J. Clin. Pathol. 39*:183–188.

Kloos, R.T., Gross, M.D., Francis, I.R., Korobkin, M., and Shapiro, B. 1995. Incidentally discovered adrenal masses. *Endocr. Rev. 16*:460–484.

Koo, B.C., Ng, C.S., U-King-Im, J., Prevost, A.T., and Freeman, A.H. 2006. Minimal preparation CT for the diagnosis of suspected colorectal cancer in the frail and elderly patient. *Clin. Radiol. 61*:127–139.

Korobkin, M., and Francis, I.R. 1997. Imaging of adrenal masses. *Urol. Clin. North. Am. 24*:603–622.

Lipscomb, G., Loughrey, G., Thakker, M., Rees, W., and Nicholson, D. 1996. A prospective study of abdominal computerized tomography and colonoscopy in the diagnosis of colonic disease in an elderly population. *Eur. J. Gastroenterol. Hepatol. 8*:887–891.

Little, J.M., Kenny, J., and Hollands, M.J. 1990. Hepatic incidentaloma: a modern problem. *World. J. Surg. 14*:448–451.

Little, J.M., Richardson, A., and Tait, N. 1991. Hepatic dystychoma: a five year experience. *H.P.B. Surg. 4*:291–297.

Luciani, L.G., Cestari, R., and Tallarigo, C. 2000. Incidental renal cell carcinoma-age and stage characterization and clinical implications: study of 1092 patients (1982–1997). *Urology 56*:58–62.

Mayo-Smith, W.W., Boland, G.W., Noto, R.B., and Lee, M.J. 2001. State-of-the-art adrenal imaging. *Radiographics 21*:995–1012.

Messersmith, W.A., Brown, D.F., and Barry, M.J. 2001. The prevalence and implications of incidental findings on ED abdominal CT scans. *Am. J. Emerg. Med. 19*:479–481.

Mills, P., Joseph, A.E., and Adam, E.J. 1989. Total abdominal and pelvic ultrasound: incidental findings and a comparison between outpatient and general practice referrals in 1000 cases. *Br. J. Radiol. 62*:974–976.

Muto, T., Bussey, H.J., and Morson, B.C. 1975. The evolution of cancer of the colon and rectum. *Cancer 36*:2251–2270.

Ng, C.S., Doyle, T.C., Courtney, H.M., Campbell, G.A., Freeman, A.H., and Dixon, A.K. 2004. Extracolonic findings in patients undergoing abdomino-pelvic CT for suspected colorectal carcinoma in the frail and disabled patient. *Clin. Radiol. 59*:421–430.

Pickhardt, P.J., Choi, J.R., Hwang, I., Butler, J.A., Puckett, M.L., Hildebrandt, H.A., Wong, R.K., Nugent, P.A., Mysliwiec, P.A., and Schindler, W.R. 2003. Computed tomographic virtual colonoscopy to screen for colorectal neoplasia in asymptomatic adults. *N. Engl. J. Med. 349*:2191–2200.

Rajapaksa, R.C., Macari, M., and Bini, E.J. 2004. Prevalence and impact of extracolonic findings in patients undergoing CT colonography. *J. Clin. Gastroenterol. 38*:767–771.

Schteingart, D.E. 2000. Management approaches to adrenal incidentalomas: a view from Ann Arbor, Michigan. *Endocrinol. Metab. Clin. North. Am. 29*:127–139, ix–x.

Sheehan, M., Latona, C., Aranha, G., and Pickleman, J. 2000. The increasing problem of unusual pancreatic tumors. *Arch. Surg. 135*:644–648; discussion 648–650.

Spreng, A., Netzer, P., Mattich, J., Dinkel, H.P., Vock, P., and Hoppe, H. 2005. Importance of extracolonic findings at IV contrast medium-enhanced CT colonography versus those at non-enhanced CT colonography. *Eur. Radiol. 15*:2088–2095.

Stevenson, G.W., Wilson, J.A., Wilkinson, J., Norman, G., and Goodacre, R.L. 1992. Pain following colonoscopy: elimination with carbon dioxide. *Gastrointest. Endosc. 38*:564–567.

Thoeni, R.F. 1997. Colorectal cancer. Radiologic staging. *Radiol. Clin. North. Am. 35*:457–485.

Thompson, G.B., and Young, W.F., Jr. 2003. Adrenal incidentaloma. *Curr. Opin. Oncol. 15*:84–90.

Vining, D., Gelfand, D., Bechtold, R., Scharling, E., Grishaw, E., and Shifrin, R. 1994. Technical feasibility of colon imaging with helical CT and virtual reality. *Am. J. Roentgenol. 62*:104.

Vinnicombe, S.J., Norman, A.R., Nicolson, V., and Husband, J.E. 1995. Normal pelvic lymph nodes: evaluation with CT after bipedal lymphangiography. *Radiology 194*:349–355.

Volk, M., Strotzer, M., Lenhart, M., Techert, J., Seitz, J., and Feuerbach, S. 2001. Frequency of benign hepatic lesions incidentally detected with contrast-enhanced thin-section portal venous phase spiral CT. *Acta Radiol. 42*:172–175.

Westbrook, J.I., Braithwaite, J., and McIntosh, J.H. 1998. The outcomes for patients with incidental lesions: serendipitous or iatrogenic? *Am. J. Roentgenol. 171*:1193–1196.

Xiong, T., Richardson, M., Woodroffe, R., Halligan, S., Morton, D., and Lilford, R.J. 2005. Incidental lesions found on CT colonography: their nature and frequency. *Br. J. Radiol. 78*:22–29.

Yee, J., Akerkar, G.A., Hung, R.K., Steinauer-Gebauer, A.M., Wall, S.D., and McQuaid, K.R. 2001. Colorectal neoplasia: performance characteristics of CT colonography for detection in 300 patients. *Radiology 219*:685–692.

Yee, J., Kumar, N.N., Godara, S., Casamina, J.A., Hom, R., Galdino, G., Dell, P., and Liu, D. 2005. Extracolonic abnormalities discovered incidentally at CT colonography in a male population. *Radiology 236*:519–526.

Zarco-Gonzalez, J.A., and Herrera, M.F. 2004. Adrenal incidentaloma. *Scandinavian J. Surg. 93*:298–301.

10

Colorectal Cancer: Magnetic Resonance Imaging–Cellular and Molecular Imaging

Jens Pinkernelle and Harald Bruhn

Introduction

When colorectal neoplasia develops, accurate diagnostic procedures are needed to guide therapeutic decisions. Since colorectal carcinomas often evolve from prior benign adenomatous polyps, colorectal screening methods are of particular interest in diagnosis to reduce arising cancer and the related economic burden.

Recently, noninvasive cross-sectional imaging techniques have been developed, and favorable results have been demonstrated. Colonography by computed tomography (CT) or magnetic resonance imaging (MRI) can be performed at a degree of sensitivity comparable to invasive endoscopy in some clinical settings. In addition, they offer an evaluation of the whole bowel anatomy, enable the visualization of tumor invasion "under the surface," and, at the same time, are suitable for screening metastases in adjacent or distant tissues. Therefore, these imaging modalities can be employed preoperatively for staging purposes in clinically proven colorectal cancer guiding further therapy.

Efforts have been made to develop fast three-dimensional techniques for high-resolution volume scanning of the colon and rectum by MRI. These imaging methods overcome the specific limitations of colorectal endoscopy such as inspection of colon sections distal from a constriction (Debatin and Lauenstein, 2003; Lauenstein *et al*., 2005a). Moreover, possible infiltration of the mesocolon and associated lymphatics can be assessed at the same time.

A few years ago adequate noninvasive imaging was considered impossible; today the quick pace of pertinent technological progress has pushed MRI toward this goal. Against that background, current growth within the field of molecular and cellular imaging can be expected to undergo a similar tantalizing development.

This chapter provides a compendium of present colorectal MRI techniques, including a critical discussion of advantages and limitations. In addition, an outline of MRI-based strategies combining cellular and molecular imaging techniques is given. Finally, the developments that are on the horizon for future clinical application are noted.

Magnetic Resonance Imaging: Basic Principles

Initially, it may be helpful to review some basic principles of MRI. Like computed X-ray tomography (CT), MRI produces cross sections of the body. Unlike CT, the MR image builds on the interaction of radio waves with paramagnetic atomic nuclei of hydrogen bound in water, lipids, and other molecules. The electromagnetic radiofrequency (rf) of MRI is about 9 orders of magnitude below the frequency of X-rays. Hence, radio waves in MRI may cause heating (not very efficient) but are far away from being able to ionize cell material as X-rays can.

If an external magnetic field is applied, then a small proportion of the protons in the body align along this magnetic field vector. While the magnetized protons are manipulated by radiofrequency pulses at specific resonant frequencies adjusted to the strength of the magnetic field (Larmor frequency), they become excited. The activated spins lose their captured energy again by a combined process of rf emission, which can be detected by appropriate radio antennas or receiver coils, and molecular interaction, which gradually decreases the emitted signal by phase dispersion within the time range of milliseconds up to a few seconds.

This relaxation process is measured in half-life periods, and the respective time constants are the relaxation times. Image contrast is based on the differences of these relaxation times because molecular interaction and mobility are variable in different tissues and anatomic structures. The relaxation processes can be modified by paramagnetic and superparamagnetic substances such as dissolved gadolinium salts or nanometer-sized iron oxides, both used as intravenous contrast material.

The instruments that make use of this radio wave imaging have become common in the industrialized world during the last 25 years. Field strengths between 0.2 and 3.0 Tesla define the clinical standard to date.

Magnetic Resonance Imaging of Colorectal Cancer in Clinical Use

MRI of the colorectum can be performed for different purposes. In addition to imaging of neoplasia, it is also used for inflammatory bowel disease such as colitis ulcerosa or Crohn's disease. In the case of cancer imaging, screening and staging have to be separated. Whereas staging has been accepted as a valuable diagnostic tool, an ambiguous view prevails regarding the value and reliability of screening. However, cross-sectional imaging for purposes of colorectal cancer screening can achieve results even for smaller lesions (< 10 mm) comparable to endoscopy, which is commonly referred to as the gold standard.

Patient Preparation for Magnetic Resonance Imaging

When considering an MRI examination, the first step is to take a detailed history of the patient to rule out specific contraindications, including medical devices (e.g., cardiac pacemakers, some aneurysm clips, shell splinters, metal-made prostheses) and metallic tattoos. While iron-containing parts will be attracted forcefully by the magnet, other metallic objects might heat up quickly leading to burns, or they will disturb the magnetic field in such a way that heavy signal extinctions and image artifacts may arise. If safety measures are not taken, then an MR examination can be life threatening for the patient.

Prior to MR examinations, a bowel cleansing is usually required to remove stool as in conventional endoscopy. This procedure is usually essential, though a fecal tagging technique has also been reported (see below). To reduce the burden of abstinence, the examination should be done in the morning. For purposes of colon distension, about 2 liters of fluid have to be instilled intraluminally. This amount of fluid should be administered warmed up and slowly in stages (> 1 minute) to avoid discomfort and bowel cramping. The instillation pressure should range at 1–1.5 meters of water column. Before commencing instillation, an intestinal relaxant such as scopolamine butylbromide (Buscopan®, 20 mg) or glucagon (1 mg) is administered intravenously to reduce colon motility. Scopolamine must not be given when the patient suffers from glaucoma. For monitoring colorectal filling, very fast two-dimensional gradient-echo imaging provides for images every second. As an alternative to fluid instillation, CO_2 insufflation may be performed in certain cases. Applying suitable rf-refocused pulse sequences, CO_2 does not itself cause significant susceptibility artifacts.

Hardware and Software Used in Magnetic Resonance Imaging

The central element of the instrumental setup is a whole-body MR scanner equipped with a powerful gradient system (maximum amplitude up to 50 mT/m to date). The magnetic field strength in clinical use usually ranges from 1.0 T to 3.0. A major advantage of a higher magnetic field is the increased signal-to-noise ratio (SNR) of the scans. Further improvements have been made regarding pulse sequences (see below), rf excitation and reception, and processing of the received signal, which in synergy provide for an overall optimization of image quality.

Phased-array coil systems, which combine up to 32 surface coil elements to date, allow for covering the whole body without repositioning the patient. These coil arrays can boost the signal yield considerably and, compared to field strength increases, are the cheaper solution toward more signal gain for fast and signal-hungry applications. Moreover, phased-array coils are the hardware basis for parallel imaging techniques, which have revolutionized the acquisition speed of MR images, allowing a certain number of phase-encoding steps to be omitted during data acquisition. While this leads to speeding up the scans two- to eightfold, the concomitant loss of signal has to be accommodated. As a general rule in MRI, the acquired signal or the gain in SNR can be traded between a higher spatial resolution or the acquisition speed. This is modified by the requirements of covering a certain anatomic region or size and of acquiring image data during a limited time period such as a breath hold.

These considerations are very important for bowel imaging. Imaging of the colon and intestines implies imaging a large body area with actively and passively moving anatomic structures. Therefore, imaging has to be spatially extended, but it should be fast enough to freeze bowel motion and fit into a breath hold. Multiple breath-hold phases compromise image quality because the inaccuracy of the breath-hold position may cause spatial inconsistencies. Navigator techniques detecting the dislocation of the diaphragm have been developed for improving this problem but, compromised by other problems, are not yet in widespread use.

Rf pulse sequences contain the parameters that determine imaging contrast. Several pulse sequences have to be combined for an imaging protocol to provide the necessary information on anatomic or pathologic contrast (Table 1). In general, it has been felt to be advantageous to get rid of the fat signal of the abdominal wall and even that of the intra-abdominal fat. This is because the high signal intensity of fat may severely degrade the images when movement cannot be completely avoided. An elegant method is the fat signal suppression by chemical shift-selective saturation

pulses, which poses no problem at field strength of 1.5 T and above, where fat and water proton resonances can be sufficiently separated. However, since the bright signal of intra-abdominal fat may provide a contrast of its own to discriminate infiltrative processes (low signal in T1-weighted MRI), the only use of fat-suppressed imaging can be misleading. Nevertheless, fat suppression is very effective in avoiding movement artifacts and to date has become indispensable in combination with high-signal contrast enhancement media.

Recently, very fast three-dimensional gradient-echo technique (e.g., dubbed volume interpolated breathhold examination (VIBEs) by Siemens and liver acquisition, LAVA, by GE) has been developed that incorporates fat suppression and can make use of parallel imaging speed-up (Fig. 1). By using this sequence, thin 3-mm sections and submillimeter in-plane resolution can be achieved in abdominal imaging within one breath hold. Its best performance is played out in combination with dynamic contrast enhancement leading to separated arterial and venous angiographic depiction of the intra-abdominal and mesenteric vessels in conjunction with contrast enhancement of the intestinal wall. Of course, the three-dimensional data matrix allows for multiplanar thin-slice reconstruction in desired orientations. T1-weighted sequences such as this gradient-echo technique play out a "dark lumen" appearance of the gas or fluid-filled intestines. To display a "bright lumen," T2-weighted sequences have to be used.

Table 1 **Typical Pulse Sequences and Protocol Parameters Used for MR Colonography with 8-Channel Phased Array Coil at 1.5 Tesla (GE TwinSpeed)**

Pulse-Sequence	Contrast	Plane	Thickness / Gap [mm]	Slices	R	Matrix	NEX	TR / TE / FA α	RBW [kHz]
BH-2D-FIESTA (True FISP)	T2 / T1	Coronal	4.5 / 0	40	2	256 × 192	2	6.4 / 1.7 / 55°	125
BH-2D-FIESTA (True FISP)	T2 / T1	Axial	4.5 / 0	60	2	256 × 256	2	6.9 / 1.7 / 55°	125
BH-3D-LAVA (VIBE)	T1fs	Coronal	3 / 0 †	48	2	256 × 256	1	3.4 / 1.6 / 15°	83.3
		Axial	3–4 / 0	50	2	256 × 256	1	3.4 / 1.6 / 15°	83.3
RT-frFSE (TSE) [ETL = 24]	T2	Coronal	6 / 0.6	22	2	352 × 352	2	3000 / 94.8 / 90°	31.2
BH-frFSE (TSE) [ETL = 24]	T2	Coronal (Sagittal)	6 / 0	9 / BH (1BH~21s)	2	224 × 160	1	2100 / 102 / 90°	31.2
RT-frFSE (TSE) [ETL = 24]	T2	Axial	5 / 0	22	2	352 × 352	1	4000 / 100eff / 90°	31.2
BH-frFSE (TSE) [ETL = 23]	T2	Axial	5 / 0	22 / BH	2	256 × 192	1	5525 / 75 / 90°	31.2
RT-ss (TSE) [ETL = 240]	T2	Axial, Coronal	8 / 0	(1BH 28s)	2	320 × 256	0.6	823 / 90°	41.7
BH- FSPGR	T1	Coronal	8 / 0	23	2	256 × 224	1	135 / 4.2 / 90°	41.7

*ZIP512; †ZIP2 (1.5–2.0 mm); ‡in-phase condition. In order to decrease motion artifacts (travelling) saturation bands cranial to transverse slices and variable bandwidth options should be applied; §multiphase option for time-resolved volume acquisitions. Acquisition times are ~ 3–4 minutes for RT-frFSE, ~ 2 minutes for BH-2D-FIESTA (6 × BH with a single BH taking 20 s), ~ 20–30 s for BH-FSPGR and BH-3D-LAVA acquisition. Note that field-of-view (FOV) depends on body size and can range from 35 to 48 cm.

[RT = respiratory triggering; BH = breath hold; NEX = number of excitations; TR = repetition time [ms]; TE = echo time [ms]; FA = flip angle; ETL = echo-train length; RBW = receiver bandwidth; R = parallel imaging factor; frFSE = fast-recovered fast spin echo; FSPGR = fast spoiled gradient echo; 2D-FIESTA = two-dimensional fast imaging employing steady-state acquisition; 3D-LAVA = three-dimensional liver acquisition with volume acceleration; ZIP512 = zero interpolation to 512 × 512 matrix; ZIP2 = zero slice interpolation to 0.5 of slice measured]

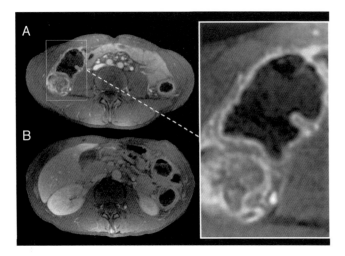

Figure 1 Very fast three-dimensional T1-weighted gradient-echo technique with thin-slice acquisition (3 mm) and fat suppression. Exact delineation of colorectal wall is achieved by this technique (**A**). Liver and kidneys can be evaluated simultaneously (**B**). Moreover, contrast-enhanced imaging provides vessel enhancement, allowing exact cancer staging of vessel involvement.

Commonly, fast spin-echo sequences with extended echo-train lengths for speeding up the data acquisition have been used in multiple respiratory triggered acquisitions or in single breath-hold scans. The requirement that high echo-trains be employed, however, causes unwanted blurring in the images. Therefore, another gradient-echo technique (dubbed True FISP by Siemens and FIESTA by GE) has gained wide acceptance. Providing a T2 over T1 contrast (T2/T1), fluid-filled intestines are also displayed with a bright lumen (Fig. 2)

as in genuine T2-weighted fast spin-echo images. The three-dimensional versions of this sequence allow for fast imaging of thin sections with high in-plane resolution. Thus, the structure of the abdominal wall can be well displayed. At 1.5 T this sequence provides for clear images that are largely free of artifacts. At 3.0 T, however, the stronger susceptibility sensitivity facing residual bowel motion and air leads to degrading artifacts all over the image. Here, the fast spin-echo T2-weighted sequences can be used more successfully (Fig. 3). The fastest of these sequences are the single-shot acquisitions (dubbed half-Fourier acquisition, HASTE, by Siemens or single-shot fast spin-echo, ssFSE, by GE), which in recent years have been successfully employed mainly for magnetic resonance cholepancreatography (MRCP). These sequences also provide a basis for real-time display of imaging data and may be used for dynamic monitoring of colorectal distension by enema.

Bright Lumen Contrast Imaging

One strategy for imaging contrast is the so-called bright (or light) lumen contrast imaging. Contrast-enhanced water serves as enema. Paramagnetic gadolinium based-contrast material (e.g., Gd-DPTA, Magnevist®) is used for that purpose. On T1-weighted (T1W) images, the filled lumen has considerably more signal intensity (bright) than the colon wall (dark) (Lauenstein *et al.*, 2005b). The image interpretation is based on intraluminal masses or structures with low signal intensity. A specific disadvantage of this strategy is that some parts of the colorectal tube may remain without fluid and display air, with low signal intensity as a

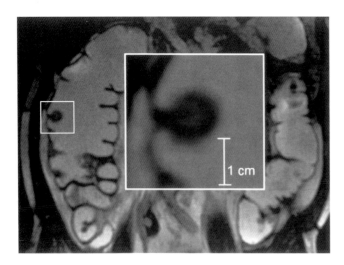

Figure 2 MR colonography with bright lumen contrast. Colorectal distension and filling are achieved by enema. Depiction of a polypous mass lesion (about 1 cm in diameter). The "bright" display of fluid is produced by T2/T1-weighted FIESTA imaging. (1.5 T, 3D-FIESTA: TR/TE = 5.9/1.8 ms, slice 6 mm.) (Courtesy of R. Roettgen, Klinik fur Strahlenheilkunde, Charite Berlin.)

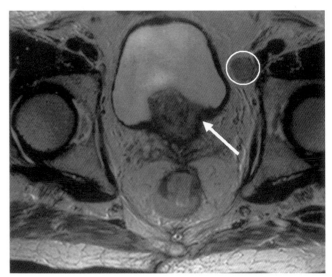

Figure 3 T2-weighted FSE image of the pelvis showing invasion of urinary bladder by a T4 rectosigmoid cancer (arrow) (1.5T, TR/TE = 4000/95 ms, 8 mm slice thickness). On both sides iliacal lymphatics are enlarged from metastasis (circle). (Courtesy of B. Gebauer, Klinik fur Strahlenheilkunde, Charite Berlin)

consequence. Therefore, the image acquisition has to be performed twice with the patient in a prone and a supine position. However, residual stool may mimic a polypous mass lesion of the colon wall.

Dark Lumen Contrast Imaging

Another technique for intestinal MRI is the so-called dark lumen contrast imaging (Goehde *et al.*, 2005). In analogy to the bright lumen modality, the colorectal tube is filled retrogradely with temperature-adjusted fluid. As a difference, contrast material is not added intraluminally but intravenously instead. In this contrast-enhanced T1W-imaging, the colon wall appears to be signal enhanced, while the lumen remains dark. A major advantage of this strategy is that polyps generally will also show contrast enhancement and, therefore, show as well delineated versus the dark lumen. Double acquisition, before and after intravenous administration of paramagnetic contrast material, may allow for subtraction of precontrast images from postcontrast images.

Fecal Tagging

In order to avoid misinterpreting feces as polyps or intraluminal mass lesions, contrast material can be administered orally (Lauenstein *et al.*, 2002). This strategy is applicable for both the bright lumen and the dark lumen imaging techniques. Here, at first, paramagnetic gadolinium-based contrast material is given orally with a meal. Major drawbacks of this antegrade intraluminal paramagnetic contrast material are high cost for and insufficient depiction of the colon wall. For dark lumen contrast, barium sulphate was successfully used to decrease the signal of feces. As a consequence, the paramagnetic-enhanced colon as well as polyps show well delineated against feces that may mimic polyps in bright lumen technique. In addition, it is considerably cheaper than gadolinium-based formulas and has an even better safety profile.

Clinical Impact of Magnetic Resonance Imaging Colonography

Conventional colonoscopy actively performed by visual inspection with a flexible endoscopic device remains the gold standard for colorectal cancer screening (Winawer *et al.*, 2003). However, evaluation by endoscopy only refers to visual inspection of intraluminal (mucosal) anatomy when no biopsy is performed. Like X-ray computed tomography colonography (as described elsewhere in this book) virtual MRI colonography is based on the acquisition of cross-sectional imaging data. A major difference between these two modalities is the avoidance of ionizing radiation using MRI. This may be an important issue, especially when colonography is considered for screening purposes in younger patients.

Furthermore, because of a more flexible modulation of MRI contrast compared to CT colonography, bowel cleansing may be avoided, particularly when using fecal tagging. Although some studies reported supportive evidence for this strategy, diagnostic accuracy still needs to be more clearly worked out in the future (Lauenstein *et al.*, 2005b).

The sensitivity and specificity of MR colonography have been shown to reach up to 100% in specific clinical settings. Most studies evaluate patients with high risk for colon carcinoma. Lesions > 10 mm in diameter can be detected as reliably as with conventional colonoscopy, as has been demonstrated by several studies (Purkayastha *et al.*, 2005). However, gross lesions may not be an adequate challenge.

Considerable uncertainty remains regarding the sensitivity towards smaller lesions. In addition, in patients with average risk for developing colorectal cancer, MR colonography was reported to perform unsatisfactorily compared to endoscopy. Since colon carcinoma arises mostly from benign adenoma and shows size progression as an important sign of malignant transformation, a high sensitivity based on improved image resolution and contrast in the submillimeter dimensions is the critical issue for detecting lesions early.

In permitting simultaneous evaluation for metastases within the bowel, the colonography has a major advantage. There is a special diagnostic value regarding carcinoma infiltration into the mesocolon and associated lymphatics. Moreover, detection of metastatic lesions in the liver or enlargement of lymph nodes may be the first clinical manifestations of a carcinoma in some cases. Furthermore, in the follow-up of patients with colorectal carcinoma, radiologic imaging modalities are essential. It was shown that tumor recurrence is not located intraluminally but rather extraluminally so that a recurrence is likely to be missed by endoscopy alone.

In addition, imaging data that are rendered from different perspectives by multiplanar or volume reconstruction allow a virtual flight through the colorectal tube and thus facilitate the evaluation of anatomical structure.

Rectosigmoidal Magnetic Resonance Imaging

The fixed sigmoid colon and the rectum are favorable imaging targets for high-resolution MRI because of less passive motion artifacts and reduced motility. Colorectal MRI is useful in showing invasiveness of a clinically detected carcinoma, especially in preoperative evaluation (Brown, 2005; Akasu *et al.*, 2005).

MRI of the rectum may replace endosonography with the need to introduce a rigid endoscopic device. This may cause pain during the examination, especially in cases of rectal constriction or obstruction caused by the carcinoma. In addition, MRI is judged superior to endosonography regarding evaluation of perirectal fatty tissue and involvement of lymph nodes, as well as arterial vessels. Even the mesorectal fascia is delineable by MRI which is of much importance for the surgeon to evaluate if total mesorectal excision (TME) will be possible or not.

Patients are prepared much as they are for colonography. For rectal imaging, however, bowel cleansing does not need to be as extensive as for colonography. A retrograde laxative given immediately before the examination is sufficient. An enema containing barium sulphate can be applied for rectal distension.

The need of an endorectal receiver coil can be avoided using modern imaging hardware at 3T, including powerful magnetic gradients and pelvic phased-array coil equipment. The recommended pulse sequences are similar to those used in colonography (Table 2). Fat-suppressed T1-weighted FSE sequences (Fig. 4) have been shown to be advantageous for thin-slice imaging before and after intravenous application of gadolinium-based contrast medium (Winter *et al.*, 2007). Axial sections are obligatory, whereas sagittal sections may help give a better spatial visualization preoperatively. In 2D sequences, intersectional gaps, error-prone to partial volume effects, can be avoided using interleaved acquisition because lesions in between cross sections cannot be missed further.

Imaging Strategies for the Future

Molecular and cellular imaging techniques are being ambitiously pursued. *In vivo* imaging modalities have developed into essential tools for basic life sciences. Nowadays, diameters of imaging targets range from centimeters to nanometers. In many studies, MRI proved to be a valuable, sensitive tool for experimental imaging of magnetically labeled cells and even molecules with a good sensitivity and an outstanding spatial resolution. Even a clinical MR imager at 3T using a simple surface coil could detect single human cells *in vitro* (Pinkernelle *et al.*, 2005). This feasibility study illuminated the promising potential of clinical MRI to detect

malignancies or to monitor therapies on the cellular level that may be carried right away to *in vivo* imaging in the future. Many studies have already demonstrated that magnetically labeled mammalian cells can be detected in animals *in vivo*. In most cases so far, MR monitoring has been applied for tracking stem cells or immune cells earlier labeled by (super-)paramagnetic substances (Fig. 5).

Cell labeling usually is achieved by nonspecific uptake from the extracellular environment. However, applying genetic engineering, we can apply the transferrin receptor system can be applied for intracellular iron-oxide uptake into a tumor cell line (Weissleder *et al.*, 2000). No significant cytotoxic effects have been detected by intracellular iron-oxide labels *in vitro* even when high iron-concentrations were present in the growth medium. Other studies demonstrated further differentiation of labeled cells without losing their labels.

Iron-oxide particles cause strong local magnetic field inhomogeneities, which produce significant signal drops in $T2^*$ weighted imaging. Even T1 relaxation time-shortening agents like paramagnetic gadolinium or manganese derivatives can be used. But the T2 time shortening effect of iron-oxide compounds is considered to be much more effective.

Superparamagnetic iron-oxide compounds with an average mean size of 10–200 nm have been used so far. However, detection of a single micron-scaled iron-oxide particle has been reported using an experimental ultra-highfield MR scanner at 11.7 T (Shapiro *et al.*, 2004). Interestingly, it seems to be more efficient to label a cell with one micron-scaled particle than with hundreds of nanoscaled particles. Another advantage may be that one big particle cannot be further diluted, whereas nanoscaled particles are equally distributed on daughter cells after cell division.

Multimodal magnetic particles may possibly be tracked in parallel by different imaging modalities such as MRI, PET, and optical imaging. Such particles consist of an iron-oxide core with a polymeric coating. Some coatings (e.g., aminosilane, citrate) offer reactive molecular groups for coupling to other signaling compounds such as isotopes or fluorescent dyes.

Table 2   **Typical Pulse Sequences and Protocol Parameters Used for MRI of Rectosigmoideum at 3.0 Tesla (GE Signa 3T)**

Pulse-Sequence	Contrast	Plane	Thickness / Gap [mm]	Slices	R	Matrix	NEX	TR / TE / FA α	RBW [kHz]
FSE-XL	T2	Axial	4 / 0	15	—	256 × 256	4	4700 / 102 / 90°	31.2
FSE-XL	T2	Sagittal	3 / 0	14	2	256 × 256	2	4500 / 99 / 90°	31.2
FSE (TSE)	T1fs	Axial	4 / 0	15	—	256 × 256	4	700 / 15 / 90°	15.6
FSE [ETL 2] (TSE)	T1fs	Sagittal	4 / 0	11	—	256 × 256	4	700 / 15 / 90°	15.6
BH-3D-LAVA (VIBE)	T1fs	Coronal	3–4 / 0†	60	2	256 × 256	1	8.9 / 1.5 / 12°	100

*ZIP512; †ZIP2 (1.5-2.0 mm); maximum acquisition times are up to ~ 5 minutes (T1-FSE).

[RT = respiratory triggering; BH = breath hold; NEX = number of excitations; TR = repetition time [ms]; TE = echo time [ms]; FA = flip angle; ETL = echo-train length; RBW = receiver bandwidth; R = parallel imaging factor; FSE = fast spin-echo; 3D-LAVA = three-dimensional liver acquisition with volume acceleration; ZIP512 = zero interpolation to 512 × 512 matrix; ZIP2 = zero slice interpolation to half of slice measured]

Note that FOV typically ranges from 140-200 mm to provide for close-up views with no phase wrap (NPW) option. In-plane resolution of 0.6-0.8 mm is the presents standard.

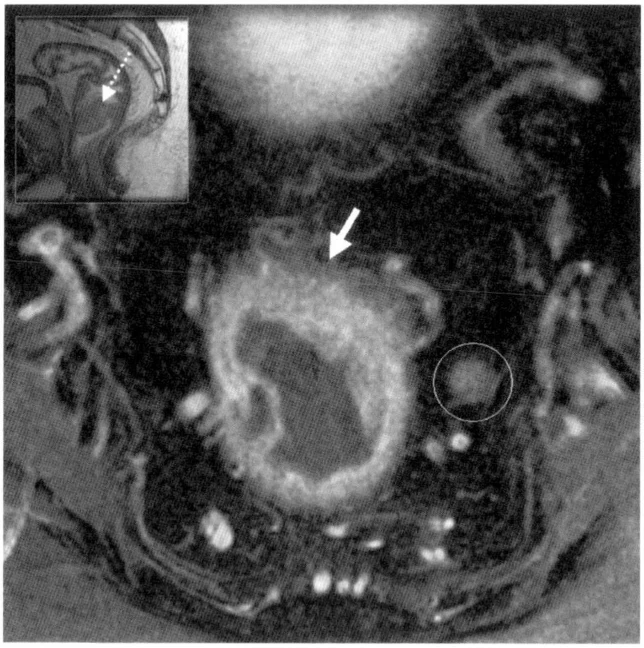

Figure 4 Axial T1-weighted image of the rectum with fat saturation and gadolinium enhancement (3T, FSE, TR/TE = 540/35 ms , spatial resolution 0.4 × 0.4 × 4 mm). A rectal carcinoma shows ventral infiltration (arrow) of perirectal fatty tissue. Pararectal contrast-enhanced lymph node (circle) is indicative for metastasis. This tumor was staged pT3 pN1 by imaging, as was confirmed by histology. In the box T2-weighted sagittal shows an exophytic tumor of rectum (TR/TE = 3800/85 ms). (Courtesy of H. Bruhn and L. Winter, Klinik fur Strahlenheilkunde, Charite Berlin.)

The specific targeting of cancer cells in a solid tumor is impaired by compartment barriers. There are several *in vitro* strategies for a more efficient transmembrane passage of iron-oxide compounds. It could be shown that transfective agents

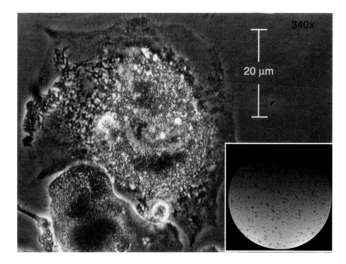

Figure 5 Intracellularly labeled human phagocytic cells (THP-1). Superparamagnetic iron oxides cause local magnetic field inhomogeneities that cause signal drops in T2-weighted imaging (box).

like peptide modification of particle coating (e.g., HIV1-tat) could increase intracellular uptake of iron-oxide compounds up to 100-fold (Zao and Weissleder, 2004). However, no efficient way for specific magnetic cell labeling *in vivo* has been identified so far. Phagocytic cells like Kupffer-Stern cells in the liver sinusoids are an exception. These cells and macrophages elsewhere take up iron-oxide particles from the circulation avidly. This can be exploited for imaging of inflammation. Another approach could be the detection of labeled tumor infiltrating lymphocytes (Kircher *et al.*, 2003). The literature reports many examples of spontaneous remission of solid tumors. Such phenomena are considered to be caused by specific immune effects like T-cell-mediated destruction of tumor cells. Therefore, in the case of immunogenic tumor material, T-cells are a favorable vehicle for distributing magnetic labels within solid tumors. Another promising strategy could be the cell-based imaging of neo-angiogenesis using labeled endothelial progenitor cells (Anderson *et al.*, 2005).

Given a suitable target molecule, solid tumors can be imaged by magnetically labeled ligands. For example, this was shown for the integrin αβ3 (a marker of neo-angiogenesis), which could be targeted by ligands linked to gadolinium (Schmieder *et al.*, 2005).

Another example is the MRI of hyaluronidase activity. Magnetic beads loaded with active hyaluronidase were shown to be detectable by MRI *in vivo* (Shiftan *et al.*, 2005). Hyaluronidase degrades peptides of the extracellular matrix, producing angiogenetic peptides. In this way cancer tumors can be imaged indirectly because of their increased neo-angiogenetic activity.

Tumor angiogenesis has also been imaged by dynamic contrast-enhanced MRI evaluating tumor vascularization directly (Marzola *et al.*, 2004). The drawbacks of such dynamic strategies are the uncertainty about the causes for diminished tumor perfusion under therapy or other clinical circumstances.

Employing MRI for molecular imaging based on contrast materials disregards the advantage of PET with respect to probe sensitivity. The sensitivity for probes is orders of magnitude higher for PET than for MRI (Table 3). The higher sensitivity when screening for small lesions has to be traded against radiation exposure.

Table 3   Outstanding Sensitivity of PET Demonstrated by Amount of Contrast Agent Applied per Patient (In contrast, MRI and CT Are Based on Amounts of Contrast Agents Which Are Orders of Magnitudes Higher)

X-ray Computed Tomography	Magnetic Resonance Imaging	Positron Emission Tomography
77,000,000 μg	4700.000 μg	0.08 μg
100 ml	10 ml	
Iodine	Gadolinium	^{18}F-deoxyglucose

Multimodal imaging combining PET sensitivity and MRI spatial resolution seems to be the most promising screening tool for cancer lesions.

Conclusion

Magnetic resonance imaging colonoscopy has gained substantial momentum in recent years. Considerable improvements in imaging hardware and software have promoted spatially and temporally high-resolution bowel imaging. Meanwhile, MRI colonoscopy is being introduced for gastrointestinal cancer screening of high-risk patients. In addition, abdominal soft tissues can be evaluated for metastases or other primary lesions. Opposite to their feelings about conventional colonoscopy, patients may feel comfortable about the fact that MRI colonoscopy requires no use of an intraluminal instrument in combination with sedation and that bowel cleansing can be avoided when contrast material is administered orally for fecal tagging. However, it is still not clear whether MRI colonoscopy can detect smaller (< 10 mm) intraluminal lesions with sufficient precision. As imaging hardware and software advance further and as experience with this imaging strategy is more widely gained, MRI colonoscopy may develop into a reliable tool for the detection of small intraluminal lesions as well. However, in the follow-up of colorectal cancer patients, radiologic imaging modalities are essential because recurrences mostly occur extraluminally.

MRI of the rectum has already become a routine procedure for preoperative staging, providing excellent highly resolved images of cancer localized in the rectum or sigmoid.

Magnetic resonance imaging of the bowel has achieved diagnostic quality brought about extensive technical innovation. This is an excellent example of the development of an imaging modality that was considered impossible a decade ago. Molecular and cellular imaging is a considerably growing field of investigation. Because of its high spatial and temporal resolution in addition to its good sensitivity, MRI seems to be a favorable tool for the imaging of iron-oxide labeled cells *in vivo*. To date, this imaging strategy is being used experimentally for monitoring labeled stem cells *in vivo* that were labeled *in vitro* before. Mammalian cells can be labeled efficiently without significant cytotoxic effects. Enhanced intracellular uptake of iron-oxide particles can be achieved by modifications of particle coatings *in vitro*. A major obstacle is still the lack of a specific magnetic cell label that could pass readily into compartment barriers *in vivo*. Presently, the most promising approach appears to be indirect imaging of tumors with the use of specific tumor-infiltrating T-cells. Detection of neo-angiogenesis was achieved with labeled endothelial progenitor cells. Even molecular markers of neo-angiogenesis can be detected by MRI opening up new lanes for MRI of tumor-induced neo-angiogenesis. The combination of MRI with PET could offer new possibilities, combining outstanding sensitivity with excellent spatial and temporal resolution. Hence, construction of combined MR-PET scanners is on the way. Although there are promising studies of molecular and cellular imaging by MRI, considerably more interdisciplinary work is needed to make these imaging strategies clinically useful.

References

Akasu, T., Iinuma, G., Fujita, T., Muramatsu, Y., Tateishi, U., Miyakawa, K., Murakami, T., and Moriyama, N. 2005. Thin-section MRI with a phased-array coil for preoperative evaluation of pelvic anatomy and tumor extent in patients with rectal cancer. *AJR Am. J. Roentgenol.* 184(2):531–538.

Anderson, S.A., Glod, J., Arbab, A.S., Noel, M., Ashari, P., Fine, H.A., and Frank, J.A. 2005. Noninvasive MR imaging of magnetically labeled stem cells to directly identify neovasculature in a glioma model. *Blood* 105(1):420–425.

Brown, G. 2005. Thin section MRI in multidisciplinary pre-operative decision making for patients with rectal cancer. *Br. J. Radiol.* 78(2): 117–127.

Debatin, J.F., and Lauenstein, T.C. 2003. Virtual magnetic resonance colonography. *Gut* 52(S4):17–22.

Goehde, S.C., Descher, E., Boekstegers, A., Lauenstein, T., Kuhle, C., Ruehm, S.G., and Ajaj, W. 2005. Dark lumen MR colonography based on fecal tagging for detection of colorectal masses: accuracy and patient acceptance. *Abdom. Imaging* 30(5):576–583.

Kircher, M.F., Allport, J.R., Graves, E.E., Love, V., Josephson, L., Lichtman, A.H., and Weissleder, R. 2003. *In vivo* high resolution three-dimensional imaging of antigen-specific cytotoxic T-lymphocyte trafficking to tumors. *Cancer Res.* 63(20):6838–6846.

Lauenstein, T.C., Ajaj, W., and Kuehle, C.A. 2005a. Virtual colonoscopy by MRI: state-of-the-art and future directions. *Gastrointest. Endosc. Clin. N. Am.* 15(4):797–811.

Lauenstein, T.C., Ajaj, W., Kuehle, C.A., Goehde, S.C., Schlosser, T.W., and Ruehm, S.G. 2005b. Magnetic resonance colonography: comparison of contrast-enhanced three-dimensional VIBE with two-dimensional FISP sequences: preliminary experience. *Invest. Radiol.* 40(2):89–96.

Lauenstein, T.C., Goehde, S.C., and Debatin, J.F. 2002. Fecal tagging: MR colonography without colonic cleansing. *Abdom. Imaging* 27(4):410–417.

Marzola, P., Degrassi, A., Calderan, L., Farace, P., Crescimanno, C., Nicolato, E., Giusti, A., Pesenti, E., Terron, A., Sbarbati, A., Abrams, T., Murray, L., and Osculati, F. 2004. *In vivo* assessment of antiangiogenic activity of SU6668 in an experimental colon carcinoma model. *Clin. Cancer Res.* 10(2):739–750.

Pinkernelle, J., Teichgraber, U., Neumann, F., Lehmkuhl, L., Ricke, J., Scholz, R., Jordan, A., and Bruhn, H. 2005. Imaging of single human carcinoma cells *in vitro* using a clinical whole-body magnetic resonance scanner at 3.0 T. *Magn. Reson. Med.* 53(5):1187–1192.

Purkayastha, S., Tekkis, P.P., Athanasiou, T., Aziz, O., Negus, R., Gedroyc, W., and Darzi, A.W. 2005. Magnetic resonance colonography versus colonoscopy as a diagnostic investigation for colorectal cancer: a meta-analysis. *Clin. Radiol.* 60(9):980–989.

Schmieder, A.H., Winter, P.M., Caruthers, S.D., Harris, T.D., Williams, T.A., Allen, J.S., Lacy, E.K., Zhang, H., Scott, M.J., Hu, G., Robertson, J.D., Wickline, S.A., and Lanza, G.M. 2005. Molecular MR imaging of melanoma angiogenesis with alphanubeta3-targeted paramagnetic nanoparticles. *Magn. Reson. Med.* 53(3):621–627.

Shapiro, E.M., Skrtic, S., Sharer, K., Hill, J.M., Dunbar, C.E., and Koretsky, A.P. 2004. MRI detection of single particles for cellular imaging. *Proc. Natl. Acad. Sci. U.S.A* 101(30):10901–10906.

Shiftan, L., Israely, T., Cohen, M., Frydman, V., Dafni, H., Stern, R., and Neeman, M. 2005. Magnetic resonance imaging visualization of hyaluronidase in ovarian carcinoma. *Cancer Res.* 65(22):10316–10323.

Weissleder, R., Moore, A., Mahmood, U., Bhorade, R., Benveniste, H., Chiocca, E.A., and Basilion, J.P. 2000. *In vivo* magnetic resonance imaging of transgene expression. *Nat. Med.* 6(3):351–355.

Winawer, S., Fletcher, R., Rex, D., Bond, J., Burt, R., Ferrucci, J., Ganiats, T., Levin, T., Woolf, S., Johnson, D., Kirk, L., Litin, S., and Simmang, C. Gastrointestinal Consortium Panel. 2003. Colorectal cancer screening and surveillance: clinical guidelines and rational—update based on new evidence. *Gastroenterology* 124(2):544–560.

Winter, L., Bruhn, H., Langrehr, J., Menhaus, P., Felix, R., and Hanninen, L.E. 2007. Magnetic resonance imaging in suspected rectal cancer determining localization, stage, and sphincter-saving respectability at 3-tesla-sustained high resolution. *Acta. Radiol.* 48:379–387.

Zhao, M., and Weissleder, R. 2004. Intracellular cargo delivery using tat peptide and derivatives. *Med. Res. Rev.* 24(1):1–12.

11

Potential New Staging Perspectives in Colorectal Cancer: Whole-Body PET/CT-Colonography

Patrick Veit-Haibach

Introduction

Colorectal cancer (CRC) continues to be the third leading cause of cancer-related mortality in Western countries, accounting for over 50,000 deaths in 2005 (Jemal *et al.*, 2005).

Despite all clinical efforts and improvements in therapeutical options, these numbers are mainly based on late diagnosis and detection of colorectal tumors. Although several screening attempts for colorectal cancer had been made to enhance early diagnosis, the majority of patients show only a moderate compliance. Therefore, early diagnosis is often not possible.

Thus, for patients with colorectal cancer, accurate tumor staging is necessary and desired for the definition of further therapy (Bipat *et al.*, 2004; Fillipone *et al.*, 2004; Neri *et al.*, 2002; Stevenson, 2000; Schofield *et al.*, 2006). In clinical routine, optical colonoscopy continues to be the standard method of choice because not only tumor detection, but also tissue sampling and therapeutic intervention are possible. Furthermore, synchronous lesions can be excluded. On the other hand, the procedure is invasive and might introduce further complications itself (e.g., bleeding or perforation). However, in addition noninvasive imaging techniques have to be performed to determine potential metastases to the lymphatic system or other organs.

For these purposes, different cross-sectional techniques have been developed in the past years. To date, MR-colonography (magnetic resonance imaging), CT-colonography (computed tomography,) as well as optimized abdominal CT protocols, are mainly used for tumor staging and detection of colorectal polyps (Ajaj *et al.*, 2005b; Lauenstein *et al.*, 2005; Jin *et al.*, 2006; Silva *et al.*, 2006; Abdel Razek *et al.*, 2005).

Within this bunch of different imaging procedures, contrast-enhanced computer tomography (CT) turned out to be one of the most commonly used modalities for staging colorectal cancer patients. Major advantages are easy to specify: it offers the possibility to visualize the primary tumor, it gives an overview of adjacent and distant organs concerning potential metastases, it is relatively easy to perform, and CT scanners are more widely available as MRI scanners. However, advantages, disadvantages, as well as technical considerations about whole-body MR and MR-colonography, are discussed in other chapters.

Overall, CT colonography and abdominal CT with bowel distension is a widely accepted technique that has been investigated for several indications (Andersen *et al.*, 2006; Park *et al.*, 2006; Fletcher *et al.*, 2002). Recent studies showed that it has a high sensitivity of detecting medium and large colorectal polyps as well as symptomatic cancer (Halligan *et al.*, 2005; Chung *et al.*, 2005). One major drawback of CT is the lack of functional data, which can potentially cause several pitfalls: the detection of small and only subtle contrast-enhancing lesions and also the evaluation of invasion or infiltration of adjacent organs and detection of metastatic spread to regional lymph nodes can be impaired on CT alone (Antoch *et al.*, 2003). [^{18}F]-Fluoro-2-deoxy-D-glucose (FDG) positron emission tomography (PET), on the other hand, can display functional information and has been found to be particularly accurate in staging primary and recurrent colorectal cancer, but has a limited anatomical resolution (Abdel-Nabi *et al.*, 1998; Kantorova *et al.*, 2003; Valk *et al.*, 1999; Cohade *et al.*, 2003; Hübner *et al.*, 2000; Rohren *et al.*, 2004).

A combination of CT and PET in a combined PET/CT scanner allows for fusion of functional and morphological data and has been used in clinical practice for several years. Since combined PET/CT scanners have been introduced into the market, different studies have shown the supremacy of integrated PET/CT over single-modality staging in different tumor entities (Antoch *et al.*, 2003, 2004b). Furthermore, recent studies demonstrated the superiority of the combined imaging modality in detection and characterization of malignant lesions when compared with CT or PET alone for colorectal cancer (Kim *et al.*, 2005). However, all of these studies evaluated non-disease-specific PET/CT protocols. Meanwhile, it has been shown that general protocols might not be specific enough to evaluate different cancer entities in all their supplementary aspects (Osman *et al.*, 2005; Schöder *et al.*, 2005; Gutman *et al.*, 2005; Israel *et al.*, 2005).

Therefore, a specific CT protocol with focus on colorectal cancer staging has been integrated in a whole-body PET/CT protocol. Initial experiences showed promising results concerning technical feasibility and tumor detection rates (Veit *et al.*, 2006). Thus, the aim of such a protocol is the enhancement of detection and characterization of colonic lesions as well as detection and characterization of distant metastases and metastatic lymph nodes. Based on such a whole-body imaging approach with an embedded colon-specific protocol, the current stepwise, multi-modality diagnostic work-up in colorectal cancer patients might be shortened. Overall, the whole-body PET/CT-colonography might be used as an "all-in-one" imaging approach in conjunction with optical colonoscopy.

Indications

Based on the only recent introduction of this protocol, only relatively small patient populations have been evaluated

with such a protocol. Furthermore, owing to the large variety of the clinical symptoms that can be caused by the different stages of colon cancer, patients generally are admitted to the hospital for a variety of examinations and are not primarily referred for a PET/CT. All patients examined so far with PET/CT-colonography received optical colonoscopy one day before the PET/CT-colonography examination and were referred for suspicion of having colorectal cancer. The main reasons for admission to the hospital were BRBPR (bright red blood per rectum), positive fecal occult blood test, long-lasting altered bowel habits and/or pain, anemia of unknown cause, and stenotic colon anastomosis in patients with already operated colon cancer. None of the patients evaluated so far suffered from a chronic inflammatory bowel disease.

Patient Preparation and Imaging Procedure

Similar to patient preparation for optical colonoscopy, all patients should receive bowel cleansing for PET/CT-colonography. In general, bowel cleansing one or two days prior to the examination is sufficient. So far polyethylene glycol-electrolytes was used one day prior to optical colonoscopy. When optical colonoscopy is performed one or two days before PET/CT, patients might stay on clear liquids afterward.

Dual-modality imaging was performed with a commercially available PET/CT system. The system used includes a dual-slice CT scanner and a full-ring PET tomograph. The PET system has an axial field-of-view of 15.5 cm per bed position and an in-plane spatial resolution of 4.6 mm. The system acquires the CT first, followed by the whole-body emission data. CT and PET data sets can be viewed separately or in fused mode on a commercially available computer workstation after the examination.

Prior to the FDG injection, blood samples should be drawn from all patients to ensure glucose levels are in normal range. If blood glucose levels are found to exceed a certain level (i.e., 120 mg/dl), patients should be treated with insulin to lower the blood glucose level and to ensure optimal imaging quality. Afterward, an adequate amount of FDG (e.g., 350 MBq, depending on national official regulation) should be administered intravenously to the patient. During the uptake time of approximately 60 minutes, an oral contrast media for small bowel distension can be administered as desired. So far, 1500 ml of a water-based, negative oral contrast agent for small bowel distension and marking showed the best results (Antoch *et al.*, 2004a). During the uptake time, the patients should rest in a relaxing position (sitting, or even better, lying) to avoid excessive muscle uptake.

The total whole-body PET/CT, which covered a field-of-view from the base of the skull to the upper thighs, was so far divided into two parts. First, data from the upper body regions (base of skull to diaphragm) were acquired in a caudo-cranial direction with the patient in a supine position using a standardized breathing protocol or in expiration if possible (Beyer *et al.*, 2003). CT images should be acquired in a full diagnostic fashion (e.g., 110 mAs, 120 kV, 5 mm slice thickness, and a 2.4 mm incremental reconstruction) to ensure reliable quality, especially in primary diagnosis cases and re-staging cases. Thus, intravenous contrast media should be used as well. The contrast media protocol itself (timing, amount of contrast media) might depend on local experience and preferences. The PET data then have to be acquired within the same field-of-view as the CT.

After this first imaging part, pharmacological bowel relaxation should be administered (N-butylscopolamin or glucagon) by bolus injection or short infusion for preparation of a rectal water enema. For this enema patients have to be positioned on the side or in prone position on the scanner table. Prone positioning is needed to achieve an optimized overview of the colon, because the small bowel cumulates at the frontal abdominal wall. Then, the water enema (2–3 liters tap water, 37° Celsius) should be performed for colonic distension. Depending of the estimated time for the abdominal scan and depending on the half-life of the used drug, an additional short intravenous infusion for pharmacological bowel relaxation might be applied for a continuous bowel relaxation during the second imaging part. For this second part of the acquisition, corresponding PET/CT data were acquired from the diaphragm to the upper thighs with the patient still in prone position. CT imaging parameters should be adjusted in order to receive full diagnostic quality in the abdomen as well. Thus, intravenous contrast is indispensable for this part as well (i.e., 120 mAs, 120 kV, 2.5–3 mm slice thickness). PET imaging should cover the same field-of-view as the abdominal CT part. Average PET acquisition time might be adjusted to 2–4 min per bed position, depending on the scanner type used. In both scan protocol portions, emission data should be corrected for scatter and attenuation based on the available CT transmission images, which offer faster imaging than with transmission sources.

Image Evaluation

First, the readers should evaluate bowel distension (small bowel and colon). For evaluation of colonic lesions, the bowel should be distended maximally, the colonic wall should barely be visible. PET/CT data sets might be reviewed side by side in addition to the fused mode and in 3D mode on a dedicated commercially available fusion workstation. Image evaluation should be done by a radiologist and a nuclear medicine specialist in consensus, or by an imaging specialist who is familiar with reading both imaging modalities and combined imaging. In cases of questionable findings, PET data sets might be evaluated with and without attenuation correction.

Contrast-enhancing, bowel wall masses in conjunction with or without focally increased glucose metabolism above the surrounding tissue level leads to the diagnosis of malignant colonic lesions. Lymph nodes should be assessed for metastatic spread based on increased glucose metabolism independent of their size on PET/CT. Furthermore, a fatty hilum as well as calcifications might indicate benign lymph nodes, whereas lymph nodes with central necroses might be evaluated as malignant, independent of their size and glucose uptake. Distant metastases should be assessed based on soft tissue, contrast-enhancing masses in different body compartments with or without focally increased glucose metabolism above the surrounding tissue level.

Clinical Experience

Most patients tolerate the procedure well. However, based on individual medical conditions and the time patients are required to remain in prone position, short and self-limiting mild nausea might occur.

PET/CT-colonography represents a new concept in colorectal cancer staging. Thus, the feasibility had to be approved first. So far, all PET/CT examinations with integrated colonography delivered fully diagnostic image quality for the colonography data sets and the whole-body tumor staging in all patients.

The average time for the combined examination amounted to approximately 33–37 minutes (+/−7 minutes), representing 7–11 bed positions per examination, depending on the patient's height. In comparison, a noncolonography PET/CT examination takes on average 30–33 minutes (+/−7 minutes) when PET and CT are acquired fully diagnostic. The pharmacological bowel relaxation, patient repositioning, new preparation of the PET/CT scanner, as well as the rectal enema caused the additional time required.

Bowel distension with tap water and pharmacological bowel relaxation so far showed highly reliable results concerning distension and relaxation. This is an indispensable precondition not only for the detection of colonic lesions, but also for artifact-free co-registration of anatomical and functional imaging.

PET/CT-colonography showed highly accurate staging results concerning the overall TNM staging: over 80% of all patients had been correctly staged with whole-body PET/CT-colonography. These included all clinical stages of colorectal cancer. The T-stages found ranged from T0-stage up to T4-stage. Over 80% of T-stages were correctly staged with PET/CT (Fig. 1). Furthermore, the patient populations evaluated so far included all N-stages, ranging from N0-stage up to the N2-stage. PET/CT was found to be correct in over 85% in N-staging so far. In addition, the M-stage can be evaluated as being highly efficient as well, based on the whole-body examination.

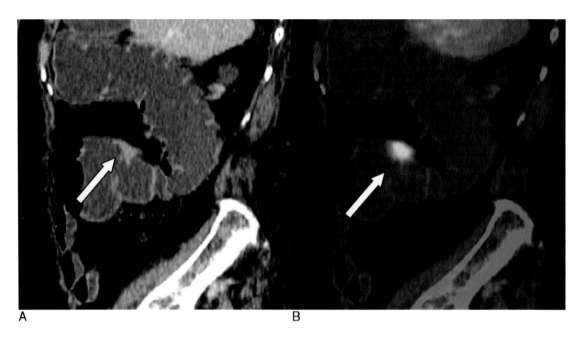

Figure 1 Sagittal CT image and corresponding PET/CT images of a patient with colon cancer at the right colonic flexure: CT shows a slightly thickened bowel wall at the right colonic flexure on CT-colonography (white arrow, **A**). Corresponding sagittal PET/CT-colonography (**B**) showed pathological glucose uptake, indicating a colorectal tumor (white arrow). Histopathological work-up confirmed the diagnosis.

It has to be added, however, that PET/CT-colonography has several drawbacks concerning T-stage as well as N-stage evaluation. This matter will be discussed in the limitations section in the conclusion of the chapter.

Several patients with incomplete optical colonoscopy due to insufficient bowel cleansing, tumor stenosis, and/or bleeding underwent PET/CT-colonography for staging as well. PET/CT was found to be accurate in the detection of additional or synchronous tumors in these patients. No experiences have been made so far in patients with rectoscopy only. However, it can be expected that PET/CT-colonography will generate accurate and reliable results in such a patient population as well.

Some patients so far were examined after endoscopical resection of large polyps and were referred based on the suspicion of residual cancer. Although reasonable results were found so far, PET/CT might not be reliable enough in these indications based on the technical background. Thus, no definite conclusion can be drawn so far from the available experiences. More details are discussed below.

Based on the whole-body concept, PET/CT was also able to detect several synchronous or secondary tumors. Thus, a whole-body PET/CT-colonography might be able to detect additional, FDG-avid tumors in one step. However, it is known that FDG-PET/CT cannot detect and characterize every tumor entity. Thus, small, non-FDG-avid tumors can be overlooked. Further research is needed in that field with more specific or combined tracers.

Perspectives and Considerations

Technical Considerations

Several aspects of such an approach, which potentially can be handled differently in other departments when pasting a dedicated colonography protocol into the whole-body PET/CT examination, have to be discussed.

Image misregistration due to bowel movements can occur during the acquisition time of approximately 15 min; therefore, bowel relaxation had to be ensured. So far, a bolus injection and, if required, a short infusion of N-butylscopolamine when exceeding 15 min acquisition time due to the drug's half-life was used, and good results could be achieved. As this drug is not FDA approved, actually no information about the use and results of glucagon, which is mainly used in the United States, in such a setting is available. Thus, further studies evaluating the use of glucagon in this modified and optimized protocol are required.

PET has been found to have higher tumor detection rates than CT, with impact on the therapy regimen (Kantorova *et al.*, 2003; Kalff *et al.*, 2002; Abdel Nabi *et al.*, 1998). However, limited anatomical information on FDG-PET often renders exact localization of lesions difficult (Nakamoto *et al.*, 2004). Thus, morphological information needs to be added to PET. An optimized abdominal CT in addition to optical colonoscopy and separate PET staging may be considered an alternative to inline PET/CT imaging. However, if CT and PET are performed separately, substantial misregistration of the bowel when correlating CT with PET must be expected due to patient movement and bowel movement between the two procedures. In addition, optimized abdominal CT for staging purposes is performed with a distended colon, while on PET alone the patient's colon is not distended. Therefore, profound image misregistration has to be expected as well.

Most experiences were obtained with tap water for colon distension. For CT-colonography or abdominal CT for colorectal cancer staging, room air or CO_2 is often used, which might upgrade patient comfort. The main reason for higher patient comfort is the significant intestinal reabsorption of the gas (Church and Delaney, 2003; Grant et al., 1986). However, gas absorption may lead to differences in bowel distension during the procedure, and therefore possible misregistration of morphological and functional data can be expected.

Only moderate experiences have been made with air insufflation in PET/CT-colonography so far. We found that the facility of inspection was inferior compared to patients with water distension, and, as expected, we found more misregistrations between morphological and functional data. In addition, based on the greater difference of Hounsfield Units between the colonic wall and the gas-filled colon, mild streak artifacts occurred at the colon wall surface. These might be particularly disturbing when looking for small or flat colonic wall lesions. So far, room air filling was performed manually, and distension was secured with a blocked rectal balloon catheter. However, an automatic insufflator with continuous pressure monitoring might help to reduce misregistration artifacts, but will further increase costs and will be more time consuming as well. Even with possibly increased misregistrations based on bowel movement due to gas reabsorption, both approaches (water versus gas filling) may not be significantly different concerning the TNM staging. Thus, further dedicated studies have to be conducted to compare both approaches in a clinical setting. However, it is the author's personal opinion that an image modality that is not presentable to the referring physicians because of misregistration artifacts will not find a find a wide clinical acceptance.

We acquired the abdominal PET/CT in prone position, albeit knowing that scanning in both positions (prone and supine) may provide better colonic distension (Yee et al., 2003; Morrin et al., 2002; Chen et al., 1999). Scanning in both positions is needed in CT-colonography to distinguish between residual stool and polyps. Those particular problems are not to be expected in PET/CT-colonography. PET/CT provides an additional functional date, which helps to distinguish between colon wall, colonic wall lesions, and stool. Since stool should not show any (or only mild) increased glucose metabolism, the "double" positioning can be avoided. Thus, the additional radiation exposure does not seem to be required, especially since previous studies show

no imperative increase in polyp detection comparing both position scans with scanning only in prone position (Yee et al., 2003). Furthermore, the added scan would additionally lengthen the already extended examination time.

The examination time in our setting was considerably prolonged due to the splitting of the protocol (separate examination of thorax and abdomen). This splitting was necessary based on the relatively slow dual-slice scanner and the needed emission time of 3 min and more per bed position. However, it can be expected that with state-of-the-art multislice scanners with new detector generations and consecutive decreased PET emission time, the PET/CT examination can be significantly shortened. Thus, a splitting of the examination may no longer be needed.

The PET/CT-colonography examinations were conducted on a dual-slice CT scanner. As mentioned earlier, Hara et al. (2001) pointed out that there may no significant difference in detection of small intestinal masses comparing single and multidetector scanners. Despite the fact that multidetector scanners provide the option of acquiring thinner slices, single-slice or dual-slice CT scanning is substantially more time consuming and may not deliver adequate resolution for artifact-free postprocessing tools. Several specific postprocessing tools and software applications for CT-colonography (i.e., virtual colonoscopy, volume-rendered images, etc.) are available from almost every major vendor (Edwards et al., 2004; Fenlon et al., 1999). Thus, data sets can be viewed and presented with different applications designed for different specific needs. For PET/CT-colonography, no equivalent software is currently commercially available (i.e., for virtual colonoscopy or preoperative planning). However, first steps have been made into this particular field of "fly-through," and "fly-around" by different groups. Quon et al. (2006) demonstrated the feasibility of such an application and also pointed out the potential usefulness for preoperative planning. Furthermore, Seemann (2007) found a statistically significant difference in detection of metastatic lymph nodes when comparing virtual PET/CT-bronchoscopy and virtual CT-bronchoscopy. Up to date, in PET/CT-colonography, evaluations were performed on fused axial images as well as 3D-MPR images. Hence, larger patient studies are needed to discover the definite clinical advantage of such post-processing tools and its potential influences on therapeutic decisions.

Staging Considerations

Overall, Tumor Node Metastases (TNM) staging in PET/CT-colonography was highly accurate in this patient population. PET/CT-colonography was statistically significant superior to CT-colonography when staging TNM. These differences were based mainly on a more accurate T-staging and a more accurate N-staging when using a threshold of 1 cm for lymph node detection in CT-colonography alone. However, in clinical routine, a 1 cm threshold seems relatively high for pericolic lymph nodes; thus a 0.7 cm threshold was established as well. In this case, no statistically significant difference could be detected. No difference was found for the M-stage as well.

There is only limited experience in preoperative TNM stage with CT alone (Fillipone *et al.*, 2004) The clinical relevance of a more accurate T-stage evaluation with PET/CT-colonography has to be considered carefully. The T-stage might be of only minor clinical relevance with regard to therapy, which will be tumor resection in most cases. However, differences of PET/CT over CT alone might arise in higher clinical stages when additional surrounding organ infiltration can be characterized by PET/CT. Furthermore, flat and/or small lesions might be more visible based on the additional functional information. However, in most other cases the clinical benefit of a more accurate assessment of the T-stage with PET/CT-colonography was small as compared to optimized abdominal CT. In patients with rectal cancer, accurate assessment of the T-stage can help to select patients with metastastic lymph nodes, which might receive neoadjuvant chemotherapy preoperatively (NCCN Guidelines for Treatment of Cancer, www.NCCN.org). Furthermore, accurate assessment of the T-stage as well as tumor size may help to decide how to access the tumor, either by laparotomy, laparoscopy, or transanally (NCCN Guidelines for Treatment of Cancer, www.NCCN.org). The literature also contains discussions about the ideal time point of resection of a colon cancer. Studies have shown that if the primary tumor has been taken out, the metastases may start to grow or an increase of metastases growth may occur after resection of the primary tumor (Peeters *et al.*, 2005, 2006). Thus, also in colon cancer, a close TNM evaluation might be helpful to define further therapy.

PET/CT had higher accuracy than CT staging when assessing the N-stage in colorectal cancer. This has been shown in several publications before (Veit *et al.*, 2006). It has to be noted that a 1 cm threshold was used in CT for most comparisons. However, as mentioned earlier, based on clinical experiences, such a threshold seems quite large for perirectal or pericolic lymph nodes, especially in areas where no lymph node chains are located. Thus, when introducing a threshold of 0.7 cm for perirectal lymph nodes, differences were no longer of statistical significance. As expected, CT's sensitivity for detection of malignant nodes increased when applying the 0.7 cm threshold instead of 1.0 cm. Interestingly, however, the specificity remained unchanged. The threshold to be applied for differentiating malignant from benign lymph nodes is controversially discussed in the literature. Hence, further studies with histopathological standard of reference are needed to clarify different CT-thresholds in different body compartments.

PET/CT detected several lesions with elevated glucose metabolism, which turned out to be adenoma with intraepithelial dysplasia. Detection and characterization of intraepithelial dysplasia with PET is a controversial topic

in the current literature, and our experience in PET/CT is actually small (Drenth *et al.*, 2001; Friedland *et al.*, 2005; Yasuda *et al.*, 2001). However, in comparison to PET alone, PET/CT can distinguish morphologically between polyps and tumorous colonic wall lesions based on the additional morphology. Furthermore, PET as well as nondisease-defined PET/CT can be impaired by unspecific focal glucose uptake (Gutman *et al.*, 2005). Due to the applied pharmacological bowel relaxation, no unspecific abdominal focal tracer uptake has been noted in our PET/CT-colonography. However, FDG has been found in the bowel lumen. It is not clear yet if it is pulled through the mucosa by an elevated osmotic level of the stool or if it is excreted actively. Obviously, this might cause additional false-positive findings. Further research on this topic is needed. Overall, if a focal glucose metabolism, whether in a polyp or colonic wall mass, is detected, further clinical work-up is indicated. PET/CT is able to provide morphological guidance to those questionable lesions.

Possible Indications and Perspectives

PET/CT-colonography is not only feasible, but also shows highly accurate tumor detection rates and promising staging results. Such a protocol may serve as a useful tool in different indications.

Patients with incomplete colonoscopy and suspected colorectal cancer may benefit from a PET/CT-colonography. It has been shown that imaging work-up in patients with incomplete colonoscopy in order to complete bowel evaluation may have a particular impact on therapeutic decisions (Ajaj *et al.*, 2005b). However, a comparison of CT-colonography, MR-colonography, and PET/CT-colonography is needed to find out the adequate modality in this indication. Such a decision might also be influenced by local evaluation protocols, reader experience, and scanner availability.

The protocol may also be used for the detection of small synchronous lesions and, of course, distant metastases. PET/CT is already known for superior detection rates concerning metastatic lymph nodes. Therefore, it might be helpful especially in rectal cancer where nodal positive patients often receive preoperative chemotherapy as discussed above.

A controversial indication might be imaging in case of suspected residual tumor after endoscopical resection. Little experience in patients with suspected residual tumor has been achieved. On CT images alone, a slightly thickened bowel wall due to granulomatous tissue would indicate a residual tumor. However, with a lack of FDG uptake, no residual tumor was suspected on PET/CT imaging. These true negative findings were confirmed by consecutive histopathology. Based on the size of the tumor resected and the texture of the colonic wall, this might be beyond the resolution of PET and PET/CT imaging. However, since detection of tumor is not only a matter of resolution but also of a tumor-to-background ratio, such an examination might be in the range of possible indications, but larger patient studies are needed for further evaluation.

At last, the protocol should also be feasible for the evaluating of local recurrence at the anastomotic site. Although this is a very rare indication, in these cases diagnosis by optical colonoscopy is often impaired due to scar stenosis or tumor growth outside the anastomosis and therefore cannot be detected and fully evaluated by optical colonoscopy. Further studies with different patient populations have to evaluate these potential benefits and the potential impact on the therapeutic decision of such a protocol.

Limitations and Conclusion

The PET/CT-colonography concept has several limitations. Based on the spatial resolution and tumor-to-background ratio, flat adenomas can be missed. For the same reasons, micrometastases cannot be detected on PET and PET/CT imaging. The image acquisition time must be considered another limitation of the combined PET/CT protocol. Compared to dedicated optimized CT protocols, the examination time is substantially longer. However, examination times were only slightly longer compared to whole-body PET/CT without colonography. Improvements might occur with the development of alternative PET detector materials and the recent introduction of new PET detectors covering a larger field-of-view. CT as well as PET/CT have clear limitations in correctly differentiating T1-tumors from T2-tumors since this requires visibility of the colon wall layers. In those cases, endoscopical ultrasound is the current procedure of choice. However, lesion access with endoscopical ultrasound can be impaired in an elongated colon or in high-grade stenoses. Further technical developments concerning CT and PET/CT resolution may improve their ability to differentiate T1 and T2 tumors. Also, SPECT/CT imaging might play a role in the near future based on the technical possibility of a very high spatial resolution.

Overall, this protocol can be used for several selected indications and points to a possible new staging concept. Within new staging algorithms, it then may help to provide the referring physician with an accurate whole-body tumor staging in one step, with or without conjointly performed optical colonoscopy, to define further therapy. However, further research has to be conducted in several study designs and selected indications as discussed earlier.

References

Abdel Razek, A.A., Abu Zeid, M.M., Bilal, M., and Abdel Wahab, N.M. 2005. Virtual CT colonoscopy versus conventional colonoscopy: a prospective study. *Hepatogastroenterology 52*:1698–1702.

Abdel-Nabi, H., Doerr, R.J., and Lamonica, D.M. 1998. Staging of primary colorectal carcinomas with fluorine-18 fluorodeoxyglucose whole-body PET: correlation with histopathologic and CT findings. *Radiology 206*:755–760.

Ajaj, W., Debatin, J.F., and Lauenstein, T. 2005a. Colonography by magnetic resonance imaging. *Eur. J. Gastroenterol. Hepatol. 17*:815–820.

Ajaj, W., Lauenstein, T.C., Pelster, G., Holtmann, G., Ruehm, S.G., Debatin, J.F., and Goehde, S.C. 2005b. MR colonography in patients with incomplete conventional colonoscopy. *Radiology 234*:452–459.

Andersen, K., Vogt, C., Blondin, D., Beck, A., Heinen, W., and Cohnen, M. 2006. Multi-detector CT-colonography in inflammatory bowel disease: prospective analysis of CT-findings to high-resolution video colonoscopy. *Eur. J. Radiology 58*:140.

Antoch, G., Kuehl, H., Kanja, J., Bauer, S., Renzing-Koehler, K., Schuette, J., Bockisch, A., Debatin, J.F., and Freudenberg, L.S. 2004a. Dual-modality PET/CT scanning with negative oral contrast agent to avoid artifacts: introduction and evaluation. *Radiology 230*:879–885.

Antoch, G., Vogt, F.M, Freudenberg, L.S., Goehde, S.C., Barkhausen, J., Dahmen, G., Bockisch, A., Debatin, J., and Ruehm, S. 2003. Whole-body dual-modality PET/CT and whole-body MRI for tumor staging in oncology. *JAMA 290*:3199–3206.

Antoch, G., Saoudi, N., Kuehl, H., Dahmen, G, Mueller, S.P., Beyer, T., Bockisch, A., Deabtin, J.F., and Freudenberg, L.S. 2004b. Accuracy of whole-body dual-modality fluorine-18-2-fluoro-2-deoxy-D-glucose positron emission tomography and computed tomography (FDG-PET/CT) for tumor staging in solid tumors: comparison with CT and PET. *J. Clin. Oncol. 22*:4357–4368.

Beyer, T., Antoch, G., Blodgett, T., Freudenberg, L.F., Akhurst, T., and Mueller, S. 2003. Dual-modality PET/CT imaging: the effect of respiratory motion on combined image quality in clinical oncology. *Eur. J. Nucl. Med. Mol. Imag. 30*:588–596.

Bipat, S., Glas, A.S., Slors, F.J.M., Zwinderman, A.H., Bossuyt, P.M.M., and Stoker, J. 2004. Rectal cancer: local staging and assessment of lymph node involvement with endoluminal US, CT, and MR imaging—a meta-analysis. *Radiology 232*:773–783.

Chen, S.C., Lu, D.S., Hecht, J.R., and Kadell, B.M. 1999. CT colonography: value of scanning in both the supine and prone positions. *AJR Am. J. Roentgenol. 172*:595–599.

Chung, D.J., Huh, K.C., Choi, W.J., and Kim, J.K. CT 2005. Colonography using 16-MDC in the evaluation of colorectal cancer. *Am. J. Roentgenol. 184*:98–103.

Church, J., and Delaney, C. 2003. Randomized, controlled trial of carbon dioxide insufflation during colonoscopy. *Dis. Colon Rectum 46*:322–326.

Cohade, C., Osman, M., Leal, J., and Wahl, R.L. 2003. Direct comparison of 18F-FDG PET and PET/CT in patients with colorectal carcinoma. *J. Nucl. Med. 44*:1797–1803.

Drenth, J., Nagengast, F., and Oyen, W. 2001. Evaluation of (pre-) malignant colonic abnormalities: endoscopic validation of FDG-PET findings. *Eur. J. N. Med. and Mol. Imag. 28*:1766.

Edwards, J.T., Mendelson, R.M., Fritschi, L., Foster, N.M., Wood, C., Murray D., and Forbes, G.M. 2004. Colorectal neoplasia screening with CT colonography in average-risk asymptomatic subjects: community-based study. *Radiology 230*:459–464.

Fenlon, H.M., Nunes, D.P., Schroy, P.C., Barish, M.A., Clarke, P.D., and Ferrucci, J.T. 1999. A comparison of virtual and conventional colonoscopy for the detection of colorectal polyps. *N. Engl. J. Med. 341*:1496–1503.

Filippone, A., Ambrosini, R., Fuschi, M., Marinelli, T., Genovesi, D., and Bonomo, L. 2004. Preoperative T and N staging of colorectal cancer: accuracy of contrast-enhanced multi-detector row CT colonography—initial experience. *Radiology 231*:83–90.

Fletcher, J.G., Johnson, C.D., and Krueger, W.R. 2002. Contrast-enhanced CT colonography in recurrent colorectal carcinoma: feasibility of simultaneous evaluation for metastatic disease, local recurrence, and metachronous neoplasia in colorectal carcinoma. *Am. J. Roentgenol. 178*:283–290.

Friedland, S., Soetikno, R., Carlisle, M., Taur, A., Kaltenbach, T., and Segall, G. 2005. 18-Fluorodeoxyglucose positron emission tomography has limited sensitivity for colonic adenoma and early stage colon cancer. *Gastroint. End. 61*:395.

Grant, D.S., Bartram, CI., and Heron, C.W. 1986. A preliminary study of the possible benefits of using carbon dioxide insufflation during double-contrast barium enema. *Br. J. Radiol. 59*:190–191.

Gutman F., Alberini, J.-L., Wartski, M., Vilain, D., Le Stanc, E., Sarandi, F., Corone, C., Tainturier, C., and Packing, A.P. 2005. Incidental colonic focal lesions detected by FDG PET/CT. *Am. J. Roentgenol. 185*:495–500.

Halligan, S., Altman, D.G., Taylor, S.A., Mallett, S., Deeks, J.J., and Atkins, W. 2005. CT colonography in the detection of colorectal polyps and cancer: systematic review, meta-analysis, and proposed minimum data set for study level reporting. *Radiology 237*:893–904.

Hara, A.K., Johnson, C.D., MacCarty, R.L., Welch, T.J., McCollough, C.H., and Harmsen, W.S. 2001. CT colonography: single- versus multi-detector row imaging. *Radiology 219*:461–465.

Hübner, R.H., Park, K.C., Shepherd, J.E., Schwimmer, J., Czernin, J., Phelps, M.E., and Gambhir, S.S. 2000. A meta-analysis of the literature for whole-body FDG PET detection of recurrent colorectal cancer. *J. Nucl. Med. 41*:1177–1189.

Israel, O., Yefremov, N., Bar-Shalom, R., Kagana, O., Frenkel, A., Keidar, Z., and Fischer, D. 2005. PET/CT detection of unexpected gastrointestinal foci of 18F-FDG uptake: incidence, localization patterns, and clinical significance. *J. Nucl. Med. 46*:758–762.

Jemal, A., Murray, T., and Ward, E. 2005. Cancer statistics. *CA Cancer J. Clin. 55*:10–30.

Jin, K.N., Lee, J.M., Kim, S.H., Shin, K.S., Lee, J.Y., Han, J.K., and Choi, B.I. 2006. The diagnostic value of multiplanar reconstruction on MDCT colonography for the preoperative staging of colorectal cancer. *Eur. Radiol. 16*:2284–2291.

Kalff, V., Hicks, R.J., Ware, R.E., Hogg, A., Binns, D., and McKenzie, A.F. 2002. The clinical impact of (18)F-FDG PET in patients with suspected or confirmed recurrence of colorectal cancer: a prospective study. *J. Nucl. Med. 43*:492–499.

Kantorova, I., Lipska, L., Belohlavek, O., Visokai, V., Trubac, M., and Schneiderova, M. 2003. Routine 18F-FDG PET preoperative staging of colorectal cancer: comparison with conventional staging and its impact on treatment decision making. *J. Nucl. Med. 44*:1784–1788.

Kim, J.-H., Czernin, J., Allen-Auerbach, M.S., Halper, B.S., Fueger, B., Ratib, O., Phelps, M.E., and Weber, W.A. 2005. Comparison between 18F-FDG PET, in-line PET/CT, and software fusion for restaging of recurrent colorectal cancer. *J. Nucl. Med. 46*:587–595.

Lauenstein, T.C., Ajaj, W., and Kuehle, C.A. 2005. Virtual colonoscopy by MRI: state-of-the-art and future directions. *Gastrointest. Endosc. Clin. N. Am. 15*:797–811.

Morrin, M., Farrell, R., Keogan, M., Kruskal, J., Yam, C.-S., and Raptopoulos, V. 2002. CT colonography: colonic distention improved by dual positioning but not intravenous glucagon. *Euro. Radiol. 12*:525.

Nakamoto, Y., Chin, B.B., Cohade, C., Osman, M., Tatsumi, M., and Wahl, R.L. 2004. PET/CT: artifacts caused by bowel motion. *Nucl. Med. Commun. 25*:221–225.

National Comprehensive Cancer Network. Guidelines for Treatment of Cancer. www.nccn.org.

Neri, E., Giusti, P., Battolla, L., Vagli, P., Boraschi, P., Lencioni, R., and Bartolozzi, C. 2002. Colorectal cancer: role of CT colonography in preoperative evaluation after incomplete colonoscopy. *Radiology 223*:615–619.

Osman, M.M., Cohade, C., Fishman, E.K., and Wahl, R.L. 2005. Clinically significant incidental findings on the unenhanced CT portion of PET/CT studies: frequency in 250 patients. *J. Nucl. Med. 46*:1352–1355.

Park, S.H., Ha, H.K., Kim, A.Y., Lee, M.J., Shin, Y.M., Yang, S.K., and Min, Y.I. 2006. Flat polyps of the colon: detection with 16-MDCT colonography—preliminary results. *Am. J. Roentgenol. 186*:1611–1617.

Peeters, C.F., de Waal, R.M., Wobbes, T., Westphal, J.R., and Ruers, T.J. 2006. Outgrowth of human liver metastases after resection of the primary colorectal tumor: a shift in the balance between apoptosis and proliferation. *Int. J. Cancer 119*:1249–1253.

Peeters, C.F., de Geus, L.F., Westphal, J.R., de Waal, R.M., Ruiter, DJ., Wobbes, T., Oyen, W.J., and Ruers, T.J. 2005. Decrease in circulating anti-angiogenic factors (angiostatin and endostatin) after surgical removal of primary colorectal carcinoma coincides with increased metabolic activity of liver metastases. *Surgery 137*:246–249.

Quon, A., Napel, S., Beaulieu, C.F., and Gambhir, S.S. 2006. "Flying through" and "flying around" a PET/CT scan: pilot study and development of 3D integrated 18F-FDG PET/CT for virtual bronchoscopy and colonoscopy. *J. Nucl. Med. 47*:1081–1087.

Rohren, E.M., Turkington, T.G., and Coleman, R.E. 2004. Clinical applications of PET in oncology. *Radiology 231*:305–332.

Schoder, H., Yeung, H.W., and Larson, S.M. 2005. CT in PET/CT: essential features of interpretation. *J. Nucl. Med. 46*:1249–1251.

Schofield, J.B., Mounter, N.A., Mallett, R., and Haboubi, N.Y. 2006. The importance of accurate pathological assessment of lymph node involvement in colorectal cancer. *Colorectal Dis. 8*:460–470.

Seemann, M.D., Schaefer, J.F., and Englmeier, K.H. 2007. Virtual positron emission tomography/computed tomography-bronchoscopy: possibilities, advantages and limitations of clinical application. *Eur. Radiol. 17*:709–715.

Silva, A.C., Vens, E.A., Hara, A.K., Fletcher, J.G., Fidler, J.L., and Johnson, C.D. 2006. Evaluation of benign and malignant rectal lesions with CT colonography and endoscopic correlation. *Radiographics 26*:1085–1099.

Stevenson, G.W. 2000. Colorectal cancer imaging: a challenge for radiologists. *Radiology 214*:615–621.

Valk, P.E., Abella-Columna, E., Haseman, M.K., Pounds, T.R., Myers, R.W., and Hofer, G.R. 1999. Whole-body PET imaging with [18F] fluorodeoxyglucose in management of recurrent colorectal cancer. *Arch. Surg. 134*:503–511.

Veit, P., Kuhle, C., Beyer, T., Kuehl, H., Herborn, C.U., Boersch, G., Stergar, C.H., Barkhausen, J., Bockisch, A., and Antoch, G. 2006a. Whole body positron emission tomography/computed tomography (PET/CT) tumour staging with integrated PET/CT colonography: technical feasibility and first experiences in patients with colorectal cancer. *Gut 55*:68–73.

Veit, P., Ruehm, S., Kuehl, H., Bockisch, A., and Antoch, G. 2006b. Lymphnode staging with dual modality PET/CT: enhancing the diagnostic accuracy in oncology. *Euro. J. Radiol. 58*:383.

Yasuda, S., Fujii, H., Nakahara, T., Nishuimi, N,. Takahashi, W., Ide, M., and Shohtsu, A. 2001. 18F-FDG PET detection of colonic adenomas. *J. Nucl. Med. 42*:989–992.

Yee, J., Kumar, N.N., Hung, R.K., Akerkar, G.A., Kumar, P.R.G., and Wall, S.D. 2003. Comparison of supine and prone scanning separately and in combination at CT colonography. *Radiology 226*:653–661.

12

Thoracic Esophageal Cancer: Interstitial Magnetic Lymphography Using Superparamagnetic Iron Oxide

Koichi Ishiyama, Satoru Motoyama, Noriaki Tomura, Ryuji Sashi, and Jun-ichi Ogawa

Introduction

Lymph node metastasis is a critical prognostic factor in patients with thoracic squamous cell esophageal cancer (Fujita *et al.*, 1995; Abo *et al.*, 1996; Motoyama *et al.*, 2006). In contrast to other gastrointestinal malignancies, thoracic squamous cell esophageal cancer shows no regularity with respect to the route or extent of lymphatic drainage, which often extends to the neck, mediastinum, and abdomen (Matsubara *et al.*, 1999, 2000). This is in large part due to the unique structure of the lymphatics around the thoracic esophagus (Murakami *et al.*, 2002). However, if the lymphatic drainage route from the tumor and the extent of the affected region could be detected before surgery in each patient, surgeons would be able to determine the appropriate minimal extent of lymphadenectomy for each patient, thereby improving the prognosis and quality of life after surgery. Unfortunately, it is too difficult to detect the lymphatic drainage route from thoracic squamous cell esophageal tumors, as is detection of lymph node micrometastasis. Furthermore, it is almost impossible to make a diagnosis based on conventional radiological examination such as computed tomography (CT) or magnetic resonance imaging

(MRI), because a majority of metastatic lymph nodes in patients with esophageal cancer shows metastases of < 10 mm in diameter. Conventional CT and MRI have a limited value due to their dependence on the native density, signal intensity, and/or size of the target (Nishimura *et al.*, 2006; Dooms and Hricak, 1986). It would, therefore, be highly desirable to develop a preoperative method to precisely map the route of lymphatic drainage from squamous cell esophageal tumors.

Two types of tracers, radioisotopes and isosulfan blue dyes, have been used previously to detect lymphatic drainage from a tumor in malignant melanoma, breast cancer, and gastric cancer (Morton *et al.*, 1992; Veronesi *et al.*, 1997; Saha *et al.*, 2000; Kitagawa and Kitajima, 2002; Arigami *et al.*, 2006). However, it is difficult to detect isosulfan blue dye in thoracic lymph nodes because of anthracosis, so this technique is useful only during surgery. Similarly, radioisotopes cannot determine an accurate lymphatic drainage route from a tumor due to the spatial resolution of scintigrams. As an alternative, we present preliminary results of interstitial MR lymphography using superparamagnetic iron oxide (SPIO), which we have performed in patients with thoracic esophageal cancer.

Method

The method of MR lymphography using SPIO is described below. We carried out endoscopic submucosal injection of ferumoxides (SPIO, Feridex; Eiken-Chemistory Co., Tokyo, Japan; diameters ranged from 70 to 140 nm; average ~ 100 nm) in patients with submucosal thoracic esophageal cancer before surgery. SPIO (2.0 ml) was injected into the submucosal layer of the peritumoral region (4 points). Immediately after injection, the patients were moved to the MR scanning room and scanned. The parameters for obtaining images were as follows, according to our phantom experiment (Ishiyama et al., 2006): fast gradient-recalled acquisition in the steady-state (FSPGR) (repetition time (TR)/echo time (TE)/flip angle: 180 msec/4.2 msec/90). Compared with the signal intensity of lymph nodes on FSPGR before injection or spin-echo T1-weighted (SET1W) images after injection, a focal low signal intensity on FSPGR images was considered to indicate influx of SPIO. We performed two studies: (1) the scan was repeated every 20 min to investigate the time course of signal intensity of lymph nodes, and (2) a wide-ranging scan (from the neck to the upper abdomen) was performed to map the lymphatic flow from the tumor.

In study 1, on MR lymphography, all cases showed influx of SPIO to the lymph nodes as decreased signal intensity at 20 min after injection. No more distal lymph nodes with influx of SPIO were observed after 40 min. In study 2, the wide-ranging MRI scan produced clear images of the lymphatic flow from the tumor, with two patients having identical patterns.

Every patient had a different pattern of lymph flow to the neck and/or abdomen. Only 1 of the 14 patients showed SPIO flow only in the neck lymph nodes, while 3 showed SPIO flow only in the abdominal lymph nodes. The other 10 patients showed SPIO flow in both the neck and abdominal lymph nodes. Some metastatic lymph nodes had influx of SPIO and some did not. The signal-to-noise ratio (SNR) of lymph nodes with influx of SPIO was significantly lower on postcontrast FSPGR images than on precontrast FSPGR images or postcontrast SET1W images. Lymph nodes with influx of SPIO appeared significantly larger on postcontrast FSPGR images than on postcontrast SET1W images. A comparison of FSPGR images with postcontrast SET1W images allowed easy identification of the influx of SPIO without precontrast images.

The following procedures and tips produced the most effective results. A gradient-echo (GRE) sequence is recommended to visualize lymph nodes with decreased signal intensity. In the present study, an FSPGR sequence (TR/TE/FA = 180 msec/4.2 msec/90°) was used. Our phantom study showed 4.2 msec of TE was the most appropriate. We also found that both GRE and SET1W images should be obtained as GRE alone makes it difficult to evaluate the signal intensity of the lymph nodes due to the small amount of SPIO influx. On FSPGR images, the lymph nodes with influx of SPIO had a lower signal intensity and larger diameter than on SET1W images. It is useful to compare GRE images with SER1W images because susceptibility artifacts are much more prominent in GRE sequences than in SE sequences. Scanning of both sequences after injection of SPIO can eliminate the need for a precontrast scan (Figs. 1 and 2).

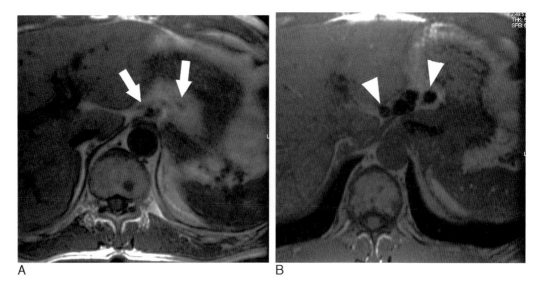

A   B

Figure 1 A 60-year-old man with lower thoracic esophageal cancer. (A) Spin-echo T1-weighted (SET1W) image of the upper abdominal level. Repetition time (TR)/echo time (TE) = 500/8 msec. Arrows show lymph nodes along the left gastric artery and the lesser curvature. (B) Fast spoiled gradient-recalled acquisition in the steady-state (FSPGR) image of the same level. TR/TE/flip anglet = 180 msec/4.2 msec/90°. Arrowheads show lymph nodes along the left gastric artery and the lesser curvature with decreased signal intensity and larger diameter than SET1W, representing influx of SPIO into the lymph nodes.

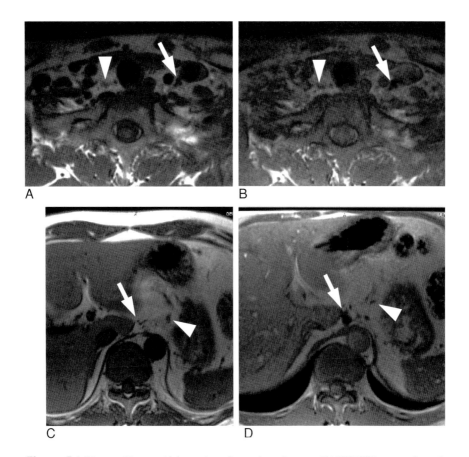

Figure 2 A 53-year-old man with lower thoracic esophageal cancer. (**A**) SET1W image at the neck level (TR/TE = 460/8 msec). Arrowhead shows right cervical paraesophageal lymph node. Arrow shows left supraclavicular lymph node. (**B**) FSPGR image of the same level (TR/TE/flip angle = 180 msec/4.2, msec/90°). Arrowhead shows right cervical paraesophageal lymph node without influx of SPIO into the lymph node. Arrow shows left supraclavicular lymph node with decreased signal intensity indicating influx of SPIO. (**C**) SET1W image of the upper abdomen. Arrow shows a lymph node along the left gastric artery. Arrowhead shows a lymph node along the lesser curvature of the stomach. (**D**) FSPGR image of the same level. Arrow shows a lymph node along the left gastric artery with decreased signal intensity indicating influx of SPIO. Arrowhead shows a lymph node along the lesser curvature without influx of SPIO.

Discussion

The sentinel lymph node (SLN) concept was first advocated by Morton *et al.* (1992) in patients with melanoma. If the concept is correct, then when a metastasis is not found in an SLN, it almost certainly will not be present in more distal lymph nodes. Although the SLN concept has recently been applied to cancer of the gastrointestinal tract, its validity in thoracic esophageal cancer remains controversial (Kitagawa *et al.*, 2002, 2004; Arigami *et al.*, 2006; Hayashi *et al.*, 2003; Kato *et al.*, 2003). Isosulfan blue dye and radionuclide-labeled colloids have also been used for intraoperative lymphatic mapping in gastroesophageal cancers (Hayashi *et al.*, 2003). However, the rapid transit of blue dye through the lymph node chain limits its utility, as the blue lymphatic vessels are often not visualized clearly during surgery. In addition, it is difficult to identify the blue-stained nodes among the mediastinal nodes with anthracosis (Kitagawa *et al.*, 2002). Favorable results have been obtained using an endoscopic scintigraphic method with radionuclide-labeled colloids and intraoperative gamma counting to identify the sentinel lymph nodes in esophageal cancer (Kitagawa *et al.*, 2002; Kato *et al.*, 2003). Unfortunately, the spatial resolution of scintigraphs is not sufficient to enable precise identification of lymph nodes. Furthermore, it is very difficult or impossible to precisely localize small lymph nodes. In contrast, interstitial MR lymphography using SPIO can precisely localize affected lymph nodes in high-resolution images (Motoyama *et al.*, 2007).

Recently, MRI using intravenous administration of ferumox-tran-10 has been useful in the identification of metastatic lymph nodes (Nishimura *et al.*, 2006). Ferumoxtran-10 particles are smaller than ferumoxide particles, enabling them to infiltrate lymph nodes after intravenous injection. However, the purpose of MRI with intravenous administration of ferumoxtran-10 is different from that of interstitial MR lymphography. Interstitial MR lymphography can provide a map of the lymphatic drainage route from the tumor to lymph nodes. Lymph nodes involving cancer cells, with micrometastases, can thereby be identified and excised.

With interstitial MR lymphography using SPIO, it is often difficult to confirm whether a lymph node is metastatic. This marker often does not flow into metastatic nodes filled with tumor cells, because (1) the lymph node is not on the lymphatic pathway from the tumor or (2) because of the high density of tumor cells. Hence, the purpose of MR lymphography is not to confirm whether the lymph node contains a metastasis but to confirm the direction and area of lymphatic flow from the tumor. Interstitial MR lymphography can determine the direction and area of the lymphatic flux, which can carry micrometastases from the tumor, allowing the surgeons to determine the precise lymphatic route from the tumor before surgery. This, in turn, might allow the performance of minimally invasive or personalized lymphadenectomies. Patients without apparent swelling of lymph nodes are good candidates for interstitial MR lymphography. However, further studies are required to compare MR lymphography with surgical findings or specimens.

There is increasing evidence of the efficacy of chemoradiation therapy in the treatment of primary squamous cell esophageal cancer (Hironaka *et al.*, 2003; Law *et al.*, 2003). The aim of radiation therapy is usually to irradiate both the tumor bed and any metastatic lymph nodes. Therefore, lymphatic mapping using interstitial MR lymphography might also be useful for determining the extent of the radiation field required.

Interstitial MR lymphography can be performed with several types of contrast media (Misselwitz, 2006), including SPIO (Vassallo *et al.*, 1994; Weissleder *et al.*, 1989; Bengele *et al.*, 1994), extracellular contrast agents (Suga *et al.*, 2003; Ruehm *et al.*, 2001; Fink *et al.*, 2002), extracellular contrast agents encapsulated in liposomes (Misselwitz and Sachse, 1997; Trubetskoy *et al.*, 1995), polymeric compounds (Harika *et al.*, 1995; Misselwitz *et al.*, 2002; Herborn *et al.*, 2003; Kobayashi *et al.*, 2003, 2004; Staatz *et al.*, 2002; Torchia and Misselwitz, 2002; Desser *et al.*, 1999), and lipophilic compounds that form aggregates or micelles (Misselwitz *et al.*, 1999; Staatz *et al.*, 2001). To our knowledge, no previous study of interstitial MR lymphography using other than SPIO has been performed in patients with esophageal cancer, and further studies are required. Contrast media with large particles such as SPIO (mean diameter = 100 nm) are expected to stay within lymph nodes for longer periods than other contrast media, which can be advan-tageous for imaging. This long stay in lymph nodes is one of the merits of SPIO. The development of a detector for a small amount of iron might make it possible to identify lymph nodes with SPIO during surgery.

This case had lymphatic flow in the left neck region. Micrometastasis was considered a possibility in that region. Lymphadenectomy found no metastases.

References

Abo, S., Kitamura, M., Hashimoto, M., Izumi, K., Minamiya, Y., Shikama, T., Suzuki, H., Temma, K., Kamata, S., and Saito, R. 1996. Analysis of results of surgery performed over a 20-year period on 500 patients with cancer of the thoracic esophagus. *Surg. Today* 26:77–82.

Arigami, T., Natsugoe, S., Uenosono, Y., Mataki, Y., Ehi, K., Higashi, H., Arima, H., Yanagida, S., Ishigami, S., Hokita, S., and Aikou, T. 2006. Evaluation of sentinel node concept in gastric cancer based on lymph node micrometastasis determined by reverse transcription-polymerase chain reaction. *Ann. Surg.* 243:341–347.

Bengele, H.H., Palmacci, S., Rogers, J., Jung, C.W., Crenshaw, J., and Josephson, L. 1994. Biodistribution of an ultrasmall superparamagnetic iron oxide colloid, BMS 180549, by different routes of administration. *Magn. Reson. Imaging* 12:433–442.

Desser, T.S., Rubin, D.L., Muller, H., McIntire, G.L., Bacon, E.R., and Hollister, K.R. 1999. Interstitial MR and CT lymphography with Gd-dTPA-co-alpha, omega-diaminoPEG(1450) and Gd-dTPA-co-1,6-diaminohexane polymers: preliminary experience. *Acad. Radiol.* 6:112–118.

Dooms, G.C., and Hricak, H. 1986. Magnetic resonance imaging of the pelvis: prostate and urinary bladder. *Urol. Radiol.* 8:156–165.

Fink, C., Bock, M., Kiessling, F., and Delorme, S. 2002. Interstitial magnetic resonance lymphography with gadobutrol in rats: evaluation of contrast kinetics. *Invest. Radiol.* 37:655–662.

Fujita, H., Kakegawa, T., Yamana, H., Shima, I., Toh, Y., Tomita, Y., Fujii, T., Yamasaki, K., Higaki, K., Noake, T., Ishibashi, N., and Mizutani, K. 1995. Mortality and morbidity rates, postoperative course, quality of life, and prognosis after extended radical lymphadenectomy for esophageal cancer. Comparison of three-field lymphadenectomy with two-field lymphadenectomy. *Ann. Surg.* 222:654–662.

Harika, L., Weissleder, R., Poss, K., Zimmer, C., Papisov, M.I., and Brady, T.J. 1995. MR lymphography with a lymphotropic T1-type MR contrast agent: Gd-DTPA-PGM. *Magn. Reson. Med.* 33:88–92.

Hayashi, H., Ochiai, T., Mori, M., Karube, T., Suzuki, T., Gunji, Y., Hori, S., Akutsu, N., Matsubara, H., and Shimada, H. 2003. Sentinel lymph node mapping for gastric cancer using a dual procedure with dye- and gamma probe-guided techniques. *J. Am. Coll. Surg.* 196:68–74.

Herborn, C.U., Vogt, F.M., Lauenstein, T.C., Goyen, M., Dirsch, O., Corot, C., Debatin, J.F., and Ruehm, S.G. 2003. Assessment of normal, inflammatory, and tumor-bearing lymph nodes with contrast-enhanced interstitial magnetic resonance lymphography: preliminary results in rabbits. *J. Magn. Reson. Imaging* 18:328–335.

Hironaka, S., Ohtsu, A., Boku, N., Muto, M., Nagashima, F., Saito, H., Yoshida, S., Nishimura, M., Haruno, M., Ishikura, S., Ogino, T., Yamamoto, S., and Ochiai, A. 2003. Nonrandomized comparison between definitive chemoradiotherapy and radical surgery in patients with T(2–3)N(any) M(0) squamous cell carcinoma of the esophagus. *Int. J. Radiat. Oncol. Biol. Phys.* 57:425–433.

Ishiyama, K., Motoyama, S., Tomura, N., Sashi, R., Imano, H., Ogawa, J., Narita, K., and Watarai, J. 2006. Visualization of lymphatic basin from the tumor using magnetic resonance lymphography with superparamagnetic iron oxide in patients with thoracic esophageal cancer. *J. Comput. Assist. Tomogr.* 30:270–275.

Kato, H., Miyazaki, T., Nakajima, M., Takita, J., Sohda, M., Fukai, Y., Masuda, N., Fukuchi, M., Manda, R., Ojima, H., Tsukada, K., Asao, T., Kuwano, H., Oriuchi, N., and Endo, K. 2003. Sentinel lymph nodes with Technetium-99 m colloidal rhenium sulfide in patients with esophageal carcinoma. *Cancer 98*:932–939.

Kitagawa, Y., and Kitajima, M. 2002. Gastrointestinal cancer and sentinel node navigation surgery. *J. Surg. Oncol. 79*:120–124.

Kitagawa, Y., Fujii, H., Mukai, M., Kubota, T., Ando, N., Ozawa, S., Ohtani, Y., Furukawa, T., Yoshida, M., Nakamura, E., Matsuda, J., Shimizu, Y., Nakamura, K., Kumai, K., Kubo, A., and Kitajima, M. 2002. Intraoperative lymphatic mapping and sentinel lymph node sampling in esophageal and gastric cancer. *Surg. Oncol. Clin. N. Am. 11*:293–304.

Kobayashi, H., Kawamoto, S., Star, R.A., Waldmann, T.A., Tagaya, Y., and Brechbiel, M.W. 2003. Micro-magnetic resonance lymphangiography in mice using a novel dendrimer-based magnetic resonance imaging contrast agent. *Cancer Res. 63*:271–276.

Kobayashi, H., Kawamoto, S., Sakai, Y., Choyke, P.L., Star, R.A., Brechbiel, M.W., Sato, N., Tagaya, Y., Morris, J.C., and Waldmann, T.A. 2004. Lymphatic drainage imaging of breast cancer in mice by micro-magnetic resonance lymphangiography using a nano-size paramagnetic contrast agent. *J. Natl. Cancer Inst. 96*:703–708.

Law, S., Kwong, D.L., Kwok, K.F., Wong, K.H., Chu, K.M., Sham, J.S., and Wong, J. 2003. Improvement in treatment results and long-term survival of patients with esophageal cancer: impact of chemoradiation and change in treatment strategy. *Ann. Surg. 238*:339–347.

Matsubara, T., Ueda, M., Kaisaki, S., Kuroda, J., Uchida, C., Kokudo, N., Takahashi, T., Nakajima, T., and Yanagisawa, A. 2000. Localization of initial lymph node metastasis from carcinoma of the thoracic esophagus. *Cancer 89*:1869–1873.

Matsubara, T., Ueda, M., Abe, T., Akimori, T., Kokudo, N., and Takahashi, T. 1999. Unique distribution patterns of metastatic lymph nodes in patients with superficial carcinoma of the thoracic oesophagus. *Br. J. Surg. 86*:669–673.

Misselwitz, B., and Sachse, A. 1997. Interstitial MR lymphography using Gd-carrying liposomes. *Acta Radiol. 38*:51–55.

Misselwitz, B., Platzek, J., Raduchel, B., Oellinger, J.J., and Weinmann, H.J. 1999. Gadofluorine 8: initial experience with a new contrast medium for interstitial MR lymphography. *MAGMA 8*:190–195.

Misselwitz, B., Schmitt-Willich, H., Michaelis, M., and Oellinger, J.J. 2002. Interstitial magnetic resonance lymphography using a polymeric T1 contrast agent: initial experience with Gadomer-17. *Invest. Radiol. 37*:146–151.

Misselwitz, B. 2006. MR contrast agents in lymph node imaging. *Eur. J. Radiol. 58*:375–382.

Morton, D.L., Wen, D.R., Wong, J.H., Economou, J.S., Cagle, L.A., Storm, F.K., Foshag, L.J., and Cochran, A.J. 1992. Technical details of intraoperative lymphatic mapping for early stage melanoma. *Arch. Surg. 127*:392–399.

Motoyama, S., Kitamura, M., Saito, R., Maruyama, K., Okuyama, M., and Ogawa, J. 2006. Outcome and treatment strategy for mid- and lower-thoracic esophageal cancer recurring locally in the lymph nodes of the neck. *World J. Surg. 30*:191–198.

Motoyama, S., Ishiyama, K., Maruyama, K., Okuyama, M., Sato, Y., Hayashi, K., Nanjo, H., Saito, H., Minayima, Y., and Ogawa, J. 2007. Preoperative mapping of lymphatic drainage from the tumor using ferumoxide-enhanced magnetic resonance imaging in clinical cubmucosal thoracic squamous cell esophageal cancer. *Surgery 141*:736–737.

Murakami, G., Abe, M., and Abe, T. 2002. Last-intercalated node and direct lymphatic drainage into the thoracic duct from the thoracoabdominal viscera. *Jpn. J. Thorac. Cardiovasc. Surg. 50*:93–103.

Nishimura, H., Tanigawa, N., Hiramatsu, M., Tatsumi, Y., Matsuki, M., and Narabayashi, I. 2006. Preoperative esophageal cancer staging: magnetic resonance imaging of lymph node with ferumoxtran-10, an ultrasmall superparamagnetic iron oxide. *J. Am. Coll. Surg. 202*:604–611.

Ruehm, S.G., Schroeder, T., and Debatin, J.F. 2001a. Interstitial MR lymphography with gadoterate meglumine: initial experience in humans. *Radiology 220*:816–821.

Ruehm, S.G., Corot, C., and Debatin, J.F. 2001b. Interstitial MR lymphography with a conventional extracellular gadolinium-based agent: assessment in rabbits. *Radiology 218*:664–669.

Saha, S., Wiese, D., Badin, J., Beutler, T., Nora, D., Ganatra, B.K., Desai, D., Kaushal, S., Nagaraju, M., Arora, M., and Singh, T. 2000. Technical details of sentinel lymph node mapping in colorectal cancer and its impact on staging. *Ann. Surg. Oncol. 7*:120–124.

Staatz, G., Nolte-Ernsting, C.C., Adam, G.B., Grosskortenhaus, S., Misselwitz, B., Bucker, A., and Gunther, R.W. 2001. Interstitial T1-weighted MR lymphography: lipophilic perfluorinated gadolinium chelates in pigs. *Radiology 220*:129–134.

Staatz, G., Spuntrup, E., Buecker, A., Misselwitz, B., and Gunther, R.W. 2002. T1-weighted MR-lymphography after intramammary administration of Gadomer-17 in pigs. *Rofo. 174*:29–32.

Suga, K., Yuan, Y., Ogasawara, N., Okada, M., and Matsunaga, N. 2003. Localization of breast sentinel lymph nodes by MR lymphography with a conventional gadolinium contrast agent. Preliminary observations in dogs and humans. *Acta Radiol. 44*:35–42.

Torchia, M.G., and Misselwitz, B. 2002. Combined MR lymphangiography and MR imaging-guided needle localization of sentinel lymph nodes using Gadomer-17. *AJR. Am. J. Roentgenol. 179*:1561–1565.

Trubetskoy, V.S., Cannillo, J.A., Milshtein, A., Wolf, G.L., and Torchilin, V.P. 1995. Controlled delivery of Gd-containing liposomes to lymph nodes: surface modification may enhance MRI contrast properties. *Magn. Reson. Imaging. 13*:31–37.

Vassallo, P., Matei, C., Heston, W.D., McLachlan, S.J., Koutcher, J.A., and Castellino, R.A. 1994. AMI-227-enhanced MR lymphography: usefulness for differentiating reactive from tumor-bearing lymph nodes. *Radiology 193*:501–506.

Veronesi, U., Paganelli, G., Galimberti, V., Viale, G., Zurrida, S., Bedoni, M., Costa, A., de Cicco, C., Geraghty, J.G., Luini, A., Sacchini, V., and Veronesi, P. 1997. Sentinel-node biopsy to avoid axillary dissection in breast cancer with clinically negative lymph-nodes. *Lancet 349*:1864–1867.

Weissleder, R., Elizondo, G., Josephson, L., Compton, C.C., Fretz, C.J., Stark, D.D., and Ferrucci, J.T. 1989. Experimental lymph node metastases: enhanced detection with MR lymphography. *Radiology 171*:835–839.

13

Esophageal Cancer: Comparison of ^{18}F-Fluoro-3-Deoxy-3-L-Fluorothymidine–Positron Emission Tomography with ^{18}F-Fluorodeoxyglucose–Positron Emission Tomography

H.L. van Westreenen, D.C.P. Cobben, L.B. Been, P.L. Jager,
P.H. Elsinga, and J.Th.M. Plukker

Introduction

Most patients with esophageal cancer are treated in specialized institutes and staged by endoscopic ultrasonography (EUS), computed tomography (CT) of the chest and abdomen, and ultrasound examination (US) of the cervical region. However, these traditional methods for staging esophageal cancer have limited sensitivity and specificity. The presence of distant metastases prior to surgery, which is not detected by conventional imaging techniques, is relatively high, as indicated by detection of metastases during operation in ~ 25% of the patients (Clements *et al.*, 2004).

Positron emission tomography (PET) using ^{18}F-fluorodeoxyglucose (FDG) is a noninvasive metabolic imaging technique, and its usefulness has been established for a number of malignancies. This is the most widely used tracer for staging tumors with PET. It is a glucose analog that enters the cells via the same membrane transporters as glucose. Glucose as well as ^{18}F-FDG are phosphorylated by the enzyme hexokinase. In contrast to glucose-6-phosphate, ^{18}F-FDG-6-phosphate is not a substrate for further metabolism in the glycolytic pathway. Therefore, ^{18}F-FDG-6-phosphate is trapped in the cells in proportion to their glycolytic activity (Phay *et al.*, 2000).

There is evidence for improved preoperative staging of esophageal cancer with ^{18}F-FDG-PET; sensitivities of 67–74% have been reported, especially with regard to the detection of nonregional lymphatic or hematogenic (van Westreenen *et al.*, 2004). Although these results may indicate an important role for ^{18}F-FDG-PET, ^{18}F-FDG is not a tumor-specific tracer and false-positive results may occur. For example, macrophages and neutrophils can demonstrate increased FDG uptake, which can lead to false-positiveresults (Strauss et al., 1996).

^{18}F-Fluoro-3′deoxy-3′-L-fluorothymidine(^{18}F-FLT), introduced as a PET proliferation tracer by Shields et al. (1998), might not have these drawbacks. ^{18}F-FLT is monophosphorylated by thymidine kinase 1 (TK1), which leads to intracellular trapping. Because the TK1 concentration is especially increased during the S phase of the cell cycle, the uptake of ^{18}F-FLT is supposed to depend on proliferation (Been et al., 2004). We investigated the feasibility of ^{18}F-FLT-PET for the detection and staging of esophageal cancer compared with ^{18}F-FDG-PET. Furthermore, the correlation between uptake of ^{18}F-FLT or ^{18}F-FDG and proliferation of the tumor was investigated.

Materials and Methods

Patients

Our prospective study consisted of ten patients with biopsy-proven malignancy of the esophagus or gastroesophageal junction. All patients were staged with multidetector CT (Somatom Sensation Siemens, Medical Systems, Erlangen, Germany) of the chest and abdomen, EUS (GF-UM20, 7.5–12 MHz, Olympus, Tokyo, Japan) and ultrasound (US) of the cervical region. Patients were included from November 2003 until February 2004. All patients gave written informed consent. Only patients with liver and kidney functions and hematological parameters (hemoglobin, hematocrit, erythrocytes, thrombocytes, leukocytes, and white cell count) within normal limits were included because of the toxicity of FLT in high concentrations. The medical ethics committee of the University Medical Center Groningen approved the study protocol.

^{18}F-FDG and ^{18}F-FLT Synthesis

^{18}F-FDG was produced according to the method described by Hamacher et al. (1986) using the coincidence ^{18}F-FDG synthesis module. Synthesis of ^{18}F-FLT was performed according to the method of Machulla et al. (2000). ^{18}F-FLT was produced by ^{18}F-fluorination of the 4,4′-dimethoxytrityl-protected anhydrothymidine, followed by a deprotection step. After purification by reversed phase high-performance liquid chromatography, the product was made isotonic and passed through a 0.22-μm filter. ^{18}F-FLT was produced with a radiochemical purity of > 95% and specific activity of > 10 TBq/mmol. The radiochemical yield was 6.7% ± 3.7% (decay corrected).

Positron Emission Tomography

The studies were performed using an ECAT EXACT HR+ (Siemens/CTI, Knoxville, TN, USA). Before PET imaging, patients were instructed to fast for at least 6 hr to keep both study protocols comparable. Patients were also instructed to drink 500 ml of water before imaging to stimulate ^{18}F-FDG and ^{18}F-FLT excretion from the renal calyces and stimulate subsequent voiding. Data acquisition started 90 and 60 min after injection of ^{18}F-FDG and ^{18}F-FLT, respectively. Scans were performed in whole-body mode for 5 min per bed position from femur to the crown. Transmission imaging was obtained for 3 min per bed position for attenuation correction. Images were reconstructed using an iterative reconstruction technique and were read from computer monitors.

Pathologic Evaluation

Tissue was fixed in 4% buffered formalin, routinely processed, and embedded in paraffin. Subsequently, 4-μm sections were cut. For morphology, slides were routinely stained with hematoxylin and eosin. Proliferating cells were detected using the monoclonal antibody MIB-1, which recognizes an epitope of the Ki-67 nuclear antigen that is present during DNA synthesis. For this immunohistochemistry, slides were pretreated for 30 min in Tris buffer (pH 9.5) at 98°C. Staining was performed using the automated immunohistochemistry slide-staining system NexES (Ventana Medical Systems Inc., Illkirch, France). As a first step, the monoclonal antibody MIB-1 (DakoCytomation BV, Heverlee, the Netherlands) detecting the cell proliferation marker Ki-67 was applied. As the second step, a basic 3,3′-diaminobenzidine detection system was used (Ventana Medical Systems Inc., Illkirch, France). All reagents and equipment were used according to the instructions of the suppliers. The MIB-1 score was estimated by counting the percentage of MIB-1-positive cell nuclei per 1000 tumor cells in the region of the tumor with the greatest density of staining, which, in most instances, corresponds to areas with the highest mitotic activity. The pathologist was unaware of the results of the PET images.

Data Analysis

Patients were staged according to the Tumor Node Metastasis (TNM) staging system of the International Union Against Cancer on the basis of CT, EUS, and US. The gold standard for the presence or absence of metastases was either histopathologic examination or follow-up. If this information was not available, other staging modalities were used as reference. Both ^{18}F-FDG-PET and ^{18}F-FLT-PET scans were interpreted independently by experienced nuclear physicians who were unaware of clinical data and information from the other PET scan.

Three-dimensional regions of interest (ROIs) were placed semiautomatically using a dedicated software program over the primary tumor on multiple slices, using a threshold of 70% of the maximum pixel value within the tumor. The maximum standardized uptake value (SUV_{max}) and mean SUV (SUV_{mean}) were calculated according to the equation:

$$SUV = \frac{C_i}{A/M}$$

Where C_i is the activity concentration, A is the injected radioactivity, and M is the body mass. SUV_{max} denotes the maximum SUV value within the tumor ROI, and SUV_{mean} denotes the mean value averaged over all voxels.

Statistical Analysis

The results of the visually interpreted PET images were compared with the histological data or dedicated radiographic imaging, which were used as standard. ^{18}F-FDG and ^{18}F-FLT uptakes were compared using the Wilcoxon signed rank test. The amount of Ki-67-positive cells and SUVs for ^{18}F-FDG and ^{18}F-FLT were compared using linear regression analysis. Two-tailed P values < 0.05 were considered significant.

Results

Patients

Ten patients were included with a median age of 61 years (range, 48–75 years). Patients received ^{18}F-FDG with a median dose of 368 MBq (range, 250–750 MBq) and received ^{18}F-FLT with a median dose of 410 MBq (range, 340–450 MBq). Eight patients underwent esophagectomy, and two patients received an expendable metal stent because of an irresectable T4 tumor on preoperative staging and an irresectable tumor encountered during surgical exploration.

Detection of Esophageal Cancer

^{18}F-FDG-PET visualized all primary tumors, whereas ^{18}F-FLT visualized 8 of 10 esophageal cancers. In patients 4 and 10, no uptake of ^{18}F-FLT could be observed. Therefore, the SUV could not be calculated for ^{18}F-FLT in these 2 patients.

Staging of Esophageal Cancer with ^{18}F-FDG-PET and ^{18}F-FLT-PET

Pathology for assessment of lymph nodes was available in 9 patients. ^{18}F-FDG PET and ^{18}F-FLT-PET were comparable with regard to the detection of regional lymph nodes. Both ^{18}F-FDG-PET and ^{18}F-FLT-PET correctly detected regional lymph node metastases in only 2 out of 8 patients. ^{18}F-FDG-PET showed false-positive uptake in the celiac trunk region in one patient, whereas all other staging modalities, including ^{18}F-FLT-PET, did not show any abnormality. Pathologic examination revealed cellular reactivity in the celiac trunk lymph nodes in this patient, and the uptake on ^{18}F-FDG-PET was scored as a false-positive result. In another patient, ^{18}F-FDG-PET and CT showed a cervical lymph node metastasis. ^{18}F-FLT-PET did not detect this metastasis and was scored as a false-negative result.

Comparison between ^{18}F-FDG and ^{18}F-FLT Uptake

The median SUV_{max} and median SUV_{mean} for ^{18}F-FDG were 7.4 and 6.0 and for ^{18}F-FLT were 4.1 and 3.4. Uptake of ^{18}F-FDG was significantly higher than ^{18}F-FLT, whether expressed in SUV_{max} ($P = 0.012$) or SUV_{mean} ($P = 0.012$). Figure 1 shows ^{18}F-FDG-PET and ^{18}F-FLT-PET of a patient.

Correlation of ^{18}F-FDG and ^{18}F-FLT Uptake with MIB-1 Score

All tissue specimens contained immunoreactivity to Ki-67 antigen. Ki-67 positivity ranged from 57 to 85%, with a median of 73%. Linear regression analysis indicated no correlation between ^{18}F-FDG SUV and Ki-67 or between ^{18}F-FLT SUV and Ki-76 (^{18}F-FDG SUV_{max} vs. Ki-67, $r = 0.14$; ^{18}F-FLT

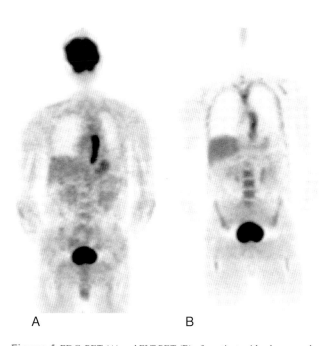

A   B

Figure 1 FDG-PET (**A**) and FLT-PET (**B**) of a patient with a long esophageal tumor.

SUV$_{max}$ vs. Ki-76, r = −0.76; ^{18}F-FDG SUV$_{mean}$ vs. Ki-67, r = 0.13; ^{18}F-FLT SUV$_{mean}$ vs. Ki-76, r = −0.74).

Additional Findings

In one patient, ^{18}F-FDG-PET showed uptake in the recto-sigmoid. However, ^{18}F-FLT-PET did not show any abnormality in that region. Additional investigation by sigmoidoscopy revealed diverticulitis. In another patient, a hypermetabolic lesion in the ascending colon was found on ^{18}F-FDG-PET and was proven to be a carcinoma by colonoscopy. However, ^{18}F-FLT-PET did not detect this synchronous neoplasm.

Discussion

This pilot study was conducted on 10 patients and showed that ^{18}F-FDG-PET could detect all esophageal cancers, whereas ^{18}F-FLT-PET visualized the tumor in 8 patients. Both ^{18}F-FDG-PET and ^{18}F-FLT-PET detected lymph node metastases in 2 out of 8 patients. The uptake of ^{18}F-FDG (median SUV$_{mean}$, 6.0; range, 3.6–11.5) in esophageal cancer was significantly higher than that of ^{18}F-FLT (median SUV$_{mean}$, 3.4; range, 2.3–4.3). Furthermore, neither ^{18}F-FDG nor ^{18}F-FLT uptake reflects proliferation as determined by Ki-67 immunostaining.

^{18}F-FDG-PET was able to detect all primary esophageal cancers, whereas ^{18}F-FLT-PET missed two of them. This fact may be related to the lower uptake of ^{18}F-FLT compared with ^{18}F-FDG, which has been reported earlier for several other tumors (Cobben *et al.*, 2004). The ^{18}F-FLT phosphorylation rate *in vitro* is known to be ~ 30% of the phosphorylation rate of serum thymidine by TK1, which could explain the low ^{18}F-FLT uptake in the tumor. Although plasma levels are low, thymidine may compete with ^{18}F-FLT for the active site of nucleoside carriers in cell membranes and also for the active site of the trapping enzyme TK1. Moreover, the affinity of human TK1 for thymidine has been reported to be four-fold higher than is the affinity for ^{18}F-FLT.

Both ^{18}F-FDG-PET and ^{18}F-FLT-PET had low sensitivity for the detection of regional lymph node metastases (2 of 8 patients). Several studies have reported the moderate sensitivity of ^{18}F-FDG-PET for detection of regional lymph node metastases, which ranges from 8 to 67%. ^{18}F-FLT-PET did not improve the regional staging of esophageal cancer. This can be explained by low-tissue uptake of ^{18}F-FLT or by the detection limit of PET for small tumor deposits.

A strong correlation between ^{18}F-FLT uptake and proliferation expressed as Ki-67-positive cells was found for lung cancer and sarcoma. However, we did not find a correlation between ^{18}F-FLT uptake and Ki-67 or between ^{18}F-FDG uptake and Ki-67. A correlation between ^{18}F-FLT

uptake and proliferation was not reported for breast cancer or thoracic tumors. The rationale of ^{18}F-FLT uptake in malignant tissue is based on TK1 dependence of proliferation. However, tumors vary in the relative contribution of *de novo* and salvage nucleotide biosynthesis. Dominance of *de novo* pathways, though uncommon, would mask proliferation-dependent increases in TK1 activity. Furthermore, in cells for which proliferation is less dependent on TK1, the correlation between tracer uptake and TK1 activity was poor. We did not obtain full kinetic parameters of ^{18}F-FLT, which might explain why a correlation between ^{18}F-FLT and proliferation was not found. For example, the correlation between the rate of phosphorylation of ^{18}F-FLT and SUV should be investigated to assess proliferation. In addition, Ki-67 is not a perfect measure of DNA synthesis because it measures the number of cells only in a proliferating state. Moreover, Ki-67 was assessed in a proliferating part of the tumor and was compared with the SUV value of a tumor volume. This comparison might be flawed.

Its small sample size and the absence of evaluation after therapy limit drawing solid conclusions from our study. ^{18}F-FDG-PET is able to identify nonresponders early during neoadjuvant chemoradiotherapy for esophageal cancer (Westerterp *et al.*, 2005). Therefore, it will be worthwhile to investigate the ability of ^{18}F-FLT PET in identifying nonresponders to neoadjuvant treatment regimens. At present, ^{18}F-FDG is the tracer of choice for the staging of esophageal cancer. Despite the lower incidence of false-positive results with ^{18}F-FLT, false-negative results will increase by using ^{18}F-FLT, which is a major disadvantage for the staging of esophageal cancer.

References

Been, L.B., Suurmeijer, A.J., Cobben, D.C., Jager, P.L., Hoekstra, H.J., and Elsinga, P.H. 2004. [18F]FLT-PET in oncology: current status and opportunities. *Eur. J. Nucl. Med. Mol. Imaging* 31:1659–1672.

Clements, D.M., Bowrey, D.J., and Havard, T.J. 2004. The role of staging investigations for oesophago-gastric carcinoma. *Eur. J. Surg. Oncol. 30*: 309–312.

Cobben, D.C., van der Laan, B.F., Maas, B., Vaalburg, W., Suurmeijer, A.J., Hoekstra, H.J., Jager, P.L., and Elsinga, P.H. 2004. 18F-FLT PET for visualization of laryngeal cancer: comparison with 18F-FDG PET. *J. Nucl. Med. 45*:226–231.

Hamacher, K., Coenen, H.H., and Stocklin, G. 1986. 2-18[F]-fluoro-2-deoxy-D-glucose using aminopolyether supported nucleophilic substitution. *J. Nucl. Med. 27*:235–238.

Machulla, H.J., Blochter, A., Kuntzsch, M., Piert, M., Wei, R., and Grierson, J.R. 2000. Simplified labeling approach for synthesizing 3'deoxy-3'-18[F]fluorothymidine. *J. Radiochem. Nucl. Chem. 243*:843–846.

Phay, J.E., Hussain, H.B., and Moley, J.F. 2000. Strategy for identification of novel glucose transporter family members by using Internet-based genomic databases. *Surgery 128*:946–951.

Shields, A.F., Grierson, J.R., Dohmen, B.M., Machulla, H.J., Stayanoff, J.C., Lawhorn-Crews, J.M., Obradovich, J.E., Muzik, O., and Mangner, T.J. 1998. Imaging proliferation *in vivo* with [F-18]FLT and positron emission tomography. *Nat. Med. 4*:1334–1336.

Strauss, L.G. 1996. Fluorine-18 deoxyglucose and false-positive results: a major problem in the diagnostics of oncological patients. *Eur. J. Nucl. Med. 23*:1409–1415.

van Westreenen, H.L., Westerterp, M., Bossuyt, P.M., Pruim, J., Sloof, G.W., van Lanschot, J.J., Groen, H., and Plukker, J.T. 2004. Systematic review of the staging performance of 18F-fluorodeoxyglucose positron emission tomography in esophageal cancer. *J. Clin. Oncol. 22*:3805–3812.

Westerterp, M., van Westreenen, H.L., Reitsma, J.H., Hoekstra, O.S., Jager, P.L., Stoker, J., Fockens, P., van Eck-Smit, B.L., Plukker, J.T., van Lanschot, J.J., and Sloof, G.W. 2005. Esophageal cancer: CT, endoscopic US, and FDG PET for assessment of response to neoadjuvant therapy—systematic review. *Radiology 236*:841–851.

14

Gastrointestinal Stromal Tumors: Positron Emission Tomography and Contrast-Enhanced Helical Computed Tomography

Niklaus G. Schaefer and Gerhard W. Goerres

Introduction

Gastrointestinal stromal tumors (GISTs) are the most common mesenchymal neoplasias of the gastrointestinal (GI) tract. Mesenchymal tumors of the GI tract represent 1% of the primary GI tumors, but most of the mesenchymal tumors fall into the GIST category. Approximately 70% of the tumors have their origin in the stomach, and 20% originate from the small intestine but can also occur in other parts of the gastrointestinal tract and are occasionally found in the omentum, mesentery, and the peritoneum. GISTs have a wide clinical spectrum from benign incidentally found lesions to large tumors. The usual presenting symptoms are gastrointestinal bleeding, anemia, abdominal pain, dyspepsia, or abdominal mass. Malignant GISTs tend to recur and metastasize, most often in the liver and peritoneum. Other metastatic sites include the lungs, pleura, retroperitoneum, bone, and subcutaneous tissues. The incidence of GISTs is 6.9 cases per million in 2002 in the United States (Perez *et al.*, 2006). The peak of incidence is 60 years, and there is a slight male predominance (Kim *et al.*, 2001).

In the past, GISTs were analyzed by their morphological features and often misclassified as leiomyomas, leiomyosarcomas, or leiomyoblastomas. However, despite the histological variety in GISTs, ~ 80% of GISTs have KIT mutations that lead to constitutive activation of the c-kit receptor (Miettinen and Lasota, 2001; Hirota *et al.*, 1998). In normal cells, the tyrosine kinase activity of c-kit is regulated by the binding of its ligand (c-kit ligand, stem-cell factor). In the gastrointestinal stromal tumor, the mutation of c-kit activates tyrosine kinase in the absence of the ligand and leads to a uncontrolled target cell proliferation.

Imaging Techniques to Localize and Monitor Gastrointestinal Stromal Tumors

Conventional radiography has no role in the small asymptomatic GIST. However, it can incidentally distinguish cases of GIST because of a possible mass effect of large abdominal lesions. Contrast studies using barium usually show the features of submucosal masses of the gastrointestinal tract. However, its use is limited to exophytic masses of a distinct region and plays a minor role in GIST staging. Transabdominal sonography helps to characterize both primary and metastatic GIST. It usually appears as a homogeneously hypoechoic mass in close relation to the gastrointestinal tract. Endoscopic sonography (EUS) can accurately diagnose and differentiate between extramural lesions, extrinsic compression, vascular lesions, and solid tumor. EUS is most useful in the esophagus, stomach, and duodenum, as well as the anorectum. Sonography, both transabdominally and endoscopically, also serves as a reliable guide for real-time biopsy. Morphological imaging with contrast-enhanced computed tomography (ceCT) is widely used to localize GIST, as well as determining the size and possibly revealing the presence of secondary localizations (Buckley and Fishman, 1998). Furthermore, ceCT is routinely used to monitor tumor response in patients with GIST (Burkill et al., 2003). Magnetic resonance imaging (MRI) offers minor additional information compared to ceCT regarding the cancer staging of GIST patients. The appearance of GIST in MRI is variable. The solid parts of GIST are typically of low signal intensity on T1-weighted images, are of high signal intensity on T2-weighted images, and are enhanced after administration of gadolinium (Levy et al., 2003). Magnetic resonance imaging provides, due to its soft tissue contrast resolution and direct multiplanar imaging, help in tumor localization and delineation of the relationships with the adjacent organs.

Use of Imatinib in Treatment of Gastrointestinal Stromal Tumors

In the past, patients with advanced GISTs had a poor prognosis due to the chemoresistance and radioresistance of the tumor cells. Surgery of individual lesions was the only curative therapy. With the recent introduction of imatinib (STI 571, Glivec, Gleevec; Novartis Pharmaceuticals), the possibilities of medical treatment of these patients have much improved. Imatinib, a tyrosine kinase inhibitor, was found to inhibit BCR-ABL, KIT, and PDGFR (Tuveson et al., 2001). The competitive interaction at the adenosine triphosphate (ATP) binding site of the c-kit receptor by imatinib leads to the suppression of uncontrolled cell proliferation in GISTs. Initial clinical studies described clinical responses and long-lasting disease stabilization in the vast majority of patients with GISTs (Joensuu et al., 2001). However, for assessing tumor response, a validated sensitive method to early evaluate tumor response is needed. Early detection of treatment success ensures effective therapy. In patients not responding to imatinib medication, tumor progression or even stable disease may require an increase in dosage or alternative strategies.

The reliability of established anatomical imaging techniques, such as ceCT and MRI, is compromised following response to treatment because metabolic improvement occurs before morphological changes. It has previously been

shown that GISTs treated with imatinib may not change their size or may even grow larger during therapy (Chen et al., 2002). The assessment of tumors responding to treatment with imatinib may show a decrease in ceCT attenuation values (Hounsfield Units, HU), but a delay of several weeks to months can be observed between the functional changes at a cellular level that are induced by an effective treatment and the macroscopic structural changes in a tumor as measured by ceCT (van den Abbeele and Badawi, 2002).

^{18}F-Fluorodeoxyglucose Positron Emission Tomography

Positron emission tomography (PET) using 18F-fluorodeoxyglucose (FDG) has been used successfully for staging and follow-up examinations in cancer patients (Juweid and Cheson, 2006). This tomography using FDG provides physiologic information that enables cancer to be diagnosed on the basis of altered tissue metabolism. Various studies have proven that FDG-PET is more accurate in staging and re-staging FDG-avid cancer than ceCT examinations (Steinert et al., 1997; Stumpe et al., 1998). Initial studies have shown high FDG uptake of untreated GIST on PET imaging (van den Abbeele and Badawi, 2002). As highlighted later, FDG-PET does not depict all GIST lesions compared to ceCT scans. However, there is a significant correlation between the FDG uptake and the mitotic index of the GIST cells (Kamiyama et al., 2005). Regarding the prognostic relevance of the mitotic index in GIST (Fletcher et al., 2002), FDG-PET can provide a significant impact on the further outcome of GIST patients.

In initial studies, FDG-PET was shown to be superior to CT in detection of the early tumor response induced by imatinib therapy (Stroobants et al., 2003). The metabolic response was already detected after one week of therapy with imatinib using the standardized uptake value (SUV) (Heinicke et al., 2005). However, in patients with initial negative FDG-PET before treatment onset, but confirmed GIST, the use of a post-treatment FDG-PET seemed futile.

The role of FDG-PET was analyzed in a comparatively large prospective study of 34 consecutive patients with proven CD117 positive GIST (Goerres et al., 2005). This study confirmed that patients responding to imatinib, as measured by normalization of initially FDG-avid areas, have a better clinical outcome than patients in whom FDG uptake was still present in the first re-staging FDG-PET. These data suggest that a single post-treatment FDG-PET scan provides prognostic information on overall survival and the time to progression (Goerres et al., 2005). In this study, more tumor lesions (45%) were found on ceCT images than on PET images, indicating that FDG-PET alone is insufficient for identifying and characterizing GIST lesions. In small

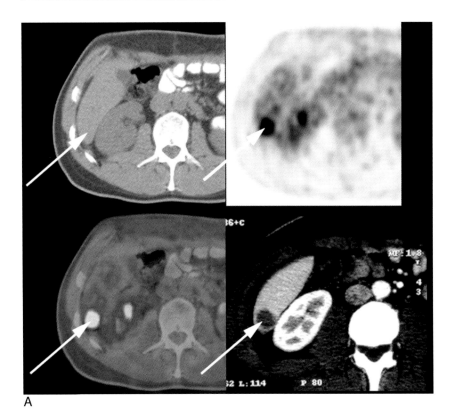

A

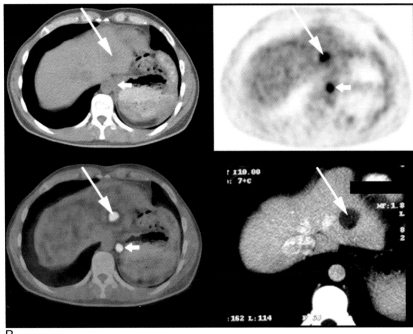

B

Figure 1 PET, CT, co-registered PET/CT and contrast-enhanced CT image of a 31-year-old male patient with a gastrointestinal stromal tumor. He underwent partial resection of the stomach and splenectomy of a large tumor, which was positive for CD 34 and CD 117. The tumor was considered to have a low-grade malignant potential based on the morphological appearance and proliferation. A PET/CT and contrast-enhanced CT routine control 2 months postoperatively revealed metastases in the liver showing avid uptake of FDG (large arrows; Fig. 1A and B). Furthermore, FDG uptake is seen in a lymph node adjacent to the gastric wall (small arrows; Fig. 1 B). The contrast-enhanced CT scan better delineates the FDG-avid lesions, which are hypodense and not clearly visible on the noncontrast-enhanced CT of PET/CT scans. The patient underwent additional surgery to remove the metastases in the left (segment II) and right liver lobe (segment VI), as well as the lymph node. In the follow-up, the patient was treated with imatinib starting with a dose of 400 mg and then increasing to 800 mg. Under this treatment, a further follow-up PET/CT scan three years later showed no areas of increased FDG uptake.

lesions, the FDG uptake was usually strong and homogeneous, but in large lesions the distribution of FDG was often heterogeneous showing areas with strong, intermediate, low, or even no uptake (corresponding to necrotic tissue). In 25 of 30 examinations of this study, at least one of the lesions was better delineated on PET/CT images than on PET and ceCT images read side by side (Goerres *et al.*, 2005). Therefore, image co-registration with PET/CT may improve delimitation of FDG-avid areas and guide surgical procedures. This is important in patients where new FDG-avid lesions arise during follow-up, which do not respond to imatinib treatment. For example, in a patient with a new single liver lesion, a precise anatomical delineation of the FDG-avid area is crucial to assess operability.

The identification of all lesions during staging and re-staging is important as surgery with complete resection is the only curative therapy, and the prognosis of a patient with GIST is excellent after complete resection (Emory *et al.*, 1998). Successful complete surgical resection is important for the control of local recurrence or concomitant and metastatic disease (DeMatteo *et al.*, 2000). Furthermore, it has recently been suggested that treatment with imatinib may improve the surgical outcome in patients with residual GIST (Hohenberger *et al.*, 2003).

Metabolic and Morphological Imaging

A combined method of metabolic and morphological imaging is available with the introduction of inline PET/CT scanners (Beyer *et al.*, 2000) as PET and CT data can be acquired at the same imaging session. Often, a noncontrast-enhanced low-dose CT is used for attenuation correction as well as image co-registration as shown in the example in Figure 1. However, the CT part of a PET/CT examination can be acquired using a regular protocol with intravenous and oral contrast application. This does not deteriorate the quality of the attenuation-corrected PET data.

PET/CT has been shown to be superior to PET, CT, or the combination of PET and CT in a range of different tumors (von Schulthess *et al.*, 2006). In a study by Antoch *et al.* (2004), PET/CT in patients with histologically proven GIST underwent 18F-FDG PET/CT imaging before and sequentially after the start of imatinib therapy. The evaluation of 20 patients showed 135 suspected GIST lesions in FDG-PET, 249 lesions with CT, 279 lesions in the side-by-side evaluation of CT and FDG-PET, and 282 lesions in the fused PET/CT images. After start of imatinib, tumor response was found on 95% of the PET/CT images after one month and 100% after three months. Positron emission tomography (PET) alone found tumor response in 85% at one month and 100% at three months after start of therapy. The CT scan was accurate in only 44% of the patients after one month, 60% at three months, and 57%

after six months (Antoch *et al.*, 2004). These data show that response of GISTs should be assessed with both functional and morphological imaging. In the above study, PET/CT in staging was slightly better than the side-by-side evaluation of FDG-PET and CT. However, the CT scan found more GIST lesions than FDG-PET. This shows that morphological imaging by CT is more important in GIST staging by evaluating a possible surgical intervention, whereas the FDG-PET imaging shows its impact on determining further management and clinical outcome after the start of imatinib (Stroobants *et al.*, 2003). This is an ideal model to underline the role of PET and the integrated PET/CT imaging for cancer staging and re-staging.

In conclusion, the combination of morphological and functional imaging, represented by CT and FDG-PET, either as inline PET/CT scanner or separated imaging modalities, is crucial for the staging and re-staging of GIST patients. Computed tomography (CT) finds more lesions than FDG-PET and is essential for planning surgical interventions. The role of FDG-PET lies clearly in its prognostic relevance, predicting the overall survival after start with imatinib. Patients not responding on the FDG-PET scan after the start of treatment have a worse prognosis, and alternative treatment or adaptation of dosage should be considered. PET/CT can help to better delineate FDG-avid lesions and thus improve assessment of operability (Table 1). This is especially important when planning a selective surgical intervention in the follow-up of a patient with otherwise stable disease under imatinib. In other words, FDG-PET is essential to assess early treatment response, and CT imaging is needed to plan surgical interventions (Table 1). These complementary methods are integrated in PET/CT, which was found to provide additional information compared with evaluation of separate PET and CT images.

Table 1 The Role of FDG-PET and PET/CT in Gastrointestinal Stromal Tumors (GISTs) Patients

Identify patients with FDG-avid GISTs, for cancer control.

Assess the prognosis, shortly after the initiation of treatment with imatinib in patients who had a pretreatment FDG-PET or FDG-PET/CT scan.

Confirm recurrent disease in patients with suspicious findings on routine CT images during follow-up, thus allowing adaptation of the dosage of imatinib.

Control, at an early point in time, the efficacy of dosage adaptation in patients in whom dosage of imatinib had been increased.

Control, at an early point in time, the efficacy of a lower dosage in patients in whom dosage of imatinib had been decreased.

Identify a lesion with increased FDG uptake in a patient with otherwise stable disease under imatinib for the planning of a selective surgical intervention.

Control the success of a surgical intervention.

References

Antoch, G., Kanja, J., Bauer, S., Kuehl, H., Renzing-Koehler, K., Schuette, J., Bockisch, A., Debatin, J.F., and Freudenberg, L.S. 2004. Comparison of PET, CT, and dual-modality PET/CT imaging for monitoring of imatinib (STI571) therapy in patients with gastrointestinal stromal tumors. *J. Nucl. Med. 45*:357–365.

Beyer, T., Townsend, D.W., Brun, T., Kinahan, P.E., Charron, M., Roddy, R., Jerin, J., Young, J., Byars, L., and Nutt, R. 2000. A combined PET/CT scanner for clinical oncology. *J. Nucl. Med. 41*:1369–1379.

Buckley, J.A., and Fishman, E.K., 1998. CT evaluation of small bowel neoplasms: spectrum of disease. *Radiographics 18*:379–392.

Burkill, G.J., Badran, M., Al-Muderis, O., Meirion, T.J., Judson, I.R., Fisher, C., and Moskovic, E. 2003. Malignant gastrointestinal stromal tumor: distribution, imaging features, and pattern of metastatic spread. *Radiology 226*:527–532.

Chen, M.Y., Bechtold, R.E., and Savage, P.D. 2002. Cystic changes in hepatic metastases from gastrointestinal stromal tumors (GISTs) treated with Gleevec (imatinib mesylate). *Am. J. Roentgenol. 179*:1059–1062.

DeMatteo, R.P., Lewis, J.J., Leung, D., Mudan, S.S., Woodruff, J.M., and Brennan, M.F. 2000. Two hundred gastrointestinal stromal tumors: recurrence patterns and prognostic factors for survival. *Ann. Surg. 231*:51–58.

Emory, T.S., and O'Leary, T.J. 1998. Prognosis and surveillance of gastrointestinal stromal/smooth muscle tumors. *Ann. Chir. Gynaecol. 87*:306–310.

Fletcher, C.D., Berman, J.J., Corless, C., Gorstein, F., Lasota, J., Longley, B.J., Miettinen, M., O'Leary T.J., Remotti, H., Rubin, B.P., Shmookler, B., Sobin, L.H., and Weiss, S.W. 2002. Diagnosis of gastrointestinal stromal tumors: a consensus approach. *Hum. Pathol. 33*:459–465.

Goerres, G.W., Stupp, R., Barghouth, G., Hany, T.F., Pestalozzi, B., Dizendorf, E., Schnyder, P., Luthi F., von Schulthess G.K., and Leyvraz, S. 2005. The value of PET, CT and in-line PET/CT in patients with gastrointestinal stromal tumors: long-term outcome of treatment with imatinib mesylate. *Eur. J. Nucl. Med. Mol. Imaging. 32*:153–162.

Heinicke, T., Wardelmann, E., Sauerbruch, T., Tschampa, H.J., Glasmacher, A., and Palmedo, H. 2005. Very early detection of response to imatinib mesylate therapy of gastrointestinal stromal tumors using 18fluoro-deoxyglucose-positron emission tomography. *Anticancer Res. 25*:4591–4594.

Hirota, S., Isozaki, K., Moriyama, Y., Hashimoto, K., Nishida, T., Ishiguro, S., Kawano, K., Hanada, M., Kurata, A.,Takeda, M., Muhammad, T.G., Matsuzawa, Y., Kanakura, Y., Shinomura, Y., and Kitamura, Y. 1998. Gain-of-function mutations of c-kit in human gastrointestinal stromal tumors. *Science 279*:577–580.

Hohenberger, P., Bauer, S., Schneider, U., Pink, D., Dirsch, O., Schuette, J., and Reichardt, P. 2003. Tumor resection following imatinib pretreatment in GI stromal tumors. *Proc. Am. Soc. Clin. Oncol. 22*: abstr. 3288.

Joensuu, H., Roberts, P.J., Sarlomo-Rikala, M., Andersson, L.C., Tervahartiala, P., Tuveson, D., Silberman, S., Capdeville, R., Dimitrijevic, S., Druker, B., and Demetri, G.D. 2001. Effect of the tyrosine kinase inhibitor STI571 in a patient with metastatic gastrointestinal stromal tumor. *N. Engl. J. Med. 344*:1052–1056.

Juweid, M.E., and Cheson, B.D. 2006. Positron-emission tomography and assessment of cancer therapy. *N. Engl. J. Med. 354*:496–507.

Kamiyama, Y., Aihara, R., Nakabayashi, T., Mochiki, E., Asao, T., and Kuwano, H. 2005. 18F-Fluorodeoxyglucose positron emission tomography: useful technique for predicting malignant potential of gastrointestinal stromal tumors. *World J. Surg. 29*:1429–1435.

Kim, C.J., Day, S., and Yeh, K.A. 2001. Gastrointestinal stromal tumors: analysis of clinical and pathologic factors. *Am. Surg. 67*:135–137.

Levy, A.D., Remotti, H.E., Thompson, W.M., Sobin, L.H., and Miettinen, M. 2003. Gastrointestinal stromal tumors: radiologic features with pathologic correlation. *RadioGraphics 23*:283–304.

Miettinen, M., and Lasota, J. 2001. Gastrointestinal stromal tumors definition, clinical, histological, immunohistochemical, and molecular genetic features and differential diagnosis. *Virchows Arch. 438*:1–12.

Perez, E.A., Livingstone, A.S., Franceschi, D., Rocha-Lima, C., Lee, D.J., Hodgson, N., Jorda, M., and Koniaris, L.G. 2006. Current incidence and outcomes of gastrointestinal mesenchymal tumors including gastrointestinal stromal tumors. *J. Am. Coll. Surg. 202*:623–629.

Steinert, H.C., Hauser, M., Allemann, F., Engel, H., Berthold, T., von Schulthess, G.K., and Weder, W. 1997. Non-small cell lung cancer: nodal staging with FDG PET versus CT with correlative lymph node mapping and sampling. *Radiology 202*:441–446.

Stroobants, S., Goeminne, J., Seegers, M., Dimitrijevic, S., Dupont, P., Nuyts, J., Martens, M., van den Borne, B., Cole, P., Sciot, R., Dumez, H., Silberman, S., Mortelmans, L., and van Oosterom, A. 2003. 18FDG-positron emission tomography for the early prediction of response in advanced soft tissue sarcoma treated with imatinib mesylate (Glivec). *Eur. J. Cancer 39*:2012–2020.

Stumpe, K.D., Urbinelli, M., Steinert, H.C., Glanzmann, C., Buck, A., and von Schulthess, G.K. 1998. Whole-body positron emission tomography using fluorodeoxyglucose for staging of lymphoma: effectiveness and comparison with computed tomography. *Eur. J. Nucl. Med. 25*:721–728.

Tuveson, D.A., Willis, N.A., Jacks, T., Griffin, J.D., Singer, S., Fletcher, C.D., Fletcher, J.A., and Demetri, G.D. 2001. STI571 inactivation of the gastrointestinal stromal tumor c-KIT oncoprotein: biological and clinical implications. *Oncogene 20*:5054–5058.

Van den Abbeele, A.D., and Badawi, R.D. 2002. Use of positron emission tomography in oncology and its potential role to assess response to imatinib mesylate therapy in gastrointestinal stromal tumors (GISTs). *Eur. J. Cancer 38*:60–65.

von Schulthess, G.K., Steinert, H.C., and Hany, T.F. 2006. Integrated PET/CT: current applications and future directions. *Radiology 238*:405–422.

15

Gastrointestinal Stromal Tumor: Computed Tomography

Hyo-Cheol Kim and Jeong Min Lee

Introduction

Gastrointestinal stromal tumors (GISTs), previously classified as leiomyomas or leiomyosarcomas, are the most common mesenchymal tumors of the gastrointestinal tract. They occur most frequently in the stomach (60–70%) but can also occur in the small bowel (20–30%), colorectum (5%), and esophagus (< 5%) (Levy *et al.*, 2003). Gastrointestinal stromal tumors rarely occur as a primary tumor of the omentum, mesentery, or retroperitoneum. Computed tomography (CT) plays an important role for the diagnosis and staging of these neoplasms because it can identify the tumor and assess for local invasion or metastasis.

Pathologic Features

Because GISTs commonly involve the muscularis propria of the intestinal wall, they have a propensity for exophytic growth. Grossly, GISTs are soft, fleshy, lobulated masses that may have internal necrosis and cystic degeneration. Mucosal ulceration of the luminal surface of the tumor is seen in up to 50% of the cases. Cavities form from extensive hemorrhage or necrosis and may communicate with the intestinal lumen. Most GISTs express a mutant form of c-kit (CD117) that can be detected with routine immunohistochemical staining,

distinguishing GISTs from true leiomyomas or leiomyosarcomas. C-kit is a growth factor receptor with tyrosine kinase activity, and its mutations cause activation of the KIT receptor tyrosine kinase and unopposed stimulus for cell growth (Hirota *et al.*, 1998). C-kit negative GISTs (2–5%) have mutations in platelet-derived growth factor receptor-α gene, which was also the product of the c-kit protooncogene (Hirota *et al.*, 2003).

Based on previous studies on GISTs, the criteria of benignity and malignancy in each anatomical region were as follows (Miettinen *et al.*, 2002). In gastric GISTs, tumors were considered probably benign if they were ≤ 5 cm in size and ≤ 5 mitoses per 50 high-power fields. Tumors were considered malignant if they were > 10 cm in size or had > 5 mitoses per 50 high-power fields. Tumors were considered to have uncertain or low malignant potential if they were > 5 cm but ≤ 10 cm in size and had ≤ 5 mitoses per 50 high-power fields. For intestinal GISTs, tumors were considered to be probably benign if they were ≤ 2 cm and had ≤ 5 mitoses per 50 high-power fields. Tumors were considered malignant if they were > 5 cm or had > 5 mitoses per 50 high-power fields. Finally, tumors were considered to be of uncertain or low malignant potential if they were > 2 cm but ≤ 5 cm and had ≤ 5 mitoses per 50 high-power fields. However, pathologists often experience the difficulty in determining tumor malignancy because the degree of mitotic activity may vary markedly within the lesion.

Clinical Features

Gastrointestinal stromal tumors account for 1–3% of gastric neoplasms, 20% of small bowel tumors, and 0.2–1% of colorectal tumors (Miettinen *et al.*, 2001). No association between geographic location, ethnicity, race, or occupation has been established. Patients with neurofibromatosis type 1 have an increased prevalence of GISTs and have multiple small intestinal GISTs. Presenting signs and symptoms depend on the size and anatomic location of the tumor. Affected individuals may present with nausea, vomiting, abdominal pain, a palpable abdominal mass, or gastrointestinal bleeding from mucosal ulceration. However, some patients with exophytic tumors may remain asymptomatic until the lesions have reached an enormous size. It is well known that biopsy of GISTs may be misleading and that excision of the tumors, if technically possible, is the best way to determine their histopathology. Moreover, mitotically inactive tumors can metastasize, which indicates that a low mitotic count does not necessarily rule out malignant behavior. In unresectable tumors, however, percutaneous biopsy is needed to confirm the immunoreactivity for CD 117 and to institute neoadjuvant therapy with imatinib.

Computed Tomography Features

On the CT scan, most GISTs seem to be well-defined exophytic masses with varying attenuation based on size; small tumors (< 5 cm) tend to appear homogeneous, while larger tumors (> 5 cm) frequently show extraluminal masses with central areas of low attenuation and peripheral enhancing viable portion (Burkill *et al.*, 2003). This description applies to GISTs in all locations.

Stomach

The stomach is the most common location for GISTs. On the CT scan, malignant GISTs commonly appear as a large well-circumscribed mass with a peripheral enhancing pattern (Fig. 1). Benign tumors usually appear as a small round intraluminal mass with the homogeneous enhancing pattern. However, no correlation between CT findings and malignant potential could be established, unless obvious local invasion or metastatic lesion was seen (Kim *et al.*, 2004a). In large tumors, the bulk of the tumor will be in an extragastric location, which makes it difficult to determine the origin of the tumor by the axial CT scan. The huge tumors may occupy most of the left upper quadrant so that the stomach can be replaced in the corner. Recently developed multidetector row CT and the three-dimensional reconstruction technology will help establish the stomach as the origin of tumors.

Some tumors may contain one or more ulcers that can cause gastrointestinal bleeding (Fig. 2). Tumors with extensive

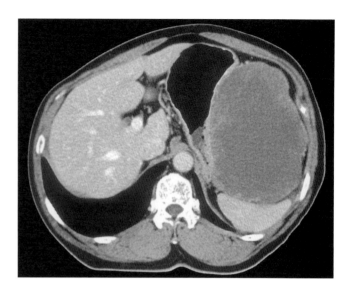

Figure 1 66-year-old man with malignant gastrointestinal stromal tumor presenting with abdominal discomfort. Contrast-enhanced CT scan shows huge well-defined exophytic gastric tumor with intact overlying mucosa.

hemorrhage or necrosis may infrequently form the large cavitary masses containing air, air-fluid levels, or oral contrast material (Burkill *et al.*, 2003). Calcification is an unusual feature, and it may occur in a punctuate pattern or show extensively throughout the tumor. Metastatic lymphadenopathy is also rare.

The differential diagnosis for gastric GISTs includes leiomyomas, leiomyosarcomas, schwannomas, neurofibromas, and neuroendocrine neoplasms. Unfortunately, all of these neoplasms have similar imaging features to those of GISTs. Gastric adenocarcinoma and lymphoma rarely form marked exophytic growth. Gastric adenocarcinomas and lymphomas commonly accompany lymphadenopathy, which is not

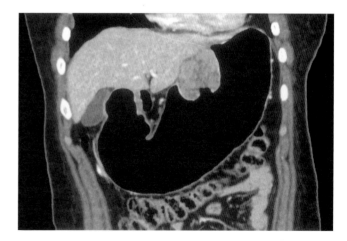

Figure 2 47-year-old woman with malignant gastrointestinal stromal tumor presenting with melena. Contrast-enhanced CT scan with coronal reformation shows endogastric mass with central ulcer.

seen in GISTs, and lymphomas usually have homogeneous enhancing patterns.

Small Intestine

The CT feature of small intestine tumors is similar to gastric tumors. As in gastric tumors, small tumors may appear as intraluminal polyps, particularly in patients with neurofibromatosis type 1 (Levy *et al.*, 2004). Large tumors are typically enhancing masses with areas of low attenuation from hemorrhage, necrosis, or cyst formation, but rarely present with the bowel obstruction. Similarly, duodenal tumors infrequently cause biliary or pancreatic duct obstruction (Kim *et al.*, 2004b). Mesenteric fat infiltration and lymphadenopathy are rarely observed. However, duodenal tumor may directly invade the adjacent organs such as the pancreas or kidney because it is located in retroperitoneal space.

The differential diagnosis for small intestinal GISTs includes lymphoma, adenocarcinoma, and metastatic neoplasms. Lymphomas may have large ulcerated or cavitating masses within the small bowel, which is indistinguishable from a GIST. In these cases, the presence of lymphadenopathy would favor the diagnosis of lymphoma. Adenocarcinoma is the most common primary malignancy of the small bowel but commonly appears as an annular lesion in the small bowel.

Colorectum

On the CT images, anorectal tumors usually appear as a well-circumscribed mural mass compressing the rectal wall. Because of their retroperitoneal location as duodenal tumors, rectal tumors may appear as soft tissue masses that extend into the ischiorectal fossa, prostate, or vagina (Levy *et al.*, 2003).

The differential diagnosis for colorectal GISTs includes adenocarcinoma, lymphoma, melanoma, carcinoid, and prostatic tumors. Adenocarcinomas tend to have irregular margins and regional lymphadenopathy, while GISTs tend to have well-defined margins and lack lymphadenopathy. GISTs with perirectal extension may be mistaken as tumors of the prostate and perineum.

Omentum and Mesentery

Primary GISTs may occur in the mesentery and omentum. They were characterized as a huge well-circumscribed mass with the large area of low attenuation (Levy *et al.*, 2003). Although tumors may appear as cystic, they do not contain an air-fluid level because they do not communicate with intestinal lumen. Gastrointestinal stromal tumors in the omentum and mesentery seem to be indistinguishable from that of other sarcomas that may arise in these locations, such as leiomyosarcoma, malignant fibrous histiocytoma, fibrosarcoma, and liposarcoma. Desmoid tumor presents as typically mesenteric masses that show homogeneous attenuation on CT images.

Metastasis

The most common site for GIST metastasis is the liver, followed by the peritoneum. The metastatic mass in the liver can be heterogeneous and peripherally enhanced, similar to primary tumor after administration of intravenous contrast (Burkill *et al.*, 2003). The low attenuation in the center of metastatic lesions often indicates central necrosis of a solid mass, and the peripheral enhanced portion represents viable solid tumor. The hepatic and peritoneal metastases resemble cystic lesions or ascites after imatinib treatment (Warakaulle and Dleeson, 2006). In patients who were treated successfully, at least initially, with imatinib mesylate, an enhancing nodule within a mass is an important sign of recurrent GISTs (Shankar *et al.*, 2005).

Conclusion

Gastrointestinal stromal tumors are mesenchymal tumors that typically arise in association with the muscularis propria of the gastrointestinal tract wall. Computed tomography can be a useful modality for the diagnosis, staging, and follow-up of patients with GISTs. Although the radiologic features of GISTs are often distinct from those of epithelial tumors, criteria to separate GISTs radiologically from other nonepithelial tumors have not yet been fully developed.

References

Burkill, G.J., Badran, M., Al-Muderis, O., Meirion, T.J., Judson, I.R., Fisher, C., and Moskovic, E.C. 2003. Malignant gastrointestinal stromal tumor: distribution, imaging features, and pattern of metastatic spread. *Radiology 226*:527–532.

Hirota, S., Isozaki, K., Moriyama, Y., Hashimoto, K., Nishida, T., Ishiguro, S., Kawano, K., Hanada, M., Kurata, A., Takeda, M., Muhammad, T.G., Matsuzawa, Y., Kanakura, Y., Shinomura, Y., and Kitamura, Y. 1998. Gain-of-function mutations of c-kit in human gastrointestinal stromal tumors. *Science 279*:577–580.

Hirota, S., Ohashi, A., Nishida, T., Isozaki, K., Kinoshita, K., Shinomura, Y., and Kitamura, Y. 2003. Gain-of-function mutations of platelet-derived growth factor receptor alpha gene in gastrointestinal stromal tumors. *Gastroenterology 125*:660–667.

Kim, H.C., Lee, J.M., Kim, K.W., Park, S.H., Kim, S.H., Lee, J.Y., Han, J.K., and Choi, B.I. 2004a. Gastrointestinal stromal tumors of the stomach: CT findings and prediction of malignancy. *Am. J. Roentgenol.183*:893–898.

Kim, H.C., Lee, J.M., Son, K.R., Kim, S.H., Lee, K.H., Kim, K.W., Lee, M., Han, J.K., and Choi, B.I. 2004b. Gastrointestinal stromal tumors ofthe duodenum: CT and barium study findings. *Am. J. Roentgenol. 183*:415–419.

Levy, A.D., Remotti, H.E., Thompson, W.M., Sobin, L.H., and Miettinen, M. 2003. Gastrointestinal stromal tumors: radiologic features with pathologic correlation. *Radiographics 23*:283–304.

Levy, A.D., Patel, N., Abbott, R.M., Dow, N., Miettinen, M., and Sobin, L.H. 2004. Gastrointestinal stromal tumors in patients with neurofibromatosis: imaging features with clinicopathologic correlation. *Am. J. Roentgenol. 183*:1629–1636.

Miettinen, M., and Lasota, J. 2001. Gastrointestinal stromal tumors—definition, clinical, histological, immunohistochemical, and molecular genetic features and differential diagnosis. *Virchows. Arch. 438*:1–12.

Miettinen, M., El-Rifai, W., Sobin, L., and Lasota, J. 2002. Evaluation of malignancy and prognosis of gastrointestinal stromal tumors: a review. *Hum. Pathol. 33*:478–483.

Shankar, S., vanSonnenberg, E., Desai, J., Dipiro, P.J., Van Den Abbeele, A., and Demetri, G.D. 2005. Gastrointestinal stromal tumor: new nodule-within-a-mass pattern of recurrence after partial response to imatinib mesylate. *Radiology 235*:892–898.

Warakaulle, D.R., and Gleeson, F. 2006. MDCT appearance of gastrointestinal stromal tumors after therapy with imatinib mesylate. *Am. J. Roentgenol. 186*:510–515.

Gastrointestinal Lipomas: Computed Tomography

Sebastian T. Schindera and William M. Thompson

Introduction

The occurrence of lipomas in the gastrointestinal tract is uncommon. Reliable radiographic diagnosis of this benign neoplastic lesion and precise differentiation from other intestinal malignant tumors are important to avoid unnecessary surgery. In this chapter, we discuss current imaging methods for gastrointestinal lipomas, particularly computed tomography (CT). Gastrointestinal lipomas are slow-growing tumors that are mainly detected in people over age 50 years, with a peak occurrence in the seventh decade. The exact etiology of this benign neoplastic lesion remains unclear. A misplacement of adipose tissue or an acquired condition is discussed as a potential cause. In 95% of cases, gastrointestinal lipomas originate in the submucosa and appear as a round, homogeneous yellow, well-circumscribed nodule on cross section (Heiken *et al.*, 1982). On cytology the tumor is composed of well-differentiated adipose tissue surrounded by a fibrous capsule.

Gastrointestinal lipomas are usually solitary and occur anywhere along the gut. The colon is the most common site for gastrointestinal lipomas (65–75%), followed by the small bowel (20–25%) and the stomach (up to 5%) (Thompson, 2005). After adenomatous polyps and gastrointestinal stromal tumors, lipomas are the second most common benign tumor in the colon and the small bowel. The cecum, the ilium, and the antrum are the most common location in the colon, small bowel, and stomach, respectively (Figs. 1–3) (Thompson, 2005).

Most intestinal lipomas are usually asymptomatic; they are discovered incidentally on imaging studies performed for unrelated causes. When the tumors are large (> 3–4 cm),

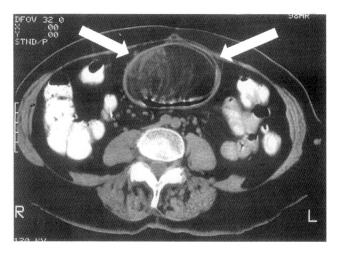

Figure 1 Gastric lipoma Axial CT scan demonstrates a low-density mass in the gastric antrum (arrows) containing some high-density stranding due to ulceration.

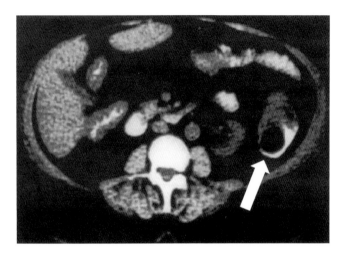

Figure 2 **Descending colon lipoma** Axial CT scan shows mass of low attenuation in the descending colon (arrow).

the most common clinical symptoms are abdominal pain and acute or chronic gastrointestinal bleeding from an ulcer (Regge *et al.*, 1999; Thompson *et al.*, 2003). Lipomas with a diameter of greater than 5 cm have a higher risk for intussusception (Fig. 3) (Buetow *et al.*, 1996).

Computed Tomography

To diagnose intestinal lipomas, CT is considered as the imaging modality of choice. Because CT permits accurate differentiation between fat and other tissues, an intestinal lipoma can be definitively diagnosed using CT. For an optimal characterization of intestinal lipomas using CT, we recommend oral and intravenous iodinated contrast administration. A positive oral contrast agent (high intraluminal density) increases the contrast between the fatty tumor and the intraluminal surrounding (Fig. 2). For patients undergoing CT examination for a suspected lipoma of the sigmoid, additional administration of rectal contrast agent is recommended. Since the peak mural enhancement of the small-bowel wall appears approximately 50 seconds after the initiation of intravenous contrast agent, this is the optimal temporal window to acquire the CT images (Schindera *et al.*, 2006). Intravenous contrast is injected via a power injector with a flow rate of 3 to 5 ml/sec. The administration of intravenous contrast agent also increases the delineation of gastrointestinal lipomas since the fatty lesion does not enhance, whereas the surrounding bowel wall clearly enhances (Figs. 1 and 3). In general, multidetector row CT should acquire the data sets with a thin collimation (< 1 mm) to allow multiplanar reconstruction. The reformat images in any desired plane are particularly valuable for displaying the entire expansion of the small bowel with its long and tortuous course.

The findings on CT are characterized by a homogeneous mass with absorption densities ranging between −80 and −120 Hounsfield Units (Figs. 1–3). Besides the uniform appearance, previous studies have demonstrated gastric lipomas with linear strands of soft tissue attenuation at the base (Taylor *et al.*, 1990; Thompson *et al.*, 2003). These tumors were associated with ulceration of the mucosa and the presence of basilar strands of nonfatty elements correlated histologically with prominent fibrovascular septa (Fig. 1).

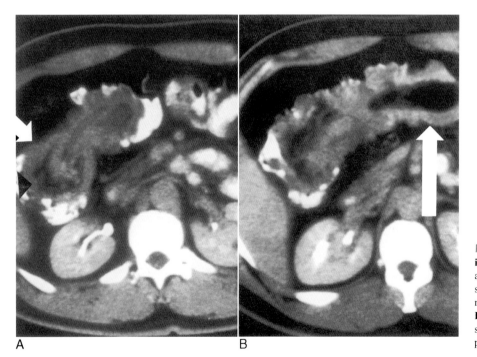

A   B

Figure 3 **Small-bowel lipoma causing intussusception A.** Axial CT through mid abdomen demonstrates an ileal-colonic intussusception (arrow). Note the classic asymmetric crescent of mesenteric fat (arrowhead). **B.** Axial CT slightly more proximal demonstrates the lipoma (arrow), which was the lead point for the intussusception.

The loss of fat density in colonic intussuscepted lipomas is also not uncommon, which directly corresponds to the degree of infarction and fat necrosis (Buetow *et al.*, 1996). The variation of the classic homogeneous appearance of a lipoma in the presence of an ulceration or infarction due to an intussusception should not be misinterpreted as a liposarcoma. This extremely rare, malignant neoplastic lesion usually manifests as an inhomogeneous mass containing large areas of nonfatty tissues.

Other Imaging Methods

Other imaging methods in diagnosing gastrointestinal lipomas include magnetic resonance imaging (MRI), barium contrast studies, and endoscopy. Since MRI with T1-weighted sequences is extremely sensitive to fat, MRI is as effective as CT in detection of fatty neoplasm along the gut (Regge *et al.*, 1999). Especially with children and patients allergic to iodinated contrast agents, MRI becomes the primary imaging tool to diagnose gastrointestinal lipomas. On barium contrast studies, the classical appearance of lipomas is a smooth, oval, or spherical mass with a very distinct margin. On palpation during fluoroscopy the lesions compress very easily. Since lipomas are hard to differentiate from other submucosal masses (e.g., gastrointestinal stromal tumor, carcinoid, leiomyoma), barium examinations are now rarely used for the diagnosis of these lesions. Characteristic endoscopic findings of a gastrointestinal lipoma include: (1) the yellow color of the lesion, (2) the indentation of the lipoma with the biopsy forceps ("cushion sign"), and (3) the easy retraction of normal mucosa overlying the lesion ("tent sign").

Although endoscopy with a possible forceps biopsy of the lipoma provides a reliable diagnosis, the technique is invasive and carries a risk of major complications, including bleeding, perforation, and infection.

Gastrointestinal lipomas have no malignant potential, and therefore surgery is only indicated in symptomatic patients or in lesions in which malignancy cannot be excluded. Patients with a submucosal mass detected on an endoscopic or upper gastrointestinal examination should undergo an abdominal CT examination since CT can specifically diagnose a lipoma. If the CT scan does show the characteristic features of a lipoma, unnecessary surgery can be avoided.

References

Buetow, P.C., Buck, J.L., Carr, N.J., Pantongrag-Brown, L., Ros, P.R., and Cruess, D.F. 1996. Intussuscepted colonic lipomas: loss of fat attenuation on CT with pathologic correlation in 10 cases. *Abdom. Imaging* *21*:153–156.

Heiken, J.P., Forde, K.A., and Gold, R.P. 1982. Computed tomography as a definitive method for diagnosing gastrointestinal lipomas. *Radiology* *142*:409–414.

Regge, D., Lo Bello, G., Martincich, L., Bianchi, G., Cuomo, G., Suriani, R., and Cavuoto, F. 1999. A case of bleeding gastric lipoma: US, CT and MR findings. *Eur. Radiol.* *9*:256–258.

Schindera, S.T., Nelson, C.R., Paulson, E.K., and DeLong, D. 2006. What is the optimal timing for imaging the small bowel with multidetector CT? Presented at the Annual Meeting of the SCBT/MR.

Taylor, A.J., Stewart, E.T., and Dodds, W.J. 1990. Gastrointestinal lipomas: a radiologic and pathologic review. *Am. J. Roentgenol.* *155*:1205–1210.

Thompson, W.M. 2005. Imaging and findings of lipomas of the gastrointestinal tract. *Am. J. Roentgenol. 184*:1163–1171.

Thompson, W.M., Kende, A.I., and Levy, A.D. 2003. Imaging characteristics of gastric lipomas in 16 adult and pediatric patients. *Am. J. Roentgenol. 181*:981–985.

17

Computed Tomography in Peritoneal Surface Malignancy

Tristan D. Yan and Paul H. Sugarbaker

Introduction

Computed tomography (CT) is the current mainstay-imaging tool for patients with peritoneal surface malignancy. With administration of adequate intravenous, oral, or rectal contrast media, the high-resolution images of CT allow more precise identification and evaluation of the peritoneal disease than those provided by sonography. Magnetic resonance imaging (MRI) provides good resolution, but requires longer scan times during which respiratory motion and bowel peristalsis can interfere with the image resolution. Positron emission tomography (PET) is useful and provides functional imaging, but the ability to detect diffuse small tumor nodules is limited. However, PET-CT is able to provide high CT resolution and simultaneous PET functional imaging. The efficacy of these radiologic modalities in the assessment of peritoneal surface malignancy remains to be evaluated.

In the past, patients with peritoneal cancer were considered preterminal and were managed with systemic chemotherapy. Surgery was selectively used to palliate patients with gastrointestinal obstruction caused by tumor progression. This management approach was traditionally agreed upon by most physicians. With better understanding of the natural history, it has been realized that the peritoneal dissemination of cancers is not systemic metastasis, but a local-regional extension of the primary tumor.

Diseases such as pseudomyxoma peritonei and diffuse malignant peritoneal mesothelioma tend to remain confined within the peritoneal cavity throughout the clinical course. Lymphatic and hematogeneous metastases are rarely seen. In patients with pseudomyxoma peritonei from appendiceal mucinous neoplasms, the median survival can be prolonged to 5 years with the traditional palliative approach because the tumors are minimally invasive, but the disease almost always recurs. Each repeat debulking procedure was associated with progressively thickened intra-abdominal scar tissues. These patients eventually die from complications of surgery or tumor progression. Prior to the year 2000, the median survival for patients with diffuse malignant peritoneal mesothelioma was < 12 months. As the large volume of ascites produced by thousands of tumor nodules accumulate, these patients develop severely debilitating symptoms before their demise.

In more aggressive gastrointestinal malignancies, such as colorectal cancer, there is a window of opportunity, where the disease remains confined within the peritoneal cavity before distant metastases develop. Colorectal cancer is the second most common cause of cancer-related deaths in the Western world. Ten percent of patients are diagnosed with synchronous peritoneal disease at the time of their primary surgery, and 25% eventually develop isolated peritoneal recurrence. As the disease advances at a rapid pace, invariably all patients die from the disease with a median survival of 6 months. Systemic chemotherapy with 5-fluorouracil, oxaliplatin, or irinotecan has not dramatically improved the prognosis of patients with colorectal metastasis in the last 40 years. Recently, a combination of these drugs with a biological agent, such as bevacizumab, reached the 20-month median survival. However, to date there is no evidence that documents the efficacy of these novel therapeutic regimens in colorectal peritoneal carcinomatosis.

An evolutionary change in the management of peritoneal surface malignancy has occurred in the last decade, which consists of cytoreductive surgery combined with perioperative intraperitoneal chemotherapy (Sugarbaker, 1995). Many studies have shown significantly improved survival as compared to the traditional approach (Sugarbaker, 2006; Glehen et al., 2004; Verwaal et al., 2003; Look et al., 2004). The intent of the combined treatment is no longer palliative, but cure in selected patients is possible. However, the survival advantage is achieved at the expense of moderate to high perioperative morbidity and mortality rates. In the current literature the morbidity rate varies from 1 to 10% and mortality ranges from 20 to 50%, depending on the extent of cytoreduction and the skill level of the surgical team (Jacquet et al., 1996; Stephens et al., 1999; Glehen et al., 2003). As a result, more emphasis has been placed on careful patient selection to identify patients groups in advance, which do not benefit from the combined treatments.

In the past decade, spiral or helical CT technology has been developed, which permits the acquisition of a volume data set from which axial slices are reconstructed. The table on which the patient lies moves at a constant speed, while the X-ray tube produces a sustained exposure. Respiratory misregistration is eliminated as the scan acquires data during a single breath hold. Scan reconstruction at intervals smaller than scan collimation produces overlapping slices, which improves the detection of smaller lesions. In addition, contrast-enhancement can be optimized due to a shorter scanning time, which, along with the development of high heat capacity tubes, allows images to be acquired in the phase of contrast enhancement most appropriate to the pathology being assessed, for example, arterial and venous phase imaging.

To a radiologist, the traditional teaching is to document the presence versus absence, as well as the characteristics of tumors seen on a CT in a systematic manner. With advances in imaging technology, these abnormalities can now be automatically and accurately quantified. Unfortunately, the majority of clinical image interpretations continue to be performed by radiologists without computerized image analysis support.

As analysis methods are becoming increasingly important and relevant, this situation is rapidly changing. However, to a surgeon, often the mere descriptions of presence versus absence, size, site, and shape of the tumors have limited clinical value in terms of diagnosis and determining whether or not a patient is a potential candidate for the novel treatment approach of cytoreductive surgery and perioperative intraperitoneal chemotherapy. This chapter will focus on CT in the diagnosis of peritoneal surface malignancy, mainly, pseudomyxoma peritonei, diffuse malignant peritoneal mesothelioma, high-grade gastrointestinal and ovarian peritoneal carcinomatosis, and peritoneal sarcomatosis as well as patient selection by CT for cytoreductive surgery and perioperative intraperitoneal chemotherapy.

Computed Tomography Diagnosis

There are distinct patterns of cancer dissemination within the peritoneal cavity, which are dependent on the degree of invasiveness of the cancer and the tendency of mucin production. First, the histologic grade or the biologic invasiveness determines the ability of free tumor emboli to adhere and implant. Low-grade cancers generally lack capability to adhere and as a result "redistribute" widely throughout the peritoneal space. Small bowel and small bowel mesentery remain free of tumor because of their active peristaltic movement, which reduces build-up of the tumor on their surfaces. Nonadherent tumor cells are carried by peritoneal fluid and accumulate at the sites of peritoneal fluid absorption, such as greater omentum and undersurfaces of the diaphragms. Whereas moderate- to high-grade cancers tend to show "randomly proximal distribution" and because of their capability to adhere and invade, peritoneal implants occur close to the site of primary tumor. The high-grade cancer may infiltrate mesentery and bowel surfaces, causing focal masses and intestinal obstruction.

The second factor that influences the patterns of peritoneal tumor spread is the extent of mucin production. Mucus tends to occupy free peritoneal space and accumulates in gravity-dependent areas, such as the pelvis, paracolic gutters, and retrohepatic and retrosplenic spaces. As the volume of mucinous ascites increases, it tends to exert pressure effects on the visceral organs, causing compression of the liver capsule and displacement of the small bowel. Invasive cancers that produce mucinous ascites may be expected to show the most extensive spread throughout the abdomen and pelvis. With these fundamental differences in characteristics of cancer dissemination, CT imaging can provide useful information in facilitating the diagnosis.

Pseudomyxoma Peritonei

Pseudomyxoma peritonei is characterized clinically by the presence of mucinous ascites throughout the abdomen in a "redistribution" pattern, which usually originates from the vermiform appendix. As the mucin escapes from the blow-out of the appendical stump, it accumulates in the pelvis, paracolic gutters, and retrohepatic and retrosplenic spaces. The phagocytic activity of the greater omentum will also take up a large volume of mucinous tumors. CT images usually show the following characteristics: (1) a periappendiceal mass, representing the primary tumor mass; (2) large quantity of mucinous tumor throughout the peritoneal cavity, especially in the pelvis, pericolic gutters, omentum, retrohepatic, and retrosplenic spaces; (3) scalloping of the liver capsule forming lenticular-shaped compression of the liver parenchyma, but no evidence of invasion; (4) compartmentalization of the small bowel, where the small bowel is displaced by large-volume mucinous ascites and omental cake to one region in the abdominopelvic cavity, and usually there is no evidence of infiltration of the bowel wall and the mesentery (Jacquet et al., 1995). When all four radiologic features are present in a patient, the diagnosis of pseudomyxoma peritonei can be made.

Diffuse Malignant Peritoneal Mesothelioma

Diffuse malignant peritoneal mesothelioma originates from the serosal lining of the peritoneal cavity. Thousands of tumor nodules produce large quantities of serous ascites. The tumor nodules may present on any peritoneal surface without a primary site of cancer origin being found. As the disease tends to be more aggressive than pseudomyxoma peritonei, it does not spare the small bowel and its mesenteric surfaces. However, despite its aggressiveness, diffuse malignant peritoneal mesothelioma rarely metastasizes to lymph nodes and distant organs. These unique clinical characteristics define the CT findings (Yan et al., 2005a). First, the disease is diffuse throughout the peritoneal cavity. Patients rarely have a large solitary mass(es) that could be misinterpreted as an epicenter of a primary abdominal or pelvic cancer. This lack of a primary site is distinctly different from gastrointestinal or gynecologic malignancies. Second, the most heavily disease-involved regions are the midabdomen and pelvis. In great contrast to pseudomyxoma peritonei or other mucinous adenocarcinomas, compartmentalization of the small bowel and a large volume of disease beneath the right hemidiaphragm are absent. Third, the presence of serous ascites rather than mucinous ascites is commonly seen with this disease. Fourth, there is a lack of extraperitoneal lymph node or distant organ metastasis. One must raise the clinical suspicion of diffuse malignant peritoneal mesothelioma when encountering these radiologic findings.

High-Grade Gastrointestinal and Ovarian Peritoneal Carcinomatosis

Usually in patients with high-grade cancers, an epicenter of the tumor is evident on CT. For gastrointestinal cancer, as full thickness invasion of the bowel wall progresses, microperforations of the serosal surface result. This will lead to the seeding of malignant cells into the free peritoneal space and/or adhering to adjacent organs and structures. Computed tomography images show that the peritoneal spread tends to be confined to the vicinity of the primary site, causing bowel obstruction, and ureteric obstruction (Archer et al., 1996). Lymph node involvement and distant organ metastases may be present. In right colon cancer, the peritoneal seeding most frequently involves the omentum, nearby loops of the terminal ileum, and the right pericolic gutter. For gastric cancer and occasionally pancreatic carcinoma, the common locations for peritoneal seeding include the lesser omentum, the omental bursa, lesser sac, and surfaces of the stomach itself. In primary ovarian cancer, the most common sites of peritoneal seeding are the cul-de-sac (pouch of Douglas), rectosigmoid colon, and the cleft between the sigmoid colon and the left pelvic sidewall. Also, tumor deposits on the dome of the bladder are frequent, as the peritoneal carcinomatosis progresses. Tumor nodules on the undersurface of the right hemidiaphragm and within the greater omentum are frequently encountered when the cancer is far advanced or has a mucinous histologic subtype.

Peritoneal Sarcomatosis

Although definitive CT diagnosis of peritoneal sarcomatosis is difficult, the difference in the morphology of a sarcomatosis versus carcinomatosis is thought to explain the difference in CT findings (Pestieau et al., 2002). The sarcoma nodules are spherical and widely distributed and reliably distort the surrounding anatomic structures. The CT density of sarcomatosis is much higher as the nodules are extremely vascular and closely resemble blood density, which results in greater contrast between sarcoma nodules and small bowel or lipose tissues.

Accuracy of Computed Tomography in Peritoneal Cancer Detection

In a number of recent series, sensitivity of CT in diagnosing peritoneal carcinomatosis varies from 60 to 90%, which is dependent on the quality of CT scans, size of tumor nodules, interpretation from a radiologist, and the abdominopelvic regions examined (Pestieau et al., 2002; Jacquet et al., 1993; de Bree et al., 2006). The size of the peritoneal tumor is an important factor for detection on CT. Sensitivity of detecting individual lesions with a maximal diameter > 5 cm was 60 to 90%, in contrast to 10 to 30% for tumors < 1 cm. There was also a great degree of variation in sensitivity for tumor detection in different areas. The sensitivity for tumor detection in the epigastrium, small-bowel region, greater omentum, pelvis, and undersurfaces of the diaphragms have been reported to be 75 to 85%, 75 to 85%, 75 to 90%, 70 to 100%, and 60 to

85%, respectively (Pestieau *et al.*, 2002; Jacquet *et al.*, 1993; de Bree *et al.*, 2006). In earlier studies on CT performance in ovarian cancer patients with peritoneal carcinomatosis, results of detection were less reliable (Forstner *et al.*, 1995). Using more advanced technology including helical CT, we can expect superior accuracy in detection of peritoneal implants with improvement of CT technology.

Computed Tomography Patient Selection

Several prognostic factors have been shown to be significant for an improved survival after cytoreductive surgery and perioperative intraperitoneal chemotherapy. These factors include extent of cytoreductive surgery, commonly represented by the peritoneal cancer index (PCI), histologic grading of the tumor, presence of lymph node or distant organ metastases, and completeness of cytoreductive surgery (CCR). The peritoneal cancer index is an assessment combining lesion size (lesion size 0 to 3) with tumor distribution, to quantify the extent of disease as a numerical score (PCI-0 to PCI-39) (Glehen *et al.*, 2003). Completeness of cytoreductive surgery measures the residual tumor volume after surgery (Glehen *et al.*, 2003). CCR-0 indicated a no visible evidence of mesothelioma. CCR-1 indicated a residual tumor nodule ≤ 2.5 mm in diameter, while CCR-2 indicated a residual tumor nodule between 2.5 mm and 2.5 cm in diameter. CCR-3 indicated residual tumor nodules > 2.5 cm in diameter or a confluence of tumor nodules present at any site. Although these parameters are prognostically significant for survival, they are not available before surgery, which means that they have limited value in the selection of patients prior to surgery.

During the cytoreductive surgery, the surgeon tries to remove all intraperitoneal tumor implants by using a series of peritonectomy procedures, including: anterior parietal peritonectomy, greater omentectomy with splenectomy, left upper quadrant peritonectomy, right upper quadrant peritonectomy, lesser omentectomy with cholecystectomy, and pelvic peritonectomy with rectosigmoid colonic resection (Sugarbaker, 1995). The visceral resections include rectosigmoidectomy, right colectomy, total abdominal colectomy, hysterectomy, and small bowel resection. These resections are performed at anatomic sites where there is visible evidence of disease.

A peritonectomy surgeon knows that presence versus absence of tumors and volume of disease in areas such as the undersurfaces of the diaphragms, omentum, pericolic gutters, and pelvis are important information to acquire preoperatively, in order to plan for the operation. However, this information has limited or is of restricted prognostic value because the disease in these areas can be readily removed with an attempt at a complete cytoreduction. With increased experience, it is realized that the volume of disease of the

small bowel and the epigastric region are very important determinants for survival. Extensive involvement of these visceral organs invariably means resection, but only limited lengths of small bowel can be resected in order to maintain a reasonable quality of life. Extensive tumor mass present in the epigastric region may be difficult to remove because the tumor almost always encases the porta hepatis and gastric vessels. The greater omentum is usually removed along with the gastroepiploic vascular arcade, which usually is one of the early procedures in the cytoreduction. The sole remaining blood supply to the stomach is the lesser omental vascular arcade composed of the right and left gastric arteries. If this vasculature is compromised, devascularization of the body of the stomach will occur. Large-volume disease in the epigastric region extensively involves the right gastric/left gastric vascular arcade. Unless the surgeon is willing to perform a total gastrectomy, this disease must not be resected. Consequently, large-volume solid tumor in the epigastric region causes a suboptimal cytoreduction to occur. On a preoperative CT, the size of tumor in the epigastric region therefore will have a significant prognostic impact (Yan *et al.*, 2005).

Interpretive Computer Tomography Classification of the Small Bowel and Its Mesentery

Interpretive CT classification of the small bowel and its mesentery has been developed, and categorized the CT appearances into four classes (Table 1) (Yan *et al.*, 2005b). These four classes represent a stepwise disease progression of peritoneal tumors, which are prognostically significant: Class 0–CT shows no ascites in the region of the small bowel; the jejunal and ileal vessels appear as round and curvilinear densities within the mesenteric fat. Class I–CT shows free intraperitoneal fluid only. The mesentery is stranded and stratified, as the fluid accumulation outlines the small-bowel mesentery. The small-bowel vessels are easily identified within the mesenteric fat (Fig. 1). Class II–CT

Table 1   Interpretative CT Classification of Small Bowel and Small-Bowel Mesentery for Diffuse Malignant Peritoneal Mesothelioma

Class	Ascites	Small Bowel and Mesentery	Mesenteric Vessel Clarity
0	No	No	No
I	Yes	No	No
II	Yes	Thickening & enhancing	No
III	Yes	Nodular thickening & segmental obstruction	Obscured

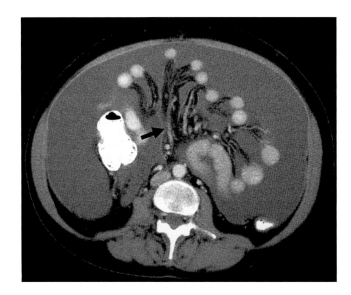

Figure 1 Computed tomography scan shows free intraperitoneal fluid only. The mesentery becomes stranded and stratified as the fluid accumulation outlines the small bowel mesentery. The small bowel vessels are identified easily within the mesenteric fat.

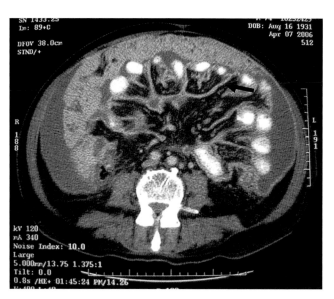

Figure 2 Computed tomography scan shows tumor involvement of the small bowel mesentery. The peritoneal lining is thickened and enhanced due to the presence of tumor nodules or plaques. There may be an increased amount of ascitic fluid. The small bowel mesenteric vessels are still identifiable.

shows tumor involvement of the small bowel and/or its mesentery. The peritoneal surfaces are thickened and enhanced due to the presence of tumor nodules (usually half-spherical bodies) or plaques (flat implants whose diameter is greater than their thickness). There may be an increased amount of ascitic fluid, and the mesentery may appear stellate or pleated. The small-bowel mesenteric vessels are still identifiable (Fig. 2). Class III–CT shows an increased solid tumor involvement, and adjacent small-bowel loops are matted together in some cuts. The configuration of the small bowel and its mesentery appears distorted and thickened. Segmental small-bowel obstruction is present. Intraperitoneal fluid may be loculated. The small-bowel mesenteric vessels are difficult to define on some cuts due to obliteration of mesenteric fat (Fig. 3).

In the performance of an adequate cytoreduction, the small-bowel mesentery is dissected. Large-volume tumor is removed, and all bowel loops and mesenteric leaves are separated to allow contact of residual tumor with the perioperative intraperitoneal chemotherapy. If adjacent intestinal and mesenteric structures are matted together, adequate tumor removal and adequate local-regional chemotherapy are not possible. Class III–CT findings of the small bowel and its mesentery have been found to be associated with inadequate surgery and reduced overall survival. Classes 0 to III represent a spectrum of disease severity. As our experience with the CT assessment of the small bowel and its mesentery increased, it became apparent that sometimes Classes I and II are not readily distinguishable, but that Classes 0, I, and II are always distinguishable from Class III.

Mere site description and volume measurements of peritoneal tumors alone are not sufficient. For example, in patients with a large volume of disease in the pelvis, the pelvic peritonectomy can almost always completely remove the disease. Therefore, a large volume of disease in the pelvis

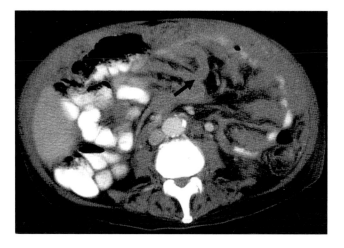

Figure 3 Computed tomography scan shows increased solid tumor involvement with adjacent bowel loops matted together The configuration of the small bowel and its mesentery is distorted and thickened. Intraperitoneal fluid may be loculated. The small bowel mesenteric vessels are difficult to define due to the obliteration of mesenteric fat density.

has no impact on survival and no prognostic implications from a preoperative CT. The same rationale applies to the extensive infiltration of the greater omentum referred to as "omental cake." The disease in the greater omentum, no matter what volume exists, can be readily resected.

A surgical finding that is of great importance in the selection of patients for attempted adequate cytoreduction is the presence versus the absence of foreshortening of the small-bowel mesentery. Although we searched for radiologic evidence of small-bowel retraction in these CT scans, we have not been able to find reliable radiologic criteria for this surgical finding. Therefore, foreshortening of the small-bowel mesentery is in our opinion difficult or impossible to visualize on the CT.

These data regarding CT findings are only meaningful for patients treated with this comprehensive approach utilizing cytoreductive surgery and perioperative intraperitoneal chemotherapy. These data used in patients managed only with systemic chemotherapy may not be valid. Also, it is probable that this CT assessment of prognosis in patients managed by debulking surgery only, without an attempt at optimal cytoreduction plus perioperative intraperitoneal chemotherapy, would have little significance.

A reality that accompanies cytoreductive surgery with perioperative intraperitoneal chemotherapy is its high morbidity and cost. An avoidance of unnecessary or low-value (in terms of survival) procedures would greatly improve the results of this new approach to peritoneal surface malignancy. In patients in whom CT suggests a poor outcome, surgery may be canceled completely. Certainly, if the patient is a poor operative risk, an aggressive approach should not occur and instead a modified, reduced risk procedure should be contemplated. In the poor prognosis group by CT criteria, the surgeon must be aware to avoid the "point of no return" in a peritoneal surface malignancy patient. This is an enterotomy above the site of partial or complete obstruction of the bowel. Repair has a high incidence of fistula formation. Multiple enterotomies may require an extensive resection to prevent postoperative complications but provide little or no survival benefit. Reliable preoperative radiological findings are of great help in the management of peritoneal surface malignancy patients.

Maximal oral barium contrast that fills the entire gastrointestinal tract is beneficial. Intrarectal contrast facilitates interpretation of the pelvic CT. Intravenous contrast injected to maximize density differences between normal tissue, tumor layered out on peritoneal surfaces as well as ascites fluid, is beneficial. The time interval between intravenous contrast infusion and spiral CT may be crucial to determination of ascites fluid versus solid tumor. A 60-second delay may be optimal in this situation. This distinction is important to separate Class I, Class II, and Class III interpretative small-bowel classification. Currently, helical CT equipment with multiple detectors is routinely used. The information regarding CT assessment of prognosis will likely increase as more modern CT technology is routinely employed in these patients. Also, gadolinium-enhanced MRI may be useful in this clinical situation. In our judgment, anatomic interpretation of CT findings preoperatively is an important aspect of patient selection when one considers the comprehensive treatment for peritoneal surface malignancy.

Acknowledgments

Tristan D. Yan, a surgical oncology research fellow, is sponsored by the Foundation for Applied Research in Gastrointestinal Oncology and Medstar Research Institute. The authors thank Ilse Sugarbaker for editing the manuscript.

References

Archer, A.G., Sugarbaker, P.H., and Jelinek, J.S. 1996. Radiology of peritoneal carcinomatosis. *Cancer Treat. Res. 82*:263–288.

de Bree, E., Koops, W., Kroger, R., van Ruth, S., Verwaal, V.J., and Zoetmulder, F.A.N. 2006. Preoperative computed tomography and selection of patients with colorectal peritoneal carcinomatosis for cytoreductive surgery and hyperthermic intraperitoneal chemotherapy. *Eur. Surg. Oncol. 32*:65–71.

Forstner, R., Hricak, H., Occhipinti, K.A., Powell, C.B., Frankel, S.D., and Stern, J.L. 1995. Ovarian cancer: staging with CT and MR imaging. *Radiology 197*:619–629.

Glehen, O., and Gilly, F.N. 2003. Quantitative prognostic indicators of peritoneal surface malignancy: carcinomatosis, sarcomatosis, and peritoneal mesothelioma. *Surg. Oncol. Clin. N. Am. 12*:649–671.

Glehen, O., Kwiatkowski, F., Sugarbaker, P.H., Elias, D., Levine, E.A., de Simone, M., Barone, R., Yonemura, Y., Cavaliere, F., Quenet, F., Gutman, M., Tentes, A.A., Lorimier, G., Bernard, J.L., Bereder, J.M., Porcheron, J., Gomez-Portilla, A., Shen, P., Deraco, M., and Rat, P. 2004. Cytoreductive surgery combined with perioperative intraperitoneal chemotherapy for the management of peritoneal carcinomatosis from colorectal cancer: a multi-institutional study. *J. Clin. Oncol. 22*: 3284–3292.

Glehen, O., Osinsky, D., Cotte, E., Kwiatkowski, F., Freyer, G., Isaac, S., Trillet-Lenoir, V., Sayag-Beaujard, A.C., Francois, Y., Vignal. J., and Gilly, F.N. 2003. Intraperitoneal chemohyperthermia using a closed abdominal procedure and cytoreductive surgery for the treatment of peritoneal carcinomatosis: morbidity and mortality analysis of 216 consecutive procedures. *Ann. Surg. Oncol. 10*:863–869.

Jacquet, P., Jelinek, J.S., Chang, D., Koslowe, P., and Sugarbaker, P.H. 1995. Abdominal computed tomography scan in the selection of patients with mucinous peritoneal carcinomatosis for cytoreductive surgery. *J. Am. Coll. Surg. 181*:530–538.

Jacquet, P., Jelinek, J.S., Steves, M., and Sugarbaker, P.H. 1993. Evaluation of computed tomography in patient with peritoneal carcinomatosis. *Cancer 72*:1631–1636.

Jacquet, P., Stephens, A.D., Averbach, A.M., Chang, D., Ettinghausen, S.E., Dalton, R.R., Steves, M.A., and Sugarbaker, P.H. 1996. Analysis of morbidity and mortality in 60 patients with peritoneal carcinomatosis treated by cytoreductive surgery and heated intraoperative intraperitoneal chemotherapy. *Cancer 77*:2622–2629.

Look, M., Chang, D., and Sugarbaker, P.H. 2004. Long-term results of cytoreductive surgery for advanced and recurrent epithelial ovarian cancers and papillary serous carcinoma of the peritoneum. *Int. J. Gynecol. Cancer 14*:35–41.

Pestieau, S.R., Jelinek, J.S., and Sugarbaker, P.H. 2002. Abdominal and pelvic CT for detection and volume assessment of peritoneal sarcomatosis. *Tumori. 88*:209–214.

Stephens, A.D., Alderman, R., Chang, D., Edwards, G.D., Esquivel, J., Sebbag, G., Steves, M.A., and Sugarbaker, P.H. 1999. Morbidity and mortality of 200 treatments with cytoreductive surgery and hyperthermic intraoperative intraperitoneal chemotherapy using the Coliseum technique. *Ann. Surg. Oncol. 6*:790–796.

Sugarbaker, P.H. 1995. Peritonectomy procedures. *Ann. Surg. 221*: 29–42.

Sugarbaker, P.H. 2006. New standard of care for appendiceal epithelial neoplasms and pseudomyxoma peritonei syndrome. *Lancet. Oncol. 7*:69–76.

Verwaal, V.J., van Ruth, S., de Bree, E., van Slooten, G.W., van Tinteren, H., Boot, H., and Zoetmulder, F.A. 2003. Randomized trial of cytoreduction and hyperthermic intraperitoneal chemotherapy versus systemic chemotherapy and palliative surgery in patients with peritoneal carcinomatosis of colorectal origin. *J. Clin. Oncol. 21*:3737–3743.

Yan, T.D., Haveric, N., Carmignani, C.P., Bromley, C.M., and Sugarbaker, P.H. 2005a. Computed tomography characterization of malignant peritoneal mesothelioma. *Tumori. 91*:394–400.

Yan, T.D., Haveric, N., Carmignani, C.P., Chang, D., and Sugarbaker, P.H. 2005b. Abdominal computed tomography scans in the selection of patients with malignant peritoneal mesothelioma for comprehensive treatment with cytoreductive surgery and perioperative intraperitoneal chemotherapy. *Cancer 103*:839–849.

18

Gastrointestinal Tumors: Computed Tomography/ Endoscopic Ultrasonography

Shiro Kikuchi, Nobue Futawatari, Masahiko Watanabe, Mayumi Sasaki, Katsumi Kubota, and Mitsuhiro Kida

Introduction

Recent advances in computer-generated image analysis technology have allowed two-dimensional data to be reconstructed into three-dimensional data. Three-dimensional imaging analyses and computer simulations have been applied to a variety of fields. In medicine, the 3D structure of organs, as well as their size and anatomical relationships with other peripheral organs, can be visualized on computer tomography (CT) and ultrasonography; computer imaging analytical techniques have been newly introduced to aid diagnosis (Kim *et al.*, 2002; Yetter *et al.*, 2003). However, in contrast to the usefulness of these techniques when dealing with the oncology of parenchymatous organs, it is difficult to determine the three-dimensional structures of gastrointestinal tumors or their size based on these conventional methods. Furthermore, the diagnostic implications of the results obtained by using these techniques are still unclear and have not yet been fully applied to clinical practice. Therefore, in tumors in the gastrointestinal tract, surface morphology, as well as the two-dimensional development of the tumors, is still primarily diagnosed by conventional radiological and endoscopic examinations. At present, the preoperative diagnosis is generally based on the information provided by these two examinations and helps determine the therapeutic strategies that will be employed.

With recent technological advances, including virtual endoscopy by three-dimensional CT (multidetector row CT: MD-CT) and three-dimensional ultrasonography (3D-EUS), the diagnosis of colonic polyps and three-dimensional images of gastrointestinal tumor lesions has become possible (Iannaccone *et al.*, 2005; Wessling *et al.*, 2005; Tsutsui *et al.*, 2005). Studies have also examined tumor volumetry (Watanabe *et al.*, 2004; Kikuchi *et al.*, 2005). In fact, it has been reported that virtual colonoscopy is as effective as conventional colonoscopy at diagnosing even small lesions (polyps > 5 mm) and is thus an excellent low-invasive screening modality (Iannaccone *et al.*, 2005; Wessling *et al.*, 2005). The major function of these technologies is to draw three-dimensional images of the gastrointestinal tumor lesions and to diagnose the presence of tumors. Many aspects of the clinical implication of being able to measure tumor volume still remain to be clarified. Currently, however, there is little physician interest in doing so.

Presently, it is thought that the depth of tumor invasion and the degree of lymph node metastasis are the most significant prognostic factors in gastrointestinal tumors (Roder *et al.*, 1993; Wu *et al.*, 1997). The size of the tumor (tumor diameter) has not been incorporated into the staging classification systems, neither in the Tumor Node Metastases (TNM) classification (Sobin and Wittekind, 2002) nor in the Japanese Classification of Gastric Cancer (JCGC) (Japanese Research Society for Gastric Cancer, 1995). However, if the three-dimensional structure of a gastric cancer and its size (volume) can be determined preoperatively, then the clinical implication of these findings needs to be clarified. Thus, the conventional concept of determining the malignant potential and the staging classification for gastrointestinal tumor is bound to change and will possibly cause a significant change in terms of making the diagnosis and determining therapeutic strategies.

Tumor Size

In general, larger solid tumors advance faster than smaller tumors. This suggests that larger tumors have a higher biological malignancy. In fact, in solid tumors of the parenchymatous organs other than in the gastrointestinal tract, tumor diameter has been employed as an index that indicates the stage of the disease.

However, gastrointestinal tumors exhibit a variety of growth types and invasion patterns. Thus, the tumor size (tumor diameter) measured with the conventional methods does not always accurately reflect the true tumor size (tumor volumes). As a result, tumor size (tumor diameter) is not considered when the tumor is staged (Kikuchi *et al.*, 2000b). On the other hand, if gastrointestinal tumor volumes could be assessed, then tumor volume could become a significant factor for determining the degree of tumor malignancy. There are several ways to reconstruct the morphology of gastrointestinal tumors into three-dimensional tumor structures and to measure tumor volume. First, the resected tumors can be used to provide two-dimensional data; in fact, the authors have reconstructed three-dimensional structures of lesions using computer graphic techniques. Subsequently, based on the three-dimensional models, the tumor volumes were determined by the surface rendering method, and the tumors were examined from a variety of angles to evaluate their clinical significance. Given our results, we concluded that tumor size in gastric cancer (tumor volume) has (1) a good correlation to the staging of the disease, including lymph node metastasis, and (2) is an important factor for determining prognosis. These results suggest that tumor volume in gastric cancer may be an important factor for determining

the degree of malignancy (Kikuchi *et al.*, 2000a; Kikuchi *et al.*, 2000c; Kikuchi *et al.*, 2001a; Kikuchi *et al.*, 2001b). Furthermore, the authors recently completed preoperative evaluations using three- dimensional endoscopic ultrasonography (3D-EUS) and three-dimensional computer tomography (3D-CT). The report also discussed the possible clinical use of these techniques for diagnosis (Kikuchi *et al.*, 2005). In the future, it would be desirable to establish an accurate diagnostic technique to routinely determine 3D tumor structure and volume using preoperative 3D-EUS and MD-CT.

Problems in Staging Classification

The two current staging classifications for gastrointestinal tumors, the TNM classification and the Japanese Classification of Gastric Cancer staging, use a combination of T (Tumor), N (Lymph Nodes), and M (Metastases). The use of these systems makes it very complicated to reach an outcome. In particular, it is difficult to accurately diagnose tumor staging and lymph node metastases preoperatively, since an objective assessment is difficult. Furthermore, standard criteria have not yet been established for classifying lymph node metastases. (The number of metastases is determined by the TNM classification, and the anatomical position of the metastases is classified by the JCGC.) Moreover, according to the current classification, tumor staging may be easily influenced by the extent of the surgical resection, especially the extent of the lymph node dissection, and by the use of different pathological tests, especially for lymph node metastases (Bodner *et al.*, 1988; Isozaki *et al.*, 1997). In order to deal with these problems, it would be ideal if the factors used to determine the degree of malignancy of a specific tumor could be assessed both pre- and postoperatively in an objective manner. The authors would suggest that if size (volume) were a significant factor with respect to the degree of malignancy, then it would be possible to create a totally new, simple, and rational staging classification for gastrointestinal tumors that was based on tumor volume. Thus a patient's treatment could be determined based on this staging.

Preoperative Three-Dimensional Structure and Volumetry of Gastrointestinal Tumors

Upper abdominal 3D-CT (MD-CT): During this examination, the patient, who is generally in a supine position, receives a contrast agent (Omnipaque, Daiichi Pharmaceutical Co., Japan) by intravenous drip infusion at a dose of 2 ml/kg. Subsequently, a gas-forming agent (Baros, Horii Co., Japan) is given, and the patient is scanned using a 32 × MD-CT (Aquilion, Toshiba Co., Japan) set at 0.5 mm slices. Three-dimensional reconstruction of the tumor is done using the 2D data of the tumor contour traced at 3-mm intervals. The imaging process and the calculation of tumor volume are performed according to the protocol of the workstation software (ZIO, AMIN, Japan).

Three-dimensional-EUS: Using an upper gastrointestinal endoscope (GIF 1T240, Olympus, Japan), a three-dimensional ultrasonography endoscope probe (DP 20-25R, Olympus, Japan) is inserted through the side channel for examination. A 3D structure of the tumor is drawn based on data obtained on scanning with a 20 MHz transducer at a 0.5-mm pitch in a scanning range of 40 mm. In order to measure the volume of the tumor, a computer imaging analysis system (Endoecho system, Olympus, Japan) reconstructed the 3D tumor image according to a protocol that is based on the two-dimensional data of the tumor contour traced at 2-mm intervals. Figure 1 shows a virtual endoscopy image and a computer gastrography image of a Borrmann type 2 advanced gastric cancer (84-year-old female patient) located in the gastric vestibular

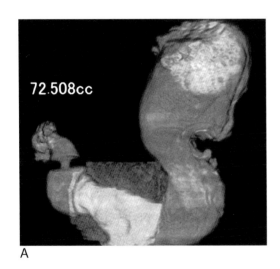

A

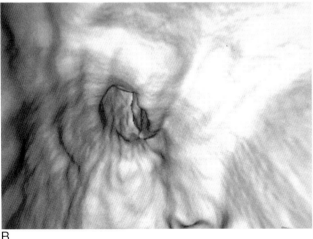

B

Figure 1 Preoperative diagnosis in an 84-year-old female with advanced gastric cancer (Borrmann type 2) on MD-CT. **(A)** The findings of the MD-CT examination (tumor volume, 72.5 cm³). **(B)** The findings on virtual gastroscopy derived by CT scans[3].

posterior wall based on the MD-CT image. The volume of the tumor was 72.5 cm³ as measured using the method that was previously described. Figure 2 shows a 2D lateral sectional image of an early gastric cancer IIa (71-year-old male patient) located in the corpus ventriculi lower vestibular based on 3D ultrasonography images. The volume of the tumor was 373.9 mm³ as measured by the method that was previously described. Based on our investigations to date, the identification and imaging of a lesion by MD-CT were found to be suitable for use in advanced gastric cancer, while 3D ultrasonography was found to be suitable for use in early-stage gastric cancer. Therefore, at present, we do 3D ultrasonography for early gastric cancer and MD-CT for advanced gastric cancer as part of our routine examinations in order to precisely measure the 3D structure of the tumor and to determine tumor volume. Given our encouraging results to date, in the future we plan to study more cases and further investigate the clinical significance of the two diagnostic methods, as well as to identify the possibe practical clinical applications of these diagnostic methods.

Future Prospects

In patients with a gastrointestinal tumor, an accurate assessment of the local stage of the lesion and the status of metastases in the surrounding area are important for determining an appropriate therapeutic strategy. Currently, gastrointestinal imaging examinations and gastrointestinal endoscopy are done to determine whether a tumor is present and to make a diagnosis (primarily with respect to gross appearances and tumor depth). Recently, ultrasonography has become useful for diagnosing the depth of tumor invasion. However, these modalities have limited diagnostic abilities. Furthermore, the assessment is largely subjective, and there are significant differences in the diagnoses made depending on the operator's degree of experience and technical skill.

Presently, the measurement of tumor volume using 3D ultrasonography and the three-dimensional reconstruction of tumors by MD-CT take the 2D data that were obtained and determine a 2D tumor contour from which a 3-D image is obtained. Thus, even these diagnostic methods also appear to be subjective assessments. With further technological advancement, however, a system in which the 2D region of the lesions can be assessed automatically could be developed based on computer image recognition functions. Thus, we can expect that the volume of gastrointestinal tumor can be assessed objectively. A new staging system for gastrointestinal tumors based on tumor volume could be the basis of an internationally common staging classification that would be much simpler and more rational than the conventional staging classification currently in use. Along with the establishment of a new diagnostic approach based on the volume of gastrointestinal tumor, a new approach will likely be found

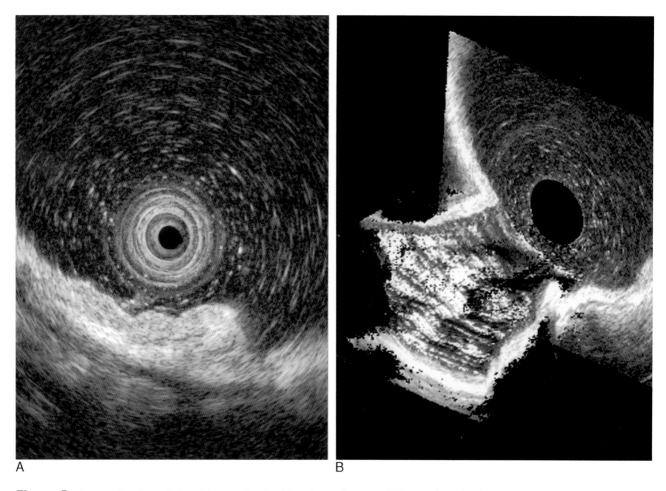

A   B

Figure 2 Preoperative diagnosis in a 77-year-old male with early gastric cancer (IIa) on endoscopic ultrasonography. (**A**) The findings on 2D endoscopic ultrasonography (image of lateral section). (**B**) The findings on 3D endoscopic ultrasonography (tumor volume, 373.9 mm³).

for treatment. We expect further progress and technological improvement in this field. In conclusion, given that the 3D structure of a gastrointestinal tumor and the tumor's volume can be measured preoperatively by 3D-EUS and MD-CT, these new diagnostic methods should be used for patient staging. This suggests the possibility of finding important new factors that could help determine both the treatment strategies and the prognosis. We are working on establishing the ability to accurately diagnose tumors by using 3D gastro-intestinal tumor images and to determine tumor volumes by using 3D-EUS and MD-CT, which are done as routine pre-operative procedures. In addition, we are working on estab-lishing the practical application of these approaches.

References

Bodner, B.E. 1988. Will Rogers and gastric carcinoma. *Arch. Surg. 123*:1023–1024.

Iannaccone, R., Catalano, C., Mangiapane, F., Murakami, T., Lamazza, A., Fiori, E., Schillaci, A., Marin, D., Nofroni, I., Hori, M., and Passariello, R. 2005. Colorectal polyps: detection with low-dose multi-detector row CT colonog-raphy versus two sequential colonoscopies. *Radiology 237*:927–937.

Isozaki, H., Okajima, K., and Fujii, K. 1997. Histological evaluation of lymph node metastasis on serial sectioning in gastric cancer with radical lymphadenectomy. *Hepatogastroenterology 44*:1133–1136.

Japanese Research Society for Gastric Cancer. 1995. *Japanese Classifica-tion of Gastric Carcinoma* (1st English ed.). Tokyo: Kanehara; 1–71.

Kikuchi, S., Sakuramoto, S., Kobayashi, N., Shimao, H., Sakakibara, Y., Sato, K., and Kakita, A. 2000a. Tumor volumetry: proposal of a new concept to predict lymph node metastasis in early gastric cancer. *Anti-cancer Res. 20*:3669–3674.

Kikuchi, S., Hiki, Y., Sakakibara, Y., Kakita, A., and Kuwao, S. 2000b. Measuring the tumor volume of gastric carcinoma by computer image analysis: clinical significance. *World J. Surg. 24*:603–607.

Kikuchi, S., Hiki, Y., Shimao, H., Sakakibara, Y., and Kakita, A. 2000c. Tumor volume: a novel prognostic factor in patients who undergo curative resection for gastric cancer. *Langenbeck's Arch. Surg. 385*:225–228.

Kikuchi, S., Matsuzaki, H., Kurita, A., Kobayashi, N., Shimao, H., Sakakibara, Y., Sato, K., and Kakita A. 2001a. Tumor volume as an indicator of nodal status in advanced gastric carcinoma. *In Vivo 15*: 295–298.

Kikuchi, S., Sakuramoto, S., Kobayashi, N., Shimao, H., Sakakibara, Y., Sato, K., and Kakita, A. 2001b. A new staging system based on tumor volume in gastric cancer. *Anticancer Res. 21*:2933–2936.

Kikuchi, S., Kida, M., Kobayashi, K., Yano, T., Sakuramoto, S., Watanabe, M., Kubota, K., and Isobe, Y. 2005. New diagnostic imaging of gastrointestinal tumors: a preliminary study of three-dimensional tumor structure and volumetry. *Anticancer Res. 25*:2935–2942.

Kim, H.C., Han, M.H., Do, K.H., Kim, K.H., Choi, H.J., Kim, A.Y., Sung, M.W., and Chang, K.H. 2002. Volume of cervical lymph nodes using 3D ultrasonography differentiation of metastatic from reactive lymphadenopathy in primary head and neck malignancy. *Acta Radiol. 43*:571–574.

Roder, J.D., Boettcher, K., Siewert, J.R., Busch, R., Hermanek, P., Meyer, H.J., and the German Gastric Carcinoma Study Group. 1993. Prognostic factors in gastric carcinoma: results of the German Gastric Carcinoma Study Group. *Cancer 72*:2089–2097.

Sobin, L.H., and Wittekind, C. 2002. *TNM Classification of Malignant Tumors* (6ᵗʰ ed.). New York: Wiley and Sons; 57–80.

Tsutsui, A., Okamura, S., Muguruma, N., Tsujigami, K., Ichikawa, S., Ito, S., and Umino, K. 2005. Three-dimensional reconstruction of endosonographic images of gastric lesions: preliminary experience. *J. Clin. Ultrasound 33*:112–118.

Watanabe, M., Kida, M., Yamada, Y., and Saigenji, K. 2004. Measuring tumor volume with three-dimensional endoscopic sonography: an experimental and clinical study. *Endoscopy 36*:976–981.

Wessling, J., Domagk, D., Lugering, N., Schierhorn, S., Heindel, W., Domschke, W., and Fischbach, R. 2005. Virtual colonoscopy: identification and differentiation of colorectal lesions using multi-detector computed tomography. *Scand. J. Gastroenterol. 40*:468–476.

Wu, C.W., Hsieh, M.C., Lo, S.S., Tsay, S.H., Li, A.F., Lui, W.Y., and P'eng, F.K. 1997. Prognostic indicators for survival after curative resection for patients with carcinoma of the stomach. *Dig. Dis. Sci. 42*:1265–1269.

Yetter, E., Acosta, K.B., Olson, M.C., and Blundell, K. 2003. Estimating splenic volume: sonographic measurements correlated with helical CT determination. *Am. J. Roentgenol. 181*:1615–1620.

19

Magnetic Resonance Cholangiopancreatography

Kevin J. Chang and Laura M. Fayad

Introduction

Magnetic resonance cholangiopancreatography (MRCP) plays an important role in the diagnosis of abnormalities of the pancreatic and biliary tract. While initially proven as the most reliable noninvasive imaging modality in depicting intraductal calculi, MRCP has also come into its own in the work-up of pancreatic and biliary malignancies. This chapter will discuss the basic principles, techniques, and pitfalls encountered in performing and reading MRCP. The findings of pancreatic neoplasms such as adenocarcinoma, islet cell and other neuroendocrine tumors, and cystic neoplasms, including serous and mucinous cystadenoma/cystadenocarcinomas as well as intraductal papillary mucinous neoplasms (IPMN), will be illustrated. Biliary tract malignancies, including gallbladder carcinoma, cholangiocarcinomas, and ampullary tumors, will also be presented. Lastly, experimental variants on MR imaging of the biliary and pancreatic tract will be discussed.

Magnetic resonance cholangiopancreatography is a relatively recent advance in pancreaticobiliary tract imaging, originally introduced in 1991, that has now found its place in oncologic imaging (Wallner *et al.*, 1991). In many cases, MRCP has supplanted endoscopic retrograde cholangiopancreatography (ERCP) and percutaneous transhepatic cholangiography (PTC) in the initial diagnostic evaluation and follow-up of diseases of the pancreas, gallbladder, and biliary tract. This is largely due to its noninvasive nature, avoiding possible complications that may occur with more invasive imaging such as pancreatitis, duodenal perforation, hemorrhage, sepsis, as well as the associated risks of sedation (Bilbao *et al.*, 1976). Overall, costs associated with MRCP are lower than those with ERCP or PTC. Magnetic resonance cholangiopancreatography does not utilize ionizing X-ray radiation like ERCP or PTC, and does not require the same degree of operator skill or patient preparation. The ductal diameter is often more accurately portrayed as the duct is not artificially distended with administered contrast. The failure rate is also much lower than that for ERCP (which is 3–10%), being limited only by factors such as patient cooperativity and ability to breath hold (Bilbao *et al.*, 1976).

Magnetic resonance cholangiopancreatography has become the technique of choice in patients with factors contributing to a high failure rate for ERCP, such as esophageal, gastric, or duodenal obstruction, stricturing or edema of the ampulla of Vater, periampullary duodenal diverticuli, or postsurgical bowel reconstruction such as choledochoenteric or pancreaticoenteric anastamoses or gastrojejunostomy (Adamek *et al.*, 1997). MRCP is especially excellent at depicting ductal anatomy beyond an obstructing lesion, which is impossible to demonstrate by ERCP. Magnetic resonance cholangiopancreatography is absolutely the test of choice in patients who have an incomplete or failed ERCP.

413

When MRCP is combined with traditional T1- and T2-weighted cross-sectional imaging sequences as well as pre- and post-gadolinium contrast imaging (as is routinely done at many institutions), extraductal disease of the liver, pancreas, or porta hepatis can also be evaluated. In fact, at our institution, an MRCP is rarely performed in the absence of traditional axial T1- and T2-weighted sequences as well as post-gadolinium contrast imaging.

Although MRCP lacks the direct therapeutic and pathologic diagnostic advantages of ERCP, MRCP can preprocedurally guide these more invasive tests. Magnetic resonance cholangiopancreatography also does not have as high a spatial resolution as ERCP and, thus, may not detect the earliest of ductal abnormalities, especially in small peripheral ducts. It may also be difficult to distinguish malignant from benign causes of obstruction using MRCP alone (which is why MRCP is often combined with traditional contrast-enhanced MRI of the abdomen for evaluation of extraductal tissues).

Principles, Techniques, and Pitfalls

Magnetic resonance cholangiopancreatography takes advantage of the inherent T2-weighted contrast that exists between intra-abdominal slow-flow fluid-containing structures and the background organs and soft tissues. Fluids in the biliary and pancreatic tree as well as the bowel have much longer T2 relaxation times than adjacent soft tissues. As a result, heavily T2-weighted sequences will depict these structures with a much higher relative signal intensity compared to background organ parenchyma and adjacent fat (which have shorter T2 relaxation times). Sequences with a particularly long TE (echo time) aid in suppressing background signal and increasing the relative contrast of fluid-containing structures (higher CNR or contrast-to-noise ratio).

A variety of approaches have been used for heavily T2-weighted imaging of the biliary and pancreatic tree, many resulting in images that mimic the appearance of a traditional ERCP or PTC. Images are typically obtained in the coronal, axial, and/or coronal oblique planes using both thick slabs (Fig. 1) and multiple contiguous adjacent thin slabs (Fig. 2). Axial scout images are typically obtained first, followed by coronal and coronal oblique planes that are prescribed from these axial images. Coronal and coronal oblique planes tend to demonstrate the hepatic biliary tree distinctly. Axial as well as coronal oblique planes are particularly clear at demonstrating the pancreatic ducts.

Thick- and thin-slab acquisitions are complementary. Approximately 30- to 80-mm thick slabs are an easily accessible way to evaluate overall ductal anatomy and to evaluate ductal caliber but may mask fine details, especially small intraductal filling defects and configuration of areas of obstruction or structuring due to obscuration by adjacent high signal intensity bile. Overlapping fluid-filled structures

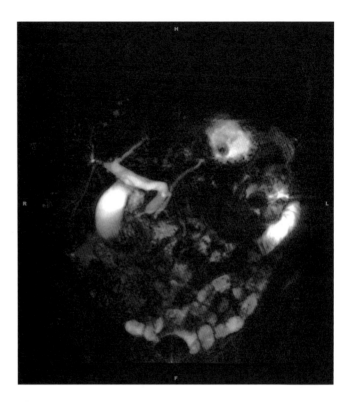

Figure 1 Thick-slab MRCP sequence performed in coronal plane shows a periampullary stricture with dilated common bile duct proximally.

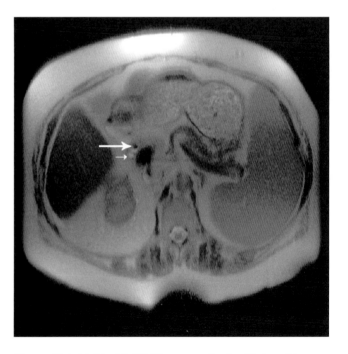

Figure 2 Axial thin-slab MRCP sequence showing dilation of the common bile duct, a low cystic duct, take-off (small arrow), and a filling defect in the common bile duct, which represents a focus of pneumobilia (long arrow).

(i.e., duodenum, stomach, renal, and hepatic cysts) may also mask an adjacent duct. Use of a long TE and/or fat saturation eliminate background signal from intra-abdominal and subcutaneous fat, resulting in fluid-only images similar to an ERCP (Fig. 1). Use of a T2 negative oral contrast agent such as ferric ammonium citrate and/or keeping the patient (Nil Per Os) for at least 4 hr may also decrease the fluid signal from the adjacent bowel. Keeping the patient NPO also aids in slowing duodenal peristalsis and promoting gallbladder filling (Vitellas *et al.*, 2000).

Multislice 2–5 mm thin-slab acquisitions using the 2D or 3D technique help to eliminate the effect of volume averaging and to define points of obstruction as to etiology (i.e., strictures vs. stones vs. extrinsic mass effect). Multislice images may also be reformatted in other planes and into maximum intensity projection (MIP) and volume-rendered projections. Imaging without fat saturation allows for evaluation of organ contours against the background of intra-abdominal fat and also allows for better visualization of periductal anatomy. As each slice is typically obtained as a sub-second acquisition, there is very little intraslice motion artifact. However, there may be slice-to-slice misregistration from respiration during two-dimensional acquisitions. Slice-to-slice misregistration may be resolved through use of respiratory triggering or gating through use of a respiratory bellows or torso strap, or through use of navigator pulses that directly monitor movement of the diaphragm. The latter technique is the one we use at our institution where a small "imaging strip" is centered over the right diaphragm, and the point at which the abdomen is most still (typically end-expiration) is the point during which the single-shot fast spin-echo sequences are triggered to be acquired.

Current techniques usually include use of ultrafast breath-hold pulse sequences such as single-shot fast spin-echo (SSFSE) and half-Fourier acquisition short TE (HASTE). These sequences allow 1–2 sec acquisitions with submillimeter resolution (256×224 matrix with 24-cm field of view). The speed of imaging "freezes" anatomic motion, decreasing the amount of artifact from peristalsis and respiration. This also allows for dynamic imaging of the biliary and pancreatic ducts, critical as a contracted sphincter of Oddi may be confused with an ampullary stricture or even tumor. Obtaining multiple coronal and/or coronal oblique images over time at the level of the ampulla of Vater increases the chances of imaging during transient relaxation of the sphincter, which excludes the presence of a stricture, obstructing mass, or sphincter of Oddi dysfunction. Dynamic imaging may also be combined with use of intravenously administered secretin to evaluate pancreatic function and excretion and aid in distension of normal pancreatic ducts (see "Experimental Techniques").

Other pulse sequences have also been used for MRCP, including two-dimensional and three-dimensional breath-averaged fast spin echo (FSE) as well as three-dimensional FSE with echo-planar imaging (EPI). Although these techniques may result in higher SNR and CNR, breath-averaging techniques remain susceptible to motion artifact from respiration and peristalsis. As previously mentioned, traditional axial T1- and T2-weighted images as well as T1-weighted gradient-echo fat-saturated images before and after gadolinium IV contrast are performed following acquisition of MRCP images. Such images are complementary and offer additional information about the parenchyma of the liver and pancreas as well as aid in evaluation of focal masses adjacent to as well as separate from the biliary and pancreatic ducts.

Pitfalls in imaging, in addition to contraction of the sphincter of Oddi, include susceptibility artifact from adjacent surgical clips (i.e., cholecystectomy clips or prior gastrointensinal or pancreatic surgery), stents, bowel gas, or pneumobilia. These materials result in loss of signal in adjacent tissues (including fluid-filled ducts) which may simulate obstruction. Correlation to plain films and/or CT as well as comparison with gradient-echo images are often helpful in confirming this cause of artifact. Pulsation artifact from adjacent vessels, biliary flow-related artifact, physiologic compression from a crossing hepatic artery, as well as intraductal debris or blood may also mimic a stenosis/stricture or stone (Fulcher and Turner, 1998; Watanabe *et al.*, 1999).

Pancreas

Pancreatic Adenocarcinoma

The major interest in performing MR pancreatography is in the evaluation of the pancreas and pancreatic duct. Adenocarcinoma represents 75 to 90% of all cases of pancreatic cancer; 70% are located in the pancreatic head, 20% in the pancreatic body, and 10% in the pancreatic tail (Molinari *et al.*, 2001; Brennan *et al.*, 1996). A common finding at MRCP is the "double duct sign" in which both the pancreatic and common bile ducts are dilated (Fig. 3). While this sign is sensitive and specific for pancreatic cancer (typically due to a mass at the head of the pancreas), this finding may be present in cases of focal pancreatitis of the pancreatic head as well as other benign causes of stricturing. "Courvoisier's sign" is another imaging finding where a distended and nontender gallbladder is present in the setting of an obstructing tumor. A focal mass typically causes a very abrupt narrowing and proximal dilatation of the common bile duct and/or pancreatic duct when the mass involves the pancreas. An obstructing stone, sludge, or debris often has a very different ductal appearance, with a "meniscus sign" or direct visualization of an intraductal calculus on MRCP images. An intraductal calculus is often easier to visualize on thin-section 3D MRCP source images in either the coronal or axial planes than on thick-slab MRCP images, as adjacent T2 hyperintense bile and pancreatic juices around the calculus may

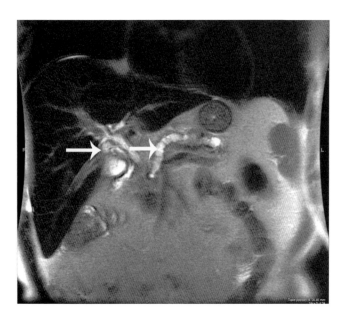

Figure 3 Coronal thin-slab MRCP sequence showing the classic double-duct sign (arrows) associated with pancreatic adenocarcinoma.

obscure the underlying hypointense stone (especially true on MIP images). Note that 20% of pancreatic adenocarcinomas may show no pancreatic ductal dilatation in the setting of biliary ductal dilatation. This tends to occur with masses in the pancreatic head proximal to the confluence of the duct of Wirsung (ventral duct) with the common bile duct at the ampulla of Vater.

The finding of a focal mass-like area of hypoenhancement in the pancreatic parenchyma with decreased T1-weighted signal intensity and variable T2-weighted signal intensity is very suggestive of a mass such as an adenocarcinoma. However, focal pancreatitis may also present in a similar way. Fat suppression on T1-weighted images aids in accentuating signal intensity differences of solid pancreatic neoplasms from normally T1 hyperintense pancreatic parenchyma. Enhancement of the tumor is delayed compared to background parenchyma and demonstrates gradual enhancement on delayed postcontrast imaging. Larger tumors may also cause focal enlargement of the pancreas or distortion of the pancreatic contour as well as textural changes in the normally "marbled" or "feathery" appearance on MR.

When there is a correlative clinical history of chronic pancreatitis or alcohol abuse, cancer and pancreatitis may be very difficult to differentiate. Findings that would suggest alcoholic chronic pancreatitis rather than cancer-causing ductal obstruction and dilatation would be the presence of irregularity in the ductal wall and caliber as well as the presence of ductal calcification (often seen as filling defects in the duct). Autoimmune pancreatitis may be present without any prior history of alcohol abuse and can manifest on imaging as main duct narrowing and focal or diffuse

parenchymal abnormality without associated ductal calcification (Salres, 1974; Van Hoe *et al.*, 1998). However, an adenocarcinoma may arise in the setting of chronic pancreatitis with pancreatic calcifications. Cancer tends to cause a smooth distension of the duct proximal/upstream to the level of obstruction and also tends to cause a larger amount of ductal distension relative to the size of the obstructing mass. A common finding with adenocarcinoma in addition to ductal dilatation is associated atrophy of the gland proximal to the level of obstruction. This manifests through decrease in the amount of parenchymal tissue as well as increase in fatty infiltration of the proximal pancreas (e.g., atrophy of the pancreatic body and tail in the case of a pancreatic head mass). The "duct penetrating sign" is a finding where a nonobstructed pancreatic duct is visualized penetrating an inflammatory pseudomass in focal pancreatitis (Ichikawa *et al.*, 2001). When these signs still cannot differentiate an adenocarcinoma from focal pancreatitis, treatment for pancreatitis followed by repeat imaging may help to document resolution of pancreatitis or interval growth of an underlying adenocarcinoma as an adenocarcinoma may arise in the setting of chronic pancreatitis or may represent the cause of an acute pancreatitis.

Factors crucial to evaluate in the setting of a suspected pancreatic adenocarcinoma are any findings that may preclude surgical resection (pancreaticoduodenectomy or Whipple procedure, or a distal pancreatectomy and splenectomy). These include vascular involvement of structures such as the celiac axis or hepatic artery, superior mesenteric artery and vein, or portal vein. Involvement of the splenic artery or vein is usually not a contraindication to a distal pancreatectomy as many surgeons will resect the splenic artery and vein in addition to performing a splenectomy when these structures are involved. More aggressive surgeons may still consider surgical resection if involvement of vessels is confined to the portal or superior mesenteric veins, as segmental resection of these veins followed by reanastamosis or reconstruction may still result in satisfactory outcomes (van Greenen *et al.*, 2001). Other contraindications to surgery include involvement of any adjacent tissues other than the duodenum (which gets resected with the pancreas during a Whipple procedure due to its shared blood supply), distant metastases such as of the liver and lymph nodes, and peritoneal or omental implants. While pancreatic adenocarcinomas may approach very close to the vicinity of a vessel due to the intimate relationship of the pancreas (especially the pancreatic head) to many of the above-mentioned vessels, actual involvement is not defined unless there has been disruption of any intervening fat planes and involvement of > 180° of the circumference of the blood vessel. Abrupt changes in the caliber of a blood vessel adjacent to a tumor are also consistent with vascular compromise.

In evaluation of the pancreas for adenocarcinoma, the MRCP protocol at our institution also includes imaging the entire liver before and after the administration of gadolinium contrast to detect metastases and local lymphadenopathy. Liver metastases may be variable in appearance but usually behave similarly to the primary pancreatic tumor, with relative hypoenhancement compared to the liver parenchyma and delayed wash-in of contrast. Cross-sectional imaging such as CT and MRI has traditionally not been very accurate in the detection and characterization of lymphadenopathy as the primary imaging criteria used in determining lymph node involvement is the size of the short axis of a node. Small nodes may still contain metastatic disease and not be detectable on anatomic imaging alone, and larger nodes may still represent reactive lymphadenopathy rather than metastasis (functional imaging may hold promise in more sensitive and specific detection of metastatic disease). Affected nodes are best detected on fat-saturated T2-weighted images, with T2 hyperintense lymph nodes measuring 1 cm or larger in short-axis dimension remaining suspicious for malignant involvement. The presence of enlarged lymph nodes is not itself a contraindication to surgical resection. As surgery is generally the patient's only chance for a complete cure, unless there are any radiologic findings that represent clear contraindications to surgery, the benefit of the doubt is usually given to the patient in staging pancreatic adenocarcinoma.

Pancreatic Neuroendocrine Tumors

The other solid pancreatic neoplasm that is much less commonly encountered than adenocarcinoma is the islet cell tumor. This tumor tends to behave much differently from adenocarcinomas in that it shows homogeneous hypervascularity and enhances to a greater degree than background pancreatic parenchyma during arterial-phase imaging. This tumor also tends to show hyperintense elements on T2-weighted images and is hypointense on T1-weighted images. Both functional and nonfunctional islet cell tumors may be identified, with most nonfunctional tumors presenting much larger and later due to lack of early warning from hormonal side effects. Overall, the most common islet cell tumor is the functional insulinoma (Fig. 4), accounting for 50% of all neuroendocrine tumors of the pancreas. Ninety percent of these are benign and, even with MRI imaging, may be difficult to detect preoperatively due to their early presentation, small size, and lack of mass effect on parenchymal contours and adjacent pancreatic duct.

Gastrinomas are the second most common neuroendocrine tumor, accounting for 30%; they appear larger at presentation than insulinomas, with an average size of 4 cm. Of these tumors, 60 to 80% are malignant, although these neoplasms tend to follow a more slowly progressive and indolent course, especially in Zollinger-Ellison syndrome. These tumors may also be found outside the pancreas in the region of the second and third portions of the duodenum, especially in cases associated with multiple endocrine neoplasia type

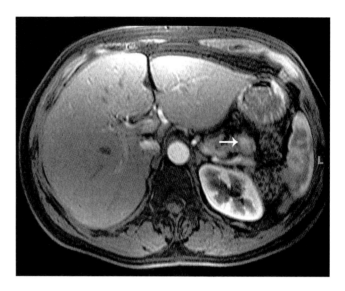

Figure 4 Axial thin-slab MRCP sequence showing an enhancing mass in the tail of the pancreas (arrow), a proven adenocarcinoma.

1 (MEN-1). This region of involvement by gastrinomas is often termed the "gastrinoma triangle" bound by the porta hepatis superiorly, and the second and third portions of the duodenum laterally and inferiorly.

Other functional islet cell neoplasms include the much less common glucagonoma, VIPoma (vasoactive intestinal polypeptide producing tumor), and somatostatinomas. These tumors typically present at 3–5 cm in size due to the nonspecific nature of their hormonal symptoms and are usually malignant.

Nonfunctional islet cell tumors either present from symptoms secondary to mass effect and pain or may be discovered incidentally. As these tumors do not secrete hormones that may cause symptoms, they often present much later in their course, and as a result often present > 6–10 cm in size. Due to their size and late presentation, these tumors are usually more heterogeneous on T2-weighted images and heterogeneous in enhancement due to areas of central necrosis and cystic degeneration. As a result, these tumors may be more difficult to differentiate from adenocarcinomas, metastases, and cystic pancreatic neoplasms (discussed below). Approximately one-half of these tumors are malignant. The second goal of imaging in cases of islet cell tumors is to metastases to the liver, lymph nodes, or bone/spine. As such, MR work-ups for islet cell tumors should include images of the entire liver. Liver metastases from islet cell tumors enhance early (arterial phase) similar to the primary tumor. Often, detection of metastases to the liver may be the initial imaging presentation prior to detection of the pancreatic primary itself.

Carcinoid Tumor

The carcinoid tumor is a neuroendocrine tumor that rarely arises from the pancreas. At presentation, they are typically very large and very heterogeneous and usually have coexistent liver metastases of variable size. While the liver metastases are typically hypervascular demonstrating early arterial-phase enhancement, the pancreatic primary may not necessarily be hypervascular. Enhancement patterns of the pancreatic primary are often more heterogeneous even when showing early arterial-phase enhancement. They are typically T1 hypointense and mildly T2 hyperintense (Semelka *et al.*, 2000).

Cystic Pancreatic Neoplasms

During the last decade, the incidence of cystic lesions detected in the pancreas has increased dramatically, most likely directly related to the increasing use of cross-sectional imaging in the abdomen. Estimates of the incidence of cystic pancreatic lesions among patients with a history of pancreatitis can be as high as 20% (Zhang *et al.*, 2002). Most of these lesions represent pseudocysts, the most common cystic mass in and around the pancreas, representing up to 90% of cystic masses in the pancreas. Their etiology is ductal disruption or microperforation of the pancreatic duct or side-branches with resulting enzymatic tissue destruction of the adjacent parenchyma and soft tissues. While many of these pseudocysts do demonstrate communication with the pancreatic duct, ERCP only detects 50% of pseudocysts; 60% of pseudocysts will eventually resolve spontaneously over time. The surgical definition of a pseudocyst has traditionally involved documenting the presence of a focal rounded/organized pancreatic or peripancreatic fluid collection for 6 weeks or longer. Surgery is generally reserved for pseudocysts that are enlarging or hemorrhaging. Hemorrhage is well demonstrated on MR as areas of T1 hyperintensity and T2 signal heterogeneity.

All cystic lesions in the pancreas demonstrate high signal intensity on T2-weighted images (including MRCP images) due to the long T2 relaxation time of fluid-containing structures and low signal intensity on T1-weighted images. Ten percent of pancreatic cystic lesions are true neoplasms, which will be classified below according to a variety of factors including location, cyst size, serous versus mucinous contents, and degree of epithelial dedifferentiation. Keep in mind, however, that other neoplasms not traditionally categorized as cystic may also develop cystic components, including adenocarcinomas. However, MRCP is an excellent technique in the detecting of the following masses, but full characterization still requires the use of pre- and postgadolinium contrast imaging of the pancreas. Aspiration of pseudocysts yields a sample rich in amylase.

Serous (Microcystic) Cystadenoma

Serous cystadenomas (see Fig. 5) are benign parenchymal tumors found anywhere throughout the pancreatic parenchyma, from head *through* tail. They represent 25% of

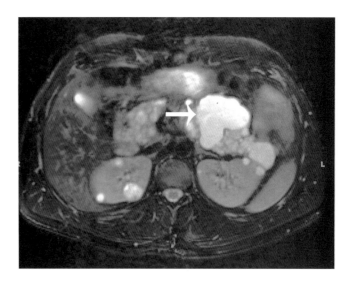

Figure 5 Axial thin-slab MRCP sequence in a patient with von Hippel-Lindau disease shows multiple pancreatic cysts as well as a pancreatic tail serous cystadenoma (arrow).

cystic neoplasms and are classically found in asymptomatic elderly females (80% > 60 years of age), though many also present in patients with von Hippel-Lindau disease. Serous cystadenomas are typically composed of at least 6 cysts each, measuring 2 cm or less in diameter, and often demonstrate a fibrous central stellate scar. This cluster of small cysts often resembles a "cluster of grapes." While typically T1 hypointense and T2 hyperintense, hemorrhagic components may result in areas of T1 hyperintensity and T2 variability. Approximately 40% of these tumors may demonstrate calcification, with 15% manifesting calcification within the central scar. These tumors may also have a very hypervascular solid soft tissue component. Percutaneous or endoscopically guided aspiration of these tumors characteristically yields large amounts of glycogen, clearly differentiating these neoplasms from the often similar-appearing mucinous cystic neoplasms.

These neoplasms do not communicate with the pancreatic duct but, if large enough, may often show enough mass effect on the adjacent duct to result in obstruction. Serous cystadenomas also do not invade vascular structures. If found to do so, then consideration should be made for the rare malignant serous cystadenocarcinoma that may not only locally invade adjacent structures but may also metastasize to distant parts of the body. Because these latter neoplasms often cannot be differentiated from cystadenomas, continued imaging surveillance or preemptive operative resection in surgical candidates may be advocated.

Mucinous (Macrocystic) Cystic Neoplasms

These cystic neoplasms are approximately half as common as serous cystadenomas and, contrary to the benign serous cystadenoma, are all either malignant or potentially malignant. These mucinous tumors range in spectrum from the "benign" mucinous cystadenoma to the malignant mucinous cystadenocarcinoma. Due to their malignant potential, however, typically these tumors are surgically excised for cure. Almost all of these tumors tend to occur in middle-aged women (the ratio of the tumor between men and women is 1:9), with tumors that histologically resemble ovarian cystadenocarcinomas in that an underlying ovarian-like stroma may demonstrate thick papillary projections. These tumors have a predilection for the pancreatic body or tail and tend to be larger than serous cystadenomas. Their typical imaging appearance differs from serous neoplasms in that they are either unilocular or contain six or fewer cysts, each measuring > 2 cm in size. Similar to serous neoplasms, areas of internal hemorrhage or proteinacious/mucinous contents within the cysts may alter their T1 and T2 signal intensity (blood manifesting as areas of T1 hyperintensity). When unilocular, serous cystadenomas/cystadenocarcinomas may be entirely indistinguishable from pseudocysts by imaging alone. Aspiration of these tumors results in mucin-rich viscous fluid with elevated CEA levels, a clearer way to differentiate these tumors from serous cystadenomas and pseudocysts.

Twenty-five percent of these tumors may demonstrate calcification (better visualized by CT), however, contrary to serous cystadenomas, the calcification is typically thin and rim-like in the periphery. If the walls and calcifications are thicker or if there are nodular mural hypovascular soft tissue components, the risk of malignancy is higher. Even more helpful is ancillary information on serum CA 19-9 and CEA levels. (The former has been shown to be 75% sensitive and 96% specific in detecting mucinous neoplasms as well as adenocarcinomas) (Sperti *et al.*, 1996).

Intraductal Papillary Mucinous Neoplasms (IPMN)

Intraductal papillary mucinous neoplasms (IPMNs) (see Fig. 6) are also mucinous cystic lesions of the pancreas, which, histologically, may range from areas of epithelial hyperplasia to areas of adenomatous change to carcinoma *in situ* to outright invasive carcinoma. Multiple other pseudonyms have been used, including intraductal papillary mucinous tumors (IPMT), ductectatic cystadenoma, and mucinous ductal ectasia. Twenty-three percent may be multiple, and, unlike other mucinous neoplasms, all communicate with the pancreatic ductal tree (Megibow *et al.*, 2001). On MRCP, IPMNs characteristically show ductal dilatation or cyst formation of either a segmental or diffuse distribution.

Intraductal papillary mucinous neoplasms are classified into two categories: main duct IPMNs and side-branch or branch-duct IPMNs. The former are generally histologically more often malignant than the latter. Unlike adenocarcinomas, ductal dilatation with IPMNs tends to be around

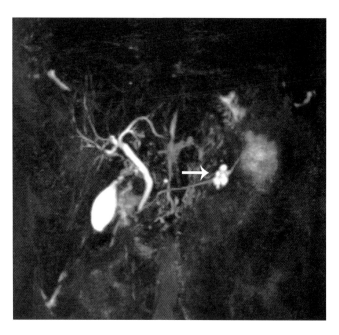

Figure 6 Coronal oblique 3D MIP MRCP image shows an IPMN as a multilobulated cystic mass (arrow) in the tail of the pancreas, associated with pancreatic ductal dilation in the tail.

and/or distal/downstream to the location of the tumor with a bulging major and/or minor papilla, a pathognomonic finding at ERCP as well as on cross-sectional imaging (though not quite as commonly seen on CT or MRI). On MRI, a T2 hyperintense and T1 variably intense papilla may protrude into the duodenal lumen similar to a choledochocele. Areas of hypointense mural filling defects seen along the duct and/or cysts on MRCP images usually indicate mural papillary projections, a finding that raises suspicion for malignancy. These papillary projections typically enhance following contrast, unlike mucinous debris, which may also manifest as hypointense filling defects within dilated ducts and cysts.

Side-branch IPMNs are located more peripherally in the pancreatic parenchyma, often in the region of the uncinate process. These IPMNs can be demonstrated to connect to the main pancreatic duct by ERCP as well as by MRCP (especially secretin-enhanced MRCP; see "Experimental Techniques" below). These types of IPMNs often strongly resemble pseudocysts in the setting of chronic pancreatitis. They are frequently confused as both their clinical and imaging findings can be very similar. However, the presence of enhancing mural nodules differentiates the IPMN from the pseudocyst. The presence of ductal dilatation distal to the IPMN, as well as communication with the duct, also aids in differentiating the IPMN from a mucinous cystic neoplasm or a necrotic/cystic adenocarcinoma.

Magnetic resonance cholangiopancreatography excels over ERCP in characterizing an IPMN. Factors that suggest malignancy are thick walls and enhancing mural nodules, both characteristics that are often easier to identify with MRCP. The size of an IPMN also directly correlates with propensity for malignancy (83% of IPMNs larger than 4 cm are malignant). In addition, the degree of ductal dilatation also correlates with malignancy, especially if there is dilatation of the main duct in a branch-type IPMN.

Management of IPMNs remains very controversial as more and more IPMNs are being incidentally detected with increasing use of MRCP and multidetector-row CTs. Although surgery has traditionally been the management option of choice, many groups have shown that small IPMNs (< 2.5 cm), especially branch-type IPMNs without any of the above factors that would suggest an increased chance of malignancy, may be followed over time without detriment, especially in older asymptomatic patients.

Biliary Tract

Gallbladder Carcinoma

Gallbladder carcinoma is the most common type of biliary malignancy and typically presents in the sixth or seventh decade of life with a mild female predominance. Magnetic resonance appearance is typically that of either irregular diffuse gallbladder wall thickening and nodularity or a focal mural-based mass protruding into or filling the entire gallbladder lumen. Often there is invasion into adjacent organs such as the liver, pancreas, and duodenum. This is the reason for their poor prognosis, as 75% of these tumors are unresectable by the time of presentation due to the presence of invasion of adjacent structures. Most of these tumors are of adenomatous origin, with a small minority related to squamous cell carcinoma.

As with most tumors, gallbladder carcinomas tend to be T1 hypointense and mildly T2 hyperintense. Unlike many tumors, however, gallbladder carcinomas are usually ill defined and poorly delineated. Gadolinium enhancement is usually very avid and heterogeneous and is the basis for evaluation of margins and degree of invasion. In the absence of imaging demonstration of organ invasion or gross lymphadenopathy, MR findings may be difficult to differentiate from complicated acute cholecystitis. Gallbladder carcinomas are best characterized through more traditional contrast-enhanced abdominal MR techniques (T1- and T2-weighted images with pre- and post-gadolinium imaging) rather than with MRCP.

Bile Ducts

Magnetic resonance cholangiopancreatography is ideally suited to the detection of biliary calculi, especially in this age of routine laparoscopic cholecystectomy where surgery may prove difficult or may be complicated by the presence of bile duct stones. While ERCP is still considered the gold standard in evaluation of the biliary system, we deem MRCP to be comparable to ERCP in the detection of common bile duct stones and even more sensitive in the detection of intrahepatic biliary ductal calculi (97% for MRCP versus 59% for ERCP) (Kim et al., 2002). Bile ducts present as a round or ovoid filling defect creating a "meniscus" margin with the proximally dilated bile duct. A major advantage of MRCP is its ability to depict the biliary system beyond an obstructing stone or calculus.

In contradistinction, a stricture or obstructing mass will cause focal extrinsic narrowing of the bile duct (Fig. 1). The presence of an obstructing mass rather than a stricture tends to cause a more focal and abrupt narrowing of the bile duct, with the appearance of "shoulders" to the contours of narrowing. Focal narrowing in the absence of a cause of stricturing (such as prior cholecystectomy or other biliary surgery) should raise the suspicion for a malignant cause of obstruction. Distinction between an obstructing mass and structuring should be made with the use of intravenous contrast. Obstructing masses of the intrahepatic and extrahepatic biliary tree tend to show early-phase hypoenhancement and late-phase hyperenhancement when compared to pancreatic and liver parenchyma. Use of fat suppression on postcontrast imaging greatly aids in making enhancing and/or thickened bile duct endothelium more conspicuous over the background of low signal fat. Other factors that are very suggestive of a malignant cause of extrahepatic biliary obstruction include long segment involvement of the biliary tree with irregular and often asymmetric margins to the narrowed biliary walls (Park et al., 2004).

Cholangiocarcinoma affects the biliary tree 90% of the time and may cause one of two different patterns; infiltrative concentric spread along the biliary tree or more focal mass-like enlargement. The more common appearance of extension along and around the central biliary tree is often difficult to visualize by cross-sectional imaging but is best characterized on MR through dynamic and delayed postcontrast imaging. As previously noted, cholangiocarcinomas are hypovascular, desmoplastic showing hypoenhancement to liver and pancreatic parenchyma with delayed interstitial enhancement, most conspicuous on 10 to 15 min delayed postcontrast images. Delayed enhancement is due to the dense scar-like composition of this tumor. On precontrast images, cholangiocarcinomas are usually mildly T1 hypointense and mildly T2 hyperintense to liver parenchyma, though infiltrative peribiliary tumors may be difficult to delineate from adjacent bile ducts and vascular structures, especially at the porta hepatis. Ten percent of cholangiocarcinomas will present as intrahepatic masses without biliary involvement and may not be obvious on traditional MRCP images. Intrahepatic cholangiocarcinomas otherwise show similar imaging characteristics as those described above and may be differentiated from hepatocellular carcinomas by their later heterogeneous enhancement pattern (hepatocellular carcinomas tend to show more brisk arterial-phase enhancement with venous phase washout), though enhancement patterns are not always specific.

Carcinomas involving the ampulla may arise from the distal common bile duct, distal pancreatic duct/parenchyma, or duodenal wall. On the whole, these tumors tend to present at a much earlier stage and with smaller size than other biliary or pancreatic ductal carcinomas due to their early presentation. Although these tumors may only measure a few millimeters at presentation, they present early with biliary and pancreatic obstructive symptoms and are surgically resectable the majority of the time (with 85% 5-year survival) (Yamaguchi and Enjoji, 1987). This is the main reason for their improved prognosis over pancreatic adenocarcinomas and cholangiocarcinomas. These tumors may often be too small to detect by cross-sectional imaging but, when identified, show similar imaging characteristics to other biliary tumors with identification of a focal hypoenhancing mildly T1 hypointense and mildly T2 hyperintense mass or region of ductal wall thickening. Metastases to the biliary tract are very rare, but when they do occur, they are usually due to breast cancer, melanoma, or lymphoma. These masses may cause biliary obstruction as well. Their imaging appearance is not usually differentiable from biliary primary malignancies unless there are concomitant liver metastases.

Experimental Techniques

Promising variations on MR cholangiopancreatography have been recently developed involving use of a stimulant to pancreatic juice excretion to aid in ductal distension and visualization as well as use of alternative contrast agents with biliary excretion. Both of these techniques add a functional component to the evaluation of the pancreatic and biliary tract.

A few minutes prior to MRCP imaging of the pancreatic tree, administration of 0.2 µg/kg of secretin intravenously over the course of 1 min in doses similar to those routinely given prior to ERCP stimulates secretion of pancreatic fluids and bicarbonate from the exocrine glands promoting pancreatic ductal distension. This aids in demonstrating pancreatic ductal anatomy as well as in resolving whether cystic lesions of the pancreas communicate with the main or side-branch pancreatic ducts (helpful in the differentiation of IPMNs and pseudocysts from cystic neoplasms) (Czako et al., 2004). During the first five minutes post-injection, concomitant sphincter contraction also helps in distending the pancreatic ducts. Continued dynamic MRCP imaging over time may be performed to observe emptying of this pancreatic fluid into the duodenum to subjectively quantify pancreatic exocrine function and evaluate for sphincter of Oddi dysfunction. As secretin is very well tolerated by most patients (with a low incidence of allergic reactions), the only drawback to this technique lies in the cost and availability of this agent.

Use of contrast agents that show biliary excretion (such as mangafodipir trisodium [Mn-DPDP, Teslascan]) can result in T1-weighted MR cholangiograms in much the same way that oral calcium ipodate was used in the past for oral cholangiographic (OCG) visualization of the bile ducts and gallbladder (Lee et al., 2001; Fayad et al., 2003). Manganese-based contrast agents are similar to gadolinium-based agents in that they demonstrate T1 shortening characteristics, but a small percentage of the agent is excreted into the hepatic biliary tree and into the gallbladder and common bile duct. Use of this agent may be supplemented to T2-weighted MRCP techniques, allowing for both anatomic and functional evaluation of biliary function; however, as this agent also tends to cause T2-shortening of bile, MRCP imaging should be performed prior to administration of Mn-DPDP. One drawback of the use of this agent is that visualization of bile ducts tends to take at least 10 min following intravenous injection in a normally functioning liver. In the presence of biliary obstruction or liver dysfunction, visualization of the bile ducts may take much longer. Use of this agent may require a significant delay to reimaging with some patients required to be brought back 1 to 24 hr later for repeat T1-weighted imaging of the bile ducts.

In conclusion, MRCP offers more than just the detection of intraductal calculi. As a noninvasive alternative to ERCP and PTC, MRCP also plays a role in detecting and characterizing malignancies of the pancreatic and biliary tracts. Short of biopsy and stenting, MR serves as a reliable and an informative step in the work-up of suspected abnormalities of the pancreaticobiliary system. When combined with the use of intravenous gadolinium-chelate contrast agents, MRCP serves as a comprehensive modality for the detection and evaluation of malignancy. MRCP is also very helpful as a guidance modality prior to tissue sampling via ERCP, endoscopic ultrasonography (EUS), or percutaneous CT or ultrasound-guided biopsy. Experimental techniques involving the use of secretin as well as contrast agents with biliary excretion offer promising future approaches to evaluation of exocrine function and improved depiction of ductal anatomy.

References

Adamek, H., Weitz, M., Breer, H., Jakobs, R., Schilling, D., and Riemann, J. 1997. Value of magnetic resonance cholangiopancreatography (MRCP) after unsuccessful endoscopic retrograde cholangiopancreatography (ERCP). *Endoscopy 29*:741–744.

Bilbao, M.K., Dotter, C.T., and Lee, T.O. 1976. Complications of endoscopic retrograde cholangiopancreatography (FRCP) study of 10,000 cases. *Gastroenterology 70*:314–320.

Brennan, M.F., Moccia, R.D., and Klimstra, D. 1996. Management of adenocarcinoma of the body and tail of the pancreas. *Ann. Surg. 223*:506–512.

Czako, L., Takacs, T., Morvay, Z., Csernay, L., and Lonovics, J. 2004. Diagnostic role of secretin-enhanced MRCP in patients with unsuccessful ERCP. *World J. Gastroenterol. 10*:3034–3038.

Fayad, L.M., Holland, G.A., Bergin, D., Iqbal, N., Parker, L., Curcillo, P.G., Kowalski, T.E., Park, P., Intenzo, C., and Mitchell, D.G. 2003. Functional magnetic resonance cholangiography (flvIRC) of the gallbladder and biliary tree with contrast-enhanced magnetic resonance cholangiography. *J. Magnetic Resonance Imaging 18*:449–460.

Fulcher, A., and Turner, M. 1998. Pitfalls of MR cholangiopancreatography (MRCP). *J. Comput. Assist Tomogr. 22*:845–850.

Ichikawa, T., Sou, H., Araki, T., Arbab, A.S., Yoshikawa, T., Ishigame, K., Haradome, H., and Hachiya, J. 2001. Duct-penetrating sign at MRCP: usefulness for differentiating inflammatory pancreatic mass from pancreatic carcinomas. *Radiology 221*:107–116.

Kim, T.K., Kim, B.S., Kim, J.H., Ha, H.K., Kim, P.N., Kim, A.Y., and Lee, M.G. 2002. Diagnosis of intrahepatic stones: superiority of MR cholangiopancreatography over endoscopic retrograde cholangiopancreatography. *AJR 179*:429–434.

Lee, V.S., Rofsky, N.M., Morgan, G.R., Teperman, L.W., Krinsky, G.A., Berman, P., and Weinreb, J.C. 2001. Volumetric mangafodipir trisodium-enhanced cholangiography to define intrahepatic biliary anatomy. *Am. J. Roentgol. 176*:906–908.

Megibow, A.J., Lombardo, F.P., Guarise, A., Carbognin, G., Scholes, J., Rofsky, N.M., Macari, M., Balthazar, E.J., and Procacci, C. 2001. Cystic pancreatic masses: cross-sectional imaging observations and serial follow-up. *Imaging 26*:640–647.

Molinari, M., Helton, W., and Espat, N.J. 2001. Palliative strategies for locally advanced unresectable and metastatic pancreatic cancer. *Surg. Clin. North Am. 81*:651–665.

Obara, T., Maguchi, H., Arisato, S., Itoh, A., Nishin, N., Ymano, M., Taruishi, M., Suzuki, H., and Watari, J. 1994. Mucin-producing tumor of the pancreas: surgery or follow-up? *Nippon Shokakibyo Gakkai Zasshi. 91*:66–74.

Park, M.S., Kim, T.K., Kim, K.W., Park, S.W., Lee, J.K., Kim, J.S., Lee, J.H., Kim, K.A., Kim, A.Y., Kim, P.N., Lee, M.G., and Ha, HK. 2004. Differentiation of extrahepatic bile duct cholangiocarcinoma from benign stricture: findings at MRCP versus FRCP. *Radiology 233*:234–240.

Salres, H.G. 1974. Chronic calcifying pancreatitis-chronic alcoholic pancreatitis. *Gastroenterology 66*:604–616.

Semelka, R.C., Custodio, C.M., Balci, C., and Voosley, J.T. 2000. Neuroendocrine tumors of the pancreas: spectrum of appearances on MRI. *Magnetic Resonance Imaging 11*:141–148.

Sperti, C., Pasquali, C., Guolo, P., Polverosi, R., Liessi, G., and Pedrazzoli, S. 1996. Serum tumor markers and cyst fluid analysis are useful for the diagnosis of pancreatic cystic tumors. *Cancer 78*:237–243.

van Greenen, R.C., ten Kate, F.J., de Wit, L.T., van Gulik, T.M., Obertop, H., and Gouma, D.J. 2001. Segmental resection and wedge excision of the portal or superior mesenteric vein during pancreatoduodenectomy. *Surgery 129*:158–163.

Van Hoe, L., Grysepeerdt, S., Ectors, N., Steenbergen, W. Van., Aerts, R., Baert, A.L., and Marchal, G. 1998. Nonalcoholic duct-destructive chronic pancreatitis: imaging findings. *Am. J. Roentgenol. 170*:643–647.

Vitellas, K., Keogan, M., Spritzer, C., and Nelson, R. 2000. MR cholangiopancreatography of bile and pancreatic duct abnormalities with emphasis on the single-shot fast spin-echo technique. *Radiographics 20*:939–957.

Wallner, B., Schumacher, K., Weidemnaier, W., and Friedrich, J. 1991. Dilated biliary tract: evaluation with MR cholangiography with a T2-weighted contrast-enhanced fast sequence. *Radiology 181*:805–808.

Watanabe, Y., Dohke, M., Ishimori, T., Amoh, Y., Okumura, A., Oda, K., Koike, S., and Dodo, Y. 1999. Diagnostic pitfalls of MR cholangiopancreatography in the evaluation of the biliary tract and gallbladder. *Radiographics 19*:415–429.

Yamaguchi, K., and Enjoji, M. 1987. Carcinoma of the ampulla of Vater: a clinicopathologic study and pathologic staging of 109 causes of carcinoma and 5 cases of adenoma. *Cancer 59*:506–515.

Zhang, X.M., Mitchell, D.G., Dohke, M., Holland, G.A., and Parker, L. 2002. Pancreatic cysts: depiction on single-shot fast spin-echo MR images. *Radiology 223*:547–553.

Occult Primary Head and Neck Carcinoma: Role of Positron Emission Tomography Imaging

Frank R. Miller, Cecelia E. Schmalbach, and Ande Bao

Introduction

The unknown primary carcinoma with involvement of cervical lymph nodes is estimated to represent 3 to 5% of all head and neck malignant neoplasms (Braams *et al.*, 1997; Miller *et al.*, 2005). Pathologically, the majority of the malignancies represent squamous cell carcinoma (> 90%), with the remainder composed of adenocarcinoma, melanoma, and other rare pathologies. The majority of these neoplastic processes are thought to arise from an occult carcinoma in the head and neck region (predominantly Waldeyer's ring, which includes the nasopharynx, tonsil, and the base of the tongue). Despite newer technology, including fiber-optic examination, biomolecular testing, positron emission tomography (PET), and PET-computed tomography (PET-CT) fusion, the detection of the occult primary tumor remains elusive in many cases (Chepea *et al.*, 2003; Ferris *et al.*, 2005).

The typical presentation is a middle-aged male with a painless neck mass that has been present for several months. Often the patient has received medical therapy in the form of antibiotics for presumed "cervical lymphadenitis." As in other squamous cell carcinomas of the upper aerodigestive tract, the major risk factor is a prior history of tobacco and alcohol use. The medical history should include a review of symptoms such as otalgia, dysphagia, odynophagia, hoarseness, respiratory difficulties, fever, night sweats, and weight loss, which may point to the area of the primary tumor. Because cutaneous cancers can metastasize to cervical lymph nodes, it is important to obtain an accurate history of previous skin cancers, "mole" removal, and skin biopsies. The review of systems should rule out a history of exposure to infectious and inflammatory agents that may produce cervical lymph node enlargement, including the history of mycobacteria, pets, and travel.

The physical examination should include a complete head and neck examination including mucosal evaluation of the nasopharynx, base of tongue, larynx, and hypopharynx using a flexible fiber-optic nasopharyngoscope, as well as a thorough cutaneous examination of the face, neck, and scalp. Several studies have demonstrated that the majority of occult primary tumors will be found in Waldeyer's ring, particularly the nasopharynx, palatine tonsils, and base of tongue (McQuone *et al.*, 1998; Mendenhall *et al.*, 1998; Miller *et al.*, 2005). Bi-manual palpation of the tonsil fossas and base of tongue may reveal an area of nodularity or induration and guide subsequent biopsies. Any suspicious areas should be noted and correlated with radiographic studies in preparation for fine needle aspiration (FNA) biopsy. The size, location (neck Level I–V), and characteristics (fixed, mobile, hard, rubbery, pulsatile, etc.) should be noted. The location of the lymph node can provide clues as to the location of the occult primary tumor (Table 1). Otologic examination should rule out an otitis media with effusion, which suggests eustachian tube dysfunction secondary to a nasopharyngeal mass. A complete cranial nerve examination should be performed. The location of the cervical lymphadenopathy heightens the suspicion for the location of the occult primary tumor. Lymph nodes located in the posterior triangle raise concern for a nasopharyngeal primary, while nodes in the upper jugular chain (Levels II–III) point toward the tonsil and base of tongue region. Isolated nodal disease low in the neck (Level IV or V) raises concern for a primary tumor arising below the clavicles from sites such as the lungs or gastrointestinal tract.

Evaluation

The initial work-up for an adult with an isolated neck mass and an otherwise normal head and neck examination includes an FNA biopsy, chest X-ray, and imaging study of the cervical region (CT versus magnetic resonance imaging [MRI]), including cuts from the skull base to the upper chest. The single most useful diagnostic test is the FNA biopsy, for it provides cytologic information that guides subsequent work-up. Nondiagnostic FNA biopsies are best repeated as this may simply represent inadequate cellular material on the first aspiration. Ultrasound guidance can be utilized to improve the diagnostic yield of the FNA biopsy. Pathologic examination, including immunohistochemistry, often confirms the specific histologic type such as squamous cell carcinoma, adenocarcinoma, and melanoma. Ultimately,

Table 1   Six Cervical Lymph Node Groups

Level	LN Group	Boundaries	Drainage Site
I			• Floor of Mouth
			• Anterior Tongue
	Submental/Submandibular	Mandible	• Lower Lip
		Digastric m.	• Mandibular
		Hyoid Bone	Alveolar Ridge
II			• Parotid
			• Nasal Cavity
		Skull Base	• Oral Cavity
	Upper Jugular Chain	Hyoid Bone	• Nasopharynx
		Stylohyoid m.	• Oropharynx
		Post. Boarder SCM	• Larynx
			• Hypopharynx
III			• Oral Cavity
		Hyoid Bone	• Nasopharynx
	Middle Jugular Chain	Cricoid	• Oropharynx
		Sternohyoid m.	• Larynx
		Post. Boarder SCM	• Hypopharynx
IV			• Larynx
		Cricoid	• Hypopharynx
	Lower Jugular Chain	Clavicle	• Thyroid
		Sternohyoid m.	• Cervical
		Post. Boarder SCM	Esophogus
V		SCM	• Nasopharynx
		Clavicle	• Oropharynx
	Posterior Triangle	Trapezius m.	• Posterior Scalp
			• Posterior Neck
VI			• Thyroid
	Anterior Compartment		• Glottis
	(Pretracheal Paratracheal Delphian Node)	Hyoid	• Subglottis
		Suprasternal Notch	• Piriform
		Common Carotid a.	• Cervical Esophogus

LN = Lymph Node
SCM = sternocleidomastoid muscle
m. = muscle
a. = artery

this diagnostic information guides the subsequent work-up and search for the occult primary tumor. The management of unknown primary tumors of each specific histologic variant is described in separate sections of this chapter.

If the complete head and neck examination is normal (i.e., there is no detectable occult primary tumor), the imaging studies are carefully reviewed. The CT or MRI imaging should be reviewed for any asymmetry in the nasopharynx, tonsil, and base of tongue. Cystic metastatic disease in the cervical region can produce controversy regarding the possibility of a primary carcinoma arising from a branchial cleft cyst (see below). Metastatic papillary thyroid cancer and tonsillar squamous cell carcinoma can also present with cystic metastatic disease. The nodal disease is staged in accordance with the American Joint Committee on Cancer Staging Classification by assessing the nodal size, location, and presence/absence of extracapsular extension. Many clinicians would include CT imaging of the chest and upper abdomen to assess for second primary tumors or evidence of distant metastatic disease. At the very least a chest X-ray should be reviewed to rule out gross metastatic disease. Positron emission tomography imaging may also be utilized as a screening tool for pulmonary disease in this patient population (Wax et al., 2002). A recent report documented that PET scanning had better accuracy than routine chest X-ray and bronchoscopy in detecting synchronous lung lesions (Wax et al., 2002; Miller et al., 2005).

Positron Emission Tomography

The next step in the diagnostic work-up, prior to proceeding with the traditional panendoscopy, should be to consider newer imaging technologies such as PET scanning to perform a total whole-body scan to detect an occult primary tumor. This imaging is a physiologic/nuclear medicine study that consists of the injection of a glucose analog (^{18}F-2-fluoro-2-deoxyglucose). The glucose analog is preferentially taken up by neoplastic cells and can guide the surgeon to potential biopsy sites during panendoscopy. The principle of PET imaging is based on the coincident detection of two opposite emitted gamma photons from the annihilation reaction between a positron (positively charged electron) and an electron. The typical positron emission radionuclides are Fluorine-18 (^{18}F), Carbon-11 (^{11}C), Nitrogen-13 (^{13}N), and Oxygen-15 (^{15}O). Since carbon, nitrogen, and oxygen are basic elements of biomolecules, and fluorine is biochemically similar to hydrogen or hydroxyl-group, PET radiopharmaceuticals display their distinct advantages in obtaining in vivo physiologic or molecular information for tumor diagnosis and for the evaluation of therapy response. Among them, ^{18}F-radiopharmaceuticals has received extensive application given its longer half-life of 110 min.

Positron emission tomography is performed in patients who have been fasting for approximately 8 hours prior to the study. The imaging study is performed after the intravenous injection of 15 mCi (543.9 MBq) of fluorodeoxyglucose F-18. Whole-body PET images are then obtained in multiple bed positions (axial, coronal, and sagittal) after a 45- to 60-minute uptake delay. Typical whole-body PET scanning includes images from the brain to the mid-thigh. The collected images are then analyzed by a nuclear medicine physician/radiologist (Miller et al., 2004, 2005; Fogarty et al., 2003; Iganej et al., 2002)

The most commonly used and clinically useful PET radiopharmaceutical is ^{18}F-2-fluoro-2-deoxyglucose (^{18}F-FDG), a glucose analog that is preferentially taken up by various types of neoplastic cells. Previous clinical studies have shown that ^{18}F-FDG-PET imaging is valuable in head and neck cancer diagnosis, cancer staging, and assessing response to therapy (Halfpenny et al., 2002; Kostakoglu and Goldsmith, 2004). Since the metabolic response of a tumor from chemotherapy or radiotherapy is earlier or more notable than tumor size change, ^{18}F-FDG demonstrates a specific advantage in assessing tumor response to therapy. In an attempt to assess the ^{18}F-FDG uptake response to various experimental treatments, researchers have utilized a xenograft nude rat model. This research has demonstrated that ^{18}F-FDG activity reflects neoplastic accumulation of ^{18}F-FDG and can be a marker to assess tumor response to a treatment protocol (Bao et al., 2006).

Several reports have suggested that 20 to 30% of occult primary tumors can be identified with PET imaging (Braams et al., 1997; Ferris et al., 2005; Miller et al., 2005; Jungehulsing et al., 2000). In a recent prospective study from our institution, the PET scan was able to identify the primary tumor site in 8 of 26 patients (30.8% detection rate), despite the lack of visible primary tumor on both office examination and CT imaging (Miller et al., 2005). Such imaging has been utilized to assess for occult primary tumors in many regions of the body and in staging various neoplasms. It is also utilized as a screening tool for pulmonary disease (Wax et al., 2002). Recent reports have documented that PET scanning can identify synchronous lung lesions with greater accuracy when compared to routine chest X-ray and bronchoscopy (Wax et al., 2002; Miller et al., 2005). The identification of these synchronous lesions is critical because it often alters the treatment plan for head and neck cancer patients.

Despite an extensive diagnostic work-up and sophisticated imaging, the ability to detect the occult tumor remains low. Overall, PET imaging identifies the primary site in ~ 30% of patients who initially present with a neck mass of unknown primary origin (Figs. 1 and 2). Tumor pathology (squamous cell carcinoma versus adenocarcinoma) and body regions (head and neck versus lung/GI tract) have not been found to impact PET sensitivity (Ghosh et al., 2005; Pavlidis et al., 2003). More recently, it has been suggested that

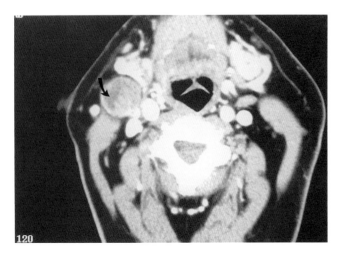

Figure 1 Axial CT scan of neck demonstrating right cervical neck mass at Level II (arrow). Fine-needle aspiration biopsy confirmed metastatic squamous cell carcinoma. A complete head and neck examination, including fiber-optic endoscopy, revealed no primary carcinoma in the head and neck region.

PET-CT fusion techniques may increase the yield and detect over 50% of occult primary tumors (Nanni *et al.*, 2005; Zimmer *et al.*, 2005).

This inability to detect the occult primary tumor, despite sophisticated pathology and radiographic imaging, has three possible explanations. First, the primary tumor has involuted and is no longer detectable, despite the presence of metastatic disease. Though uncommon, spontaneous tumor regression has been described in several tumors (Ghosh *et al.*, 2005).

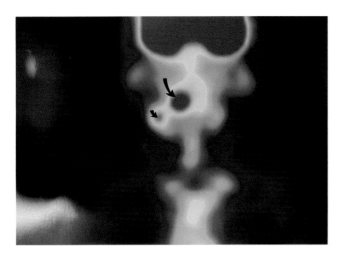

Figure 2 Same patient as Figure 1. Positron emission tomography (coronal view) obtained 6o minutes after injection with 15 mCi of ^{18}F-2-fluoro-deoxy-glucose. Cervical lymph node with fine-needle biopsy-proven squamous cell carcinoma is noted (small arrow) along with suspicious occult primary tumor in right tonsil (large arrow). Right tonsillectomy confirmed occult primary submucosal squamous cell carcinoma of the right tonsil (size 1.2 cm). Final pathologic staging T1N1 squamous cell carcinoma of the right tonsil.

The second explanation is that the malignant phenotype and genotype of the primary tumor favor metastatic biologic behavior over local tumor growth. In this situation, a slow-growing primary tumor might produce early metastatic disease whose growth surpasses that of the primary parent tumor. The third explanation is that our current technology (including PET imaging) lacks the resolution to detect tumors < 5 mm to 10 mm in size. Studies have demonstrated that PET fails to detect occult carcinoma < 5 mm in size (Chepea *et al.*, 2003; Zimmer *et al.*, 2005). In this scenario it is possible to have a small, nondetectable occult tumor in the head and neck region that does not enhance on the PET study secondary to limitations in the technology. This limitation has been further demonstrated in a recent study in which four PET scans failed to identify the occult primary tumor that was ultimately diagnosed on panendoscopy and biopsy (Miller *et al.*, 2005). All four false-negative PET studies demonstrated a small focus of occult primary tumors measuring 0.8 mm, 1 mm, 2 mm, and 5 mm, respectively.

Panendoscopy

The final step in the diagnostic work-up includes a panendoscopy (direct laryngoscopy, bronchoscopy, esophagoscopy) and examination under anesthesia with directed biopsies of the "at-risk" primary tumor sites, including the base of tongue, nasopharynx, hypopharynx, and bilateral tonsillectomy. If detected, the majority of primary tumors will be in the tonsil fossa or base of tongue. Mendenhall *et al.* (1998) successfully identified a primary head and neck cancer in 58 of 140 (43% detection rate) individuals initially presenting with unknown primary carcinoma. Of the 58 tumors detected, 48 (82%) were detected in the tonsil fossa and base of tongue. Several other reports have confirmed the high incidence of occult cancer in the tonsil fossa. For this reason, many surgeons have recommended bilateral tonsillectomy as opposed to incisional tonsil biopsies (McQuone *et al.*, 1998; Miller *et al.*, 2005, In press). The authors generally perform directed biopsies of the base of tongue, nasopharynx, and bilateral tonsillectomy. Hypopharyngeal biopsies are done if enhancement is seen on the PET or if suspicious findings on endoscopy are noted. If the primary tumor is detected at endoscopy, the tumor is staged and appropriate treatment is selected based on the location and staging.

Treatment

Despite an extensive work-up, the majority (50 to 70%) of primary occult tumors are not detected. In these circumstances, the clinician must formulate a rational treatment plan. The stage of the neck disease dictates the overall prognosis for patients with carcinoma of the cervical lymph nodes in the absence of a known primary tumor. Multiple retrospective studies have demonstrated a better 5-year survival for N1 (65 to 80%) versus. N2 (40 to 60%), and N3 disease (15 to 30%) (Colletier *et al.*, 1998; Coster *et al.*, 1992; Harper *et al.*, 1990; Maulard *et al.*, 1992; Nguyen *et al.*, 1994). Traditionally, the treatment of the N1 neck consists of a modified radical neck dissection followed by postoperative radiotherapy to the neck and any potential primary tumor sites. This aggressive approach has yielded high loco-regional control rates (> 75%) for the N1 neck. In selected patients, some clinicians have advocated neck dissection alone for the isolated N1 neck in the absence of aggressive prognostic markers such as extracapsular extension (ECS). In a retrospective experience from the Mayo Clinic (1965 to 1987), 24 patients with N1 and N2 neck disease underwent neck dissection but refused postoperative radiation therapy (Coster *et al.*, 1992). There were no recurrences in the subset of N1 patients without ECS. Current indications for postoperative radiation therapy following neck dissection include multiple positive nodes, bulky N2+ neck stage, or the presence of ECS on the pathology report.

In select cases where the patient has undergone open biopsy of a single node and the pathology reveals squamous cell carcinoma, the clinician is confronted with a decision to return to the operating room for a formal neck dissection versus radiotherapy. In a retrospective experience from M.D. Anderson Cancer Center (1968 to 1992), 39 patients underwent an excisional neck node biopsy only, followed by definitive post-biopsy XRT to the neck and potential primary tumor sites (Colletier *et al.*, 1998). There were no regional/cervical relapses in these 39 patients. The presence of multiple nodes and ECS portended a worse survival. Overall, patients with a single node measuring < 3 cm in size and no ECS have an excellent prognosis for long-term loco-regional control. Our preference is to perform the work-up discussed above, including PET imaging, followed by panendoscopy with directed biopsies and bilateral tonsillectomy. If no primary occult tumor is identified, a comprehensive neck dissection (Levels I–V) is performed. The preservation of the internal jugular vein, sternocleidomastoid muscle, and spinal accessory nerve is dictated by the extent of disease at the time of surgery. The final pathology report includes information regarding the number of positive lymph nodes, levels of lymph node involvement, size of the lymph nodes, presence/absence of ECS, and presence/absence of angio-invasion and perineural invasion. This information is used to identify patients who may benefit from postoperative adjuvant therapy (primarily postoperative XRT +/− chemotherapy). Postoperative radiation therapy traditionally consists of 5000 to 6000 cGy administered to the neck, with radiation ports also including the potential primary sites such as the nasopharynx, oropharynx, and hypopharynx.

More extensive neck disease (N2 or N3) portends a worse prognosis. Several retrospective series have shown 5-year survival rates of 40 to 60% for N2 neck stage, and 18 to 35% for N3 neck stage (Colletier *et al.*, 1998; Miller *et al.*, In press). The treatment of the patient with more advanced neck disease (N2 or N3) generally consists of combined therapy utilizing surgery, radiation therapy, and, in selected cases, chemotherapy. Our preferred approach in the N2 or N3 neck is to consider primary surgery to the neck in the form of a comprehensive neck dissection (Levels I to V) with preservation of the internal jugular vein, spinal accessory nerve, and sternocleidomastoid muscle as dictated by the extent of the disease. Postoperative radiation therapy (5000 to 6000 cGy) to the neck and potential primary tumor sites is then administered. In the event of multiple positive nodes and/or extracapsular spread, the radiation oncologist may consider a boost to selected neck regions. More recently, there is emerging evidence that the addition of postoperative chemotherapy (concurrent chemoradiotherapy) improves the rates of loco-regional control and disease-free survival in patients with head and neck squamous cell carcinoma.

In the select group of patients with advanced unresectable neck disease (N3 with invasion of the carotid artery, pre-vertebral muscle invasion, or extension into the cervical spine), our preference is to consider primary concurrent XRT and chemotherapy. After completion of the treatment, the neck is restaged and assessed for surgical salvage. Definitive treatment may necessitate an extended radical neck dissection that includes resection of additional structures such as neck musculature and cranial nerves intimately involved with tumor.

Unknown Primary Adenocarcinoma

As discussed earlier, one of the critical early steps in the assessment of the patient with a neck mass is an accurate pathologic diagnosis. While the majority of unknown primary tumors in the head and neck region consist of squamous cell carcinoma, small subsets are adenocarcinoma (Chorost *et al.*, 2001). This small percentage is in contrast to other lymphatic regions where adenocarcinoma is the most common histologic finding for patients with an unknown primary carcinoma (Chorost *et al.*, 2001; Ghosh *et al.*, 2005; Pavlidis *et al.*, 2003).

Fine needle aspiration biopsy in combination with immunohistochemistry may raise suspicion for the occult primary tumor. However, in many cases an open biopsy is required to ascertain the true histology and to provide adequate material for immunohistologic testing (Ghosh *et al.*, 2005). Immunohistology, along with microscopic analysis, guides the surgeon to the primary tumor site (Table 2).

Along with the utilization of FNA and immunohistology, the location of the node can guide the surgeon to the potential primary tumor location. Supraclavicular lymph nodes harboring adenocarcinoma should raise a high degree of

Table 2   Immunohistology Staining Techniques

Stain or Histologic Feature	Suggested Primary Site or Neoplasm
Thyroglobulin	Thyroid carcinoma
Calcitonin	Medullary carcinoma of the thyroid
PSA/prostatic acid phosphatase	Prostate
Alpha-fetoprotein	Liver, stomach, germ cell
CEA	Carcinoma
Estrogen/progesterone receptor	Breast
Psammoma bodies	Ovary, thyroid carcinoma
Signet ring cells	Stomach
Cytokeratin	Squamous cell carcinoma
Epithelial membrane antigen	Squamous cell carcinoma
Melan-A (MART 1)	Melanoma
HMB-45/S-100	Melanoma

suspicion for a primary tumor below the clavicles. Particular emphasis must be paid to the chest and abdomen (i.e., lung and GI tract including pancreas). In addition, mammography should be considered for a woman as a means to assess occult breast cancer, especially if a personal or family history exists. In men, serologic testing, including prostate specific antigen, should be performed to rule out prostate carcinoma, and a complete examination is required to palpate the prostate as well as the testicles. Positron emission tomography imaging may prove valuable in this group of patients both as a means of identifying the occult primary tumor and of ruling out additional metastatic disease. Recent data would suggest that PET and PET-CT fusion imaging can detect the occult primary tumor in selected patients. Nanni *et al.* (2005) reported 12 occult primary adenocarcinomas identified in a series of 25 patients (detection rate of 57%) using PET-CT fusion techniques. Other reports (Ghosh *et al.*, 2005; Pavlidis *et al.*, 2003) suggest that PET may detect an occult adenocarcinoma in 25 to 30% of patients.

If the metastatic lymph node is located along the jugular chain (Levels I to III), a head and neck primary cancer must be considered. Emphasis must be given to the salivary glands (particularly the parotid) and the thyroid gland. Imaging studies and immunohistologic analysis can rule out an occult well-differentiated cancer that carries an excellent prognosis versus metastatic disease from below the clavicle, which portends a poor prognosis.

Small subsets of patients with metastatic adenocarcinoma have a favorable prognosis (thyroid and testicular primaries). Unfortunately, the majority of the patients presenting with metastatic adenocarcinoma in the neck suffer from disseminated disease portending a poor prognosis. Early referral to a medical oncologist is in the best interest of the patient (Ghosh *et al.*, 2005; Pavlidis *et al.*, 2003). Combinations of chemotherapy may be considered, including taxol, carboplatin, and etoposide. Despite aggressive treatment in this setting, the median survival remains a dismal 10 months (Chorost *et al.*, 2001).

Melanoma of Unknown Primary Tumor

Primary melanoma of the head and neck represents ~ 25 to 30% of all melanoma (Lentsch and Myers, 2001). Rarely, melanoma is identified in cervical or parotid lymph nodes without evidence of a primary tumor. It is important to obtain a detailed history of any previous skin lesions that disappeared or were removed. Many authors think that the metastatic melanoma in the cervical lymph node represents metastases from a primary tumor that has undergone spontaneous regression. Pathology slides of all previously excised "benign skin lesions" must be reviewed by an experienced dermatopathologist.

Like all new onset neck masses, an FNA biopsy is often the initial step that leads to a diagnosis of melanoma. Melanoma-specific immunohistologic staining such as Melan-A (MART-1), HMB-45, and S-100 may help confirm the histologic diagnosis. Once the histology is confirmed, one should search for an occult melanoma primary lesion. This evaluation includes a complete dermatologic skin examination as well as a search for the rare occult visceral melanoma (mucosal, eyes, adrenal, etc.). If no primary occult melanoma is detected, the treatment plan must focus on the cervical disease and the possibility of distant metastatic disease.

The role of whole-body PET imaging in melanoma is under debate (Wagner *et al.*, 2005; Garbe, 2005). In the initial evaluation of early stage cutaneous melanoma, PET imaging has not proven efficient. In a recent study, Wagner *et al.* (2005) prospectively evaluated the impact of PET imaging on the detection of occult lymph node metastases and distant metastases. The sensitivity of this scan was 0.21, and specificity was 0.97 in detecting occult metastatic disease in patients with early stage melanoma. Other researchers have suggested that PET imaging may be a valuable adjunct to stage patients with recurrent melanoma or more advanced stage tumors (Garbe, 2005).

Cervical melanoma of unknown primary origin remains a surgical disease. Patients presenting with jugular chain involvement require a modified radical neck dissection (Levels I–V), sparing all vital structures not involved with disease. The surgeon must consider a posterior-lateral neck dissection for treatment of metastatic melanoma in Level V, the postauricular, and the occipital nodal basins. Interferon alpha 2-b remains the only FDA-approved adjuvant therapy for melanoma. All patients with cervical metastasis (N1 disease or greater) are candidates. In addition, patients with stage III disease in the setting of multiple positive nodes or ECS have gained increased locoregional control with the administration of postoperative hypofractionated radiotherapy (30 Gy in five fractions) (Lentsch and Myers, 2001). Alternative systemic treatments, including gene therapy and biochemotherapy, are available within the context of clinical trials.

Cystic Metastatic Disease in the Neck

The presence of a primary carcinoma arising from a branchial cleft remnant continues to generate controversy (Ferris *et al.*, 2005; Briggs *et al.*, 2002). Given that a primary occult squamous cell carcinoma arising from Waldeyer's ring (nasopharynx, tonsil, and base of tongue) can generate cystic metastatic disease in 33 to 50% of cases, strict criteria for branchial cleft carcinoma have been suggested. The criteria to make a diagnosis of branchial cleft carcinoma include (1) location of the tumor along the anterior border of the sternocleidomastoid muscle, (2) histologic findings consistent with the presence of a branchial cleft cyst, (3) histologic findings consistent with the carcinoma arising within the branchial cleft cyst wall, and (4) no evidence of a primary squamous cell carcinoma arising in the upper aerodigestive tract for a minimum 5-year follow-up period (Miller *et al.*, 2005). As a general rule, any adult with a cystic neck mass that resembles a branchial cleft cyst should undergo an appropriate work-up, including imaging and FNA biopsy to rule out malignancy. A recent report from the University of Pittsburgh (Ferris *et al.*, 2005) analyzed 40 adult patients who presented with cystic neck masses. In this study, PET imaging faired no better than traditional CT scan in the identification of malignancy. The authers' conclusions were that a thorough clinical evaluation by an experienced head and neck surgeon, in conjunction with contrast-enhanced CT and FNA biopsy, is sufficient to evaluate patients with a cystic cervical neck mass.

Given these strict criteria, the clinician cannot confirm the possibility of a branchial cleft carcinoma until five or more years of follow-up. In the majority of cases, the carcinoma is thought to represent metastases from a primary occult carcinoma (particularly in Waldeyer's ring). The work-up and treatment should proceed as outlined for any unknown primary carcinoma.

In addition to cystic metastatic squamous cell carcinoma, other primary tumors can present with cystic metastatic lesions in the cervical region. Foremost among these is papillary carcinoma of the thyroid gland. A lateral neck mass may be the initial presenting finding, and early utilization of FNA biopsy will confirm the thyroid carcinoma and direct subsequent work-up and treatment.

Conclusions/Future Direction

The role of PET imaging in the management and staging of head and neck oncology patients continues to evolve. The PET study can identify the occult primary tumor in ~ 30% of patients who present with an unknown primary tumor and have no detectable tumor using conventional methods including fiber-optic endoscopy and CT/MRI imaging. New-generation PET scanners and PET-CT fusion may increase the accuracy and effectiveness in head and neck cancer patients. The fused PET-CT has been shown to be superior to either modality alone in the assessment of head and neck malignancies (Zimmer *et al.*, 2005). The ability to identify the occult primary tumor is imperative because it allows site-specific therapy in a more directed fashion and avoids the side effects of wide field radiation.

The future of PET imaging in head and neck cancer is likely to mature with the development of new PET tracers that allow for more accurate tumor detection with less uptake by the normal tissue. The new PET tracer carbon-11-choline (CHOL) detects squamous cell carcinoma with the accuracy equivalent to FDG-PET but has the advantage of less muscle uptake and shorter examination times (Zimmer *et al.*, 2005) Another area of development will include the use of monoclonal antibodies directed against tumor-specific antigens in PET imaging. Tumors as small as 36 mg can be detected with 89Zr-labeled antibodies in tumor-bearing nude mice (Zimmer *et al.*, 2005). Current research is promising and will ultimately define the future role of PET imaging in the evaluation of unknown primary head and neck cancers.

References

American Joint Commission on Cancer (AJCC). 2002. Cancer Staging Manual.

Bao, A., Phillips W.T., Goins, B., McGuff, H.S., Zheng, X., Woolley, F.R., Natarajan, M., Santoyo, C., Miller, F.R., and Otto, R.A. 2006. Setup and characterization of a human head and neck squamous cell carcinoma xenograft model in nude rats. *Otolaryngol Head Neck Surg.* 135: 853–857.

Braams, J.W., Pruim, J., Kole, A.C., Nikkels, G.J., Vaalburg, W., Vermey, A., and Roodenburg, L.N. 1997. Detection of unknown primary head and neck tumors by positron emission tomography. *Int. J. Oral Maxillofac. Surg.* 26:112–115.

Briggs, R.D., Pou, A.M., and Schnadig, V.J. 2002. Cystic metastases versus branchial cleft carcinoma: a diagnostic challenge. *Laryngoscope 112*:1010–1014.

Chepea, D., Koch, W., and Pitman, K. 2003. Management of unknown primary tumor. *Head Neck 25*:499–504.

Chorost, M.I., McKinley, B., and Tschoi, M. 2001. The management of the unknown primary. *J. Am. College Surgeons* 193:666–677.

Colletier, P.J., Garden, A.S., Morrison, W.H., Goepfort, H., Geara, F., and Ang, K.K. 1998. Postoperative radiation for squamous cell carcinoma metastatic to cervical lymph nodes from an unknown primary site: outcomes and patterns of failure. *Head Neck 20*:674–681.

Coster, J.R., Foote, R.L., Olsen, K.D., Jack, S.M., Schaid, D.J., and DeSanto, L.W. 1992. Cervical nodal metastases of squamous cell carcinoma of unknown origin: indications for withholding radiation therapy. *Int. J. Radiation Oncology Biol. Phys.* 23:743–749.

Ferris, R.L., Branstetter, B.F., and Nayak, J.V. 2005. Diagnostic utility of positron emission tomography-computed tomography for predicting malignancy in cystic neck masses in adults. *Laryngoscope 115*:1979–1982.

Fogarty, G.B., Peters, L.J., Stewart, J., Scott, C., Rischin, D., and Hicks, R.J. 2003. The usefulness of fluorine 18-labelled deoxyglucose positron emission tomography in the investigation of patients with cervical lymphadenopathy from an unknown primary tumor. *Head Neck 25*:138–145.

Garbe, C. 2005. Cutaneous melanoma: baseline and ongoing laboratory evaluation. *Dermatologic Therapy 18*:413–421.

Ghosh, L., Dahut, W., Kakar, S., Posades, E.M., Torres, C.G., Cancel-Santiago, R., and Ghosh, B.C. 2005. Management of patients with metastatic cancer of unknown primary. *Curr. Probl. Surg 42*:12–66.

Halfpenny, W., Hain, S.F., Biassoni, L., Maisey, M.N., Sherman, J.A., and McGurk, M. 2002. FDG-PET: a possible prognostic factor in head and neck cancer. *Br. J. Cancer 86*:512–516.

Harper, C.S., Mendenhall, W.M., Parsons, J.T., Stringer, S.P., Cassisi, N.J., and Million, R.R. 1990. Cancer in neck nodes with unknown primary site: role of mucosal radiotherapy. *Head Neck 12*:463–469.

Iganej, S., Kagan, R., Anderson, P., Rao, A., Tome, M., Wang, R., Dowlatshai, M., Cosmatos, H., and Morgan, T. 2002. Metastatic squamous cell carcinoma of the neck from an unknown primary: management options and patterns of relapse. *Head Neck 24*:236–246.

Jungehulsing, M., Scheidhauer, K., Damm, M., Pietrzyk, U., Eckel, H., Schicha, H., and Stennert, E. 2000. 2 (18F)flouro-deoxy-D-glucose positron emission tomography is a sensitive tool for the detection of occult primary cancer (carcinoma of unknown primary syndrome) with head and neck lymph node manifestation. *Otolaryngol Head Neck Surg. 123*:294–301.

Kostakoglu, L., and Goldsmith, S.J. 2004. PET in the assessment of therapy response in patients with carcinoma of the head and neck and esophagus. *J. Nucl. Med. 45*:56–68.

Lentsch, E.J., and Myers, J.N. 2001. Melanoma of the head and neck: current concepts in diagnosis and management. *Laryngoscope 111*:1209–1222.

Maulard, C., Housse, M., Brunel, P., Huart, J., Ucla, L., Rozec, C., Delanian, S., and Baillet, F. 1992. Postoperative radiation therapy for occult cervical lymph node metastases from an occult squamous cell carcinoma. *Laryngoscope 102*:884–890.

McQuone, S.J., Eisle, D.W., Lee, D., Westra, W.H., and Koch, W.M. 1998. Occult tonsillar carcinoma in the unknown primary. *Laryngoscope 108*:1605–1610.

Mendenhall, W.M., Mancus, A.A., Parsons, J.T., Stringer, S.P., and Cassisi, N.J. 1998. Diagnostic evaluation of squamous cell carcinoma metastatic to cervical lymph nodes from an unknown head and neck primary site. *Head Neck 20*:739–744.

Miller, F.R. 2004. Adult with a left sided neck mass. Patient of the month program. American Academy of Otolaryngology-Head Neck Surgery Foundation. Volume 34:2.

Miller, F.R., Hussey, D., Beeram, M., Eng, T., McGuff, H.S., and Otto, R.A. 2005. Positron emission tomography in the management of unknown primary head and neck carcinoma. *Arch. Otolaryngol. Head Neck Surg. 131*:626–629.

Miller, F.R., Karnad, A., Eng, T., Hussey, D., McGuff, H.S., and Otto, R.A. Management of the unknown primary carcinoma; the long term follow-up on a negative PET scan. *Head Neck.* In press.

Nanni, C., Rubello, D., Castelluci, P., Farsad, M., Franchi, R., Toso, S., Barile, C., Rampin, L., Nibale, O., and Fanti, S. 2005. Role of 18 F-FDG PET-CT imaging for the detection of an unknown primary tumor: preliminary results in 21 patients. *European J. Nuclear Medicine Molecular Imaging 32*:589–592.

Nguyen, C., Shenouda, G., Black, M.J., Vuong, T., Donath, D., and Yassa, M. 1994. Metastatic squamous cell carcinoma to cervical lymph nodes from unknown primary mucosal sites. *Head Neck 16*:58–63.

Pavlidis, N., Briasoulis, E., Hainsworth, J., and Greco, F.A. 2003. Diagnostic and therapeutic management of an unknown primary. *European Journal Cancer 39*:1990–2005.

Wagner, J.D., Schauwecker, D., Davidson, D., Logan, T., Coleman, J.J., Hutchins, G., Love, C., Wenck, S., and Daggy, J. 2005. Inefficiency of F-18 flourodeoxy-D-glucose-positron emission tomography scans for initial evaluation in early stage cutaneous melanoma. *Cancer 104*:570–579.

Wax, M.K., Myers, L.L., Gabalski, E.C., Husain, S., Gona, J.M., and Nabi, H. 2002. Positron emission tomography in the evaluation of synchronous lung lesions in patients with untreated head and neck cancer. *Arch. Otolaryngol. Head Neck Surg. 128*:703–707.

Zimmer, L.A., Branstetter, B.F., Nayak, J.V., and Johnson, J.T. 2005. Current use of 18-f-flourodeoxyglucose positron emission tomography and combined positron emission tomography and computed tomography in squamous cell carcinoma of the head and neck. *Laryngoscope 115*:2029–2034.

21

Benign and Malignant Nodes in the Neck: Magnetic Resonance Microimaging

Misa Sumi and Takashi Nakamura

Introduction

The presence of metastatic lymph nodes in the neck of patients with head and neck cancer is an important prognostic determinant in staging the cancer and in planning the patient's surgery and chemo- and radiotherapy. Therefore, metastatic nodes should be effectively differentiated from benign lymphadenopathies. The cervical lymph nodes are also the sites where other benign and malignant diseases occur, including infectious diseases and malignant lymphomas. Imaging examinations are expected to provide clues to differentiate between the benign and malignant nature in order to determine treatment planning.

We propose a high-resolution MR technique using a microscopy coil (MR microimaging) to differentiate between malignant and benign nodes in the neck. Detailed assessment of the affected nodes using high-resolution MR images could greatly improve the diagnostic performance of MR imaging in terms of detecting metastatic cervical nodes. Furthermore, assessment of the structural changes in the nodes by using the MR microimaging technique may be useful in differentiating between metastatic lymph nodes, nodal lymphomas, and benign lymphadenopathies.

Technical Details

The MR microimaging system used in this study is composed of a 1.5-T MR imager (Gyroscan Intera 1.5T Master; Philips Medical Systems) and a microscopy coil with a diameter of 47 mm. The 47-mm microscopy allows local acquisition of the MR signals with a high signal-to-noise ratio. This critical property of the microscopy coil, coupled with a field-of-view (FOV) of a small size and thin image sections, allows the achievement of high-resolution MR images. For example, when a 160×128 matrix size for a 7-cm FOV, 2-mm image thickness, and 0.2-mm interslice gap are used, MR images with a $0.438\,\text{mm} \times 0.547\,\text{mm} \times 2\,\text{mm}$ measured voxel size can be obtained. This resolution is much higher than those ranging from $0.7\,\text{mm} \times 0.7\,\text{mm} \times 4\,\text{mm}$ to $1\,\text{mm} \times 1\,\text{mm} \times 6\,\text{mm}$ that are obtained using other coils.

An inherent property of these coils of a small size is a low signal yield at increasingly greater distances from them. To overcome the image intensity inhomogeneity, the contrast-level appearance (CLEAR) postprocessing technique (Philips Medical Systems) is routinely used. This technique uses the premeasured sensitivity profile of the coil to calculate the compensation needed to apply to the pixel intensities so that even image intensity can be achieved. The 47-mm microscopy coil is positioned so that the nodes remain under the coil; the coil is secured using an adhesive tape and a band.

Axial fat-suppressed spectral presaturation with inversion recovery (SPIR) T2 images and axial T1-weighted spin-echo images, both obtained using the CLEAR technique, are useful for assessing the internal nodal architecture. T1-weighted imaging after an intravenous injection of a gadolinium-based contrast agent, such as gadopentetate dimeglumine, can provide additional information regarding the changes to the nodal vascularity. The acquisition time for each sequence is < 4 min for 15 slices.

Anatomy of the Lymph Node

A lymph node consists of four structural and functional components: (1) the cortex with its germinal center, where the B-cell system develops; (2) the medullary zone in which most of the plasma cells reside and the B-cell system exerts its secretory functions; (3) the paracortex lying between the germinal centers in which most T-cells reside; and (4) the sinuses, which contain macrophages and other mononuclear phagocytes.

The capsule of the lymph node is interrupted at various places by afferent lymphatics that transport lymph into the marginal sinus. The marginal sinus continues into the cortical or trabecular sinuses that traverse the paracortex and then enter the medullary cords; here the sinus (medullary sinus) becomes wider and more tortuous.

Almost all blood vessels enter lymph nodes through the hilum. The larger arterial branches initially run within the trabeculae; then they abruptly enter the medullary cords to supply their capillary network. Next, the arteries reach the cortex where they distribute to capillary plexuses of the cortical parenchyma and the germinal centers. In the paracortex, the capillary branches give rise to the high endothelial venules, which are characteristic of this region, and transport circulating lymphocytes, predominantly T-cells, to the paracortex.

Metastatic Nodes

Metastatic Focus and Nodal Necrosis

Cervical lymph node metastasis may occur in patients with both squamous and nonsquamous cell carcinomas of the head and neck. Lymph node metastasis leads to drastic changes in the components and structures of the nodes. A metastatic focus first appears in the cortical portion of the node. The focus continues to grow and gradually displaces the surrounding lymphoid tissues of the node. In conjunction with the growth of the metastatic focus, the metastatic

node becomes larger, and the metastatic cancer cells rupture the nodal capsule and, eventually, extend outward beyond the capsule (extranodal spread, ENS). The extranodal cancer cells may occasionally invade the surrounding structures such as the blood vessels, muscles, and skin, worsening the patient's prognosis.

Nodal necrosis may associate with nodal metastasis as cancer cells infiltrate into the medullary portion of the nodes and surpass the available blood supply, and is considered to be a pathognomonic feature of metastatic nodes in patients with squamous cell carcinomas of the head and neck. The nodal necrosis is also one of the most reliable imaging findings of metastatic nodes. It was reported to occur in 56–63% and 10–33% of metastatic nodes > 1.5 cm and < 1 cm in diameter, respectively (King *et al.*, 2004b). Conventional MR imaging is unable to detect the necrotic foci that were < 3 mm (van den Brekel *et al.*, 1990). In addition, small metastatic foci do not always cause enlargement of the affected nodes. In fact, 71% of metastatic nodes were smaller than 1 cm in minimal axial diameter (Castelijns and van den Brekel, 2002). Therefore, a small metastatic node with a necrotic focus that is < 3 mm may often be misinterpreted as a nonmetastatic node on conventional MR images.

Metastatic foci may exhibit, in addition to cancer cell nests and keratinization, either liquefaction necrosis or coagulation necrosis, or both (Nakamura and Sumi, 2007). On gadolinium-enhanced T1-weighted images, necrosis in the node is identified as a noncontrast-enhancing area (focal defect). On fat-suppressed T2-weighted images, the metastatic focus is most frequently identified as an area with high signal intensity; this corresponds to liquefaction necrosis. However, the metastatic focus may contain coagulation necrosis, which is demonstrated on fat-suppressed T2-weighted images as an area with lower signal intensity when compared with the residual normal lymphoid tissue (Fig. 1).

Keratinization is depicted as areas with remarkably low signal intensity on fat-suppressed T2-weighted and contrast-enhanced T1-weighted images. On T1-weighted images, however, keratinization may often be depicted as high signal intensity areas reflected in keratin protein. Cancer cell nests can be observed as low signal intensity areas on fat-suppressed T2-weighted images when compared with the residual normal lymphoid tissue. However, they are enhanced on gadolinium-enhanced T1-weighted images.

Magnetic resonance microimaging using a microscopy coil can potentially facilitate the detection of a metastatic lymph node in its early stages. Using MR microimaging, we were able to effectively distinguish metastatic nodes that harbored metastatic foci as small as 1.5 mm in diameter (Sumi *et al.*, 2006). Magnetic resonance microimaging can be coupled with other magnetic resonance imaging sequences; for example, diffusion-weighted imaging is used to evaluate water diffusibility in nodes with or without metastasis. In this regard, the apparent diffusion coefficients (ADCs) are

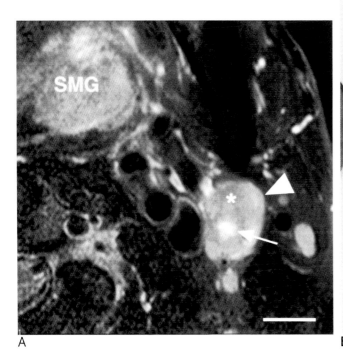
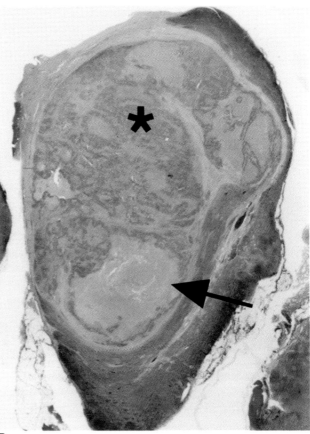

A

B

Figure 1 56-year-old man with tongue squamous cell carcinoma. (**A**) Axial fat-suppressed T2-weighted images shows a metastatic node (arrowhead) at level II of the neck. The node contains hyperintense focus (arrow) in a relatively hypointense area (*). SMG, submandibular gland. Scale bar = 10 mm. (**B**) Photomicrograph of the excised metastatic node in (**A**) shows large cancer nests (*) associated with liquefaction necrosis (arrow), which corresponds to the hyperintense focus in (**A**). Cancer nests consist mainly of proliferating cancer cells and coagulation necrosis.

significantly greater in the metastatic nodes than those in the benign nodes of the patients with head and neck carcinoma (Sumi *et al.*, 2006). Therefore, a combined use of these magnetic resonance microscopic criteria on nodal architectures and ADCs may be a promising technique for discriminating metastatic nodes.

Loss of Hilar Structure

As the metastasized cancer cell nest continues to increase in size and volume, the hilum becomes obliterated and the node eventually loses its bean-shaped contour. The presence of a normal hilum, and parenchymal homogeneity is suggestive of nonmetastatic nodes. The hilum is best depicted by ultrasonography (US) and can be identified as a highly echogenic structure in the central part of the node. The lack of the normal hilar echogenicity is one of the US criteria for the diagnosis of metastatic lymph nodes (Sumi *et al.*, 2001).

With regard to conventional MR imaging, little has been discussed on the appearance of the hilar structure; this is mainly because of the low spatial resolution.

High-resolution MR microimaging, on the other hand, can readily depict the normal hilum structure as a concavity of the nodes that is filled with fatty tissue. The hilar fat is depicted as a high-intensity area on T1-weighted images and as a low-intensity area on fat-suppressed T2-weighted images. The vessels in the hilum may also be depicted as a high-intensity area on both fat-suppressed T2- and contrast-enhanced T1-weighted images. The hilar fat is lost at a high rate in the metastatic lymph nodes (92%); however, such absence may also be noted in nodal lymphomas (79%) and even in benign lymphadenopathy (46%) (Sumi *et al.*, 2006). In the early stages of nodal metastasis, when the metastatic cancer nest is still very small, the hilar structures are intact. Missing hilar structure can also be observed in benign nodes as stated above. Therefore, although the findings on the hilar structures are helpful in differentiating between metastatic and benign nodes, they are not as predictive as the findings on focal defects with or without nodal necrosis.

Extranodal Spread

Extranodal spread (ENS) is a significant factor affecting the treatment plan and patients' prognosis. Therefore, sensitive detection of the ENS is mandatory for predicting poor treatment outcome and deciding whether regional and systemic adjuvant therapy should be considered. For detection of the advanced stages of ENS, we strongly recommend investigating the presence of lymph edema around the metastatic node. The nodes with ENS are frequently associated with high-intensity signals in the interstitial tissues. These signals can be observed around the metastatic nodes and appear to extend from them (flare sign) (unpublished observation).

The detection of ENS in its early stages by conventional MR imaging is difficult owing to its low spatial resolution. Even with MR microimaging, it is very hard to detect slight changes in the nodal capsule or minimal extensions of cancer cells into the surrounding fatty tissues. However, in relatively advanced stages, MR microimaging can depict an irregular margin blending into the surrounding tissues as an important finding suggestive of the ENS (Sumi *et al.*, 2006). Therefore, MR microimaging could detect early stages of ENS in the neck more readily than conventional MR imaging.

Nodal Lymphomas and Infectious Lymphadenopathy

Nodal Lymphomas

When a patient with an unknown primary neoplasm has cervical lymphadenopathy, differential diagnosis between metastatic lymph node and nodal lymphoma should be considered. Nodal lymphomas are generally well circumscribed and exhibit a homogeneous parenchyma on both T1- and fat-suppressed T2-weighted images (Fig. 2). Furthermore, the ADC of the lymphomas is significantly lower than that of the benign nodes and metastatic nodes (Sumi *et al.*, 2006). Therefore, it is not difficult to differentiate nodal lymphoma from nodal metastasis.

However, nodal necrosis is never uncommon in Hodgkin's and non-Hodgkin's Lymphomas, in particular, the diffuse large B-cell lymphomas (King *et al.*, 2004a; Sumi *et al.*, 2006). In such cases, nodal lymphomas may be reminiscent of metastatic nodes with a necrotic focus, and the differentiation between these two entities may be difficult. In addition, the presence of a necrotic area within the lymphoma would affect the ADC levels of the lesion. It is noteworthy that the nodal necrosis in lymphomas seems to differ from

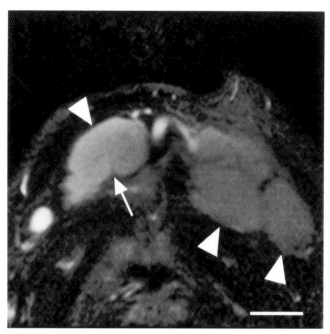

Figure 2 43-year-old man with non-Hodgkin's Lymphoma (mantle cell lymphoma). Axial fat-suppressed T2-weighted image shows multiple, enlarged nodes (arrowheads) with homogeneous areas of high signal intensity at level IA of the neck. Narrowed hilum (arrow) is seen in one of the nodal lymphomas. Scale bar = 10 mm.

that in metastatic nodes in that the former frequently occupies almost the entire node with minimal loss of the hilar structures. Moreover, it may appear as a hypointense focus on fat-suppressed T2-weighted images.

Infectious Lymphadenopathy

Infectious lymphadenopathies are very common and are in most cases caused by bacterial, mycobacterial, or viral infection. The presence of a normal hilum and homogeneous parenchyma suggests benign lymphadenopathy. However, in the inflammatory nodes, such as those in bacterial adenitis and cat-scratch disease, the nodal parenchyma is heterogeneous on MR microimages. This may be due to the pus formation, which is pathognomonic of the condition; it may also be due to the dilated blood vessels and the increased number of blood vessels. On fat-suppressed T2-weighted images, hyperintense radiating streaks representing blood vessels (Fig. 3), or a central hypointense core representing the flow-void phenomenon, are highly indicative of inflammatory nodes.

Imaging Strategy for Diagnosing Lymphadenopathy in the Neck

MR microimaging has some disadvantages. First, MR microimaging requires additional time for examination. Second, the small field-of-view makes observing

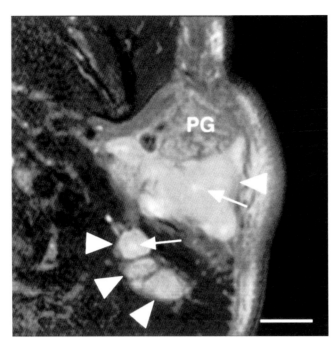

Figure 3 16-year-old girl with lymphadenitis in parotid nodes. Axial fat-suppressed T2-weighted image shows enlarged nodes (arrowheads) in and around the parotid gland (PG). Some of the nodes contain hyperintense areas (arrows) suggestive of enlarged blood vessels. Scale bar = 10 mm.

the surrounding structures difficult. Third, the technique does not apply to deep nodes. Therefore, the MR technique is not suitable for imaging the whole neck. A rapid and sensitive MR technique such as a coronal turbo STIR sequence would be useful for surveying suspected nodes in the whole of the neck before undertaking MR microimaging. When nodes are superficially located (within 6–7 cm from the neck surface) and a detailed examination of the nodes is required for purposes such as differential diagnosis of metastatic lymph nodes, nodal lymphomas, or benign lymphadenopathies, or for examining the presence or absence of extranodal spread, MR microimaging is recommended.

References

Castelijns, J.A., and van den Brekel, M.W.M. 2002. Imaging of lymphadenopathy in the neck. *Eur. Radiol. 12*:727–738.

King, A.D., Lei, K.I., and Ahuja, A.T. 2004a. MRI of neck nodes in non-Hodgkin's Lymphoma of the head and neck. *Br. J. Radiol. 77*:111–115.

King, A.D., Tse, G.M.K., Ahuja, A.T., Yuen, E.H.Y., Vlantis, A.C., To, E.W.H., and van Hasselt, A.C. 2004b. Necrosis in metastatic neck nodes: diagnostic accuracy of CT, MR imaging, and US. *Radiology 230*:720–726.

Nakamura, T., and Sumi, M. 2007. Nodal imaging in the neck: recent advances in US, CT, and MR imaging of metastatic nodes. *Eur. Radiol. 17*:1235–1241.

Sumi, M., Ohki, M., and Nakamura, T. 2001. Comparison of sonography and CT for differentiating benign from malignant cervical lymph nodes in patients with squamous cell carcinoma of the head and neck. *AJR Am. J. Roentgenol. 176*:1019–1024.

Sumi, M., Van Cauteren, M., and Nakamura, T. 2006. MR microimaging of benign and malignant nodes in the neck. *AJR Am. J. Roentgenol. 186*:749–757.

van den Brekel, M.W.M., Stel, H.V., Castelijns, J.A., Nauta, J.P.N., Van, der, Waal, I., Valk, J., Meyer, C.J.L.M., and Snow, G.B. 1990. Cervical lymph node metastasis: assessment of radiologic criteria. *Radiology 177*:379–384.

22

Oral Squamous Cell Carcinoma: Comparison of Computed Tomography with Magnetic Resonance Imaging

Akiko Imaizumi and Tohru Kurabayashi

Introduction

Malignant tumors of the oral cavity account for 2 to 3% of all malignancies. Histopathologically, ~ 90% of oral malignancies are squamous cell carcinomas (SCCs), and the other 10% include malignant lymphoma, mucoepidermoid carcinoma, and adenoid cystic carcinoma. Oral SCCs tend to occur in aged persons and are more common in males than in females. Tobacco smoking and alcohol are major risk factors for oral SCCs. Because of heavier tobacco and alcohol use, the incidence of oral SCCs is higher in males than in females. Tobacco chewing is also apparently associated with the development of oral SCCs. Actually, oral SCC is one of the most common cancers in India and South-East Asia, where the habit of chewing tobacco is seen. There are also special factors that are found primarily in the oral cavity. These include chronic irritation from jagged teeth and restorations, and ill-fitting dentures. Squamous cell carcinomas may occur anywhere in the oral cavity, including the lip, buccal mucosa, upper and lower alveolar ridges, retromolar trigone, floor of the mouth, hard palate, and oral tongue (anterior two-thirds of the tongue). Among these, the most

common site is the oral tongue, where more than 50% of oral SCCs occur, followed by the floor of the mouth. According to the histopathological findings, SCCs are classified into three types: well-, moderately, and poorly differentiated types. A well-differentiated SCC is a tumor that is mature and closely resembles the tissue of origin. In contrast, a poorly differentiated SCC is a tumor with much cellular and nuclear pleomorphism and numerous mitoses but little or no keratinization. Most oral SCCs are the moderately differentiated type.

Treatment of oral SCC includes surgical resection, radiation therapy, chemotherapy, or a combination of these approaches. The choice of treatment usually depends on many factors: the location and size of primary tumor, the tumor extent into surrounding tissues, and the presence or absence of lymph node and distant metastases. Thus, tumor staging is crucial for treatment planning. Tumor Node Metastasis (TNM) classification by the International Union Against Cancer (UICC) or the American Joint Committee on Cancer (AJCC) is most commonly used for staging. The T-stage, which has a strong influence on treatment planning, is stratified as follows:

T1: The greatest diameter of tumor is 2 cm or less.

T2: The greatest diameter of tumor is > 2 cm but not > 4 cm.

T3: The greatest diameter of tumor is > 4 cm.

T4: Tumor with invasion into adjacent structures including the medullary bone, extrinsic muscle of the tongue, maxillary sinus, and skin.

Although lesions in the oral cavity can easily be detected and palpated, the extent of tumor invasion into deep tissues is difficult to assess by clinical examination alone. However, imaging can clearly show the extent of tumor and its relationship to adjacent structures. Such imaging information is useful for accurate tumor staging, and helps surgeons and radiologists determine adequate resection margins and irradiation fields. Particularly in surgical planning, resection margins must be adequately defined, as neither too much nor too little, because excessive resection in the head and neck region will cause significant functional impairment of speech, chewing and swallowing, as well as aesthetic damage. Various imaging techniques, including conventional radiography, bone scintigraphy, computed tomography (CT), magnetic resonance imaging (MRI), and ultrasonography (US), have been used for patients with oral SCC. Among these techniques, currently CT and MRI are most commonly used.

When CT is applied to patients with oral SCC, the extracranial head and neck, from the skull base to the thoracic inlet, should be entirely scanned after contrast medium administration. Slice thickness should not exceed 5 mm. For evaluating bone invasion, a thinner slice is needed. After scanning, the images should be reconstructed with both soft tissue and bone algorithms. On CT images, oral SCC is depicted as a soft tissue mass with ill-defined border and irregular shape, and shows contrast enhancement. However, sufficient contrast between the tumor and surrounding soft tissues may not be obtained on CT, limiting the delineation of tumor extent in the surrounding soft tissues. Another limitation of CT is that bulky metal artifacts from dental restorations frequently hamper image interpretation (Fig. 1). However, CT is reported to be a reliable technique for assessing bone destruction and lymph node metastases.

The scanning range of MRI is the same as that of CT; thus, coils for the head and neck region should be used. The basic pulse sequences for oral SCCs comprise unenhanced and contrast-enhanced T1-weighted sequences and T2-weighted sequence. In addition to basic axial images, coronal images should be obtained to assess the supero-inferior extent of tumor. In the case with midline lesion, sagittal images might be useful. Slice thickness including interslice gap should be 3–5 mm. On T2-weighted and contrast-enhanced T1-weighted images, the use of fat-suppression techniques increases the contrast between tumor and surrounding tissues, resulting in improvement of tumor detectability. Similar to that on CT images, oral SCC is depicted as a soft tissue mass with an ill-defined border and irregular shape on MR images. On unenhanced T1-weighted images, the tumor shows homogeneous, isointensity in comparison with muscles. On T2-weighted images, the tumor mostly shows heterogeneous, high signal intensity. On contrast-enhanced T1-weighted images, the tumor shows contrast enhancement, and the enhancement pattern is mostly heterogeneous (Fig. 1). Heterogeneity increases by means of intratumorous hemorrhage or necrosis. It is obvious that MRI is superior to CT in demonstrating the tumor extent in soft tissues because of its excellent contrast resolution and multiplanar facility. On MR images, metal artifact is less harmful than that on CT. However, the images may be severely distorted by motion artifact because of the prolonged scanning time. To minimize patient movement, the radiology staff should carefully instruct the patient to remain still during the imaging. The use of fast imaging techniques reducing the scanning time is also considered useful.

Because oral SCC frequently arises close to the mandible, one of the most important roles of imaging is to assess the presence or absence of tumor invasion into the mandible. This is especially true of the tumors arising from the lower gingiva, retromolar trigone, floor of the mouth, and buccal mucosa. When the tumor extends to the mandible, marginal or segmental mandibulectomy must be performed, depending on its extent of invasion. When marginal mandibulectomy is performed, although the superior portion of the mandible is excised, the inferior portion is left intact and mandibular continuity is preserved. However, when segmental mandibulectomy is performed, the entire portion of the mandible is resected, resulting in mandibular discontinuity. Thus, segmental mandibulectomy causes more severe damage to postoperative function and aesthetics than marginal mandibulectomy. Although the final determination regarding the extent of resection will be made intraoperatively, preoperative imaging examinations are helpful for surgeons in planning either a marginal or a segmental mandibulectomy.

Many studies have reported the diagnostic accuracy of CT and MRI in evaluating mandibular invasion of oral SCC. Among them, Mukherji et al. (2001) used 3-mm-thick bone algorithm CT images and reported a sensitivity of 96% and a specificity of 87%. They concluded that CT was a reliable imaging modality for evaluating mandibular invasion when appropriate CT techniques were used. On the other hand, MRI was reported by some researchers to be highly sensitive but have a low positive predictive value for evaluating mandibular invasion. However, Bolzoni et al. (2004) recently reported a high diagnostic accuracy of MRI, a sensitivity of 93%, and a specificity of 93%, and considered that the specificity of MRI might be superior to that of CT. Most of the previous studies, including these reports, evaluated either CT or MRI alone and did not compare these two imaging modalities simultaneously. Only a few studies performed a

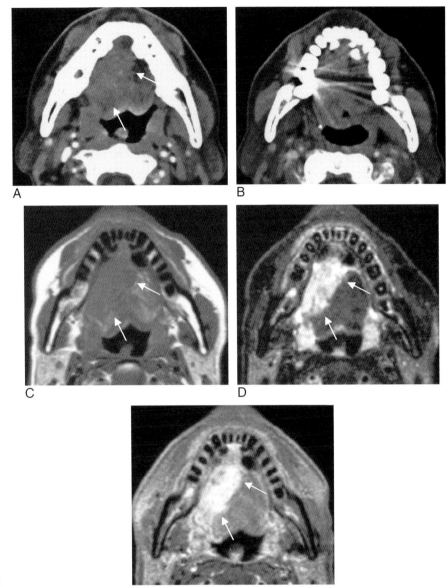

Figure 1 56-year-old man with right tongue carcinoma. (**A**), (**B**) Contiguous axial contrast-enhanced CT images reconstructed with soft tissue algorithm. (C) Axial T1-weighted MR image. (D) Axial T2-weighted MR image with fat saturation. (E) Axial contrast-enhanced T1-weighted MR image with fat saturation. Tumor of the right tongue is depicted as an inhomogeneously enhanced soft tissue mass with ill-defined border and irregular shape on CT image (A: arrows). However, contrast between the tumor and surrounding soft tissues is not enough; therefore, it is difficult to delineate the tumor margins precisely. The image is severely hampered by metal artifacts from dental restorations, which is a major drawback of CT for oral tumors (B). MR images provide better contrast between tumor and surrounding soft tissues and are superior to CT in delineating the tumor extent. The tumor shows homogeneous isointensity in comparison with muscles on unenhanced T1-weighted image (C: arrows) and heterogeneous, high signal intensity on T2-weighted image (D: arrows). On post-contrast image, the tumor is inhomogeneously enhanced (E: arrows). The tumor margins can be better delineated on T2-weighted and post-contrast T1-weighted images than on precontrast T1-weighted image.

direct comparison of CT and MRI. Once study showed that the respective sensitivity and specificity were 94% and 73% for MRI and 64% and 89% for CT, and that neither of these two imaging modalities was accurate enough. However, it seems that CT images used in the study were not optimal for the evaluation. Although Wiener *et al.* (2006) compared the diagnostic accuracy of 16-multidetector CT and that of MRI and reported that MRI was superior to CT in evaluating bone invasion, there was no statistically significant difference due to a limited number of cases. Others stated that CT depicts cortical bone invasion better and that the extent of medullary bone invasion is better defined with MRI; however, no evidence was provided that supported their views.

Thus, it is still controversial as to which modality has more advantages for evaluating mandibular invasion. Under these backgrounds, we directly compared the diagnostic accuracy of MRI and that of CT for assessing the presence and extent of mandibular invasion by oral SCCs.

Methods

Patients

Our study included 60 patients with SCC of the oral cavity clinically suspected of having mandibular invasion who were examined by both MRI and CT examinations prior to surgery. The patients comprised 44 males and 16 females with a mean age of 64 years (range 37 to 84 years). The primary site of the carcinoma was gingival mucosa in 31 patients, floor of the mouth in 22 patients, and buccal mucosa in 7 patients. After MRI and CT examinations, all patients underwent marginal ($n = 28$) or segmental ($n = 32$) mandibulectomy. Of the 60 patients, 30 patients had undergone some form of preoperative treatment: radiation therapy ($n = 8$), chemotherapy ($n = 9$), or radiation and chemotherapy ($n = 13$). None of the patients had undergone mandibular surgery before MRI or CT.

Imaging Protocol

Magnetic resonance images were obtained using a 1.5-T unit with a head and neck coil. In axial planes, T1-weighted spin-echo images (TR/TE = 500–700/14 ms) and T2-weighted fast spin-echo images (3000–5000/90; echo-train length, seven) with fat saturation were obtained in all 60 patients. In coronal planes, T1-weighted (500–700/14) and/or T2-weighted images (3000–5000/90) were obtained in all patients. In 48 out of 60 patients, axial and coronal T1-weighted spin-echo images (500–700/14) with fat saturation after intravenous administration of 0.1 mmol/kg of body weight of gadolinium contrast agent were also obtained. All images were obtained with 3–4-mm slice thickness, a 0.3–1-mm interslice gap, a field-of-view (FOV) of 173 × 230 mm, and a matrix of 154 × 256 (phase × frequency). Thus, we used a rectangular FOV technique to save measurement time while maintaining the same spatial resolution as in a square image. For axial imaging, superior and inferior presaturation pulses were applied.

For CT examination, spiral CT scanner was used. In all patients, 5-mm-thick axial spiral scan was performed from the skull base to the thoracic inlet after intravenous administration of 60–100 ml of iodine contrast agent, and contiguous 5-mm-thick axial images were reconstructed with both soft tissue and bone algorithms. In 41 cases in which the presence or extent of bone invasion was difficult to evaluate with the axial images alone, 1-mm-thick axial spiral scan for the mandible was added, and dental CT-reformatted images were also obtained using the Dental CT software, a CT software program that provides multiple panoramic and cross-sectional images of the jaw bone (Brockenbrough et al., 2003).

The average interval between MRI and CT was 12 days (range, 0–79 days; median, 6 days). In 82% of the cases (49/60), the interval was within 20 days. The average interval between the day when both imaging examinations were completed and that of surgery was 10 days (range, 1–73 days; median, 6 days). In 85% of the cases (51/60), the interval was within 20 days.

Imaging Assessment

Two radiologists who were not given any information regarding the tumor except for the primary site reviewed MR and CT images independently. The images were evaluated for the presence or absence of [A] mandibular cortical invasion, [B] bone marrow involvement, and [C] inferior alveolar canal involvement by tumor. The observers were first asked to evaluate [A]. When [A] was regarded as positive, then [B] was evaluated. Likewise, when [B] was regarded as positive, then [C] was evaluated. When the tumor was regarded as negative for [A], it was also regarded as negative for [B] and [C] without further assessment of images.

The diagnostic criteria of MRI and CT were as follows:

[A] mandibular cortical invasion
    MRI, CT: defect of the cortical bone adjacent to the tumor mass
[B] bone marrow involvement
    MRI: abnormal signal intensity of bone marrow* contiguous to the cortical defect
    CT: trabecular disruption contiguous to the cortical defect
[C] inferior alveolar canal involvement
    MRI, CT: bone marrow involvement reaching the inferior alveolar canal

Magnetic resonance images used for the evaluation of [A] were axial and coronal T1-weighted images, which are known to visualize the cortical bone most clearly. In six cases in which coronal T1-weighted images were not obtained, instead coronal T2-weighted images were used. For the evaluation of [B] and [C], all of T1-, T2-, and contrast-enhanced T1-weighted images were used. On the other hand, for CT evaluation, bone algorithm axial images were used in all cases. In addition, dental CT-reformatted images were also used in 41 cases. When disagreement existed between the assessments of two observers, a consensus was reached by discussion. Interobserver agreement was evaluated with κ statistics.

Pathological Assessment

The presence and extent of bone invasion by tumor were definitively determined by histopathological findings, which were used as the gold standard for this study. After fixation, mandibulectomy specimens were cut in the coronal plane at 5-mm intervals so as to include the deepest area of the tumor invasion. Then, after decalcification, the specimens were sectioned and stained with hematoxylin and eosin. Microscopic examinations were performed by one pathologist, who was unaware of imaging findings.

---

*Hypointense on T1-weighted and hyperintense on fat-suppressed T2-weighted image, with enhancement after contrast administration

Statistical Analysis

Magnetic resonance imaging and CT findings were correlated with histopathological findings. Sensitivity, specificity, positive and negative predictive values, and accuracy of each modality were calculated. To compare these two modalities for sensitivity and specificity, the McNemar test was used. A p-value less than 0.05 was considered to indicate a statistically significant difference. The κ values were calculated for interobserver agreement. A κ value of less than 0.40 was considered to indicate poor agreement; that of 0.40–0.59, fair agreement; that of 0.60–0.74, good agreement; and that of 0.75–1.00, excellent agreement.

Results

Thirty-two (53%) of the 60 tumors had histopathological evidence of mandibular invasion, whereas the remaining 28 had no evidence of invasion. In all 32 cases with invasion, the tumor involved both the cortex and the bone marrow. In 9 of those, the tumor was histopathologically confirmed to involve the inferior alveolar canal. Interobserver agreement was good or excellent for both MRI and CT. In the assessment of mandibular cortical invasion, bone marrow involvement, and inferior alveolar canal involvement, the κ values for MRI were 0.67, 0.83, and 0.90, respectively; and those for CT were 0.83, 0.79, and 1.00, respectively.

Mandibular Cortical Invasion

Of the 32 tumors with histopathologically positive results, 31 were true positive with both modalities. The remaining one was true positive with CT but false negative with MRI. This was a case of gingival carcinoma, which slightly involved the alveolar crest. The sensitivity of MRI and CT was 97% and 100%, respectively, and the difference was not significant (McNemar test, $p > 0.05$) (Table 1).

On the other hand, of the 28 tumors with histopathologically negative results, 14 were true negative and four were false positive with both modalities. The remaining 10 tumors were true negative with CT but false positive with MRI (Fig. 2). The specificity of MRI and CT was 50% and 86%, respectively (Table 1). The specificity of MRI was significantly lower than that of CT ($p = 0.002$). Eight of the 10 tumors in which only MRI showed false-positive results were anterior floor-of-mouth carcinomas. The misclassification of these eight cases with MRI seemed to be attributed to chemical shift artifacts induced by bone marrow fat. Namely, it was considered that the black line of the cortex adjacent to the tumor mass was obscured by spatial misplacement of fat (Fig. 2). The other false-positive cases, including two cases with only MRI and four with both modalities, were attributed to severe periodontal disease or secondary changes from tooth extraction. Such misclassification was found in both modalities, although more common with MRI than with CT.

Bone Marrow Involvement

The results with CT for bone marrow involvement were the same as those for cortical invasion. As to MRI, all of the eight cases that showed false-positive results for cortical invasion due to chemical shift artifacts had true-negative results for bone marrow invasion. The sensitivity of MRI and CT was 97% and 100%, respectively, and the difference was not significant ($p > 0.05$) (Table 1). The specificity of MRI and CT was 82% and 86%, respectively, and the difference was not significant ($p > 0.05$) (Table 1).

Table 1 Diagnostic Accuracy of MRI and CT in Evaluating Bone Invasion

	TP	TN	FP	FN	Sensitivity	Specificity	PPV	NPV	Accuracy
	(No. of cases)						(%)		
Mandibular cortical invasion									
MRI	31	14	14	1	97	50*	69	93	75
CT	32	24	4	0	100	86*	89	100	93
Bone marrow involvement									
MRI	31	23	5	1	97	82	86	96	90
CT	32	24	4	0	100	86	89	100	93
Inferior alveolar canal involvement									
MRI	9	35	16	0	100	69**	36	100	73
CT	9	47	4	0	100	92**	69	100	93

TP: true positive, TN: true negative, FP: false positive, FN: false negative, PPV: positive-predictive value, NPV: negative-predictive value.
*$p = 0.002$, **$p = 0.002$ (McNemar test).

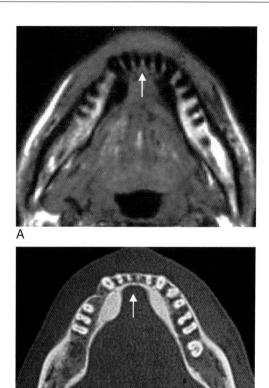

Figure 2 49-year-old man with anterior floor-of-mouth carcinoma showing a false-positive result with MRI and true-negative result with CT for cortical invasion. **(A)** Axial T1-weighted MR image. **(B)** Axial CT image reconstructed with bone algorithm. The lingual cortex is suspected to be involved by the tumor mass on T1-weighted MR image (A: arrow), whereas it is intact on CT (B: arrow). Histopathological examination after marginal mandibulectomy confirmed no tumor invasion into the mandible. Chemical shift artifacts induced by bone marrow fat are considered to account for the false-positive result with MRI. That is, the black line of the cortex adjacent to the tumor mass is thought to be obscured by spatial misplacement of bone marrow fat (A).

Inferior Alveolar Canal Involvement

Both MRI and CT correctly diagnosed the nine tumors with histopathological evidence of inferior alveolar canal involvement, providing the sensitivity of 100% (Table 1). On the other hand, the number of false-positive cases was 16 with MRI, whereas it was four with CT. Thus, the specificity of MRI was significantly lower than that of CT (69% for MRI and 92% for CT, $p = 0.002$) (Table 1). Magnetic resonance imaging often showed the tumor and the surrounding inflammation in the bone marrow with similar signal intensity, resulting in overestimation of the tumor extent. When the 30 patients who received preoperative radiation and/or chemotherapy were excluded from the study, the specificity

of MRI was still significantly lower than that of CT (69% for MRI and 96% for CT, $p = 0.039$).

Discussion

Because of their close anatomical relationship to the mandible, SCCs of the oral cavity have a high tendency to invade the mandible. Thus, for those tumors clinically close to the mandible, one of the most important roles of imaging is to evaluate accurately the presence and extent of tumor invasion into the mandible. Various imaging techniques, including conventional radiographs, bone scintigraphy, CT, and MRI, have been used for this purpose. Among them, conventional radiographs cannot reveal bone invasion in detail. Bone scintigraphy has been reported to have considerable false-positive rates, although being highly sensitive.

Computed tomography is the imaging technique that is most commonly used to evaluate mandibular invasion. The diagnostic accuracy of CT in detecting mandibular invasion varies widely depending on the researchers. Some studies reported > 30% false-positive and/or false-negative rates for CT, but these results are considered to be due to inappropriate CT techniques that were used. Mukherji *et al.* (2001) used 3-mm-thick bone algorithm CT images and reported a sensitivity of 96% and specificity of 87%. Similarly, the studies in which overlapping 5-mm-thick bone algorithm images or dental CT-reformatted images were used showed a high diagnostic accuracy of CT. Thus, as indicated by Mukherji *et al.* (2001), CT seems to be a reliable imaging modality for evaluating mandibular invasion when appropriate CT techniques are used.

On the other hand, the number of studies focusing on MRI is relatively limited. Among them, some researchers reported a high rate of false-positive studies with MRI. One study showed that a positive-predictive value of MRI was 67% for evaluating mandibular invasion. Similarly, others reported that a positive-predictive value of MRI was < 70% for evaluating cortical invasion and < 50% for medullary invasion. However, Bolzoni *et al.* (2004) recently reported a high diagnostic accuracy of MRI for detecting mandibular invasion, a sensitivity of 93%, and a specificity of 93%. Therefore, it is still controversial as to which modality is better in evaluating the presence and extent of mandibular invasion by tumor. For this purpose, we directly compared the diagnostic accuracy between MRI and CT.

We used the imaging criteria similar to those in most previous studies for evaluating mandibular invasion. When evaluating CT, bone algorithm axial images were used in all cases. In addition, in more than two-thirds of the cases in which the presence and/or extent of mandibular invasion was unclear on axial images, dental CT-reformatted images were also obtained and used. It is difficult to evaluate the presence of the slight invasion of tumor into the alveolar crest or the supero-inferior extent of tumor invasion into the mandible with axial CT alone. In our study, dental CT-reformatted images were obtained in all cases in which such evaluation was needed. For evaluating MRI, we used unenhanced axial and coronal T1-weighted images to detect mandibular cortical invasion, because those images are known to demonstrate cortical destruction most clearly. On the other hand, we used all MR images to detect tumor invasion into the bone marrow. Namely, in our study, bone marrow fat replacement on T1-weighted images alone was not regarded as medullary invasion, because such finding can be found in reactive bone sclerosis and idiopathic dense bone island, which are conditions commonly seen in the mandible.

In the evaluation of mandibular cortical invasion, we found one false-negative study with MRI. In this case, dental CT-reformatted images were useful in detecting slight invasion of a gingival carcinoma into the alveolar crest. We used a single helical CT with 1-mm-thick sections to reconstruct dental CT. The diagnostic accuracy may be further improved by using multidetector CT with thinner slice thickness or cone beam CT with a minute voxel of an isotropic cube with a side of ~ 0.125 mm. On the other hand, we found four false-positive studies with both modalities and ten with only MRI. The specificity of MRI was significantly lower than that of CT (50% for MRI and 86% for CT, $p = 0.002$). It has been reported that false-positive cases could be created by inflammatory odontogenic disease, postextraction bone defect, osteoradionecrosis, some normal variations of the cortex, and partial-volume effect. In our study also, some false-positive cases were attributed to severe periodontal disease or secondary changes from tooth extraction. Although such misclassification occurred in both modalities, it was more common with MRI than with CT. The bone defects due to these benign processes tend to show smooth margins on images, in contrast to those by malignant lesions generally showing irregular or ill-defined margins. Therefore, they may be differentiated to some extent, on the basis of the imaging features. It seemed that CT was superior to MRI in evaluating the contours of bone resorption in detail.

In addition to the well-known conditions simulating tumor invasion, our study showed that chemical shift artifact was a possible cause of false-positive results with MRI. Eight of the ten tumors in which only MRI showed false-positive results were anterior floor-of-mouth carcinomas. In these cases, the lingual cortex adjacent to the tumor mass was lost by spatial misplacement of bone marrow fat on MR images, while it was completely intact on CT (Fig. 2).

To confirm our hypothesis that chemical shift artifact might obscure the lingual cortex of the midline mandible, we performed the validation study in which MRI was performed in a normal volunteer. In the study, the mandible was imaged by the three different methods of T1-weighted spin-echo sequence: T1-weighted image with ordinary setting of phase- and frequency-encoding directions; T1-weighted

image in which phase- and frequency-encoding directions are swapped; and T1-weighted image with fat saturation. The study showed that the lingual cortex was lost on the ordinary T1-weighted image, whereas it remained intact when phase- and frequency-encoding directions were swapped or when fat saturation pulse was used. These findings confirmed our hypothesis.

The hydrogen protons in fat process at 3.5 ppm lower frequency than those in water, resulting in a spatial misplacement of the fat signal to the lower level along the frequency-encoding direction. The difference corresponds to 220 Hz when 1.5-T unit is used. Considering other parameters in our study, including bandwidth of 32 kHz, FOV of 230 mm, and matrix of 256 pixels in the frequency-encoding direction (y-axis direction), the misplacement of fat is calculated as follows:

$$220 \text{ Hz} / (32 \text{ kHz}/256 \text{ pixels}) = 1.8 \text{ pixels}$$
$$1.8 \text{ pixels} \times 230 \text{ mm}/256 \text{ pixels} = 1.6 \text{ mm}$$

This amount of the shift is thought to be large enough to obscure the black line of the cortex. When obtaining axial MR images in the head and neck region, it is recommended to set the phase- and the frequency-encoding directions along x- and y-axes, respectively, in order to minimize the effect of motion artifacts by globe movement or arterial blood flow. In addition, if a rectangular FOV technique is applied, the frequency-encoding direction must be set along the y-axis because an image is longer in y-axis than in x-axis direction. If lower frequencies are inferior, spatial misplacement of bone marrow fat will obscure the lingual cortex on MR images. Similarly, when superior, the fat will obscure the labial cortex. In both occasions, chemical shift artifacts can be a potential pitfall of MRI for assessing mandibular invasion by tumor.

As to the tumor extent within the mandible, we evaluated both bone marrow involvement and inferior alveolar canal involvement. In this regard, we evaluated the presence or absence of tumor invasion reaching the inferior alveolar canal, and we found that it tended to be overestimated with MRI. One study reported that MRI could clearly reveal the tumor in the bone marrow with different signal intensity and was considered superior to CT in evaluating the pathologic change in this location. However, our results were not compatible with that study. In evaluating inferior alveolar canal involvement, the specificity of MRI was significantly lower than that of CT (69% for MRI and 92% for CT, $p = 0.002$). Even in cases that were true negative with MRI, it often showed greater extent of the tumor than CT and pathologic specimens. Comparing imaging with histopathological features, we found that inflammatory changes (i.e., peritumoral edema, reactive changes, fibrosis, etc.) in the surrounding bone marrow could show abnormal signal intensity similar to that of tumor, resulting in the overestimation of the tumor extent. In addition, regardless of the presence or absence of tumor mass, severe dental caries and periodontal disease can easily cause chronic inflammation of the mandible. Therefore, such abnormal signal in the bone marrow is more commonly found in the mandible compared with other bones of the body. This will also account for the low specificity of MRI. Dynamic MRI may be useful to distinguish tumor from inflammatory changes; however, further investigation will be needed to determine whether this technique is valuable in evaluating the tumor extent in the bone marrow.

Our study had some limitations that should be addressed. The first limitation was the difference of spatial resolution between both modalities. Magnetic resonance imaging had apparently lower resolutions than 1-mm-thick CT. Recently, several investigations have reported the usefulness of high-resolution MRI with small-diameter surface coils in the diagnosis of the head and neck region (Kress et al., 2004; Wiener et al., 2005). Although only conventional MR images were evaluated in our study, such high-resolution images might have shown further details of the mandible and improved the diagnostic accuracy of MRI. The second limitation was the preoperative treatment with radiation and/or chemotherapy in half the patients, which could affect the bone marrow signal of MRI. We confirmed that the specificity of MRI was still lower than that of CT, when those patients were excluded from the study. However, such pretreatment may account for some of the cases that were false positive with MRI but true negative with CT in the assessment of inferior alveolar canal involvement. Finally, SCC might invade into the mandibular bone marrow without cortical destruction, although such cases were not encountered in this series. Bolzoni et al. (2004) reported a case in which mandibular involvement by neoplastic vascular embolization into the bony lacunae was histopathologically confirmed with absence of direct cortical invasion. If such a case had been encountered in our study, it would have been misclassified with both CT and MRI because of the lack of evidence of cortical invasion.

Conclusion

For assessing the presence and extent of mandibular invasion in oral SCC, the specificity of MRI was significantly lower than that of CT. The false-positive cases of MRI in the evaluation of mandibular cortical invasion were due mostly to chemical shift artifact by bone marrow fat, which obscured the black line of the cortex. On the other hand, those cases

in evaluating inferior alveolar canal involvement were due to the fact that MRI showed the tumor and the surrounding inflammation with similar signal intensity, resulting in overestimation of the tumor extent in the bone marrow.

On the basis of our results, we would propose an imaging protocol for oral SCC as follows:

1. Magnetic resonance imaging is recommended as the basic imaging modality for primary tumor in the oral cavity. This modality can depict the tumor infiltration into deep tissues that is easily missed by clinical examinations. Unenhanced and contrast-enhanced T1-weighted sequences and T2-weighted sequences are mandatory, and, if possible, fat-suppression techniques should be applied to T2-weighted and contrast-enhanced T1-weighted imaging.

2. When mandibular invasion by tumor is suspected on MR images, CT should be added. Thin-slice bone algorithm images are most suitable for evaluating tumor invasion into the mandible. If possible, Dental CT-reformatted images should be used for assessing the supero-inferior tumor extent or detecting small alveolar bone destruction.

3. When only MRI can be used for the evaluating of the tumor invasion into the mandible, radiologists should know the potential pitfall of MRI shown in our study, causing a significant number of false-positive cases.

References

Bolzoni, A., Cappiello, J., Piazza, C., Peretti, G., Maroldi, R., Farina, D., and Nicolai, P. 2004. Diagnostic accuracy of magnetic resonance imaging in the assessment of mandibular involvement in oral-oropharyngeal squamous cell carcinoma: a prospective study. *Arch. Otolaryngol. Head Neck Surg.* 130:837–843.

Brockenbrough, J.M., Petruzzelli, G.J., and Lomasney, L. 2003. DentaScan as an accurate method of predicting mandibular invasion in patients with squamous cell carcinoma of the oral cavity. *Arch. Otolaryngol. Head Neck Surg.* 129:113–117.

Kress, B., Gottschalk, A., Anders, L., Stippich, C., Palm, F., Bahren, W., and Sartor, K. 2004. High-resolution dental magnetic resonance imaging of inferior alveolar nerve responses to the extraction of third molars. *Eur. Radiol.* 14:1416–1420.

Mukherji, S.K., Isaacs, D.L., Creager, A., Shockley, W., Weissler, M., and Armao, D. 2001. CT detection of mandibular invasion by squamous cell carcinoma of the oral cavity. *Am. J. Roentgenol.* 177:237–243.

Wiener, E., Kolk, A., Neff, A., Settles, M., and Rummeny, E. 2005. Evaluation of reconstructed orbital wall fractures: high-resolution MRI using a microscopy surface coil versus 16-slice MSCT. *Eur. Radiol.* 15:1250–1255.

Wiener, E., Pautke, C., Link, T.M., Neff, A., and Kolk, A. 2006. Comparison of 16-slice MSCT and MRI in the assessment of squamous cell carcinoma of the oral cavity. *Eur. J. Radiol.* 58:113–118.

23

Computed Tomography in Renal Cell Carcinoma

Eduard Ghersin, Marco A. Amendola, and Ahuva Engel

Introduction

Renal cell carcinoma was estimated to account for > 35,000 new diagnoses and > 12,000 cancer-related deaths in the United States in 2005, making it the most common and most lethal genitourinary malignancy (Lane and Kattan, 2005; Sheth *et al.*, 2001). As such, early diagnosis and accurate characterization and staging of renal cell carcinoma are of paramount importance for treatment triage and patient survival. The present widespread use of cross-sectional imaging in general and multidetector computed tomography (MDCT) in particular enables radiologists and clinicians to refine diagnostic work-up, treatment, and follow-up of renal cell carcinoma.

Multidetector Computed Tomography Technique

Among the prominent advantages of recent MDCT technology over previous single-detector-row CT are markedly improved speed and volume coverage as well as submillimeter collimation. These features are responsible for marked improvement in spatial, contrast, and temporal resolutions, allowing fast, multiphasic volumetric data acquisition of the entire kidney as well as urinary tract. These unique capabilities encouraged radiologists to design a single comprehensive imaging protocol to thoroughly evaluate the entire urinary tract. As a result, MDCT urography emerged as a real one-stop-shop imaging modality (Caoili *et al.*, 2002; Lang *et al.*, 2003).

In the context of renal cell carcinoma, all reported MDCT protocols share one common characteristic: multiphasic scanning of the entire kidney. Many of these protocols include an unenhanced scan, a corticomedullary–late arterial phase, a nephrographic–parenchymal phase, and a urographic–excretory phase. Each phase has its distinctive values and limitations, and only their combination achieves the goal of accurate imaging of renal cell carcinoma.

Unenhanced Computed Tomography Scan

Most renal cell carcinomas are solid lesions with attenuation values of 20 Hounsfield Units (HU) or greater at unenhanced CT (Fig. 1A). Small tumors tend to have a homogeneous appearance, while larger lesions tend to be more heterogeneous owing to hemorrhage or necrosis (Sheth *et al.*, 2001). Unenhanced scans provide a reference attenuation map of the entire kidney volume from which to measure the enhancement within the lesion after the administration of intravenous contrast material. Commonly being a hypervascular tumor, conventional (clear cell) renal cell carcinomas are enhanced significantly following administration of contrast material, with mean enhancement values of 106 HU and 62 HU during corticomedullary and excretory phases, respectively (Kim *et al.*, 2002). This feature aids in the differential diagnosis between hyperdense renal cysts and renal cell carcinomas. Enhancement values below 15–20 HU are considered "pseudoenhancement" and are the result of overcorrection for beam hardening in the reconstruction algorithm. However, enhancement values of > 15–20 HU are considered true enhancements and raise suspicion for malignancy (Foley, 2003; Israel and Bosniak, 2005). The presence of true enhancement cannot be overemphasized, and it is regarded as the most important criterion used in the differentiation of surgical from nonsurgical renal masses (Israel and Bosniak, 2005). Unenhanced scans are also valuable in demonstrating calcifications, which are found in 11 to 38% of renal cell carcinomas (Kim *et al.*, 2002). Dense calcifications may interfere with contrast-enhancement detection, especially if prior unenhanced scans are not available for correlation.

Corticomedullary–Late Arterial Phase

This phase starts at 25–40 sec following initiation of contrast material injection. During this phase there is primary enhancement of the renal cortex, whereas the renal medulla enhances insignificantly (Fig. 1B). This enhancement pattern is the result of preferential arterial blood flow to the cortex and rapid glomerular filtration. This phase is essential for accurate staging and surgical planning of renal cell carcinoma since it provides adequate opacification of both renal veins and arteries. Furthermore, hypervascular renal metastases to solid abdominal organs (liver, spleen, and pancreas) will be more conspicuous during this phase.

Though essential for imaging, radiologists should be aware of several potential pitfalls in the CT appearance of renal cell carcinoma during the corticomedullary phase (Sheth *et al.*, 2001). The most common pitfall leading to false-negative readings occurs when centrally located small renal cell carcinomas are mistaken for normal hypodense renal pyramids. Additional less common pitfalls occur when heterogeneously enhancing medulla is mistaken for a small centrally located renal cell carcinoma or when a small peripherally located renal cell carcinoma enhances to the same degree as the normal adjacent renal cortex, leading, respectively, to false-positive and false-negative readings.

Nephrographic–Parenchymal Phase

This phase starts at 80 sec and lasts up to 180 sec following initiation of contrast material injection. During this phase there is homogeneous enhancement of the renal parenchyma, including cortex and medulla. This enhancement pattern is the result of slower medullary blood supply and continuous propagation of the filtered contrast material through nephrons' tubular system, eventually filling the loops of Henle and collecting tubules, which are located in the renal medulla.

This phase is invaluable regarding renal cell carcinoma detection (Fig. 1C) (Sheth *et al.*, 2001). During this phase there is maximal discrepancy between the heterogeneous enhancement of renal cell carcinoma and the homogeneous enhancement of normal renal parenchyma, thus avoiding many of the pitfalls described during the corticomedullary phase. Suh *et al.* (2003) demonstrated that enhancement values, together with enhancement heterogeneity patterns evaluated during the nephrographic phase, can identify renal cell carcinoma from high-attenuation renal cysts with substantial accuracy. They concluded that attenuation values > 70 HU or the presence of moderate or marked internal heterogeneity was an accurate sign of renal cell carcinoma, with a sensitivity of 91% and a specificity of 84–92% (Suh *et al.*, 2003). This information is of particular importance to radiologists since nowadays with the widespread use of computed tomography up to 61% of renal cell carcinomas are asymptomatic and are discovered incidentally during routine abdominal CT performed only in the nephrographic phase of contrast material enhancement.

Urographic–Excretory Phase

This phase starts at 180 sec following initiation of contrast material injection; however, many researchers use prolonged delays of 5–8 min to ensure adequate opacification of renal collecting systems and ureters (Caoili, 2002; Catalano *et al.*, 2003; Gray Sears *et al.*, 2002; McTavish *et al.*, 2002). During this phase, the homogeneous enhancement of the renal parenchyma progressively diminishes together with dense opacification of renal collecting systems and ureters. This enhancement pattern is the result of continuous contrast material excretion through the collecting tubules into the renal collecting systems (Fig. 1D). In the context of centrally located renal cell carcinomas, this phase provides valuable delineation of potential involvement of renal calyces or renal pelvis.

Based on a recent updated literature review, most dedicated MDCT protocols for diagnosis and staging of previously identified or suspected renal cell carcinomas include all four phases of renal enhancement as described previously, despite the added radiation exposure (Table 1) (Catalano *et al.*, 2003; Lang *et al.*, 2003; Sheth *et al.*, 2001). Nonetheless, some authors do not routinely include the urographic–excretory phase of enhancement, unless delineation of potential involvement of renal calyces or renal pelvis by a centrally located renal cell carcinoma is required (Israel and Bosniak, 2005). Contrast enhancement is achieved using 120–150 ml of nonionic iodinated contrast material, injected via an 18-gauge peripheral venous access at a rate of 3–4 ml/sec.

Role of Image Reconstruction

Image reconstruction using multiplanar reformats, maximal intensity projections, and volume-rendering algorithms

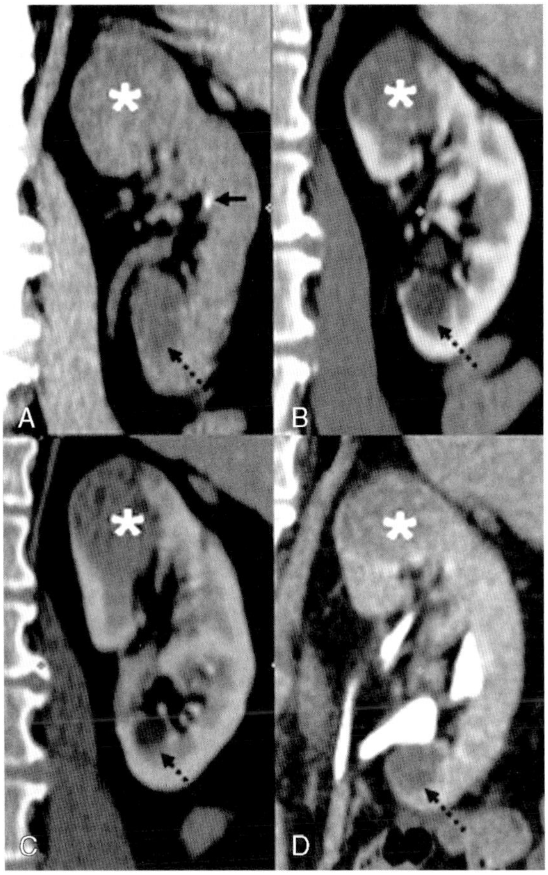

Figure 1 A 56-year-old man, with an upper pole left renal mass, initially depicted during urinary tract calculi assessment using an unenhanced CT scan. Coronal oblique reformats from a dedicated multiphasic MDCT scan clearly show a 5-cm upper pole renal mass (*). The mass demonstrates marked heterogeneous enhancement, with attenuation values of 20–25 HU on unenhanced scan (A), 70–145 HU on corticomedullary–late arterial phase scan (B), 91–163 HU on nephrographic–parenchymal phase scan (C), 56–80 HU on urographic–excretory phase scan (D). Also noted are simple nonenhancing renal cyst in the lower pole (dotted black arrows) and tiny calculus in the middle calyx (solid black arrow). This mass was correctly staged as a T1b renal cell carcinoma. Final pathological diagnosis revealed clear cell renal cell carcinoma.

are essential for establishing tumor size, location and relationship to renal surface, collecting system, vascular pedicle, and adjacent organs. It also helps to delineate the uppermost extension of inferior vena cava thrombotic involvement, essential information for planning the surgical approach.

Staging of Renal Cell Carcinoma

Radical cancer surgery remains the only curative treatment in localized and advanced renal cell carcinoma. Therefore, accurate staging is one of the main roles of imaging, since it predicts outcome and helps triaging appropriate treatment (Heidenreich and Ravery, 2004). In that con-

text, multidetector CT has a reported accuracy of 83–91% (Hallscheidt et al., 2004; Sheth et al., 2001).

The anatomic spread of renal cell carcinoma at the time of diagnosis was found to be the most reliable single prognostic factor, with a reported 5-year survival of 71–97% in patients with renal confined disease compared to 5–10% in patients with distant metastatic disease (Frank et al., 2005; Sheth et al., 2001).The specific histological tumor type is another factor that affects patients' survival. For example in papillary and chromophobe renal cell carcinomas, only 10% and 16.6% of tumors, respectively, demonstrate extrarenal extension at the time of diagnosis, compared to 49% of clear cell renal cell carcinomas (Bonsib, 2005).

There are two commonly used staging systems, the older Robson classification (Robson, 1982) and the more recent Tumor Node Metastases (TNM) classification, which was updated by the American Joint Committee on Cancer in 2002 (Frank et al., 2005). Although the TNM classification is more complex, it predicts to a better extent curative surgical resectability as well as patient survival. Both classifications with their corresponding multidetector CT findings are presented in Table 2.

Tumors Confined within the Renal Capsule

Patients with renal cell carcinomas limited to the kidney, consistent with stage T1a-b and T2 or I according to TNM and Robson classifications, respectively, have a better prognosis, with a 5-year survival of 71–97% following curative surgical resection (Frank et al., 2005). With the present widespread use of cross-sectional imaging, as many as 30–61% of renal tumors are discovered incidentally, and many lesions can be appropriately treated with nephron sparing surgery and maximal preservation of the surrounding unaffected parenchyma (Catalano et al., 2003; Suh et al., 2003). This surgical approach can only be contemplated pending imaging documentation of tumor organ confinement without evidence of perinephric fat infiltration. Using thin, 1-mm collimated, MDCT scan during the nephrographic–parenchymal phase of enhancement, Catalano et al. (2003) were able to diagnose organ confinement with a sensitivity, specificity, accuracy, positive-predictive value, and negative-predictive value of 96, 93, 95, 100, and 93, respectively. They used the presence of a pseudocapsule (a thin band of fibrous tissue and compressed renal parenchyma surrounding the lesion) coupled with lack of perinephric fat infiltration as the MDCT sign of tumor organ confinement.

Tumor Invasion of Perinephric Fat

Patients with renal cell carcinoma invasion of the perinephric fat, consistent with stage T3a or II according to TNM and Robson classifications, respectively, have an intermediate prognosis with a 5-year survival of 53% following

Table 1   Suggested Multidetector CT Protocols for the Diagnosis and Staging of Renal Cell Carcinoma

Imaging Parameters / Enhancement Phase	Unenhanced	Corticomedullary	Nephrographic	Urographic
Scanning delay (seconds)	0	22–40	60–140	180–480
Detector collimation (mm)	1.5–2.5	0.75–1	1–2.5	1–2.5
Section thickness (mm)	3–5	1–1.25	1.25–3	1.25–3
Reconstruction interval (mm)	3–5	1	1–3	1–3
Area scanned	Lower thorax—lower pole of kidneys	Diaphragm—lower pole of kidneys	Diaphragm—lower pole of kidneys	Upper pole of kidneys—ischial tuberosity
Image reconstruction	MPR	MPR MIP projections VR	MPR	MPR MIP projections VR

Note: MPR—multiplanar reformatted images, MIP—projection maximum intensity projections; VR—volume-rendering reformatted images.

curative surgical resection (Frank *et al.*, 2005). The reported MDCT signs of perinephric tumor spread are the presence of perinephric fat stranding, perinephric collateral vessels, and perinephric enhancing soft tissue masses. The last finding is regarded as the most specific sign, although its sensitivity is only 46% (Sheth *et al.*, 2001). Since the presence of perinephric fat stranding and perinephric collateral vessels is not specific of tumor infiltration and may result from edema, vascular engorgement, or previous inflammation, several authors reported sensitivity and specificity values of ~ 50% in diagnosing renal cell carcinoma invasion of the perinephric fat by MDCT (Sheth *et al.*, 2001). Although yet to be proven by a larger series of patients, application of thin 1-mm collimated CT scans may significantly improve the sensitivity and specificity of MDCT in diagnosing perinephric fat infiltration (Catalano *et al.*, 2003). Accurate preoperative identification of perinephric fat spread is of paramount importance because it modifies the surgical approach from conservative to radical nephrectomy.

Tumor Involvement of the Ipsilateral Adrenal Gland

Patients with renal cell carcinoma involvement of the ipsilateral adrenal gland are still consistent with stage T3a or II according to TNM and the Robson classifications, respectively, and are candidates for curative aggressive surgery, including adrenalectomy. Nonetheless, several investigators suggest that ipsilateral adrenal gland involvement should be regarded as a more advanced stage since it is associated with an extremely dismal prognosis with a reported 5-year survival of 20% following curative surgical resection (Thompson *et al.*, 2005). The likelihood of ipsilateral adrenal involvement increases with large and advanced stage renal cell carcinomas and with renal cell carcinomas of the upper

pole of the kidney. In that context, MDCT was found to be very efficient in excluding ipsilateral adrenal involvement by demonstrating the normal ipsilateral adrenal gland, giving a negative-predictive value of 100%. In addition, application of very thin 1-mm collimated CT scans resulted in a sensitivity of 100% in preoperative detection of ipsilateral adrenal involvement (Catalano *et al.*, 2003). These findings support the present accepted surgical approach allowing an adrenal sparing approach in the case of unsuspicious findings on MDCT (Heidenreich and Ravery, 2004).

Tumor Venous Spread

Patients with renal cell carcinoma invasion into the renal vein and inferior vena cava, consistent with stage T3b-c or IIIA according to TNM and the Robson classifications, respectively, is relatively common, occurring in 23% and 4–10% of patients, respectively (Sheth *et al.*, 2001). Nevertheless, these patients are still candidates for curative aggressive surgical resection pending absence of venous wall invasion and nodal or distant metastases, with a reported 5-year survival of 37–44% (Frank *et al.*, 2005). In that context, the most important task for preoperative imaging is accurate depiction of the superior extent of inferior vena cava thrombotic involvement in renal cell carcinoma. This information is crucial for surgeons to plan their surgical approach to ensure complete resection and to avoid intraoperative tumoral embolism. The accepted surgical approaches are abdominal for renal vein and infrahepatic inferior vena cava spread, right thoracoabdominal for intrahepatic inferior vena cava spread, and cardiopulmonary bypass for suprahepatic inferior vena cava or right atrial spread (Sheth *et al.*, 2001).

Several researchers have demonstrated that the extent of venous thrombi can be accurately diagnosed with MDCT, with reported accuracies similar to contrast-enhanced MRI,

Table 2   TNM and Robson Staging Systems of Renal Cell Carcinomas and Their Corresponding Multidetector CT Findings

Tumor Extension	TNM Stage	Robson Stage	Multidetector CT Findings
Limited to kidney	T1a Tumor 4 cm or less T1b Tumor 4–7 cm T2 Tumor larger than 7 cm	I	Heterogeneously enhancing soft tissue mass with possible central necrosis when large Organ confinement can be validated by presence of a pseudocapsule and absence of perinephric fat infiltration
Extension beyond renal capsule but not beyond Gerota fascia	T3a Direct invasion of ipsilateral adrenal gland, perinephric fat, or renal sinus fat T3b Extension into renal veins (main and segmental) and infradiaphragmatic inferior vena cava T3c Extension into supradiaphragmatic inferior vena cava	II IIIA	Adrenal soft tissue masses or adrenal obscuration. Presence of perinephric fat stranding, perinephric collateral vessels, and perinephric enhancing soft tissue masses Heterogeneously enhancing venous hypodense filling defects representing tumor thrombi
Extension beyond renal Gerota fascia	T4 Direct extension beyond renal Gerota fascia to involve adjacent organs and tissues	IVA	Loss of separating tissue planes and irregular contours between renal tumor and adjacent organs
Regional lymph node metastases	N0 No regional lymph nodes metastases N1 Metastasis in a single regional lymph node N2 Metastasis in more than one regional lymph node	IIIB	Hilar and retroperitoneal nodal enlargement greater than 1 cm in short-axis diameter
Distant metastases	M0 No distant metastases M1 Distant metastases	IVB	Frequently to the lungs and mediastinum, bones, and liver. Less commonly to the contralateral kidney, adrenal gland, brain, pancreas, mesentery, and abdominal wall

ranging between 78% and 100% (Gupta *et al.*, 2004; Hallscheidt *et al.*, 2005; Lawrentschuk *et al.*, 2005). Although most venous extensions are following blood flow direction in the inferior vena cava, retrograde venous spread into the opposite renal vein, hepatic veins, and right gonadal vein have been reported with MDCT (Ghersin *et al.*, 2005). Hence, meticulous evaluation of the inferior vena cava and its branches is necessary to ensure complete thrombus resection. Venous invasion is best depicted during the corticomedullary–late arterial phase of enhancement when maximal renal vein enhancement occurs. During this phase, radiologists should assess the presence of heterogeneously enhancing venous hypodense filling defects (Fig. 2). This finding is the most

specific diagnostic sign of a tumoral thrombus on MDCT. Focal or diffuse dilatation of the renal vein is not adequate for diagnosing venous invasion by renal cell carcinoma, and whenever solely present correlation with color-Doppler ultrasound or MRI is recommended.

Regional Lymph Node Spread

Patients with renal cell carcinoma invasion of regional lymph nodes, consistent with stage N1 or N2 or IIIB according to TNM and Robson classifications, respectively, have a poorer prognosis, with a 5-year survival of 18% following radical surgical resection (Terrone *et al.*, 2006). Identification

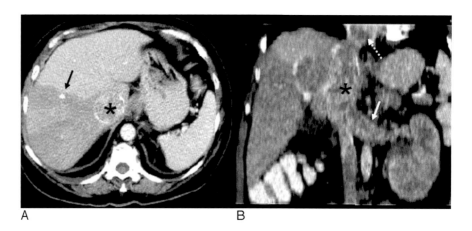

Figure 2 A 67-year-old woman, with painless macrohematuria and a lower pole left renal mass (not shown), depicted during dedicated multiphasic MDCT scan. Axial image at the level of the intrahepatic inferior vena cava (**A**) and coronal oblique reformat (**B**) of the corticomedullary–late arterial phase scan clearly depicts a heterogeneously enhancing venous tumoral thrombus involving and dilating the left renal vein (white solid arrow), the infrahepatic, intrahepatic, and supradiaphragmatic inferior vena cava, (*) and the right atrium (white dotted arrow). Secondary to thrombus extension into the right hepatic vein are transient hepatic attenuation differences between segment 7 (black solid arrow) and the rest of the liver parenchyma, consistent with secondary Budd-Chiari syndrome. This mass was correctly staged as a T3c renal cell carcinoma. Final pathological diagnosis revealed clear cell renal cell carcinoma.

of lymph node metastases still relies on nodal enlargement > 1 cm in short-axis diameter. Using solely the size criteria, we see that diagnosing lymph node involvement with MDCT remains a problem since it will result in a false-negative rate of ~ 10%, especially in the presence of micrometastases and a false-positive rate of 3–43%, mainly due to reactive hyperplasia (Heidenreich and Ravery, 2004). Hence, patients with regional nodal enlargements are still candidates for radical surgical resection, unless there is cytological confirmation of nodal spread via fine needle aspiration.

Although application of 2-[fluorine-18] fluoro-2-deoxy-D-glucose-PET in patients with renal cell carcinoma is still under initial investigation, Kang *et al.* (2004) reported sensitivity and specificity values of 75% and 100%, respectively, in diagnosing retroperitoneal lymph node metastases. It is our belief that hybrid imaging with PET and contrast-enhanced MDCT holds the potential of further improvement in the reported sensitivity and specificity values of either MDCT or PET in diagnosing regional lymph node spread.

Local Spread and Distant Metastases

Patients with renal cell carcinoma extension beyond the boundaries of Gerota fascia, involving neighboring organs, consistent with stage T4a or IVB according to TNM and Robson classifications, respectively, have a poor prognosis, with a 5-year survival of 20% following radical surgical resection (Frank *et al.*, 2005). Identification of the involvement of adjacent organs is based on the loss of separating tissue planes and irregular contours between the renal tumor and the adjacent organ. In that context, MDCT technology with narrower submil-

limeter collimation effectively reduces partial-volume effects and corresponding artifacts, resulting in significant improvement in quality of three-dimensional reformats. As a result, we may anticipate an improvement in assessing the involvement of adjacent organs as suggested by Catalano *et al.* (2003).

Renal cell carcinoma metastasizes most frequently to the lungs and mediastinum, bones, and liver. Less common sites include the contralateral kidney, adrenal gland, brain, pancreas, mesentery, and abdominal wall (Sheth *et al.*, 2001). Since most renal cell carcinomas are hypervascular, assessment of liver and other abdominal parenchymal metastases should include a dual MDCT scan during both late arterial and portal phases of enhancement. Accurate mapping of visceral metastases using MDCT of the chest and abdomen appears to be crucial since it has been shown that even patients with metastatic disease limited to lymph nodes and lungs might benefit from radical nephrectomy followed by systemic immunotherapy in the case of a good performance status (Heidenreich and Ravery, 2004). Nonetheless, generally speaking, patients with metastatic renal cell carcinoma have a poor prognosis, with a 5-year survival of 5–10% (Sheth *et al.*, 2001).

Role of Multidetector Computed Tomography in Conservative Treatment of Renal Cell Carcinoma

During the past three decades, the surgical approach to small organ-confined renal cell carcinomas evolved gradually toward a more conservative approach termed *nephron sparing surgery*. This approach includes complete resection of tumor including a tumor-free surgical margin of at least 0.5 cm, instead of radical nephrectomy. This method is usually reserved for relatively small tumors of up to 4 cm in their maximal diameter, located in the renal poles, sufficiently apart from the renal hilum and renal collecting system (Sheth et al., 2001). The reported 5- and 10-year survival rates of nephron sparing surgery are 97.8% and 95.8%, respectively (Becker et al., 2005).

Based on the encouraging results of nephron sparing surgery, application of image-guided radiofrequency tumor ablation was introduced as an optional minimally invasive treatment of renal cell carcinoma (Hines-Peralta and Goldberg, 2004; Slabaugh and Ogan, 2005; Wagner et al., 2005). Radiofrequency tumor ablation involves tumor coagulation using heating of a short duration (< 15 min) by directly applying temperatures > 50°C via needle electrodes. This therapy is indicated mainly for patients with known contraindications to partial or complete nephrectomy as a result of comorbid conditions or advanced age, patients with a predisposition for multiple renal cell carcinomas such as von Hippel-Lindau syndrome, and patients with renal cell carcinoma in a solitary kidney. This treatment is usually reserved for small renal cell carcinomas (< 3 cm) sufficiently distant from the renal hilum, central collecting system, and upper ureter. Although the present accumulated data demonstrate > 90% efficacy of radiofrequency ablation of primary renal cell carcinomas < 3 cm, it is clear that essential 5-year outcome data are still unavailable. Imaging in general and MDCT in particular have an important role in management of potential candidates for conservative treatments of renal cell carcinoma. First, to ensure optimal patient selection, abdominal and nonabdominal imaging should accurately identify all present tumors and the actual extent of the disease. In addition, imaging (usually ultrasound or CT) provides guidance for optimal radiofrequency electrode placement during the ablation procedure. Eventually, postprocedural imaging, typically by multidetector CT at least 1 month after treatment, monitors treatment success. On CT, viable residual tumor maintains its enhancement (> 10 HU) after contrast injection, whereas successfully ablated tumor loses its attenuation.

Multidetector Computed Tomography of Cystic Renal Cell Carcinoma

Approximately 10% of renal cell carcinomas manifest primarily as a fluid-filled unilocular or multiloculated cystic mass (Hartman et al., 2004). As such, imaging in general and MDCT in particular play an important role in differentiating these renal cell carcinomas from simple renal cysts and, more importantly, from benign renal cysts complicated with hemorrhage, infection, inflammation, or ischemia. These complicated benign cysts and cystic renal cell carcinomas may have identical macroscopic gross features. On MDCT,

either cystic renal cell carcinomas or benign complicated renal cysts are characterized by one or more of the following features: calcification, high attenuation (> 20 HU) at unenhanced CT scan, septations, multiple locules, enhancement, wall thickening, or nodularity.

In an attempt to differentiate between cystic renal cell carcinomas and complicated benign renal cysts, based on CT imaging features, Bosniak (1986) developed a classification that was further revised by Israel and Bosniak (2003). This revised classification includes five categories of cystic renal masses (Israel et al., 2004). Category I lesions are benign simple cysts with hairline-thin walls without evidence of septa, calcifications, solid components, or enhancement after intravenous contrast material administration. Category II lesions are benign minimally complicated cysts that may contain one to four hairline-thin septations, fine calcification, or a short segment of slightly thickened calcification in the walls or septa of such lesions. Cysts with uniformly high attenuation that are < 3 cm in diameter and do not enhance are included in this category. These lesions do not demonstrate any measurable contrast enhancement, although minimal perceived enhancement of a hairline-thin smooth septum or wall can be present. These lesions are considered nonsurgical and require no further attention. Category IIF lesions are more complex cysts that require continuous follow-up, since the risk of malignancy in these lesions is ~ 5% (Hartman et al., 2004; Israel and Bosniak, 2003). These cysts may contain an increased number of hairline-thin septations (5 to 9) or have minimal but smooth thickening of the wall or septa. The wall and/or septa may contain calcifications that may be thick and nodular. Similar to category II lesions these lesions do not demonstrate any measurable contrast enhancement, although minimal perceived enhancement of a hairline-thin smooth septum or wall can be present. Cysts with uniformly high attenuation that are > 3 cm in diameter and do not enhance are also classified as category IIF lesions.

Category III lesions are indeterminate renal lesions with an ~ 50% risk of being malignant renal cell carcinomas (Hartman et al., 2004). As such, these lesions are considered surgical and should be removed. They can have thickened irregular walls or septa, which can enhance following intravenous contrast material administration. Category IV lesions are malignant cystic renal cell carcinomas and should be removed surgically. They have similar features to those seen in Category III masses but also have an enhancing soft tissue component adjacent to, but independent of, the wall or septum.

Although the Bosniak classification relies primarily on the CT features of cystic renal lesions, ultrasound and MRI can be employed for additional characterization of complex cystic masses with ambiguous CT features. An example for such a lesion is a cystic renal mass that demonstrates borderline enhancement of 10–15 HU. Ultrasound and MRI can differentiate between pseudoenhancement due to volume averaging, imperfect placement of the region of interest, motion, or streak artifacts and between true border-line enhancement of a slow, minimally enhancing renal neo-plasm such as papillary renal cell carcinoma. Furthermore, Israel *et al.* (2004) have demonstrated that MRI findings, when compared to CT findings of 69 cystic renal lesions, led to a cyst classification upgrade of seven lesions, from category II to IIF ($n = 2$), IIF to III ($n = 3$), or III to IV ($n = 2$). This discrepancy resulted from the improved con-trast resolution of MRI, which enabled depiction of addi-tional septations, thickening of the wall and/or septa, and enhancement. Thus, MRI findings may lead to an upgraded Bosniak cyst classification and can affect case management. One potential limitation of this study is the use of various nonstandardized CT protocols with a variable slice thick-ness of 2.5–7 mm. It is our belief that application of MDCT using thinner overlapping (1 mm thick with 0.5-mm overlap) sections holds the potential to improve CT characterization of complex cystic masses. Nonetheless, it is important that radiologists will use additional imaging modalities when the CT findings are borderline–nonconclusive, and when there are conflicting findings at evaluation with different imaging modalities, the mass should be managed according to the most aggressive finding.

Multidetector Computed Tomography Features of Specific Subtypes of Renal Cell Carcinoma

Although the CT findings of different types of renal cell carcinomas are nonspecific and do not allow definite pre-operative diagnosis, some histological subtypes may have distinctive CT findings, and the familiarity with them is important to suggest an appropriate differential diagnosis. The importance of such differential diagnosis is augmented by the fact that distinct histological subtypes have varying degrees of local and metastatic spread that can affect imag-ing follow-up strategies as well as therapy and prognosis.

Clear Cell Renal Cell Carcinoma

Conventional clear cell renal carcinoma, which originates from the proximal convoluted tubule, contributes 60–62% of all renal cell carcinomas. On MDCT these tumors are char-acterized by strong enhancement of 106 +/− 48 HU (mean +/− SD) in the corticomedullary phase and 62 +/− 25 HU in the excretory phase (Kim *et al.*, 2002). The enhancement pattern is mostly heterogeneous, predominantly peripheral in 55–84%. Cystic degeneration is relatively common, while calcifications are relatively uncommon in only 11% of cases (Fig. 3A) (Kim *et al.*, 2002; Sheir *et al.*, 2005).

The reported metastatic relapse rate and 5- and 10-year actuarial disease-free survival following curative surgery

for conventional clear cell renal cell carcinoma are 11.9%, 73.3%, and 50.8%, respectively (Beck *et al.*, 2004).

Papillary Renal Cell Carcinoma

Papillary renal cell carcinoma, which probably origi-nates from the distal convoluted tubule, stands for 7–14% of all renal cell carcinomas. On MDCT these tumors are characterized by weak, mostly homogeneous enhancement (Sheir *et al.*, 2005; Tsuda *et al.*, 2005). Calcifications are relatively more common in 32% of cases (Figs. 3B & C) (Kim *et al.*, 2002). The reported metastatic relapse rate and 5- and 10-year actuarial disease-free survival following curative surgery for papillary renal cell carcinoma are 9%, 81.7%, and 67.6%, respectively (Beck *et al.*, 2004).

Chromophobe Renal Cell Carcinoma

Chromophobe renal cell carcinoma, which probably origi-nates from the intercalated cells, stand for 6–11% of all renal cell carcinomas. On MDCT, these tumors are characterized by weak homogeneous enhancement (Sheir *et al.*, 2005). Calcifications are relatively more common in 38% of cases (Kim *et al.*, 2002). The reported metastatic relapse rate and 5- and 10-year actuarial disease-free survival following cura-tive surgery for chromophobe renal cell carcinoma are 6%, 80.1%, and 80.1%, respectively (Beck *et al.*, 2004).

Collecting Duct Carcinoma of the Kidney

Collecting duct carcinoma is a rare type of renal cell car-cinoma that originates from the collecting duct (of Bellini). It affects younger patients, and is associated with aggres-sive regional and distant spread (Chao *et al.*, 2002). These tumors are characterized on MDCT by medullary location, weak and heterogeneous enhancement, involvement of the renal sinus, infiltrative growth, preserved renal contour, and presence of a cystic component (Fig. 3D) (Yoon *et al.*, 2005). The reported average survival of these patients is 11.5 months (Chao *et al.*, 2002).

Differential Diagnosis of Renal Cell Carcinoma with Multidetector Computed Tomography

Although any solid enhancing renal mass should be con-sidered a potential renal neoplasm, not all these masses should be treated surgically. Imaging in general and MDCT in par-ticular can be valuable in differentiating renal neoplasms that require surgical resection, including renal cell carcinoma, transitional cell carcinoma, and oncocytoma, from renal neoplasms that do not routinely require surgical resection, such as angiomyolipoma, lymphoma, and metastatic disease.

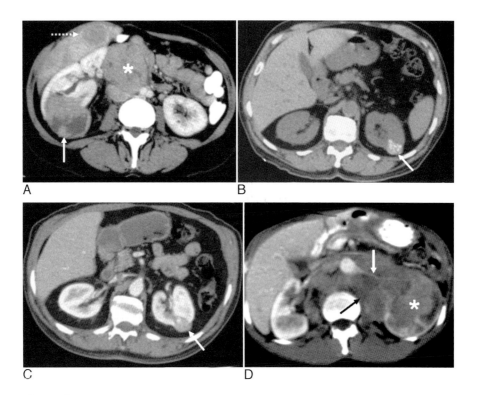

Figure 3 (**A**) A 43-year-old woman, with painless macrohematuria. Axial image from the nephro-graphic–parenchymal phase scan, at the level of the lower right renal pole, clearly depicts a heterogeneously partially cystic, 5-cm right renal mass (white solid arrow), prominent retroperitoneal lymphadenopathy (*), and a liver metastasis (white dotted arrow). This mass was correctly staged as an N2, M1 renal cell carcinoma. Final pathological diagnosis revealed clear cell renal cell carcinoma. (**B&C**) A 74-year-old man, with a 2.5-cm interpolar left renal mass, initially depicted during MDCT scan for staging of a known urinary bladder transitional renal cell carcinoma. Note the small, well-defined, hyperdense renal mass on the unenhanced scan (**B**) due to multiple minute calcifications (white solid arrow). On the corticomedullary–late arterial phase scan, the mass is hypodense relative to the adjacent normal renal parenchyma; however, accurate attenuation measurements demonstrate mild contrast enhancement of 20 HU. This mass was correctly staged as a T1a renal cell carcinoma. Final pathological diagnosis revealed papillary renal cell carcinoma. (**D**) A 57-year-old man with macrohematuria. Axial image from the corticomedullary–late arterial phase scan, at the level of the left renal hilum, demonstrates a sinus centered mildly heterogeneous left renal mass (*). Also noted were prominent hilar and retroperitoneal lymphadenopathy (black solid arrow) engulfing the left renal artery (white solid arrow), and liver metas-tases (not shown). This mass was correctly staged as a N2, M1 renal cell carcinoma. Final pathological diagnosis revealed collecting duct carcinoma.

The diagnosis of an angiomyolipoma is made primarily by demonstrating any amount of fat within a solid renal mass, in the absence of tumor calcifications. This approach is jus-tified because the great majority of renal angiomyolipomas contain a measurable amount of intratumoral fat without calcifications, whereas renal cell carcinomas rarely contain intratumoral fat and calcifications (Hammadeh *et al.*, 1998; Kim *et al.*, 2004). Therefore, meticulous evaluation of all solid renal masses, using an unenhanced dedicated MDCT examination, for the presence of fat is mandatory to avoid misdiagnosing an angiomyolipoma as renal cell carcinoma.

Renal lymphoma can have variable appearances, but most frequently it is manifested by bilateral solid renal masses. Additional manifestations include solitary renal mass or a homogeneous infiltrating renal mass, which can enlarge the kidney. Whenever a patient with known systemic lym-phoma presents with a questionable renal mass, biopsy of the mass is required prior to systemic therapy for lymphoma. The same approach is justified whenever a patient without known systemic lymphoma presents with renal mass fea-tures characteristic of renal lymphoma such as bilateral solid renal masses or an infiltrating renal mass.

Metastatic disease to the kidney typically manifests as multiple bilateral renal masses, often associated with meta-static disease to other organs. When appropriate clinical his-tory is available, the diagnosis is straightforward. However, in a patient with a solitary renal mass or an infiltrating renal mass and history of previous malignancy (especially carci-noma of the lung), percutaneous renal biopsy is required for definitive diagnosis (Israel and Bosniak, 2005).

Transitional cell carcinoma of the kidney is usually diagnosed by detecting an enhancing filling defect in the collecting system and is best imaged using CT or MR urography (Caoili *et al.*, 2002; Zielonko *et al.*, 2003). However, uncommonly transitional cell carcinomas are anaplastic and infiltrate the kidney parenchyma and renal sinus. The differential diagnosis of such an appearance also includes renal cell carcinoma, lymphoma, and metastasis. As such, whenever imaging or urine cytology findings are nonconclusive, tissue diagnosis is required, to triage an appropriate surgical treatment, which in the case of transitional cell carcinoma is nephroureterectomy.

Oncocytomas, which are benign renal neoplasms, may correspond to up to 10% of solid renal tumors. Basically, they are indistinguishable from renal cell carcinomas at imaging, although Eiss *et al.* (2005) found that in two-thirds of cases large oncocytomas (> 3 cm) showed a hypodense scar-like nonenhancing region, central or eccentric in location, and surrounded by homogeneously enhancing tumoral tissue on postcontrast images. This finding is in contrast to renal cell carcinomas, which may demonstrate central scar-like regions, but these are usually surrounded by heterogeneously enhancing tumoral tissue due to focal areas of necrosis (Eiss *et al.*, 2005). Nonetheless, for practical purposes, renal oncocytomas should be treated surgically as renal cell carcinomas.

Radiation Dose Associated with Multidetector Computed Tomography of Renal Cell Carcinoma

Because of the repeated acquisitions during a dedicated multiphasic MDCT scan for the assessment of renal cell carcinoma, the patient may receive a radiation dose that is as much as three to four times that from a typical abdominal CT examination. Nawfel *et al.* (2004) have demonstrated that a multiphasic MDCT urography protocol, which includes three scans of the abdomen and pelvis using a collimation of 1 and 2.5 mm, incorporates a mean effective dose for patients of 14.8 mSv, versus 9.7 mSv for a conventional urography. Thus, patient dose estimates should be taken into consideration when imaging protocols are established for renal cell carcinoma. In an attempt to address this issue, vendors of MDCT equipment developed automatic radiation exposure control systems, which are based on both angular (*x-y* axis) and *z*-axis online tube current modulations. Mulkens *et al.* (2005) evaluated such a system and found that a mean dose reduction of 38% can be achieved for upper abdominal scans with preservation of diagnostic image quality. Nevertheless, further research is needed to validate the diagnostic performance of such automatic radiation exposure control systems in the specific assessment of renal cell carcinoma.

References

Beck, S.D., Patel, M.I., Snyder, M.E., Kattan, M.W., Motzer, R.J., Reuter, V.E., and Russo, P. 2004. Effect of papillary and chromophobe cell type on disease-free survival after nephrectomy for renal cell carcinoma. *Ann. Surg. Oncol. 11*:71–77.

Becker, F., Siemer, S., Humke, U., Hack, M., Ziegler, M., and Stockle, M. 2005. Elective nephron sparing surgery should become standard treatment for small unilateral renal cell carcinoma: long-term survival data of 216 patients. *Eur. Urol. 49*:308–313.

Bonsib, S.M. 2005. T2 clear cell renal cell carcinoma is a rare entity: a study of 120 clear cell renal cell carcinomas. *J. Urol. 174*:1199–11202.

Bosniak, M.A. 1986. The current radiological approach to renal cysts. *Radiology 158*:1–10.

Caoili, E.M. 2002. Imaging of the urinary tract using multidetector computed tomography urography. *Semin. Urol. Oncol. 20*:174–179.

Caoili, E.M., Cohan, R.H., Korobkin, M., Platt, J.F., Francis, I.R. Faerber, G.J., Montie, J.E., and Ellis, J.H. 2002. Urinary tract abnormalities: initial experience with multi-detector row CT urography. *Radiology 222*:353–360.

Catalano, C., Fraioli, F., Laghi, A., Napoli, A., Pediconi, F. Danti, M., Nardis, P., and Passariello, R. 2003. High-resolution multidetector CT in the preoperative evaluation of patients with renal cell carcinoma. *AJR Am. J. Roentgenol. 180*:1271–1277.

Chao, D., Zisman, A., Pantuck, A.J., Gitlitz, B.J., Freedland, S.J., Said, J.W., Figlin, R.A., and Belldegrun, A.S. 2002. Collecting duct renal cell carcinoma: clinical study of a rare tumor. *J. Urol. 167*:71–74.

Eiss, D., Larousserie, F., Mejean, A., Ghouadni, M., Merran, S., Correas, J.M., and Helenon, O. 2005. Renal oncocytoma: CT diagnostic criteria revisited. *J. Radiol. 86*:1773–1782.

Foley, W.D. 2003. Renal MDCT. *Eur. J. Radiol. 45* (Suppl. 1):S73–S78.

Frank, I, Blute, M.L., Leibovich, B.C., Cheville, J.C., Lohse, C.M., and Zincke, H. 2005. Independent validation of the 2002 American Joint Committee on cancer primary tumor classification for renal cell carcinoma using a large, single institution cohort. *J. Urol. 173*:1889–1892.

Ghersin, E., Leiderman, M., Meretik, S., Kaftori, J.K., Amendola, M.A., and Engel, A. 2005. Renal cell carcinoma invading the right ovarian vein: multidetector computed tomography and ultrasound Doppler findings. *J. Comput. Assist. Tomogr. 29*:472–474.

Gray Sears, C.L., Ward, J.F., Sears, S.T., Puckett, M.F., Kane, C.J., and Amling, C.L. 2002. Prospective comparison of computerized tomography and excretory urography in the initial evaluation of asymptomatic microhematuria. *J. Urol. 168*:2457–2460.

Gupta, N.P., Ansari, M.S., Khaitan, A., Sivaramakrishna, M.S., Hemal, A.K., Dogra, P.N., and Seth, A. 2004. Impact of imaging and thrombus level in management of renal cell carcinoma extending to veins. *Urol. Int. 72*:129–134.

Hallscheidt, P.J., Bock, M., Riedasch, G., Zuna, I., Schoenberg, S.O., Autschbach, F., Soder, M., and Noeldge, G. 2004. Diagnostic accuracy of staging renal cell carcinomas using multidetector-row computed tomography and magnetic resonance imaging: a prospective study with histopathologic correlation. *J. Comput. Assist. Tomogr. 28*:333–339.

Hallscheidt, P.J, Fink, C., Haferkamp, A., Bock, M., Luburic, A., Zuna, I., Noeldge, G., and Kauffmann, G. 2005. Preoperative staging of renal cell carcinoma with inferior vena cava thrombus using multidetector CT and MRI: prospective study with histopathological correlation. *J. Comput. Assist. Tomogr. 29*:64–68.

Hammadeh, M.Y., Thomas, K., Philp, T., and Singh, M. 1998. Renal cell carcinoma containing fat mimicking angiomyolipoma: demonstration with CT scan and histopathology. *Eur. Radiol. 8*:228–229.

Hartman, D.S., Choyke, P.L., and Hartman, M.S. 2004. From the RSNA refresher courses: a practical approach to the cystic renal mass. *Radiographics 24* (Suppl. 1):S101–S115.

Heidenreich, A., and Ravery, V. 2004. Preoperative imaging in renal cell cancer. *World J. Urol. 22*:307–315.

Hines-Peralta, A., and Goldberg, S.N. 2004. Review of radiofrequency ablation for renal cell carcinoma. *Clin. Cancer Res. 10*:6328S–6334S.

Israel, G.M., and Bosniak, M.A. 2003. Follow-up CT of moderately complex cystic lesions of the kidney (Bosniak category IIF). *AJR Am. J. Roentgenol. 181*:627–633.

Israel, G.M., and Bosniak, M.A. 2005. How I do it: evaluating renal masses. *Radiology 236*:441–450.

Israel, G.M., Hindman, N., and Bosniak, M.A. 2004. Evaluation of cystic renal masses: comparison of CT and MR imaging by using the Bosniak classification system. *Radiology 231*:365–371.

Kang, D.E., White, R.L., Jr., Zuger, J.H., Sasser, H.C., and Teigland, C.M. 2004. Clinical use of fluorodeoxyglucose F 18 positron emission tomography for detection of renal cell carcinoma. *J. Urol. 171*:1806–1809.

Kim, J.K., Kim, T.K., Ahn, H.J., Kim, C.S., Kim, K.R., and Cho, K.S. 2002. Differentiation of subtypes of renal cell carcinoma on helical CT scans. *AJR Am. J. Roentgenol. 178*:1499–1506.

Kim, J.K., Park, S.Y., Shon, J.H., and Cho, K.S. 2004. Angiomyolipoma with minimal fat: differentiation from renal cell carcinoma at biphasic helical CT. *Radiology 230*:677–684.

Lane, B.R., and Kattan, M.W. 2005. Predicting outcomes in renal cell carcinoma. *Curr. Opin. Urol. 15*:289–297.

Lang, E.K., Macchia, R.J., Thomas, R., Watson, R.A., Marberger, M. Lechner, G., Gayle, B., and Richter, F. 2003. Improved detection of renal pathologic features on multiphasic helical CT compared with IVU in patients presenting with microscopic hematuria. *Urology 61*:528–532.

Lawrentschuk, N., Gani, J., Riordan, R., Esler, S., and Bolton, D.M. 2005. Multidetector computed tomography vs magnetic resonance imaging for defining the upper limit of tumour thrombus in renal cell carcinoma: a study and review. *BJU. Int. 96*:291–295.

McTavish, J.D., Jinzaki, M., Zou, K.H., Nawfel, R.D., and Silverman, S.G. 2002. Multi-detector row CT urography: comparison of strategies for depicting the normal urinary collecting system. *Radiology 225*:783–790.

Mulkens, T.H., Bellinck, P., Baeyaert, M., Ghysen, D., Van D, X., Mussen, E., Venstermans, C., and Termote, J.L. 2005. Use of an automatic exposure control mechanism for dose optimization in multi-detector row CT examinations: clinical evaluation. *Radiology 237*:213–223.

Nawfel, R.D., Judy, P.F., Schleipman, A.R., and Silverman, S.G. 2004. Patient radiation dose at CT urography and conventional urography. *Radiology 232*:126–132.

Robson, C.J. 1982. Staging of renal cell carcinoma. *Prog. Clin. Biol. Res. 100*:439–445.

Sheir, K.Z., El-Azab, M., Mosbah, A., El-Baz, M., and Shaaban, A.A. 2005. Differentiation of renal cell carcinoma subtypes by multislice computerized tomography. *J. Urol. 174*:451–455.

Sheth, S., Scatarige, J.C., Horton, K.M., Corl, F.M., and Fishman, E.K. 2001. Current concepts in the diagnosis and management of renal cell carcinoma: role of multidetector CT and three-dimensional CT. *Radiographics 21 Spec No*:S237–S254.

Slabaugh, T.K., and Ogan, K. 2005. Renal tumor radiofrequency ablation. *Minerva Urol. Nefrol. 57*:261–269.

Suh, M., Coakley, F.V., Qayyum, A., Yeh, B.M., Breiman, R.S., and Lu, Y. 2003. Distinction of renal cell carcinomas from high-attenuation renal cysts at portal venous phase contrast-enhanced CT. *Radiology 228*:330–334.

Terrone, C., Cracco, C., Porpiglia, F., Bollito, E., Scoffone, C., Poggio, M., Berruti, A., Ragni, F., Cossu, M., Scarpa, R.M., and Rossetti, S.R. 2006. Reassessing the current TNM lymph node staging for renal cell carcinoma. *Eur. Urol. 49*:324–331.

Thompson, R.H., Leibovich, B.C., Cheville, J.C., Lohse, C.M., Frank, I. Kwon, E.D., Zincke, H., and Blute, M.L. 2005. Should direct ipsilateral adrenal invasion from renal cell carcinoma be classified as pT3a? *J. Urol. 173*:918–921.

Tsuda, K., Kinouchi, T., Tanikawa, G., Yasuhara, Y., Yanagawa, M., Kakimoto, K., Ono, Y., Meguro, N., Maeda, O., Arisawa, J., and Usami, M. 2005. Imaging characteristics of papillary renal cell carcinoma by computed tomography scan and magnetic resonance imaging. *Int. J. Urol. 12*:795–800.

Wagner, A.A., Solomon, S.B., and Su, L.M. 2005. Treatment of renal tumors with radiofrequency ablation. *J. Endourol. 19*:643–652.

Yoon, S.K., Nam, K.J., Rha, S.II., Kim, J.K., Cho, K.S., Kim, B., Kim, K.H., and Kim, K.A. 2005. Collecting duct carcinoma of the kidney: CT and pathologic correlation. *Eur. J. Radiol. 57*:453–460.

Zielonko, J., Studniarek, M., and Markuszewski, M. 2003. MR urography of obstructive uropathy: diagnostic value of the method in selected clinical groups. *Eur. Radiol. 13*:802–809.

24

Renal Cell Carcinoma Subtypes: Multislice Computed Tomography

Khaled Z. Sheir

Introduction

Malignant tumors of the kidney represent 2 to 3% of all human neoplasia. Renal cell carcinoma (RCC) accounts for 85 to 90% of all kidney tumors (McClennan and Deyoe, 1994). Renal cell carcinoma is a term commonly used to describe renal epithelial tumors with malignant potential. It is becoming apparent that RCC is a heterogeneous disease from its very inception and is best considered a family of neoplasms rather than a single entity. The differences among the various types of RCC are related to the oncogenic molecular events and the epithelial site targeted by these events, leading to distinct morphologic, antigenic, and immunophynotypic patterns. These differences are reflected in the clinical course of RCC and the variable prognosis in the affected individuals (Uzzo et al., 2003).

In the United States, there has been a steady rise in the rates of RCC of 2.3 to 4.3% annually (Chow et al., 1999). This rise can be attributed in part to increased detection through the widespread use of noninvasive imaging techniques. However, a significant improvement in the overall 5-year survival has been noted owing to early detection and advances in the surgical management of the disease. A delay in diagnosis may result from the ability of the retroperitoneal space occupying lesion to become large before causing local symptoms. Moreover, the manifestations of RCC are protean and may give rise to a constellation of nonspecific symptoms (Uzzo et al., 2003). So, the development of diagnostic noninvasive approaches for early detection of RCC is imperative.

Renal Cell Carcinoma Subtypes

The classification of RCC into subtypes has become of great interest because of the association with prognosis. It can be classified into clear cell, papillary, chromophobe, collecting duct, and unclassified subtypes (Bostwick and Eble, 1999). Although most cases are sporadic (96%), several distinct syndromes have been described to predispose to RCC in a hereditary manner (Pavlovich et al., 2003).

Sporadic Renal Cell Carcinoma

Conventional (Clear Cell) Renal Cell Carcinoma

Conventional (clear cell) renal cell carcinoma (CCRCC) is the most commonly found subtype and accounts for 70 to 80% of renal neoplasms (Storkel et al., 1997). It can be an aggressive tumor and, when advanced, most commonly metastasizes to lung, bone, lymph nodes, and adrenal gland (Renshaw and

Richie, 1999). There is no cure when this tumor is metastatic, which underscores the role of surgical removal at an early stage. Bilateral or multifocal CCRCC is rare in nonhereditary situations, occurring at a rate of 3.2% and 11%, respectively (Reuter and Presti, 2000). The overall 5-year survival rate for CCRCC is 44 to 54% (Amin *et al.*, 1997).

Conventional (clear cell) renal cell carcinoma is most likely of proximal tubular origin and is usually found as a sporadic solitary tumor in the sixth and seventh decades of life (Reuter and Presti, 2000; Amin *et al.*, 2002). Tumors predominantly consist of cells with clear cytoplasm, although cells with eosinophilic cytoplasm are common (Fig. 1A & B). The architecture is commonly solid and cystic, with a characteristic delicate branching vascular component. Sarcomatoid change occurs in 5% of these tumors (Storkel *et al.*, 1997).

Papillary Renal Cell Carcinoma

Papillary renal cell carcinoma (PRCC) is the second most common subtype, accounting for 15 to 20% of renal neoplasms (Amin *et al.*, 1997). It appears to be less aggressive stage-for-stage than CCRCC. Nevertheless, it has metastatic potential and a predilection for lymph nodes, liver, bone, and brain (Renshaw and Richie, 1999; Amin *et al.*, 2002). Papillary renal cell carcinomas are most often sporadic solitary tumors found in patients with advanced age (Reuter and Presti, 2000). Although PRCCs are more often multifocal than CCRCC, multifocal PRCC is rare in nonhereditary situations. They are the most common subtype of RCC found in patients with acquired cystic kidney disease secondary to chronic renal failure (Pavlovich *et al.*, 2003). The overall 5-year survival rate for PRCC is 82 to 90%, which is higher than that for CCRCC (Amin *et al.*, 1997; Cheville *et al.*, 2003).

As is true for CCRCC, PRCC is thought to be of renal proximal tubular origin, although owing to a different gene defect. It is morphologically and cytogenetically distinct from other subtypes. The architecture of PRCCs may be papillary, tubular, tubular papillary, and solid, and is defined as papillary when 75% of the tumor has a papillary or tubular papillary architectural pattern (Thoenes *et al.*, 1986; Amin *et al.*, 1997; Renshaw *et al.*, 1997). Papillary renal cell carcinomas have variable cytoplasmic and nuclear staining, and are subdivided into eosinophil, basophile, and duophil (Thoenes *et al.*, 1986). Basophilic tumors consist of small cells with scanty amphophilic cytoplasm and small low-grade nuclei. Eosinophilic tumors have large cells with abundant eosinophilic cytoplasm and usually large nuclei. Duophilic tumors are a mixture of eosinophilic and basophilic cells. Another classification was proposed to consider basophilic tumors as type I and eosinophilic as type II (Fig. 1C & D). Type I occurs about twice as frequently as type II (Delahunt and Eble, 1997; Delahunt *et al.*, 2001).

Chromophobe Renal Cell Carcinoma

Chromophobe renal cell carcinoma (ChRCC) accounts for 5% of renal neoplasms (Crotty *et al.*, 1995). It generally has a slowly progressive and locally invasive course, although metastatic progression has been noted. These tumors tend to be manifested at a slightly larger size than CCRCC and PRCC at an average size of 7 to 9 cm; however, their overall course is more benign (Reuter and Presti, 2000; Amin *et al.*, 2002). Metastases from ChRCC, although exceedingly rare, tend to be found in the liver (Renshaw and Richie, 1999). The overall 5-year survival rate for ChRCC is 78 to 92% (Thoenes *et al.*, 1988; Cheville *et al.*, 2003).

The presumed progenitor cells for ChRCC are the intercalated cells of the collecting duct (Pavlovich *et al.*, 2003). Chromophobe renal cell carcinoma is characterized by a compact growth pattern of large polygonal cells with pale reticular cytoplasm and prominent cell membranes. These cells have low glycogen content compared to CCRCC (Thoenes *et al.*, 1988; Crotty *et al.*, 1995). Another diagnostic hallmark is the lack of cytoplasmic coloring with routine dyes but a diffuse and strong staining with Hale's colloid iron stain, which is suggested to be characteristic of ChRCC (Tickoo *et al.*, 1998). However, this tumor may be composed of so-called eosinophilic chromophobe cells, which have a large number of mitochondria and few vesicles in the cytoplasm (Fig. 1E and F).

Collecting Duct Renal Cell Carcinoma

Collecting duct renal cell carcinoma (CDRCC) represents a minority of renal neoplasms, ranging from 0.4 to 2.6% (Thoenes *et al.*, 1986; Storkel *et al.*, 1997). It is of high malignant potential and is more often found in younger patients than the other RCC subtypes. A particularly malignant and invariably fatal variant of CDRCC, known as medullary RCC, has been found exclusively in black patients with sickle cell anemia with mean age at presentation of 22 years (Davis *et al.*, 1995; Pavlovich *et al.*, 2003). Its behavior is more aggressive than that of previous RCC subtypes. Extension into the perinephric fat and invasion of the renal pelvis, and regional spread with infiltration of adrenal glands and lymph node metastases, are common (Rumpelt *et al.*, 1991). It was found that 35 to 40% of patients presented with metastatic disease, and 67% of them were dead of disease within 2 years of diagnosis (Kontak and Campbell, 2003). The average survival for patients with medullary CDRCC is only 15 weeks (Davis *et al.*, 1995). Other than surgery, which is rarely curative, no treatments have proven efficacious in controlling these highly malignant tumors (Avery *et al.*, 1996).

Collecting duct renal cell carcinoma is thought to arise from the medullary collecting ducts (Rumpelt *et al.*, 1991). Tumors are located mainly in the medulla or central part of the kidney, are white gray, and show tubular papillary growth combined with a microcystic and solid pattern. Microscopically, high-grade cytological atypia, stromal desmoplasia, and associated dysplastic changes in the neighboring medullary renal tubules as well as strong positivity for intracytoplasmic mucin with staining characterize CDRCC (Fig. 1G) (Rumpelt *et al.*, 1991). Medullary CDRCC exhibits a reticular, yolk

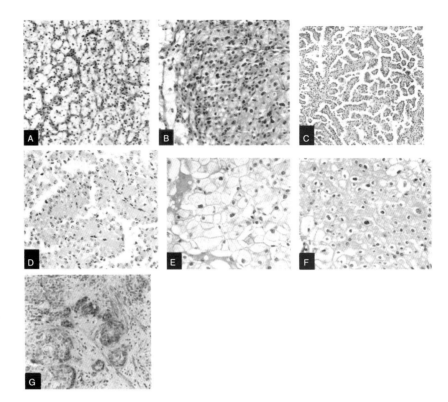

Figure 1 Histopathological appearance of various RCC subtypes. (**A**) Typical CCRCC with clear cytoplasm delicate fine vascularity. (**B**) CCRCC with eosinophilic (granular) cytoplasm (low power). (**C**) Type I PRCC with basophilic cytoplasm. (**D**) Type II PRCC with eosinophilic (granular) cytoplasm. (**E**) Typical ChRCC composed predominantly of clear cells with distinct cell border. (**F**) ChRCC composed predominantly of eosinophilic cells. (**G**) CDRCC, the characteristic dense desmoplasia with clusters of tumor cells and solid nests of tumors. All are H (Hematoxylin) and E (Eosin) at low power.

sac-like or adenoid cystic appearance, often with poorly differentiated areas in a highly desmoplastic stroma admixed with neutrophils and usually marginalized lymphocytes, peripheral satellites in the renal cortex, and pelvic soft tissues as well as venous and lymphatic invasion are usually present (Davis *et al.*, 1995; Avery *et al.*, 1996).

Unclassified Renal Cell Carcinoma (URCC)

In some surgical series, URCC comprised 2.8 to 5% of cases (Zisman *et al.*, 2002). These carcinomas are aggressive tumors and typically present with significantly larger size than CCRCC, and 94% of patients present with regional lymph node or distant metastasis. Compared with CCRCC there is significantly increased propensity for URCC to involve local invasion of the adrenal gland and adjacent organs as well as metastatic involvement of the bone and regional or nonregional lymph nodes (Zisman *et al.*, 2002). Unclassified renal cell carcinoma has a dismal prognosis when compared stage-for-stage with other classifiable subtypes, with overall 5-year survival of 24% (Amin *et al.*, 2002). The overall median survival in one series was 4.3 months. Nephrectomy combined with immunotherapy confers some survival advantages; patients who received immunotherapy had significantly improved survival, with a median of 11.1 months compared to 2.9 for those who did not (Zisman *et al.*, 2002).

Renal cell carcinoma is categorized as unclassified when it does not meet the histological criteria of the recognized variations of established RCC subtypes. URCC may have the feature

of undifferentiated carcinoma with pleomorphic or anaplastic nuclear morphology, or features of pure sarcomatoid or mixed sarcomatous and anaplastic tumors (Zisman *et al.*, 2002).

Hereditary Renal Cell Carcinoma

von Hippel-Lindau Syndrome

The ophthalmologists von Hippel and Lindau first described retinal angiomas as a hallmark of this syndrome, which is a constellation of systemic manifestations that are a result of germline mutation or deletion of the VHL gene in the region of the short arm of chromosome 3. The syndrome is transmitted in autosomal dominant fashion, and its incidence is 1 case per 36,000 population (Pavlovich *et al.*, 2003).

The manifestations include tumors of the blood vessels of the retinas and central nervous system (hemangioblastomas), pheochromocytoma, CCRCCs, and renal cysts, pancreatic cysts and neuroendocrine tumors, endolymphatic sac (inner ear) tumors, and broad ligament (female) and epididymal (male) papillary cystadenomas. The wide variety of tissues suggests a common dependence on the VHL gene or its protein products. All of these structures share in common the process of tubularization at day 21 in embryogenesis and the fact that a faulty VHL gene precludes such normal organ development (Pavlovich *et al.*, 2003).

Kidney lesions are always CCRCC and cysts. Biopsies demonstrating multifocal tumors other than CCRCC rule out von Hippel-Lindau disease. Clear cell renal cell carcinoma in von Hippel-Lindau disease presents earlier than in sporadic CCRCC, 37 years versus 61 years, respectively, and can metastasize early, especially when tumor growth has exceeded 3 cm (Amin *et al.*, 2002).

Hereditary Papillary Renal Cell Carcinoma (HPRCC)

This syndrome was described in families in which the predisposition to develop multiple bilateral PRCC was transmitted in an autosomal dominant fashion. HPRCC is characterized by late onset and papillary renal tumors that are often detected incidentally in asymptomatic family members or during screening of at-risk family members. The male-to-female ratio of affected members is 2:1 (Zbar *et al.*, 1995). Genetic linkage analysis has localized the responsible gene to chromosome 7q31 (Schmidt *et al.*, 1997).

Unlike von Hippel-Lindau disease, no common extrarenal manifestations of HPRCC have been documented. The renal tumors are multiple and bilateral. Patients in HPRCC families have previously been reported to have renal cancer as an average in the sixth decade of life. However, in a recent report, individuals in HPRCC families are at risk in the second decade. This report emphasized that HPRCC can be a lethal disease because a number of affected individuals in these families died of metastatic disease (Schmidt *et al.*, 2004). The diagnosis of HPRCC is confirmed by germline mutational analysis of patients in HPRC families or patients who present with multiple or bilateral PRCC inherited in autosomal dominant fashion (Pavlovich *et al.*, 2003). Once diagnosis is confirmed, annual abdominal CT is recommended. Contrast-enhanced CT is preferable to ultrasonography in HPRCC because the lesions are hypovascular and difficult to differentiate from renal parenchyma owing to their similar ultrasonographic echogenicities (Schmidt *et al.*, 2004). Histologically, while all tumors were classified as papillary type I, areas of clear cell differentiation were seen in some individuals with extensive necrosis (Schmidt *et al.*, 2004).

Birt-Hogg-Dubé (BHD) Syndrome

This syndrome was originally described in Canadian kindred in 1977 by Birt, Hogg, and Dubé (Schmidt *et al.*, 2005) as an inherited autosomal genodermatosis characterized by the development of benign tumors of the hair follicle (fibrofolliculomas), which present as multiple skin papules about the face, neck, back, and chest appearing after puberty. Birt-Hogg-Dubé syndrome is inherited in an autosomal dominant manner and has been reported to be associated with renal tumors, spontaneous pneumothorax, colon polyps, and colon carcinomas (Schmidt *et al.*, 2005). Risk assessment study of BHD-affected patients concluded that a diagnosis of BHD conferred a 7-fold increased risk of developing renal neoplasia and a 50-fold increased risk of spontaneous pneumothorax but no increased risk of colon polyps or colon cancer (Zbar *et al.*, 2002). Males develop

renal tumor 2.5-fold more often than females. Tumors may develop bilaterally with multiple foci or unilaterally with single focus. Genetic linkage analysis in nine kindreds with BHD localized the disease locus to chromosome 17p11.2 (Schmidt *et al.*, 2005). The average onset of renal tumors in BHD syndrome may be slightly later than seen in VHL syndrome (Pavlovich *et al.*, 2003). The frequency of renal tumors among BHD-affected individuals who were evaluated by CT scan is 29% (Schmidt *et al.*, 2005).

Birt-Hogg-Dubé syndrome patients develop a variety of histological types of renal tumors, including CCRCC, ChRCC, PRCC type I, and benign renal oncocytoma. The most common form is oncocytic hybrid tumor with microscopic features of ChRCC and oncocytoma. These different histologies suggest that a germline BHD gene mutation is not exclusively associated with the development of a particular tumor type but is related to a predisposition to a variety of renal epithelial neoplasms (Pavlovich *et al.*, 2003, 2005).

Multislice Computerized Tomography

Multislice computed tomography is the most recent advance in CT technology, also known as multichannel, multisection, or multidetector CT (MDCT). It uses a multiple-row detector array instead of the single-row detector array used in helical CT (McCollough and Zink, 1999). The main advantages of MDCT are *faster scanning time*, *increased volume coverage*, and *improved spatial and temporal resolution* (Rydberg *et al.*, 2003).

The faster scanning time is due to the very fast gantry rotation time of 0.4 sec or less for one 360° rotation that allows 2 to 25 times faster scanning time than helical CT with the same or better image quality. These faster scanning times result in decreased breath-hold time with reduced motion artifact, increased coverage along the *z*-axis, and more diagnostic images (Kocakoc *et al.*, 2005). The number of slices obtained per unit time depends on the scanner's number of rows and on the gantry rotation time. So, as MDCT uses multiple rows of detectors, it allows for the registration of more than one channel per gantry rotation (while it is one channel for single detector helical CT). The number of slices obtained per second can be as many as 38 for a 16-slice CT with 0.4-sec rotation time (Rydberg *et al.*, 2003).

Increased volume coverage is combined with thinner slice thickness to obtain better quality volume data sets for workstation analysis, either in 2D axial, multiplanar reformation, or 3D imaging. Moreover, different image thicknesses can be obtained from the same acquisition data set (Kocakoc *et al.*, 2005). Multidetector CT allows images to be obtained in multiple phases of renal parenchymal enhancement and excretion in the collecting system after administration of a single bolus of intravenous (IV) contrast material. Therefore, detection and characterization of small renal masses, display of the arterial and venous supply of the kidney similar to conventional angiography, and demonstration of the collecting system's abnormalities using different 3D display techniques are possible.

Differentiation of RCC Subtypes by MDCT

As discussed earlier, the prognosis of RCCs depends on tumor subtypes. The behavior of RCC depends on its subtype, and accordingly precise prediction of the subtype may be helpful for treatment planning, such as determining the degree of preoperative evaluation and the appropriate extent of surgery. A patient with a subtype that does not tend to metastasize or recur, such as the ChRCC, may not need to undergo a complex metastasis survey and unnecessary wide resection may be avoided, thereby decreasing postoperative morbidity or mortality. The differentiation of renal cell carcinoma subtypes by imaging modalities is still a well-known challenge. In the following sections, studies by Sheir *et al.* (2005) will be discussed in comparison to the few other published studies concerning this issue.

We compared MDCT findings in different subtypes of RCC and investigated its role in differentiating subtypes. Between January 2001 and March 2004, 98 patients underwent radical nephrectomy for renal cell carcinoma. Eleven patients were excluded because they did not undergo the same CT protocol. Therefore, 87 patients, including 46 men and 41 women with a mean age of 55 years (range 22 to 75), of whom each had one tumor, were included in this study. Of these patients 37 had the clear cell subtype, 26 had the papillary subtype, and 24 the chromophobe subtype.

MDCT Examination Protocol

All CT examinations were performed using a multislice CT scanner (LightSpeed Plus, General Electric Medical Systems, Milwaukee, Wisconsin). Scans were obtained with certain parameters for imaging acquisition, including scan type helical/full/0.8 sec, gantry tilt $0°$, 120 kV, 220 mA, slice thickness 2.5 mm, table speed 7.5 mm per rotation, reconstruction interval 2.5 mm, and large field-of-view. Images were reconstructed on a 512×512 matrix. All patients received 500 to 1000 ml oral contrast material 30 min before CT and 120 ml contrast material (iopamidol) injected intravenously into the antecubital vein using a mechanical injector at a rate of 3.0 ml per sec.

All patients underwent biphasic CT, including unenhanced, corticomedullary phase (CMP) and excretory phase (EP) scanning. Computed tomography of the entire kidney was performed in every phase during 20 to 23 sec of patient breath-holding. Scanning for the corticomedullary and excretory phases was started 30 and 300 sec after contrast injection, respectively. Immediately after scanning for the

excretory phase, scanning covering the lower abdomen and pelvis was performed.

Image Analysis

An experienced radiologist blinded to RCC subtype reviewed CT images at a special workstation (Advantage Window 4.1, GE Medical Systems). The length and CT number of the lesion in a particular region of interest were measured. We assessed tumor size, enhancement degree and pattern (homogeneous, heterogeneous, and predominantly peripheral), the presence or absence of calcification or cystic degeneration (necrotic or hemorrhagic areas within the tumor), and tumor spreading patterns (perinephric change, venous invasion, and lymphadenopathy).

To evaluate the degree of tumor enhancement, we measured the attenuation of three separate regions of interest and calculated the mean of these three values. One location for measuring the attenuation value was the solid enhancing area in the excretory phase. A region of interest cursor was placed over an enhanced area, which was consistent in location during all CT phases. We tried to exclude areas of calcification from the region of interest. The tumor enhancement pattern was classified as homogeneous when most tumor areas showed a uniform degree of enhancement, predominantly peripheral when most tumor portions were not enhanced, and only the peripheral rim or septa showed enhancement. The pattern was classified as heterogeneous in the remaining cases. To eliminate the effect of tumor size on enhancement pattern and cystic degeneration, we classified tumors into two groups according to maximum diameter, namely, 5 cm or less and greater than 5 cm. Perinephric changes were indicated when there was evidence of strands of soft tissue attenuation or parasitized vessels in the perinephric area and thickening of Gerota's fascia. Venous invasion was indicated when the lumen of the renal vein or inferior vena cava was replaced by tumor. Lymphadenopathy was defined as a lymph node enlarged to more than 1 cm.

Statistical Analysis

Statistical comparisons were performed for various CT findings of different RCC subtypes. Group comparison was done with the Kruskal-Wallis test for CT attenuation values at different phases, patient age, and tumor size. When ANOVA was statistically significant, pairwise comparisons were made with the Mann-Whitney U test. The distribution of patient sex, enhancement pattern frequency, presence of calcification or cystic degeneration, tumor-spreading patterns, and tumor vascularity were compared using the Chi square test. Test results were considered significant at $p > 0.05$. An investigator blinded to cohort identity performed the statistical analysis. To evaluate the diagnostic validity of the attenuation value in different RCC subtypes, we generated receiver operating characteristic (ROC) curves and analyzed them to determine the cutoff value for the differentiation with the highest accuracy.

Results

Mean age ± SD was 54 ± 7 years (range 37 to 75) in patients with the clear cell subtype, 52 ± 10 years (range 37 to 71) in those with the papillary subtype, and 47 ± 9 (range 22 to 66) in those with the chromophobe subtype ($p = 0.03$). Pairwise analysis revealed a statistically significant difference between the clear cell and chromophobe subtypes only ($p = 0.005$). The male-to-female ratio was 0.5:1 for the clear cell, 1.6:1 for the papillary, and 1.2:1 for the chromophobe subtype ($p = 0.09$). Mean tumor diameter was 9 ± 3.8 cm (range 3.5 to 20) for the clear cell subtype, 7.9 ± 2.8 cm (range 3 to 15) for the papillary subtype, and 8.1 ± 3.6 cm (range 3 to 14) for the chromophobe subtype ($p = 0.3$). There were 6 clear cell, 4 papillary, and 6 chromophobe cases with a tumor of 5 cm or less ($p = 0.6$).

Table 1 lists attenuation values of the three subtypes. Clear cell, chromophobe, and papillary subtype pre-enhancement attenuation values did not differ ($p = 0.07$), (Fig. 2, IA, IIA, and IIIA). On CMP and EP images, attenuation values were higher for the clear cell subtype than for the chromophobe and papillary subtypes ($p = 0.001$) (Fig. 2, IB, IC, IIB, IIC, IIIB, and IIIC). Pairwise comparisons showed significantly different attenuation values for the clear cell and papillary subtypes on CMP only ($p = 0.001$). Significant differences in attenuation values were seen on CMP and EP between the clear cell or papillary and chromophobe subtypes ($p = 0.001$).

The ROC curves showed that the area under the curve (Az value) for CMP enhancement was 0.94 (95% CI 0.887 to 0.993) with high statistical significance ($p = 0.001$) and highest accuracy at cut-off value of 83.5 HU, and the area under the curve (Az value) for EP enhancement was 0.74 (95% CI 0.635 to 0.841) with high statistical significance ($p = 0.001$) and highest accuracy at cut-off value of 64.5 HU.

The enhancement patterns of the three subtypes had no statistically significant differences among all subtypes even when classified according to tumor size. Calcification within the tumor was noted in 8 patients (21.6%) with CCRCC, in 6 (23.1%) with PRCC, and in 6 (25%) with ChRCC ($p > 0.05$).

Cystic degeneration (necrotic or hemorrhagic areas within the tumor) was more evident in the clear cell subtype than in the other subtypes regardless of tumor size ($p = 0.001$). A hypervascular pattern (higher tumor enhancement after contrast medium injection due to higher vascularity) was observed in 48.6% of the CCRCC in comparison to 15.4% of the PRCC and 4.2% of the ChRCC ($p = 0.001$).

When evaluating tumor spreading patterns, we observed perinephric changes in 15 clear cell (40.5%), 5 papillary (19.2%), and 7 chromophobe (29.2%) cases. Venous invasion was noted in 10 clear cell (27%), 4 papillary (15.4%), and 2 chromophobe (8.3%) cases. These cases were also confirmed at pathological examination. Lymphadenopathy was noted in 7 clear cell (18.9%), 5 papillary (19.2%), and 5 chromophobe (20.8%) cases. Statistical analysis revealed that the frequency of perinephric changes, venous invasion, and lymphadenopathy in the different subtypes did not differ significantly ($p > 0.05$). The computed tomography stage according to the American Joint Committee on Cancer system (Russo, 2000) was I (T1 N0 M0) in 71 patients (clear cell in 29, papillary in 21, and chromophobe in 21), II (T2 N0 M0) in 15 (clear cell in 7, papillary in 5, and chromophobe in 3), and IV (T1–3b N2 M0) in only 1 with the clear cell subtype.

In this study it was found that the degree of enhancement is the most valuable parameter for differentiating among renal cell carcinoma subtypes. The presence or absence of cystic degeneration, tumor vascularity, and enhancement patterns can serve a supplemental role in the differentiation of renal cell carcinoma subtypes. Computed tomography findings could help in preoperative identification of the renal cell carcinoma subtype and influence the degree of preoperative evaluation and extent of surgery, resulting in less aggressive surgery in patients with a subtype that does not tend to metastasize or recur, such as chromophobe subtype. Thus, postoperative morbidity and mortality would be decreased, particularly in elderly patients or in patients with significant comorbidities.

Discussion

Until recently, the differentiation of renal cell carcinoma subtypes has been attempted on CT in only five series. Wildberger *et al.* (1997) evaluated CT findings, including tumor

Table 1 Computed Tomography Attenuation for the Three Subtypes of Renal Cell Carcinoma

	Conventional $N = 37$	Papillary $N = 26$	Chromophobe $N = 24$	p
Pre-enhancement	29.9 (7.0)	32.9 (3.0)	33.6 (3.7)	0.07
CMP	138.2 (38.0)	89.2 (31.4)	55.17 (24.0)	0.000
EP	73.0 (17.6)	70.0 (10.4)	33.9 (12.1)	0.000

Data presented as mean (SD).
Comparisons were done using the Kruskal-Wallis test.

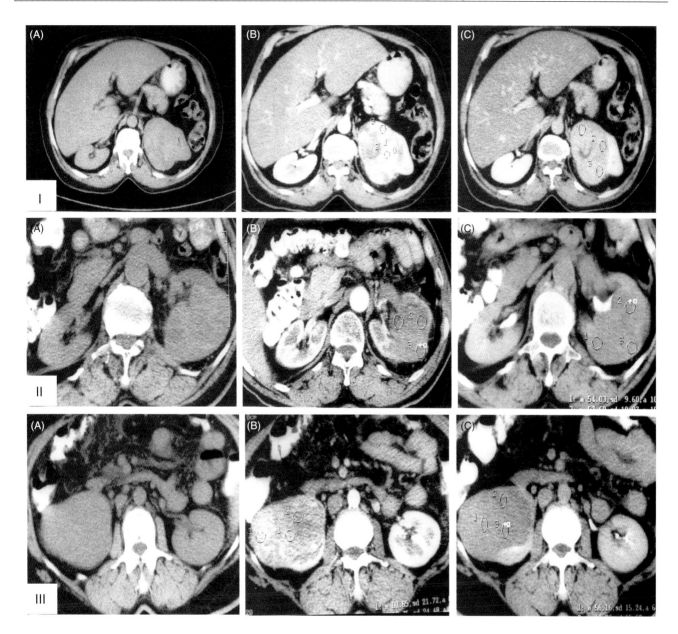

Figure 2 MDCT images for various RCC subtypes. I. A male patient 53 years old with *conventional (clear cell) renal carcinoma*. **Unenhanced CT scan (A)** shows well-demarcated oval parenchymal mass with 7.7-cm diameter and 35-H attenuation value in left kidney. The mass showed heterogeneous enhancement on contrast-enhanced CT scans (obtained at the same level) measured 152 H in *corticomedullary phase (B)*, and 99 H in *excretory phase (C)*. **II.** A male patient 75 years old with *chromophobe renal carcinoma*. **Unenhanced CT scan (A)** shows a fairly defined mass with 8.1-cm diameter and 33-H attenuation value in left kidney. The mass shows homogeneous enhancement on contrast-enhanced CT scans (obtained at same level) that measured 63 H in *corticomedullary phase (B)* and 35 H in *excretory phase (C)*. **III.** A female patient 54 years old with *papillary renal carcinoma*. **Unenhanced CT scan (A)** shows well-demarcated mass with 8.7-cm diameter and 36-H attenuation value in right kidney. The mass shows heterogeneous enhancement on contrast-enhanced CT scans (obtained at the same level) that measured 86 H in *corticomedullary phase (B)* and 52 H in *excretory phase (C)*.

nodule, margin, shape, and enhancement, to differentiate various subtypes. They found that the sensitivity for differentiating the clear cell subtype was 72%. Fujimoto *et al.* (1999) analyzed the enhancement pattern of RCCs > 5 cm on contrast-enhanced helical CT. They reported that strong enhancement equal to the renal cortex was noted only in the clear cell

subtype (75% of cases) and not in the other subtypes. Jinzaki *et al.* (2000) found that the enhancement pattern in double-phase helical CT was different among the subtypes of RCC, and correlated with microvessel density or the existence of intratumoral necrosis or hemorrhage. All CCRCC showed a peak attenuation value in the CMP > 100 HU, all ChRCC showed a peak attenuation value in the CMP < 100 HU, and all PRCC showed a gradual enhancement with an attenuation value in the CMP < 100 HU. However, they could not differentiate between RCC and other solid benign tumors. Kim *et al.* (2002) observed that the sensitivity and specificity for differentiating the clear cell subtype from the other subtypes were 74% and 100% at a cut-off of 84 HU on CMP, and 84% and 91% at a cut-off of 44 HU for EP, respectively. Kitamura *et al.* (2004) evaluated the diagnostic accuracy of dynamic CT and color Doppler ultrasound for preoperative diagnosis of renal solid tumors. They found that most PRCC and all ChRCC (only two cases were included in the study) show hypovascularity and lower enhancement in the CMP than CCRCC. However, in all of these studies the nonclear cell subtypes could not be predicted by CT criteria, and they found no difference in attenuation values of EP (except Kim *et al.*, 2002) between the different subtypes. Another two studies that evaluated the CT characteristics of the hereditary or sporadic PRCC reported that this subtype is typically hypovascular and homogeneous (Choyke *et al.*, 1997; Herts *et al.*, 2002).

In the author's study, it was found that the attenuation value is the most useful parameter for differentiating renal cell carcinoma subtypes, especially the clear cell versus the other subtypes, with high validity (Az value > 0.94 on CMP and 0.74 on EP). The clear cell subtype showed stronger enhancement than the other subtypes on CMP and EP, and tumors with attenuation values more than 83.5 HU on CMP and 64.5 HU on EP were likely to be clear cell renal carcinoma. Although strong enhancement of the clear cell subtype has been observed in previous reports, the actual enhancement values for differentiating it from nonconventional subtypes have only been reported by Kim *et al.* (2002). Strong enhancement of the clear cell subtype is caused by its rich vascular network and alveolar architecture on histological examination. Moreover, in this study differentiation between the PRCC and ChRCC was possible in both CMP and EP as the enhancement of the PRCC was significantly higher than that of ChRCC.

The author's study revealed that the enhancement pattern, the presence or absence of calcification, and the tumor-spreading pattern overlap among RCC subtypes. There were no statistically significant differences among all subtypes, even when they were further classified according to tumor size. However, the clear cell (70.3%) and papillary (69.2%) subtypes tended to show heterogeneous or predominantly peripheral enhancement, whereas the chromophobe subtype (75%) usually showed homogeneous enhancement. These findings are in agreement with those reported by Jinzaki *et al.* (2000) and Kim *et al.* (2002). Different enhancement patterns of renal cell carcinoma subtypes are supported by findings on pathological examination. The chromophobe subtype, which tends to demonstrate homogeneous enhancement on CT, shows a homogeneous cut surface without hemorrhage or necrosis and a solid growth pattern on patho-

logical examination. In contrast, the clear cell subtype, which usually shows heterogeneous or predominantly peripheral enhancement on CT, commonly has hemorrhage or necrosis within the tumor on pathological examination.

In the author's study of the overall frequency of perinephric changes, venous invasion and lymphadenopathy were lower than those documented in previous reports (McClennan and Deyoe, 1994; Bonsib, 1999). This finding might be attributable to the fact that the increased use of CT has resulted in the earlier detection of renal cell carcinoma than in the past, and the use of contrast-enhanced multislice CT has been beneficial for differentiating malignant tumors from unenhanced benign cysts.

Limitations of These Studies and Ideas for Potential Advancement

Renal cell carcinoma enhancement may be variable according to the contrast injection parameters and scan delay time. In the study of Birnbaum *et al.* (1996) using different contrast injection protocol, the degree of enhancement was stronger on EP than on CMP, which was dramatically different from our study. Therefore, our tumor enhancement criterion is applicable only to cases in which the contrast injection protocol and scan time are similar to those in our study. Jinzaki *et al.* (2000) found that the pattern of attenuation value of one oncocytoma showed a similar pattern as ChRCC, and two metanephric adenomas showed a similar pattern as PRCC. This overlap is very interesting. Oncocytoma is known to be phenotically closely related to ChRCC and is often difficult to differentiate from ChRCC. A recent report suggests that oncocytoma and ChRCC may arise from a common progenitor lesion (Tickoo *et al.*, 1999). Metanephric adenoma is suggested to be genetically related to PRCC (Brown *et al.*, 1997). The similarity of attenuation value patterns in double-phase helical CT was consistent with the similarities of phenotic or genetic findings. In other words, the similarity of attenuation value patterns may support these hypotheses.

The mechanism of iodine contrast media enhancement is related to a variety of factors, which include microvessel density, size of the abnormal vessels, and the permeability of those vessels. Thus, the degree of enhancement in the CMP does not completely correlate with microvessel density, and the analysis of the size of the abnormal vessels or permeability of tumor vessels on imaging modality will be required in the future (Jinzaki *et al.*, 2000). The rarity of CDRCC and URCC makes it difficult to define the criteria of differentiation between them and other subtypes. So, further studies in a larger population are necessary to validate the accuracy of the MDCT protocol of the previous studies in differentiation of the three major subtypes and to include a larger number of patients with the rare subtypes.

References

Amin, M.B., Tamboli, P., Javidan, J., Stricker, H., de-Peralta Venturina, M., Deshpande, A., and Menon, M. 2002. Prognostic impact of histologic subtyping of adult renal epithelial neoplasms: an experience of 405 cases. *Am. J. Surg. Pathol. 26*:281–291.

Amin, M.B., Corless, C.L., Renshaw A.A, Tickoo, S.K., Kubus, J., and Schultz, D.S. 1997. Papillary (chromophil) renal cell carcinoma: histomorphologic characteristics and evaluation of conventional pathologic prognostic parameters in 62 cases. *Am. J. Surg. Pathol. 21*:621–635.

Avery, R.A, Harris, J.E., Davis, C.J. Jr., Borgaonkar, D.S, Byrd, J.C., and Weiss, R.B. 1996. Renal medullary carcinoma: clinical and therapeutic aspects of a newly described tumor. *Cancer 78*:128–132.

Birnbaum, B.A., Jacobs, J.E., and Ramchandani, P. 1996. Multiphasic renal CT: comparison of renal mass enhancement during the corticomedullary and nephrogenic phases. *Radiology 200*:753–758.

Bonsib, S.M. 1999. Risk and prognosis in renal neoplasms: a pathologist's prospective. *Urol. Clin. N. Am. 26*:643–660.

Bostwick, D.G., and Eble, J.N. 1999. Diagnosis and classification of renal cell carcinoma. *Urol. Clin. N. Am. 26*:627–635.

Brown, J.A., Anderl, K.L., Borell, T.J., Qian, J., Bostwick, D.G., and Jenkins, R.B. 1997. Simultaneous chromosome 7 and 17 gain and sex chromosome loss provide evidence that renal metanephric adenoma is related to papillary renal cell carcinoma. *J. Urol. 158*:370–374.

Cheville, J.C., Lohse, C.M., Zincke, H., Weaver, A.L., and Blute, M.L. 2003. Comparison of outcome and prognostic features among histologic subtypes of renal cell carcinoma. *Am. J. Surg. Pathol. 27*:612–624.

Chow, W.H., Devesa, S.S, Warren, J.L, Fraumeni, J.F., Jr. 1999. Rising incidence of renal cell cancer in the United States. *JAMA 281*:1628–1632.

Choyke, P.L., Walther, M.M., Glenn, G.M., Wagner, J.R., Venzon, Zbar, B., and Linehan, W.M. 1997. Imaging features of hereditary papillary renal cancers. *J. Comput. Assist. Tomogr. 21*:737–741.

Crotty, T.B., Farrow, G.M., and Lieber, M.M. 1995. Chromophobe renal cell carcinoma: clinicopathological features of 50 cases. *J. Urol. 154*:964–967.

Davis, C.J., Mostofi, F.K., and Sesterhenn, I.A. 1995. Renal medullary carcinoma: the seventh sickle cell nephropathy. *Am. J. Surg. Pathol. 19*:1–11.

Delahunt, B., and Eble, J.N. 1997. Papillary renal cell carcinoma: a clinicopathologic and immunohistochemical study of 105 tumors. *Mod. Pathol. 10*:537–544.

Delahunt, B., Eble, J.N., McCredie, M.R., Bethwaite, P.B., Stewart, J.H., and Bilous, A.M. 2001. Morphologic typing of papillary renal cell carcinoma: comparison of growth kinetics and patient survival in 66 cases. *Hum. Pathol. 32*:590–595.

Fujimoto, H., Wakao, F., Moriyama, N., Tobisu, K., Sakamoto, M., and Kakizoe, T. 1999. Alveolar architecture of clear cell renal carcinoma (< or = 5.0 cm) show high attenuation on dynamic CT scanning. *Jpn. J. Clin. Oncol. 29*:198–203.

Herts, B.R, Coll, D.M., Novick, A.C., Obuchowski, N., Linnell, G., Wirth, S.L., and Baker, M.E. 2002. Enhancement characteristics of papillary renal neoplasms revealed on triphasic helical CT of the kidneys. *AJR 178*:367–372.

Jinzaki, M., Tanimoto, A., Mukai, M., Ikeda, E., Kobayashi, S., Yuasa, Y., Narimatsu, Y., and Murai, M. 2000. Double-phase helical CT of small renal parenchymal neoplasms: correlation with pathologic findings and tumor angiogenesis. *J. Comput. Assist. Tomogr. 24*:835–842.

Kim, J.K, Kim, T.K., Ahn, H.J., Kim, C.S., Kim, K.R., and Cho, K.S. 2002. Differentiation of subtypes of renal cell carcinoma on helical CT scans. *AJR 178*:1499–1506.

Kitamura, H., Fujimoto, H., Tobisu, K., Mizuguchi, Y., Maeda, T., Matsuoka, N., Komiyama, M., Nakagawa, T., and Kakizoe, T. 2004. Dynamic computed tomography and color Doppler ultrasound of renal parenchymal neoplasms: correlation with histopathological findings. *Jpn. J. Clin. Oncol. 34*:78–81.

Kocakoc, E., Bhatt, S., and Dogra, V.S. 2005. Renal multidetector row CT. *Radiol. Clin. N. Am. 43*:1021–1047.

Kontak, J.A., and Campbell, S.C. 2003. Prognostic factors in renal cell carcinoma. *Urol. Clin. N. Am. 30*:467–480.

McClennan, B.L., and Deyoe, L.A. 1994. The imaging evaluation of renal cell carcinoma: diagnosis and staging. *Radiol. Clin. N. Am. 32*:55–69.

McCollough, C.H., and Zink, F.E. 1999. Performance evaluation of a multislice CT system. *Med. Phys. 26*:2223–2230.

Pavlovich, C.P., Grubb, R.L. IIIrd, Hurley, K., Glenn, G.M., Toro, J., Schmidt, L.S., Torres-Cabala, C., Merino, M.J., Zbar, B., Choyke, P., Walther, M.M., and Linehan, W.M. 2005. Evaluation and management of renal tumors in the Birt–Hogg–Dubé syndrome. *J. Urol. 173*:1482–1486.

Pavlovich, C.P., Schmidt, L.S., and Phillips, J.L. 2003. The genetic basis of renal cell carcinoma. *Urol. Clin. N. Am. 30*:437–454.

Renshaw, A.A., Zhang, H., Corless, C.L., Fletcher, J.A., and Pins, M.R. 1997. Solid variants of papillary (chromophil) renal cell carcinoma: clinicopathologic and genetic features. *Am. J. Surg. Pathol. 21*:1203–1209.

Renshaw, A.A., and Richie, J.P. 1999. Subtypes of renal cell carcinoma: different onset and sites of metastatic disease. *Am. J. Clin. Pathol. 111*:539–543.

Reuter, V.E., and Presti, J.C., Jr. 2000. Contemporary approach to the classification of renal epithelial tumors. *Semin. Oncol. 27*:124–137.

Rumpelt, H.J., Storkel, S., Moll, R., Scharfe, T., and Thoenes, W. 1991. Bellini duct carcinoma: further evidence for this rare variant of renal cell carcinoma. *Histopathology 18*:115–122.

Russo, P. 2000. Renal cell carcinoma: presentation, staging, and surgical treatment. *Semin. Oncol. 27*:160–176.

Rydberg, J.L., Liang, Y, and Teague, S.D. 2003. Fundamentals of multichannel CT. *Radiol. Clin. N. Am. 41*:465–474.

Schmidt, L., Duh, F.M., Chen, F., Kishida, T., Glenn, G., Choyke, P., Scherer, S.W., Zhuang, Z., Lubensky, I., Dean, M., Allikmets, R., Chidambaram, A., Bergerheim, U.R., Feltis, J.T., Casadevall, C., Zamarron, A., Bernues, M., Richard, S., Lips, C.J., Walther, M.M., Tsui, L.C., Geil, L., Orcutt, M.L., Stackhouse, T., Lipan, J., Slife, L., Brauch, H., Decker, J., Niehans, G., Hughson, M.D., Moch, H., Storkel, S., Lerman, M.I., Linehan, W.M., and Zbar, B. 1997. Germline and somatic mutations in the tyrosine kinase domain of the MET proto-oncogene in papillary renal carcinomas. *Nat. Genet. 1*:68–73.

Schmidt, L.S., Nickerson, M.L., Angeloni, D., Glenn, G.M., Walther, M.M., Albert, P.S., Warren, M.B., Choyke, P.L., Torres-Cabala, C.A., Merino, M.J., Brunet, J., Bérez, V., Borràs, J., Sesia, G., Middelton, L., Phillips, J.L., Stolle, C., Zbar, B., Pautler, S.E., and Linehan, W.M. 2004. Early onset hereditary papillary renal carcinoma: germline missense mutations in the tyrosine kinase domain of the met proto-oncogene. *J. Urol. 172*:1256–1261.

Schmidt, L.S., Nickerson, M.L., Warren, M.B., Glenn, G.M., Toro, J.R., Merino, M.J., Turner, M.L., Choyke, P.L., Sharma, N., Peterson, J., Morrison, P., Maher, E.R., Walther, M.M., Zbar, B., and Linehan, W.M. 2005. Germline BHD-mutation spectrum and phenotype analysis of a large cohort of families with Birt–Hogg–Dubé Syndrome. *Am. J. Hum. Genet. /6*:1023–1033.

Sheir, Z.K., El-Azab, M., Mosbah, A., El-Baz, M., and Shaaban, A.A. 2005. Differentiation of renal cell carcinoma subtypes by multislice computerized tomography. *J. Urol. 174*:451–455.

Storkel, S., Elbe, J.N, Adlakha, K., Amin, M., Blute, M.L., Bostwick, D.G., Darson, M., Delahunt, B., and Iczkowski, K. 1997. Classification of renal cell carcinoma: Workgroup No. 1. Union Internationale Contre le Cancer (UICC) and the American Joint Committee on cancer (AJCC). *Cancer 80*:987–989.

Thoenes, W., Storkel, S., and Rumpelt, H.J. 1986. Histopathology and classification of renal tumors (adenomas, oncocytomas, and carcinomas). The basic cytological and histopathological elements and their use for diagnosis. *Path. Res. Pract. 181*:125–143.

Thoenes, W., Storkel, S., Rumpelt, H.J., Moll, R., Baum, H.P., and Werner, S. 1988. Chromophobe cell renal carcinoma and its variants—a report on 32 cases. *J. Pathol. 155*:277–287.

Tickoo, S.K., Amin, M.B., and Zarbo, 1998. Colloidal iron staining in renal epithelial neoplasms, including chromophobe renal cell carcinoma: emphasis on technique and patterns of staining. *Am. J. Surg. Pathol. 22*:419–424.

Tickoo, S.K., Reuter, V.E., Amin, M.B., Srigley, J.R., Epstein, J.I., Min, K.W., Rubin, M.A., and Ro, J.Y. 1999. Renal oncocytosis: a morphologic study of fourteen cases. *Am. J. Surg. Pathol. 23*:1094–1101.

Uzzo, R.G., Cairns, P., Al-Saleem, T., Hudes, G., Haas, N., Greenberg, R.E., and Kolenko, V. 2003. The basic biology and immunobiology of renal cell carcinoma: considerations for the clinician. *Urol. Clin. N. Am. 30*:423–436.

Wildberger, J.E., Adam, G., Boeckmann, W., Munchau, A., Brauers, A., Gunther, R.W., and Fuzesi, L. 1997. Computed tomography characterization of renal cell tumors in correlation with histopathology. *Invest. Radiol. 32*:596–601.

Zbar, B., Glenn, G., Lubensky, I., Choyke, P., Walther, M.M., Magnusson, G., Bergerheim, U.S.R., Pettersson, S., Amin, M., Hurley, K., and Line-han, W.M. 1995. Hereditary papillary renal cell carcinoma: clinical studies in 10 families. *J. Urol. 153*:907–912.

Zbar, B., Alvord, W.G., Glenn, G., Turner, M., Pavlovich, C.P., Schmidt, L., Walther, M., Choyke, P., Weirich, G., Hewitt, S.M., Duray, P., Gabril, F., Greenberg, C., Merino, M.J., Toro, J., and Linehan, W.M. 2002. Risk of renal and colonic neoplasms and spontaneous pneumothorax in the Birt–Hogg–Dubé syndrome. *Cancer Epidemiol. Biomarkers Prev. 11*:393–400.

Zisman, A., Chao, D.H., Pantuck, A.J., Kim, H.J., Wieder, J.A, Figlin, R.A., Said, J.W., and Belldegrun, A.S. 2002. Unclassified renal cell carcinoma: clinical features and prognostic impact of new histological subtype. *J. Urol. 168*:950–955.

25

Renal Impairment: Comparison of Noncontrast Computed Tomography, Magnetic Resonance Urography, and Combined Abdominal Radiography/Ultrasonography

Ahmed A. Shokeir

Introduction

The ureter can be obstructed due to intramural, mural, or extramural diseases. Intramural obstruction is most commonly caused by stones and other rare causes, including blood clots, fungus balls, and ureteral polyps. Infiltrative ureteral carcinoma is the most common intrinsic cause of ureteral obstruction. Inflammatory ureteral disorders such as tuberculosis and schistosomiasis may cause ureteral strictures. Extrinsic involvement of the ureter can result from a variety of pathologic processes that cause obstruction by direct invasion (e.g., bladder carcinoma and extravesical extension of prostatic carcinoma), pressure (e.g., pelvic neoplasm, pelvic abscess, retroperitoneal tumors, pancreatic carcinoma, lymphoma, and abdominal adenopathies from any malignant tumors), or constriction (e.g., retroperitoneal fibrosis).

Bilateral ureteral obstruction or obstruction of a solitary kidney will result in renal impairment. Under such conditions, the conventional excretory urography (IVP) and contrast-enhanced computed tomography (CT) are contraindicated. In patients with renal impairment, the traditional methods of diagnosing the cause of ureteral obstruction start with the noninvasive plain abdominal X-ray (KUB) combined with abdominal gray-scale ultrasonography (US). Alternative methods of visualizing the upper urinary tract (e.g., retrograde or antegrade pyelography or ureteropyeloscopy) are invasive. In the last few years, some recent noninvasive investigations have been introduced for the diagnosis of ureteral obstruction, for example, noncontrast computed tomography (NCCT) and magnetic resonance urography (MRU).

In the present chapter we will focus on the role of non-invasive imaging modalities, including NCCT, MRU, and combined KUB and US, in the diagnosis of the cause of ureteral obstruction in patients with renal impairment. The diagnostic accuracy, advantages, and limitations of each imaging modality will be discussed, and special emphasis will be placed on imaging of ureteral obstruction due to malignant disorders. The author's experience will be presented and discussed with the results of similar other studies.

Combined Plain Abdominal Radiography and Ultrasonography

Traditionally, the combination between KUB and gray-scale US is the first step used by most radiologists and urologists to diagnose the cause of ureteral obstruction. Plain abdominal radiography alone is not sufficient to diagnose stone disease, giving a sensitivity of 45–59% (Shokeir, 2002). It is limited by the superimposed bowel and bone, and inability to visualize radiolucent stones and pelvic phleboliths may be mistaken as stones in the pelvic part of the ureter. Apart from urolithiasis, KUB has almost no role in the diagnosis of other causes of ureteric obstruction.

Gray-scale US has many advantages in the diagnosis of obstructive uropathy. It is noninvasive, quick, portable, repeatable, and inexpensive, and it does not use ionizing radiation or contrast materials. Therefore, it is very attractive especially in pregnancy and in patients with renal impairment. Gray-scale US can visualize stones located in renal calcies, renal pelvis, pelviureteric junction, and most proximal and distal parts of ureter. Nevertheless, stones located in the middle part of the ureter are difficult to be seen by US because of the superimposed bones and gas. The presence of pyelocaliectasis stimulates urologists and radiologists to differentiate between dilated obstructed and dilated nonobstructed kidneys. Under such conditions, the use of Doppler US with measurement of renal resistive index and ureteric jets is of great clinical importance (Shokeir, 2002).

Ultrasound is not as sensitive as CT in identifying or characterizing renal masses; as CT urography emerges as an initial imaging investigation for hemsturia, US will likely play a limited diagnostic role in the future. Ultrasound can be useful in patients with renal functional impairment or allergy to iodinated contrast material, although MR imaging is becoming established as the investigation of choice in these patients. Ultrasound can also allow assessment of the degree of hydronephrosis and guide interventional procedures in the setting of acute obstruction.

At US, renal pelvic transitional cell carcinoma (TCC) typically appears as a central soft tissue mass in the echogenic renal sinus, with or without hydronephrosis (Fig. 1). This carcinoma is usually slightly hyperechoic relative to surrounding renal parenchyma; occasionally, high-grade TCC may show areas of mixed echogenicity. Infundibular tumors may cause focal hydronephrosis. Although lesions may extend into the renal cortex and cause focal contour distortion, typically TCC is infiltrative and does not distort the renal contour (Browne *et al.*, 2005). Ultrasound has a limited role in the evaluation of ureteric TCC as the ureters

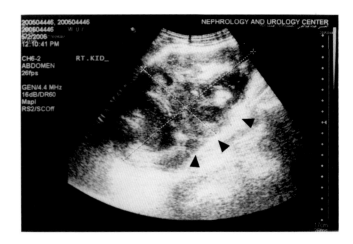

Figure 1 Sagittal gray-scale US scan in a case of right renal transitional cell carcinoma shows a tumor (arrows) in the echogenic renal sinus.

are rarely visualized in their entirety, even if dilated. If visualized, these tumors are typically intraluminal soft tissue masses with proximal distension of the ureter (Jung *et al.*, 2000). Ultrasound also allows limited assessment of periureteric tissues. Recent development in high-resolution endoluminal US performed during ureterorenoscopy have shown promise in evaluation of upper tract TCC, offering potential advantages over other imaging techniques, and may assume a more prominent role in future diagnosis (Kirkali and Tuzel, 2003).

Bladder tumor may invade one or both ureteric orifices and may cause renal impairment due to obstructive uropathy. Sonography is not routinely used for staging cancer of the urinary bladder. If the tumor is found incidentally, it often appears as a polypoid or plaquelike, hypoechoic lesion that may project into the bladder (Fig. 2). Calcifications or fibrosis produces an increase in echogenicity. Blood

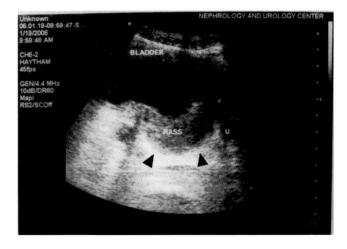

Figure 2 Axial gray-scale US scan in a case of urinary bladder tumor shows an echogenic posterior wall mass (arrows) encroaching upon the orifices of the dilated ureters (u).

flow can be shown in tumors on Doppler US (Kundra and Silverman, 2003).

Noncontrast Computed Tomography

Noncontrast computed tomography is the procedure of choice for diagnosis of stone disease, giving a sensitivity of 98% and a specificity of 100% (Shokeir *et al.*, 2002). In this setting, NCCT carries several advantages, including no use of contrast materials and time saving because the procedure requires only 5 min. Except for indinavir urolithiasis, all stones are visible on NCCT. In addition, several secondary NCCT signs of ureteral obstruction are often present, which are useful when a stone is not readily identified. The ability to diagnose a wide range of disease entities that result in obstructive uropathy is an advantage of NCCT. It is accurate in identifying extrinsic causes of ureteric obstruction. Moreover, NCCT can easily visualize nonorgan-confined bladder or prostate cancer, causing bilateral hydroureteronephrosis due to infiltration of the distal parts of both ureters (Fig. 3A, B). In addition, the attenuation values of nonopaque filling defects in the intramural ureter aid in confirming lesion location and nature. On NCCT, TCC is typically hyperattenuating (5–30 HU) to urine and renal parenchyma, but less attenuating than other pelvic filling defects such as clot (40–80 HU) or calculus (> 100 IIU).

Magnetic Resonance Urography

T2-weighted MRU is an option in patients who have contrast allergy because it does not require the administration of any gadolinium. It also eliminates the need for costly nonionic-iodinated compounds or prophylaxis against an allergic reaction with steroids. Administration of intravenous contrast to diabetic patients can be avoided because these patients may have compromised renal function secondary to impaired glomerular filtration and nephrosclerosis. T2-weighted MRU is safe during pregnancy; therefore, it potentially has the ability to differentiate physiologic dilatation in pregnancy from pathologic dilatation (Spencer *et al.*, 2000). Dilatation of the urinary tract facilitates the diagnosis by T2-weighted MRU, because the fluid in the upper tract is visualized. Several studies have shown that T2-weighted MRU can correctly determine the grade of dilatation and location of obstruction, although identifying the underlying abnormality may be missed in up to one-half of the cases (Shokeir *et al.*, 2004).

The addition of an axial T2-weighted sequence requires only an extra 3 to 4 min but easily allows the combination of MRU and conventional axial MR pulse sequences, offering " a one-stop shopping" diagnostic procedure that is well suited for the assessment of intrinsic and extrinsic ureteral disorders. Such sequences can help to distinguish a soft tissue

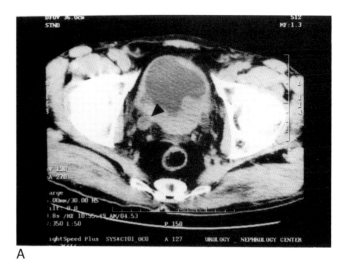

A

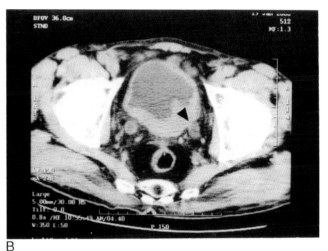

B

Figure 3 Axial noncontrast CT scan of the pelvis in a case of urinary tumor shows a posterior wall hyperdense mass encroaching upon the right ureter (**A**) and left ureter (**B**) [arrows].

mass from blood clots or calculi, which display a signal void. Transitional cell carcinoma displays a more heterogeneous signal morphology, including hyperintense and cystic-like areas on T2-weighted spin echo images (Nolte-Ernsting *et al.*, 2001).

Previous investigators have shown that gadolinium on T1-weighted images can be used in conjunction with MRU to further characterize renal neoplasms or other causes of noncalculus obstruction (Shokeir *et al.*, 2004). In partially obstructed kidneys with minimal dilation, gadolinium-enhanced MRU can give functional information in the same way as IVP enables more accurate evaluation of the degree and cause of obstruction. The whole urinary tract, including nondilated ureters, can be visualized. However, gadolinium-enhanced MRU is not recommended for the evaluation of pregnant women. Furthermore, gadolinium-enhanced MRU is of limited value in poorly functioning kidneys with long-standing obstruction. It seems logical that the kidney must have some residual function to allow excretion of gadolinium. The critical value of this function has to be determined in additional studies. A good visualization of gadolinium was obtained with serum creatinine as high as 2.5 mg/dl.

In the side-by-side comparison with IVP, gadolinium-enhanced MRU provides particularly impressive accuracy in the examination of the ureters and their pathologic abnormalities. This implies that the MRU technique may have the potential to become the preferred imaging modality for the diagnosis of any suspected ureteral disease. In one series, almost all patients, even those with moderately reduced excretory function, the combined use of gadolinium and low-dose furosemide resulted in complete visualization of the ureters with a markedly high signal intensity (Nolte-Ernsting *et al.*, 1998). Superimposed intestinal gas and fluid collections, which are a common problem in radiography, US, and, at times, T2-weighted MRU, never degrade the conspicuity of the ureters at T1-weighted diuretic-enhanced excretory MRU. Furthermore, pelvic phleboliths are not visible on MR images and, therefore, cannot be misinterpreted (Nolte-Ernsting *et al.*, 1998). Magnetic resonance urography is not without limitations: It is contraindicated in very old patients or young children who do not or cannot cooperate. Patients who have metallic implants or pacemakers are absolute contraindications. Moreover, gadolinium injection is not recommended in pregnant patients (Shokeir *et al.*, 2004).

Transitional cell carcinoma has lower signal intensity than the normally high-signal-intensity urine on T2-weighted images, permitting good demonstration of tumor in a dilated collecting system (Fig. 4). However, TCC is nearly isointense to renal parenchyma on T1- and T2-weighted images, meaning that gadolinium contrast material is necessary for accurate assessment of tumor extent (Browne *et al.*, 2005). Although TCC is a hypovascular tumor, moderate enhancement is seen with gadolinium contrast material, although

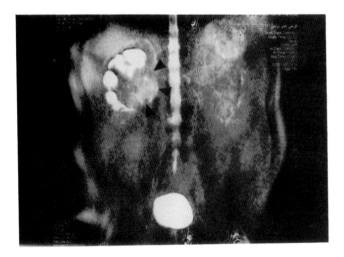

Figure 4 Coronal heavily T2W MRU in a case of right renal transitional cell carcinoma shows hydronephrotic changes with large hypointense mass (arrows) at the dilated right pelvis and middle calyces.

not to the same degree as renal parenchyma. Postcontrast imaging may be performed by using three-dimensional (3D) sequences to allow dynamic evaluation of the kidney. This allows assessment of the renal vasculature in arterial and venous phases and the renal parenchyma in cortico-medullary and nephrographic phases. Vascular invasion of the renal vein or inferior vena cava, although rare, may be demonstrated without gadolinium contrast material by using T2-weighted or gradient-echo flow-sensitive sequences (Browne *et al.*, 2005).

Ureteric TCC is isointense to muscle on T1-weighted images and slightly hyperintense on T2-weighted images (Blandino *et al.*, 2002). At MRU, ureteric TCC typically appears as an irregular mass (Fig. 5A), whereas calculi appear as sharply delineated filling defects (Fig. 5B), although differentiation between small calculi and tumor may be difficult. Tumor enhancement after administration of gadolinium contrast material can also help distinguish it from calculi. Soft tissue stranding in the periureteric fat is suggestive of periureteric extension, although prior surgery, radiation, and inflammation can also give these appearances. Magnetic resonance urography may help differentiate these entities; however, fibrosis will appear hyperintense on T2-weighted images, particularly in long-standing cases (Browne *et al.*, 2005).

The signal intensity of TCC usually differs sufficiently from that of other causes of ureteral filling defects, such as stones and blood clots, to suggest an accurate diagnosis. Stones are the most common cause of ureteral filling defects. Both in hydrographic and excretory MRU, a ureteral stone appears as a round or ovoid signal void filling defect that causes a variable degree of dilatation of the urinary tract (Fig. 5B). Because small calculi may be obscured by hyperintense urine on maximum-intensity projection (MIP) images in both excretory and multislice HASTE MRU, evaluation of the source images is essential to confirm the presence of stones (Nolte-Ernsting *et al.*, 1998).

Surgery, diagnostic or therapeutic procedures, or gas-producing infections of the urinary tract can be the source of intraluminal gas bubbles that appear as a single or, more frequently, multiple round or oval sharply delineated signal void filling defects creating a typical string-of-pearls appearance. Characteristically, the gas bubbles float into the mid-ureter, which in a patient who is in the supine position is the uppermost part of the excretory urinary tract (Blandino *et al.*, 2002). Finally, a rare cause of ureteral filling defect is coagulum, which is typically hyperintense on T1-weighted MRU (Blandino *et al.*, 2002). Magnetic resonance urography is of particular importance in the staging of bladder cancer in patients with compromised renal function when contrast-enhanced CT is contraindicated. The accuracy of MR imaging for the staging of bladder cancer ranges from 72 to 96% (Kundra and Silverman, 2003). Staging is improved with gadolinium enhancement.

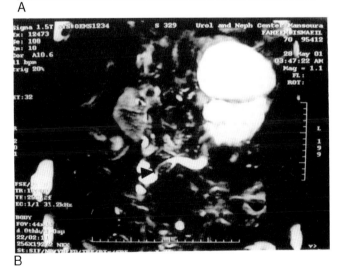

A

B

Figure 5 (A) Coronal heavily T2W MRU shows irregular low-signal-intensity tumor in the distal left ureter with secondary hydroureteronephrosis. (B) Coronal heavily T2W MRU in a case of urinary diversion with left hydroureteronephrosis secondary to a signal void stone at the lower end of the ureter (arrow)

mediate signal, slightly higher than that of the bladder wall (Fig. 6). Fat has a low signal but may have a high signal if faster sequences, such as fast spin echo, are used. Urine has a high signal. On T1-weighted sequences, the tumor has an intermediate signal and contrasts with the high signal in fat. In addition, urine in the bladder has a lower signal than the tumor. T1 sequences are helpful for evaluating spread into the perivesical fat. Cancer of the urinary bladder enhances after gadolinium injection. Peak enhancement is earlier than that of the bladder wall, which may be helpful if dynamic imaging is performed. Enhancement with or without fat saturation can show invasion into adjacent organs. Coronal and sagittal planes can also be useful in identifying perivesical invasion, particularly at the dome and at the base of the bladder. Synchronous or metachronous lesions in the ureter may also be detected on MR imaging (Kundra and Silverman, 2003).

Materials and Methods

We performed a prospective study that included 149 consecutive patients, of whom 110 had bilateral ureteral obstruction and 39 had obstruction of a solitary kidney (Shokeir *et al.*, 2003). Therefore, the total number of renal units was 259. All patients had renal impairment with serum creatinine > 2.5 mg/dl. Therefore, IVP and contrast-enhanced CT were contraindicated. The mean age was 51 years (range 21 to 72), and there were 99 males and 55 females. Besides history, routine clinical examination, and biochemical profile, patients underwent combined

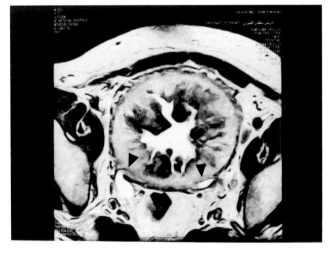

Figure 6 Axial T2W MRI of the pelvis in a case of urinary bladder tumor shows a large heterogeneous mass encircling the bladder wall and infiltrating ureteric orifices (arrows).

As with CT, MR imaging cannot depict the depth of bladder wall invasion, but it is used for stage T3b disease and beyond. On T2-weighted imaging, tumor has an inter-

KUB and US as well as NCCT and MRU using heavily T2-weighted sequences.

We used certain diagnostic criteria to differentiate the intrinsic from the extrinsic cause of ureteral obstruction. An abrupt change in ureteral caliber on axial as well as reconstructed images was suggestive of intraluminal lesions, while gradual tapering of the ureter with no intraluminal masses or filling defects was indicative of mural or extra-urinary causes. On NCCT a hyperdense focus within the ureter was diagnostic of a calculus, while an intraluminal mass of soft tissue density was considered a sign of tumor. On MRU, a well circumscribed filling defect signal void within the high intensity of the urine represented criteria for stone (Fig. 5B), while a more heterogeneous signal intensity lesion was indicative of neoplasm (Fig. 5A). Extraureteral lesions were diagnosed according to the mass effect, and specific density and signal intensity on NCCT and MRU. The gold standard for diagnosis of the cause of obstruction was retrograde or antegrade ureterogram, ureteroscopy, and/or open surgery. The sensitivity, specificity, and overall accuracy of NCCT, MRU, and combined KUB and US in the diagnosis of ureteral obstruction were calculated in comparison with the gold standard.

Techniques of Noncontrast Computed Tomography

Noncontrast computed tomography was performed with a light-speed plus scanner (General Electric, Milwaukee, Wisconsin). No oral or intravenous contrast material was used. Spiral scans were performed from the top of the kidney to the bladder base, with a table feed rate of 22.5 mm per rotation and a nominal section thickness of 5 mm (pitch = 6). Image reconstruction was routinely performed at 4-mm increments with 360° interpolation. When a calcific density was seen along the course of the ureter, additional evaluation of this region was performed with retrospective reconstruction in 2-mm increments. In some patients, reformatted images were also obtained with overlapped sections at 2-mm intervals to create images similar to those obtained with MRU.

Techniques of Magnetic Resonance Urography

Static, heavily T2-weighted MRU was performed using 1.5 Tesla scanner (Signa Horizon LX, EchoSpeed; GE Medical System, Milwaukee, Wisconsin). Coronal, two-dimensional, fast spin-echo sequences using a body coil were done. The scanning parameters were repetition time 9900 ms (12,000 according to respiratory trigger); echo time 250 ms; slice thickness, 4 mm; matrix 256 × 128; acquisition time 2 min. Gadolinium-enhanced dynamic MRU was not used. Maximal-intensity-projection images and, occasionally, multiplanar reconstruction and original source images were available on films for evaluation.

We also performed a standard axial T2-weighted fast spin-echo sequence (repetition time/echo time 6000 ms/85 ms; echo-train length 12) at the level of obstruction. For the analysis of MRU, we included the axial T2-weighted images and the original source images of MRU and did not rely exclusively on the maximal-intensity-projection images. Noncontrast computed tomography and MRU were interpreted by two different radiologists, who were unaware of the definitive diagnosis. Each radiologist read only one type of study.

Results

The causes of ureteral obstruction were classified as calculous in 146 (56%) and noncalculous in 113 (44%). The stones were located in the lumbar ureter in 63, iliac ureter in 20, and pelvic ureter in 63 renal units. The causes of noncalculous ureteral obstruction were ureteral stricture in 65 renal units, bladder tumors invading the lower end of the ureters in 37, ureteral tumors in 6, retroperitoneal pelvic collections following pelvic surgery in 3, and retroperitoneal fibrosis in 2. Compared to the gold standard, the site of stone impaction was identified in all 146 renal units by NCCT (100% sensitivity), in 101 by MRU (69.2% sensitivity), and in 115 by combined KUB and US (78.7% sensitivity), a difference of significant value in favor of NCCT ($p < 0.001$).

Ureteral strictures were identified by NCCT in 18 of 65 cases (28%) and by MRU in 54 of 65 (83%). Bladder and ureteral tumors causing ureteral obstruction could be diagnosed in approximately half of the patients by NCCT (22 of 43) and in all except 1 patient by MRU (42 of 43). Noncontrast computed tomography and MRU could identify all extraurinary causes of obstruction. Overall, of the 113 kidneys with noncalculous obstruction, the cause could be identified by MRU in 101 (89% sensitivity), by NCCT in 45 (40% sensitivity), and by combined KUB and US in only 20 (18% sensitivity), a difference of significant value in favor of MRU ($p < 0.001$).

Discussion and Conclusion

In our series, NCCT identified 100% of calculous causes of obstruction. Similar results were reported by several previous studies (Dalrymple et al., 1998). The ability to diagnose a wide range of disease entities that result in obstructive uropathy was suggested as an advantage of NCCT. However, 188 of 417 patients (45%) with flank pain reported by Dalrymple et al. (1998) were found to have ureteral stone disease. Of the remaining 229 cases, a correct alternative diagnosis was made or suggested by CT in only 65 (27%). These diagnoses included entities related and unrelated to the urinary tract. Similarly, in the current series, noncalculous obstruction was found in 113 renal units (44%), of which NCCT identified the cause of obstruction in only 45 (40%). This finding means that the sensitivity of NCCT for identifying noncalculous obstruction is not as good as that in the setting of calculous obstruction.

The current study demonstrates that the sensitivity of MRU for detecting urinary stones is ≈ 70%. Several previous studies have shown that small stones are difficult to visualize by MRU (Jung *et al.*, 2000; Sudah *et al.*, 2001). Detecting urinary stones by MRU depends on secondary signs because stones are not represented directly, as on KUB or CT. Hence, it is impossible to detect parenchymal stones by MRU, but pelvic or ureteral stones can be visualized because they are surrounded by fluid and produce a filling defect within the high signal intensity of the urine. These filling defects may be mimicked by physiological peristalsis of the ureter (Jung *et al.*, 2002). With improving MRI resolution and software, the stone detection rate may likely improve.

References

Blandino, A., Gaeta, M., Minutoli, F., Salamone, I., Magno, C., Scribano, E., and Panadolfo, I. 2002. MR urography of the ureter. *Am. J. Roentgenol. 179*:1307–1314.

Browne, R.F.J., Meehan, C.P., Colville, J., Power, R., and Torreggiani, W.C. 2005. Transitional cell carcinoma of the upper urinary tract: spectrum of imaging findings. *RadioGraphics 25*:1609–1627.

Dalrymple, N.C., Verga, M., Adersen, K.R., Bove, P., Covey, A.M., and Rosenfield, A.T. 1998. The value of unenhanced helical computerized tomography in the management of acute flank pain. *J. Urol. 159*:735–740.

Jung, P., Brauers, A., Nolte-Ernsting, C.A., Jakse, G., and Gunther, R.W. 2000. Magnetic resonance urography enhanced by gadolinium and diuretic: a comparison with conventional urography in diagnosing the cause of ureteric obstruction. *B.J.U. Int. 86*:960–965.

Kirkali, Z., and Tuzel, E. 2003. Transitional cell carcinoma of the ureter and renal pelvis. *Crit. Rev. Oncol. Hematol. 47*:155–169.

Kundra, V., and Silverman, P.M. 2003. Imaging in oncology from the University of Texas M.D. Anderson Cancer Center. *Am. J. Roentgenol. 180*:1045–1054.

Nolte-Ernsting, C.C.A., Bucker, A., and Adam, G.B. 1998. Gadolinium-enhanced excretory MR urography after low-dose diuretic injection: comparison with conventional excretory urography. *Radiology 209*:147–157.

Nolte-Ernsting, C.C.A., Adam, G.B., and Gunther, R.W. 2001. MR urography: examination techniques and clinical application. *Eur. Radiol. 11*:355–372.

Shokeir, A. 2002. Renal colic: new concepts related to pathophysiology, diagnosis and treatment. *Curr. Opin. Urol. 12*:263–269.

Shokeir, A.A., El-Diasty, T., Essa, W., Mosbah, A., Abou El-Ghar, M., Mansour, O., Dawaba, M., and El-Kappany, H. 2003. Diagnosis of ureteral obstruction in patients with compromised renal function: the role of noninvasive imaging modalities. *J. Urol. 171*:2303–2306.

Shokeir, A.A., El-Diasty, T., Essa, W., Mosbah, A., Mohsen, T., Mansour, O., Dawaba, M., and El-Kappany, H. 2004. Diagnosis of noncalcareous hydronephrosis: role of magnetic resonance urography and noncontrast computed tomography. *Urology 63*:225–229.

Spencer, J.A., Tomlinson, A.J., Weston, M.J., and Lloyd, S.N. 2000. Early comparison of breath-hold MR excretory urography, Doppler ultrasound and isotope renography in evaluation of symptomatic hydronephrosis in pregnancy. *Clin. Radiol. 55*:446–453.

26

Renal Lesions: Magnetic Resonance Diffusion-Weighted Imaging

Maria Assunta Cova, Alexia Rossi, and Fulvio Stacul

Introduction

The technique of diffusion-weighted imaging (DWI) is one of the most recent products of the evolution of magnetic resonance imaging (MRI) (Mori and Barker, 1999). Diffusion is one of the three flow parameters of the MR signal, together with macroscopic flow and perfusion, which introduces new elements to the MR study (Colagrande *et al.*, 2005). Molecular diffusion refers to the random translational motion of molecules, also called Brownian motion, that results from the thermal energy carried by these molecules (Le Bihan *et al.*, 2001).

The phenomenon of diffusion is usually described with the use of Fick's laws, which describe the behavior of a solute that moves along a concentration gradient. In other words, in those systems where the concentration of particles is not uniform, diffusion occurs macroscopically like a flow of particles from the region of high concentration toward the region of lower concentration. In this case the diffusion coefficient can be defined as macroscopic quantity, which characterizes the phenomenon and which reflects the constant of proportionality that links the flow of particles to the concentration gradient. If, on the other hand, the concentration is the same at all points (homogeneous fluid), even though the particles continue to diffuse, macroscopic flow

is no longer observed, and it is therefore no longer possible to define a diffusion coefficient as described above. In this case, Fick's laws do not apply, and instead reference needs to be made to a probabilistic model to describe the motion of the molecules. This means that instead of knowing the precise position of a particle, the phenomenon is described with a function indicating the probability that a particle travels a given distance in a given time (Colagrande *et al.*, 2005).

Magnetic resonance imaging is the only means we have to observe diffusion *in vivo* noninvasively. Furthermore, MRI provides access to both superficial and deep organs with high resolution and does not interfere with the diffusion process itself: diffusion is an intrinsic physical process that is totally independent of the MR effect or the magnetic field (Le Bihan *et al.*, 2001).

Diffusion MRI imaging as a technique was pioneered in 1986 by Le Bihan *et al.* (1986) and in 1990 by Moseley (Moseley *et al.*, 1990a). The most successful application of diffusion MRI since the early 1990s has been brain ischemia, following the finding by Moseley *et al.* (1990b) that water diffusion drops at a very early stage of the ischemic event in the cat brain. Diffusion MRI provides some patients with the opportunity to receive suitable treatment at a stage when brain tissue might still be salvageable (Le Bihan *et al.*, 2001).

At the same time, new fields of application developed in neuroradiology, including the study of brain masses to differentiate solid and cystic lesions and recently the study of demyelinizating lesions.

Technique

It is necessary to present some principles of the formation of MRI signal to understand how MRI allows the diffusion study. The precession frequency of the spins in a magnetic field is given by the Larmor equation

$$f = \gamma B_0$$

where f is the precession frequency, γ is the specific gyromagnetic constant for each nucleus, and B_0 is the intensity of the static magnetic field. If the magnetic field is uniform, all of the spins will have the same precession frequency. On the other hand, in the presence of a magnetic field gradient (e.g., applied along the x-axis) the precession frequency depends on the position of the spins and is described by

$$f = \gamma B_0 + \gamma(Gx)$$

where G is the magnetic field gradient along the x-axis and x is the position of the spin along the same axis. Applying a constant gradient G for a time δ, the spins will accumulate a phase:

$$\Phi = \gamma G \delta x$$

The key to sensitizing the MR sequences to diffusion, so as to render the phenomenon of diffusion evident and measurable, was historically the introduction of pulse gradients. The first to apply two short-duration gradients rather than a single-gradient constant over time were Stejskal and Tanner (Stejskal and Tanner, 1965). If we apply two gradients of opposite polarities, of equal intensity and duration, separated by a time interval Δ, the phase accumulated by the spins is given by

$$\Phi = \gamma G \delta (x_0 - x_i)$$

where x_0 is the position of the spins at the time of the application of the first gradient, whereas x_i is the position of the spins at the time of the application of the second gradient. The phase therefore depends on the movements of the spins, which occur in the time interval between the application of the first and second gradients.

If the movement is random, as occurs with Brownian motion, the different spins acquire different phase variations, resulting in a loss of signal. The loss of signal due solely to diffusion is described by the equation

$$S = S_0 e^{-bD}$$

where S and S_0 are the signal intensities with and without diffusion sensitization, respectively, and D is the diffusion coefficient. The b-factor expresses the level of sensitization to diffusion of the sequence.

It is, therefore, clear how diffusion-weighted images can be obtained. They are not only influenced by T1 and T2, but also to a large extent by the degree of water diffusion: low diffusion corresponds, therefore, to lower signal loss, while high diffusion corresponds to a higher signal loss (Colagrande et al., 2005). Diffusion is truly a three-dimensional process. Hence, molecular mobility in tissues may not be the same in all directions. This anisotropy may result from a peculiar physical arrangement of the medium (such as in liquid crystals) or from the presence of obstacles limiting molecular movements in some directions. Only molecular displacements that occur along the direction of the gradient are visible. The effect of diffusion anisotropy can then easily be detected by observing variations in the diffusion measurements when the direction of the gradient pulses is changed. This is a unique, powerful feature not found with usual MRI parameters, such as T1 or T2 (Le Bihan et al., 2001).

Diffusion anisotropy was observed long ago in the muscles (Cleveland et al., 1976). With the advent of diffusion MRI, anisotropy was also detected in vivo at the end of the 1980s in the spinal cord (Moseley et al., 1990a) and in the brain white matter (Chenevert et al., 1990). More recently, diffusion anisotropy has also been seen in rat brain gray matter (Hoehn Berlage et al., 1999) and in human brain of neonates. Diffusion anisotropy in the white matter is related to its specific organization in bundles of more or less myelinated axonal fibers running in parallel: diffusion in the direction of the fibers is faster than in the perpendicular direction (Le Bihan et al., 2001).

Because of the need to consider this feature, the diffusion coefficient D is substituted with an apparent diffusion coefficient (ADC) and the expression that describes the signal loss becomes:

$$S = S_0 e^{-b\text{ADC}}$$

Indeed, the ADC is so called because the measured quantity only partially describes a more complex event. The ADC characterizes the molecular movements in a single direction and therefore is not able to describe the three-dimensional movements of the molecules in nonisotropic systems. It corresponds to the diffusion coefficient in homogeneous and isotropic media, but it is unable to fully describe diffusion in anisotropic media. A scalar quantity such as ADC, therefore, cannot be used to fully describe diffusion in all situations. However, not even a vector quantity (characterized by three components in space) is sufficient. Indeed, even measuring the ADCs along three orthogonal directions and combining the three components would produce a result dependent on the choice of the system of orthogonal axes. This occurs because in anisotropic systems the diffusion motions in orthogonal directions are correlated among themselves. A crucial factor for describing the phenomenon mathematically is the tensor, which is an operator capable of taking into consideration the correlations between the orthogonal directions (Colagrande *et al.*, 2005).

Technically, the MR examination should be performed with a high-field superconductive magnet (1.5 T) equipped with 23–30 mT/m intensity gradients, a slew rate of 150 mT/m/s, and phased-array surface coils. All sequences are acquired in breath hold to reduce respiratory artifacts. Chemical-shift artifacts are reduced by systematically using fat presaturation. In addition, where possible, the use of parallel imaging, a technique capable of reducing acquisition time or increasing the matrix—and therefore the spatial resolution without altering the acquisition time and without significant loss in image quality (sensitivity encoding, SENSE)—can be an advantage (Colagrande *et al.*, 2006).

Diffusion-weighted images are acquired using a variation of the spin-echo (SE) sequences (the Stejskal and Tanner sequence) performed with the single-shot echo-planar technique. Conventional SE sequences have the major disadvantage of lasting several minutes, and when they are used to acquire diffusion-weighted images, the patient is required to remain motionless. Clearly, if the signal loss in diffusion-weighted images is produced by the Brownian motion of the water molecules, macroscopic motion, such as heartbeat and respiration, conceals the microscopic variations of the diffusivity of the various tissutal components. Macroscopic motion is, therefore, exceedingly deleterious to the signal of diffusion-weighted images and may almost completely cancel the signal itself. The use of increasingly powerful and actively shielded gradients has enabled the passage from conventional SE sequences to echo-planar imaging (EPI) sequences. This technique is capable of acquiring "instantaneous" images with a temporal resolution below 200 ms, which eliminates the deleterious effect of macroscopic motion (Colagrande *et al.*, 2005), thus allowing use of DW MR in extracranial organs and functional evaluation of different abdominal organs (Thoeny *et al.*, 2005).

Diffusion-weighted images are influenced by limitations of EPI sequences that are associated with the high velocity of acquisition: low spatial resolution (as a consequence, this type of sequence cannot be used to obtain T2-weighted images) and high sensitivity to magnetic susceptibility. This entails a classic spin-echo sequence characterized by two successive radiofrequency impulses at 90° and 180°, to which two additional gradients known as motion-probing gradients (MPGs) equal in breadth and duration but opposite in direction are added immediately before and after the 180° impulse (Colagrande *et al.*, 2006).

The other parameters of the sequence generally used are: TR 1800–5000 ms, 60 < TE < 120, matrix 128 × 128–256,

number of measurements 1, indicative bandwidth 2080 Hz/pixel, number of sections acquired 12–20, slice thickness 5–8 mm, and field-of-view (FOV) variable based on the size of the patient (Colagrande *et al.*, 2006). Using these sequences with these characteristics, we can acquire DW images. These images provide qualitative information on the diffusion of water molecules in a region (high or low diffusion), and they permit study of the anisotropy of the region under evaluation (Colagrande *et al.*, 2005).

With the acquisition of at least two images with different degrees of diffusion weighting, that is, with different b values (e.g., 0 and 1000 s/mm^2), ADC maps and mean diffusivity can be obtained. ADC maps are quantitative maps where the signal intensity of each voxel represents the mean diffusivity (along the direction selected by the gradient) in the voxel itself. Tracing regions of interest on these maps enables the measurement of the ADC along various axes, in different tissues, and the comparison of possible variations over time of pathological processes. The formula to calculate the ADC value is:

$$ADC = (\ln S_0 - \ln S) / b$$

To better understand the signal of DW images, we need to bear in mind all of the effects that contribute to its formation and therefore reassess the T2 shine-through phenomenon and introduce a pseudodiffusion D*, with which we mean the totality of nondiffusional intravoxel incoherent motion (IVIM), or that derived from perfusion and circulatory, respiratory, and peristaltic motion.

With regard to T2 shine-through, it should be borne in mind that the long TR/TE times that enable the activation of the supplementary dephasing/rephasing gradient render the DW image heavily weighted in T2. Therefore, when considering a high signal, we need to question whether the signal is related to reduced diffusion or to high T2 (shine-through effect); in the same way, a low signal can be related to high diffusion or to a reduced T2 signal intensity.

In contrast to the DW images, the ADC maps are not "contaminated" by the effects of T2, even though they remain dependent on the alterations deriving from the pseudodiffusion. Observing the equation

$$ADC = (\ln S_0 - \ln S) / b$$

we can see that the dependence on T2 is reduced because the term in T2 is contained in both S_0 and S. The ADC measures all the IVIM, incorporating both the diffusion and the pseudodiffusion (that is, the IVIM dependent on diffusion and not dependent) and is equal to the real diffusion only when the latter is the only present motion, as in a test tube containing saline solution. In living tissue, the ADC has a higher value than would otherwise be expected owing to perfusion and other nondiffusional IVIM.

With an increase in the value of *b*, the intensity of the signal in DW is reduced. Structures that present high ADC values display low signal in the DW images. In the ADC map, a hyperintense image indicates high IVIM, and a hypointense image low IVIM, the opposite occurring in DW images where hyperintensity corresponds to low IVIM and hypointensity to high IVIM. For low values of *b*, the obtained ADC values are markedly influenced by D^*. In addition, high *b* values (> 100) almost completely eliminate the effects induced by nondiffusional IVIM and therefore for those values the weight of D^* is equal to zero. To obtain a truly expressive image of diffusion, the *b* values should be 1200 and ADC should be calculated: the high *b* values increase the weighting in diffusion and cancel the effects of D^* and weighting in T2, while the ADC eliminates the shine-through effects (Colagrande *et al.*, 2005).

Renal Diffusion

The kidney could be a particularly interesting organ to study by means of diffusion imaging because of its high blood flow and water transport function. Although the kidneys constitute only about 0.5% of total body weight, they receive about 25% of the cardiac output, which represents perfusion of more than $400\,ml/min^{-1}/g^{-1}$. Moreover, renal water content (83%) is higher than water content in any other organ (Muller *et al.*, 1994a). Since water transport is the predominant renal function because of the kidney's role in water reabsorption and concentration-dilution, the diffusion characteristics of the kidney may provide information on the mechanism of various renal diseases (Jones and Grattan-Smith, 2003). The application of diffusion imaging techniques to the kidney has been hindered by several problems, notably the extreme motion sensitivity, especially to respiratory motion and arterial pulsation, of diffusion sequences and the anisotropic nature of renal diffusion (Jones and Grattan-Smith, 2003), reflecting the radial-oriented structures in the kidney, such as renal vessels and tubules (Fukuda *et al.*, 2000).

Renal Normal Parenchyma

ADC values of renal normal parenchyma are higher when compared with those of the other abdominal parenchymas. The first mean ADC value of renal parenchyma reported in the literature is $3.54 \times 10^{-3}\,mm^2/s$ (Muller *et al.*, 1994b). The same authors also assessed the ADC value in initially dehydrated and then rehydrated patients, and measured higher mean values by around 25% in condition of hydration than in dehydration ($3.56 \times 10^{-3}\,mm^2/s$ versus $2.88 \times 10^{-3}\,mm^2/s$, respectively). In each case, dehydration and hydration were confirmed by determination of urine osmolality. The increase of ADC with rehydration could be due to an increase in water content, plasma volume, and glomerular filtration rate (Muller *et al.*, 1994a).

The degree of renal perfusion influences the ADC values as well. In an animal study a transitional reduction of ADC values, in both the cortex and medulla, after intravenous administration of high-viscosity nonionic contrast material, was shown and related to a contrast material-induced reduction of renal perfusion (Laissy *et al.*, 2000). It is important to remember that the contribution of perfusion to ADC value is fully eliminated with the use of high MPGs because capillary perfusion is markedly faster than water diffusion and the occurring signal intensity loss is related more to perfusion than to diffusion (Fukuda *et al.*, 2000). The ADC values change according to different measurement sites.

The ADC values of the cortex are different from the ADC values of the medulla, but in the literature conflicting opinions are reported. In one study (Thoeny *et al.*, 2005), the ADCs values of healthy volunteers calculated with all *b*-factor values and with high *b*-factor values (500, 750, or $1000\,s/mm^2$) are significantly higher in the cortex than in the medulla. When comparing ADC values with a low *b*-factor and ADC values with high *b*-factor of the cortex and the medulla, a significant difference could not be observed with low *b*-factor (0, 50, or $100\,s/mm^2$). The difference in ADC values with a high *b*-factor is probably due to the presence of more free diffusion-inhibiting structures in the medulla than in the cortex. However, the lack of difference of the ADC values between the cortex and the medulla when the *b*-factor was low might occur because the effect of higher true diffusion in the cortex is largely canceled by the greater anisotropy due to the radial orientation of the structures in the medulla (Thoeny *et al.*, 2005). On the other hand, another study shows ADC values of the medulla to be higher than those of the cortex (Nanimoto *et al.*, 1999).

A study (Fukuda *et al.*, 2000) showed that the ADC value at the upper pole was significantly higher than at the central portion using low *b*-factor values whereas no significant differences were obtained with high *b*-factor values. This is explained by anisotropic diffusion, as structures in the polar regions are oriented parallel to the gradients, whereas in the central portion they are perpendicular. Furthermore, there is a greater amount of cortex than medulla in the renal poles, and it should be borne in mind that blood flow in the cortex is about ten times greater than that in the medulla. High ADC values at the poles are therefore justified by the higher perfusion, an effect noted when low *b* values are used, whereas with high *b* values such an effect is almost entirely eliminated (Fukuda *et al.*, 2000). The capabilities of DWI are also studied in various pathological conditions such as functional alterations, kidney infections, hydro/pyonephrosis, and tumors.

Functional Alterations

In patients with renal artery stenosis (RSA), there is a reduction of ADC values, especially in the cortex, because there is a reduction of the renal perfusion (Nanimoto *et al.*,

1999). Also, in chronic renal failure (CRF) we can observe a reduction of ADC values because this pathological condition is characterized by a loss of nephrons and by fibrosis. Due to fibrosis in CRF kidneys, the water transport functions are reduced, and as a result there is a restriction of molecule motion (Nanimoto et al., 1999). In acute renal failure (ARF), the ADC values of the cortex and the medulla are lower than that in the normal parenchyma, but they are always higher than those of CRF kidneys (Nanimoto et al., 1999). A study carried out on rats demonstrates that the decrease of ADC values in renal failure might be attributed to renal ischemia and to accumulation of diffusion-restricted water in the intracellular space. In the same study, a decreased renal perfusion and a reduced glomerular plasma flow are seen in ARF. So, both tubular and vascular events contribute to reduce ADC values in both the cortex and the medulla. Apparent diffusion coefficient values in the medulla are poorly related to elevated level of serum creatinine; a more sensitive indicator of a renal dysfunction is the ADC value of the cortex (Vexler et al., 1996).

Hydronephrosis, Pyonephrosis, and Renal Infection

Inflammation appears to reduce ADC values; this has been found in cases of pyelonephritis and renal abscess or abscessed renal cyst (Cova et al., 2004). DWI can have a role in the differential diagnosis between hydronephrosis and pyonephrosis. Hydronephrosis is defined as a dilatation of the renal collecting system due to obstruction of the urinary tract, while pyonephrosis is described as a collection of purulent material within the collecting system of the kidney associated with destruction of renal parenchyma and loss of renal function.

Prompt differential diagnosis between these entities has a vital clinical significance; in fact, if an urgent percutaneous drainage is not performed, pyonephrosis will rapidly progress to septicemia. The traditional MR sequences are not useful for the differentiation because both pathological conditions appear hypointense on T1-weighted images and hyperintense on T2-weighted images unless the dependent portion of the collecting system contains high-protein content material or debris. Moreover the administration of contrast material does not give helpful information (Chan et al., 2001).

In a study carried out on 12 patients (Chan et al., 2001), on DWI with b-factor equal to $1000\,s/mm^2$, the renal pelvis of the hydronephrotic kidney ($n = 8$) is hypointense while the renal pelvis of the pyonephrotic kidney ($n = 4$) is markedly hyperintense. The mean ADC of the hydronephrotic renal pelvis is $(2.98 \pm 0.65) \times 10^{-3}\,mm^2/s$, while the mean ADC of the pyonephrotic renal pelvis is $(0.64 \pm 0.35) \times 10^{-3}\,mm^2/s$. The ADCs of the pyonephrotic kidneys are significantly lower than those of the hydronephrotic kidneys.

The collecting system of a pyonephrotic kidney is filled with purulent material, which is a thick, yellowish brown, adhesive fluid with a very high viscosity and cellularity that provides very low ADC values that account for its signal hyperintensity on diffusion-weighted images and signal hypointensity on ADC maps (Chan et al., 2001). Another study confirming the different ADC values between hydronephrotic and pyonephrotic renal pelvis has been reported. In this DWI is acquired with a b-factor of $500\,s/mm^2$: the ADC value of hydronephrotic pelvis is $(3.7 \pm 0.08) \times 10^{-3}\,mm^2/s$, while in pyonephrotic pelvis it is $(0.96 \pm 0.09) \times 10^{-3}\,mm^2/s$ (Cova et al., 2004). Therefore, lower ADC values in the pyonephrotic pelvis are confirmed.

Renal Masses

Diffusion-weighted imaging can have great capabilities in the study of focal renal lesions even if there are few works on this topic in literature. In fact, the signal intensity on DWI is closely related to the cellular density of the evaluated tissue. The mobility of water molecules is reduced in tissues that are characterized by high cellularity, such as tumors with quick growth, and for this reason there is a reduction of the diffusion. On the contrary, cystic lesions and tumors with high necrotic component, where there is a destruction of part of the tumoral tissue, are characterized by a great mobility of water molecules and therefore by an increased diffusion of these molecules.

Renal Cystic Lesions

Bosniak's classification of renal cystic masses was introduced in 1986. It is based on CT features, and it subdivides the cystic lesions into definitely benign lesions (class I and class II), lesions requiring a follow-up to prove their benignity (class IIF), and lesions requiring the surgical treatment because of their eventual or established malignant nature. This classification is used for the radiological diagnosis and affects the therapeutic management of cystic renal lesions (Bosniak, 1986; Israel and Bosniak, 2003).

In the study by Cova et al. (2004), the difference of ADC values between normal renal parenchyma and cystic lesions was evaluated. The mean ADC value of simple cysts (Bosniak I) is $(3.65 \pm 0.09) \times 10^{-3}\,mm^2/s$; this value is significantly higher compared to the normal parenchyma, which is $(2.19 \pm 0.17) \times 10^{-3}\,mm^2/s$.

Because Bosniak's classification provides information on the treatment the patient should undergo, future studies on different DWI patterns of lesions belonging to different Bosniak classes can be an appealing idea (Fig. 1). Actually, it would be very interesting to differentiate, for instance, between cystic tumors and complex cysts. No studies in the literature have considered this topic so far.

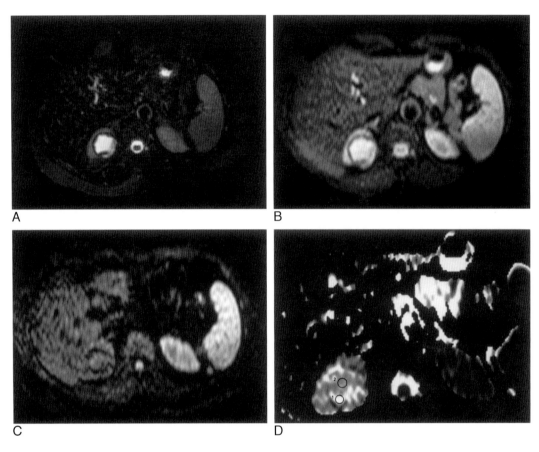

Figure 1 Complex cyst of the right kidney. (**A**) Axial turbo spin-echo (TSE) T_2-weighted image with fat saturation. The lesion is hyperintense with a thick wall and thick septum. (**B**) Diffusion-weighted spin-echo echo-planar imaging (SE EPI) image with $b = 0\,\mathrm{s/mm^2}$. The complex cyst is highly hyperintense in the fluid component. (**C**) Diffusion-weighted spin-echo echo-planar imaging (SE EPI) image with $b = 500\,\mathrm{s/mm^2}$. The cyst is isointense in the fluid component. (**D**) Apparent diffusion coefficient map (ADC). The ADC value measured in the fluid component is $(3.64 \pm 0.44) \times 10^{-3}\ \mathrm{mm^2/s}$, while the ADC value measured in the cyst thick wall is $(2.68 \pm 0.15) \times 10^{-3}\ \mathrm{mm^2/s}$.

Solid Renal Lesions

Solid renal lesions can be benign or malignant. We will briefly describe the anatomopathological characteristics of these lesions because they can be related to aspects of the lesions in DWI. In the group of benign lesions, oncocytomas and angiomyolipomas are more frequent. The oncocytoma is an epithelial tumor that is thought to originate from type A intercalated cell of the collecting duct (Cohen and McGovern, 2005). It is usually isolated and unilateral (in more than 95% of the cases), well circumscribed, nonencapsulated without gross necrosis; hemorrhage or cystic degeneration can occur. Only in the large lesions (about 50% of the cases) is there a characteristic central stellate fibrous scar. Usually, it shows an acinar or trabecular growth pattern, in an edematous, vascular stroma (Linder *et al.*, 2003). The angiomyolipomas of the kidney are a hamartoma with coexistence of blood vessels, smooth muscle, and fatty tissue. Its diagnosis rests on detecting macroscopic fat within a renal mass (Israel *et al.*, 2005). It is a well-circumscribed lesion, not encapsu-

lated, compressing the surrounding structures; hemorrhage is a common finding (Linder *et al.*, 2003).

Among malignant masses, the most frequent type is the renal cell carcinoma (RCC), a tumor arising from the renal epithelium (Cohen and McGovern, 2005). In 1997, the Union International Contre le Cancer (UICC) and the American Joint Committee on Cancer proposed a new, simplified classification of the RCC (Storkel *et al.*, 1997):

1. Clear cell carcinoma
2. Papillary cell carcinoma
3. Chromophobe cell carcinoma
4. Collecting duct carcinoma
5. Unclassified carcinoma

The *clear cell carcinoma* (Fig. 2) is the most common cell type among RCCs, accounting for 70% of all RCCs (Yoshimitsu *et al.*, 2004). Most of these tumors are isolated (4% of multifocality in one kidney and 0.5 to 3% of bilateralism). The clear cell carcinoma has often a pseudocapsule, and the large tumors can present a considerable amount of necrosis.

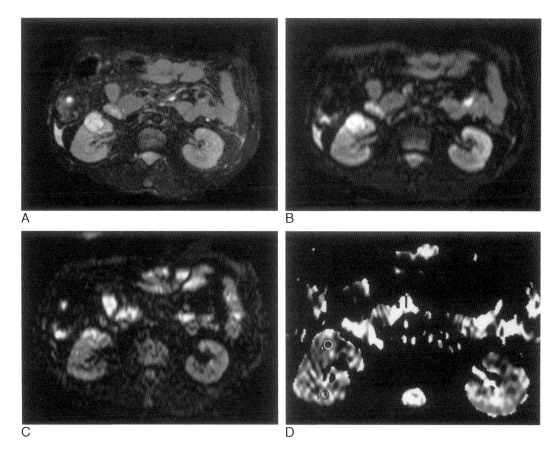

Figure 2 Clear cell carcinoma of the right kidney. (**A**) Axial turbo spin-echo (TSE) T_2-weighted image with fat saturation. The lesion is inhomogeneously hyperintense. (**B**) Diffusion-weighted spin-echo echo-planar imaging (SE EPI) image with $b = 0\,\text{s/mm}^2$. The lesion is slightly hyperintense and inhomogeneous. (**C**) Diffusion-weighted spin-echo echo-planar imaging (SE EPI) image with $b = 500\,\text{s/mm}^2$. The lesion is partly iso- and partly slightly hyperintense. (**D**) Apparent diffusion coefficient map (ADC). The ADC value measured in the adenocarcinoma is $(2.03 \pm 0.18) \times 10^{-3}\,\text{mm}^2/\text{s}$, while the ADC value measured in the normal parenchyma is $(2.61 \pm 0.44) \times 10^{-3}\,\text{mm}^2/\text{s}$.

Sometimes a pseudocystic aspect or hemorrhage or fibrosis and calcification occur. The architectural pattern could be acinar, tubular, cystic, or solid in a poor stroma but with a very characteristic rich vasculature (Linder *et al.*, 2003). The RCC of this cell type has a moderate prognosis, about 50–60% 5-year survival rate (Yoshimitsu *et al.*, 2004).

The *papillary cell carcinoma* is the second most frequent carcinoma of the kidney, accounting for 10 to 15% of cases. This type of RCC is well circumscribed by a thick pseudocapsule. Compared to other types of RCCs it is more frequently multifocal (39%), whereas it is seldom bilateral (4%). It has a predominant papillary or tubulo-papillary architecture; the papillae consist of delicate fibrovascular cores covered by a single layer of carcinomatous cells (Linder *et al.*, 2003). The 5-year survival rate is ~ 90% (Yoshimitsu *et al.*, 2004).

The *chromophobe cell carcinoma* accounts for 5% of RCCs in surgical series (Linder *et al.*, 2003). It is thought to originate from type B intercalate cells of collecting ducts (Cohen and McGovern, 2005). Often unilateral, the tumor is well circumscribed, lacking necrosis or hemorrhage. Solid architecture is

the most common. It has a better prognosis than other variants of RCC (Linder *et al.*, 2003).

Only two studies considered the features of focal renal lesions with DWI.

In the study by Cova *et al.* (2004), the mean ADC value of solid renal lesions ($n = 7$) was $(1.55 + 0.20) \times 10^{-3}\,\text{mm}^2/\text{s}$. In this study, the low number of solid lesions prevented a distinction between benign and malignant masses on the basis of DWI. The mean ADC value of the renal tumors was significantly lower than that of normal renal parenchyma, which is $(2.19 \pm 0.17) \times 10^{-3}\,\text{mm}^2/\text{s}$.

In the literature only one article considers a possible correlation between ADC values, tumoral cellularity, and tumoral histotype (Squillaci *et al.*, 2004). In this study they showed a significant difference between ADC values of the normal renal parenchyma and ADC values of 18 renal tumors: $(2.23 \pm 0.20) \times 10^{-3}\,\text{mm}^2/\text{s}$ versus $(1.72 \pm 0.46) \times 10^{-3}\,\text{mm}^2/\text{s}$, respectively. The authors showed a different ADC value for the different tumoral histotypes. In clear cell carcinoma, the mean ADC value was $(1.5 \pm 0.8) \times 10^{-3}\,\text{mm}^2/\text{s}$. The histopathologic differential diagnosis between granular cell carcinoma and oncocytoma is very difficult: it is only possible to evaluate the different numbers of mitochondria with electron microscopy. Both lesions are characterized by a high cellularity, but they showed different ADC values: 2.67×10^{-3} mm^2/s for the granular cell carcinoma ($n = 1$) and $(1.7 \pm 0.3) \times 10^{-3}$ mm^2/s for the oncocytomas ($n = 2$). Angiomyolipomas ($n = 4$) showed a low ADC value: $(1.46 \pm 0.09) \times 10^{-3}$ mm^2/s (Squillaci et al., 2004). According to the UICC system, all of these granular cell carcinomas can be classified as either oncocytoma, chromophobe RCC, papillary RCC, collecting duct carcinoma, or epithelioid angiomyolipoma (Storkel et al., 1997).

The clear cell carcinoma grows forming homogeneous and uniform sheets of neoplastic cells, which can justify the low ADC value. In contrast, the granular cell carcinoma and the oncocytomas have higher ADC values than the clear cell carcinoma probably because these lesions grow building trabecular structures and cell nidus, which are divided by wide interstitial spaces where water molecules are free to move. The angiomyolipoma has an important compound of collagen stroma that can be responsible for the low ADC value. Actually, the collagen stroma can reduce the diffusion velocity of water molecules. The authors suggested that the ADC values of solid renal lesions are not correlated with the cellularity of the lesions but with their histological architecture; for this reason, extracellular water diffusion has the potential to be considered as a sensitive and specific tool for the classification of renal masses. We can consider water diffusion as an indirect sign of the complexity of the intra- or extracellular space, of the histological architecture, of the tumoral share of free or binding water, and of the modality of growth of the renal tumors (Squillaci et al., 2004).

In our personal experience we studied the features of renal solid masses, histologically documented, with DWI. The mean ADC value of angiomyolipomas ($n = 2$) was $(1.71 \pm 0.36) \times 10^{-3}$ mm^2/s. The mean ADC value of clear cell carcinoma ($n = 8$) was higher, $(2.27 \pm 0.13) \times 10^{-3}$ mm^2/s, while the mean ADC value of papillary cell carcinoma ($n = 8$) was lower, $(1.67 \pm 0.09) \times 10^{-3}$ mm^2/s. The chromophobe cell carcinoma ($n = 1$) had an ADC value of 1.22×10^{-3} mm^2/s.

It is necessary to investigate a larger number of patients to reinforce these data; only afterwards will a correlation between ADC values and histotype be possible. The current treatment strategy for resectable RCC is radical nephrectomy, in which the whole kidney is resected, along with Gerota's fascia and the ipsilateral adrenal gland. Preoperative knowledge of the cell type would not change the treatment strategy in these operable patients, and thus it is not important. The prediction of cell types may be of value in patients for whom radical surgery is not indicated. For instance, patients who will be kept under "watchful waiting" without any specific treatment, typically elderly patients or those who are at risk, may benefit from cell-type prediction. Recently, percutaneous treatments, including radiofrequency ablation, cryotherapy, and nephron-sparing nephrectomy, have been introduced as alternative therapeutic choices for patients at risk for radical surgery. In these procedures, the possibility of tumor dissemination during the procedure is not completely excluded; therefore, the knowledge that the tumor has a relatively good prognosis may further justify these procedures (Yoshimitsu et al., 2004). These comments underscore the notion that therapeutic choices can be influenced by the assessment with DWI in cases where it can predict the tumoral histotype with reasonable accuracy.

Therefore, the DW sequence could be a promising technique, and it is worthwhile considering that its acquisition time is only 17 sec with our unit. It can have an important role in the characterizing of the renal masses, provide information on the nature of complex cystic lesions, differentiate benign and malignant solid lesions, and suggest the histotype of malignant lesions. For these reasons, in our department this sequence is presently integrated in the MR protocol for the study of renal lesions. Nevertheless, much research is no doubt still required to clarify the reliability of this technique.

References

Bosniak, M.A. 1986. The current radiological approach to renal cyst. Radiology 158:1–10.

Chan, J.H.M., Tsui, E.Y.K., Luk, S.H., Fung, S.L., Cheung, Y.K., Chan, M.S.M., Yuen, M.K., Mak, S.F., and Wong, K.P.C. 2001. MR diffusion-weighted imaging of kidney: differentiation between hydronephrosis and pyonephrosis. Clin. Imaging 25:110–113.

Chenevert, T.L., Brunberg, J.A., and Pipe, J.G. 1990. Anisotropic diffusion within human white matter: demonstration with NMR techniques in vivo. Radiology 177:401–405.

Cleveland, G.G., Chang, D.C., and Hazelwood, C.F. 1976. Nuclear magnetic resonance measurements of skeletal muscle. Biophys. J. 16:1043–1053.

Cohen, H.T., and McGovern, F.J. 2005. Renal-cell carcinoma. N. Engl. J. Med. 353:2477–2490.

Colagrande, S., Carbone, F., Carusi, L.M., Cova, M., and Villari, N. 2006. Magnetic resonance diffusion-weighted imaging: extraneurological application. Radiol. Med. 111:392–420.

Colagrande, S., Pallotta, S., Vanzulli, A., Napoletano, M., and Villari, N. 2005. Il parametro "Diffusione" in Risonanza Magnetica: elementi di fisica, tecnica e semeiotica. Radiol. Med. 109:1–16.

Cova, M., Sqillaci, E., Stacul, F., Manenti, G., Gava, S., Simonetti, G., and Pozzi Mucelli, R. 2004. Diffusion-weighted MRI in the evaluation of renal lesions: preliminary results. Br. J. Radiol. 77:851–857.

Fukuda, Y., Ohashi, I., Hanafusa, K., Nakagawa, T., Ohtani, S., An-naka, Y., Hayashi, T., and Shibuya, H. 2000. Anisotropic diffusion in kidney: apparent diffusion coefficient measurements for clinical use. J. Magn. Reson. Imaging 11:156–160.

Hoehn Berlage, M., Eis, M., and Schmitz, B. 1999. Regional and directional anisotropy of apparent diffusion coefficient in rat brain. Magn. Reson. Med. 38:662–668.

Israel, G.M., and Bosniak, M.A. 2003. Follow-up CT studies for moderately complex cystic renal masses (Bosniak category IIF). Am. J. Roentgenol. 181:627–633.

Israel, G.M., Hindman, N., Hecht, E., and Krinsky, G. 2005. The use of opposite-phase chemical shift MRI in the diagnosis of renal angiomyolipomas. Am. J. Roentgenol. 184:1868–1872.

Jones, R.A., and Grattan-Smith, J.D. 2003. Age dependence of the renal apparent diffusion coefficient in children. *Pediatr. Radiol. 33*:850–854.

Laissy, J.P., Menegazzo, D., Dumont, E., Piekarski, J.D., Karila Cohen, P., Chillon, S., and Schouman-Claeys, E. 2000. Hemodynamic effect of iodinated high-viscosity contrast medium in the rat kidney: a diffusion weighted MRI feasibility study. *Invest. Radiol. 35*:647–665.

Le Bihan, D., Breton, E., Lallemand, D., Grenier, P., Cabanis, E., and Laval-Jeantet, M. 1986. MR imaging of intravoxel incoherent motions: application to diffusion and perfusion in neurologic disorders. *Radiology 161*:401–407.

Le Bihan, D., Mangin, J.-F., Poupon, C., Clark, C.A., Pappata, S., Molko, N., and Chabriat, H. 2001. Diffusion tensor imaging: concepts and applications. *J. Magn. Reson. Imaging 13*:534–546.

Linder, V., Lang, H., and Jacqmin, D. 2003. Pathology and genetics in renal cell cancer. *EAU Update Series 1*:197–208.

Mori, S., and Barker, P.B. 1999. Diffusion magnetic resonance imaging: its principles and application. *Anat. Rec. 257*:102–109.

Mosely, M.E., Cohen, Y., Kucharczyk, J., Mintorovitch, J., Asgari, H.S., Wendland, M.F., Tsuruda, J., and Norman, D. 1990a. Diffusion-weighted MR imaging of anisotropic water diffusion in cat central nervous system. *Radiology 176*:439–445.

Mosely, M.E., Cohen, Y., and Mintorovitch, J. 1990b. Early detection of regional cerebral ischemic injury in cats: evaluation of diffusion and T2-weighted MRI and spectroscopy. *Magn. Reson. Med. 14*:330–346.

Muller, M.F., Prasad, P.V., Bimmler, D., Kaiser, A., and Edelman, R.R. 1994a. Functional imaging of the kidney by means of measurement of the apparent diffusion coefficient. *Radiology 193*:711–715.

Muller, M.F., Prasad, P.V., Siewert, B., Nissenbaum, M.A., Raptopoulos, V., and Edelaman, R.R. 1994b. Abdominal diffusion mapping with use of a whole-body echo-planar system. *Radiology 190*:475–478.

Nanimoto, T., Yamashita, Y., Mitsuzaki, K., Nakayama, Y., Tang, Y., and Takahashi, M. 1999. Measurement of the apparent diffusion coefficient in diffuse renal disease by diffusion-weighted echo-planar MR imaging. *J. Magn. Reson. Imaging 9*:832–837.

Squillaci, E., Manenti, G., Cova, M., Di Roma, M., Miano, R., Calmieri, G., and Simonetti, G. 2004. Correlation of diffusion-weighted MR imaging with cellularity of renal tumors. *Anticancer Res. 24*:4175–4180.

Stejskal, E.O., and Tanner, J.E. 1965. Spin diffusion measurements: spin echoes in the presence of time-dependent field gradient. *J. Chem. Phys. 42*:288–292.

Storkel, S., Eble, J.N., Adlakha, K., Amin, M., Blute, M.L., Bostwick, D.G., Darson, M., Delahunt, B., and Iczkowskik, K. 1997. Classification of renal cell carcinoma. *Cancer 80*:987–989.

Thoeny, H.C., De Keyzer, F., Oyen, R.H., and Peeters, R.R. 2005. Diffusion-weighted MR imaging of kidneys in healthy volunteers and patients with parenchymal diseases: initial experience. *Radiology 235*:911–917.

Vexler, V.S., Roberts, T.P., and Rosenau, W. 1996. Early detection of acute tubular injury with diffusion-weighted magnetic resonance imaging in a rat model of myohemoglobinuric acute renal failure. *Ren. Fail. 18*:41–57.

Yoshimitsu, K., Hiroyuki, I., Tajima, T., Nishie, A., Asayama, Y., Hirakawa, M., Nakayama, T., Kakihara, D., and Honda, H. 2004. MR imaging of renal cell carcinoma: its role in determining cell type. *Radiat. Med. 22*:371–376.

Malignant Lymphoma: ^{18}F-Fluorodeoxyglucose-Positron Emission Tomography

Stefano Fanti, Roberto Franchi, and Paolo Castelluci

Introduction

The management of Hodgkin's disease (HD) and non-Hodgkin's Lymphoma (NHL) relies on the clinical staging of the disease, classification of histologic subtype, and identification of established prognostic factors. The contribution of diagnostic imaging has been related mainly to computed tomography (CT), especially for staging. Despite its important role, CT imaging has limitations, for example in determining the presence of disease within residual masses. Therefore, functional imaging techniques such as gallium-67 scan and, more recently, Fluorine-18 fluorodeoxyglucose (FDG) positron emission tomography (PET) may have an advantage over anatomical imaging. The potential of FDG as an agent for the detection of lymph node involvement in lymphoma using PET scanning was suggested more than 15 years ago by Wahl *et al.* (1990), and in the last decade a number a studies demonstrated the effectiveness of FDG-PET in patients affected by lymphoma. This method has been proven to be more accurate than other conventional imaging modalities and provides important information with direct impact on patient management (Hoskin, 2003).

The effectiveness of PET is due to its capability of identifying active disease. For example, after therapy completion,

FDG-PET affects patient management by differentiating patients with residual lymphoma (nonresponders or partial responders) from those without viable tumor (complete responders). Similarly, in cases of relapse, early identification of disease recurrence may influence the success rate of therapy by allowing earlier treatment. Several indications for FDG-PET have been suggested in patients with malignant lymphoma: a useful role has been established for staging, for evaluating early response to chemotherapy, and for assessing end response to therapy, especially in the presence of residual masses. Other suggested indications are evaluation before transplantation, radiation therapy and radioimmunotherapy planning, and during follow-up.

Principle and Methods

It is well known that malignant lymphoma demonstrates increased uptake of the glucose analog FDG. Therefore, the detection of active lymphoma by PET is based on the degree of FDG uptake. Although most lymphomas can be successfully imaged by FDG-PET, a few cases lacking FDG uptake have been reported. While 100% of HD, large B-cell lymphoma, follicular lymphoma, mantle cell lymphoma, and other less

---

Cancer Imaging: Instrumentation and Applications

485

frequent subtypes were demonstrated to be FDG-avid (Elstrom *et al.*, 2003), a significant number of false-negative PET studies were observed in marginal zone lymphoma, peripheral T-cell lymphoma, and cutaneous B-cell lymphoma. In these infrequent histologies, PET may therefore be less accurate. Positron emission tomography scanning in a lymphoma patient does not pose any particular problem as a method, requiring standard doses, uptake time, and duration of scanning. The use of dedicated hybrid PET-CT tomography may result in increased accuracy by reducing the number of false-positive studies. Nevertheless, the great majority of PET scans carried out in lymphoma patients can be adequately reported without the need for anatomical information given by PET-CT. Overall, the use of PET-CT in lymphoma patients can be reasonably considered useful but not mandatory.

Interpretation of PET scanning in lymphoma requires the identification of areas of increased FDG uptake in sites different from areas of known physiologic uptake. Potential sources of pitfalls are well recognized, including thymic hyperplasia (common in post-chemotherapy), diffuse bone marrow activity (after therapy), and inflammation, which can cause increased FDG uptake. Therefore, misinterpretation of images is possible because PET can demonstrate high radiotracer concentration unrelated to lymphoma, but the incidence of false-positive reports is acceptably low, inferior to 5% (Castellucci *et al.*, 2005).

Positron Emission Tomography and Staging

Correct staging of lymphoma is important for selecting the appropriate treatment. Diagnosis and staging of both HD and NHL depend to a large degree on imaging studies, including CT, MR, PET, and other modalities, as well as on history, physical examination, laboratory data, bone marrow biopsy, and tissue biopsies. Among imaging modalities, CT is definitely the most widely used in lymphoma patients, and its efficacy and effectiveness have been reported. Nevertheless, CT has a major limitation for staging, namely, the fact that recognition of nodal involvement depends almost entirely on the size of lymph nodes. Thus, CT has a limited accuracy in identifying disease in lymph nodes of normal size, as well as in excluding disease in non-malignant enlarged lymph nodes. Molecular imaging using PET may overcome the problem, and a number of published studies confirmed the usefulness of FDG-PET for staging malignant lymphoma (Kumar *et al.*, 2004).

The different nature of information provided by CT and PET is related with different performances of these imaging methods. However, in almost all studies, most lesions will remain without tissue verification for obvious ethical and practical reasons; therefore, true sensitivity, specificity, and accuracy cannot be assessed. Most reported studies directly compare the results of CT with PET and describe concordance of findings, thus allowing an indirect assessment of accuracy. Overall, the sensitivity of PET is about 15% higher than that of CT, whereas the specificity is the same for both imaging modalities (Schiepers *et al.*, 2003).

Regarding different anatomic regions, PET has shown a higher sensitivity in the neck and thorax (> 90%) and lower in the infradiaphragmatic lesions (~ 80%), with peripheral disease involvement diagnosed with a sensitivity of approximately 85%. Some body parts, such as the central nervous system and urinary system, are not properly evaluable by FDG-PET, but the involvement of these organs with lymphoma is rare. Several investigators have reported a high accuracy of PET for determining bone marrow involvement in lymphoma patients, but it cannot replace bone marrow biopsy. The diffusion of the disease to the spleen can also be accurately documented by PET (Rini *et al.*, 2003).

A number of publications have raised the relevant question of what impact FDG-PET has on the staging of malignant lymphoma. Whether or not PET staging may lead to changes in therapy approach or patient management is very important (Fig. 1). Data from the literature indicate that change of stage attributable to PET findings is observed in 20 to 40% of patients, with a relevant variability due to differences in study design. For example, one of the first trials to evaluate the impact of PET on initial staging and management of lymphoma compared 129 sites of disease in 45 patients (Delbeke *et al.*, 2002). This system correctly modified staging in 16% of cases, leading to a change of therapy in 13%. A recent study prospectively evaluated 88 patients with Hodgkin's disease at presentation (Naumann *et al.*, 2004): 18 patients (20%) had the stage changed by PET, and in 16 cases (18%) management of the disease would have been changed. Positron emission tomography more frequently upstages than downstages disease, but this modification of staging does not necessarily imply a modification in treatment strategy. Available data on therapy modification by PET indicate that treatment was changed in 5 to 40% of all patients, with most consisting series suggesting a determinant impact of PET on 20% of cases.

Positron Emission Tomography and Early Response to Therapy

Lymphomas are a heterogeneous group of diseases that differ in clinical behavior, response to therapy, and final outcome. In patients with curable subtypes of lymphoma, it is critical to assess the response to treatment. Several studies have suggested that patients with rapid response to induction therapy are more likely to have a better and more durable response. Therefore, it is important to distinguish between responders to standard approaches and nonresponders who may benefit from an early change to an alternative treatment.

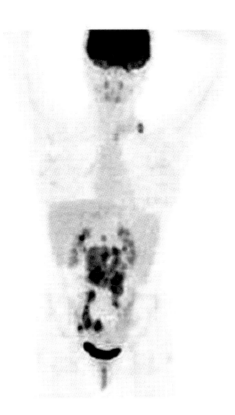

Figure 1   Non-Hodgkin's Lymphoma at presentation. PET confirms abdominal involvement, already documented at CT but demonstrated also supradiaphragmatic disease, at retroclavear node level. This finding upstaged patients from stage II to stage III and may lead to a change in therapy.

The FDG-PET method has the capability of providing information about the metabolic behavior of the disease independent of morphological criteria, and thus seems to be the ideal tool for the early evaluation of treatment response (Spaepen *et al.*, 2001).

Several investigators have documented the relationship between early changes in FDG metabolism and final response to chemotherapy: in both HD and NHL, persistent FDG uptake was a strong predictor of treatment failure. Furthermore, interim PET showed a high predictive value for identifying relapse, with an early negative PET resulting in prolonged complete remission (2-year progression-free survival (PFS) rate of 60–80%), whereas the relapse rate in early positive PET was 80–100%. The capability of the PET scan to predict response to treatment was demonstrated as early as after the first cycle of therapy (Kostakoglu *et al.*, 2001) in both HD and NHL, but most of the studies were carried out after two to four cycles. The high prognostic value of early PET scan suggests the potential use of this method for early assessing the response to treatment. Efforts are directed toward improving the outcome of patients who do not achieve a complete remission with aggressive therapy,

and the clinical challenge is to incorporate the PET information into patient management. At present, several clinical trials are investigating this issue.

Post-Therapy Positron Emission Tomography

Review of the literature reveals that the majority of studies have evaluated the ability of FDG-PET to accurately monitor response to therapy after completion. The response to treatment is assessed by clinical, imaging, and histopathologic criteria. The imaging modality most commonly used for this purpose has long been CT. A decrease in the size of lymphomatous mass is considered a response to treatment, but the decrease in size may take a long time to become evident on CT, or the decrease may be partial. Furthermore, the evaluation of residual masses on CT imaging is a major problem in a number of patients with malignant lymphoma. The residual masses are present in the majority of patients treated for HD and in about half of those treated for NHL; most masses are constituted by fibrotic and necrotic tissue, and only a small percentage contain residual disease. Anatomic imaging methods, including CT and MR, cannot reliably differentiate active disease from fibrosis and necrosis, and thus functional imaging (such as gallium-67 scintigraphy) has been proposed. Gallium-67 scintigraphy, however, is hampered by limited resolution and nonspecific uptake in bowel and benign lesions, and has progressively been replaced by FDG-PET.

A number of studies have demonstrated the effectiveness of PET in the assessment of treatment response. Progression-free survival rates at 2 years for patients with positive PET findings at therapy completion range from 0 to 5%, indicating a very high positive-predictive value (Kumar *et al.*, 2004). In PET negative patients, the PFS rate was 80 to 95%, with a good but not absolute negative-predictive value. In other words, a negative post-treatment PET scan has a good prognostic value but cannot rule out relapse; however, in predicting disease-free survival PET showed better accuracy than CT.

FDG uptake is strongly suggestive of a residual disease, but is not definitely specific for tumoral tissue. In particular, when abnormal FDG uptake is observed outside the initially involved sites, other causes and especially inflammation have to be excluded. Therefore, it is always indicated to correlate PET findings with clinical data, other imaging modalities, and, if necessary, a biopsy. On the other hand, a negative FDG-PET cannot exclude minimal residual disease, possibly leading to relapse. Jerusalem *et al.* (2005), in a recent review of 17 studies, were able to calculate an overall sensitivity of 79%, a specificity of 94%, a positive-predictive value of 82%, a negative-predictive value of 93%, and an accuracy of 91%.

The importance of accurate identification of insufficient treatment response is due to the characteristics of lymphoma, which, in contrast to many solid tumors, is highly sensitive to several therapeutic agents. Prediction of disease control has a direct influence on the choice of treatment modalities; such prediction is especially important because maximizing disease remission and minimizing toxicity are key management goals. Furthermore, an increasing number of treatment modalities are available for lymphoma patients, including chemotherapy, radiotherapy, immunotherapy, immunoradiotherapy, and stem-cell transplantation, offering an effective possibility of long-term remission even in patients who relapse after first-line therapy. At present, the PET scan carried out at the end of treatment plays a pivotal role in accurate assessment of response and, therefore, in patient management. A definitely positive PET study is highly suggestive for persistent disease, thus prompting further aggressive treatment (Fig. 2). On the other hand, an equivocal PET scan or a faintly positive PET, especially if located in a site different from presentation, should be assessed with caution and eventually confirmed with biopsy or strict follow-up.

Positron Emission Tomography before Transplantation

High-dose chemotherapy with autologous stem-cell transplantation (ASCT) has been shown to be an effective therapeutic option in patients who have relapsed from lymphoma, and during recent years, ASCT has become a front-line therapy in patients with high-risk disease. Prognostic factors allowing prediction of the final outcome at the time of transplantation would be helpful, and FDG-PET has been

suggested as a potential tool to predict early relapse (Filmont *et al.*, 2003). Recent data indicate that FDG-PET imaging performed before transplantation has a high predictive value: patients with a negative PET showed a good overall survival rate, and most remained in complete remission (65–75%). PET is usually carried out after salvation chemotherapy and before ASTC, and all data confirm the poor outcome of patients with a positive PET: relapse rates are in the range of 90 to 100% within one year. The impressive positive-predictive value of the FDG-PET scan before ASCT will probably translate into changes in patient management. In fact, the risk of treatment failure is so high in the presence of positive PET that these patients will be candidates for alternative therapy.

Positron Emission Tomography and Radiotherapy and Radioimmunotherapy

While PET is gaining a relevant role for radiotherapy planning in different solid tumors, presently the potential use of FDG-PET data to determine the volumes for radiation therapy in lymphoma patients has not been assessed. Radioimmunotherapy (RIT) is a promising approach for the treatment of NHL. The antitumor mechanisms of RIT are independent of those of most chemotherapeutic agents, and the role of RIT is rapidly growing. Initial reports are investigating the feasibility of FDG-PET in monitoring response to RIT, and reports show that PET data after RIT correlated well with the ultimate response of NHL to RIT. For both radiotherapy planning and response assessment after radioimmunotherapy, further studies are warranted before FDG-PET can be suggested for routine use.

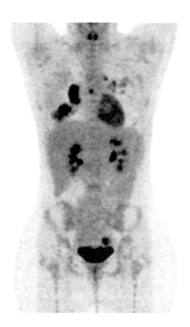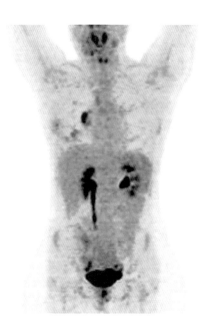

Figure 2 Non-Hodgkin's Lymphoma at presentation (left) and after completion of chemotherapy. PET indicates bilateral thoracic involvement, with good response to therapy but persistence of residual disease, thus requiring further treatment.

Positron Emission Tomography and Relapse

Malignant lymphomas are highly responsive to therapy; nevertheless, relapse occurs in approximately 20 to 30% of HD patients and up to 50% of NHL patients, usually in the first years after treatment. Early diagnosis of disease recurrence is important for successful treatment, before lymphoma spreads extensively. Relapse is usually identified as a result of the investigation of symptoms rather than by routine screening of asymptomatic patients, although regular radiological studies may be useful. A few studies have investigated the value of FDG-PET for the detection of preclinical relapse in the follow-up of patients with lymphoma. Available data indicate that FDG-PET can be positive several months before histological confirmation of an asymptomatic relapse. On the other hand, a number of false-positive cases have been reported (Jerusalem *et al.*, 2003). It is clear that PET is more sensitive than routine visits, laboratory tests, and radiological studies, but FDG is not an absolute tumor-specific tracer, and thus histological or other evidence of disease recurrence should be obtained before the start of salvage therapy. Positron emission tomography plays a significant role in the follow-up of lymphoma patients, and its use has been suggested in a proposed algorithm for appropriate use of FDG-PET, taking into account that even the value of CT has not yet been evaluated in routine follow-up after treatment for lymphoma. The current strategy recommends follow-up PET scans for several years in patients at high risk of relapse, namely, NHL and HD stage III and IV.

In conclusion, in the field of malignant lymphomas FDG-PET has gained widespread acceptance as a fundamental clinical tool, supported by a robust literature. Several indications can be considered as definitely established:

1. **Staging**: PET is useful and may detect sites of disease missed by conventional imaging techniques. PET data, however, will not necessarily modify patient management; therefore, PET is complementary to CT and is recommended only in selected cases or when a baseline scan is necessary for further evaluation.

2. **Early therapy monitoring**: PET results correlate with patient outcome and have a strong prognostic value but at present no clinical application. Data regarding the use of early PET for modifying therapy before completion are expected very soon.

3. **End of treatment evaluation**: PET is the most useful noninvasive imaging modality for response assessment; therefore, it is mandatory in almost all cases of lymphoma at the end of treatment.

4. **Follow-up and relapse**: In case of clinical or CT suspect of relapse, PET is recommended for appropriate re-staging.

The use of PET for routine follow-up of lymphoma patients is debatable and may be suggested in high-risk patients.

References

Castellucci, P., Zinzani, P., Pourdehnad, M., Alinari, L., Nanni, C., Farsad, M., Battista, G., Tani, M., Stefoni, V., Canini, R., Monetti, N., Ribello, D., Alavi, A., Franchi, R., and Fanti, S. 2005. 18F-FDG-PET in malignant lymphoma: significance of positive findings. *Eur. J. Nucl. Med. Mol. Imag.* 32:749–756.

Delbeke, D., Martin, W.H., Morgan, D.S., Kinney, M.C., Feurer, I., Kovalsky, E., Arrowsmith, T., and Greer, J.P. 2002. 2-deoxy-2-(F-18) fluoro-D-glucose imaging with positron emission tomography for initial staging of Hodgkin's disease and lymphoma. *Mol. Imag. Biol.* 4:104–114.

Elstrom, R., Guan, L., Baker, G., Nakhoda, K., Vergilio, J.A., Zhuang, H., Pitsilos, S., Bagg, A., Downs, L., Mehrotra, A., Kim, S., Alavi, A., and Schuster, S.J. 2003. Utility of FDG-PET scanning in lymphoma by WHO classification. *Blood 15*:101:3875–3876.

Filmont, J.E., Czernin, Y., Yap, C., Silverman, D.H., Quon, A., Phelps, M.E., and Emmanoulides, C. 2003. Value of F-18 fluorodeoxyglucose positron emission tomography for predicting the clinical outcome of patients with aggressive lymphoma prior to and after autologous stem-cell transplantation. *Chest 124*:608–613.

Hoskin, P.J. 2003. PET in lymphoma: what are the oncologist's needs? *Eur. J. Nucl. Med. Mol. Imag. 30*:S37–S41.

Jerusalem, G., Hustinx, R., Beguin, Y., and Fillet, G. 2005. Evaluation of therapy for lymphoma. *Semin. Nucl. Med. 35*:186–196.

Jerusalem, G., Beguin, Y., Fassotte, M.F., Belhocine, T., Hustinx, R., Rigo, P., and Fillet, G. 2003. Early detection of relapse by whole-body positron emission tomography in the follow-up of patients with Hodgkin's disease. *Ann. Oncol. 14*:123–130.

Kostakoglu, L., Coleman, M., Leonard, J.P., Kuji, I., Zoe, H., and Goldsmith, S.J. 2002. PET predicts prognosis after 1 cycle of chemotherapy in aggressive lymphoma and Hodgkin's disease. *J. Nucl. Med. 43*:1018–1027.

Kumar, R., Maillard, I., Schuster, S.J., and Alavi, A. 2004. Utility of fluorodeoxyglucose-PET imaging in the management of patients with Hodgkin's and non-Hodgkin's Lymphomas. *Radiol. Clin. North Amer. 42*:1083–1100.

Naumann, R., Beuthien-Baumann, B., Reiss, A., Schultze, H., Hanel, A., Bredow, J., Kuhnel, G., Kropp, J., Hanel, M., Laniado, M., Kotzerke, J., and Ehningen, G. 2004. Substantial impact of FDG-PET imaging on the therapy decision in patients with early-stage Hodgkin's Lymphoma. *Br. J. Cancer. 90*:620–625.

Rini, J.N., Leonidas, J.C., Tomas, M.B., and Palestro, C.J. 2003. 18F-FDG PET versus CT for evaluating the spleen during initial staging of lymphoma. *J. Nucl. Med. 14*:1072–1074.

Schiepers, C., Filmont, J.E., and Czernin, J. 2003. PET for staging of Hodgkin's disease and non-Hodgkin's Lymphoma. *Eur. J. Nucl. Med. Mol. Imag. 30*:S82–S88.

Spaepen, K., Stroobants, S., Dupont, P., Thomas, J., Vandeberghe, P., Balzarini, J., DeWolf-Peeters, C., Mortelmans, L., and Verhoef, G. 2001. Can positron emission tomography with (18F)-fluorodeoxyglucose after first-line treatment distinguish Hodgkin's disease patients who need additional therapy from others in whom additional therapy would mean avoidable toxicity? *Br. J. Haematol. 115*:272–278.

Wahl, R.L., Kaminski, M.S., Ethier, S.P., and Hutchins, G.D. 1990. The potential of 2-deoxy-2(18F)fluoro-D-glucose (FDG) for the detection of tumor involvement in lymph nodes. *J. Nucl. Med. 31*: Nov; 1831–1835.

28

Malignant Melanoma: Positron Emission Tomography

Paul McQuade

Introduction

Malignant melanoma are tumors derived from melanocyte cells which are present within the epidermis layer of the skin. Their function is to produce melanin, the pigment that gives skin its color. As a consequence, melanoma are often black or brown in appearance. It is one of the most aggressive forms of skin cancer, and can be broken down into four main subtypes (Swetter *et al.*, 2005). The most common is superficial spreading melanoma (SSM), which accounts for around 70% of all diagnosed cases and typically arises from a preexisting pigmented benign lesion. Nodular melanoma (NM) is the next most common subtype and is typically found on the trunk, head, or neck. Unlike SSM, NM lesions can form from normal skin with no history of benign lesions. Patients diagnosed with NM typically have a lower cure rate than those diagnosed with SSM, as the lesions tend to invade the body more rapidly, increasing the risk of metastatic sites. Of the two remaining main subtypes, lentigo maligna melanoma (LMM) is most common in older patients with a history of sun overexposure, while acral lentiginous melanoma (ALM) is most commonly found in dark-skinned populations, occurring primarily on the palms of the hands or soles of the feet.

The number of new cases of melanoma reported in the United States has been increasing steadily for decades. However, the rate of increase for new cases has slowed in recent years. Overall, the American Cancer Society estimated that in 2006 there would be 62,190 new cases of melanoma in the United States, with 7910 deaths. Melanoma is also a disease that affects ethnicities to a significantly different extent, with whites being 10 times more likely to develop lesions than blacks. However, blacks diagnosed with melanoma are more frequently diagnosed with an advanced disease state and as a consequence show dramatically lower long-term survival rates. One reason for this is that the most common type of melanoma found in dark skinned populations (ALM) is one of the most aggressive forms of melanoma (Rahman and Taylor, 2001).

Early detection of melanoma is essential unless the primary tumor is excised, typically through surgery, as patient prognosis is poor (Eberle and Froidevaux, 2003). This can be exemplified when the 5-year survival rate of 96% for localized melanoma is compared to the 14% seen when distal metastasis are found. Since 1998, however, the number of deaths in white males diagnosed with melanoma has decreased, while in white females a decrease in the mortality rate has been observed since 1988 (Edwards *et al.*, 2005). This improvement in patient prognosis is due to earlier detection of both primary and secondary tumor sites in part due to Positron Emission Tomography (PET) imaging and improved treatment protocols.

The physiological location of PET radionuclides can be determined due to the formation of two 511 keV gamma rays produced from the annihilation reaction between a positron emitted from the nucleus of a PET radioisotope and an electron. These gamma rays are emitted at 180° to each other and can then be detected externally using a PET camera. Several reviews have been published that give a more detailed explanation of this process (Tai and Laforest, 2005; Talbot *et al.*, 2003). For PET imaging to be successful, the characteristics of the pharmaceutical and radionuclide used must be compatible to allow suitable time for significant localization in target tissue along with clearance from the circulation and normal tissue, generating suitable contrast between target and non-target tissue.

Positron Emission Tracers

2-Deoxy-2-^{18}F-Fluorodeoxyglucose

At present the compound most commonly used for diagnosing and staging of cancer via PET is 2-deoxy-2-^{18}F-fluorodeoxyglucose (FDG). Tumor uptake of FDG is not due to binding to any specific antigen present on the cell surface or newly formed vasculature, but rather to the fact that cancerous cells are metabolically more active than surrounding tissue. Accumulation of FDG results from a trapping mechanism, where uptake is initiated by transport into tumor cells by means of the glucose transporter protein (GLUT) and, once there, it is phosphorylated by hexokinase (HK) to FDG-6-phosphate. Until this point FDG behaves similarly to glucose; however, unlike glucose-6-phosphate, FDG-6-phosphate cannot be metabolized further and becomes trapped within the cell (Kumar and Alavi, 2005). Although the mechanism of FDG uptake and retention is known, the correlation between GLUT expression, HK activity, and the levels of FDG uptake is still unclear. The reason for this uncertainty is that early work showed that FDG uptake in tumor cells was directly correlated with both GLUT expression and HK activity (Haberkorn *et al.*, 1994). However, conflicting reports have since indicated that FDG uptake is correlated with only HK activity (Burt *et al.*, 2001) or GLUT expression levels (Brown *et al.*, 2002). Recently, work in both human and murine melanoma cell lines showed that there was no correlation between GLUT expression and FDG uptake. Instead, it is the combination of cell viability, proliferation rate, and HK activity that determined FDG uptake (Yamada *et al.*, 2005).

The progression of melanoma can be broken down into four stages, with patient prognosis deteriorating as the stages progress (Kumar and Alavi, 2005). The accuracy of FDG in locating melanoma lesions is strongly dependent on the disease stage at the time of diagnosis. Stage I is diagnosed if the lesion is ulcerated and < 1.0 mm thick or below 2 mm if no ulceration is observed. Progression to stage II occurs if the ulcerated lesions are over 1 mm in thickness or 2 mm

if no ulceration is present. At stage III the primary tumor has metastasized to regional lymph nodes; stage IV is diagnosed upon conformation of distal metastases. For patients with stage I–II primary melanoma tumors, the use of FDG is unwarranted as the size of these lesions is smaller than the resolution obtained with current clinical PET scanners (~ 5 mm). Also, imaging is unwarranted as lesions can be detected by physical examination and treated by removal of diseased tissue.

A similar argument could also be applied to stage III melanoma patients containing micrometastases. This was illustrated when FDG and PET imaging was used in 48 patients with confirmed stage I and II primary malignant melanoma to detect any regional lymph node metastases present. These results were then compared to sentinel lymph node biopsy (SNB), the accepted reference standard for detecting such metastases (Fink *et al.*, 2004). Of the 48 patients enrolled, the breakdown in melanoma subtypes was 52% NM, 13% ALM, 29% SSM, and 6% LMM. In total, 8 patients (16.7%) were found to have a positive SNB; with an average metastasis size of 3.35 mm. FDG detected lymph node metastases in only 1 patient, also detected by SNB, meaning that FDG demonstrated a sensitivity of 13% and a specificity of 100%. This metastasis was detected because of its 11 mm size.

In an analogous study containing 38 patients, 56 lymph node basins containing 647 lymph nodes were removed and analyzed histologically. Prior to the surgical removal, FDG had been administered and PET images obtained (Crippa *et al.*, 2000). Examination of the basins showed the presence of metastatic tumor sites in 114 of the lymph nodes (17.6%), with sizes ranging from 0.3 to 45 mm. Analysis of the PET images showed that positive identification could be broken down in relation to the size of the metastases, with 100% of metastases > 10 mm and 83% of the metastases between 6 and 10 mm detected. This high sensitivity was dramatically reduced with lesions < 5 mm in size, with only 23% being detected. These findings were repeated in numerous other studies that found that FDG is insensitive in determining regional lymph node metastases when compared to sentinel node biopsy (Libberecht *et al.*, 2005; Wagner *et al.*, 2005).

In an analytical study, data obtained from 13 institutions were combined to obtain a total of 17,600 patients in which a complete set of clinical, pathologic, and follow-up data were available (Balch *et al.*, 2001). In total, 604 patients (3.4%) were found to have clinically detectable regional lymph node metastasis at the time of their first surgery, while 1158 patients (6.6%) were found to have distant metastases. As discussed, FDG has its limitations detecting regional lymph node lesions. SNB however gives no direct information on possible distant metastases. It is therefore in the detection of these metastases that FDG finds its optimum use. But again, the size of these lesions must be greater than 4–5 mm in diameter for detection.

Another question that must be addressed is how PET imaging compares to more conventional imaging techniques such as CT or MRI. In one study, a review was performed on 104 patients with primary or recurrent melanoma and the use of PET or whole-body CT imaging in the detection of metastatic lesions (Swetter *et al.*, 2002). In total, 157 PET and 70 CT images were analyzed, with an average patient follow-up of 24 months. Of the 104 patients enrolled, each received at least one PET scan that detected 167 of the 199 metastatic sites (84% sensitivity), with a 97% specificity (3 false positives). Of these false positives, 2 were located in bone, with the final one in the liver, and were identified as such either histologically or by other imaging modalities. In contrast, CT images obtained in 54 patients that had been previously analyzed by PET detected only 77 of 133 metastatic sites (58% sensitivity), with 70% specificity (9 false positives). As before, false positives were confirmed either by other imaging modalities or histologically. The sensitivity with CT could be increased to ~ 70% if areas not routinely evaluated were excluded. This, however, caused no change in specificity. In further analysis, 66 consecutive PET/CT scans were performed on 53 of the original 104 patients. In this cohort, 30 patients had a combined total of 132 metastases, with 107 (81%) and 75 (57%) detected by PET and CT, respectively. The data presented in this study showed that PET outperformed CT in the detection of metastatic sites in all regions. Exceptions were the brain in which both methods had no selectivity and the kidneys/adrenal with 73% and 82% of sites being detected by PET and CT, respectively. To detect brain metastases, MR imaging was performed on 43 patients. A total of 7 metastases in 3 individuals were discovered, representing both a 100% selectivity and sensitivity. FDG could not detect these lesions because of the high metabolic rate found in the brain, resulting in low tumor-to-background ratios.

In a further comparative study, FDG was compared against CT and MR imaging in 18 patients with confirmed stage IV metastatic melanoma (Finkelstein *et al.*, 2004). The location of the metastatic tumor sites varied, but patients with brain metastases were excluded. Analysis of PET images generated similar results to those obtained via CT/MRI, with each having sensitivities of 79% and 76% respectively, the specificity of both was identical at 87%. In a patient-by-patient analysis, it was found that PET had a higher accuracy in detecting lesions in 3 patients (16.7%), was similar in 10 (55.6%), and less accurate in 5 (27.8%) when compared to CT/MRI. Although the predictive nature of these images was acceptable, it was believed that further improvements could be made. In an attempt to do so, images obtained from PET were co-registered with those obtained by CT/MRI and analyzed for lesion sites. This was done independently in all 18 patients. By analyzing the co-registered images, identification of positive tumor sites improved, demonstrating the advantages of combining PET with an imaging modality that provides anatomical information.

In a recent study, PET/CT was used in the staging of melanoma in 250 patients (Reinhardt *et al.*, 2006). In total, 243

(97.2%) were staged correctly by PET/CT, compared to only 232 patients (92.8%) by PET and 197 patients (78.8%) by CT. If the patient population is broken down further and only 78 patients with regional metastases are examined, PET/CT gave a more accurate analysis with no overstaging and only 4 occurrences of understaging. In contrast, PET alone caused the overstaging in 4 patients and the understaging of 6. Analysis of CT images was even more problematic, with 22 patients overstaged and 12 understaged. When this analysis was done on the 84 patients with distal metastatic sites, it was found that PET/CT yielded similar results, with 4 patients overstaged and 1 understaged. By way of comparison, analysis of PET images caused the overstaging of 8 patients and the understaging of an additional 9. Again CT was more inaccurate with 20 and 21 patients over- and understaged, respectively. Further analysis showed that of the 670 metastases identified, PET/CT detected 661 (98.7%), significantly higher than either PET (595, 88.8%) or CT (467, 69.7%).

As described earlier, the use of FDG and PET imaging compares very favorably with other imaging techniques in regards to disease staging and metastatic lesion detection. As a result, the use of FDG can affect treatment protocols for patients with varying stages of melanoma. An excellent example is in the previously described study, where the use of PET/CT resulted in a change of treatment in 121 of the 250 patients (48.4%) (Reinhardt *et al.*, 2006). In fact, PET does not have to be coupled to a secondary imaging modality for these changes in treatment therapies to occur. Several studies have reported that imaging only with PET via FDG has led to changes in planned treatment regiments of between 15% and 40% of patients (Harris *et al.*, 2005; Mijnhout *et al.*, 2002; Tyler *et al.*, 2000).

3'-^{18}F-Fluoro-3'-Deoxy-L-Fluorothymidine

A major disadvantage with FDG is that, although most melanoma cells have high glucose utilization as shown by *in vitro* experiments (Wahl *et al.*, 1991), uptake is non-specific. Therefore, inflammation and infection, which also have an increased metabolic rate when compared to normal cells will also show elevated FDG uptake, resulting in false positives (Zhuang *et al.*, 2003). Another hindrance to the use of FDG is that substantial reductions in tumor uptake can result in patients with elevated glucose blood levels as seen in hyperglycemia (Dave *et al.*, 2002). In an attempt to address these issues, PET tracers such as 3'-^{18}F-fluoro-3'-deoxy-L-fluorothymidine (FLT), a cell proliferation tracer, have been evaluated as possible oncological PET ligands (Been *et al.*, 2004). It functions by being taken up by cells either by passive diffusion or direct transport by Na$^+$-dependent carriers. Once in a cell, it is phosphorylated by the enzyme thymidine kinase 1 (TK$_1$), which leads to intracellular trapping. The amount of TK$_1$ present is directly related to the level of proliferation, with TK$_1$ levels increasing when a cell is actively proliferating. Thus, the level of trapped FLT is directly related to TK$_1$

and a measure of cell proliferation. As a consequence, FLT would not have the same disadvantages that are associated with FDG, with the added advantage of being able to detect brain metastases due to the low proliferation rates found in normal brain cells.

In an initial clinical study, 10 patients with clinically confirmed stage III melanoma were imaged with FLT to test its accuracy in correctly staging melanoma and to see if it could be used to detect previously undetected lesion sites (Cobben *et al.*, 2003). The study reported that the sensitivity for detecting lymph node metastatic disease was 88%, with a specificity of 60% due to the three true-negative and two false-positive results obtained. The detection limit for lesions was ∼ 6 mm, which is in the range typically observed for FDG and is a consequence of the resolution of current PET cameras. In addition, use of FLT resulted in 11 additional lesions being detected and 2 patients having their disease state upstaged. The results indicated that the use of FLT in this study is at least comparable to results obtained with FDG in similar patient populations, and that further work is required to gauge whether FLT is a suitable alternative to FDG in the staging of metastatic melanoma.

Receptor-Specific PET Tracers

Although tracers such as FDG and FLT can be used to detect metastatic melanoma lesions, their mode of uptake is nonspecific. As a consequence, both tracers can exhibit elevated uptake in nontarget tissue, resulting in poor signal-to-background ratios. There is therefore a need for agents that could specifically target cell-surface receptors present on melanoma cells, or the newly formed vasculature of a growing tumor.

Alpha vs. Beta 3 Integrin

One moiety receiving particular interest is the integrin *alpha vs. beta 3* ($\alpha_v\beta_3$). It is found on endothelial cells lining newly formed blood vessels at a higher density than mature ones, with studies showing that there may be as many as 500,000 $\alpha_v\beta_3$ receptors per cell in cultured human umbilical vein endothelial cells (HUVEC) (Byzova *et al.*, 1998). The formation of new vasculature (angiogenesis) is essential for the expansion of tumors beyond a few cubic millimeters (Folkman, 1971), thus $\alpha_v\beta_3$ would be a good indicator for expanding tumors. The first ligand found to bind to $\alpha_v\beta_3$ was vitronectin, but since this discovery other ligands, including fibrinogen and von Willebrand factor, have also been found to bind (McQuade and Knight, 2003). The amino acid sequence responsible for $\alpha_v\beta_3$ binding is Arg-Gly-Asp (RGD), which is also responsible for binding to other integrins, including $\alpha_3\beta_1$, $\alpha_5\beta_1$, and $\alpha_{IIb}\beta_3$ (McQuade and Knight, 2003). Use of RGD containing ligands has been shown to

prevent angiogenesis by blocking $\alpha_v\beta_3$ receptors, resulting in apoptosis of the actively proliferating vascular cells but not mature vascular cells, indicating the selectivity of this targeting approach (Brooks *et al.*, 1994).

In addition to being overexpressed in newly formed vasculature, $\alpha_v\beta_3$ and other integrins including $\alpha_1\beta_1$, $\alpha_3\beta_1$, and $\alpha_5\beta_1$ are also found on the surface of certain cancer cells, including melanoma, glioblastoma, and osteosarcoma (Johnson, 1999). With melanoma cells, expression of $\alpha_v\beta_3$ is closely associated with tumor progression and subsequent metastases development (Nip and Brodt, 1995). The reason for this is that expression of β_3 integrins is restricted to cells in the vertical growth phase (Albelda *et al.*, 1990), which is directly related to metastatic capacity making $\alpha_v\beta_3$ a good indicator for patient prognosis (Hieken *et al.*, 1999).

Numerous ligands have been developed to target $\alpha_v\beta_3$, ranging from small-molecular-weight compounds to monoclonal antibodies. Some of the most commonly examined ligands are cyclized peptides containing the RGD sequence, whose advantage is the rapid uptake coupled with the relatively fast clearance. This enables radiolabeling with short-lived radioisotopes such as ^{18}F via prosthetic groups, including *N*-succinimidyl 4-[^{18}F]fluorobenzoate. In one study the mono-, di-, and tetrameric RGD peptides were fluorinated, with studies carried out on nude mice implanted subcutaneously with both M21 (high $\alpha_v\beta_3$ expression) and M21-L (low $\alpha_v\beta_3$ expression) human melanomas (Poethko *et al.*, 2004). *In vitro* binding assays showed that the $\alpha_v\beta_3$ IC_{50} values for the monomer, dimer, and tetramer were 20 nM, 3 nM, and 0.2 nM, respectively, with biodistribution data at 120 min showing that both the dimer and tetramer had substantially higher uptake in the $\alpha_v\beta_3$ positive tumor than the monomer. All three species, however, had significantly higher uptake in the $\alpha_v\beta_3$ positive tumor as compared to the $\alpha_v\beta_3$ negative tumor. MicroPET images obtained with the tetramer showed that the M21 tumor was clearly visible after 90 min, as was the M21-L tumor, though considerably less intense. Uptake in both tumors could be blocked by co-infusion of 360 μg of the $\alpha_v\beta_3$-specific peptide c(RGDfV), demonstrating tumor specificity. Specific uptake in the M21-L xenograft is a result of binding to the low levels of $\alpha_v\beta_3$ present on the cell surface along with $\alpha_v\beta_3$ integrins present in the immature tumor vasculature.

Although clearance of these cyclized RGD containing peptides is rapid, the pharmacokinetics was further improved upon when the $\alpha_v\beta_3$ selective peptide c(RGDfK) had a sugar conjugated at the lysine position (Haubner *et al.*, 2001). The radiolabeled product, [^{18}F]Galacto-c(RGDfK), had a 5 nM affinity for $\alpha_v\beta_3$. The *in vivo* characteristics of this tracer were analyzed on nude mice bearing either M21 or M21-L human melanoma xenografts. In the study, accumulation in the M21 xenograft was two-fold higher than seen for M21-L after only 10 min, increasing to four-fold by 60 min. Tumor uptake could also be blocked by co-infusion of excess $\alpha_v\beta_3$-specific peptide. MicroPET images showed that the M21 xenograft was clearly visible after 90 min, with a tumor-to-background ratio of 5.7. By contrast, uptake in the M21-L xenograft was only 1.2 times higher than background tissue.

[^{18}F]Galacto-c(RGDfK) was investigated further in a clinical setting (Beer *et al.*, 2005). In total, 19 patients were enrolled, 7 of whom had malignant melanoma, the remainder having sarcomas (10) or osseous metastases (2). As predicted from animal experiments, the tracer showed rapid clearance from the blood pool, with renal excretion the major mode of clearance. Maximum tumor uptake occurred early and remained consistent throughout the course of the experiment. In total, lesions were positively identified in 17 patients (89.4%), with 23 of 29 known lesions detected (79.3%). As tumor uptake remained constant, tumor-to-background ratios improved over time, with tumor-to-blood and tumor-to-muscle ratios of 3.3 ± 2.2 and 7.7 ± 5.4 achieved at 72 min, respectively. However, large variations in tumor uptake were observed, this being indicative of the wide range of $\alpha_v\beta_3$ expression levels seen in naturally occurring tumors.

SPECT isotopes have been used to image $\alpha_v\beta_3$ integrin expressing tumors. For example, ^{99m}Tc was used to label the linear peptide RGDSCRGDSY, which was then used in 14 patients diagnosed with malignant melanomas (Sivolapenko *et al.*, 1998). The overall sensitivity of this labeled peptide in detecting known lymph node metastases was 77.3%, which rose to 90% for lesions greater than 2 cm. ^{111}In has also been used to label the cyclic peptides c(KRGDf) and c(ERGDf), with the radiolabeled peptides used to image melanoma xenografts implanted in mice (Wang *et al.*, 2005).

Melanocortin-1 Receptors

$\alpha_v\beta_3$ is not the only receptor that has been found to be overexpressed on melanoma cells. Melanocortin-1 receptors (MC1R), expressed on the surface of melanocytes, are also overexpressed on melanoma cells (Froidevaux *et al.*, 2004). α-Melanotropin-stimulating hormone (α-MSH) has been found to bind avidly to MC1R, with structure-bioactivity studies of α-MSH showing that the amino acid sequence His-Phe-Arg-Trp (HFRW) is sufficient for receptor recognition (Cornish *et al.*, 2003). Peptide analogs containing this core sequence have been prepared, with some analogs possessing subnanomolar affinities for MC1R while being internalized rapidly upon binding (Cheng *et al.*, 2004).

One such peptide examined was the cyclic species DOTA-[Re-Cys^{3,4,10}, Phe^7, Arg^{11}]α-MSH$_{3-13}$ [DOTA-ReCCMSH (Arg^{11})], which in one study was labeled with both ^{64}Cu and ^{86}Y, and the pharmacokinetics investigated in mice implanted subcutaneously with B16-F1 murine melanoma xenografts (McQuade *et al.*, 2005). For both tracers, maximum tumor uptake was achieved 30 min post-injection, with values of 9.7 ± 1.5 %ID/g (^{64}Cu) and 11.9 ± 3.3 %ID/g (^{86}Y) achieved. Tumor uptake was shown to be specific as when co-infused, with excess unlabeled peptide tumor uptake

was reduced to fourfold for ^{64}Cu, while for the ^{86}Y labeled species, there was an almost 19-fold decrease. In general, ^{86}Y-DOTA-ReCCMSH(Arg^{11}) demonstrated lower non-target tissue accumulation than that of its ^{64}Cu analog, the one exception being the kidneys. These differences can be attributed in part to both the radioligand charge and the *in vivo* stability of the metal chelate, which has been shown to alter pharmacokinetics (Froidevaux *et al.*, 2002). MicroPET images obtained with both ^{64}Cu- and ^{86}Y-DOTA-ReCCMSH(Arg^{11}) showed the tumor could be visualized after 30 min and could still be delineated out to 24 hr. It was also evident from the ^{86}Y images that lower background accumulation was observed, consistent with the biodistribution data. The uptake of these tracers was compared to FDG. By 2 hr, tumor uptake for FDG was 5.1 ± 1.1 %ID/g, which was twofold lower than that seen for both ^{64}Cu and ^{86}Y labeled DOTA-ReCCMSH(Arg^{11}). Non-target tissue uptake of FDG was also substantially higher in all organs examined compared to the ^{86}Y-labeled species, the kidneys again being the only exception. This increase in non-target accumulation was evident when the tumor-to-blood and tumor-to-muscle ratios of FDG, 21 and 1 respectively, were compared to the value of 164 obtained for both ratios with the ^{86}Y-labeled peptide. By way of comparison, ^{64}Cu-DOTA-ReCCMSH(Arg^{11}) had tumor-to-blood and tumor-to-muscle ratios of 12 and 18, respectively, at 2 hr.

Conclusion

At present, the invasive procedure known as sentinel node biopsy is the most accurate method for detecting regional metastases caused by melanoma. This technique, however, cannot locate distant metastatic sites, which is where PET imaging finds its greatest use. As such PET imaging, in particular with FDG, has helped improve the diagnosis of patients with melanoma by either indicating the presence of distal metastatic sites or providing information leading to modification of treatment protocols. The overall sensitivity and selectivity for detecting lesions can be improved further by fusing together PET images with anatomical images obtained from modalities such as MR or CT. Further research is also continuing into new agents capable of targeting these lesions. To this end, pharmaceuticals are being developed that can target cell-surface receptors found only on cancerous cells or at a higher concentration than normal cells. As a result, these radiotracers differ from FDG, which instead targets cells with high metabolic activity. Two antigens that have received particular attention are *alpha vs. beta* 3 integrin, which is expressed on the majority of melanoma tumors, as well as the newly formed vasculature and melanocortin-1 receptors, which is also overexpressed on melanoma cells. To target these antigens, small-molecular-weight peptide mimics of larger naturally occurring species have been developed. Data obtained from these agents are promising, but further work is required to see if these agents can be transferred successfully to a clinical setting.

References

Albelda, S.M., Mette, S.A., Elder, D.E., Stewart, R., Damjanovich, L., Herlyn, M., and Buck, C.A. 1990. Integrin distribution in malignant melanoma: association of the beta 3 subunit with tumor progression. *Cancer Res.* 50:6757–6764.

Balch, C.M., Soong, S.J., Gershenwald, J.E., Thompson, J.F., Reintgen, D.S., Cascinelli, N., Urist, M., McMasters, K.M., Ross, M.I., Kirkwood, J.M., Atkins, M.B., Thompson, J.A., Coit, D.G., Byrd, D., Desmond, R., Zhang, Y., Liu, P.Y., Lyman, G.H., and Morabito, A. 2001. Prognostic factors analysis of 17,600 melanoma patients: validation of the American Joint Committee on Cancer melanoma staging system. *J. Clin. Oncol.* 19:3622–3634.

Been, L.B., Suurmeijer, A.J., Cobben, D.C., Jager, P.L., Hoekstra, H.J., and Elsinga, P.H. 2004. [18F]FLT-PET in oncology: current status and opportunities. *Eur. J. Nucl. Med. Mol. Imaging* 31:1659–1672.

Beer, A.J., Haubner, R., Goebel, M., Luderschmidt, S., Spilker, M.E., Wester, H.J., Weber, W.A., and Schwaiger, M. 2005. Biodistribution and pharmacokinetics of the alpha v beta3-selective tracer 18F-galacto-RGD in cancer patients. *J. Nucl. Med.* 46:1333–1341.

Brooks, P.C., Clark, R.A., and Cheresh, D.A. 1994. Requirement of vascular integrin alpha v beta 3 for angiogenesis. *Science* 264:569–571.

Brown, R.S., Goodman, T.M., Zasadny, K.R., Greenson, J.K., and Wahl, R.L. 2002. Expression of hexokinase II and Glut-1 in untreated human breast cancer. *Nucl. Med. Biol.* 29:443–453.

Burt, B.M., Humm, J.L., Kooby, D.A., Squire, O.D., Mastorides, S., Larson, S.M., and Fong, Y. 2001. Using positron emission tomography with [(18)F]FDG to predict tumor behavior in experimental colorectal cancer. *Neoplasia* 3:189–195.

Byzova, T.V., Rabbani, R., D'Souza, S.E., and Plow, E.F. 1998. Role of integrin alpha(v)beta3 in vascular biology. *Thromb. Haemost.* 80:726–734.

Cheng, Z., Chen, J., Quinn, T.P., and Jurisson, S.S. 2004. Radioiodination of rhenium cyclized alpha-melanocyte-stimulating hormone resulting in enhanced radioactivity localization and retention in melanoma. *Cancer Res.* 64:1411–1418.

Cobben, D.C., Jager, P.L., Elsinga, P.H., Maas, B., Suurmeijer, A.J., and Hoekstra, H.J. 2003. 3′-18F-fluoro-3′-deoxy-L-thymidine: a new tracer for staging metastatic melanoma? *J. Nucl. Med.* 44:1927–1932.

Cornish, J., Callon, K.E., Mountjoy, K.G., Bava, U., Lin, J.M., Myers, D.E., Naot, D., and Reid, I.R. 2003. Alpha-melanocyte-stimulating hormone is a novel regulator of bone. *Am. J. Physiol. Endocrinol. Metab.* 284:E1181–1190.

Crippa, F., Leutner, M., Belli, F., Gallino, F., Greco, M., Pilotti, S., Cascinelli, N., and Bombardieri, E. 2000. Which kinds of lymph node metastases can FDG PET detect? A clinical study in melanoma. *J. Nucl. Med.* 41:1491–1494.

Dave, N.N., Walia, R., Shor, M., and Ali, A. 2002. Effect of hyperglycemia on tumoral uptake of F-18 FDG. *Clin. Nucl. Med.* 27:682–683.

Eberle, A.N., and Froidevaux, S. 2003. Radiolabeled alpha-melanocyte-stimulating hormone analogs for receptor-mediated targeting of melanoma: from tritium to indium. *J. Mol. Recognit.* 16:248–254.

Edwards, B.K., Brown, M.L., Wingo, P.A., Howe, H.L., Ward, E., Ries, L.A., Schrag, D., Jamison, P.M., Jemal, A., Wu, X.C., Friedman, C., Harlan, L., Warren, J., Anderson, R.N., and Pickle, L.W. 2005. Annual report to the nation on the status of cancer, 1975–2002, featuring population-based trends in cancer treatment. *J. Natl. Cancer Inst.* 97:1407–1427.

Fink, A.M., Holle-Robatsch, S., Herzog, N., Mirzaei, S., Rappersberger, K., Lilgenau, N., Jurecka, W., and Steiner, A. 2004. Positron emission tomography is not useful in detecting metastasis in the sentinel lymph node in patients with primary malignant melanoma stage I and II. *Melanoma Res.* 14:141–145.

Finkelstein, S.E., Carrasquillo, J.A., Hoffman, J.M., Galen, B., Choyke, P., White, D.E., Rosenberg, S.A., and Sherry, R.M. 2004. A prospective analysis of positron emission tomography and conventional imaging for detection of stage IV metastatic melanoma in patients undergoing metastasectomy. *Ann. Surg. Oncol.* 11:731–738.

Folkman, J. 1971. Tumor angiogenesis: therapeutic implications. *N. Engl. J. Med.* 285:1182–1186.

Froidevaux, S., Calame-Christe, M., Schuhmacher, J., Tanner, H., Saffrich, R., Henze, M., and Eberle, A.N. 2004. A gallium-labeled DOTA-alpha-melanocyte-stimulating hormone analog for PET imaging of melanoma metastases. *J. Nucl. Med.* 45:116–123.

Froidevaux, S., Eberle, A.N., Christe, M., Sumanovski, L., Heppeler, A., Schmitt, J.S., Eisenwiener, K., Beglinger, C., and Macke, H.R. 2002. Neuroendocrine tumor targeting: study of novel gallium-labeled somatostatin radiopeptides in a rat pancreatic tumor model. *Int. J. Cancer.* 98:930–937.

Haberkorn, U., Ziegler, S.I., Oberdorfer, F., Trojan, H., Haag, D., Peschke, P., Berger, M.R., Altmann, A., and van Kaick, G. 1994. FDG uptake, tumor proliferation and expression of glycolysis associated genes in animal tumor models. *Nucl. Med. Biol.* 21:827–834.

Harris, M.T., Berlangieri, S.U., Cebon, J.S., Davis, I.D., and Scott, A.M. 2005. Impact of ^{18}F-fluorodeoxyglucose positron emission tomography on the management of patients with advanced melanoma. *Mol. Imaging Biol.* 7:304–308.

Haubner, R., Wester, H.J., Weber, W.A., Mang, C., Ziegler, S.I., Goodman, S.L., Senekowitsch-Schmidtke, R., Kessler, H., and Schwaiger, M. 2001. Noninvasive imaging of alpha(v)beta3 integrin expression using 18F-labeled RGD-containing glycopeptide and positron emission tomography. *Cancer Res.* 61:1781–1785.

Hieken, T.J., Ronan, S.G., Farolan, M., Shilkaitis, A.L., and Das Gupta, T.K. 1999. Molecular prognostic markers in intermediate-thickness cutaneous malignant melanoma. *Cancer* 85:375–382.

Johnson, J.P. 1999. Cell adhesion molecules in the development and progression of malignant melanoma. *Cancer Metastasis Rev.* 18:345–357.

Kumar, R., and Alavi, A. 2005. Clinical applications of fluorodeoxyglucose—positron emission tomography in the management of malignant melanoma. *Curr. Opin. Oncol.* 17:154–159.

Libberecht, K., Husada, G., Peeters, T., Michiels, P., Gys, T., and Molderez, C. 2005. Initial staging of malignant melanoma by positron emission tomography and sentinel node biopsy. *Acta Chir. Belg.* 105:621–625.

McQuade, P., and Knight, L.C. 2003. Radiopharmaceuticals for targeting the angiogenesis marker alpha(v)beta(3). *Q. J. Nucl. Med.* 47:209–220.

McQuade, P., Miao, Y., Yoo, J., Quinn, T.P., Welch, M.J., and Lewis, J.S. 2005. Imaging of melanoma using [64]Cu- and [86]Y-DOTA-ReCCMSH(Arg[11]), a cyclized peptide analogue of alpha-MSH. *J. Med. Chem.* 48:2985–2992.

Mijnhout, G.S., Comans, E.F., Raijmakers, P., Hoekstra, O.S., Teule, G.J., Boers, M., De Gast, G.C., and Ader, H.J. 2002. Reproducibility and clinical value of 18F-fluorodeoxyglucose positron emission tomography in recurrent melanoma. *Nucl. Med. Commun.* 23:475–481.

Nip, J., and Brodt, P. 1995. The role of the integrin vitronectin receptor, alpha v beta 3 in melanoma metastasis. *Cancer Metastasis Rev.* 14:241–252.

Poethko, T., Schottelius, M., Thumshirn, G., Herz, M., Haubner, R., Henriksen, G., Kessler, H., Schwaiger, M., and Wester, H.-J. 2004. Chemoselective pre-conjugate radiohalogenation of unprotected mono- and multimeric peptides via oxime formation. *Radiochimica Acta* 92:317–327.

Rahman, Z., and Taylor, S.C. 2001. Malignant melanoma in African Americans. *Cutis.* 67:403–406.

Reinhardt, M.J., Joe, A.Y., Jaeger, U., Huber, A., Matthies, A., Bucerius, J., Roedel, R., Strunk, H., Bieber, T., Biersack, H.J., and Tuting, T. 2006. Diagnostic performance of whole body dual modality 18F-FDG PET/CT imaging for N- and M-staging of malignant melanoma: experience with 250 consecutive patients. *J. Clin. Oncol.* 24:1178–1187.

Sivolapenko, G.B., Skarlos, D., Pectasides, D., Stathopoulou, E., Milonakis, A., Sirmalis, G., Stuttle, A., Courtenay-Luck, N.S., Konstantinides, K., and Epenetos, A.A. 1998. Imaging of metastatic melanoma utilising a Technetium-99m labelled RGD-containing synthetic peptide. *Eur. J. Nucl. Med.* 25:1383–1389.

Swetter, S.M., Boldrick, J.C., Jung, S.Y., Egbert, B.M., and Harvell, J.D. 2005. Increasing incidence of lentigo maligna melanoma subtypes: northern California and national trends 1990–2000. *J. Invest. Dermatol.* 125:685–691.

Swetter, S.M., Carroll, L.A., Johnson, D.L., and Segall, G.M. 2002. Positron emission tomography is superior to computed tomography for metastatic detection in melanoma patients. *Ann. Surg. Oncol. 9:*646–653.

Tai, Y.C., and Laforest, R. 2005. Instrumentation aspects of animal PET. *Annu. Rev Biomed. Eng. 7:*255–285.

Talbot, J.N., Petegnief, Y., Kerrou, K., Montravers, F., Grahek, D., and Younsi, N. 2003. Positron emission tomography with [18F]-FDG in oncology. *Nuclear Instruments & Methods in Physics Research, Section A: Accelerators, Spectrometers, Detectors, and Associated Equipment. 504:*129–138.

Tyler, D.S., Onaitis, M., Kherani, A., Hata, A., Nicholson, E., Keogan, M., Fisher, S., Coleman, E., and Seigler, H.F. 2000. Positron emission tomography scanning in malignant melanoma. *Cancer 89:*1019–1025.

Wagner, J.D., Schauwecker, D., Davidson, D., Logan, T., Coleman, J.J., 3rd, Hutchins, G., Love, C., Wenck, S., and Daggy, J. 2005. Inefficacy of F-18 fluorodeoxy-D-glucose-positron emission tomography scans for initial evaluation in early-stage cutaneous melanoma. *Cancer 104:*570–579.

Wahl, R.L., Hutchins, G.D., Buchsbaum, D.J., Liebert, M., Grossman, H.B., and Fisher, S. 1991. ^{18}F-2-deoxy-2-fluoro-D-glucose uptake into human tumor xenografts. Feasibility studies for cancer imaging with positron-emission tomography. *Cancer 67:*1544–1550.

Wang, W., McMurray, J.S., Wu, Q., Campbell, M.L., and Li, C. 2005. Convenient solid-phase synthesis of diethylenetriaminepenta-acetic acid (DTPA)-conjugated cyclic RGD peptide analogues. *Cancer Biother. Radiopharm. 20:*547–556.

Yamada, K., Brink, I., Bisse, E., Epting, T., and Engelhardt, R. 2005. Factors influencing [F-18] 2-fluoro-2-deoxy-D-glucose (F-18 FDG) uptake in melanoma cells: the role of proliferation rate, viability, glucose transporter expression and hexokinase activity. *J. Dermatol. 32:*316–334.

Zhuang, H., Yu, J.Q., and Alavi, A. 2005. Applications of fluorodeoxyglucose-PET imaging in the detection of infection and inflammation and other benign disorders. *Radiol. Clin. North Am. 43:*121–134.

Multiple Myeloma: Scintigraphy Using Technetium-99m-2-Methoxyisobutylisonitrile

Jaroslav Bacovsky and Miroslav Myslivecek

Introduction

Multiple myeloma (MM) is a clonal B-lymphocyte neoplasm of plasma cells. It accounts for 1% of all malignant diseases and represents 10% of hematologic malignancies. The hallmark of MM is the presence of a monoclonal protein (MIG), produced by the abnormal plasma cells in the blood or urine. Once the diagnosis is suspected, a radiographic skeletal survey (XR), bone marrow aspiration, and biopsy are performed. The effects of abnormal plasma cells proliferation are excessive bone resorption and inhibition of bone formation.

To evaluate the extent of MM and follow-up on the disease, a routine practice covers the determination of hemoglobin (Hb), biopsy of bone marrow with percentage determination of plasma cells (Pb), assessment of monoclonal immunoglobulin concentration (MIG) in the serum or urine, and XR. Biological activity of MM has been routinely assessed by the examination of beta-2-microglobulin in the serum (B_2M), albumin in the serum, serum thymidinekinase (sTK), C-reactive protein (CRP), LDH, evaluation of free light chains in serum, and biochemical markers of bone resorption carboxyterminal telopeptide of type I collagen (ICTP).

The clinical presentations of MM include bone pain, severe osteopenia, and skeletal fractures, including multilevel spinal cord compression fractures. In clinical practice of myeloma patients, imaging is complementary to measurements of biochemical markers of bone turnover. The biochemical markers were reported to reflect the disease activity in bone and the extent of disease and to be helpful in identifying patients likely to respond to biphosphonate treatment .

The purpose of imaging is to identify bone involvement as early as possible, to determine the full extent of disease, to evaluate the presence of complications that may accompany malignant bone involvement (including pathologic fractures and spinal cord compression), to monitor response to therapy, and occasionally to guide biopsy if histologic confirmation is indicated.

A radiographic skeletal survey is the primary imaging modality for detecting bone changes in MM and is included in the Durie-Salmon clinical staging criteria of newly diagnosed MM. Its main limitation is that 50% bone destruction must occur before there is radiographic evidence of a bone lesion. Four distinct forms of myeloma have been described on XR: a solitary lytic lesion (plasmocytoma), diffuse skeletal involvement (myelomatosis) presenting as osteolytic lesions with discrete margins, diffuse skeletal osteopenia without well-defined lytic lesions, and rare sclerosing myeloma. Conventional radiography XR will detect involvement in 75–95% of cases and with 80% sensitivity. Discrimination between new active osteolytic areas and persisting osteolytic lesions using radiography is not possible. These techniques have some limitations. In particular, the persistence of radiological abnormalities cannot be considered evidence of active disease because they may represent residual osteolysis in the absence of plasma cell proliferation.

Computed tomography (CT) is a sensitive tool for detecting the bone-destructive effects of MM. Multiple myeloma findings that can be detected on CT include lytic lesions, lesions with soft tissue masses, diffuse osteopenia, and fractures. Magnetic resonance imaging (MRI) has recently been used in patients with MM for assessment of the actual tumor burden in the marrow and the presence of accompanying complications. Spinal compression fractures caused by bone destruction or by a mass occur in 60 to 70% of patients with MM. The image features of MM on MRI, however, are not specific and can also be found in other disease processes, such as drug-induced reactive marrow or increased hematopoiesis in patients with severe anemia.

Several radionuclide procedures have been used in patients with multiple myeloma. Conventional bone scintigraphy with Tc-99m-MDP (Technetium-99m methylene diphosphonate) is considered less sensitive than XR and CT due to the presence of only minimal osteoblastic activity in most myeloma lesions, which are predominantly osteolytic. Almost half of the abnormal sites of disease identified radiographically are overlooked by bone scintigraphy. Scintigraphic abnormalities associated with myeloma may appear as increased sites of Tc-99m-MDP uptake, mainly in the presence of fractures, or as "cold" lesions. Soft tissue uptake may be detected in association with calcification within a plasmocytoma or secondary amyloidosis. Presently, bone scintigraphy with Tc-99m-MDP is rarely performed because of its low sensitivity compared with plain radiography (XR). Similarly, gallium-67-citrate scans also do not belong to the imaging technique of choice at present.

Experience with fluorine-18 fluorodeoxyglucose positron emission tomography (18F-FDG-PET) in patients with MM is rapidly expanding. Previous reports have shown that 18F-FDG-PET can detect unexpected medullary and extramedullary sites of disease missed by XR, CT, and Technetium-99m-MDP bone scintigraphy. A sensitivity of 93% has been reported for detection of osteolytic MM by 18F-FDG-PET. Durie et al. (2002) assessed the role of 18F-FDG-PET in 66 patients with MM and monoclonal gammopathy of undetermined significance (MGUS). Their results suggest that positive 18F-FDG-PET reliably detects active MM, whereas a negative study strongly supports the diagnosis of MGUS. The authors concluded that detection of extramedullary sites of disease and residual 18F-FDG uptake on a follow-up study after stem-cell transplantation are poor prognostic factors.

Recently, Technetium-99m-2-methoxyisobutylisonitrile (Tc-99m-MIBI, Tc-99m-sestamibi) has been proposed as a potential tracer for imaging and identifying patients with active multiple myeloma. Tc-99m-MIBI is well characterized metallopharmaceutically, and is currently in clinical use for the assessment of myocardial perfusion. A number of studies have also reported the successful use of Tc-99m-MIBI for the detection of primary and metastatic sites of a variety of neoplastic diseases, including breast, lung, brain, thyroid and parathyroid tumors, musculoskeletal sarcomas, and low-grade lymphomas.

Although several hypotheses have been proposed to explain the increased accumulation of Tc-99m-MIBI in malignant tumors, the exact uptake mechanism of this tracer has not been completely elucidated. A number of studies have documented the passive influx of this lipophilic cation in relation to high negative transmembrane potentials and a reversible accumulation within mitochondria of both normal and malignant cells. In agreement with these findings, malignant tumors are reported to be associated with increased mitochondrial and plasma transmembrane potentials, a phenomenon resulting from their increased metabolic requirements. However, when mitochondrial density and other inherent histological factors, such as mitotic activity and neo-angiogenesis, were evaluated in solid malignant tumors, controversial results were obtained, and no definite correlation with Tc-99m-MIBI uptake was found.

In the study of Fonti et al. (2001), bone marrow samples obtained from 24 multiple myeloma patients, three patients with monoclonal gammopathy of undetermined significance, and two healthy donors were studied for evaluation of in vitro uptake in order to estimate quantitatively Tc-99m-MIBI bone marrow uptake and to verify the intracellular localization of the tracer. No specific tracer uptake was found in bone marrow samples obtained from the two healthy donors. Microautoradiography showed localization of Tc-99m-MIBI inside the plasma cells infiltrating the bone marrow. Fonti et al. concluded that the degree of tracer uptake both in vitro and in vivo is related to the percentage of infiltrating plasma cells that accumulate the tracer in their inner compartment. Therefore, Tc-99m-MIBI scintigraphy can be considered a useful tool in the diagnosis and monitoring of patients with multiple myeloma.

Technetium-99m-MIBI Scintigraphy

Technique

Tc-99m-MIBI scintigraphy is usually performed using a dual-head gamma camera equipped with low-energy, high-resolution, parallel hole-collimators. Anterior and posterior whole-body scans are obtained 10 min after the IV injection of 740 MBq Tc-99m-MIBI because the accumulation of tracer within mitochondria has very rapid kinetics, allowing maximum tumor uptake to be achieved within such a short time. However, Tc-99m-MIBI is also reported to be a substrate for P-glycoprotein, and a reduced net tracer uptake has been shown in resistant cultured tumor cells as a consequence of the enhanced P-glycoprotein-dependent outward transport. Overexpression of P-glycoprotein is one of the primary mechanisms of multidrug resistance in multiple myeloma. Thus, it can be hypothesized that Tc-99m-MIBI uptake could be influenced by P-glycoprotein expression. It has been indeed shown that delayed MIBI uptake ratio (i.e., tumor-to-background ratio at one or more hours after tracer injection) is reduced in resistant tumors as compared with sensitive counterparts. However, when measured on early images (i.e., 10 min after tracer application), tumor-to-background ratios were not found to be significantly different in P-glycoprotein-overexpressing tumors as compared with P-glycoprotein-negative tumors. Therefore, early Tc-99m-MIBI scintigraphy performed within 10 min of injection is not likely to be affected by the multidrug resistant phenotype.

Evaluation of Tc-99m-MIBI Scintigraphy

Tc-99m-MIBI is physiologically accumulated in salivary and thyroid glands, heart, and spleen, and because the main route of its excretion is the liver and hepatobiliary system, a large amount of Tc-99m-MIBI radioactivity is usually seen in the bowels. The physiological radioactivity is also present in kidneys and urinary bladder. Homogeneous mild diffuse uptake of Tc-99m-MIBI was observed in 90% of the group of 124 control patients with presumed normal bone and bone marrow.

One of the very useful semiquantitative Tc-99m-MIBI scan classifications has been proposed by Pace *et al.* (1998). According to their scoring, the scans are classified as pattern N, when only physiological uptake of Tc-99m-MIBI is present; pattern D, when diffuse bone marrow uptake is observed; pattern F, when areas of focal uptake of the radiotracer are evident; and pattern D + F, when both patterns are observed. The diffuse bone marrow uptake is graded according to extension (E) and intensity (I) of the uptake (Tables 1 and 2). E-score: E0 = no evidence of marrow uptake; E1 = spine and pelvis uptake; E2 = uptake by spine, pelvis, and ribs or proximal humeral and femoral epiphyses; E3 = uptake by spine, pelvis, ribs, and distal and femoral epiphyses. I score: I0 = no evidence of marrow uptake; I1 = bone marrow uptake less than myocardium; I2 = bone marrow uptake equal to myocardium; I3 = bone marrow uptake higher than myocardium. In addition, a summed score (SS = E + I) can be computed for each patient.

Clinical Applications of Tc-99m-MIBI Scintigraphy

The diagnostic value of Tc-99m-MIBI scintigraphy in the detection of bone marrow and extramedullar involvement has been evaluated in several studies. Alexandrakis *et al.* (2002), in a study with 35 MM patients, found that the activity of MM

was directly related to the grade of Tc-99m-MIBI uptake in bone marrow. Similarly, Balleari *et al.* (2001) reported on the high sensitivity and specificity of Tc-99m-MIBI scintigraphy for MM activity in bone marrow and considered this imaging method to be a reliable examination at the staging and follow-up of patients with MM. Svaldi *et al.* (2001), in their study with MM patients, described a diffuse pattern of Tc-99m-MIBI scan that reflected a higher percentage of bone marrow plasma cells, and considered Tc-99m-MIBI scintigraphy as an effective method for discrimination of the biologically active myeloma. Pace *et al.* (1998) concluded that Tc-99m-MIBI scintigraphy appeared to be a highly sensitive method for identification of patients with active disease, selection of patients requiring therapy, and discrimination of patients in remission from patients with recurrent disease. They also proved a correlation with the clinical stage of the disease.

Significant statistical correlation was found between the grade of Tc-99m-MIBI uptake expressed by summary score SS of Tc-99m-MIBI scintigrams and known markers of disease activity (beta2-microglobulin, monoclonal immunoglobulin level, serum thymidinkinase, CRP, cross-linked carboxyterminal telopeptide of type I collagen, and bone marrow plasmocytosis). A significant negative correlation was recorded between summary score (SS) and hemoglobin (Bačovský *et al.*, 2005). These results suggest more extensive disease activity, as determined by high levels of markers correlating with a higher uptake of the radiotracer (Fig. 1).

The results of several studies suggest a relevant potential role of Tc-99m-MIBI scintigraphy in patients with

Table 1   Semiquantitative Scoring of 99mTc-MIBI Bone Marrow Uptake According to Its Extension (E-score)

E Score	Extension of 99mTc-MIBI Bone Marrow Uptake
E0	No evidence of marrow uptake
E1	Spine and pelvis uptake
E2	Uptake by spine, pelvis, and ribs or proximal humeral and femoral epiphyses
E3	Uptake by spine, pelvis, ribs, and distal and femoral epiphyses

Table 2   Semiquantitative Scoring of 99mTc-MIBI Bone Marrow Uptake According to Its Intensity (I-score)

I Score	Intensity of 99mTc-MIBI Bone Marrow Uptake
I0	No evidence of marrow uptake
I1	Bone marrow uptake less than myocardium
I2	Bone marrow uptake equal to myocardium
I3	Bone marrow uptake higher than myocardium

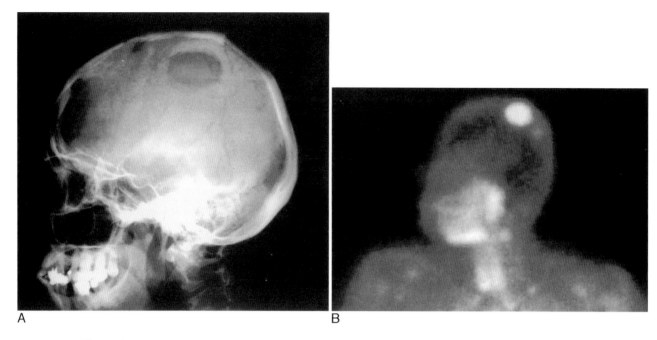

Figure 1 Multiple myeloma IgG kappa III A. XR of skull-osteolytic lesion. MIBI scintigraphy—focal uptake on skull.

multiple myeloma, both as a prognostic tool and for monitoring the disease course (Table 3). The findings of focal uptake of Tc-99m-MIBI in baseline scintigrams before therapy (scintigraphy pattern F or F + D) is a negative-predictive factor for response to conventional chemotherapy. Tc-99m-MIBI uptake can be modified by the presence of a 170 KDa P-glycoprotein encoded by the MDR-1 gene (Del Vecchio et al., 1997). This protein functions as an efflux energy-dependent pump. Other studies have shown that Tc-99m-MIBI is a transport substrate recognized by the human MDR-1P-glycoprotein, which recognizes and transports a large group of cytotoxic substances out of plasma cells. Because P-glycoprotein overexpression is one of the primary mechanisms of multidrug resistance in multiple myeloma, some studies tested whether Tc-99m-MIBI could be used as an indicator of Pgp overexpression. The potential role of Tc-99m-MIBI washout measuring in predicting response to chemotherapy in patients with multiple myeloma has been suggested. Disease-free survival (or EFS—event-free survival) was significantly better in patients with lower washout of Tc-99m-MIBI.

A recent study by Koutsikos et al. (2005) determined the role of combined use of Tc-99m-MIBI and Tc-99m-pentavalent dimercaptosuccinic acid scintigraphy in evaluating the effectiveness of chemotherapy in patients with multiple myeloma. Combined use of the two agents allowed the effectiveness of chemotherapy to be evaluated through a comparison of nonactive additional lesions/total number of positive lesions ratios even in the absence of a baseline study. Tc-99m-MIBI scintigraphy has high sensitivity and specific-

ity in tracing active nonsecretory multiple myeloma lesions. It should be considered complementary to another conventional imaging (XR, CT, or MRI) for monitoring this type of disease. Tc-99m-MIBI scintigraphy can detect bone marrow lesions in myeloma patients, which cannot be detected by other imaging methods and which it can be useful especially in solitary myeloma to exclude other involved sites.

Table 3   Use of Tc-99m-MIBI Scintigraphy in Multiple Myeloma

— MIBI is a tool for diagnosing, staging, and following up focal myeloma lesions in the bone as well as in soft tissues.

— MIBI is more specific than conventional XR in identifying sites of active disease.

— MIBI detects lesions that are negative by plain radiography (XR).

— MIBI is a useful tool for evaluating the extension and activity of myeloma, especially where MRI is not available.

— MIBI is a useful additional diagnostic tool for detecting otherwise occult sites of myeloma.

— The use of MIBI or PET should particularly be considered in the evaluation of a patient with an early-stage plasma cell dyscrasia to exclude the presence of more extensive disease.

— MIBI may be helpful in evaluating the presence of ongoing disease activity in previously irradiated sites that remain abnormal on skeletal survey following treatment. This may be relevant for follow-up of patients who have received radiotherapy to an isolated plasmacytoma, or for assessment of patients who continue to have pain at a previously irradiated site.

— Combined use of MIBI and 99mTc-V-DMSA scanning during chemotherapy allows evaluation of the effectiveness of the administered chemotherapy.

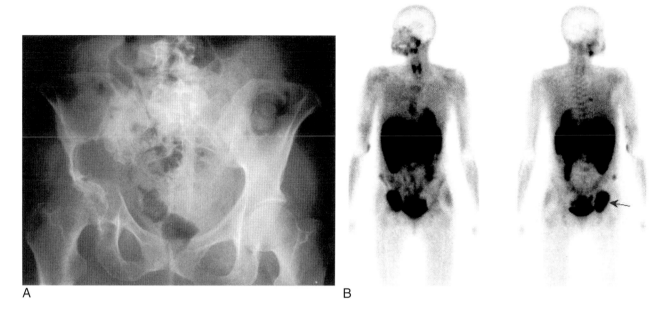

Figure 2 Nonsecretory multiple myeloma XR of pelvis—osteolytic lesion of right hip. MIBI scintigraphy—focal uptake in right part of pelvis.

Myslivecek *et al.* (2003) investigated the validity of Tc-99m-MIBI scintigraphy and MRI in the diagnosis and prediction of therapy response in patients with multiple myeloma. It was found that Tc-99m-MIBI scintigraphy and MRI are equally sensitive methods for detecting multiple myeloma lesions and complement each other. The advantages of Tc-99m-MIBI scintigraphy are whole-body examination and faster detection of response to therapy, while the advantages of MRI are exact detection of epidural masses and vertebral compressions influencing the therapeutical strategy.

Few authors have reported the potential value of fluorine-18 fluorodeoxyglucose positron emission tomography (FDG-PET) in the evaluation of multiple myeloma. Both the Tc-99m-MIBI scintigraphy and FDG-PET scans are useful in evaluation of the disease. In comparison with Tc-99m-MIBI scintigraphy, FDG-PET can detect more lesions. However, both methods are useful additional diagnostic tools for detecting otherwise occult sites of myeloma.

Use of FDG-PET should particularly be considered in evaluating patients with an early-stage plasma cell dyscrasia to exclude the presence of more extensive disease. Both FDG-PET and Tc-99m MIBI scans have been reported to identify sites of disease. They are useful in evaluating patients with MM, particularly for detecting otherwise occult sites of myeloma. However, FDG-PET can detect more lesions than the Tc-99m MIBI scintigraphy. Uptake on MIBI reflects both activated mitochondria and the density of malignant plasma cells. Fluorine-18 FDG is a glucose analog, radiolabeled with fluorine-18. Cellular uptake occurs via the glucose transporter protein, GLUT-1. FDG is then phosphorylated and remains trapped in the cell. Consequently, higher uptake is seen in tumor cells because they have increased glucose metabolism. Like MIBI, FDG-PET can detect skeletal and extra-osseous myeloma involvement. A focal or mixed focal/diffuse FDG-PET uptake pattern exhibited a higher positive-predictive value for active disease compared with diffuse uptake pattern (100% and 75%, respectively). In a recent report, Mileshkin *et al.* (2004) compared the utility of MIBI with FDG-PET in the evaluation of bony disease in myeloma. Overall, they found that in the patient cohort that was investigated by both MIBI and FDG-PET, MIBI detected additional sites to FDG-PET in 52% of cases. Moreover, the extent of skeletal involvement by MIBI, but not by FDG-PET, demonstrated a positive correlation with plasma cell infiltrate in the bone marrow.

In conclusion, whole-body scintigraphy using Tc-99m-MIBI seems to be an easy, sensitive, and available parameter of biological activity of multiple myeloma (MM). Individual patterns of Tc-99m-MIBI uptake in MM patients showed a close association with the grade of disease activity, and correlation with the clinical stage of the disease and allowed with high sensitivity the discrimination of patients in remission from those with recurrent disease. Patients with MGUS had a mostly physiological pattern of Tc-99m-MIBI uptake, or only a very low activity of diffuse pattern. Tc-99m-MIBI scintigraphy can be used in MM for determining the optimal site for punction biopsy, especially in cases of suspected involvement of soft tissues. Some preliminary findings in our study indicate that Tc-99m-MIBI scintigraphy may play a predictive role in the follow-up of patients with MM in clinical stage IA according to Durie-Salmon.

References

Alexandrakis, M.G., Kyriakou, D.S., Passam, F.H., Malliaraki, N., Christophoridou, A.V., and Karkavitsas, N. 2002. Correlation between the uptake of Tc-99m-sestaMIBI and prognostic factors in patients with multiple myeloma. *Clin. Lab. Haematol. 24*:155–159.

Bačovský, J., Scudla, V., Myslivecek, M., Nekula, J., and Vytrasova, M. 2005. 99mTc-MIBI scintigraphy—sensitive parameter of biologic activity of multiple myeloma. *Neoplasma 52*:302–306.

Balleari, E., Villa, G., Garre, S., Ghirlanda, P., Agnese, G., Carletto, M., Clavio, M., Ferrando, F., Gobbi, M., Mariani, G., and Ghio, R. 2001. Technetium-99m-sestamibi scintigraphy in multiple myeloma and related gammopathies: a useful tool for the identification and follow-up of myeloma bone disease. *Haematologica 86*:78–84.

Del Vecchio, S., Ciarmello, A., and Potena, M.I. 1997. *In vivo* detection of multidrug-resistant (MDRI) phenotype by Tc-99m-sestaMIBI scans in untreated breast cancer patients. *Eur. J. Nucl. Med. 24*:150–159.

Durie, B.G.M., Waxman, A.D., D'Agnolo, A., and Williams, C.M. 2002. Whole-body 18F-FDG-PET identifies high-risk myeloma. *J. Nucl. Med. 43*:1457–1463.

Fonti, R., Del Vecchio, S., Zannetti, A., De Renzo, A., Di Gennaro, F., Catalano, L., Califano, C., Pace, L., Rotoli, B., and Salvatore, M. 2001. Bone marrow uptake of ^{99m}Tc-MIBI in patients with multiple myeloma. *Eur. J. Nucl. Med. 28*:214–220.

Koutsikos, J., Athanasoulis, T., Anagnostopoulos, A., Velidaki, A., Passadi, M., Dimopoulos, M.A., and Zerva, C. 2005. Combined use of 99mTc-sestamibi and 99mTc-V-DMSA in the assessment of chemotherapy effectiveness in patients with multiple myeloma. *J. Nucl. Med. 46*:978–982.

Mileshkin, L., Blum, R., Seymour, J.F., Patrikeos, A., Hicks, R.J., and Prince, H.M. 2004. A comparison of fluorine-18 fluorodeoxyglucose PET and technetium-99m sestamibi in assessing patients with multiple myeloma. *Eur. J. Haematol. 72*:32–37.

Myslivecek, M., Bacovsky, J., Koranda, P., Vytrasova, M., Kaminek, M., Husák, V., Scudla, V., and Nekula, J. 2003. Technetium-99m-MIBI scintigraphy in patients with multiple myeloma: a role of the examination in the follow-up and its prognostic value. *Eur. J. Nucl. Med. 30*:S284.

Pace, L., Catalano, L., Pinto, A.M., De Renzo, A., Di Gennaro, F., Califano, C., Del Vecchio, S., Rotoli, B., and Salvatore, M. 1998. Different patterns of technetium-99m sestamibi uptake in multiple myeloma. *Eur. J. Nucl. Med. 25*:714–720.

Svaldi, M., Tappa, C., Gebert, U., Bettini, D., Fabris, P., Franzelin, F., Osele, L., and Mitterer, M. 2001. Technetium-99m-sestamibi scintigraphy: an alternative approach for diagnosis and follow-up of active myeloma lesions after high-dose chemotherapy and autologous stem cell transplantation. *Ann. Hematol. 80*:393–397.

30

Nasopharyngeal Carcinoma: ^{18}F-Fluorodeoxyglucose-Positron Emission Tomography

Shu-Hang Ng, Sheung-Fat Ko, and Tzu-Chen Yen

Introduction

Nasopharyngeal carcinoma (NPC) is an epithelial malignancy that occurs worldwide with particularly high frequency in southern China, parts of Southeast Asia, Northern Africa, and Alaska. The etiological factors for endemic NPC include Epstein-Barr virus, environmental factors, and genetic susceptibility. The incidence rate begins to rise at the early age of 20, reaching a plateau between 35 and 64 years and declining thereafter. Men are more often afflicted than women.

This carcinoma is diagnosed primarily with endoscopy. The mainstay of treatment is radiotherapy, but chemotherapy is also needed in advanced disease. Imaging is used to delineate the tumor extent to facilitate treatment planning. Magnetic resonance imaging (MRI) currently is the preferred imaging modality over computed tomography (CT) in evaluating NPC. It provides an accurate assessment of the local tumor extent and, in turn, the T-stage of NPC. Magnetic resonance imaging is also sensitive in detecting radiation-induced complications. However, MRI has some limitations in identifying nodal metastasis of NPC and in accurately differentiating post-radiation changes from tumor recurrence. It also has difficulty in assessing the distant metastasis in the whole body in a single session of the examination.

Positron emission tomography (PET) is a whole-body functional imaging technique that provides information about tissue metabolism. By pinpointing at the regions of accelerated glucose metabolism using the radionuclide ^{18}F-fluorodeoxyglucose (FDG), FDG-PET has shown promise in the evaluation of head and neck malignancy. It can reveal metastatic deposits in the lymph nodes of a normal size. It also facilitates the identification of viable tumors within the fibrotic areas in the irradiated field, and helps to differentiate tumor recurrence from post-treatment inflammation. Since FDG-PET can scan the whole body, it has another advantage of disclosing distant metastasis in a single session. However, due to its inherent relatively poor anatomic resolution, FDG-PET cannot accurately define the local anatomic extent of the tumor and thus cannot be used in isolation for tumor staging. The present resolution of PET scanners is ~ 3 mm^3, and thus, a negative FDG-PET does not completely rule out the presence of tumor. This technique is also known to have limitations for the detection of nodal micrometastases as well as largely necrotic metastatic nodes. In addition, FDG-PET may occasionally have false-positive results for malignancy due to a benign inflammatory process. Because FDG-PET is an expensive imaging modality, it should be used judiciously. This chapter addresses the role of FDG-PET in the evaluation of NPC.

Pretreatment Evaluation

Primary Tumor

Nasopharyngeal carcinoma usually originates from the lateral wall of the nasopharynx, particularly the fossa of Rosenmuller. A superficial mucosal tumor may be difficult to distinguish from adenoidal tissue radiographically, and one early feature of malignant disease is invasion to the musculo-fascial planes around the levator and tensor palatini muscles. NPC often shows a high degree of aggressive regional invasion at presentation and spreads along well-defined routes. NPC often spreads anteriorly into the nasal fossa, laterally to the parapharyngeal space, posteriorly to the pre-vertebral muscles, inferiorly spread to the oropharynx, or superiorly to the skull base, sphenoid sinus floor, and intracranial areas. It is well recognized that MRI is better than CT in demonstrating these locoregional tumor extents (Ng *et al.*, 1997).

FDG-PET can readily detect the primary tumor of NPC. In the study by Yen *et al.* (2005d), the sensitivities of both FDG-PET and MRI for detection of the primary NPC at the nasopharynx were 100%. FDG-PET can also be useful in demonstrating a nasopharyngeal primary tumor in patients with cervical metastatic adenopathy of unknown primary cancer. However, due to its relatively poor anatomic resolution and moderate specificity, FDG-PET alone cannot map exactly the locoregional extent of NPC. Contiguous paranasal sinusitis may mimic tumor invasion into the paranasal sinus (Chan *et al.*, 2005). In the clinical setting where distinct tumor staging is required, the limited anatomical information provided by FDG-PET assigns it in a complementary position. Rather, the definition of tumor-bearing tissues provided by FDG-PET can greatly assist CT/MRI in precise tumor delineation for the planning of radiotherapy, particularly intensity-modulated radiotherapy. Imaging fusion between FDG-PET and MRI/CT has been reported to be useful in the determining gross tumor volume for three-dimensional conformal radiotherapy of NPC, leading to the sparing of irradiation to adjacent normal tissues for the majority of the cases (Nishioka *et al.*, 2002). In their study, image fusion was performed in 9 patients with NPC by using a plastic, custom-made head/neck support and localizer systems for immobilization and by taking images with standardized body posture. At present, a hybrid PET/CT scanner has become available and can provide more accurate information about tissue characterization and the exact extent of tumor tissue in one imaging procedure. The potential of PET/CT in delineating tumor-bearing tissues for planning of radiotherapy of NPC is of interest and needs further validation.

Nodal Spread

The patterns of nodal spread of NPC greatly influence the planning of radiotherapy portals. It has been reported that 60 to 80% of patients have regional nodal metastases at presentation (Ng *et al.*, 1997; King *et al.*, 2000). Accurate depiction of nodal spread is important when radiotherapy is the primary treatment and no histopathology is available. For the identification of metastatic adenopathy from NPC, MRI can demonstrate nodes in both the neck and retropharyngeal region well. In clinical practice, nodal metastasis is usually considered to be present when the shortest axial diameter of the cervical nodes is at least 10 mm (except in the case of jugulodigastric nodes, where the minimum diameter is 11 mm) or the shortest axial diameter of the retropharyngeal nodes is at least 5 mm. A cluster of three borderline-sized nodes is another imaging criterion for malignancy. Central necrosis and extracapsular spread are also indicators of metastasis (van den Brekel *et al.*, 1990). However, MRI may not be able to identify metastatic lesions in nodes of a normal size, and it cannot distinguish enlarged reactive nodes from malignant nodes with certainty. In interpreting MR images of NPC, lymph nodes of borderline size, without nodal necrosis or extracapsular spread, always pose a diagnostic challenge.

For NPC, FDG-PET has proven to be significantly superior to CT and MRI in identifying neck nodal metastasis (Kao *et al.*, 2000; Nishioka *et al.*, 2002; Yen *et al.*, 2005d). This technique has another advantage in that it can simultaneously reveal distant nodal metastases. However, owing to its poor anatomic resolution, FDG-PET may not differentiate primary tumor extension from contiguous metastatic lymph nodes, particularly those in the retropharyngeal and carotid sheath spaces (Ng *et al.*, 2004a). It may even show false negatives for metastatic nodes with small size or cystic necrosis. In addition, FDG-PET may occasionally have difficulties in differentiating pathological nodes from physiologic uptakes in normal organs such as muscle, salivary glands, tonsils, vocal cords, supraclavicular fat, and mucous membranes. Some reactive or inflammatory nodes may mimic metastatic nodes on FDG-PET images.

Occasionally, discrimination of nodal metastasis from reactive nodal hyperplasia on FDG-PET is difficult by visual inspection. Standardized uptake value (SUV) has been used as an important reference to differentiate benign from malignant lesions (Lapela *et al.*, 1995). There were many exceptions, however. A dual time point FDG-PET imaging technique was then considered feasible in differentiating malignancy from inflammation and normal tissue in the head and neck lesions (Hustinx *et al.*, 1999). However, its application for NPC appears to be unnecessary. Yen *et al.* (2005b) have employed the dual-phase technique, which includes a delayed FDG-PET scan (scan at 3 hr after the intravenous injection of FDG) in addition to a conventional FDG-PET scan (scan at 40 min after injection) to examine NPC patients, but unfortunately, the results showed that the additional 3-hr FDG-PET scan contributed no further information in the diagnostic accuracy of locoregional metastatic nodal detection.

For identifying nodal metastases of NPC, MRI and FDG-PET appear to complement each other well. In a series of

101 patients, ~ 40% of patients have discordant results between FDG-PET and MRI (Ng *et al*., 2004a). The majority of discordant results were due to the superior capability of FDG-PET over MRI in the assessment of nodal metastasis. These included revelation of metastatic cervical nodes that did not meet the morphologic criteria of metastasis, exclusion of borderline-sized retropharyngeal nodes from tumor involvement, and disclosure of distant metastatic nodes in the mediastinum and abdomen. Other discordant results stemmed from the inferior capability of FDG-PET to MRI in identifying those metastatic nodes that merged with primary tumor or dental caries. A few cervical and mediastinal benign reactive nodes with fatty hila were well demonstrated on MRI but were falsely misinterpreted as metastatic nodes on FDG-PET.

FDG-PET, in conjunction with MRI, can clearly demonstrate the patterns of nodal spread of NPC (Ng *et al*., 2004a). Nodal metastases of NPC principally affected neck level II nodes, from which lymphatic spread extended caudally to involve level III, level IV, and the supraclavicular fossa nodes, or extended posteriorly to involve level V nodes. The frequency of skip metastases was ~ 8% of patients. Distant spread to mediastinal or abdominal nodes was found in 3–5% of patients, usually associating with supraclavicular nodal metastases. The patterns of nodal spread in NPC have an important clinical impact on the treatment planning. For disease without distant nodal metastasis, primary gross tumor areas and the positive nodal areas are irradiated with the radical dose up to 70–76 Gy, while the negative nodal areas in the neck are irradiated with the prophylactic dose of 45–50 Gy.

For disease with distant nodal metastasis, chemotherapy is the primary treatment mode, and then palliative radiotherapy will be performed if good response to chemotherapy is attained. Because NPC is treated primarily by radiotherapy and no neck dissection is performed, there arises a problem about the actual sensitivity for negative nodes on both MRI and FDG-PET. However, because such nodes were controlled by irradiation with prophylactic doses without recurrence, the tumor deposit within such nodes seemed to be zero or microscopic. Another problem is that in a few cases the location of the FDG uptake could not exactly match with that of MRI by meticulous side-by-side visual correlation or even co-registration by a computer algorithm owing to variations in the neck position. With the advance in FDG-PET technology, integrated PET/CT can provide accurate fused data of FDG-PET and CT simultaneously, and may be the most convenient and accurate imaging modality for evaluating the nodal spread of NPC.

Distant Metastasis

Of all the squamous cell carcinomas of head and neck origin, NPC is one of the highest incidences for distant metastasis. Generally, 30% of NPC patients will eventually develop distant metastasis, but only one-sixth (5%) of those are diagnosed with metastatic cases at their initial diagnosis by conventional staging work-up, with one-third (10%) identified within 3 months after diagnosis (Teo *et al*., 1996; Lee *et al*., 1992). In other words, 10 to 20% of NPC is understaged at the initial work-up because distant metastasis is already present but not detected. The conventional staging work-up for NPC, including chest radiography, abdominal sonography, and skeletal scintigraphy, does not appear not to be sensitive enough to detect early distant metastasis of NPC. Because FDG-PET can reveal distant metastases in the bones, liver, and chest within the large field-of-view with high sensitivity, it appears to be clinically valuable for changing the treatment regimen from aggressive curative intended locoregional treatment to palliative systemic treatment.

The role of FDG-PET in distant metastasis of NPC has recently been investigated. The results published by Yen *et al*. (2005a) showed that FDG-PET disclosed distant metastasis in 13% of NPC patients with an initial stage of M0. Advanced nodal status ($N = 3$) was the only statistically significant variable associated with development of distant metastases. The patient-based sensitivity and specificity of FDG-PET for distant metastases were 100% and 87%, respectively. Similar high sensitivity was reported in another series of 95 patients with NPC (Chang *et al*., 2004). Their results showed that 14 patients (15%) had distant metastasis, in whom 10 patients (11%) were exclusively disclosed by FDG-PET. Of these 10 patients, 8 had a single metastasis, which might reflect a low metastatic tumor burden. This study confirmed that NPC has a higher probability of occult distant metastasis at presentation than previously expected, and FDG-PET is sensitive enough to detect most of them, obviating conventional tumor staging work-up. Thus, the indication of whole-body FDG-PET is highly justified for imaging NPC with advanced nodal disease, particularly those with N3 diseases who are at greatest risk of distant metastasis (Fig. 1). However, the drawback of relatively poor specificity of FDG-PET should be recognized. A substantial number of false-positive results occurred in the lung and mediastinum, particularly in those areas, such as Taiwan, with a high incidence of tuberculosis (Chang *et al*., 2004).

A comparative study about the capability of FDG-PET and conventional skeletal scintigraphy for detecting bone metastasis of NPC has recently been published (Liu *et al*., 2006). At initial staging, the sensitivity and accuracy of FDG-PET were significantly higher than those of skeletal scintigraphy for the detection of bone metastasis (70% vs. 37%; 98% vs. 89%, respectively). Among 30 patients who were found to have bone metastasis, 11 were detected by FDG-PET rather than skeletal scintigraphy, while only one patient with a solitary rib metastasis was missed by FDG-PET but was detected by skeletal scintigraphy, presumably because of the narrow marrow space that might confine the number of proliferating tumor cells at the early phase of metastasis.

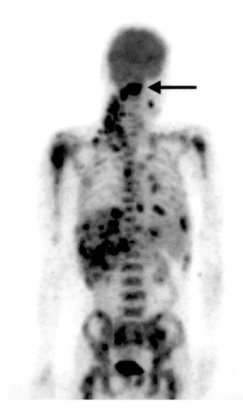

Figure 1 Nasopharyngeal carcinoma with widespread nodal, pulmonary, hepatic, and sketelal metastases. The coronal FDG-PET scan shows abnormal FDG uptake in the nasopharynx (arrow), bilateral cervical nodes, right supraclavicular nodes, lung, liver, and skeleton.

Analysis of these results showed that advanced nodal stage was the only significant risk factor for bone metastasis, and coexistence of hepatic metastasis was a prognosticator of poor survival.

Post-Treatment Tumor Evaluation

Nasopharyngeal carcinoma is highly radiosensitive, and most NPC tumors regress within 3 months following radiotherapy. A persistent tumor is defined as a tumor that does not regress completely in 6 months, and a tumor recurrence is defined as a lesion detected after a documented tumor-free period. Detection of early recurrence is important because it can result in the prompt institution of appropriate therapy.

Post-treated NPC is generally evaluated by conventional methods, including physical examination, endoscopy, CT, and MRI. Although flexible endoscopy is generally more sensitive than imaging in identifying mucosal recurrence, post-radiation mucositis, crusting, or varying degrees of trismus may hamper endoscopy. Magnetic resonance imaging, by virtue of its high contrast resolution and multiplanar capability, is superior to CT in assessing morphologic changes of NPC after irradiation. However, it still cannot reliably assess the cancer viability in post-treatment masses because the

morphological changes of tumors after therapy usually progress rather slowly. In addition, MRI cannot always help in differentiating post-radiation changes from residual/recurrent tumor (Ng *et al.*, 1999). The presence of soft tissue lesions in the irradiated nasopharynx or neck seen on MRI always poses a diagnostic question whether or not the lesion harbors viable tumor. This difficult problem is generally managed with a biopsy or by a "wait-and-see" policy with serial follow-up clinical/imaging examinations. However, biopsy of previously irradiated tissues cannot be done with impunity because it carries a significant risk of bleeding and infection, while a "wait-and-see" policy may result in the progression of disease and delay in the initiation of salvage treatment.

FDG-PET is thought to be a sensitive and specific approach for the prediction of therapeutic response because it can estimate interval functional changes that are expected to precede morphological changes. *In vitro* studies have suggested that the population size and growth rate of viable tumor cells can be reflected in FDG uptake (Higashi *et al.*, 1993). *In vivo* cellular glycolysis in malignant tissues, detected by FDG uptake, has been documented to be significantly reduced when cytotoxic treatment is effective. The histopathological response to a therapy is well correlated with the changes in FDG uptake before and after the therapy (Smith *et al.*, 2000).

Response to Radiotherapy

After radiotherapy, a rapid reduction in tumor FDG uptake generally indicates a good radiation response, whereas a persistent high tumor uptake of FDG generally suggests the presence of residual cancer. However, the time interval between the completion of therapy and FDG-PET study is important. The clinical usefulness of FDG-PET for evaluating the radiation effect in patients with NPC was first recorded by Mitsuhashi *et al.* (1998). They also found that decreased levels of FDG uptake in FDG-PET scans obtained 1–3 months after radiotherapy did not accurately reflect the status of the disease. In the early post-radiation period, inflammation caused by irradiation is usually severe and can cause more false-positive FDG-PET results. Greven *et al.* (2001) performed serial FDG-PET scans in 45 patients with head and neck cancers following completion of radiotherapy at 1 month, 4 months, 12 months, and 24 months. Most of the false-negative FDG-PET findings were found at the 1-month post-radiation scan, as the metabolic mechanism of the residual tumor tissue may be temporarily inhibited by irradiation, the so-called stunning effect. FDG-PET scans thus might be inaccurate for predicting the presence of cancer at an early post-radiation period, whereas an FDG uptake 4 months after radiotherapy could predict the response better.

In a series of 46 patients with NPC treated by radiotherapy studied by Peng *et al.* (2000), the sensitivity and specificity of FDG-PET to detect residual or recurrent lesions in patients with FDG-PET 6 months after radiation therapy were 92% and 100%, respectively, considerably higher than the overall sensitivity and specificity of 80% and 87%, respectively. They claimed that the optimal timing in assessing residual tumor or tumor recurrence in post-radiation patients should be 6 months or later. In line with these findings, the majority of false-positive FDG-PET results were found to occur during the early post-therapy period in another series of 37 patients using FDG-PET for assessing recurrent NPC (Ng et al., 2004b). Therefore, FDG-PET before 6 months from treatment should be read with caution. However, a surveillance program is designed to identify recurrent disease as soon as possible because the lower the stage at the time of diagnosis of recurrent NPC, the better the overall prognosis (Chang et al., 2000). Therefore, the 6-month interval may be too lengthy and may miss the treatment window of opportunity for salvaging early residual or recurrent disease. In clinical practice, FDG-PET is commonly performed at 4 months after completion of radiotherapy. The frequency of further follow-up FDG-PET depends on the presence of any predictors of high risk for recurrence.

Response to Chemotherapy

One promising clinical application for FDG-PET is noninvasive monitoring in patients who are treated with chemotherapy. Accurate assessment of tumor response to chemotherapy is crucial in formulating the treatment strategy as it permits effective tailoring of subsequent treatment. The nonresponders may benefit from an early switch

to alternative treatments, thereby avoiding the unnecessary side effects of chemotherapy. The usefulness of FDG-PET for monitoring for NPC after induction chemotherapy is currently being investigated. Yen et al. (2005a) studied 50 patients with locoregionally advanced NPC by FDG-PET after completion of one or two courses of chemotherapy with mitomycin, epirubicin, cisplatin, fluorouracil, and leucovorin, and documented that FDG-PET was useful for predicting both the therapeutic response and the outcome after the first or second course of induction therapy.

Re-staging FDG-PET images provided valuable information for fine tuning subsequent treatment regimens by localizing any surviving tumor cell population and concentration. Only 1 of 23 major responders subsequently developed local recurrence, while 15 of the 27 nonmajor responders had recurrent/metastatic NPC. The survival rate was significantly higher in the major responder group than in the nonmajor responder group. Treatment response between the primary tumor and metastatic lymph nodes was similar in all cases except in one woman in the nonmajor responder group, probably due to the heterogeneity of the tumors. Obviously, FDG-PET appears to have great potential for evaluating the early response of NPC to chemotherapy. However, further accumulation of data is needed before any conclusions can be drawn.

The shortcoming of FDG-PET due to poor anatomical detail restricts its role in tumor re-staging. In nonmajor responders who show persistently high FDG uptake in the primary tumor after induction chemotherapy, it is difficult to evaluate the extension of residual tumor in order to determine the T-stage precisely. However, the newly developed inte-

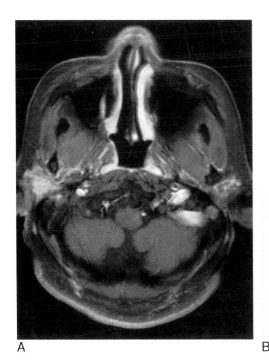

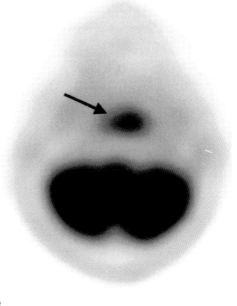

A   B

Figure 2 Residual nasopharyngeal carcinoma tumor detected by FDG-PET but missed by MRI. (A) Contrast-enhanced T1-weighted MR image shows mild mucosal thickening, falsely interpreting as post-radiation mucositis. (B) True-positive FDG-PET findings that show strong uptake in the nasopharynx (arrow). Histopathologic findings show residual cancer cells in the nasopharynx.

grated PET/CT can overcome this shortcoming and has significantly better spatial resolution, facilitating localization
and determination of the extension of focal uptake.

Residual or Recurrent Tumor

FDG-PET can identify a viable tumor on the basis of
higher glycolytic rates in neoplasms than in necrotic or reactive tissues. It has great potential in detecting recurrent NPC
when the MRI findings are questionable (Fig. 2). High efficacy of FDG-PET in the detection of locally recurrent NPC
was demonstrated in several studies (Kao *et al.*, 1998; Tsai
et al., 2002; Yen *et al.*, 2003), in which the sensitivity was
consistently 100%, whereas the specificity ranged from 92
to 96%. Yen *et al.* (2005b) also demonstrated that the presence of FDG hypermetabolism was significantly correlated
with the survival time of recurrent NPC patients. Despite
these encouraging results of FDG-PET, it is unlikely that
small recurrent NPC can be completely excluded by FDG-
PET alone. In one series of 37 NPC patients in whom post-
treatment MRI showed questionable findings for recurrence
(Ng *et al.*, 2004b), FDG-PET showed 1 false negative and 6
false positives at primary sites, resulting in a sensitivity of
92% and a specificity of 76%. The single false negative was
due to small tumor recurrence at the nasopharyngeal mucosa,
indicating that continued clinical follow-up of patients with
negative FDG-PET is mandatory and FDG-PET should not
obviate regular endoscopic examination with biopsy. The
false positives were mostly related to the radiation-induced
inflammation. Indeed, specificity of FDG-PET for recurrent
NPC may also be related to the initial T-stage of the patients
and the treatment mode of radiotherapy they received.

A recent comparative study of FDG-PET and MRI showed
that FDG-PET had significantly higher specificity than that
by MRI in detecting residual tumors among NPC patients
with advanced disease, but the reverse occurred among
those with T_{1-2} tumor treated with intracavitary brachytherapy (Chan *et al.*, 2006). Intracavitary brachytherapy boost
after completion of external radiotherapy may improve local
control in patients with T_{1-2} tumor but may complicate with
severe mucositis, ulceration, or necrosis in the nasopharynx.
Thus, FDG-PET seems to be superior to MRI in the identification of treatment response in NPC patients with initial
advanced T-stage, but may be limited in evaluation of those
patients who had initial early T-stage tumor and had received
intracavitary brachytherapy.

Nodal recurrence of NPC can occur in isolation or be associated with local or distant recurrences. FDG-PET should be
a sensitive tool in detecting residual or recurrent nodes in
NPC. In the study by Ng *et al.* (2004b), the sensitivity and
specificity of FDG-PET have been reported to be 90% and
89%, respectively. It was particularly useful in disclosing
clinically unexpected metastatic adenopathy. However, one

false-negative result due to small cervical nodes of 0.5-cm
diameter and 3 false-positive results due to reactive hyperplasia were also found. Therefore, further confirmatory procedures should be pursued to avoid understaging or overstaging
of recurrent disease.

Recurrent NPC may be manifested as distant metastasis
alone or with locoregional recurrence. Because FDG-PET
can easily scan the whole body, it can disclose unexpected
tumor recurrence outside the head and neck region. This
method can detect distant recurrence of NPC with high sensitivity (Ng *et al.*, 2004b). However, the distant site FDG
uptake must be viewed with caution, as three of the eight
FDG-PET positive scans in this series were false positives,
including granulomatous axillary adenitis, reactive mediastinal nodal hyperplasia, and a posttraumatic effect in
the humerus, respectively. In addition, FDG-PET underestimated the number of lung metastases in one case due to
small tumor size. Despite a considerable false-positive rate,
FDG-PET is of clinical value if it averts the aggressive salvage treatment of recurrent NPC by early detection of concomitant distant metastases.

The results published by Yen *et al.* (2005a) showed that
FDG-PET was able to change treatment regimen by revelation of distant metastasis in 18% (4/22) of patients with recurrent NPC. In another study by Yen *et al.* (2005b), FDG-PET
missed two distant metastases. One false-negative finding
in the lung was presumably due to small size of the lesion
beyond the detection threshold of FDG-PET scanner, while
the other false-negative findings in the pericardium were
plausibly explained by the fact that intense FDG uptake in the
contiguous myocardium interfered with abnormal pericardial
metabolism. This indicates that a conventional cross-sectional
imaging examination is still needed in order to exclude the
small metastatic foci in the lung or elsewhere contiguous to
normal organs with vivid physiological FDG uptake.

The published data (Ng *et al.*, 2004b) showed that the
overall sensitivity of FDG-PET was high but that the specificity was only moderate for detecting recurrent NPC. The
high sensitivity to residual or recurrent disease is very useful
in aiding early detection, because it enables the timely institution of appropriate management. When FDG-PET results
are negative, the probability of having residual/recurrent
disease is very low. The moderate specificity may be associated with additional costs of an unnecessary conventional
cross-sectional imaging or biopsy; the clinician should be
well aware of this problem.

The clinical implications of FDG-PET in NPC patients in
whom MRI findings are questionable for recurrence have been
reported (Ng *et al.*, 2004b). FDG-PET provided useful information in about half of such patients by exclusion of viable
tumors, revealing unexpected small metastatic lymphadenopathy and disclosing distant metastatic foci. On the other hand,
FDG-PET provided no additional significant information in a
quarter of the patients and even caused additional perplexity of

the patients or extra cost of the confirmatory examinations in the remaining quarter due to false-positive and false-negative findings. To determine the optimized utilization of FDG-PET in the post-treatment surveillance of NPC patients, further cost-effectiveness analysis of FDG-PET in combination with conventional management is warranted.

Are SUV quantification and dual-phase technique necessary in the post-treatment FDG-PET scanning? Ng et al. (2004b) used SUV as an accessory reference to assist visual interpretation in differentiating residual/recurrent NPC from post-radiation change. The mean SUV of the true positive lesions at the primary site was significantly higher than that of the false-positive lesions, suggesting that SUV might be of clinical benefit in lesion discrimination. However, it should be noted that both true-positive and false-positive uptakes had a wide range of SUV values that partially overlap with each other. Thus, their differentiation could not entirely be based on a single SUV figure on a lesion-by-lesion basis. The clinical usefulness of SUV quantification at the regional lymph nodes and the distant sites was small because the difference of SUVs between true-positive and false-positive lesions was statistically insignificant. A dual-phase technique with scanning at 40 min and 3 hr was also performed in an attempt to enhance the diagnostic accuracy of visual interpretation of FDG-PET in the detection of recurrent NPC. However, it appeared to be unhelpful in such treated NPC patients and might even result in more false positives. Indeed, more data are needed to determine the optimal cut-off level of FDG uptake and the optimal time of dual-phase technique for better differentiation between tumor recurrence and treatment-induced inflammation.

Radiation-Induced Complications

Radiation-induced complications may occur in NPC patients after radiotherapy, including cerebral or spinal cord necrosis, cranial nerve paralysis, masticator space fibrosis, osteoradionecrosis, and radiation-associated tumor. Magnetic resonance imaging plays an important role in detecting post-radiation complications of NPC, but it has limitations in distinguishing osteoradionecrosis from skull base recurrence. FDG-PET has been thought to be helpful in differentiation between these two entities; however, false-positive results with high SUV did occur (Liu et al., 2004; Hung et al., 2005). Therefore, the positive FDG-PET findings in the skull base of NPC patients after irradiation should be read with caution, and histological proof is still needed to decide further management.

Conclusion

FDG-PET is a unique imaging modality for functional evaluation of NPC. However, because of its inherent relatively poor anatomic resolution, it is generally used in conjunction with conventional cross-sectional imaging rather than in isolation. FDG-PET has a role in accurate mapping of nodal spread and in delineating tumor-bearing tissue for the planning of conformal radiotherapy. By virtue of its high sensitivity in disclosing unexpected distant metastasis, FDG-PET is most feasible in NPC patients with advanced nodal stage.

In the surveillance of NPC after treatment, FDG-PET facilitates the identification of viable tumors within the fibrotic areas in the irradiated field. FDG-PET is more effective when performed about 4 months after completion of radiotherapy in order to minimize false negatives due to the "stunning" effect in the early radiotherapy period and false positives due to transient tracer accumulation in acute reactive tissues. Regardless of whether early changes in the tracer uptake of NPC after radiotherapy can predict the treatment response, rapid changes in tumor FDG uptake after the first or second course of induction chemotherapy correlate well with treatment response and prognosis.

For the detection of recurrent NPC, FDG-PET has high sensitivity but only moderate specificity. Questionable MRI or CT findings for tumor recurrence can better be characterized after FDG-PET scan. A negative FDG-PET scan virtually, though not absolutely, excludes gross tumor recurrence. However, positive FDG-PET findings may be due to recurrent tumor or post-treatment inflammation. Osteoradionecrosis and postbrachytherapy mucositis may mimic tumor recurrence. Thus, positive FDG uptakes should be viewed with caution, and histopathological confirmation should be performed whenever possible before further treatment strategy starts. SUV can be used as an accessory reference to assist visual interpretation in differentiating residual/recurrent NPC at the primary site from post-radiation changes. This might not be so for the nodal and distant sites. Dual-phase technique with scanning at 40 min and 3 hr appears to give no further advantage over the conventional single-phase technique. Recently, integrated PET/CT scanner has become available, which can provide accurately fused functional PET and morphological CT data in a single examination session. Initial studies evaluating this new imaging tool show promising results in staging oncological diseases when compared with FDG-PET alone. Whether PET/CT can be employed as a first-line imaging modality for NPC warrants further investigation.

References

Chan, S.C., Ng, S.H., Yen, T.C., Chang J.T., and Chen, T.M. 2005. False-positive findings on F-18 fluoro-2-deoxy-D-glucose positron emission tomography in a patient with nasopharyngeal carcinoma and extensive sinusitis. Clin. Nucl. Med. 30:62–63.

Chan, S.C., Ng, S.H., Chang, J.T., Chen, Y.C., Lin, C.Y., Chang, Y.C., Hsu, C.L., Wang, H.M., Liao, C.T., Wu, Y.F., and Yen, T.C. 2006. Advantages and pitfalls of PET in detecting residual or recurrent nasopharyngeal carcinoma: comparison with MRI. Eur. J. Nucl. Med. Mol. Imaging 33:1032–1040.

Chang, J.T., See, L.C., Liao, C.T., Ng, S.H., Wang, C.H., Chen, I.H., Tsang, N.M., Tseng, C.K., Tang, S.G., and Hong, J.H. 2000. Locally recurrent nasopharyngeal carcinoma. *Radiotherapy Oncol. 54*:135–142.

Chang, T.C., Chan, S.C., Yen, T.C., Liao, C.T., Lin, C.Y., Lin, K.J., Chen, I.H., Wang, H.M., Chen, T.M., and Ng, S.H. 2004. Nasopharyngeal carcinoma staging by (18) F-fluorodeoxyglucose positron emission tomography. *Int. J. Radiat. Oncol. Biol. Phys. 62*:501–507.

Greven, K.M., Williams, D.W., III, McGuirt, W.F., Harkness, B.A., D'Agostion, R.B., Keyes, J.W., Jr, and Watson, N.E., Jr. 2001. Serial positron emission tomography scans following radiation therapy of patients with head and neck cancer. *Head Neck 23*:942–946.

Higashi, K., Anaira, C.C., and Wahl, R.L. 1993. Does FDG uptake measure proliferative activity of human cancer cells? *In vitro* comparison with DNA flow cytometry and tritiated thymidine uptake. *J. Nucl. Med. 34*:414–419.

Hung, G.U., Tasi, S.C., and Lin, W.Y. 2005. Extraordinarily high F-18 FDG uptake caused by radiation necrosis in a patient with nasopharyngeal carcinoma. *Clin. Nucl. Med. 30*:558–559.

Hustinx, R., Smith, R.J., Benard, F., Rosenthal, D.I., Machtay, M., Farber, L.A., and Alavi, A. 1999. Dual time point fluorine-18 fluorodeoxyglucose positron emission tomography: a potential method to differentiate malignancy from inflammation and normal tissue in the head and neck. *Eur. J. Nucl. Med. 26*:1345–1348.

Kao, C.H., ChangLai, S.P., Chieng, P.U., Yen, R.F., and Yen, T.C. 1998. Detection of recurrent or persistent nasopharyngeal carcinomas after radiotherapy with 18F-2-fluoro-2-deoxyglucose positron emission tomography and comparison with computed tomography. *J. Clin. Oncol. 16*:3550–3555.

Kao, C.H., Hsieh, J.F., Tsai, S.C., Ho, Y.J., Yen, R.F., ChangLai, S.P., and Chieng, P.U. 2000. Comparison of 18F-2-fluoro-2-deoxyglucose positron emission tomography and computed tomography in detection of cervical lymph node metastases of nasopharyngeal carcinoma. *Ann. Otol. Rhinol. Laryngol. 109*:1130–1134.

Kao, C.H., Shiau, Y.C., Shen, Y.Y., and Yen, R.F. 2002. Detection of recurrent or persistent nasopharyngeal carcinomas after radiotherapy with Technetium-99m methoxyisobutylisonitrile single photon emission computed tomography and computed tomography: comparison with 18-fluoro-2-deoxyglucose positron emission tomography. *Cancer 94*:1981–1986.

King, A.D., Ahuja, A.T., Leung, S.F., Lam, W.W., Teo, P., Chan, Y.L., and Metreweli, C. 2000. Neck node metastases from nasopharyngeal carcinoma: MRI of patterns of disease. *Head Neck 22*:275–281.

Lapela, M., Grenman, R., Kurki, T., Joensuu, H., Leskinen, S., Lindholm, P., Haaparanta, M., Ruotsalainen, U., and Minn, H. 1995. Head and neck cancer: detection of recurrence with PET and 2-[F-18] fluoro-2-deoxy-D-glucose. *Radiology 197*:205–211.

Lee, A.W., Poon, Y.F., Foo, W., Law, S.C., Cheung, F.K., Chan, D.K., Tung, S.Y., Thaw, M., and Ho, J.H. 1992. Retrospective analysis of 5037 patients with nasopharyngeal carcinoma treated during 1976–1986: overall survival and patterns of failure. *Int. J. Radiat. Oncol. Biol. Phys. 23*:261–270.

Liu, F.Y., Chang, J.T., Wang, H.M., Liao, C.T., Ng, S.H., and Yen, T.C. 2006. 18F-FDG PET is more sensitive than skeletal scintigraphy for detecting bone metastasis in endemic nasopharyngeal carcinoma at initial staging. *J. Clin. Oncol. 24*:599–604.

Liu, S.H., Chang, J.T., Ng, S.H., Chan, S.C., and Yen, T.C. 2004. False positive fluorine-18 fluorodeoxy-D-glucose positron emission tomography finding caused by osteoradionecrosis in nasopharyngeal carcinoma patient. *Brit. J. Radiol. 77*:257–260.

Mitsuhashi, N., Hayakawa, K., Hasegawa, M., Furuta, M., Katano, S., Sakurai, H., Akimoto, T., Takahashi, T., Nasu, S., and Niibe, H. 1998. Clinical FDG-PET in diagnosis and evaluation of radiation response of patients with nasopharyngeal tumor. *Anticancer Res. 18*:2827–2832.

Ng, S.H., Chang, T.C., Ko, S.F., Yen, P.S., Wan, Y.L., Tang, L.M., and Tsai, M.H. 1997. Nasopharyngeal carcinoma: MRI and CT assessment. *Neuroradiology 39*:741–746.

Ng, S.H., Chang, T.C., Ko, S.F., Wan, Y.L., Tang, L.M., and Chan, M.C. 1999. MRI in recurrent nasopharyngeal carcinoma. *Neuroradiology 41*:855–862.

Ng, S.H., Liu, H.M., Ko, S.F., Hao, S.P., and Chong, V.F. 2002. Posttreatment imaging of the nasopharynx. *Eur. J. Radiol. 44*:82–95.

Ng, S.H., Chang, J.T.C., Chan, S.C., Ko, S.F., Wang, H.M., Liao, C.T., Chang ,Y.C., and Yen, T.C. 2004a. Nodal metastases of nasopharyngeal carcinoma: patterns of disease on MRI and FDG PET. *Eur. J. Nucl. Med. Mol. Imaging 31*:1073–1080.

Ng, S.H., Chang, T.C., Chan, S.C., Ko, S.F., Wang, H.M., Liao, C.T., Chang, Y.C., Lin, W.J., and Yen, T.C. 2004b. Clinical usefulness of FDG PET in nasopharyngeal carcinoma patients with questionable MRI findings for recurrence. *J. Nucl. Med. 45*:1669–1676.

Nishioka, T., Shiga, T., Shirato, H., Tsukamoto, E., Tsuchiya, K., Kato, T., Ohmori, K., Yamazaki, A., Aoyama, H., Hashimoto, S., Chang, T.C., and Miyasaka, K. 2002. Image fusion between 18FDG-PET and MRI/CT for radiotherapy planning of oropharyngeal and nasopharyngeal carcinomas. *Int. J. Oncology Biol. Phys. 53*:1052–1057.

Peng, N., Yen, S., Liu, W., Tsay, D., and Liu, R. 2000. Evaluation of the effect of radiation therapy to nasopharyngeal carcinoma by positron emission tomography with 2-F-[18]-fluoro-2-deoxy-D-glucose. *Clin. Positron. Imaging 3*:51–56.

Smith, I.C., Welch, A.E., Hutcheon, A.W., Miller, I.D., Payne, S., Chilcott, F., Waikar, S., Whitaker, T., Ah-See, A.K., Eremin, O., Heys, S.D., Gilbert, F.J., and Sharp, P.F. 2000. Positron tomography using [18F]-fluorodeoxy-D-glucose to predict the pathologic response of breast cancer to primary chemotherapy. *J. Clin. Oncol. 18*:1679–1688.

Teo, P.M., Kwan, W.H., Lee, W.Y., Leung, S.F., and Johnson, P.J. 1996. Prognosticators determining survival subsequent to distant metastasis from nasopharyngeal carcinoma. *Cancer 77*:2423–2431.

Tsai, M.H., Shiau, Y.C., Kao, C.H., Shen, Y.Y., Lin, C.C., and Lee, C.C. 2002. Detection of recurrent nasopharyngeal carcinomas with positron emission tomography using 18-fluoro-2-deoxyglucose in patients with indeterminate MRI findings after radiotherapy. *J. Cancer Res. Clin. Oncol. 128*:279–282.

Tsai, M.H., Huang, W.S., Tsai, J.J., Chen, Y.K., Changlai, S.P., and Kao, C.H. 2003. Differentiating recurrent or residual nasopharyngeal carcinomas from post-radiotherapy changes with 18-fluoro-2-deoxyglucose positron emission tomography and thallium-201 single photon emission computed tomography in patients with indeterminate computed tomography findings. *Anticancer Res. 23*:3513–3516.

van den Brekel, M.W., Stel, H.V., Castelijns, J.A., Nauta, J.J., van der Waal, I., Valk, J., Meyer, C.J., and Snow, G.B. 1990. Cervical lymph node metastasis: assessment of radiologic criteria. *Radiology 177*:379–384.

Yen, R.F., Hung, R.L., Pan, M.H., Wang, Y.H., Huang, K.M., Lui, L.T., and Kao, C.H. 2003. FDG PET in detecting residual/recurrent NPC and comparison with MRI. *Cancer 98*:283–287.

Yen, R.F., Chen, T.H., Ting, L.L., Tzen, K.Y., Pan, M.H,. and Hong, R.L. 2005a. Early restaging whole-body (18)F-FDG PET during induction chemotherapy predicts clinical outcome in patients with locoregionally advanced nasopharyngeal carcinoma. *Eur. J. Nucl. Med. Mol. Imaging 32*:1152–1159.

Yen, R.F., Hong, R.L., Tzen, K.Y., Pan, M.H., and Chen, T.H. 2005b. Whole-body 18F-FDG PET in recurrent or metastatic nasopharyngeal carcinoma. *J. Nucl. Med. 46*:770–774.

Yen, T.C., Chang, J.T., Ng, S.H., Chang, Y.C., Chan, S.C., Lin, K.J., and Lin, C.Y. 2005c. The value of 18F-FDG PET in the detection of stage M0 carcinoma of the nasopharynx. *J. Nucl. Med. 46*:405–410.

Yen, T.C., Chang, Y.C., Chan, S.C., Chang, T.C., Hsu, C.H., Lin, K.J., Lin, W.J., Fu, Y.K., and Ng, S.H. 2005d. Are dual-phase 18F-FDG PET scans necessary in nasopharyngeal carcinoma to assess the primary tumour and loco-regional nodes? *Eur. J. Nucl. Med. Mol. Imaging 32*:541–548.

31

Nasopharyngeal Carcinoma for Staging and Re-Staging with ^{18}F-FDG-PET/CT

Yen-Kung Chen

Introduction

The epidemiology of nasopharyngeal carcinoma (NPC) suggests multiple determinants including diet, viral agents, and genetic susceptibility. Endemic areas include Southern China, North Africa, and regions within the far Northern Hemisphere. The World Health Organization has divided NPC into three types: type 1, keratinizing squamous cell carcinoma; type 2, nonkeratinizing carcinoma; and type 3, the undifferentiated carcinoma. Type 3 is the most frequently identified neoplasm. It characteristically is associated with a lymphoid infiltrate that accounts for its more familiar description, lymphoepithelioma. Additional cancer types noted include lymphoma, juvenile angiofibroma, plasmacytoma, and adenocarcinomas. Adenocarcinomas are of minor salivary gland origin.

The nasopharyngeal cavity is the uppermost part of the aerodigestive tract. The nasopharynx is a cuboidal structure covered by stratified mucociliary columnar epithelium. Anteriorly, it is in continuity with the nasal cavity by way of the posterior choanae. The roof is downward sloping and is formed cranially to caudally by the basisphenoid, the basiocciput, and the anterior aspect of the first two cervical vertebrae. The lateral walls of the nasopharynx contain the eustachian tube openings, which lie within the elevations of the torus tubarii. Behind the torus is the lateral pharyngeal recess or fossa of Rosenmüller, which is the most common site of NPC development. The floor of the nasopharynx is the upper surface of the soft palate. Lymphatic drainage from the nasopharynx encompasses all levels within the neck as it proceeds along the jugular vein and spinal accessory nerve. Extensive lymphatics within the nasopharynx also drain into the retropharyngeal nodes medial to the carotid artery. Involvement of these nodes can rarely be detected clinically. Radiologic assessment, either PET/CT or magnetic resonance imaging (MRI), is the most sensitive diagnostic technique for detecting retropharyngeal node enlargement.

Nasopharyngeal carcinoma grows either by infiltration or by expansion with the former growth pattern predominating. Mucosal abnormalities frequently reflect only a small portion of tumor extent. On occasion, no abnormalities of the mucosa are identifiable. In such instances, tumors may exist submucosally and extend into sites outside the confines of the nasopharynx. The most common presenting complaint of NPC is a mass in the neck occurring in ~ 90% of patients. Additional frequently encountered symptoms include alterations in hearing associated with serous otitis media, tinnitus, nasal obstruction, and pain. Patients may present with symptoms that reflect growth of the disease into the many significant surrounding anatomic structures. Tumors can access the parapharyngeal space through the sinus of Morgagni, an opening in the lateral nasopharyngeal wall through which the eustachian tube courses. Infiltration laterally into paranasopharyngeal space may lead to pterygoid muscle involvement and trismus. Frequently, cranial nerve involvement is manifested with more extensive growth into the skull base. Under such circumstances growth into the cavernous sinus can lead to impairment of cranial nerves II to VI. In addition, cancer may break through the pharyngobasilar fascia and spread along vascular sheaths. Disease extending along these planes may also extend within the skull base and lead to cranial nerve involvement.

Methods: Positron Emission Tomography/Computed Tomography Imaging Protocol

Our PET center was opened in February 2001 with a Siemens (ECAT EXACT HR+, model 962, Knoxville, Tennessee) whole-body scanner and a GE minitrace cyclotron. The second scanner, a PET-CT system (Discovery LS, GE Medical Systems, Waukesha, Wisconsin), was added to the center in March 2002. Patients were required to fast for at least 8 hr before the PET scan. Furthermore, they had to be well hydrated, and they were instructed to avoid strenuous work or exercise for 24 hr before the scan. They were scanned in as many sequential images as necessary to include the entire head, thorax, abdomen, and pelvis. Transmission images were obtained for 2 min per bed position to correct for photon attenuation using a germanium 68 line source. In the PET/CT scanner, the PET attenuation correction factors were calculated from the CT images. Computed tomography was performed using a multidetector helical CT scanner. Acquisitions occurred at 5–7 bed positions and had the following parameters: 140 kV, 40 mA, 0.8 s per CT rotation, a pitch of 6, a table speed of 22.5 mm/s, coverage of 722.5–1011.5 mm, and an acquisition time of 31.9–37 sec. Computed tomography was performed before the emission acquisition. Computed tomography data were resized from a 512×512 matrix to a 128×128 matrix to match the PET data so that the images could be fused and CT transmission maps generated. The transaxial resolution (full width at half maximum) of PET and PET/CT were 4.58 mm and 4.8 mm, respectively. After intravenous administration of 370 MBq (10 mCi) of 2-[Fluorine-18]fluoro-2-deoxy-D-glucose (FDG), emission images were acquired for 5 min per bed position. The uptake period between the FDG injection and the beginning of the emission scan was 60 plus/minus 10 min (range 50 to 70). Accurate positioning of the patient between transmission and emission scans was performed using laser marks. With the use of camera-based PET/CT, acquisition of FDG and low-dose CT were both performed during normal breathing. Image data sets were obtained using iterative reconstruction (ordered-subset expectation maximization method). The standardized uptake value (SUV) is calculated as follows: SUV = (mean ROI activity in mCi/ml) / (injected dose in mCi/patient's weight in kg).

Results and Discussion

Normal FDG Distribution Patterns in the Head and Neck

To interpret PET images accurately, it is essential to be fully familiar with the normal patterns, intensities, and frequencies of 2-[Fluorine-18]fluoro-2-deoxy-D-glucose (FDG) distribution in the head and neck area. Combined PET/CT scanners enable a highly precise localization of the metabolic abnormalities seen on PET.

At the nasopharyngeal level of the border between the hard and soft palates, the inferior concha generally shows low-uptake activity (mean SUV 1.56 ± 0.37). The uptake in the parotid glands is variable (mean SUV 1.90 ± 0.68). In 14% of the patients, intense FDG uptake is seen in the parotid glands without specific symptoms (Nakamoto et al., 2005). The uptake in the lateral pharyngeal recess of the bilateral nasopharynx shows no or mild FDG uptake (mean SUV 1.36 ± 0.28). Then, symmetrical increased or intense FDG uptake is seen without symptoms of lymphoid hyperplasia or inflammatory process. The adenoids, or pharyngeal tonsils, are lymphatic tissue located in the midline roof of the nasopharynx. Prominent adenoids are typically present in children, and the maximal size of the adenoids occurs at ~ 5 years of age. Gradual adenoidal involution normally begins near the time of puberty. However, normal adenoidal tissue may occasionally be seen in adults in their fourth, fifth, and even sixth decade of life. If such a nasopharyngeal mass is seen in an older patient, clinical correlation should be sought.

Intense FDG uptake (mean SUV 3.13 ± 0.78) is observed at the oropharyngeal level of the soft palate in 72% of the patients. The palatine and lingual tonsils also commonly show intense FDG uptake, which is seen in 80% and 74% of the patients, respectively. The mean SUV is 3.48 ± 1.30 for the palatine tonsils and 3.1 ± 1.06 for the lingual tonsils. In contrast, the tongue has no or mild accumulation of FDG in 99% of the patients. The palatine tonsils are usually largest in individuals aged 5–7 years; then they typically become smaller with age. Thus, for the palatine tonsils, the time course of involution of physiologic tonsilar size may partly explain the results.

At the hypopharyngeal level, the mean SUV is 2.11 ± 0.57 for the submandibular glands and 2.93 ± 1.39 for the sublingual glands, respectively. The vocal cords and thyroid gland show no or mild uptake; the mean SUV is 1.77 ± 0.69 and 1.3 ± 0.30, respectively. Occasionally, differentiation between normal and abnormal FDG uptake may be difficult on PET alone; therefore, PET/CT may be valuable in such situations by accurately localizing increased FDG uptake.

Primary Tumors

Small tumors in the nasopharynx seldom result in symptoms, and are clinically inaccessible; hence, prompt diagnosis is difficult. In addition, primary malignancies of the nasopharynx are often understaged by clinical examination. Five percent of patients with head and neck squamous cell carcinoma are present with metastatic cervical nodes without an identifiable primary site at clinical examination. 2-[Fluorine-18]fluoro-2-deoxy-D-glucose-positron emission tomography has been shown to be able to reveal unknown primary tumors in ~ 30–50% of patients who had metastatic disease to the lymph nodes in the neck and no detectable primary tumor at clinical examination (AAssar et al., 1999). However, in FDG-PET images, tumor size may be overestimated due to the scatter phenomenon of radiation. Also, intense FDG uptake may obscure the uptake by adjacent enlarged lymph nodes, thereby resulting in false-negative results. In our study of using PET/CT on 20 newly diagnosed NPC patients for primary tumor staging, five patients were found with primary tumor of nasopharynx in the absence of FDG uptake. In 5 out of 20 patients, no definite mucosal change of nasopharynx was found in their CT images. In 3 out of 20 patients, intense FDG uptakes without mucosal change in the nasopharynx were observed. In addition, 3 out of 20 patients showed mucosal thickening without FDG uptake in the nasopharynx. Finally, in 2 out of 20 patients, no FDG uptake and mucosa change were found in the nasopharynx. This study suggests that CT and PET are complementary for the initial evaluation. Positron emission tomography, however, is more efficient for the evaluation of treatment efficiency and detection of relapses. Therefore, the combination of PET/CT is a more accurate tumor staging tool than PET or CT alone (Schoder et al., 2004; Rusthoven et al., 2005; Branstetter et al., 2005).

Accurate diagnosis of tumor extent is important in three-dimensional conformal radiotherapy. Fusion images of FDG-PET and MRI/CT may provide for better target delineation in radiotherapy planning of head and neck cancers. Gross tumor volume (GTV) is commonly determined based on clinical examination and FDG uptake on the fusion images. Clinical target volume (CTV) is determined following the usual pattern of lymph node spread for each disease entity, along with the clinical presentation of each patient. The preliminary study shows that image fusion of FDG-PET and MRI/CT is useful in GTV and CTV determination in conformal radiotherapy, thus sparing normal tissues (Nishioka et al., 2002; Rusthoven et al., 2005).

False-negative results with FDG-PET/CT may occur in the following conditions: (1) early scan performed shortly after completion of chemotherapy or radiation therapy;

(2) malignancy present in structures with a physiologically elevated metabolism; (3) tumor size below the resolution of current PET/CT scanner; and (4) tumor with low cell density or low metabolic rate of FDG. Delayed view with a prolonged emission time may be helpful in detecting tumors and avoiding false-negative results (Chen and Kao, 2005).

In general, false-positive results may occur on FDG-PET because of infections; physiologically increased uptake in structures such as tonsils, salivary glands, and muscles; uptake in reactive nonneoplastic lymph nodes; and, if after recent surgery, noninfectious inflammation and granulation at the surgical site (Nakamoto et al., 2005). The major advantage of CT is its help in correctly differentiating physiologic uptake that would otherwise be mistaken for tumor on PET alone. Co-registered images with FDG-PET/CT allow direct correlation between FDG metabolic uptake and anatomic structures thus reducing false-positive results. Standardized uptake values (SUVs) may be useful in distinguishing between malignant and benign FDG uptake. However, there is an overlapping zone between them. Therefore, it is important to evaluate patients' clinical history and physical findings to make an accurate distinction between benign and malignant condition. The superiority of PET/CT to whole-body MRI in overall Tumor Node Metastases (TNM) staging (Antoch et al., 2003) supports the usefulness of FDG-PET/CT as a possible first-line modality for whole-body tumor staging.

Nodal Metastases of Nasopharyngeal Carcinoma

The patterns of nodal spread of NPC have an important influence on treatment planning. In the literature, 60 to 90% of patients have nodal spread at the time of initial diagnosis, and nearly 50 to 80% of patients have bilateral disease (Ng et al., 2004). The presence of lymph node enlargement, however, has no relationship to the size of the primary tumor. Retropharyngeal nodes (Fig. 1) have been reported to be the first-echelon nodes for NPC, with involvement in 94% of patients with nodal metastases (King et al., 2000). However, other findings show that the retropharyngeal nodes are involved in 64 to 82% of the NPC patients with nodal metastases (Sun et al., 2004; Ng et al., 2004). In general, nodal metastases principally affect level II (upper jugular) nodes, from which lymphatic spread extends down in an orderly manner to involve level III (middle jugular), level IV (lower jugular), and the supraclavicular fossa nodes, or extended posteriorly to involve level V nodes. Using the posterior edge of the sternocleidomastoid muscle as the cut-off line, nodes lying anteriorly are categorized as internal jugular nodes (levels II, III, or IV), while those situated posteriorly are categorized as level V nodes. The frequency of skip metastases

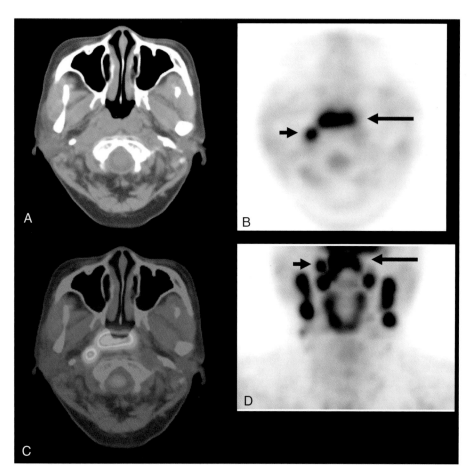

Figure 1 A 71-year-old woman with newly diagnosed NPC underwent PET/CT scan for staging. Transverse CT (**A**), PET (**B**), fused PET/CT (**C**), and PET maximal intensity projection (**D**) images of the head and neck structures and metabolism are showed. Increased FDG uptakes in the primary tumor (long arrow), right retropharyngeal (short arrow), and bilateral neck lymph nodes in the transaxial (B) and projection (D) images are observed.

is 2.3 to 7.9%. Distant spread to mediastinal or abdominal nodes is found in 3–5% of patients, usually in association with supraclavicular nodal metastases. Level I nodes and occipital nodes typically become affected only after alteration of the primary lymphatic drainage, as found following radiation therapy.

2-[Fluorine-18]fluoro-2-deoxy-D-glucose-positron emission tomography is superior to CT or MRI for detecting cervical lymph nodal metastases (Kao *et al.*, 2000; Nishioka *et al.*, 2002). The diagnostic accuracy of FDG-PET for detecting regional lymph node metastases is superior to that of conventional modalities, with a sensitivity and a specificity of up to 90% and 94%, respectively, compared with CT values of up to 82% and 85%, respectively, and MRI values of up to 88% and 79% (Adams *et al.*, 1998; Kau *et al.*, 1999). However, FDG-PET has poor anatomical resolution and cannot accurately assess lymph node size. Although PET is better for the assessment of metastasis in lymph nodes that appear morphologically normal according to size criteria, CT is more accurate for assessing the level and size of nodes, the number of nodes in conglomerate nodal masses, and the presence of extracapsular

spread. Therefore, a combination of PET/CT is likely to result in more accurate nodal staging than that on PET or CT alone.

Distant Metastases

Nasopharyngeal carcinoma shows a high frequency of distant metastasis compared to other tumors of the head and neck. The frequency of distant spread varies between 5% and 41%, compared with 5 to 24% for other head and neck tumors. Patients with low cervical lymphadenopathy, especially in the supraclavicular fossa, have a significantly higher risk of distant metastasis. Distant metastases often are present as mediastinal lymph node metastases, while lung, bone, and liver metastases occur later in the stage of disease. Although the 5-year survival rate for overall NPC patients is high, ~ 90% of patients with distant metastases will die within 1 year. Thus, detection of distant metastases enables a different or more aggressive management. Compared to PET alone, PET/CT may provide more valuable information for judging whether the focus is metastasis and whole-body metastases of NPC (Yu *et al.*, 2004).

In one of our retrospective studies, 86 studies of FDG-PET/CT were performed on 70 patients with NPC. Each study was interpreted in three ways: PET images in the absence of CT data, CT images in the absence of PET data, and fused PET/CT images. Fused PET/CT images correctly characterized the Tumor Node Metastases system stage in 82 out of 86 studies (95.4%). Side-by-side PET and CT were found to be accurate in 71 out of 86 studies (82.6%) and 63 out of 86 studies (73.3%), respectively. Furthermore, differences between PET/CT and either PET alone or CT alone are statistically significant ($p < 0.05$). Overall, the study-based analysis of FDG-PET/CT for detecting TNM stage and restage of NPC demonstrated 48 true-positive, 2 false-negative, 34 true-negative, and 2 false-positive studies. The sensitivity, specificity, accuracy, positive-predictive value, and negative-predictive value of FDG-PET/CT studies for detecting the TNM stage and re-stage of NPC were 96%, 94.4%, 95.4%, 96%, and 94.4%, respectively.

Local Recurrence

Nasopharyngeal carcinoma is very radiosensitive, and most NPC tumors regress within 3 months after radiotherapy. A persistent tumor is defined as a tumor that does not regress completely within 6 months, and tumor recurrence is defined as a lesion detected after a documented tumor-free period. Detection of early recurrence is important because it allows for a prompt institution of appropriate therapy.

The mainstay of treatment is radiotherapy; however, post-radiotherapy changes such as edema, loss of tissue planes, fibrosis, and scarring may obscure the detection of tumor recurrence by conventional methods. Not all asymmetry of the nasopharyngeal mucosal outline, presence of mass lesions, abnormal enhancement, or unusual signal change in MRI are signs of tumor recurrence. MRI still presents some difficulty in differentiating post-radiation changes from residual or recurrent tumor (Yen *et al.*, 2003). Soft tissue seen in the irradiated nasopharynx or neck on MRI always poses a diagnostic question of whether the lesion harbors viable tumor. This difficult problem is generally managed by biopsy or by a wait-and-see policy with serial clinical or imaging follow-up examinations. However, biopsy of previously irradiated tissues cannot be done with impunity because it carries a significant risk of bleeding and infection, whereas a wait-and-see policy may result in disease progression and delayed salvage treatment. As a functional imaging technique that provides information about tissue metabolism, PET with FDG has shown extremely high sensitivity (91.6 to 100%) in the detection of recurrent NPC at the primary site by identifying regions of accelerated glucose metabolism (Tsai *et al.*, 2003; Ng *et al.*, 2004). Also, PET with FDG has proved useful in detecting recurrent NPC at nodal and distant sites (Ng *et al.*, 2004).

Published literature suggests that FDG-PET is more specific than MRI or CT in detecting residual or recurrent nodal metastasis in head and neck malignancies, with specificities ranging from 77 to 100% (Fischbein *et al.*, 1998; Wong *et al.*, 1997). On the other hand, PET has been considered to have limitations for the detecting nodal micrometastases and tiny or necrotic metastatic nodes (Fischbein *et al.*, 1998). Ng *et al.* (2004) suggest that FDG-PET has a high sensitivity, but only a moderate specificity, for detection of recurrent NPC in patients with equivocal MRI findings. However, PET/CT images may increase the specificity of recurrent NPC detection (Fig. 2).

Secondary Tumors

Primary tumor at a second site, either synchronous or metachronous, is not an unusual finding in head and neck cancer. Synchronous tumors are defined as tumors that are diagnosed within six months of each other, and metachronous tumors are tumors that are diagnosed with an interval more than six months. These lesions are usually situated in the head and neck, lung, or esophagus. Two theories have been proposed about the etiology of secondary primary tumor (SPT): (1) a single cell is transformed and through migration (for instance, through the submucosa or lymphatic system) of daughter cells gives rise to genetically related tumors with a common clonal origin; (2) the new tumor has developed from independent foci, which evolve from exposure to the same carcinogens, such as tobacco and alcohol. The second type of tumor will probably be of polyclonal origin and can develop any time after the index tumor (or may be present at the same time; see Scholes *et al.*, 1998). The aspect of a possible difference in the time period after the index tumor between the two SPT types may give clues about the clonality of the first and second tumors. To exclude the possibility that an SPT is in fact a recurrence or a metastasis, a borderline of 3 years after the index tumor may be warranted. The importance of a borderline of 3 years between the tumors for the "real" SPTs of polyclonal origin is in line with the present study. It is concluded that, conditional on an SPT-free survival of at least 3 years, a high mutagen sensitivity greatly increases the risk of developing SPT.

2-[Fluorine-18]fluoro-2-deoxy-D-glucose-positron emission tomography has shown high sensitivity not only for tumors arising in the head and neck but also for tumors in most other sites in the upper aerodigestive tract, including the lung and esophagus. The greater accuracy of whole-body PET/CT imaging may also prove useful for detection of synchronous tumors and for surveillance of metachronous lesions. In addition, FDG-PET appears to be a promising imaging modality for the detection of simultaneous tumors in head and neck cancer patients (Nishiyama *et al.*, 2005).

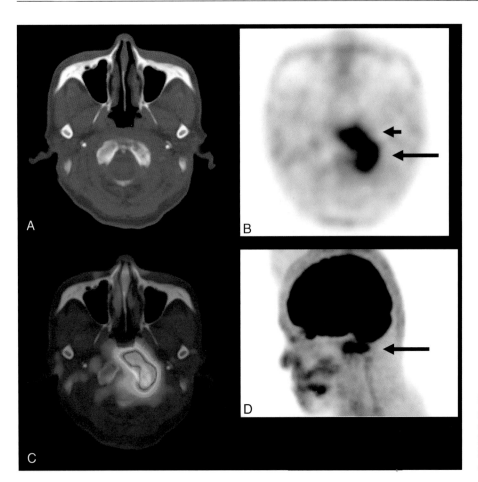

Figure 2 A 47-year-old man received radiotherapy for NPC 4 years ago and underwent PET/CT scan for recurrence detection. PET images show increased FDG uptakes in the left nasopharynx (short arrow) and C-1 level of spine (long arrow).

Unknown Primary Tumor

Squamous cell carcinoma metastatic to mediastinal and cervical lymph nodes can have a primary site in the lung, the upper portion of the esophagus, skin, thymus, anus, and head and neck region, including the larynx and pharynx. When upper and middle cervical lymph node involvement is present, the primary site usually is in the head and neck region. When the lower cervical and supraclavicular nodes are involved, lung cancer becomes a more plausible suspected primary site. However, even in these cases, of the 10 to 60% of patients in whom the primary tumor is identified, the majority of the primary tumors are in the head and neck region (Schoder and Yeung, 2004).

Nasopharyngeal carcinoma is distinct from other squamous cell tumors of the head and neck in that it shows aggressive infiltration locally and often has a high degree of regional spread at presentation, even though the primary tumor may have the appearance of a small or early lesion. In ~ 5% of cases, regional nodal metastasis is the presenting feature, and the primary tumor is not identified by standard techniques. Patients with unknown primary sites present a diagnostic and therapeutic dilemma. When no primary site can be identified, more generalized radiation therapy to include all likely sites

of origin, including the nasopharynx, oropharynx, and hypopharynx, is usually chosen. Patients with unknown primary tumors have a poor median survival of 3 to 4 months, with less than 25% of patients alive 1 year after diagnosis and less than 10% alive at 5 years (Braams *et al.*, 1997).

The usual work-up of these patients includes a complete physical examination, including triple endoscopy. Because by definition these examinations do not reveal an obvious tumor, random biopsies of multiple likely sites of origin, including tongue base, tonsils, piriform sinuses, and nasopharynx, are usually included. Biopsies performed without accompanying imaging studies typically have a yield of only ~ 10%. With the aid of CT or MR imaging, the yield may increase to ~ 20%. The reasons for these low yields are uncertain, but they probably relate to small primary tumor or a submucosal location that is not evident on direct inspection. In some cases, the primary tumor may have spontaneously regressed.

FDG-PET's good sensitivity for detecting tumors in the head and neck suggests that this technique may improve the detection rate for occult primary tumors. Following negative conventional evaluations, PET has identified the unknown primary tumors in 20–50% of cases (Safa *et al.*, 1999; AAssar *et al.*, 1999; Jungehulsing *et al.*, 2000). For negative

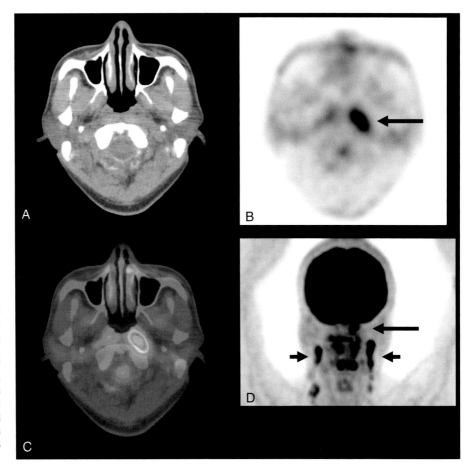

Figure 3 A 41-year-old man with bilateral neck lymphadenopathy is diagnosed with poorly differentiated squamous cell carcinoma from unknown origin and underwent PET/CT scan for primary tumor and staging. Transverse CT (**A**), PET (**B**), fused PET/CT (**C**), and PET maximal intensity projection (**D**) images of the head and neck structures and metabolism are showed. Increased FDG uptakes in the primary tumor (long arrow) and bilateral neck lymph nodes (short arrow) in the transaxial (B) and projection (D) images are observed.

PET results, tumor differentiation may be more of a limiting factor than tumor size. 2-[Fluorine-18]fluoro-2-deoxy-D-glucose consumption tends to be lower in well-differentiated tumors, as is reflected by the lower glucose metabolic rate in several types of tumors. Therefore, a small, high-grade tumor may be visualized clearly, whereas a larger, low-grade tumor may be shaded by its surrounding tissue. Recently, fused FDG-PET and CT images (Fig. 3) have increased the sensitivity of detecting carcinoma of unknown primary tumors compared to CT alone, but not to FDG-PET alone or FDG-PET and CT read side by side. Hence, accurate fusion of functional and morphologic data by FDG-PET/CT is a promising imaging modality in the clinical work-up of patients with cervical carcinoma of unknown primary tumors (Freudenberg et al., 2005).

Several reasons have been postulated for not being able to locate the primary tumor. For example, (1) spontaneous regression, (2) immune-modulated destruction of the primary cancer, (3) faster proliferation rate of the lymph node metastases, (4) removal of the primary site by sloughing of a necrotic tumor from the gastrointestinal tract, and (5) branchiogenic carcinoma mistaken for a lymph node metastasis

could also be an explanation for an unsuccessful primary search (Jungehulsing et al., 2000).

Therapy Monitoring

Most NPCs are both radio- and chemosensitive. For patients with advanced disease, induction chemotherapy followed by concurrent chemoradiotherapy has been the preferred therapeutic regimen. In the study of Klabbers et al. (2003), patients were re-staged after chemotherapy induction according to results of the PET studies. Major responders are patients who were downstaged to stage I or II, whereas nonmajor responders are patients classified as stage III or IV. The early re-staging by a single whole-body FDG-PET scan after the first or second course of induction chemotherapy is useful in detecting response to induction chemotherapy and in predicting therapy outcome for locoregionally advanced NPC patients. The nonmajor responders may benefit from early PET re-staging by switching to an alternative treatment to avoid the unnecessary side effect of chemotherapy or by fine-tuning the subsequent treatment modalities (Klabbers et al., 2003).

Conventional anatomic imaging modalities, such as CT and MRI, have only limited ability to differentiate residual or recurrent tumor from tumor necrosis and tissue fibrosis after radiotherapy. Therefore, it has been proposed that FDG-PET, a whole-body imaging technology based on glucose metabolism, can be useful to differentiate viable tumor from necrosis or fibrosis. 2-[Fluorine-18]fluoro-2-deoxy-D-glucose-positron emission tomography has a high sensitivity in detecting recurrence or residual malignancy, cervical lymph node metastases, distant metastases, and secondary primary cancer and it also has a high specificity in predicting the absence of malignancy. Yen et al. (2005) have demonstrated that there is a significant correlation between the presence of FDG hypermetabolism and the survival time of NPC patients. Tumors having high FDG uptakes are at greater risk of failure and should be considered for more aggressive multimodality therapy (Allal et al., 2004).

The outcome of locally advanced head and neck cancer often is poor. An important determinant of treatment failure is tumor hypoxia arising from an inappropriate blood supply. Quantitation of the hypoxic fraction and blood flow in vivo may provide prognostic information and a means to target specifically tumor cells resistant to conventional treatment. Tumor blood flow is measured using the $[^{15}O]H_2O$ autoradiographic technique followed by evaluation of oxygenation status using $[^{18}F]$fluoroerythronitroimidazole ($[^{18}F]$FETNIM). In addition, the PET tracer ^{18}F-fluoromisonidazole (FMISO) also allows noninvasive assessment of tumor hypoxia. High tumor blood flow predicts for a poor response to RT in the head and neck cancer. PET with $[^{15}O]H_2O$ or $[^{18}F]$FETNIM may become useful in clinical trials in which novel therapeutic agents targeting tumor vasculature or hypoxia are evaluated (Lehtio et al., 2004). The outcome after radiotherapy can be predicted on the basis of the kinetic behavior of FMISO in tumor tissue (Eschmann et al., 2005).

Radiation necrosis is the most severe form of radiation injury. Most commonly, it arises as a single lesion at the site of the original primary tumor. Other patterns include multiple lesions, lesions in the contralateral hemisphere or remote from the primary site, and subependymal lesions. As radiation necrosis progresses with tumor-like growth, white matter and cortex shrink, and brain atrophy occurs. 2-[Fluorine-18]fluoro-2-deoxy-D-glucose-positron emission tomography can be used to separate viable tumor from radiation-induced temporal lobe necrosis if radiologic findings are equivocal (Hustinx et al., 2005). There are considerably lower levels of FDG in areas of radiation-induced necrosis compared with those that have recurrent tumor. The amount of intracellular FDG is proportionate to the rate of glucose transport and intracellular phosphorylation. Malignant cells have high rates of glucose metabolism, whereas low-grade gliomas and some metastases have metabolic rates less than normal cortex. However, radiation-induced necrosis may sometimes appear hypermetabolic. Thallium 201 SPECT can also be used to separate these entities (New, 2001).

Most NPCs are both radio- and chemosensitive. Initiation of a stage-adapted therapy is known to improve patient survival for a variety of malignant tumors. Computed tomography imaging provides mainly anatomical information on the extent of primary site and regional metastases. 2-[Fluorine-18]fluoro-2-deoxy-D-glucose-positron emission tomography provides functional data on tumor metabolism. With the introduction of dual-modality PET/CT, which combined functional and structural data, FDG-PET/CT becomes a valuable imaging tool in patients for initial staging and re-staging diagnosis of NPC. The false-negative and false-positive rate may be decreased by using a combined FDG-PET/CT. The sensitivity and specificity of this dual system are better than those of PET alone. FDG-PET/CT hence is strongly recommended as a standard clinical imaging modality in the staging of NPC, and in the detection of recurrent disease after radiotherapy. In addition, FDG-PET/CT also provides valuable information in localizing primary tumor in patients with neck nodal metastases from an unknown primary tumor.

References

AAssar, O.S., Fischbein, N.J., Caputo, G.R., Kaplan, M.J., Price, D.C., Singer, M.I., Dillon, W.P., and Hawkins, R.A. 1999. Metastatic head and neck cancer: role and usefulness of FDG PET in locating occult primary tumors. Radiology 210:177–181.

Adams, S., Baum R.P., Stuckensen, T., Bitter K., and Hor, G. 1998. Prospective comparison of ^{18}F-FDG PET with conventional imaging modalities (CT, MRI, US) in lymph node staging of head and neck cancer. Eur. J. Nucl. Med. 25:1255–1260.

Allal, A.S., Slosman, D.O., Kebdani, T., Allaoua, M., Lehmann, W., and Dulguerov, P. 2004. Prediction of outcome in head-and-neck cancer patients using the standardized uptake value of 2-[^{18}F]fluoro-2-deoxy-D-glucose. Int. J. Radiat. Oncol. Biol. Phys. 59:1295–1300.

Antoch, G., Vogt, F.M., Freudenberg, L.S., Nazaradeh, F., Goehde, S.C., Barkhausen, J., Dahmen, G., Bockisch, A., Debatin, J.F., and Ruehm, S.G. 2003. Whole-body dual-modality PET/CT and whole body MRI for tumor staging in oncology. JAMA 290:3199–3206.

Braams, J.W., Pruim, J., Kole, A.C., Nikkels, P.G., Vaalburg, W., Vermey, A., and Roodenburg, J.L. 1997. Detection of unknown primary head and neck tumors by positron emission tomography. Int. J. Oral Maxillofac. Surg. 26:112–115.

Branstetter, B.F., IV, Blodgett, T.M., Zimmer, L.A., Snyderman, C.H., Johnson, J.T., Raman, S., and Meltzer, C.C. 2005. Head and neck malignancy: is PET/CT more accurate than PET or CT alone? Radiology 235:580–586.

Chen, Y.K., and Kao, C.H. 2005. Metastatic hepatic lesions are detected better by delayed imaging with prolonged emission time. Clin. Nucl. Med. 30:455–456.

Eschmann, S.M., Paulsen, F., Reimold, M., Dittmann, H., Welz, S., Reischl, G., Machulla, H.J., and Bares R. 2005. Prognostic impact of hypoxia imaging with ^{18}F-misonidazole PET in non-small cell lung cancer and head and neck cancer before radiotherapy. J. Nucl. Med. 46:253–260.

Fischbein, N.J., AAssar, O.S., Caputo, G.R., Kaplan, M.J., Singer, M.I., Price, D.C., Dillon, W.P., and Hawkins, R.A. 1998. Clinical utility of positron emission tomography with ^{18}F-fluorodeoxyglucose in detecting residual/recurrent squamous cell carcinoma of the head and neck. A.J.N.R. 19:1189–1196.

Freudenberg, L.S., Fischer, M., Antoch, G., Jentzen, W., Gutzeit, A., Rosenbaum, S.J., Bockisch, A., and Egelhof, T. 2005. Dual modality of ^{18}F-fluorodeoxy glucose-positron emission tomography/computed tomography in patients with cervical carcinoma of unknown primary. *Med. Princ. Pract. 14*:155–160.

Hustinx, R., Pourdehnad, M., Kaschten, B., and Alavi, A. 2005. PET imaging for differentiating recurrent brain tumor from radiation necrosis. *Radiol. Clin. North Am. 43*:35–47.

Jungehulsing, M., Scheidhauer, K., Damm, M., Pietrzyk, U., Eckel, H., Schicha, H., and Stennert, E. 2000. 2[F]-fluoro-2-deoxy-D-glucose positron emission tomography is a sensitive tool for the detection of occult primary cancer (carcinoma of unknown primary syndrome) with head and neck lymph node manifestation. *Otolaryngol. Head Neck Surg. 123*:294–301.

Kao, C.H., Hsieh, J.F., Tsai, S.C., Ho, Y.J., Yen, R.F., ChangLai, S.P., and Chieng, P.U. 2000. Comparison of 18-fluoro-2-deoxyglucose positron emission tomography and computed tomography in detection of cervical lymph node metastases of nasopharyngeal carcinoma. *Ann. Otol. Rhinol. Laryngol. 109*:1130–1134.

Kau, R.J., Alexiou, C., Laubenbacher, C., Werner, M., Schwaiger, M., and Arnold, W. 1999. Lymph node detection of head and neck squamous cell carcinomas by positron emission tomography with fluorodeoxy-glucose F 18 in a routine clinical setting. *Arch. Otolaryngol. Head Neck Surg. 125*:1322–1328.

King, A.D., Ahuja, A.T., Leung, S.F., Lam, W.W., Teo, P., Chan, Y.L., and Metreweli, C. 2000. Neck node metastases from nasopharyngeal carcinoma: MRI of patterns of disease. *Head Neck. 22*:275–281.

Klabbers, B.M., Lammertsma, A.A., and Slotman, B.J. 2003. The value of positron emission tomography for monitoring response to radiotherapy in head and neck cancer. *Mol. Imaging. Biol. 5*:257–270.

Lehtio, K., Eskola, O., Viljanen, T., Oikonen, V., Gronroos, T., Sillanmaki, L., Grenman, R., and Minn, H. 2004. Imaging perfusion and hypoxia with PET to predict radiotherapy response in head-and-neck cancer. *Int. J. Radiat. Oncol. Biol. Phys. 59*:971–982.

Nakamoto, Y., Tatsumi, M., Hammoud, D., Cohade, C., Osman, M.M., and Wahl, R.L. 2005. Normal FDG distribution patterns in the head and neck: PET/CT evaluation. *Radiology 234*:879–885.

New, P. 2001. Radiation injury to the nervous system. *Curr. Opin. Neurol. 14*:725–734.

Ng, S.H., Chang, J.T., Chan, S.C., Ko, S.F., Wang, H.M., Liao, C.T., Chang, Y.C., and Yen, T.C. 2004. Nodal metastases of nasopharyngeal carcinoma: patterns of disease on MRI and FDG PET. *Eur. J. Nucl. Med. Mol. Imaging 31*:1073–1080.

Ng, S.H., Joseph, C.T., Chan, S.C., Ko, S.F., Wang, H.M., Liao, C.T., Chang, Y.C., Lin, W.J., Fu, Y.K., and Yen, T.C. 2004. Clinical usefulness of ^{18}F-FDG PET in nasopharyngeal carcinoma patients with questionable MRI findings for recurrence. *J. Nucl. Med. 45*:1669–1676.

Nishioka, T., Shiga, T., Shirato, H., Tsukamoto, E., Tsuchiya, K., Kato, T., Ohmori, K., Yamazaki, A., Aoyama, H., Hashimoto, S., Chang, TC., and Miyasaka, K. 2002. Image fusion between ^{18}FDG-PET and MRI/CT for radiotherapy planning of oropharyngeal and nasopharyngeal carcinomas. *Int. J. Radiat. Oncol. Biol. Phys. 53*:1051–1057.

Nishiyama, Y., Yamamoto, Y., Yokoe, K., Miyabe, K., Ogawa, T., Toyama, Y., Satoh, K., and Ohkawa, M. 2005. FDG PET as a procedure for detecting simultaneous tumours in head and neck cancer patients. *Nucl. Med. Commun. 26*:239–244.

Rusthoven, K.E., Koshy, M., and Paulino, A.C. 2005. The role of PET-CT fusion in head and neck cancer. *Oncology (Huntington) 19*:241–253.

Safa, A.A., Tran, L.M., Rege, S., Brown, C.V., Mandelkern, M.A., Wang, M.B., Sadeghi, A., and Juillard, G. 1999. The role of positron emission tomography in occult primary head and neck cancers. *Cancer J. Sci. Am. 5*:214–218.

Schoder, H., and Yeung, H.W. 2004. Positron emission imaging of head and neck cancer, including thyroid carcinoma. *Semin. Nucl. Med. 34*: 180–197.

Schoder, H., Yeung, H.W., Gonen, M., Kraus, D., and Larson, S.M. 2004. Head and neck cancer: clinical usefulness and accuracy of PET/CT image fusion. *Radiology 231*:65–72.

Scholes, A.G., Woolgar, J.A., Boyle, M.A., Brown, J.S., Vaughan, E.D., Hart, C.A., and Jones, S.A. 1998. Synchronous oral carcinomas: independent or common origin? *Cancer Res. 58*:2003–2006.

Sun, Y., Ma, J., Lu, T.X., Wang, Y., Huang, Y., and Tang, L.L. 2004. Regulation for distribution of metastatic cervical lymph nodes of 512 cases of nasopharyngeal carcinoma. *Ai Zheng. 23*:1523–1527.

Tsai, M.H., Huang, W.S., Tsai, J.J., Chen, Y.K., Changlai, S.P., and Kao, C.H. 2003. Differentiating recurrent or residual nasopharyngeal carcinomas from post-radiotherapy changes with 18-fluoro-2-deoxyglucose positron emission tomography and thallium-201 single photon emission computed tomography in patients with indeterminate computed tomography findings. *Anticancer Res. 23*: 3513–3516.

Wong, W.L., Chevretton, E.B., McGurk, M., Hussain, K., Davis, J., Beaney, R., Baddeley, H., Tierney, P., and Maisey, M. 1997. A prospective study of PET-FDG imaging for the assessment of head and neck squamous cell carcinoma. *Clin. Otolaryngol. 22*:209–214.

Yen, R.F., Hung, R.L., Pan, M.H., Wang, Y.H., Huang, K.M., Lui, L.T., and Kao, C.H. 2003. 18-fluoro-2-deoxyglucose positron emission tomography in detecting residual/recurrent nasopharyngeal carcinomas and comparison with magnetic resonance imaging. *Cancer 98*:283–287.

Yen, R.F., Hong, R.L., Tzen, K.Y., Pan, M.H., and Chen, T.H. 2005. Whole-body ^{18}F-FDG PET in recurrent or metastatic nasopharyngeal carcinoma. *J. Nucl. Med. 46*:770–774.

Yu, D.F., Zuo, C.T., Dai, J.Z., Dong, M.J., Zhao, J., Lin, X.T., and Guan, Y.H. 2004. Application of ^{18}F-FDG PET/CT scan in following-up of nasopharyngeal carcinoma after radiotherapy. *Ai Zheng. 23*:1538–1541.

32

Ovarian Sex Cord-Stromal Tumors: Computed Tomography and Magnetic Resonance Imaging

Seung Eun Jung

Introduction

Ovarian sex cord-stromal tumors constitute a heterogeneous group of rare tumors that develop from stromal cells and primitive sex cords in the ovary. Stromal cells consist of fibroblasts, theca cells, and Leydig cells, and primitive sex cords contain granulosa cells in the normal ovary, Sertoli cells in the testis, and Sertoli cells in ovarian tumors. These tumors comprise ~ 8% of all primary ovarian neoplasms and affect all age groups. They account for most of the hormonally active ovarian tumors that show estrogenic effects or virilization (Outwater et al., 1998).

Ovarian sex cord-stromal tumors are classified as granulosa-stromal cell tumors, Sertoli-stromal tumors, and steroid cell tumors. Granulosa-stromal cell tumors include granulosa cell tumors, fibrothecoma, and sclerosing stromal tumor. Sertoli-stromal tumors consist of Sertoli-Leydig cell tumors (Jung et al., 2002). These tumors differ from the more common epithelial neoplasms in clinical and radiologic aspects. Clinically, ~ 70% of patients with these tumors are stage I lesion at presentation, whereas ~ 75% of common epithelial tumors are stage III or IV at diagnosis. Consequently, sex cord-stromal tumors are primarily treated surgically and have generally good prognosis (Jung et al., 2002). In addition, these tumors may have characteristic imaging features and differential points from more common ovarian epithelial tumors. Understanding the clinical and imaging features of ovarian sex cord-stromal tumors is helpful in specific diagnosis of ovarian tumors.

Computed tomography and magnetic resonance imaging can both provide the valuable information needed to evaluate the ovarian masses. Because MR imaging has high-contrast resolution, it allows confirmation of fat, blood, fluid, or fibrous tissue. Contrast-enhanced images are highly accurate for characterization of complex adnexal masses because of improved visualization of intratumoral configuration. Computed tomography has been used for staging and treatment planning of ovarian malignancy and is recommended for evaluating peritoneal implants. Recent advances in CT technology, with use of multiplanar reformatting, improving spatial resolution, and reduced artifact, have increased the accuracy of CT for detection and characterization of ovarian masses. However, the MR image is still used as a problem-solving modality in the assessment of complex adnexal masses because of tumor characterization of MR image over CT and potential risk in patient dose of CT.

Granulosa Cell Tumors

Granulosa cell tumors of the ovary represent the most common malignant sex cord-stromal tumor as well as the most common clinically estrogenic ovarian tumor. These tumors constitute ~ 5% of all malignant ovarian tumors. Adult granulosa cell tumors appear more often than the juvenile type and occur usually in postmenopausal women. They can reveal with abnormal vaginal bleeding and can be associated with endometrial hyperplasia, polyp, and carcinoma (3–25% of cases). Granulosa cell tumors have potential for clinically malignant behavior. Although prognosis correlates with stage and age at the time of the diagnosis, most patients with these tumors have an excellent prognosis. They have a tendency of late recurrence, even 10 to 20 years after diagnosis (Kim and Kim, 2002).

Adult granulosa cell tumors present a variety of imaging findings, from solid masses to tumors with cystic or hemorrhagic changes (Fig. 1), to multilocular cystic lesions (Fig. 2), and to completely cystic tumors. These variable imaging findings are due to various histologic appearances and various arrangements of tumor cells. Heterogeneity of tumor is caused by intratumoral bleeding, infarct, fibrous degeneration, or irregularly arranged tumors cells. In contrast to the more common epithelial tumors, granulosa cell tumors are confined to the ovary at the time of diagnosis with less propensity for peritoneal seeding, and they are only rarely bilateral. They may rupture and result in the hemoperitoneum (Jung *et al.*, 2005).

Fibroma, Fibrothecoma, and Thecoma

Fibroma, fibrothecoma, and thecoma are a spectrum of benign ovarian sex cord-stromal tumor, according to the proportion of theca cells and fibroblasts. Fibroma originating

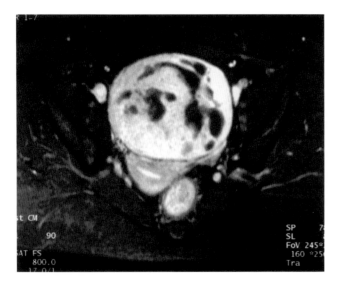

Figure 1 35-year-old woman with a granulosa cell tumor. Axial T1-weighted image after gadolinium administration shows marked enhancement of the solid portions with multiple small cystic or hemorrhagic areas within the tumor.

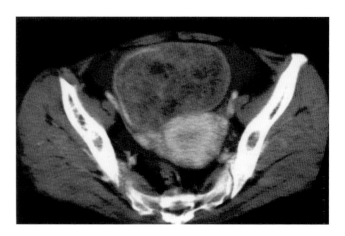

Figure 2 45-year-old woman with a granulosa cell tumor. Contrast-enhanced CT scan shows a large, complex mass with multiple cystic areas, resulting in "spongy-like" appearance.

from nonfunctioning stroma exhibits no estrogenic activity, but thecoma composed of swollen lipid-laden stromal cells can show estrogenic activity. Ovarian fibromas are the most common solid primary ovarian tumors (~ 4% of wall ovarian tumors) and the most common sex cord-stromal tumor. They are often found incidentally in both pre- and postmenopausal women. Fibromas can be associated with Meigs' syndrome characterized by an ovarian tumor, ascites, and a right-sided pleural effusion (Troiano *et al.*, 1997).

Because fibromas and fibrothecomas have abundant collagen and fibrous contents, these tumors show relatively diagnostic imaging findings. The mass appears as a homogeneous solid tumor with delayed enhancement on CT scan and as a hypointense mass on T1-weighted MR image with very low signal intensity on T2-weighted image (Fig. 3). Ovarian fibromas may calcify or exhibit cystic degeneration. Dense calcifications are often seen. On T2-weighted MR images, large fibrothecoma has internal high signal intensity areas, which are caused by edema or cystic degeneration.

The differential diagnosis includes pedunculated uterine fibroid and solid ovarian neoplasms, such as Brenner tumor and Sertoli-Leydig cell tumor (Jung *et al.*, 2005).

Sclerosing Stromal Tumor of Ovary

Sclerosing stromal tumors are rare, benign ovarian sex cord-stromal tumors that affect mainly young women. The most common clinical symptom is menstrual irregularity, although a few cases manifest clinical signs related to androgenic or estrogenic activity. Ascites may be seen but rarely. Surgical removal of the tumor is curative, and there is no local or distant recurrence (Kim *et al.*, 2003).

These tumors appear as a large mass with hyperintense cystic components, or a heterogeneous solid mass of intermediate to high signal intensity on T2-weighted MR imaging. Because

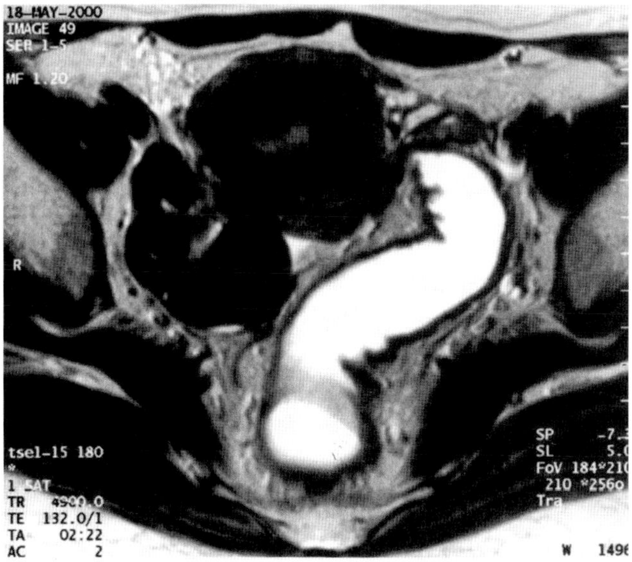

Figure 3 52-year-old woman with a fibroma. Multilobulated low signal intensity mass is noted in the right adnexal region on T2-weighted images. The mass has typical dark signal intensity.

the tumor is slowly growing, the ovarian cortex is compressed, showing thick peripheral hypointense rim on T2-weighted MR image. Striking contrast enhancement of tumor is a characteristic finding of these tumors. On dynamic contrast-enhanced images, the tumors show early peripheral enhancement with centripetal progression. Striking early enhancement reflects the cellular areas with their prominent vascular network, and an area of prolonged enhancement in the inner portion of the mass represents the collagenous hypocellular area. These findings can be useful in differentiating sclerosing stromal tumor from fibroma because fibroma shows absence of early enhancement and delayed accumulation of the contrast material (Jung et al., 2005).

Sertoli-Leydig Cell Tumor

Sertoli-Leydig cell tumors are very rare (< 0.5% of ovarian tumors). They usually occur in young women. Approximately one-third of patients reveal virilization. They are microscopically divided into four subtypes: well differentiated, intermediately differentiated, poorly differentiated, and retiform (Tanaka et al., 2004). Prognosis correlates with degree of differentiation and stage. Most of these tumors diagnose as stage I disease and usually behave in a benign fashion. In contrast to granulosa cell tumors, Sertoli-Leydig cell tumors tend to recur relatively soon after initial diagnosis. They are almost always unilateral tumors that can be solid, solid and cystic, and cystic, or even papillary. The mass appears as a well-defined, enhancing solid mass with intratumoral cysts on CT scan and

hypointense with multiple cystic areas of variable size on MR imaging. Low signal intensity on T2-weighted images depends on extent of fibrous stroma. Multicystic areas are developed due to heterologous elements (Jung et al., 2005).

Steroid Cell Tumor

Steroid cell tumors are very rare ovarian tumors and composed of lutein cells, Leydig cells, and adrenocortical cells. Stromal luteoma, Leydig cell tumor, and steroid cell tumor not otherwise specified are included in this tumor group. They affect patients from a wide range of ages but usually those in the fifth or sixth decade of life. The majority of steroid cell tumors are virilizing, and rare cases are associated with Cushing syndrome. Approximately one third of these tumors behave in a clinically malignant fashion. Steroid cell tumors are usually small (< 3 cm) nodules and always almost unilateral. The tumor appears as a small mass with hyperintense area on T1-weighted MR image due to abundant intracellular lipid and intense enhancement due to rich vascularity (Tanaka et al., 2004).

Summary

Ovarian sex cord-stromal tumors are rare ovarian neoplasms that arise from stromal cells and primitive sex cords in the ovary. These tumors may have characteristic clinical and imaging features. They affect all age groups and account for most of the hormonally active ovarian tumor. Most of them are stage I lesions at presentation with good prognosis. Granulosa cell tumors are usually large multiloculated cystic masses with variable solid portions. The tumors are associated with endometrial abnormalities. Fibromas, fibrothecoma, and thecomas manifest usually as solid masses with dark signal intensity on T2-weighted MR image and variable extent of calcification edema or cystic degeneration. Sclerosing stromal tumors demonstrate typical early peripheral enhancement with centripetal progression. Sertoli-Leydig cell tumors appear as well-defined, enhancing solid masses with variable-sized intratumoral cysts. Steroid cell tumor shows a small heterogeneous solid mass with internal areas of intracellular lipid. Clinical and radiologic clues are useful in differential diagnosis from the more common epithelial tumors of ovary.

References

Jung, S.E, Lee, J.M., Rha, S.E., Byun, J.Y., Jung, J.I., and Hahn, S.T. 2002. CT and MR imaging of ovarian tumors with emphasis on differential diagnosis. *RadioGraphics 22*:1305–1325.

Jung, S.E., Rha, S.E., Lee, J.M., Park, S.Y., Oh, S.N., Cho, K.S., Lee, E.J., Byun, J.Y., and Hahn, S.T. 2005. CT and MRI findings of sex cord-stromal tumor of the ovary. *AJR Am. J. Roentgenol. 185*:207–215.

Kim, S.H., and Kim, S.H.. 2002 Granulosa cell tumor of the ovary: common findings and unusual appearances on CT and MR. *J. Comput. Assist. Tomogr. 26*:756–761.

Kim, J.Y., Jung, K., Chung, D.S., Kim, O.D., Lee, J.H., and Youn, S.K. 2003. Sclerosing stromal tumor of the ovary: MR-pathologic correlation in three cases. *Korean J. Radiol. 4*:194–199.

Outwater, E.K., Wagner, B.J., Mannion, C., McLarney, J.K., and Kim, B. 1998. Sex cord-stromal and steroid cell tumors of the ovary. *Radio-Graphics 18*:1523–1546.

Tanaka, Y.O., Tsunoda, H., Kitagawa, Y., Ueno, T., Yoshikawa, H., and Saida, Y. 2004. Functioning ovarian tumors: direct and indirect findings at MR imaging. *RadioGraphics 24*:S147–S166.

Troiano, R.N., Lazzarini, K.M., Scoutt, L.M., Lange, R.C., Flynn, S.D., and McCarthy, S. 1997. Fibroma and fibrothecoma of the ovary: MR imaging findings. *Radiology 204*:795–798.

Malignant Germ Cell Tumors: Computed Tomography and Magnetic Resonance Imaging

Marc Bazot

Introduction

Germ cell tumors represent 20 to 30% of all ovarian tumors in adults (Scully *et al.*, 1998) and are classified according to the World Health Organization classification. These tumors are benign in 95% of cases and consist mainly of mature cystic teratomas (Talerman, 1995). In children and adolescents, > 60% of ovarian neoplasms are of germ cell origin, and one-third of those are malignant (Talerman, 1995). Although most types of germ cell tumors occur in pure form, each of them may also be mixed with one or more other types. The prognosis of a mixed germ cell tumor generally reflects that of its most malignant element, but a small focus of high malignancy does not influence the prognosis as adversely as a large component (Scully *et al.*, 1998).

Dermoid Cyst with Malignant Transformation

Malignant transformation with mature cystic teratoma is very rare and accounts for 0.17% of all dermoid cysts (Comerci

et al., 1994). These tumors are detected after the age of 30 years with a mean age of 59 years (Scully *et al.*, 1998). Dermoid cyst with malignant transformation is unilateral and tends to be larger than benign ovarian dermoid cyst (Scully *et al.*, 1998; Talerman, 1995). It is typically associated with dermoid cysts larger than 6 cm in diameter. In most cases, malignancy arises mainly in the dermoid plug, so careful pathologic examination of this area is of particular interest. This malignant transformation can also occur in other parts of the tumor, specifically in the wall cyst. Malignant transformation appears as cauliflower-like masses protruding into the cavity of the cyst, as a mural plaque or a nodule, or, if extensive, as a solid tumor mass that almost obliterates the cyst. Foci of hemorrhage and necrosis within the malignant component are common. Invasion of the wall tends to perforate. Small cancers may not be visible on gross examination. Approximately three-fourths of these tumors are squamous cell carcinomas, almost always invasive, sometimes *in situ*. Carcinoids, adenocarcinomas, undifferentiated carcinomas, various types of sarcomas, and melanomas can also be encountered (Scully *et al.*, 1998). Squamous cell carcinoma antigen (SCCA), CA-125, and CA-19-9 are useful markers that suggest diagnosis (Scully *et al.*, 1998).

Imaging Findings

As previously suggested by Buy *et al*. (1989), CT is very useful for detecting a malignant transformation either in the Rokitansky protuberance or in the cyst wall. Some features are of particular interest, including large size of the tumor (> 5 cm), protuberance with a cauliflower shape, irregular borders, formation of obtuse angles with the inner wall of the cyst, and significant contrast uptake with tumoral vessels on the dynamic incremental CT scanner, mass arising in the wall with extracapsular extension, peritoneal, or hematogeneous extension features (e.g., liver metastasis).

No MR imaging case has been reported to our knowledge. In a personal case (not published), MR imaging displayed a unilateral nonspecific solid-cystic mass containing a small area of fat.

Immature Teratoma

Immature teratomas represent < 1% of all ovarian cancers. In contrast to mature cystic teratomas, which occur at all ages, immature teratomas are most common during the two first decades (Scully *et al*., 1998). They are composed of variable amounts of immature tissue, differentiating toward any or all of the three germ layers (Talerman, 1995). Mature elements are also present in most cases (Scully *et al*., 1998). The immature teratoma is a malignant neoplasm, and a histological grading system has been proposed for prognostic and therapeutic purposes (Norris *et al*., 1976). To investigate the relationship between immature teratomas and dermoid cysts, 350 immature teratomas were recently studied; 26% of the immature teratomas contained at least one grossly visible dermoid cyst, 10% were associated with a contralateral dermoid cyst, and 2.6% occurred in patients with a history of resection of an ipsilateral dermoid cyst (Yanai-Inbar and Scully, 1987). The same investigators analyzed 10 dermoid cysts with microscopic foci of immature tissue and concluded that a patient with a history of resection of a dermoid cyst was at a slightly increased risk for subsequent development of an immature teratoma in the same ovary, and that a history of multiplicity and rupture of a dermoid cyst might further increase the risk. Immature teratomas usually appear as predominantly unilateral solids, lobulated masses that contain numerous small cysts. Soft tissue corresponding to immature neural tissue is often conspicuous and may be the site of necrosis and hemorrhage. Occasionally, it may be mainly cystic, unilocular or multilocular, with solid areas present in the cyst wall corresponding to the Rokitansky protuberance (Fig. 1).

The two most common important factors of prognosis are the stage and the histologic grade. Alpha-foeto-protein (AFP) is a very useful tumor marker for the diagnosis and management of immature teratomas (Kawai *et al*., 1990).

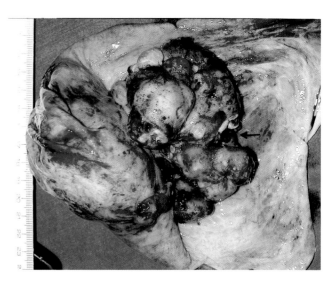

Figure 1 Macroscopic specimen shows immature teratoma (grade 2) with a large irregular Rokitansky protuberance (arrow).

Imaging Techniques

On CT scan, calcifications scattered throughout the tumor and small amount of adipose tissue can be displayed and highly suggest the diagnosis of immature teratoma. When the tumor is predominantly solid, it contains solid portions of soft tissue density with less dense areas and foci of denser areas related to hemorrhage. In solid-cystic lesion, diffuse calcifications or fat are found within a large irregular Rokitansky protuberance (Bazot *et al*., 1999). On dynamic CT scan, typical tumoral vessels at the arterial phase and contrast uptake at the parenchymal phase strongly suggest the diagnosis of malignant ovarian tumor (Fig. 2) (Bazot *et al*., 1999).

In the predominantly solid form, besides the usual findings of a mixed mass, the advantage of MRI is to better display the areas of hemorrhage on T1-weighted images. In the predominantly cystic form, differential diagnosis with other multiloculated cystic masses, especially mucinous borderline or carcinoma, can be difficult. In a large series of 10 patients, Yamaoka *et al*. (2003) reported that all lesions appeared to be fat-containing tumors with solid components consisting of numerous cysts of various sizes (Fig. 3). Solid tissue exhibited a wide variety of signal intensities on T2-weighted imaging. Punctate foci of fat were present in all lesions. No correlation was found between the amount of solid tissue and the tumor grade in their series.

Rarely, immature teratomas are associated with peritoneal implants composed exclusively or mainly of mature glial tissue (peritoneal gliomatosis) (Brammer *et al*., 1990). These implants can be extensively calcified. Similar glial tissue is sometimes encountered in pelvic and para-aortic lymph nodes. Metastatic liver lesions may contain fat and calcification (Lentini *et al*., 1986). After chemotherapy, retroconversion of immature to mature tissue in metastasis has

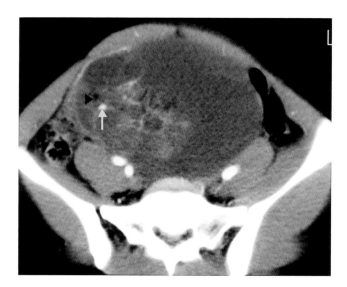

Figure 2 Immature teratoma (grade 2): Axial dynamic incremental CT scanner at the arterial phase shows arterial vessels within a large irregular Rokitansky protuberance. Note the presence of associated fat (arrowhead) and calcifications (arrow).

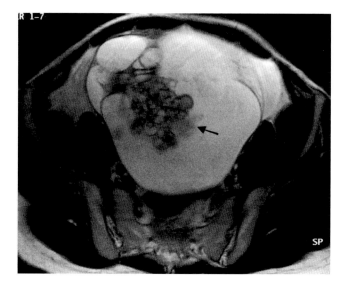

Figure 3 Immature teratoma (grade 2): Axial turbo spin-echo T2-weighted image shows a huge multilocular cyst containing a large irregular Rokitansky protuberance (arrow).

been described (Lentini *et al.*, 1986; Moskovic *et al.*, 1991). The lesions can increase in size and have been described as the growing teratoma syndrome (Nimkin *et al.*, 2004). The margins of the lesions become better circumscribed. Calcification with fatty areas and cystic changes can appear.

Dysgerminoma

The dysgerminoma is the homolog of the testicular seminoma. Eighty percent of dysgerminomas occur during the

second and third decades of life. The great majority of dysgerminomas develop on a normal gonad or are sometimes associated with gonadal dysgenesis. In the latter case, most dysgerminomas develop from a gonadoblastoma which is an unusual gonadal neoplasm composed of germ cell and stromal elements (Scully *et al.*, 1998). Symptoms are related to an abdominal mass. Loss of weight may also be an accompanying symptom. The tumor when small can be found incidentally. Occasionally, menstrual and endocrine abnormalities may be the presenting symptoms; this tends to be more common in patients with dysgerminoma associated with other primitive germ cell tumors, especially choriocarcinoma. In children, precocious sexual development may occur.

Lactic deshydrogenase is elevated in up to 95% of patients, with the level varying with the size and stage of the tumor. Determination of this marker may also be useful in detecting recurrent tumor and monitoring response to therapy (Scully *et al.*, 1998). Dysgerminomas form solid masses and range up to 50 cm in size. The external surfaces are typically bosselated but may be smooth. The stroma is characteristically lobulated separated by fibrovascular septa, which can be broad or fine (Talerman, 1995). Cysts may be encountered, rarely attaining a diameter of 15 cm. Areas of necrosis and hemorrhage are occasionally observed. Minute foci of calcification are rarely present and strongly suggest an underlying gonadoblastoma. Bilaterality is found in 5 to 10% of cases.

Imaging Techniques

On CT, calcifications can be visualized with a speckled pattern (Brammer *et al.*, 1990). Recently, Tanaka *et al.* (1994) reported CT and MR findings of three patients with ovarian dysgerminoma. The tumors were divided into lobules by septa that were hypointense or isointense on T2-weighted imaging and showed marked enhancement on gadolinium enhanced T1-weighted imaging and contrast-enhanced CT. These septa corresponded to fibrovascular bundles at histological examination. The authors concluded that CT and MR findings characteristic of fibrovascular septa within solid ovarian masses should raise the possibility of dysgerminomas (Tanaka *et al.*, 1994). Even though 70% of dysgerminomas are stage 1 tumors at the time of discovery, they can sometimes metastasize. When lymphatic spread occurs, it usually spreads through the lymphatic system to iliac and more frequently aortic lymph nodes and subsequently to the mediastinum and supraclavicular fossa (Gallion *et al.*, 1988). On CT and MR, these lymph nodes are diagnosed when their short axis is larger or equal to 10 mm. Hematogeneous metastases are rare, occurring most commonly in the liver.

Endodermal Sinus Tumor

Endodermal sinus tumor (EST) is also known as yolk sac tumor because it resembles, on histology, the endodermal sinuses of the rat yolk sac (Kurman and Norris, 1978). Endodermal sinus tumors are most common in patients in the second and third decades of life. Patients usually present with abdominal pain, frequently of sudden onset, and a large abdominal or pelvic mass. The tumors are typically large, with a median diameter of 15 cm (Scully *et al.*, 1998). The typical neoplasm is predominantly solid, but cystic areas are also commonly found (Kurman and Norris, 1978). Extensive areas of hemorrhage and necrosis are frequent. A honeycomb appearance due to many small cysts, or rarely an entirely cystic tumor, may be observed (Scully *et al.*, 1998). Gross incidence of other germ cell elements, most commonly a dermoid cyst, is seen in 15% of cases. On histology, these cystic areas are either epithelial-lined cysts produced by the EST itself or, less commonly, cysts of coexisting mature teratoma. As with the other malignant germ cell tumors, EST may be associated with ascites and peritoneal implants (Kurman and Norris, 1978). Extension to the peritoneum, retroperitoneal lymph modes, or both is seen in 30 to 70% of the cases (Scully *et al.*, 1998).

Endodermal sinus tumor is a highly malignant neoplasm metastasizing early and invading the surrounding structures and organs. The tumor is very aggressive locally, spreads beyond the ovary, and is observed in a number of patients at operations (Kurman and Norris, 1978). Endodermal sinus tumor metastasizes first via the lymphatic system to the para-aortic and common iliac lymph nodes and then to the mediastinal and supraclavicular lymph nodes (Talerman, 1995). There is a hematogeneous spread in the lungs, liver, and other organs (Talerman, 1995). Alfa-foeto-protein is very often much elevated. Though not specific, the diagnosis of EST is suggested when the level is > 1000 mg/ml (Scully *et al.*, 1998).

Imaging Findings

On CT scan, the tumor is partly cystic and partly solid. A significant contrast uptake is visualized in the wall and septa (Levitin *et al.*, 1996). On MR imaging, Yamaoka *et al.* (2000) reported that endodermal sinus tumors were predominantly solid, with cystic degeneration, necrosis, and findings suggestive of hemorrhage on T1-W images. They were shown as well-enhancing solid tumors on both CT and MR studies and were associated with prominent signal voids on MRI.

Choriocarcinoma

Primary pure ovarian choriocarcinoma (PPOC) accounts for < 1% of ovarian malignant tumors (Scully *et al.*, 1998). Shiromizu *et al.* (1991) recently studied 467 ovarian germ cell tumors, and found only one choriocarcinoma. Choriocarcinoma is an aggressive tumor occurring during or outside of pregnancy. Gestational choriocarcinoma of the ovary can be primitive, associated with ovarian pregnancy, or metastatic, arising from a primary gestational choriocarcinoma occurring in the uterus. Nongestational choriocarcinoma of the ovary can be pure but is more frequently associated with other germ cell tumors (Talerman, 1995). In most cases, the plasma human chorionic gonadotropin (HCG) level is markedly elevated.

Imaging Findings

In our study, unenhanced CT revealed a latero-uterine mass, without fat (Bazot *et al.*, 2004). A large vascularized ovarian pedicle and huge and irregular arterial vessels were seen at the periphery of the mass during the arterial phase of dynamic CT. These findings were typical of a malignant tumor, although the presence of very large vessels restricted to the periphery was unusual for a malignant epithelial tumor. Significant contrast uptake was observed in the peripheral solid portion of the mass. Abdomino-pelvic examination showed no extra-ovarian dissemination. Abnormal vessels and small cystic cavities in the irregular peripheral solid portion were displayed on T2-weighted MR images. High signal intensity foci in the solid portion and a large central area with high and intermediate signal intensities were suggestive of hemorrhage on T1-weighted images. Significant gadolinium uptake in the solid portion was suggestive of a highly vascularized tumor. These features were well correlated with gross appearance of the tumor, which contained multiple cystic cavities with hemorrhagic content seen in the peripheral solid portion, and a large central necrotic and hemorrhagic area. Microscopic examination showed thick, highly vascularized fibrovascular septa highly correlated with the highly vascularized nature of this mass (Bazot *et al.*, 2004).

Embryonal Carcinoma

This malignant germ cell tumor is very rare. In the largest series of 15 embryonal carcinomas reported by Kurman and Norris (1976), the tumors were described as being predominantly solid, with areas of extensive necrosis and hemorrhage. Serum level of HCG and AFP may occasionally be elevated. No radiological features are reported to our knowledge.

Malignant Mixed Germ Cell Tumors

Mixed tumors contain at least two different malignant germ cell components. It has been stated that mixed tumors account for 8% of the malignant germ cell tumors of the ovary. The appearance of a malignant mixed germ cell tumor varies according to its individual constituents, but it is generally a complex, predominantly solid tumor, as are the other germ cell tumors (Brammer *et al.*, 1990).

References

Bazot, M., Cortez, A., Sananes, S., Boudghene, F., Uzan, S., and Bigot, J.M. 1999. Imaging of dermoid cysts with foci of immature tissue. *J. Comput. Assist. Tomogr. 23*:703–706.

Bazot, M., Cortez, A., Sananes, S., and Buy, J.N. (2004). Imaging of pure primary ovarian choriocarcinoma. *AJR Am. J. Roentgenol. 182*: 1603–1604.

Brammer, H.M., III, Buck, J.L., Hayes, W.S., Sheth, S., and Tavassoli, F.A. 1990. From the archives of the AFIP: malignant germ cell tumors of the ovary: radiologic-pathologic correlation. *Radiographics 10*:715–724.

Buy, J.N., Ghossain, M.A., Moss, A.A., Bazot, M., Doucet, M., Hugol, D., Truc, J.B., Poitout, P., and Ecoiffier, J. 1989. Cystic teratoma of the ovary: CT detection. *Radiology 171*:697–701.

Comerci, J.T., Jr., Licciardi, F., Bergh, P.A., Gregori, C., and Breen, J.L. 1994. Mature cystic teratoma: a clinicopathologic evaluation of 517 cases and review of the literature. *Obstet. Gynecol. 84*:22–28.

Gallion, H.H., Van, N.J., Jr, Donaldson, E.S., and Powell, D.E. (1988). Ovarian dysgerminoma: report of seven cases and review of the literature. *Am. J. Obstet. Gynecol. 158*:591–595.

Kawai, M., Furuhashi, Y., Kano, T., Misawa, T., Nakashima, N., Hattori, S., Okamoto, Y., Kobayashi, I., Ohta, M., and Arii, Y. 1990. Alpha-fetoprotein in malignant germ cell tumors of the ovary. *Gynecol. Oncol. 39*:160–166.

Kurman, R., and Norris, H.J. 1976. Embryonal carcinoma of the ovary: a clinicopathologic entity distinct from endodermal sinus tumor resembling embryonal carcinoma of the adult testis. *Cancer 38*:2420–2433.

Kurman, R.J., and Norris, H.J. 1978. Germ cell tumors of the ovary. *Pathol. Annu. 13*:291–325.

Lentini, J.F., Love, M.B., Ritchie, W.G., and Sedlacek, T.V. 1986. Computed tomography in retroconversion of hepatic metastases from immature ovarian teratoma. *J. Comput. Assist. Tomogr. 10*:1060–1062.

Levitin, A., Haller, K.D., Cohen, H.L., Zinn, D.L., and O'Connor, M.T. 1996. Endodermal sinus tumor of the ovary: imaging evaluation. *AJR Am. J. Roentgenol. 167*:791–793.

Moskovic, E., Jobling, T., Fisher, C., Wiltshaw, E., and Parsons, C. 1991. Retroconversion of immature teratoma of the ovary: CT appearances. *Clin. Radiol. 43*:402–408.

Nimkin, K., Gupta, P., McCauley, R., Gilchrist, B.F., and Lessin, M.S. 2004. The growing teratoma syndrome. *Pediatr. Radiol. 34*:259–262.

Norris, H.J., Zirkin, H.J., and Benson, W.L. 1976. Immature (malignant) teratoma of the ovary: a clinical and pathologic study of 58 cases. *Cancer 37*:2359–2372.

Scully, R.E., Young, R.H., and Clement, P.B. 1998. In: Rosai, J. (Ed.), *Tumors of the Ovary and Maldeveloped Gonads, Fallopian Tube, and Broad Ligament*, Vol. 23. Washington, DC Armed Forces Institute of Pathology, pp. 226–299.

Shiromizu, K., Kawana, T., Sugase, M., Izumi, R., and Mizuno, M. 1991. Clinicostatistical study of ovarian tumors of germ cell origin. *Asia Oceania J. Obstet. Gynaecol. 17*:207–215.

Talerman, A. 1995. Germ cell tumors of the ovary. In: Kurman, R. (Ed.), *Blaustein's Pathology of the Female Genital Tract*, Vol. 1. New York: Springer-Verlag, pp. 849–914.

Tanaka, Y. O., Kurosaki, Y., Nishida, M., Michishita, N., Kuramoto, K., Itai, Y., and Kubo, T. 1994. Ovarian dysgerminoma: MR and CT appearance. *J. Comput. Assist. Tomogr. 18*:443–448.

Yamaoka, T., Togashi, K., Koyama, T., Fujiwara, T., Higuchi, T., Iwasa, Y., Fujii, S., and Konishi, J. 2003. Immature teratoma of the ovary: correlation of MR imaging and pathologic findings. *Eur. Radiol. 13*:313–319.

Yamaoka, T., Togashi, K., Koyama, T., Ueda, H., Nakai, A., Fujii, S., Yamabe, H., and Konishi, J. 2000. Yolk sac tumor of the ovary: radiologic-pathologic correlation in four cases. *J. Comput. Assist. Tomogr. 24*:605–609.

Yanai-Inbar, I., and Scully, R.E. 1987. Relation of ovarian dermoid cysts and immature teratomas: an analysis of 350 cases of immature teratoma and 10 cases of dermoid cyst with microscopic foci of immature tissue. *Int. J. Gynecol. Pathol. 6*:203–212.

34

Ovarian Small Round Cell Tumors: Magnetic Resonance Imaging

Yumiko Oishi Tanaka

Introduction

The utility of magnetic resonance imaging (MRI) in differential diagnosis in adnexal masses has been established. Its excellent contrast resolution enables radiologists to make tissue characterization (Siegelman and Outwater, 1999). Radiologists can also make a specific diagnosis based on tissue characterization with MRI, clinical presentation, and patients' age, even though many kinds of tumors affect the female genital tract. In this chapter, we will show the MRI characteristics of ovarian small, round cell tumors, including granulocytic sarcoma and lymphoma, based on our experience and literature review.

Neoplasms arising from a hematopoietic organ (i.e., lymphoma, leukemia, and myeloma) are sometimes categorized under the general term of *small round cell tumors*. Malignant lymphoma usually appears as the solid tumors of nodal or extranodal diseases; however, they rarely begin as adnexal masses (Monterroso *et al.*, 1993). Myeloma occasionally creates an extraskeletal mass called plasmacytoma, which is extremely rare in the female genital system, and only seven cases of ovarian plasmacytoma have been reported (Emery *et al.*, 1999). Solid tumors composed of malignant myeloid precursor cells, named chloroma or granulocytic sarcoma and primary ovarian lymphoma, are also considered to be extremely rare (Oliva *et al.*, 1997). In lymphoma,

the most common histologic type is the small noncleaved cell, Burkitt's type, followed by the diffuse large B-cell type (Monterroso *et al.*, 1993). Burkitt's lymphoma usually affects patients of younger age (Osborne and Robboy, 1983). Secondary involvement in systemic disease occasionally occurs in lymphoma (McCarville *et al.*, 2001). Most of the reported granulocytic sarcomas of the ovary appear at the time of relapse of acute myelogenous leukemia (Oliva *et al.*, 1997; Yamamoto *et al.*, 1991).

Imaging Findings

No specific imaging features of the ovarian involvement of small round cell tumors have been reported; however, homogeneous structures without calcification, hemorrhage, or necrosis are frequently seen in ovarian lymphoma on ultrasound or computed tomography (CT). Ovarian plasmacytoma showing large solid mass has been reported in pathology literature. However, there is no published study on the imaging of ovarian plasmacytoma. On the other hand, there are several reports on the MR findings of ovarian lymphoma or granulocytic sarcoma (Ferrozzi *et al.*, 2000; Jung *et al.*, 1999; McCarville *et al.*, 2001; Mitsumori *et al.*, 1999). One of these articles, Mitsumori *et al.* (1999), reported a case of

B-cell-type non-Hodgkin's Lymphoma, which showed hyper-intense septal structures on T2-weighted images. McCarville *et al.* (2001) also reported two cases of Burkitt's lymphoma that had well-enhanced septal structures on CT. The septal structures observed in ovarian involvement in lymphoma are thought to be a useful characteristic of the disease.

Primary ovarian involvement in Burkitt's lymphoma is relatively common in younger patients (Osborne and Robboy, 1983), whom ovarian dysgerminoma also frequently affects. Ovarian dysgerminoma has been reported to be characterized by fibrovascular septa on MR (Tanaka *et al.*, 1994). Therefore, dysgerminoma may be a tumor that should be differentiated from ovarian lymphoma. Ferrozzi *et al.* (2000) reported a cerebroid appearance in some cases of ovarian lymphoma. The cerebroid appearance is made up of a relatively large, lobulated homoge-neous mass without hemorrhage or necrosis. This homogeneous appearance is consistent with the reported sonographic or CT findings. Regarding pathological findings of ovarian lymphoma or granulocytic sarcoma, the external surface of the involved ovaries has been reported as lobulated or nodular (Osborne and Robboy, 1983). Microscopically, the tumors had the appearance of a monotonous cellular infiltrate. The cerebroid appearance may correspond to these external surface structures.

The signal intensity of the tumors was varying in reported cases; however, they often show lower signal intensity on T2-weighted MR images (Jung *et al.*, 1999; Tanaka *et al.*, 2006). Koeller *et al.* (1997) reported dense cellularity of the tumor, explaining its typical hypointensity on T2-weighted MR images in primary lymphoma of the central nervous system (CNS). As virtually all primary CNS lymphomas are composed of B-cells, this may explain why ovarian small round cell tumors show low signal intensity on T2-weighted MR images. Another cause of T2 shortening has been reported by Parker *et al.* (1996) in a case with granulocytic sarcoma of CNS. They reported that the lesion's tendency to remain hypointense on T2-weighted images is presumably attributable to the presence of myeloperoxidase, an iron-containing enzyme normally found in white blood cells.

We (2006) have found small cystic structures at the periph-ery of the tumors in patients with ovarian lymphoma and leukemia who had a normal menstrual cycle. Such a finding was also observed in previously published works (Ferrozzi *et al.*, 2000; Jung *et al.*, 1999; Mitsumori *et al.*, 1999). Jung *et al.* (1999) reported a case of granulocytic sarcoma in which multiple small cystic areas within the solid component corre-sponded to ovarian follicles. Monterroso *et al.* (1993) reported that lymphoma cells grow within the ovary, sparing the ovar-ian follicles in diffuse large-cell lymphoma. We could not find any normal ovarian tissue such as theca interna or stratum granulosum in surgically removed specimens of our own case,

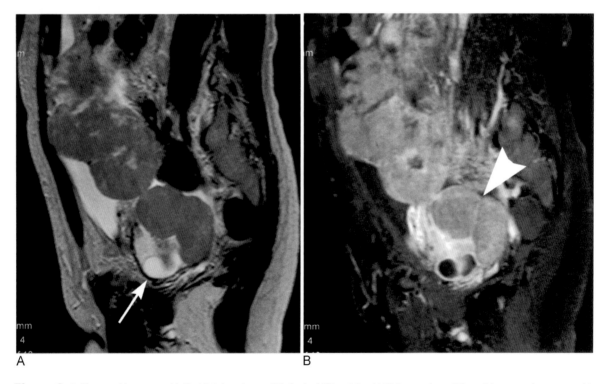

Figure 1 A 41-year-old woman with Burkitt's lymphoma. (**A**) Sagittal T2-weighted MR image shows bilateral large ovarian tumor with relatively low signal intensity. There are several small hyperintense round structures at the periphery of the masses (arrow). (**B**) The masses show a cerebroid appearance made up of nodules divided by a well-enhanced septal structure (arrowhead) on the sagittal contrast-enhanced T1-weighted MR image.

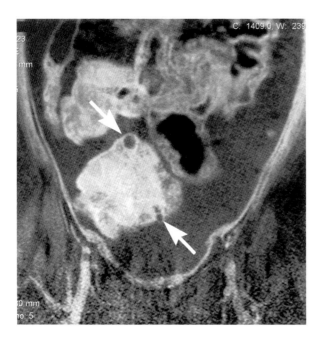

Figure 2 A 20-year-old woman with diffuse large B-cell lymphoma. Coronal contrast-enhanced T1-weighted MR image shows a large ovarian tumor with homogeneous contrast enhancement. There are several small unenhanced round structures at the periphery of the mass (arrows).

as tumor cells diffusely proliferated and replaced the normal ovarian tissue. However, the cystic structure was located in the cortical areas of the ovaries, and it was not observed in a postmenopausal patient. Therefore, the cystic structure might correspond to preserved follicles. The preservation of ovarian follicles at the periphery of the large lobulated mass with a cerebroid appearance is not observed in any other malignant solid ovarian tumors. This seems to be characteristic of ovarian round cell tumors.

Multiple nonenlarged cortically located ovarian follicles in a diffusely enlarged ovary are reported in a case of massive ovarian edema (Kramer *et al.*, 1997). Massive ovarian edema is the result of the partial intermittent torsion of the meso-ovarium, and it usually appears as acute abdomen. Lymphomatous involvement of the ovary usually shows no specific symptoms (Monterroso *et al.*, 1993). Therefore, we believe that these two conditions can be distinguished from each other in the clinical setting. In conclusion, the preserva-

tion of ovarian follicles at the periphery of the large lobulated mass with cerebroid appearance seems to be a characteristic of ovarian round cell tumors. In addition, they tend to show low signal intensity on T2-weighted imaging, reflecting the higher cellularity or rich intracytoplasmic myeloperoxidase.

References

Emery, J.D., Kennedy, A W., Tubbs, R.R., Castellani, W.J., and Hussein, M.A. 1999. Plasmacytoma of the ovary: a case report and literature review. *Gynecol. Oncol. 73*:151–154.

Ferrozzi, F., Tognini, G., Bova, D., and Zuccoli, G. 2000. Non-Hodgkin Lymphomas of the ovaries: MR findings. *J. Comput. Assist. Tomogr. 24*:416–420.

Jung, S.E., Chun, K.A., Park, S.H., and Lee, E.J. 1999. MR findings in ovarian granulocytic sarcoma. *Br. J. Radiol. 72*:301–303.

Koeller, K.K., Smirniotopoulos, J.G., and Jones, R.V. 1997. Primary central nervous system lymphoma: radiologic-pathologic correlation. *Radiographics 17*:1497–1526.

Kramer, L.A., Lalani, T., and Kawashima, A. 1997. Massive edema of the ovary: high resolution MR findings using a phased-array pelvic coil. *J. Magn. Reson. Imag. 7*:758–760.

McCarville, M.B., Hill, D.A., Miller, B.E., and Pratt, C.B. 2001. Secondary ovarian neoplasms in children: imaging features with histopathologic correlation. *Pediatr. Radiol. 31*:358–364.

Mitsumori, A., Joja, I., and Hiraki, Y. 1999. MR appearance of non-Hodgkin's Lymphoma of the ovary. *AJR Am. J. Roentgenol. 173*:245.

Monterroso, V., Jaffe, E.S., Merino, M.J., and Medeiros, L.J. 1993. Malignant lymphomas involving the ovary: a clinicopathologic analysis of 39 cases. *Am. J. Surg. Pathol. 17*:154–170.

Oliva, E., Ferry, J.A., Young, R.H., Prat, J., Srigley, J.R., and Scully, R.E. 1997. Granulocytic sarcoma of the female genital tract: a clinicopathologic study of 11 cases. *Am. J. Surg. Pathol. 21*:1156–1165.

Osborne, B.M., and Robboy, S.J. 1983. Lymphomas or leukemia presenting as ovarian tumors: an analysis of 42 cases. *Cancer 52*:1933–1943.

Parker, K., Hardjasudarma, M., McClellan, R.L., Fowler, M.R., and Milner, J.W. 1996. MR features of an intracerebellar chloroma. *AJNR Am. J. Neuroradiol. 17*:1592–1594.

Siegelman, E.S., and Outwater, E.K. 1999. Tissue characterization in the female pelvis by means of MR imaging. *Radiology 212*:5–18.

Tanaka, Y.O., Kurosaki, Y., Nishida, M., Michishita, N., Kuramoto, K., Itai, Y., and Kubo, T. 1994. Ovarian dysgerminoma: MR and CT appearance. *J. Comput. Assist. Tomogr. 18*:443–448.

Tanaka, Y.O., Yamada, K., Oki, A., Yoshikawa, H., and Minami, M. 2006. Magnetic resonance imaging findings of small round cell tumors of the ovary: a report of 5 cases with literature review. *J. Comput. Assist. Tomogr. 30*:12–17.

Yamamoto, K., Akiyama, H., Maruyama, T., Sakamaki, H., Onozawa, Y., and Kawaguchi, K. 1991. Granulocytic sarcoma of the ovary in patients with acute myelogenous leukemia. *Am. J. Hematol. 38*:223–225.

Ovarian Borderline Serous Surface Papillary Tumor: Magnetic Resonance Imaging

Sun Ho Kim and Seung Hyup Kim

Introduction

Primary ovarian tumors are classified based on cell origin, and epithelial cell tumors are the most common. Serous tumor is the most common type of the ovarian epithelial tumor, and 25% of them are malignant. Fifteen percent of serous tumors are "borderline malignancies" in which more proliferation and possible metastasis distinguish them from benign tumors. They are also different from malignant tumors in that the invasion to the ovarian stroma is not present, which is the most important histologic feature. Most borderline tumors are found in mucinous or serous tumors, although they can occur with any epithelial cell types (Moon, 2005).

Serous tumors, whether benign or malignant, usually form cystic masses and are named pathologically as cystadenoma or cystadenocarcinoma. Solid components in these cystic tumors are strong indicators of borderline or malignant tumors. *Papillary projection* is the term used to describe this characteristic solid component pathologically and on radiologic imaging. In many cases, the differentiation between borderline and malignant tumors is difficult or impossible on imaging, although a borderline tumor can be suggested according to the amount and invasiveness of solid components and the degree of peritoneal seeding or metastasis.

In some serous tumors, cyst formation is poor and the solid component is dominant. When these solid components show papillary growth pattern, serous papillary tumor can be a pathologic diagnosis. If the tumor lacks a papillary growth pattern, the term *serous adenocarcinoma* can be used. Papillary growth pattern can be recognized both on gross and microscopic examinations, and is also visible on magnetic resonance (MR) imaging.

Serous surface papillary tumor is a rare, but distinct, subtype of serous tumors. Serous surface papilloma and serous surface papillary carcinoma (SSPC) belong to this entity. Characteristic pathologic features of these tumors are papillary masses present only on the ovarian surface without stromal invasion (Mills *et al.*, 1988). Therefore, peritoneal seeding and ascites can be prominent, although ovarian masses are very small or even inconspicuous on CT and MR imaging.

Serous surface papillary carcinoma has been regarded as a peritoneal carcinoma (SSPC of the peritoneum) in many literatures, because the pathologic features are almost identical, and multifocal SSPCs may be found in both the peritoneum and the ovary (Mulhollan *et al.*, 1994). Ovarian surface epithelium is considered as modified peritoneum, and the origin of this tumor is controversial. Common histologic appearance is identified in both SSPC of the ovary and SSPC of the peritoneum, and the treatment plan and responsiveness to surgery and chemotherapy are also the same. Radiologic imaging findings are also similar. Therefore, in most cases, differentiation of SSPC of the ovary from SSPC of the peritoneum is impossible radiologically and pathologically (Liapis *et al.*, 1996).

Some reports, however, have described SSPC of the ovary as a distinct subtype of serous papillary carcinoma that originates from the ovarian surface epithelium rather than a peritoneal carcinoma with ovarian surface involvement (Gooneratne *et al.*, 1982). A possible solution to this confusing description is to understand these two entities as a spectrum, and the difference lies in the proportion of ovarian masses to the peritoneal seeding.

"Surface" of SSPC should also be used in limited cases. Pathologically, the tumor in SSPC should be located on the ovarian surface without stromal invasion. However, a mild degree of ovarian stromal invasion is difficult to detect radiologically, especially on CT imaging. Ovaries of normal size are suggestive findings, but on pathologic examination stromal invasion may be found even in these cases. Practically, many tumors diagnosed as SSPCs on radiologic imaging are revealed as merely serous papillary carcinomas pathologically. Therefore, the term *surface* should be used only when the official pathologic diagnosis includes "surface" in the name of an ovarian tumor.

Discussion

Reported CT imaging findings of SSPCs are a large amount of ascites with extensive peritoneal seeding masses and no or subtle lesions in the ovary without enlargement (normal-looking ovaries) (Chopra *et al.*, 2000). These find-

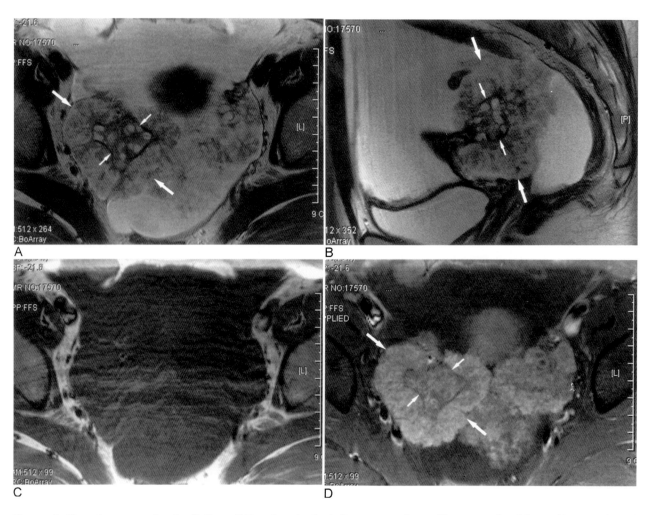

Figure 1 Magnetic resonance imaging findings of bilateral ovarian borderline serous surface papillary tumors in a 26-year-old woman. (**A and B**) On T2-weighted axial (3977/99, A) and sagittal (4072/99, B; left ovary) MR images, bilateral ovarian masses (large arrows) show multilobulated appearances and have internal branching patterns. Normal-looking ovaries (small arrows) with distorted shape are well delineated inside the masses by the dark-signal-intensity of ovarian capsule and contain multiple follicular cysts. (**C and D**) On T1-weighted axial MR image (741/14, C), the masses and ovaries are not discriminated from surrounding ascites. However, the masses (large arrows) are well enhancing on contrast-enhanced T1-weighted axial MR image (836/14, D), and the ovary (small arrows) is clearly visible inside the mass.

ings are not specific for SSPCs, and the most important differential diagnosis is peritoneal carcinomatosis from another primary malignancy. Because the findings are similar or even indistinguishable, thorough assessment of major abdominal organs, including stomach, colon, and pancreas, should be made so as not to miss primary malignancies. However, small foci of malignancy may not be identified or may be overlooked on CT imaging. Therefore, the absence of a visible primary tumor on CT cannot exclude the possibility of peritoneal carcinomatosis from another primary malignancy. In these cases, high elevation of serum level of tumor markers such as CA-125 may be helpful in the diagnosis of SSPC because the serum CA-125 level is not as high in peritoneal carcinomatosis from a primary malignancy as with ovarian malignancies (Furukawa *et al.*, 1999). A report has described the presence of marked calcifications in extensive peritoneal and omental masses as a distinct CT feature of SSPCs (Stafford-Johnson *et al.*, 1998). However, another report showed no extensive calcification in their series of SSPCs (Kim *et al.*, 2004). Although a "normal-looking ovary" is a feature of SSPC on CT, some patients may have relatively large ovarian masses (Zissin *et al.*, 2001; Kim *et al.*, 2004). In these cases, SSPC of the ovary is not easily differentiated from other ovarian malignancies with peritoneal seeding.

Magnetic resonance imaging can offer outstanding soft tissue contrast compared with CT and may depict more subtle ovarian lesions in SSPCs. However, reported MR imaging findings were also nonspecific: small nodularities might be found on the ovarian surface, uterus, and pelvic peritoneum, but discrete, large mass was not found (Kim *et al.*, 1997). In our daily practice, it is also difficult to find specific MR imaging findings of ovaries involved by SPCC. However, in one case we encountered MR imaging findings that could be considered characteristic and specific for SSPC (Kim *et al.*, 2005). Bilateral ovarian masses were detected by sonography in a 26-year-old woman, in whom the serum level of CA-125 was elevated. Computed tomography revealed poorly defined, solid-looking ovarian masses, accompanied by a large amount of ascites. These findings raised the possiblity of primary ovarian cancers with peritoneal seeding, although no detectable peritoneal seeding mass was identified except for mild septations in the ascites and omental infiltration. On MR imaging (Fig. 1), the ovarian masses showed papillary appearances with internal branching patterns. The most characteristic finding was a normal-looking ovary inside the mass, which contained multiple follicles and was outlined by a well-preserved ovarian capsule. The capsule could be discriminated most clearly as a dark-signal-intensity rim on T2-weighted images, and all tumors were located outside this capsule. Contrast-enhanced images showed clear enhancement of the tumors and the ovaries, preserving sharp demarcations between them. Large amounts of ascites were present, but no discrete peritoneal seeding mass was detected on MR imaging. The tumors were confirmed pathologically as ovarian borderline serous surface papillary tumors.

In this case, MR imaging findings are quite different from those described in previous reports: large ovarian masses were main lesions, and the findings suggestive of peritoneal seeding were minimal. We tried to explain these differences on the basis that this tumor was a borderline malignancy and well differentiated. This imaging could demonstrate characteristic imaging findings of these ovarian masses clearly owing to good soft tissue contrast. The findings are very striking and impressive, and are seldom found in other ovarian diseases or tumors. In summary, although SSPCs usually have subtle or no ovarian lesions compared with extensive peritoneal seeding on CT and MR imaging, ovarian masses may be main lesions in limited cases of low-grade and well-differentiated malignancies. Preserved normal ovaries inside the masses and papillary appearances may be clearly visible on MR imaging due to outstanding soft tissue contrast in these cases.

References

Chopra, S., Laurie, L.R., Chintapalli, K.N., Valente, P.T., and Dodd, G.D., III. 2000. Primary papillary serous carcinoma of the peritoneum: CT-pathologic correlation. *J. Comput. Assist. Tomogr.* 24:395–399.

Furukawa, T., Ueda, J., Takahashi, S., Higashino, K., Shimura, K., Tsujimura, T., and Araki, Y. 1999. Peritoneal serous papillary carcinoma: radiological appearance. *Abdom. Imaging* 24:78–81.

Gooneratne, S., Sassone, M., Blaustein, A., and Talerman, A. 1982. Serous surface papillary carcinoma of the ovary: a clinicopathologic study of 16 cases. *Int. J. Gynecol. Pathol.* 1:258–269.

Kim, H.J., Kim, J.K., and Cho, K.S. 2004. CT features of serous surface papillary carcinoma of the ovary. *Am. J. Roentgenol.* 183:1721–1724.

Kim, S.H., Cho, J.Y., Park, I.A., Kang, S.B., Lee, H.P., and Han, M.C. 1997. Radiological findings in serous surface papillary carcinoma of the ovary. Case reports. *Acta Radiol.* 38:847–849.

Kim, S.H., Yang, D.M., and Kim, S.H. 2005. Borderline serous surface papillary tumor of the ovary: MRI characteristics. *Am. J. Roentgenol.* 184:1898–1900.

Liapis, A., Condi-Paphiti, A., Pyrgiotis, E., and Zourlas, P.A. 1996. Ovarian surface serous papillary carcinomas: a clinicopathologic study. *Eur. J. Gynaecol. Oncol.* 17:79–82.

Mills, S.E., Andersen, W.A., Fechner, R.E., and Austin, M.B. 1988. Serous surface papillary carcinoma: a clinicopathologic study of 10 cases and comparison with stage III-IV ovarian serous carcinoma. *Am. J. Surg. Pathol.* 12:827–834.

Moon, M.H. 2005. Epithelial tumors of the ovary. In: Kim, S.H., McClennan, B.L., and Outwater, E.K. (Eds.), *Radiology Illustrated: Gynecologic Imaging* (1st ed.). Philadelphia: Elsevier Saunders, pp. 501–502.

Mulhollan, T.J., Silva, E.G., Tornos, C., Guerrieri, C., Fromm, G.L., and Gershenson, D. 1994. Ovarian involvement by serous surface papillary carcinoma. *Int. J. Gynecol. Pathol.* 13:120–126.

Stafford-Johnson, D.B., Bree, R.L., Francis, I.R., and Korobkin, M. 1998. CT appearance of primary papillary serous carcinoma of the peritoneum. *Am. J. Roentgenol.* 171:687–689.

Zissin, R., Hertz, M., Shapiro-Feinberg, M., Bernheim, J., Altaras, M., and Fishman, A. 2001. Primary serous papillary carcinoma of the peritoneum: CT findings. *Clin. Radiol.* 56:740–745.

36

Chronic Pancreatitis versus Pancreatic Cancer: Positron Emission Tomography

Yukihiro Yokoyama, Masato Nagino, and Yuji Nimura

Introduction

Early diagnosis and accurate staging of pancreatic cancer is critical in determining the treatment of choice. Differential diagnosis between benign and malignant pancreatic tumors is particularly important because the prognosis of malignant pancreatic tumor is very poor, and it is curable only by surgical resection in its early stage.

Recent advances in imaging techniques have contributed to an early and accurate diagnosis of pancreatic cancer. Computed tomography (CT), endoscopic ultrasonography (EUS), endoscopic retrograde cholangiopancreatography (ERCP), and magnetic resonance cholangiopancreatography (MRCP) are commonly used imaging modalities in detecting pancreatic cancer. Fluorine-18 deoxyglucose positron emission tomography (FDG-PET) has evolved as an additional modality, which sensitively detects the pancreatic cancer using different metabolic status of cancer tissue. FDG, a glucose analog, is highly metabolized in tumor cells as an energy source and a carbon backbone for DNA and RNA synthesis (Bares et al., 1993). Therefore, it is suitable to detect a tumor with a high proliferation rate. Although CT and MR imaging are advantageous in providing precise anatomical delineation of pancreatic lesions, they are less specific in differentiating malignant

and benign lesions (Ho et al., 1996). In contrast, FDG-PET has been shown to be useful in detecting altered metabolic activity in malignant tumors (Delbeke et al., 1999), although it is less sensitive in detecting anatomical localization of the tumor.

Despite numerous reports describing the usefulness of PET with its high sensitivity and specificity (Koyama et al., 2001) in detecting pancreatic malignancies, differential diagnosis of inflammatory lesions from malignant lesions is challenging (Kasperk et al., 2001). A variety of clinical manifestations of pancreatic disease make the diagnosis more difficult. Inflammatory pancreatic disease includes chronic pancreatitis, acute pancreatitis, pancreatic abscess, pancreatic pseudocysts, and mass-forming autoimmune pancreatitis. Pancreatic neoplasms include various clinicopathologic types such as invasive ductal carcinomas, intraductal papillary and mucinous neoplasms (IPMNs), mucinous cystic tumors, serous cystic tumors, and endocrine tumors. Moreover, the coexistence of benign and malignant pancreatic lesions is commonly observed and makes the diagnosis more difficult. This chapter describes the usefulness and limitations of FDG-PET in differentiating inflammatory pancreatic disease and pancreatic cancer, which is one of the most controversial issues in pancreatic cancer imaging.

Usefulness of FDG-PET

A number of reports have shown the advantages of FDG-PET in diagnosing pancreatic tumor. Overall sensitivity and specificity of FDG-PET in detecting pancreatic cancer have been reported as being 94 to 96% and 78 to 88%, respectively (Delbeke *et al.*, 1999; Zimny *et al.*, 1997), which are superior to those of CT. Especially for the lesion < 2 cm in diameter, the sensitivity of PET is superior to that achieved with other imaging modalities. Positron emission tomography is also useful in detecting recurrent pancreatic carcinoma, even in a patient with anatomic alteration after surgery.

Pancreatic cancer includes not only a solid lesion but also a cystic lesion. Intraductal papillary mucinous neoplasms (IPMNs) of the pancreas frequently reveal a cystic lesion and contain various histological types, ranging from malignant to benign neoplasms. Differential diagnosis between benign and malignant IPMN is crucial because treatment varies depending on the histological malignancy. FDG-PET was shown to be more accurate than CT in identifying and managing these pancreatic cystic lesions (Sperti *et al.*, 2001). Sperti *et al.* (2001) performed FDG-PET in addition to CT scanning for 56 patients with a suspected cystic tumor of the pancreas. Sensitivity, specificity, and positive-and negative-predictive values for FDG-PET and CT scanning in detecting malignant cystic tumors were 94%, 97%, 94%, and 97% and 65%, 87%, 69%, and 85%, respectively. These results indicate that a positive result on FDG-PET strongly suggests malignancy, whereas a negative result suggests a benign tumor. Another report from Japan showed the usefulness of FDG-PET in diagnosing malignant IPMN even when it has no solid component (Yoshioka *et al.*, 2003).

FDG-PET has other advantages. It is superior to conventional radiographic modalities in predicting the survival of patients with pancreatic carcinoma who are subjected to chemotherapy. A report showed that patients who experienced a diminished or reduced FDG uptake after chemotherapy had a significantly better overall survival in comparison to patients who had unchanged FDG uptake (Maisey *et al.*, 2000). Another report showed that the median survival among patients with low FDG uptake was longer than patients with high uptake, indicating that the results of FDG-PET provide additional prognostic information in patients with pancreatic carcinoma (Zimny *et al.*, 2000).

Limitations of FDG-PET

Despite the above-mentioned usefulness, FDG-PET has several limitations. It cannot accurately detect local invasion of adjacent visceral structures because of limited spatial resolution. Fused images from CT (especially when multidetector-row CT is used) and FDG-PET allow precise anatomical assessment and could resolve this problem. However, these modalities are available in only a few institutions.

Patients with high serum glucose levels that are competitors for FDG receptor showed high false-negative results due to decreased FDG uptake by tumors (Zimny *et al.*, 1999). The detection rates and mean uptake values for pancreatic malignancies were lower if fasted plasma glucose levels were high (> 130 mg/dl or with a diagnosis of diabetes mellitus). Therefore, negative PET results with elevated plasma glucose should be interpreted with caution. One of the most important challenges in imaging pancreatic tumor is how to accurately delineate active inflammatory lesions from malignant lesions. This issue is discussed in the following section.

Differential Diagnosis between Pancreatic Cancer and Inflammatory Pancreatic Lesions

A semiquantitative index called the standardized uptake value (SUV) is the most commonly used index in FDG-PET, which provides objective quantification of FDG accumulation in the lesion (Delbeke *et al.*, 2001). The SUV is derived by the following formula:

$$\text{Standardized uptake value} = \frac{\dfrac{\text{tissue radioactivity concentration (MBq/ml)}}{\text{injected dose (MBq)} \times \text{body weight (g)}}}{\dfrac{1}{\text{decay factor of }^{18}\text{F}}}$$

Several reports have shown that mean SUV for pancreatitis is significantly lower than that for pancreatic cancer (Ho *et al.*, 1996; Zimny and Buell, 1997; Friess *et al.*, 1995; Kato *et al.*, 1995; Keogan *et al.*, 1998; Imdahl *et al.*, 1999). However, mean SUV for pancreatitis and pancreatic cancer ranges widely depending on the report (Table 1), and recommended SUV cut-off level in differentiating malignant lesion is variable (1.5 to 4.0). Shreve *et al.* (1998) reported a difficulty in differentiating pancreatic cancer from inflammatory pancreatic disease by FDG-PET. Among 42 patients studied by FDG-PET for pancreatic disease, 12 showed focal FDG uptake in the pancreas, which was ultimately found to be related to inflammation rather than neoplasm. The SUV ranged from 3.4 to 11.2 on FDG-PET in these cases. Drawbacks of PET in this regard include relatively wide overlap in SUV between cancers and inflammatory lesions.

Some researchers have described the usefulness of kinetic analysis of FDG uptake in differentiating benign and malignant lesions (Nakamoto *et al.*, 2000). The retention index of FDG, calculated by dividing the increase in the SUV between 1 hr and 2 hr post-injection by the SUV at 1 hr post-injection, was significantly higher in malignant

Table 1 Comparison of Mean SUV for Pancreatitis and Pancreatic Carcinoma

Author	Pancreatitis (*)	Carcinoma (*)
Friess, H. et al. (1995)	0.9 (32)	3.1 (42)
Kato, T. et al. (1995)	2.8 (9)	4.6 (15)
Ho, C.L. et al. (1996)	2.2 (6)	4.1 (8)
Zimny, M. et al. (1997)	3.6 (32)	6.4 (74)
Keogan, M.T. et al. (1998)	1.9 (12)	5.1 (25)
Imdahl, A. et al. (1999)	3.5 (12)	7.3 (27)

(*) Number of patients.

lesions than in benign lesions, indicating that a malignant lesion tends to progressively retain FDG more than a benign lesion. However, images at 3 hr post-injection usually were not helpful in differentiating further between malignant lesions and benign lesions. Combining this retention index with the SUV at 2 hr post-injection provided a > 90% diagnostic accuracy. Another report showed a different FDG kinetics between pancreatitis and pancreatic carcinoma (Nitzsche et al., 2002). The shape of the time-activity curve was different between pancreatitis and pancreatic carcinoma even within 1 hr post-injection, although no significant difference existed between chronic pancreatitis and acute pancreatitis. Specificity of this kinetic analysis in differentiating pancreatic carcinoma from pancreatitis was superior to semiquantitative uptake value analysis.

Mass-forming autoimmune pancreatitis is one of the phenotypes of chronic pancreatitis and should be kept in mind when making a differential diagnosis of pancreatic cancer with the assistance of FDG-PET. Reske et al. (1997) reported that the SUVs of FDG in patients with pancreatic cancer and mass-forming pancreatitis were 2.98 ± 1.23 and 1.25 ± 0.51, respectively. This difference may not be enough to clearly delineate these two lesions.

Patients with an acute exacerbation of chronic pancreatitis (Imdahl et al., 1999; Yokoyama et al., 2005) may have an increased SUV with ranges similar to those for patients with pancreatic carcinoma. Differential diagnosis is difficult in such a case even with concomitant analysis of serum amylase, serum lipase, and other serological tests. There might be a correlation between the stage of inflammatory process and the level of SUV. Figure 1 presents a representative case of chronic pancreatitis superimposed by degenerative necrosis, which showed intense signal by FDG-PET in the granulation tissue and was difficult to differentiate from a malignant tumor even after laparotomy. In this case, it was speculated that the amount of granulation tissue actively repairing degenerative necrosis was correlated to the level of signal by FDG-PET. This speculation is supported by a report of pancreatic tuberculosis, in which noncaseating pancreatic granuloma showed high SUV (= 4.09) (Sanabe et al., 2002). Different results could be expected if FDG-PET was

performed later when the degenerative necrosis is replaced by fibrous granulation tissue through its repairing process. This case suggests a limitation of FDG-PET in distinguishing malignant lesions in the pancreas especially from acute inflammatory change in chronic pancreatitis. It also suggests the need to repeat examination of FDG-PET for an accurate diagnosis of inflammatory lesions.

Is There Any Better Tracer Than FDG?

The problem of differential diagnosis between inflammatory lesion and malignant lesion may be alleviated by performing multitracer studies. Many tracers detect different metabolic aspects of pancreatic tumors and pancreas with chronic pancreatitis, although the usefulness of these tracers is still controversial.

L-[methyl-11C] methionine (11C-Met) is a useful tracer for pancreatic imaging with PET. This tracer accumulates very rapidly in the pancreas after intravenous administration (Takasu et al., 1999). The drawbacks include a short half-life and high physiological accumulation in the abdominal organs. 11C-Met-PET can be used for quantitative analysis of amino acid metabolism and thus is useful for evaluating pancreatic exocrine function in chronic pancreatitis (Takasu et al., 2001). The radioactivity ratio of the pancreas to that of the liver in patients with chronic pancreatitis was significantly lower than that of healthy subjects after radioactive methionine injection. This method may differentiate chronic pancreatitis not only from normal pancreas, but also from malignant pancreatic lesion. However, pancreatic cancer with obstruction of the main pancreatic duct frequently accompanies upstream pancreatitis. This may make the diagnosis more difficult.

[18F]fluorophenylalanine (18F-Phe), which shares the same amino acid transport system with Met, seems to be a potentially useful amino acid tracer for tumor imaging with a longer half-life and with higher tumor contrast in the abdomen than 11C-Met (Kubota et al., 1996). However, accumulation of 18F-Phe in the pancreas is not efficient compared to other organs, and therefore the sensitivity to detect a pancreatic tumor is not high.

Protein synthesis and amino acid transport are enhanced in most tumor cells, whereas those are less affected in inflammation. In this regard, it was expected that 2-(18)F-fluoro-L-tyrosine (18F-TYR), an amino acid tracer, could be superior in visualizing cancer lesions to FDG PET. However, unexpectedly, clinical studies using 18F-TYR-PET did not show any superiority to 18F-FDG-PET (Hustinx et al., 2003).

[11C]choline (CH) is a sensitive tracer and allows detection of smaller lesions (< 5 mm). It is very useful particularly if it is combined with FDG-PET. However, the pancreas is one of the organs that showed high uptake to this tracer

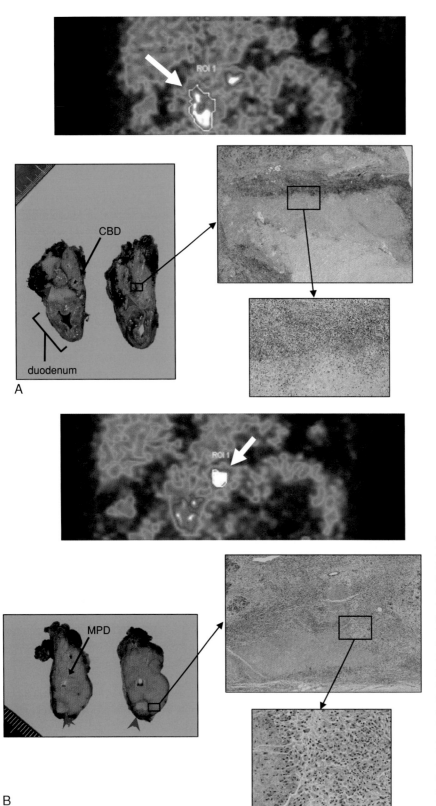

Figure 1 A 66-year-old male with sudden onset of epigastralgic pain was admitted to the hospital. FDG-PET was performed to rule out the possibility of pancreatic cancer. It showed intense FDG accumulation in the head (**A**) (SUV = 4.1) and body (**B**) (SUV = 6.7) of the pancreas (white arrows), which are correlated to the tumors detected by CT and US. Because of the findings of FDG-PET, he was diagnosed as having two malignant pancreatic tumors, and pancreatoduodenectomy was performed. In macroscopic and microscopic (hematoxylin-eosin staining) view, two tumorous lesions consisted of degenerative necrosis surrounded by granulation tissue. The tumor in the pancreatic head (SUV; 4.1) (A) consisted of a large amount of degenerative necrosis, which was surrounded by granulation tissue. The granulation tissue was observed mainly at the rim of the necrosis. In the pancreatic body tumor (SUV; 6.7) (B), in contrast, the proportion of degenerative necrosis was smaller, and it predominantly consisted of granulation tissue. CBD = common bile duct; MPD = main pancreatic duct.

and may not be feasible for detecting pancreatic tumors. Although some authors claimed that better discrimination between proliferative tissue and inflammation is possible with 11C-CH-PET than with 18F-FDG-PET (Sasaki, 2004; Khan *et al.*, 2004), the results are still controversial.

1-[11C]-acetate (11C-acetate-PET) promptly accumulates in the normal pancreas (as early as 2 min post-injection), and subsequent clearance of the tracer from the pancreas is slow relative to the adjacent organs. Pancreatic uptake of 1-[11C]-acetate was unaffected by pancreatic endocrine insufficiency, but is absent in chronic pancreatitis complicated by exocrine insufficiency. The level of tracer accumulation was substantially reduced in mass-forming chronic pancreatitis. Therefore, it was tried to differentiate mass-forming chronic pancreatitis from adenocarcinoma by taking advantage of their metabolic differences. However, it did not provide additional diagnostic benefits in a clinical study (Rasmussen *et al.*, 2004). Taken together, FDG-PET is the most useful and commonly used tracer, and presently no other tracer seems to be superior to FDG.

Conclusions and Future Perspective

Because many of the pancreatic cancers are difficult to cure by surgical resection, preoperative evaluation of curability is essential. Factors that may preclude a curative resection include invasion of major vessels, involvement of neural plexus around the celiac axis and superior mesenteric artery, invasion of adjacent organs, and distant metastasis. The use of thin-slice helical CT and 3D-CT angiography is superior to PET in precluding these factors. Positron emission tomography, at best, is complementary in this regard. Accumulating data, however, showed that PET is superior to CT or MRI in differentiating malignant pancreatic lesions from inflammatory lesions. Differentiation could be more objective by using semiquantitative SUV. Functional imaging using FDG-PET is especially useful when the images are fused with those obtained with CT and MRI. However, relatively wide overlap in SUV between malignant lesions and inflammatory lesions is one of the major problems. This problem can be resolved by performing multitracer PET, which detects different metabolic aspects of the pancreatic tumor. However, presently there is no reliable tracer for the pancreatic lesions other than the FDG. Further case accumulation and establishment of better analytic method, which allow more sensitive differentiation between cancers and inflammation, are necessary in the future.

References

Bares, R., Klever, P., Hellwig, D., Hauptmann, S., Fass, J., Hambuechen, U., Zopp, L., Mueller, B., Buell, U., and Schumpelick, V. 1993. Pancreatic cancer detected by positron emission tomography with 18F-labelled deoxyglucose: method and first results. *Nucl. Med. Commun.* 14:596–601.

Delbeke, D., and Martin, W.H. 2001. Positron emission tomography imaging in oncology. *Radiol. Clin. North. Am. 39*:883–917.

Delbeke, D., Rose, D.M., Chapman, W.C., Pinson, C.W., Wright, J.K., Beauchamp, R.D., Shyr, Y., and Leach, S.D. 1999. Optimal interpretation of FDG PET in the diagnosis, staging and management of pancreatic carcinoma. *J. Nucl. Med. 40*:1784–1791.

Friess, H., Langhans, J., Ebert, M., Beger, H.G., Stollfuss, J., Reske, S.N., and Buchler, M.W. 1995. Diagnosis of pancreatic cancer by 2[18F]-fluoro-2-deoxy-D-glucose positron emission tomography. *Gut 36*: 771–777.

Ho, C.L., Dehdashti, F., Griffeth, L.K., Buse, P.E., Balfe, D.M., and Siegel, B.A. 1996. FDG-PET evaluation of indeterminate pancreatic masses. *J. Comput. Assist. Tomogr. 20*:363–369.

Hustinx, R., Lemaire, C., Jerusalem, G., Moreau, P., Cataldo, D., Duysinx, B., Aerts, J., Fassotte, M.F., Foidart, J., and Luxen, A. 2003. Whole-body tumor imaging using PET and 2-18F-fluoro-L-tyrosine: preliminary evaluation and comparison with 18F-FDG. *J. Nucl. Med. 44*:533–539.

Imdahl, A., Nitzsche, E., Krautmann, F., Hogerle, S., Boos, S., Einert, A., Sontheimer, J., and Farthmann, E.H. 1999. Evaluation of positron emission tomography with 2-[18F]fluoro-2-deoxy-D-glucose for the differentiation of chronic pancreatitis and pancreatic cancer. *Br. J. Surg. 86*:194–199.

Kasperk, R.K., Riesener, K.P., Wilms, K., and Schumpelick, V. 2001. Limited value of positron emission tomography in treatment of pancreatic cancer: surgeon's view. *World J. Surg. 25*:1134–1139.

Kato, T., Fukatsu, H., Ito, K., Tadokoro, M., Ota, T., Ikeda, M., Isomura, T., Ito, S., Nishino, M., and Ishigaki, T. 1995. Fluorodeoxyglucose positron emission tomography in pancreatic cancer: an unsolved problem. *Eur. J. Nucl. Med. 22*:32–39.

Keogan, M.T., Tyler, D., Clark, L., Branch, M.S., McDermott, V.G., DeLong, D.M., and Coleman, R.E. 1998. Diagnosis of pancreatic carcinoma: role of FDG PET. *Am. J. Roentgenol. 171*:1565–1570.

Khan, N., Oriuchi, N., Ninomiya, H., Higuchi, T., Kamada, H., and Endo, K. 2004. Positron emission tomographic imaging with 11C-choline in differential diagnosis of head and neck tumors: comparison with 18F-FDG PET. *Ann. Nucl. Med. 18*:409–417.

Koyama, K., Okamura, T., Kawabe, J., Nakata, B., Chung, K.H., Ochi, H., and Yamada, R. 2001. Diagnostic usefulness of FDG PET for pancreatic mass lesions. *Ann. Nucl. Med. 15*:217–224.

Kubota, K., Ishiwata, K., Kubota, R., Yamada, S., Takahashi, J., Abe, Y., Fukuda, H., and Ido, T. 1996. Feasibility of fluorine-18-fluorophenylalanine for tumor imaging compared with carbon-11-L-methionine. *J. Nucl. Med. 37*:320–325.

Maisey, N.R., Webb, A., Flux, G.D., Padhani, A., Cunningham, D.C., Ott, R.J., and Norman, A. 2000. FDG-PET in the prediction of survival of patients with cancer of the pancreas: a pilot study. *Br. J. Cancer. 83*:287–293.

Nakamoto, Y., Higashi, T., Sakahara, H., Tamaki, N., Kogire, M., Doi, R., Hosotani, R., Imamura, M., and Konishi, J. 2000. Delayed (18)F-fluoro-2-deoxy-D-glucose positron emission tomography scan for differentiation between malignant and benign lesions in the pancreas. *Cancer 89*:2547–2554.

Nitzsche, E.U., Hoegerle, S., Mix, M., Brink, I., Otte, A., Moser, E., and Imdahl, A. 2002. Non-invasive differentiation of pancreatic lesions: is analysis of FDG kinetics superior to semiquantitative uptake value analysis? *Eur. J. Nucl. Med. Mol. Imaging 29*:237–242.

Rasmussen, I., Sorensen, J., Langstrom, B., and Haglund, U. 2004. Is positron emission tomography using 18F-fluorodeoxyglucose and 11C-acetate valuable in diagnosing indeterminate pancreatic masses? *Scand. J. Surg. 93*:191–197.

Reske, S.N., Grillenberger, K.G., Glatting, G., Port, M., Hildebrandt, M., Gansauge, F., and Beger, H.G. 1997. Overexpression of glucose transporter 1 and increased FDG uptake in pancreatic carcinoma. *J. Nucl. Med. 38*:1344–1348.

Sanabe, N., Ikematsu, Y., Nishiwaki, Y., Kida, H., Murohisa, G., Ozawa, T., Hasegawa, S., Okawada, T., Toritsuka, T., and Waki, S. 2002. Pancreatic tuberculosis. *J. Hepatobiliary Pancreat. Surg. 9*:515–518.

Sasaki, T. 2004. [11C]choline uptake in regenerating liver after partial hepatectomy or CCl4-administration. *Nucl. Med. Biol. 31*:269–275.

Shreve, P.D. 1998. Focal fluorine-18 fluorodeoxyglucose accumulation in inflammatory pancreatic disease. *Eur. J. Nucl. Med. 25*:259–264.

Sperti, C., Pasquali, C., Chierichetti, F., Liessi, G., Ferlin, G., and Pedrazzoli, S. 2001. Value of 18-fluorodeoxyglucose positron emission tomography in the management of patients with cystic tumors of the pancreas. *Ann. Surg. 234*:675–680.

Takasu, A., Shimosegawa, T., Shimosegawa, E., Hatazawa, J., Kimura, K., Fujita, M., Koizumi, M., Kanno, I., and Toyota, T. 1999. 11C-methionine uptake to the pancreas and its secretion: a positron emission tomography study in humans. *Pancreas 18*:392–398.

Takasu, A., Shimosegawa, T., Shimosegawa, E., Hatazawa, J., Nagasaki, Y., Kimura, K., Fujita, M., and Toyota, T. 2001. [11C]methionine positron emission tomography for the evaluation of pancreatic exocrine function in chronic pancreatitis. *Pancreas 22*:203–209.

Yokoyama, Y., Nagino, M., Hiromatsu, T., Yuasa, N., Oda, K., Arai, T., Nishio, H., Ebata, T., and Nimura, Y. 2005. Intense PET signal in the degenerative necrosis superimposed on chronic pancreatitis. *Pancreas 31*:192–194.

Yoshioka, M., Sato, T., Furuya, T., Shibata, S., Andoh, H., Asanuma, Y., Hatazawa, J., and Koyama, K. 2003. Positron emission tomography with 2-deoxy-2-[(18)F] fluoro-d-glucose for diagnosis of intraductal papillary mucinous tumor of the pancreas with parenchymal invasion. *J. Gastroenterol. 38*:1189–1193.

Zimny, M., Bares, R., Fass, J., Adam, G., Cremerius, U., Dohmen, B., Klever, P., Sabri, O., Schumpelick, V., and Buell, U. 1997. Fluorine-18 fluorodeoxyglucose positron emission tomography in the differential diagnosis of pancreatic carcinoma: a report of 106 cases. *Eur. J. Nucl. Med. 24*:678–682.

Zimny, M., and Buell, U. 1999. 18FDG-positron emission tomography in pancreatic cancer. *Ann. Oncol. 10 Suppl 4*:28–32.

Zimny, M., Fass, J., Bares, R., Cremerius, U., Sabri, O., Buechin, P., Schumpelick, V., and Buell, U. 2000. Fluorodeoxyglucose positron emission tomography and the prognosis of pancreatic carcinoma. *Scand. J. Gastroenterol. 35*:883–888.

Pancreatic Cancer: p-[^{123}I]Iodo-L-Phenylalanine Single Photon Emission Tomography for Tumor Imaging

Samuel Samnick and Marcus Menges

Introduction

Pancreatic cancer is associated with the worst 5-year survival rate of any human cancer. This high mortality rate is due, in part, to difficulties in establishing early and accurate diagnosis. Because most tumors share the ability to accumulate amino acids more effectively than normal tissues and any other pathology, assessment of amino acid metabolism in tumor cells using radiolabeled amino acids has become one of the most promising tools for tumor imaging. This study investigated the potential of the iodine-123 labeled amino acid p-[^{123}I]iodo-L-phenylalanine (IPA) for detection of pancreatic cancer by single photon emission tomography. The affinity of IPA for pancreatic tumor was investigated in human PaCa44 and PanC1 pancreatic adenocarcinoma cells, following by analysis of the underlying mechanisms of tracer accumulation in neoplastic cells. Thereafter, IPA was evaluated for targeting of pancreatic cancer using severe combined immunodeficient

(SCID) mice engrafted with primary human pancreatic adenocarcinoma, as well as in acute inflammation models in immunocompetent mice and rats. The *in vivo* evaluation included measurements of the kinetics of tumor and organ uptake by dynamic imaging using a high-resolution gamma-camera and by gamma-counting of the organs of interest after dissection.

p-[^{123}I]iodo-L-phenylalanine accumulated intensively in human pancreatic tumor cells. Radioactivity accumulation in tumor cells following a 30-min incubation at 37°C/pH 7.4 varied from 41 to 58% of the total loaded activity per 10^6 cells. The cellular uptake was predominantly mediated by specific carriers for neutral amino acids, namely, the sodium-independent and L-leucine-preferring (L-system) transporter and by alanine-, serine-, and cysteine-preferring (ASC-system) transporter. Protein incorporation was less than 8%. Biodistribution studies showed rapid localization of the tracer to tumors, reaching $10 \pm 2.5 - 15 \pm 3\%$ of the injected dose per gram (I.D./g) in heterotopic tumors compared with 17 ± 3.5 to $22 \pm 4.3\%$

I.D./g in the orthotopic tumors, at 60 and 240 min post-injection of IPA, respectively. In contrast, IPA uptake in the gastrointestinal tract and areas of inflammation remained moderate and decreased with time. Excellent tumor detection was obtained by gamma-camera imaging. The specific and high-level targeting of IPA to tumor and the negligible uptake into gastrointestinal tract and areas of inflammation indicate that p-[^{123}I]iodo-L-phenylalanine single photon emission tomograpy is a promising tool for differential diagnosis of pancreatic cancer.

Of all gastrointestinal tumors, pancreatic cancer has one of the worst prognoses. This poor prognostic results from difficulty in early detection, lack of effective treatment, and limited knowledge of the biological characteristic of the disease (Warshaw and Fernandez-del Castillo, 1992; Faivre et al., 1998). At present, only radical resection of the tumor with surrounding lymph nodes provides a curative chance for patients. Unfortunately, this option is limited to only 10–20% of patients because the majority of cases are diagnosed at late stages of disease (Schafer et al., 2002; Trumper et al., 2002). At time of diagnosis the tumor is often already large, with invasion of surrounding tissue or metastasis to distant organs. Therefore, besides substantial attempts to improve our understanding of the malignancy, major efforts need to be directed toward earlier and more accurate diagnosis of the disease, with a view to improving the outcome in patients with pancreatic cancer. But even hopeful new strategies to establish an earlier diagnosis of pancreatic cancer have been disappointing when tested in a prospective manner under clinical conditions. Therefore, intensive efforts have been made to explore imaging methods for the detection and staging of pancreatic carcinomas. However, the differential diagnosis of pancreatic cancer by current imaging techniques and especially accurate differentiation between inflammatory (i.e., acute or chronic pancreatitis) and neoplastic masses remain uncertain (Grino et al., 2003; Diederichs et al., 2000; Nitzsche et al., 2002). One promising approach that appears more sensitive than other imaging modalities, including computed tomography (CT), magnetic resonance imaging (MRI), ultrasonography (US) and positron emission tomography (PET) with [^{18}F]fluoro-2-deoxy-D-glucose (FDG), is the use of tumor-affine radiolabeled amino acids to study the physiological processes associated with the high utilization of amino acids in malignant cells noninvasively (Laverman et al., 2002; Jager et al., 2001).

Previous investigations have demonstrated that tumor imaging with amino acid tracers is less influenced by inflammation due to the generally low accumulation of amino acids into inflammatory cells (Jager et al., 2001; Laverman et al., 2002; Rau et al., 2002; Hellwig et al., 2005). This indicates that amino acid tracers with high affinity for pancreatic cancer are potentially more tumor-specific and therefore more suitable for differentiating between viable neoplastic tissues and inflammatory lesions. However, development of amino acid-based tracers for pancreatic tumor diagnosis has not been the subject of intensive study in the past decade. As part of our effort to explore radiolabeled amino acids for noninvasive diagnosis of pancreatic cancer, we developed a series of tumor-affine radioiodinated amino acids. Among them, the L-phenylalanine derivative, IPA, showed a marked affinity for pancreatic tumors in previous investigations (Samnick et al., 2001; Hellwig et al., 2005). In this report, we studied the uptake characteristics of IPA in human pancreatic adenocarcinoma cells, followed by investigation of the mechanisms promoting the cellular uptake. Thereafter, IPA was validated in in vivo models of human pancreatic carcinoma in SCID mice, and in inflammation models in immunocompetent mice and rats in comparison with the clinically established FDG, in order to assess its suitability as a radiotracer to target pancreatic tumor specifically by routine single photon emission tomography.

Materials and Methods

Reagents

Sodium [^{123}I]iodide for radiolabeling and FDG were obtained commercially from Forschungszentrum Karlsruhe (Karlsruhe, Germany). L-alanine, L-phenylalanine, L-tyrosine, L-serine, L-cysteine, L-leucine and their D-isomers, as well as 2-amino-2-norbornane-carboxylic acid (BCH), α-(methylamino)-iso-butyric acid (MeAIB), nigericin, valinomycin, 4-bromo-L-phenylalanine, and non-radiolabeled 4-iodo-L-phenylalanine ("cold" IPA), were from Sigma-Aldrich (Deisenhofen, Germany). Concanavalin A (ConA) for induction of acute inflammation was purchased from ICN (Eschwede, Germany). Concanavalin A was dissolved in PBS (pH = 7) for injection. Unless otherwise stated, all other solvents were of analytical or clinical grade and were obtained either from Merck (Darmstadt, Germany) or purchased via the local university hospital pharmacy. Radioactivity in tissues, blood, and tumor was measured on a Berthold LB 951 G scintillation counter (Berthold, Wildbad, Germany) after reference samples (triplicates) of the injected dose had been prepared as standards.

Preparation of p-[^{123}I]Iodo-L-Phenylalanine

p-[^{123}I]iodo-L-phenylalanine was prepared by nonisotopic Cu(II)-assisted [^{123}I]iodo-debromination of p-bromo-L-phenylalanine in the presence of ascorbic acid. IPA was isolated from unreacted starting materials and radioactive impurities by HPLC, and the fraction containing the radiopharmaceutical was collected into a sterile tube, buffered with PBS (pH 7.0), and sterile-filtered through a 0.22 μm filter into an evacuated sterile tube prior to studies. IPA used in the present study was obtained in 90 ± 5 radiochemical yield after HPLC isolation. A radiochemical purity of > 99% was obtained. Details concerning the radiosynthesis and formulation have been described previously (Samnick *et al.*, 2001; Hellwig *et al.*, 2005).

Cell Cultures

The human pancreatic adenocarcinoma PaCa44 (established by Dr. M. v. Bülow, Mainz, Germany) and PanC-1 (American Type Culture Collection, Rockville, Maryland) cell lines were provided by the oncological research laboratory of the University Center of Saarland (Homburg, Germany). Cells were cultivated in RPMI-1640 medium containing 10% (v/v) heat-inactivated fetal calf serum (FCS), penicillin (50 U/ml), streptomycin (50 µg/ml), and 50 µL insulin (10 µL/ml) (PromoCell, Heidelberg, Germany). The cells were incubated in a humidified 5% CO$_2$ incubator at 37°C. Cells were passaged routinely every five days. Before the experiment, subconfluent cell cultures were trypsinized with a solution of 0.05% trypsin in PBS without Ca^{2+} and Mg^{2+} and containing 0.02% EDTA. Cells were washed with medium and placed in PBS shortly before implantation or uptake experiments after counting by vital staining on a hemocytometer. Cells were free of mycoplasms. Viability of the cells was assessed by trypan blue and was > 95%.

Cell Uptake Experiments

To assess nonspecific binding of the tracer to plastic tubes, they were presaturated with 1% bovine serum albumin in 0.1 M PBS (pH 7.4), followed by addition of freshly prepared IPA. The solution was maintained in an incubator at 37°C for 30–180 min, followed by treatment with ice-cold PBS at the end of the experiment. The radioactivity binding to plastic tubes was less than 0.5% of total loaded radioactivity for incubation periods up to 180 min.

All experiments were performed fourfold, simultaneously with 250,000, 500,000, and 10^6 freshly resuspended human pancreatic tumor cells. Before experiments, subconfluent cells were trypsinized as described above. The suspension was mixed thoroughly, and transferred to a 50-ml centrifuge tube (Falcon®, Becton Dickinson, USA). Cells were centrifuged for 5 min at 200 × *g*; the resulting supernatant was removed and the pellet re-suspended in serum-free Dulbecco's Mod Eagle medium and then transferred to Eppendorf tubes at concentrations of 10^6 cells/ml for the uptake investigations. Before the incubation with IPA, the pancreatic tumor cells were preincubated for 15 min in 500 µL medium at 37°C in 1.5-ml Eppendorf centrifuge tubes. Aliquots of 30–50 µL (10^6 – 1.5 × 10^6 cpm) freshly prepared IPA were added, and cells were incubated at 37°C for 1, 2, 5, 15, 30, 60, 90, and 120 min while shaking. Uptake was stopped with 500 µL ice-cold PBS (pH 7.4) and an additional 3 min in an ice bath, the cells were centrifuged for 2 min at 300 × *g*, the supernatant was removed, and the pellet was washed three times with ice-cold PBS. Cell pellets were counted for radioactivity together with 3 aliquots of standards on a Berthold LB951 gamma counter. The percentage of binding of IPA was calculated by the formula: (cpm cell pellet/mean cpm radioactive standards) × 100. The results were expressed either as a percentage of the applied dose per 10^6 cells or as cpm/1000 cells for better comparison.

In separate experiments, IPA uptake into tumor cells was investigated at different temperatures (4, 20, and 37°C, pH 7.4) and pH (5.0–9.0, 37°C), as well as in sodium-containing and in high K$^+$ medium (135 mm KCl). Furthermore, the contribution of the mitochondria on the cellular uptake was assessed in the presence of valinomycin and nigericin (1 mmol/L, 100 µL), known to disrupt the metabolism of mitochondria. Radioactivity retained in tumor cells was determined as described above after a 30-min incubation at 37°C/pH 7.4.

Investigation of the Mechanisms Underlying the Uptake for IPA in Tumor Cells

Competitive inhibition experiments were carried out to characterize the mechanisms promoting the uptake of IPA into pancreatic carcinoma cells. For this purpose, suspensions containing 10^6 tumor cells/ml were pre-incubated with 100 µL of specific inhibitors for amino acid transport and with selected neutral L- and D-amino acids with known carrier system. Aliquots of 30–50 µL (10^6 – 1.5 × 10^6 cpm) freshly prepared IPA were added, followed by an incubation of the mixture at 37°C/pH 7.4 for 30 min. At the end of the incubation, 0.5 ml ice-cold PBS (pH 7.4) was added to stop the reaction. Cell pellets were isolated after centrifugation, and radioactivity was retained in tumor cells determined on a γ-counter as described above.

The following specific amino acid carrier inhibitors and neutral amino acids were used: BCH, MeAIB and alanine-serine-cysteine (1:1:1), L-leucine, L-phenylalanine, L-tyrosine, and L-proline. The concentration of the inhibitors used was 1 and 5 mmol/L. A parallel experiment was performed with increasing concentrations of unlabeled 4-iodo-L-phenylalanine to assess the capacity of the transport system. In addition, the fraction of IPA incorporated into protein was determined by acid precipitation, using 10% trichloroacetic acid, as described previously (Hellwig *et al.*, 2005).

Animals

All animal experiments were conducted in accordance with the *Guide for the Care and Use of Laboratory Animals* published by the U.S. National Institutes of Health (NIH Publication No. 85-23, revised 1996) and in compliance with the German animal protection law. Experiments were approved by the local district government (Saarpfalz-Kreis, AZ: K 110/180-07, January 22, 2004).

Pathogen-free mice (age: 7 to 8 weeks; strain: CB-17-scid/IcrCrl of both sexes) were obtained from Charles River (Sulzfeld, Germany). They were maintained under sterile conditions in the animal facility of the Saarland University Medical Center at the Institute of Clinical and Experimental Surgery. After a period of adaptation, implantations were performed in SCID mice, which were 8–10 weeks old at the time of cell inoculation. In addition, immunocompetent CD rats (230–300 g) and ICR mice (25–32 g) (Charles River, Sulzfeld, Germany) were used to induce acute inflammation, because SCID mice lack the ability to develop inflammation after ConA inoculation, as confirmed in a control experiment.

Tumor Implantation and Induction of Inflammation

Two different tumor implantation methods were conducted in this study, including a heterotopic implantation by subcutaneous (sc) injection of primary human pancreatic tumor cells into the flank of SCID mice and an orthotopic inoculation of tumor cells into the pancreas of the animals.

A first group of mice ($n = 36$) received subcutaneous injections into the right flank of 2.0–2.5×10^6 human pancreatic adenocarcinoma PaCa44 or PanC-1 cells in 35–60 µL PBS. For the orthotopic implantation, animals ($n = 36$) were anesthetized by intraperitoneal administration of a mixture of ketamine (70 mg/kg) and xylazine (Rompun® 2%, 20 mg/kg). Thereafter, laparotomy was performed by a midline incision, and the spleen and distal pancreas were mobilized. Then 1.5–2.0×10^6 tumor cells in a volume of 20–25 µL PBS were injected into the proximal part of the exposed pancreas. After cell inoculation, the incision was closed in two layers using continuous vicryl suture (Metric 1.5, Norderstedt, Germany). After tumor implantation, the animals were inspected daily for complications and checked for tumor formation both visually and by palpation. Tumor size was calculated by the following formula: tumor volume (cm^3) = $W^2 \times L \times \frac{1}{2}$, where L is the length (cm) and W the width (cm) of the tumor (Adachi *et al.*, 1997). Tumor growth was also monitored noninvasively by magnetic resonance imaging, starting 15 days after implantation. Inflammation was induced by injection of a solution of ConA (150 µg in 100 µL PBS) into the right posterior foot pad of male immunocompetent rats and mice ($n = 15$) as described elsewhere (Rau *et al.*, 2002).

Magnetic Resonance Imaging

Magnetic resonance imaging was performed using a 2.4-Tesla small-animal magnetic resonance tomograph (Brucker Biospec 2.4, Karlruhe, Germany). This system was equipped with a mouse coil to fix the animal and transmit homogeneous signals. All SCID mice were imaged while under ketamine/xylazine anesthesia. Multiple axial and coronal images (T1- and T2-weighted) were acquired for 20 min without contrast media. The parameters used were: T1-weighted (TR = 100 msec, TE = 6.5 msec, flip angle 30°, FOV = 2×2 cm, $256 \times 128 \times 64$ matrix) and T2-weighted (TR = 500 msec, TE = 17.5 msec, 1 acquisition, RARE factor 16, FOV = 2×2 cm, $256 \times 256 \times 32$ matrix, slap-thickness 16 mm). The size of the detected tumors was calculated from the multislice T2-weighted images by counting the total number of tumor voxels in each tumor-containing slice and multiplying by the voxel size (0.1 mm^3), as described previously (Schneider *et al.*, 2002).

Biodistribution Studies, Gamma-Camera, and PET Imaging

Biodistribution studies were carried out in SCID mice 4–5 weeks after tumor implantation to assess tumor and organ uptake of IPA quantitatively. To this end, tumor-bearing mice were anesthetized by ketamine/xylazine as described earlier. Thereafter, freshly prepared IPA (2–3 MBq in 0.1–0.2 ml injectable solution) was administered via a tail vein, and the animals were held in metabolic cages. Four mice per group were sacrificed 15, 60, and 240 min after injection. The abdomen and thoracic cavity of the animals were examined systematically for the presence of tumor and metastases. Samples of blood were obtained by heart puncture. Tumors and various organs were excised and weighed. Radioactivity concentration in organs and tumors was determined by gamma counting. After correction for physical decay, percent injected dose per gram tissue (% I.D./g) was calculated for each tissue. At the end of the experiment, tumor mass and organs of interest, including the lung, kidneys, pancreas, spleen, stomach, liver, intestine, and bladder, were examined histopathologically. ICR mice and rats with acute inflammations received i.v. injections of IPA (2–4 MBq) in the same manner 24 hr after ConA inoculation, while under pentobarbital (50 mg/kg, i.p.) narcosis. Four animals per time point were sacrificed at 15, 60, and 240 min after injection of the tracer. Radioactivity accumulation in organs and inflammatory lesions was determined by gamma counting as described above, followed by histopathological examinations of the tissues.

In separate experiments, whole-body distribution of the tracer in tumor-bearing SCID mice and in rats presenting acute inflammation was visualized at different time points after intravenous administration of 8–10 MBq of IPA. Images were acquired over 20 min using a single-head gamma-camera (APEX SPX 4, Elscint Medical Systems, former Elscint Ltd, Haifa, Israel). The camera was equipped with low-energy, high-resolution parallel-hole collimators (APC-45S, Elscint), and a 20% energy window was used, centered on the 159-keV photopeak of iodine-123. At the end of the gamma scintigraphy, rats with induced acute inflammation were subsequently injected with 10 MBq of FDG, and PET imaging was performed at 60 min post-injection on an ECAT

ART PET Scanner (Siemens/CTI, USA). Attempts to acquire the whole-body distribution of FDG in SCID mice (25–30 g) accurately by means of PET were unsuccessful owing to the low resolution of our PET scanner.

Histological Examination

Tumors and tissues from experimental animals were fixed in 4% neutral buffered formalin and embedded in paraffin wax. Sections were stained with hematoxylin-eosin and Verhoeff-van Gieson and examined histopathologically.

Statistical Analysis

The statistical significance of differences among experimental groups was determined by Student's t-test. A p value less than 0.05 was considered significant.

Results

Cell Uptake and Mechanisms for the IPA Accumulation in Tumor Cells

The uptake kinetic of IPA into primary human pancreatic adenocarcinoma PaCa44 and PanC1 cells and results of inhibition experiments are given in Figure 1. IPA showed high accumulation in pancreatic tumor cells. The IPA uptake into tumor cells was rapid and linear in the first 7 min. More than 70% of the total radioactivity binding in cells, as determined over 120 min, occurred within the first 5 min of incubation. The uptake kinetic increased slowly from 15 min onward. Radioactivity accumulation in pancreatic tumor cells following a 30-min incubation at 37°C/pH 7.4 varied from 41 to 58% of the total loaded activity per 10^6 cells (490–610 and 570–820 cpm/1000 cells for PaCa44 and PanC1, respectively). Compared with the uptake at 37°C, that at 4°C was reduced by up to $90 \pm 5\%$ ($p < 0.01$). Cell precipitation with trichloroacetic acid after an incubation with IPA for 30 min demonstrated that IPA incorporation into protein is relatively low, with $7 \pm 3\%$ of the radioactivity in the acid-precipitable fraction. While lowering the medium pH (from 7.4 to 5.0) resulted in a reduction of the cellular uptake by $40 \pm 10\%$, neither depolarizing membrane potential in high K$^+$ buffer nor increasing the sodium concentration affected the accumulation of IPA in tumor cells significantly < 25% (Fig. 1B). Valinomycin and nigericin, which are known to influence cellular mitochondrial activity, induced a slight alteration in the cellular uptake of the tracer, suggesting that membrane and mitochondrial potentials play a minor role in the cellular uptake. In contrast, preloading tumor cells with BCH and L-alanine-serine-cysteine, as well as with the neutral L-amino acids L-leucine, L-alanine, L-phenylalanine and L-tyrosine, affected the uptake of IPA by up to $95 \pm 3\%$,

($p < 0.01$). In contrast, MeAIB, the selective inhibitor of the amino acid transport system A, L-proline and neutral D-amino acids induced no significant alteration in the accumulation of IPA in human pancreatic tumor cells.

Animal Models and In Vivo Validation of p-[^{123}I]Iodo-L-Phenylalanine

All SCID mice developed a pancreatic tumor within 5 weeks after implantation of primary human adenocarcinoma cells. The heterotopically implanted tumors were accurately detected noninvasively by MRI and confirmed histologically ($n = 36$, tumor = 100%). The heterotopic PaCa44 tumors were palpable 14 to 18 days after subcutaneous cell inoculation. In comparison, accurate detection of the heterotopic PanC1 tumors by palpation was possible from 3 weeks upward. Tumor size, as calculated by the method described by Adachi et al. (1997) was $0.75 \pm 0.35\,\text{cm}^3$ by 3.5–4 weeks after subcutaneous injection of tumor cells, compared with $0.62 \pm 0.27\,\text{cm}^3$ by MRI determination. Figure 1C shows an example of T1-weighted coronal MRI of an heterotopic PaCa44 tumor xenograft. The corresponding whole-body scintigraphies with a gamma-camera at 120 min (Fig. 1D) and 18 hr (Fig. 1E) after injection of IPA demonstrate a specific uptake of the amino acid tracer into tumor tissues and an excellent visualization of the tumor masses. Magnetic resonance imaging was only true positive in 70% and 90% of the histologically confirmed orthotopic PanC1 and PaCa44 tumor xenograft, respectively. Most of the orthotopic xenotransplanted tumors could not be confirmed by palpation. The size of tumors, as determined by MRI at 4 weeks after cell inoculation into the pancreas, ranged from 0.230 to $0.675\,\text{cm}^3$.

The heterotopic xenotransplanted tumors showed only local invasion into adjacent muscle. No distant metastases were macroscopically or histologically determined in the abdomen or thoracic cavity even 4 weeks after subcutaneous implantation of human PaCa44 and PanC1 pancreatic tumor cells. In contrast, most of the orthotopically implanted tumors grew beyong the pancreas, with invasion of adjacent organs and metastases in different abdominal sites.

Biodistribution results for IPA in human pancreatic tumor-bearing SCID mice are summarized in Figure 2. IPA showed high accumulation in engrafted tumors following intravenous administration. Tumor uptake increased gradually with time, while accumulation in muscle, spleen, kidney, stomach, pancreas, intestine, and liver remains moderate and decreases over time. Comparison of the two implantation models shows that uptake of IPA by the heterotopic tumors was lower than that by the orthotopic tumors ($p < 0.02$). At 60 and 240 min post-injection of IPA, radioactivity binding in tumor amounted to, respectively, $10 \pm 2.5\%$ and $15 \pm 3\%$ of the injected dose per gram tumor (I.D./g) in heterotopic tumors (Fig. 2A–B) compared with 17 ± 3.5 and $22 \pm 4.3\%$ I.D./g in

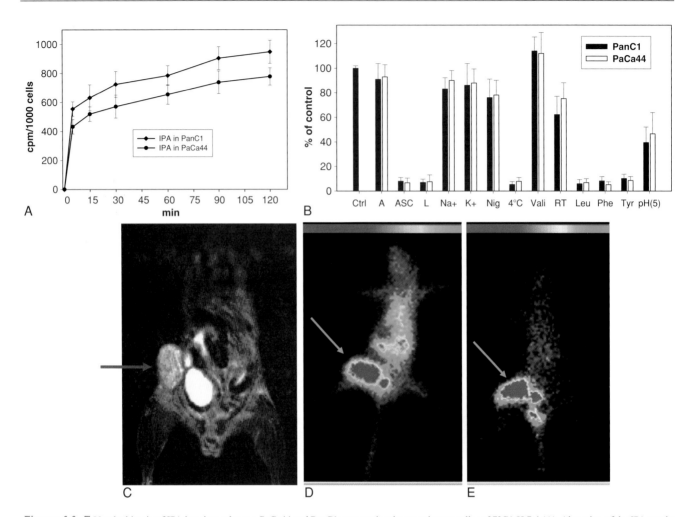

Figure 1A–E Uptake kinetic of IPA in primary human PaCa44 and PanC1 pancreatic adenocarcinoma cells at 37°C/pH 7.4 (**A**). Alteration of the IPA uptake in tumor cells by α-(methylamino)isobutyric acid (*A*), L-alanine/L-serine/L-cysteine (*ASC*), 2-amino-2-norbornane-carboxylic acid (*L*), sodium (Na+), KCl (*K*+), nigericin (*Nig*), valnomycin (*Vali*), room temoperature (*RT*), L-leucine (*leu*), L-phenylalanine (*Phe*), and L-tyrosine (*Tyr*) after co-incubation for 30 min is given a percentage of the control (*Ctrl*). The influence of temperature and pH is also shown (**B**). (*n* = 4, mean ± SD). T2-weighted coronal MRI (**C**) of a heterotopic human pancreatic adenocarcinoma PaCa44 xenograft, demonstrating tumor in the flank of the SCID mouse. Corresponding whole-body gamma-camera imaging at 120 min (**D**) and 18 hr (**E**) after injection of IPA (10 MBq) demonstrates high and specific uptake of the radiopharmaceutical by the tumor and a renal excretion, while uptake in the gastrointestinal tract and the remaining body was qualitatively insignificant over time (**E**). *Arrows* indicate the tumor location.

the orthotopic tumors (Fig. 2C–D). The corresponding mean tumor-to-organ ratios for heterotopic and orthotopic tumors at 60 and 240 min were 2.2 ± 0.7 and 6.4 ± 1.6 (tumor/blood), 3.4 ± 1.1 and 6.7 ± 1.5 (tumor/spleen), 2.1 ± 0.7 and 4.4 ± 1.6 (tumor/pancreas), 3.8 ± 1.1 and 7.6 ± 1.3 (tumor/intestine), 3.4 ± 1.3 and 7.2 ± 1.5 (tumor/liver), and 6.1 ± 1.4 and 11.5 ± 1.6 (tumor/muscle), respectively.

Gamma-camera imaging of a rat presenting an acute inflammation at 60 min after injection of IPA and the PET images of the same rat following FDG administration are shown in Figure 3. FDG uptake was significantly increased in areas of acute inflammation (> 500%). The ratio between the uptake of FDG in inflammatory lesions and that into the healthy opposite left thigh was at least 5:1 (*n* = 4). In comparison, gamma-camera imaging demonstrated that the increase in IPA in inflammation was relatively moderate, at 10–20%. At 15, 60, and 240 min, the radioactivity accumulation in ConA induced inflammation in immunocompetent mice was 2.5 ± 1.2, 2.4 ± 1.1, and 1.9 ± 0.7% I.D./g, respectively, versus 2.2 ± 0.5, 2.0 ± 0.6, and 1.6 ± 0.7% I.D./g into the opposite left foot of the mouse, which served as control (data not shown). The resulting ratio between the uptake of IPA into areas of acute inflammation and that into the healthy skeletal muscle of immunocompetent mice amounts to 1.1–1.2. Histological analysis of the inflammatory lesions demonstrated the presence of lymphohistiocytic cells and scattered plasma cells, as well as granulocytes and macrophages.

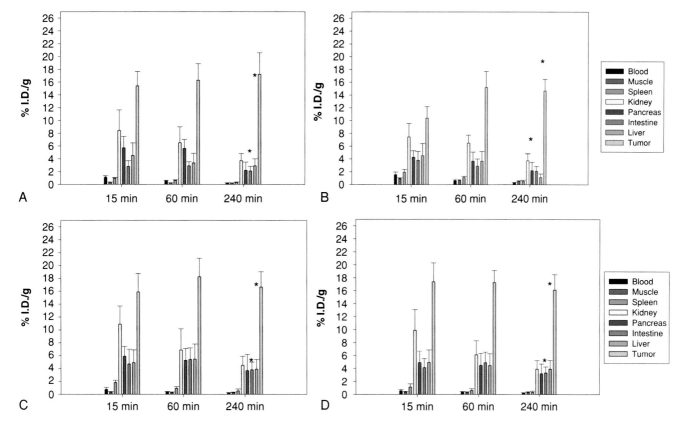

Figure 2A–D Biodistribution of IPA in heterotopic (**A, B**) and orthotopic (**C, D**) human pancreatic carcinoma PaCa44 (**A** and **C**) and PanC1 (**B** and **D**)-bearing SCID mice at 15, 60, and 240 min after intravenous injection of 2–4 MBq of the radiopharmaceutical. Uptakes are expressed as percentages of injected dose/g tissue (% I.D./g), (median, $n = 4$).

Discussion

Because there is no highly sensitive clinical test for the diagnosis of pancreatic cancer, intensive efforts have been undertaken to improve both the sensitivity and the specificity of imaging techniques for detecting and staging pancreatic carcinomas. Although the detection of the tumor has been considerably improved using current imaging techniques, including computer tomography, ultrasonography, magnetic resonance imaging, and positron emission tomography with [^{18}F]fluoro-2-deoxy-D-glucose, differential diagnosis of pancreatic cancers remains a challenge, especially in the early stage of the disease (Nitzsche et al., 2002; Diederichs et al., 2000; Obuz et al., 2001; DiMagno et al., 1999). The aim of this study was to assess experimentally the ability of the novel amino acid tracer IPA to detect pancreatic carcinomas. IPA was found to exhibit high uptake in human pancreatic tumor cells with a continuous increase over the investigation time of 120 min. This result provides evidence of the high affinity of IPA for pancreatic cancer. A major point of discussion is the underlying mechanisms of tumor uptake. It is assumed that the amino acid transport may be more important for tumor imaging than the incorporation of the amino

acid tracers into proteins (Laverman et al., 2002; Langen et al., 2002; Miyagawa et al., 1998). Thus, we investigated the transport mechanisms responsible for the uptake of IPA into pancreatic tumor cells. Several studies have characterized a number of distinct systems for the transport of amino acids inside mammalian cells (Saier et al., 1988; Segel et al., 1989; Barker et al., 1999).

Analogous to these experiments, we investigated the cellular uptake of IPA by competitive inhibition, using substrates known to be specific inhibitors for the amino acid transport. We found that accumulation of IPA in human pancreatic tumor cells was predominantly mediated by the L and ASC transport pathways. This finding was also confirmed by the strong inhibition of the tracer uptake by neutral L-amino acids known to be solely transported by L- and ASC-system (Segel et al., 1989; Parker et al., 1999). In contrast, neutral D-amino acids do not affect the IPA uptake into cells significantly, indicating the stereospecificity of the tracer uptake in tumor cells. Importantly, the protein incorporation of IPA was less than 8% in our study. Therefore, the high accumulation of IPA in pancreatic cancer cells could be primarily associated with the increased amino acid transport activity in the neoplastic cells.

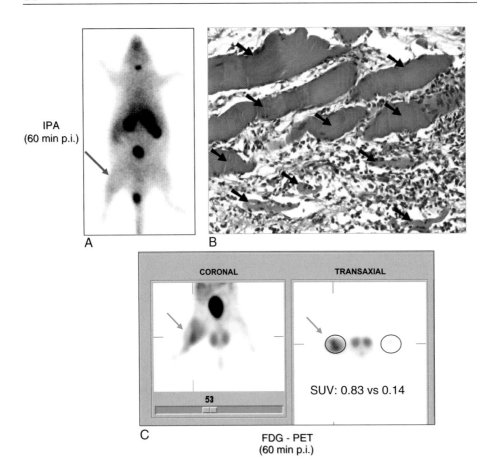

IPA
(60 min p.i.)

A

B

CORONAL   TRANSAXIAL

53

SUV: 0.83 vs 0.14

C

FDG - PET
(60 min p.i.)

Figure 3A–C Representative whole-body image of an immunocompetent rat with a ConA-induced inflammation in the right foot (*arrow*), 60 min after i.v. injection of IPA (10 MBq). The gamma-camera image showed qualitatively no significant differences in the uptake of IPA in areas of inflammation and in the unaffected left foot, used as a control (**A**). Histomorphological analysis of the corresponding skeletal muscle demonstrated acute inflammatory changes composed mainly of lympho-histiocytic cells and scattered plasma cells, as well as granulocytes and macrophages; H&E, original magnification ×200 (**B**). In comparison, the subsequent FDG-PET images of the same animal 60 min after injection of FDG shows high FDG accumulation in areas of inflammation (**C**). *Arrows* indicate inflammation location.

The second goal of this study was to evaluate the ability of IPA to target pancreatic carcinomas *in vivo* and thereby to assess its potential as a tracer for diagnosis of pancreatic cancer by means of single photon emission computed tomography (SPECT). We used SCID mice engrafted with primary human pancreatic adenocarcinoma cells as an animal model. Magnetic resonance imaging, autopsy, and histopathological analysis demonstrated that human pancreatic carcinomas engrafted into SCID mice disseminated in a pattern analogous to human disease, including invasion by the tumor into adjacent organs and formation of metastases in different sites of the abdomen. Thus, our model fulfills the major requirements as an *in vivo* model of human pancreatic cancer and can be used for preclinical evaluations. IPA was found to accumulate intensively in implanted pancreatic tumors, in agreement with results obtained in *in vitro* experiments. Importantly, the IPA uptake by the lung, liver, kidney, liver, stomach, and intestine remained moderate and diminished considerably with time, resulting in an excellent contrast between tumor and organs, especially from 120 min upward. The ability of SPECT with IPA to detect pancreatic cancer was impressively confirmed by gamma-camera imaging (Fig. 1). From 360 min onward

only tumor tissues were demonstrated scintigraphically. This result indicated that IPA is a highly selective tracer for noninvasive diagnosis of pancreatic cancer.

As yet, accurate clinical differentiation between inflammation and neoplastic tissues is not possible. Consequently, we also examined the uptake of IPA in areas of inflammation in comparison with the uptake by normal tissue and tumor. Inflammation was induced by inoculation of concanavalin (ConA) into the right foot of immunocompetent rats and mice. The most prominent inflammatory reactions occurred 12 to 24 hr after ConA injection. Accumulation of IPA in areas of inflammation was moderate and comparable with the uptake by the unaffected skeletal muscle of immunocompetent animals, and significantly lower than that in tumors ($p < 0.01$). In comparison, the uptake of FDG increased by up to 700% in inflammatory lesions (Fig. 3). This important finding indicates that IPA is a valuable tracer for differentiation between neoplastic masses and inflammation *in vivo*.

In conclusion, the radioiodinated amino acid IPA inhibits high affinity for human pancreatic cancer. Its marked accumulation in tumor reflects the increased amino acid transport in neoplastic cells and is predominantly mediated by the L and ASC carrier pathways. In addition to its high tumor accumulation, the uptake of IPA into the gastrointestinal tract and areas of inflammation is moderate or decreases rapidly with time, resulting in sufficiently high tumor-to-background contrast for clinical applications with SPECT. These data indicate that IPA is a very promising radiopharmaceutical for noninvasive imaging of pancreatic carcinomas by routine SPECT.

Acknowledgments

The authors express their deep appreciation to Miss Elisabeth Gluding for her expertise in animal care, Mrs. Claudia Schormann for cell cultures, and Mrs. D. Wagner and Katja Fischer for their technical support in the performance of scans with MRI and the gamma-camera.

References

Adachi, T., Hinoda, Y., Nishimori, I., Adachi, M., and Imai, K. 1997. Increased sensitivity of gastric cancer cells to natural killer and lymphokine-activated killer cells by antisense suppression of N-acetylgalactosaminyltransferase. *J. Immunol.* *159*:2645–2651.

Barker, G.A., Wilkins, R.J., Golding, S., and Ellory, J.C. 1999. Neutral amino acid transport in bovine articular chondrocytes. *J. Physiol.* *514*:795–808.

Diederichs, C.G., Staib, L., Vogel, J., Glasbrenner, B., Glatting, G., Brambs, H.J., Beger, H.G., and Reske, S.N. 2000. Values and limitations of ¹⁸F-fluorodeoxyglucose-positron-emission tomography with preoperative evaluation of patients with pancreatic masses. *Pancreas 20*:109–116.

DiMagno, E.P., Reber, H.A., and Tempero, M.A. 1999. AGA technical review on the epidemiology, diagnosis, and treatment of pancreatic ductal adenocarcinoma. American Gastroenterological Association. *Gastroenterology 117*:1464–1484.

Faivre, J., Forman, D., Esteve, J., Obradovic, M., and Sant, M. 1998. Survival of patients with primary liver cancer, pancreatic cancer and biliary tract cancer in Europe. *Eur. J. Cancer 34*:2184–2190.

Grino, P., Martinez, J., Grino, E., Carnicer, F., Alonso, S., Perez-Berenguer, H., and Perez-Mateo, M. 2003. Acute pancreatitis secondary to pancreatic neuroendocrine tumors. *Journal of Pancreas 4*:104–110.

Hellwig, D., Menges, M., Schneider, G., Moellers, M.O., Romeike, F.M., Menger, M.D., Kirsch, C.M., and Samnick, S. 2005. Radioiodinated phenylalanine derivatives to image pancreatic cancer: a comparative study with [¹⁸F]fluoro-2-deoxy-D-glucose in human pancreatic carcinoma xenografts and in inflammation models. *Nucl. Med. Mol. 32*:137–145.

Jager, P.L., Vaalburg, W., Pruim, J., de Vries, E.G., Langen, K.J., and Piers, D.A. 2001. Radiolabeled amino acids: basic aspects and clinical applications in oncology. *J. Nucl. Med. 42*:432–445.

Langen, K.J., Pauleit, D., and Coenen, H.H. 2002. 3-[(123)I]iodo-alpha-methyl-ʟ-tyrosine: uptake mechanisms and clinical applications. *Nucl. Med. Biol. 29*:625–631.

Laverman, P., Boerman, O.C., Corstens, F.H., and Oyen, W.J. 2002. Fluorinated amino acids for tumor imaging with positron emission tomography. *Eur. J. Nucl. Med. Mol. Imaging 29*:681–690.

Miyagawa, T., Oku, T., Uehara, H., Desai, R., Beattie, B., Tjuvajev, J., and Blasberg, R. 1998. "Facilitated" amino acid transport is upregulated in brain tumors. *J. Cereb. Blood Flow Metab. 18*:500–509.

Nitzsche, E.U., Hoegerle, S., Mix, M., Brink, I., Otte, A., Moser, E., and Imdahl, A. 2002. Non-invasive differentiation of pancreatic lesions: is analysis of FDG kinetics superior to semiquantitative uptake value analysis? *Eur. J. Nucl. Med. 29*:237–242.

Obuz, F., Dicle, O., Coker, A., Sagol, O., and Karademir, S. 2001. Pancreatic adenocarcinoma: detection and staging with dynamic MR imaging. *Eur. J. Radiol. 38*:146–150.

Rau, F.C., Weber, W.A., Wester, H.J., Herz, M., Becker, I., Kruger, A., Schwaiger, M., and Senekowitsch-Schmidtke, R. 2002. O-(2-[(18)F]Fluoroethyl)-ʟ-tyrosine (FET): a tracer for differentiation of tumor from inflammation in murine lymph nodes. *Eur. J. Nucl. Med. Mol. Imaging 29*:1039–1046.

Saier, M.H., Daniels, G.A., Boerner, P., and Lin, J. 1988. Neutral amino acid transport systems in animal cells: potential targets of oncogene action and regulators of cellular growth. *J. Membr. Biol. 104*:1–20.

Samnick, S., Schaefer, A., Siebert, S., Richter, S., Vollmar, B., and Kirsch, C.M. 2001. Preparation and investigation of tumor affinity, uptake kinetic and transport mechanism of iodine-123-labelled amino acid derivatives in human pancreatic carcinoma and glioblastoma cells. *Nucl. Med. Biol. 28*:13–23.

Schafer, M., Mullhaupt, B., and Clavien, P.A. 2002. Evidence-based pancreatic head resection for pancreatic cancer and chronic pancreatitis. *Ann. Surg. 236*:137–148.

Segel, G.B., Woodlock, T.J., Murant, F.G., and Lichtman, M.A. 1989. Photoinhibition of 2-amino-2-carboxybicyclo[2,2,1]heptane transport by O-diazoacetyl-ʟ-serine: an initial step in identifying the ʟ-system amino acid transporter. *J. Biol. Chem. 264*:16399–16402.

Schneider, G., Fries, P., Wagner-Jochem, D., Thome, D., Laurer, H., Kramann, B., Mautes, A., and Hagen, T. 2002. Pathophysiological changes after traumatic brain injury: comparison of two experimental animal models by means of MRI. *Magnetic Resonance Materials in Physics, Biology and Medicine 14*:233–241.

Trümper, L., Menges, M., Daus, H., Kohler, D., Reinhard, J.O., Sackmann, M., Moser, C., Sek, A., Jacobs, G., Zeitz, M., and Pfreundschuh, M. 2002. Low sensitivity of the ki-ras polymerase chain reaction for diagnosing pancreatic cancer from pancreatic juice and bile: a multicenter prospective trial. *J. Clin. Oncol. 21*:4331–4337.

Warshaw, A.W., and Fernandez-del Castello, C. 1992. Pancreatic carcinoma. *N. Engl. J. Med. 326*:455–465.

38

Pancreatic Islet Cell Tumors: Endoscopic Ultrasonography

Koichi Aiura and Tomotaka Akatsu

Introduction

Pancreatic islet cell tumors (pancreatic endocrine tumors in the World Health Organization histological classification) are relatively rare tumors with a reported incidence of < 10 per million per year in the general population (Eriksson and Öberg, 2000). In spite of a low incidence, islet cell tumors require resection after diagnosis in patients without metastases because of clinical symptoms due to excessive hormone production or frequent malignancy. Complete surgical resection is essential for a successful outcome. The prognosis of patients after complete removal of islet cell tumors is much better than that of pancreatic adenocarcinoma.

Preoperative imaging is important in planning the therapeutic strategy. Accurate localization of islet cell tumors facilitates successful curative surgical resection. Although ultrasound (US), computed tomography (CT), and magnetic resonance imaging (MRI) have become standard imaging modalities for islet cell tumors, these techniques lack the sensitivity to detect small endocrine tumors of the pancreas. In contrast, endoscopic ultrasonography (EUS) is gaining widespread acceptance for even localizing islet cell tumors of a small size because of high resolution and very little acoustic obstruction. This method plays a pivotal role in depicting the precise location and number of lesions, and in differentiating between benign and malignant tumor characteristics.

Classification of Islet Cell Tumors

Islet cell tumors are classified as functioning or nonfunctioning. Functioning islet cell tumors cause clinical symptoms related to uncontrolled hormone production. These tumors are subclassified according to the hormone they produce. Insulinomas and gastrinomas are the most common neuroendocrine tumors of the pancreas. These tumors are usually small in size, measuring < 20 mm in diameter (Outwater and Siegelman, 1996). Furthermore, tumors measuring < 10 mm are common. Approximately, one-third to one-half of gastrinomas are located outside the pancreas (Outwater and Siegelman, 1996; Norton et al., 1986). Other functioning islet cell tumors of the pancreas include glucagonomas, VIPomas, somatostatinomas, and carcinoid tumors, which are often large by the time of diagnosis. Each of these tumors may be benign adenoma or malignant neoplasm.

In addition to functioning tumors, approximately one-third to two-thirds of pancreatic islet cell tumors are thought to be nonfunctioning (Lo et al., 1996; Kent et al., 1981). Nonfunctioning islet cell tumors usually become large before diagnosis due to the lack of endocrine symptoms, and have a high malignancy rate of up to 92% (Kent et al., 1981). However, the chance of the incidental discovery of small nonfunctioning islet cell tumors has recently increased in asymptomatic patients.

Cancer Imaging: Instrumentation and Applications

Most islet cell tumors occur sporadically, but a minority of patients with islet cell tumors have an inherited disorder such as von Hippel-Lindau disease or multiple endocrine neoplasia (MEN) type I. In addition, multiple occurrences of pancreatic islet cell tumors are not unusual. Therefore, accurate preoperative imaging of islet cell tumors of a small size is needed for determining appropriate treatment. Endoscopic ultrasonography (EUS) is very useful for the detection and localization of pancreatic islet cell tumors in this regard. Furthermore, EUS provides important information regarding tumor shape, margin, echogenicity, and echotexture. Morphologically, nonfunctioning islet cell tumors are indistinguishable from functioning tumors; thus, EUS cannot discriminate between functioning and nonfunctioning tumors.

Detection and Localization by Endoscopic Ultrasonography

Although transabdominal US can identify large-size tumors of the pancreas, it is difficult to visualize tumors of a small size (< 20 mm in diameter) because of the presence of a blind spot and bowel gas, with a detection rate of only 20 to 60% (Galiber et al., 1988; Gorman et al., 1986). Endoscopic ultrasonography is superior to transabdominal US for scanning the entire pancreas with high resolution and little noise interference. It has been reported that the overall sensitivity of EUS for localizing pancreatic islet cell tumors is 93% (Anderson et al., 2000). Furthermore, the sensitivity of EUS for detecting pancreatic islet cell tumors in patients with negative transabdominal US and CT was reported to be 82% (Rösch et al., 1992). These observations suggest that EUS is more sensitive for detecting tumors than transabdominal US, CT, and angiography, especially tumors < 20 mm in diameter (Anderson et al., 2000). It is also possible that EUS could detect pancreatic lesions as small as 6 mm (Glover et al., 1992).

Though more sensitive than other imaging modalities, EUS may have a blind spot in the region of the splenic hilum, because the sensitivity of 60% for tumors in the tail was less than the 95% and 78% sensitivity for tumors of the head and body of the pancreas, respectively (Rösch et al., 1992). Moreover, EUS was not reliable for localizing extrapancreatic tumors (Anderson et al., 2000). Approximately one-third to one-half of gastrinomas are extrapancreatic and are frequently located in the wall of the duodenum and lymph nodes in some cases. Extrapancreatic sites of endocrine tumors are difficult to visualize by EUS. Conversely, in the case of gastrinomas, a negative EUS of the pancreas reliably predicted the presence of an extrapancreatic gastrinoma (Anderson et al., 2000; Thompson et al., 1994). In addition to high sensitivity, the specificity of EUS for islet cell tumors is also quite high (95%) (Anderson et al., 2000; Rösch et al., 1992). However, it is possible that EUS could recognize hyperplastic lymph nodes of the parapancreas as pancreatic islet cell tumors (Rösch et al., 1992; Glover et al., 1992).

Endoscopic Ultrasonographic Findings of Islet Cell Tumors

As islet cell tumors originate as a solid mass and grow expansively, they typically appear as well-defined, smoothly surfaced, and round to oval, or sometimes lobular lesions on EUS. Echogenicity of islet cell tumors usually appears on EUS as homogeneously hypoechoic masses or hypoechoic masses with a central echogenic area compared with the surrounding normal pancreatic parenchyma (Glover et al., 1992). As most of the tumors are encapsulated, the distinct margin was visualized in spite of tumor size. However, the internal echo patterns of islet cell tumors, such as echogenicity and echotexture, are highly variable. Histopathological findings of islet cell tumors are variable, and each EUS feature corresponds to a pathological feature of the tumor. Internal echo findings of tumors depend on the arrangement of tumor cells, quantity of fibrous stroma, and the existence of hyalinosis, calcification, microcysts, hemorrhage, and necrosis within the mass (Akatsu et al., 2004a; Yamada et al., 1991). Homogeneously hypoechoic tumors indicate that tumor cells are densely arranged with a small amount of stroma (Fig. 1). In contrast, hyperechoic tumors are comprised of tumor cells that are roughly textured with abundant stroma (Fig. 2). Rösch and his colleagues have reported in their study from six centers that pancreatic endocrine tumors were visualized as homogeneously hypoechoic in 69% (22/32) of cases, homogeneously isoechoic in 6% (2/32), and homogeneously hyperechoic in 6% (2/32) (inhomogeneous in 19%) (Rösch et al., 1992).

Furthermore, echotexture of islet cell tumors also reflects the histopathological findings within the tumors. The small islet cell tumors usually consisted of an orderly cell arrangement without calcification or necrosis, showing a homogeneous or regular central echogenic pattern. However, even a small, benign tumor could show a heterogeneous mass due to the existence of hyalinosis, small calcification, and microcysts (Yamada et al., 1991) (Fig. 3). In addition, irregular central echogenic areas also correspond to a disarrangement of tumor cells in the nests, hemorrhage, necrosis, and/or cystic degeneration in malignant tumors (Akatsu et al., 2004a; Yamada et al., 1991). Strong echo spots within the tumor represent calcification, and focal lesions of necrosis are visualized as irregular central echogenic or echo-free areas.

Microcysts within the tumor tend to increase in number and size in large-sized tumors. The frequency of both tumor calcification and cystic degeneration resulting from hemorrhage or necrosis also increases with tumor size, suggesting that irregular internal echotexture is more frequent in large- than in small-size tumors. Tumor size has been reported to

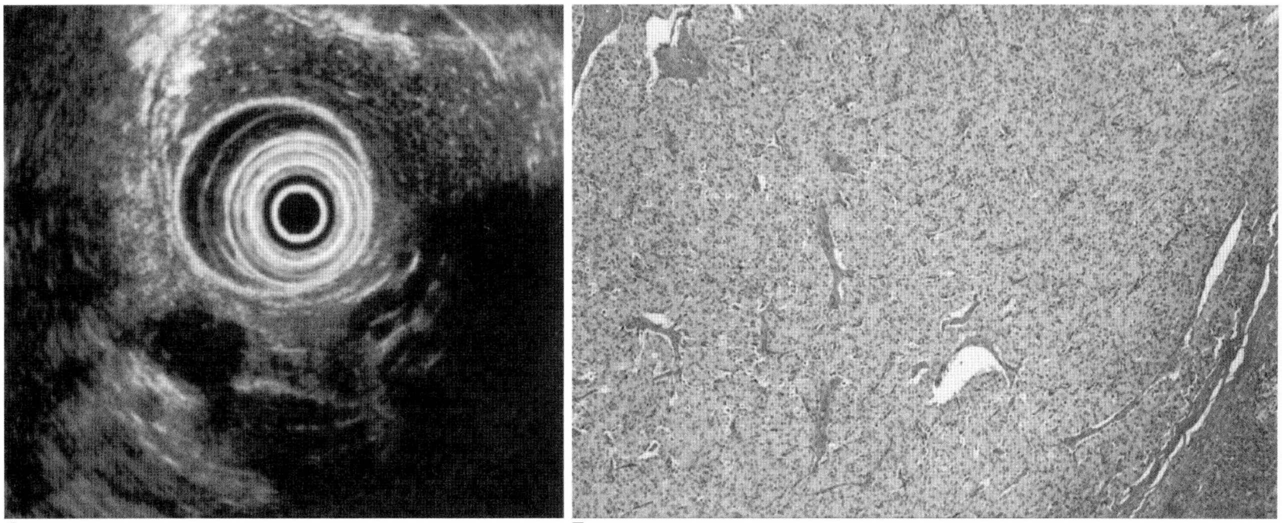

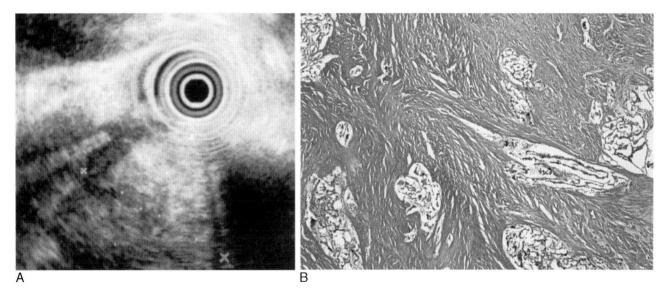

Figure 1 (**A**) Endoscopic ultrasonography of a benign insulinoma, 12 × 11 mm in size, showing a round, well-defined, and homogeneous hypoechoic mass. (**B**) Histological examination revealing dense arrangement of tumor cells with small amounts of stroma (H&E stain, ×50).

Figure 2 (**A**) Endoscopic ultrasonography of a malignant nonfunctioning pancreatic islet cell tumor, 39 × 38 mm in size, showing a hypoechoic mass with irregular central hyperechoic portions. (**B**) Histological examination demonstrating tumor cells roughly textured with abundant fibrous stroma (H&E stain, ×40).

be one of the important predictors of malignancy, and larger tumors are more associated with malignant behavior in islet cell tumors (Buetow *et al.*, 1995). These findings suggest that the irregularity of internal ultrasonographic features could be closely related to the malignancy of islet cell tumors. In support of this concept, Akatsu *et al.* (2004a) reported that all malignant nonfunctioning islet cell tumors appeared as a heterogeneous mass with an irregular internal structure, although benign tumors did not show such an EUS pattern. Moreover, malignant pancreatic islet cell tumors of a small size (20 mm or less in diameter) were also visualized as

hypoechoic masses with irregular central echogenic portions due to the disarrangement of cells in nests or necrotic foci (Yamada *et al.*, 1991).

The microscopic assessment of malignancy in primary pancreatic islet cell tumors is based on the presence of angio-invasion, capsular invasion, perineural invasion, or mitotic rates. However, it is difficult to determine malignant behavior even microscopically, and the most reliable evidence of malignancy is metastasis to the liver and/or the regional lymph nodes. Therefore, it is very useful for a conclusive diagnosis if some predictive factors suggest malignancy. It

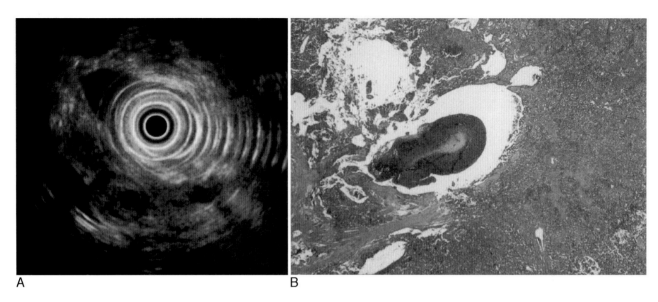

A   B

Figure 3 (**A**) Endoscopic ultrasonography of a benign nonfunctioning pancreatic islet cell tumor, 18 × 14mm in size, showing a round, well-defined, and hypoechoic mass with echogenic portions and a cystic area. (**B**) Histological examination revealing cystic formation and hialinosis within the tumor (H&E stain, ×20).

is possible that internal EUS irregularity could be one of the preoperative indicators of malignant islet cell tumors.

Atypical Manifestations and Differential Diagnosis

As islet cell tumors grow larger, cystic degeneration may occur, causing cysts of variable size within the tumor. The cystic changes are usually solitary because they are thought to result from relative ischemia and hemorrhagic necrosis (Fig. 4). However, a rare case of an islet cell tumor showing

a microcystic honeycomb appearance consisting of multicystic lesions has been reported in which the EUS findings mimicked serous cystadenoma (Imaoka *et al.*, 2005; Gerke *et al.*, 2004).

The main pancreatic ducts in cases with islet cell tumors were usually normal on EUS. However, EUS could demonstrate the involvement of the main pancreatic duct in malignant tumors and sometimes the dilatation of the distal portion of the main pancreatic duct (Fig. 5). Malignancy should be strongly suspected in cases with complete obstruction of the main pancreatic duct (Akatsu *et al.*, 2004a). In addition, it has been reported that intraductal growth of an

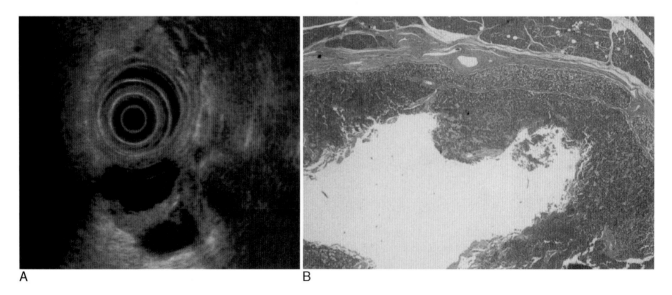

A   B

Figure 4 (**A**) Endoscopic ultrasonography of a malignant nonfunctioning pancreatic islet cell tumor showing a cystic mass with irregularly thick septum and wall. (**B**) Microphotograph revealing intratumoral cystic formation (H&E stain, ×15).

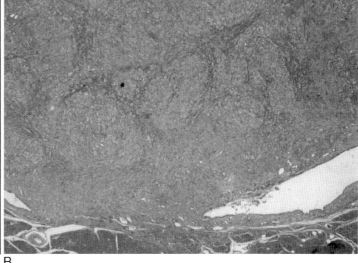

A   B

Figure 5 (**A**) EUS of a malignant nonfunctioning pancreatic islet cell tumor (T) involving the main pancreatic duct (+ − +). (**B**) Histological examination demonstrating exposure of the tumor cells into the main pancreatic duct (H&E stain, ×15).

islet cell tumor in the proximal direction appeared on EUS in a case with a malignant nonfunctioning tumor (Akatsu *et al.*, 2004b), although intraductal tumors of the pancreas are generally referred to as intraductal papillary mucinous neoplasms. Another pancreatic tumor displaying an unusual intraductal growth pattern has been reported in acinar cell carcinoma (Hashimoto *et al.*, 2003) and metastatic renal cell carcinoma (Yachida *et al.*, 2002).

Metastatic renal cell carcinoma is well known to be hypervascular and to often develop late solitary metastasis to the pancreas, even more than 20 years after manifestation of the primary tumor (Wente *et al.*, 2005). It should be noted

that the imaging characteristics of pancreatic metastases from hypervascular tumors, particularly renal cell carcinomas, are similar to those of islet cell tumors. Furthermore, von Hippel-Lindau disease, which results from mutation of the tumor suppressor VHL gene, produces brain and spinal cord hemangioblastomas, retinal angiomas, renal cell carcinomas, pancreatic neuroendocrine tumors, and microcystic serous adenomas. Clear cell endocrine pancreatic tumors closely mimicking renal cell carcinoma have been reported to be distinctive neoplasms of von Hippel-Lindau disease (Hoang *et al.*, 2001) (Fig. 6). The EUS characteristics of renal cell carcinoma and clear cell endocrine tumors are similar; therefore, EUS is not useful for

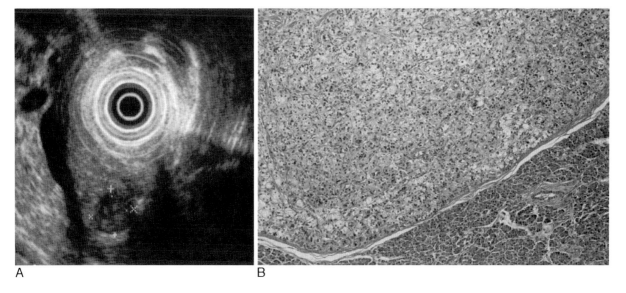

A   B

Figure 6 (**A**) Endoscopic ultrasonography of a pancreatic islet cell tumor associated with von Hippel-Lindau disease. (**B**) Histological examination demonstrating neoplastic clear cells with positive immunoreactivity for chromogranin and synaptophysin (H&E stain, ×80).

discriminating between these two types of tumors. When renal and pancreatic clear cell tumors coexist either synchronously or metachronously in patients with von Hippel-Lindau disease, the pancreatic tumor has the possibility of both metastatic renal cell carcinoma and primary endocrine tumor.

In conclusion, accurate localization of islet cell tumors is pivotal for successful surgical resection. Endoscopic ultrasonography plays an important role as a primary diagnostic modality in the evaluation and management of patients with islet cell tumors of the pancreas. This method is more sensitive in detecting small-sized pancreatic tumors compared with transabdominal US and CT. Furthermore, detailed EUS findings such as echogenicity and echotexture could provide additional information useful in differential diagnosis and in assessing the malignant potential of a tumor.

References

Akatsu, T., Aiura, K., Shimazu, M., Ueda, M., Wakaayashi, G., Tanabe, M., Kawachi, S., Hayashida, T., Kameyama, K., Sakamoto, M., and Kitajima, M. 2004a. Endoscopic ultrasonography of nonfunctioning pancreatic islet cell tumors with histologic correlation. *Hepato-Gastroenterology 51*:1590–1594.

Akatsu, T., Wakabayashi, G., Aiura, K., Suganuma, K., Takigawa, Y., Wada, M., Kawachi, S., Tanabe, M., Ueda, M., Shimazu, M., Sakamoto, M., and Kitajima, M. 2004b. Intraductal growth of a nonfunctioning endocrine tumor of the pancreas. *J. Gastroenterol. 39*:584–588.

Anderson, M.A., Carpenter, S., Thompson, N.W., Nostrant, T.T., Elta, G.H., and Scheiman, J.M. 2000. Endoscopic ultrasound is highly accurate and directs management in patients with neuroendocrine tumors of the pancreas. *Am. J. Gastroenterol. 95*:2271–2277.

Buetow, P.C., Parrino, T.V., Buck, J.L., Pantongrag-Brown, L., Ros, P.R., Dachman, A.H., and Cruess, D.F. 1995. Islet cell tumors of the pancreas: pathologic-imaging correlation among size, necrosis and cysts, calcification, malignant behavior, and functional status. *AJR Am. J. Roentgenol. 165*:1175–1179.

Eriksson, B., and Öberg, K. 2000. Neuroendocrine tumours of the pancreas. *Br. J. Surg. 87*:129–131.

Galiber, A.K., Reading, C.C., Charboneau, J.W., Sheedy, P.F., II, James, E.M., Gorman, B., Grant, C.S., van Heerden, J.A., and Telander, R.L. 1988. Localization of pancreatic insulinoma: comparison of pre- and intraoperative US with CT and angiography. *Radiology 166*:405–408.

Gerke, H., Byrne, M.F., Bill Xie, H., Paulson, E.K., Tyler, D.S., Baillie, J., and Jowell, P.S. 2004. A wolf in sheep's clothing: a non-functioning islet cell tumor of the pancreas masquerading as a microcystic (serous cystic) adenoma. *J. Pancreas 5*:225–230.

Glover, J.R., Shorvon, P.J., and Lees, W.R. 1992. Endoscopic ultrasound for localisation of islet cell tumors. *Gut 33*:108–110.

Gorman, B., Charboneau, J.W., James, E.M., Reading, C.C., Galiber, A.K., Grant, C.S., van Heerden, J.A., Telander, R.L., and Service, F.J. 1986. Benign pancreatic insulinoma: preoperative and intraoperative sonographic localization. *AJR Am. J. Roentgenol. 147*:929–934.

Hashimoto, M., Matsuda, M., Watanabe, G., Mori, M., Motoi, N., Nagai, K., and Ishibashi, M. 2003. Acinar cell carcinoma of the pancreas with intraductal growth: report of a case. *Pancreas 26*:306–312.

Hoang, M.P., Hruban, R.H., and Albores-Saavedra, J. 2001. Clear cell endocrine pancreatic tumor mimicking renal cell carcinoma. *Am. J. Surg. Pathol. 25*:602–609.

Imaoka, I., Yamao, K., Salem, A.A., Sawaki, A., Takahashi K., Mizuno, N., Kawai, H., Tajika, M., Isaka, T., Okamoto, Y., Shimizu, Y., and Yanagisawa, A. 2005. Pancreatic endocrine neoplasm can mimic serous cystadenoma. *Int. J. Gastrointest. Cancer 35*:217–220.

Kent, R.B., III., van Heerden, J.A., and Weiland, L.H. 1981. Nonfunctioning islet cell tumors. *Ann. Surg. 193*:185–190.

Lo, C.Y., van Heerden, J.A., Thompson, G.B., Grant, C.S., Soreide, J.A., and Harmsen, W.S. 1996. Islet cell carcinoma of the pancreas. *World J. Surg. 20*:878–883.

Norton, J.A., Doppman, J.L., Collen, M.J., Harmon, J.W., Maton, P.N., Gardner, J.D., and Jensen, R.T. 1986. Prospective study of gastrinoma localization and resection in patients with Zollinger-Ellison syndrome. *Ann. Surg. 204*:468–479.

Outwater, E.K., and Siegelman, E.S. 1996. MR imaging of pancreatic disorders. *Topics Magn. Res. Imaging 8*:265–289.

Rösch, T., Lightdale, C.J., Botet, J.F., Boyge, G.A., Sivak, Jr., M.V., Yasuda, K., Heyder, N., Palazzo, L., Dancygier, H., Schusdziarra, V., and Classen, M. 1992. Localization of pancreatic endocrine tumors by endoscopic ultrasonography. *N. Engl. J. Med. 326*:1721–1726.

Thompson, N.W. Czako, P.F., Fritts, L.L., Bude, R., Bansal, R., Nostrant, T.T., and Scheiman, J.M. 1994. Role of endoscopic ultrasonography in the localization of insulinomas and gastrinomas. *Surgery 116*:1131–1138.

Wente, M.N., Kleeff, J., Esposito, I., Hartel M., Müller, M.W., Fröhlich, B.E., Büchler, M.W., and Friess, H. 2005. Renal cancer cell metastasis into the pancreas—a single-center experience and overview of the literature. *Pancreas 30*:218–222.

Yachida, S., Fukushima, N., Kanai, Y., Nimura, S., Shimada, K., Yamamoto, J., and Sakamoto, M. 2002. Pancreatic metastasis from renal cell carcinoma extending into the main pancreatic duct: a case report. *Jpn. J. Clin. Oncol. 32*:315–317.

Yamada, M., Komoto, E., Naito, Y., Tsukamoto, Y., and Mitake, M. 1991. Endoscopic ultrasonography in the diagnosis of pancreatic islet cell tumors. *J. Ultrasound Med. 10*:271–276.

39

Parotid Gland Tumors: Advanced Imaging Technologies

Hasan Yerli and A. Muhtesem Agildere

Introduction

The parotid gland is located in the parotid space, and this small space includes the facial nerve, Stenson's duct, lymph nodes, and vessels as well as the parotid gland. Evaluation of parotid masses poses a significant problem in radiological and clinical practice. Different types of tumoral and non-tumoral masses may be detected by swelling in the parotid gland. Clinical palpation is nonspecific, and conventional imaging methods include ultrasonography (US), computed tomography (CT), and magnetic resonance imaging (MRI). Even US-guided fine needle aspiration biopsy might be nonspecific.

Preoperative imaging of suspicious parotid masses is important in determining whether the mass has an intraglandular or extraglandular location. Radiologic examination can also demonstrate additional clinically silent tumors in the same lobe or in the contralateral parotid gland, and these findings are important for surgical planning. Another important factor related to surgical procedure is preoperative diagnosis of the tumor type. Benign tumors of the parotid, such as pleomorphic adenomas and basal cell adenomas (BCA), are usually treated with local excision by applying superficial parotidectomy or subtotal parotidectomy, whereas most malignancies are excised via total parotidectomy with or without facial nerve removal (Rehberg *et al.*, 1998; Koyuncu *et al.*, 2003). Successful treatment of parotid tumors is related not only to tumor type but also to correct location and its relationship with facial nerve. Inaccurate diagnosis may lead to inappropriate management of tumors. It can therefore be difficult to decide on appropriate surgical management.

Magnetic resonance imaging, CT, and US are commonly used in the characterization of parotid tumors. However, the limitations of these conventional imaging methods are well known. To improve diagnostic accuracy, alternative methods, including diffusion weighted MRI (DWMRI), positron emission tomography (PET), proton magnetic resonance spectroscopy imaging (^{1}H-MRS), and Tc-99m pertechnetate scintigraphy were also studied.

The main imaging modalities used to evaluate parotid gland tumors are MRI and CT. Computed tomography has a few limitations, including the administration of nephrotoxic contrast material with large volume and lower resolution than MRI (Rubin, 2003). Other limitations are use of the X-ray and inability to demonstrate facial nerve relationship to the tumor. Ultrasonography is a noninvasive, feasible, and cost-effective method for initial evaluation of suspected superficial parotid masses. Whether the lesion is intraglandular or extraglandular and a pure cystic lesion can be determined with great accuracy by using US (Gritzmann, 1989). However, US cannot evaluate tumors located in the deep parotid lobe, parapharyngeal region, and pedunculated parotid tumors. Another limitation of US is that the evaluation is dependent on the operator's experience. MRI has a higher soft tissue resolution than other imaging techniques, which is helpful in identifying the location of parotid tumors (deep or superficial lobe), the precise extent of their involvement (muscle and parapharyngeal space), and the relationship between the tumor and the facial nerve; MRI also has the capability of multiplanar imaging.

The conventional imaging characteristics of parotid tumors are nonspecific. Most parotid tumors are solid and usually have regular contours. Indistinct margins are not important findings that distinguish malignant tumors from benign tumors. Malignant tumors and complicated Warthin's tumors may have rough contours. Both acinic cell carcinoma and Whartin's tumors have focal low-attenuating areas on CT, which is seen as a microcyst or necrosis on pathologic examination (Suh *et al.*, 2005). The signal intensity of a parotid mass on T2-weighted images is greater than that of cerebrospinal fluid; this indicates mostly pleomorphic adenoma. However, Motoori *et al.* (2004) determined a characteristic bright signal on T2-weighted images in only 3 of 11 pleomorphic adenomas. Also, acinic cell carcinoma can show bright high signal intensity similar to that in pleomorphic adenoma. Metastasis in the regional lymph nodes may not be seen on malignant parotid tumors (Suh *et al.*, 2005). Multinodular enhancement is not specific for any parotid tumor. Pleomorphic adenomas, BCAs, and recurrent tumors can be multinodular (Yerli *et al.*, 2007). Furthermore, the presence of intratumoral calcifications, internal hemorrhage, bilateral occurrence, or multiplicity does not help in the differential diagnosis of parotid tumor. Both malignant tumors and benign tumors of the parotid gland can show intense vascularity at color Doppler US (Martinoli *et al.*, 1994). Unfortunately, there is no patognomonic conventional MRI or CT finding that identifies tumor types of the parotid. Alternative imaging methods are needed for better preoperative evaluation of parotid tumors (King *et al.*, 2005).

In this chapter, imaging findings of parotid tumors in advanced imaging techniques, including dynamic contrast-enhanced multislice CT (CEMSCT), dynamic contrast-enhanced MRI (CEMRI), DWMRI, ^{1}H-MRS, and others are presented, and an evaluation is made on whether these methods are valuable for diagnosing parotid tumors, or narrowing in the differential diagnosis of these tumors.

Dynamic Contrast-Enhanced Imaging

Dynamic contrast-enhanced imaging provides images at different time points and time-enhancement curves secondary to intravascular or extravascular accumulation of contrast material in the tissue after the intravenous application of contrast media. Rapid enhancement of the lesion is defined as washin, and rapid decrease of enhancement is defined as washout (Som *et al.*, 1985). Time-contrast enhancement curves on dynamic CECT or CEMRI examinations are useful for pathologic diagnosis of parotid tumors (Fig. 1). Magnetic resonance imaging is more commonly used due to higher contrast resolution and the lack of X-ray. Dynamic MRI images are obtained every 30 seconds after application of intravenous contrast material. Thus, a lot of dynamic images are provided by MRI, but limited dynamic images are provided by dynamic CT due to ionization radiation. The degree of enhancement for each phase of the tumors is calculated at each phase using the region of interest (ROI). The examiner should be careful in locating ROI. The ROI should be placed to cover only the solid portion of the tumor during the measurement. Obvious cystic areas and vessels should be excluded from the ROI (Choi *et al.*, 2000). The contrast-enhancement features of the tumors are related mostly to solid components reflecting histopathologic character and vascularity.

Parotid tumors usually show four types of time-enhancement curves on dynamic CECT and CEMRI (Fig. 1) (Yabuuchi

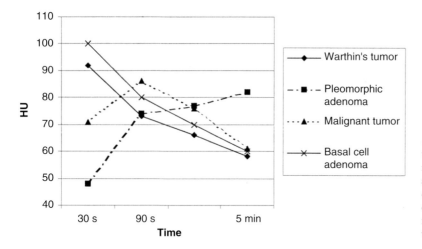

Figure 1 Time-HU (Hounsfield Unit) curves of contrast-enhanced dynamic CT for four of the tumor categories reveal rapid contrast enhancement of Warthin's tumors and basal cell adenomas (strong at 30 sec) and reduction of enhancement from the first to the late phase; increased enhancement through the phases for pleomorphic adenomas; and peak enhancement at 90 sec for the malignant tumors (Min: minutes).

et al., 2003). The type A curve shows gradual enhancement, and the type B and C curves show rapid peak enhancement between 30 and 120 sec after IV contrast material. The washout ratio of the type B curve is higher than that of the type C curve. Type D is a flat curve. Pleomorphic adenomas usually show gradual enhancement. Both malignant tumors and Warthin's tumors show mostly rapid enhancement (type B and C curves), but Warthin's tumors show a higher washout ratio than do malignant tumors. Yabuuchi *et al.* (2003) pointed out that a washout ratio of 30% can differentiate Warthin's tumors from malignant tumors. They also emphasized that peak contrast enhancement at 120 sec might be able to differentiate malignant tumors from pleomorphic adenoma at dynamic CEMRI.

The presence of ferromagnetic devices in a patient, relatively high cost, and sometimes extended imaging time are the well-known limitations of MRI imaging (Koyuncu *et al.*, 2003). If any MRI limitation is present in a patient with parotid tumor, dynamic CT is a reliable alternative diagnostic method to dynamic MRI (Choi *et al.*, 2000). Intensive research has been done on conventional and dynamic MRI findings that differentiate various types of parotid tumors, but very little has been published about dynamic CECT imaging findings for this purpose. Dynamic spiral computed tomography has increased the efficiency of CT in detecting and characterizing tumors. Moreover, multidetector technology has made spiral CT a valuable method for examining parotid tumors. Dynamic study of tumors with MSCT is more practical owing to the high gantry speed compared with single-slice CT (Yerli *et al.*, 2007). Timing for contrast-enhancement optimization with MSCT is also better than single-slice CT. Faster scanning prevents images from being corrupted by motion (Rubin, 2003). In our department we are using three-phase dynamic CT, with images obtained at 30 sec, 90 sec, and 5 min. Because peak contrast enhancement at 30 sec might be optimal for identifying Warthin's tumors, peak enhancement at 90 sec might be optimal for diagnosing malignant tumors, and delayed enhancement is an indicator for diagnosing pleomorphic adenomas (Yerli *et al.*, 2007). To decrease patient exposure to X-rays, we are performing a complete neck study at 30 sec, and then we are scanning at the level of the tumor at 90 sec and 5 min.

Diffusion Weighted Magnetic Resonance Imaging and Apparent Diffusion Coefficient Calculation

The measurement of free molecular diffusion by DWMRI mainly reflects the random thermal motion of molecules in tissues and, to a lesser extent, the micromotion of molecules in capillaries. This is why measured molecular diffusion is defined as the "apparent" diffusion coefficient. Quantification of diffusivity is possible by using ADC (apparent diffusion coefficient) maps created from diffusion-weighted images. Diffusion weighted MRI is sensitive to the diffusion of water molecules, and it is used mainly as a routine imaging sequence of cranial MRI in stroke patients. Echoplanar MRI has a low signal-to-noise ratio, and DWMRI of the parotid region can be seriously distorted due to susceptibility effects and motion artifacts (Fig. 2) (Sumi *et al.*, 2002). It is possible, however, to measure the ADC of parotid gland tissue and lesions within this region (Wang *et al.*, 2001). To increase the signal-to-noise ratio, a large number of excitations should be used. A thinner slice can be used in cases with marked distortion artifacts. Wang *et al.* (2001) suggested that an anti-susceptibility device could be used to reduce susceptibility artifacts. We apply an echoplanar spin-echo sequence in the axial plane with *b*-values of 0, 500, and 1000 mm²/s, and we use a phase-encoding matrix with 128 × 128 slice thickness with 5 mm and 5 excitations.

A few reports have suggested that ADC calculation might be helpful in diagnosing parotid tumors (Motoori *et al.*, 2004, 2005; Wang *et al.*, 2001; Ikeda *et al.*, 2004). Different types of parotid tumors have different histologic structures, a consideration that may dictate different ADC values. The movement of water protons is relatively free in the fluid than in those of solid tissues. Therefore, it is well known that increased water content is associated with higher ADC, although the differences in ADC values among cystic lesions can change according to the protein level of the lesions. So, ADC value of solid portion in the tumor should be measured.

Proton Magnetic Resonance Spectroscopy Imaging (^{1}H-MRS)

^{1}H-MRS provides metabolite data related to biochemical changes in the tissues. Choline (Cho) is known as a metabolite reflecting membrane turnover, and creatine (Cr) is a metabolite that has a function in the cell energy system. ^{1}H-MRS has been commonly used to characterize neurologic diseases such as brain tumors and multiple sclerosis. The value of ^{1}H-MRS in head and neck tumors has also been researched in a new study. The importance of metabolite ratios for tumors of the parotid gland was researched by King *et al.* (2005). In this initial study, King *et al.* pointed out that ^{1}H-MRS may be used to characterize parotid tumors. They determined only lipid peak in normal parotid glands, but they demonstrated both Cho and Cr peaks in benign and malignant tumors and calculated Cho/Cr and Cho/water ratios by using with Cho, Cr, and water peak amplitudes for differentiation of parotid tumors. They observed significant differences between Warthin's tumors and pleomorphic adenomas and between benign tumors and malignant tumors. The most important potential limitation of this method is that ^{1}H-MRS cannot be performed in tumors of small size due to contamination problems.

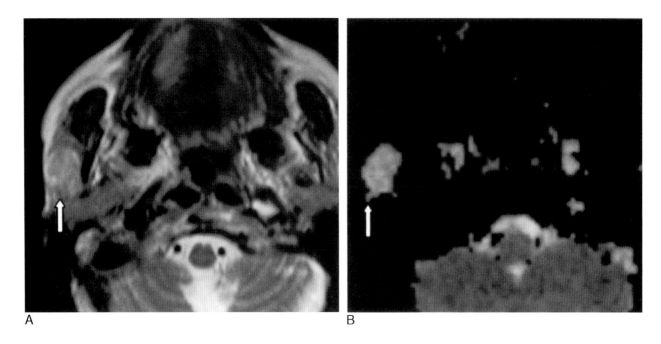

A   B

Figure 2 A pleomorphic adenoma located in the superficial lobe of the right parotid gland. (**A**) An axial T2-weighted image (3800/90, TR/TE) shows a mass lesion that is hyperintense (arrow) compared to muscle. (**B**) An ADC map shows a solid lesion (arrow) with a high ADC (1.68×10^{-3} mm²/s) and helps to establish the diagnosis (pathologic diagnosis was obtained after total excision).

Positron Emission Tomography and Scintigraphy

Nuclear medical diagnosis methods, including PET with F-18 fluorodeoxyglucose (FDG) and Tc-99m pertechnetate scintigraphy, have lower spatial and contrast resolution than CT and MRI and are not useful to demonstrate the tumor morphology and their relation to adjacent structures. Positron emission tomography and Tc-99m pertechnetate scintigraphy provide mainly metabolic information and limited morphological information for tumors. These methods employ positron-releasing radionuclides with ultra-short half-lives, and they measure the standardized uptake values (SUVs) of tumors quantitatively. Positron emission tomography reflects biological information for tumors associated with glucose metabolism (Matsuda *et al.*, 1998).

The differentiation of benign and malignant parotid tumors is limited by using Tc-99m pertechnetate scintigraphy or PET methods due to a relatively high false-positive rate (Okamura *et al.*, 1998; Uchida *et al.*, 2005). These methods are also not as cost-effective as other imaging techniques. However, PET has higher sensitivity and specificity for detecting lymph node metastases of the head and neck than to CT and MRI. Besides, parotid gland scintigraphy using Tc-99m pertechnetate scintigraphy is useful for the diagnosis of Warthin's tumors (Uchida *et al.*, 2005). Warthin's tumors show mostly high uptake, but other benign parotid tumors and malignant tumors reflect a cold scan on Tc-99m pertechnetate scintigraphy. Malignant parotid tumors show almost higher FDG accumulation than benign tumors except Warthin's tumor (Uchida *et al.*, 2005).

Benign Parotid Tumors

Most benign tumors of the parotid gland are small and unilateral, and are round or slightly oval in shape with well-circumscribed borders. Lobulated contours are also seen. A freely moving, painless, slowly enlarging mass is the most common clinical symptom (Howlett *et al.*, 2002). These tumor groups exhibit heterogeneous or homogeneous enhancement following contrast administration with CT and MRI. Images obtained in the axial planes from the skull base to the hyoid bone are satisfactory for evaluating benign parotid tumors.

Pleomorphic Adenoma

Eighty percent of parotid tumors are benign, and the most common benign parotid tumor, which is thought to arise from myoepithelial cells, is pleomorphic adenoma. Pleomorphic adenomas can be seen in adults, adolescents, and children in the ages 15 to 70 years, and it more likely affects women (Howlett *et al.*, 2002). Pleomorphic adenomas are commonly encapsulated, and the lobulation at the contour can be seen. Most pleomorphic adenomas grow gradually, and some of them undergo malignant transformation. The risk of recurrence is approximately 15% in long-term follow-up. Preoperative diagnosis of the pleomorphic adenoma without biopsy is important because needle biopsy will open the capsule of the tumor and thereby increase risk of recurrence (Motoori *et al.*, 2004).

Histopathologically, pleomorphic adenomas have an adenomatous biphasic appearance that reflects the admixture of epithelium and myxoid stroma. The rates of epithelial and myxoid tissue in the tumor vary in each tumor. Pleomorphic adenomas usually show low or intermediate signal on T1-weighted images and extremely high signal intensity on T2-weighted images. This signal intensity, which reflects myxoid tissue in tumor, is higher than that of cerebrospinal fluid. However, pleomorphic adenomas with abundant cellular component and less myxoid tissue do not show bright signal intensity on T2-weighted images (Fig. 2A) (Motoori *et al.*, 2004). The tumor capsule is seen as a low-signal intensity rim surrounding the tumor on T2-weighted images. T1-weighted images do not clearly show a low-intensity capsule as do the T2-weighted images. Dystrophic calcifications rarely occur and are best visualized with CT (Som *et al.*, 1985).

Dynamic Contrast-Enhanced Imaging

Yabuuchi *et al.* (2003) examined 12 pleomorphic adenomas of the parotid gland with dynamic CEMR imaging at 30, 60, 90, 120, 150, 180, 240, and 300 sec after contrast material application. Pleomorphic adenomas were enhanced gradually in 75% of their cases. They observed that the typical histopathologic features in pleomorphic adenomas are large myxoid matrix, rare epithelial components, and a low microvessel count. The gradual enhancement of pleomorphic adenoma may be attributed to the slow leakage of contrast material to vascular spaces and myxoid matrix from the low number of microvessels (Yerli *et al.*, 2007). Choi *et al.* (2000) examined 35 pleomorphic adenomas with dynamic helical CECT at 30 sec and 120 sec, and also examined images at different times during the late phase (6–25 min). They determined increased attenuation in 30 (86%) pleomorphic adenomas. The finding of delayed enhancement is sensitive in the diagnosis of pleomorphic adenoma (Fig. 1). The main differential diagnosis for pleomorphic adenoma based on dynamic imaging findings is salivary duct carcinoma of the parotid. As opposed to pleomorphic adenoma, the gradual enhanced foci of salivary duct carcinoma show lower signal intensity on T2-weighted images. It is thought that these areas are associated with desmoplasia. Moreover, the ADC value of salivary duct carcinomas is lower than that of pleomorphic adenoma (Motoori *et al.*, 2005).

Diffusion Weighted Magnetic Resonance Imaging

The two basic components of pleomorphic adenomas reflect the difference in ADC values. However, the ADC value

of total tumor mass in the parotid gland is usually higher than that of malignant tumors and Warthin's tumors. Most of the epithelial components of the tumor are of glandular nature. We thought that water protons move relatively freely in the glandular areas of pleomorphic adenomas. Abundant extracellular fluid, adenomatous nature, and myxoid tissue of the tumor may account for the higher ADC values (Fig. 2). We found that the mean ADC for the eight pleomorphic adenomas ($1.78 \pm 0.39 \times 10^{-3}$ mm²/s) was significantly higher than the corresponding values for the Warthin's tumors ($0.90 \pm 0.16 \times 10^{-3}$ mm²/s) and the malignant tumors ($0.88 \pm 0.27 \times 10^{-3}$ mm²/s) (Yerli *et al.*, 2005).

Other Advanced Imaging Techniques

Pleomorphic adenomas have higher Cho/Cr ratios than malignant tumors, but lower than Warthin's tumors. King *et al.* (2005) found that the average Cho/Cr at an echo time of 136 msec and 272 msec for the pleomorphic adenomas were 3.46 ± 0.84 and 3.67 ± 1.23, respectively. The mean Cho/water ratios for the pleomorphic adenomas at an echo time of 136 msec and 272 msec were 0.71 ± 0.35 and 1.61 ± 1.21, respectively.

Although pleomorphic adenomas show mostly low uptake by PET-FDG, they also exhibit a wide range of FDG accumulations (Uchida *et al.*, 2005). The SUV of pleomorphic adenomas does not correlate with the proportion of epithelial or myxoid component of the tumor (Matsuda *et al.*, 1998). However, there is a positive correlation between tumor size and SUV. Pleomorphic adenomas with large size can show relatively high SUV levels similar to that in malignant tumors. FDG-PET provides quantitative information associated with the growth capacity of tumors. Matsuda *et al.* (1998) thought that a large pleomorphic adenoma tended to have greater growth capacity, which might cause recurrence following surgical treatment.

Pleomorphic adenomas show a cold scan on Tc-99m pertechnetate scintigraphy similar to that in malignant tumors. Therefore, the differentiation of pleomorphic adenomas from other benign and malignant tumors by Tc-99m pertechnetate scintigraphy is difficult (Uchida *et al.*, 2005). In summary, high signal intensity on T2-weighted images, gradual enhancement curves on dynamic CECT or MRI images, and high ADC values on DWI are clues in the diagnosis of pleomorphic adenoma.

Warthin's Tumor

The second most common parotid tumor, Whartin's tumor—also called papillary cystadenoma lymphomatosum or adenolymphoma—originates from heterotropic parotid tissue located within parotid lymph nodes. These tumors are bilateral or multiple in 10 to 15% of cases and are the most common bilateral and multifocal parotid neoplasms.

Warthin's tumors account for 5 to 10% of tumors in the parotid and are more common in middle-aged and advanced-age males. Warthin's tumor is one of the tumor types that is composed of oncocytes. Microscopically, lymphoid tissue is prominent, often with germinal centers. This lymphoid stroma is predominantly composed of B lymphocytes. Covering the surface of this lymphoid tissue are large epithelial cells with oncocytic features. These cells are arranged in two layers, and some of the apical cells may be ciliated (Howlett et al., 2002).

Warthin's tumors have low intensity or isointensity compared with muscle on T1-weighted images. Small, high signal intensity focuses associated with complicated cysts filled with proteinous material or focal hemorrhage can be determined in the tumor area on T1-weighted images. Microcystic areas appear as a low attenuating focus on CT. These tumors show iso- or hyperintensity on T2-weighted images and may have a thin capsule that cannot be demonstrated by MRI.

Dynamic Contrast-Enhanced Imaging

The characteristic dynamic imaging findings of Warthin's tumors have been reported as quick contrast enhancement in early phases and as decreasing enhancement with a high washout ratio (> 30%) in late phases (Fig. 1). Yabuuchi et al. (2003) reported that Warthin's tumors, with high microvessels and hypercellular stroma, had a high washout ratio. A 30% washout ratio has been accepted as a useful threshold in predicting Warthin's tumor. We determined that Warthin's tumors might show earlier intense contrast enhancement than malignant tumors at 30 sec on CECT (Yerli et al., 2007). The high micovessel count causes earlier peak enhancement time than the enhancement pattern for other benign tumors.

Diffusion Weighted Magnetic Resonance Imaging

The ADC values of Warthin's tumors tend to be lower than ADCs for parotid carcinomas and pleomorphic adenomas. Ikeda et al. (2004) have suggested that the lower ADC values of Warthin's tumors can be explained by the higher protein content in their cystic portions. These tumors have the highest microvessel count of all parotid gland tumors, and they also exhibit high cellularity. The typical microscopic appearance of a Warthin's tumor is abundant lymphoid sheets with conspicuous follicles and germinal centers. Thus, the mean ADCs for Warthin's tumors and lymphomas are lower than the corresponding means for the pleomorphic adenomas and carcinomas (Table 1). The lower ADC values for Warthin's tumors also reflect inhibited movement of water protons in the hypercellular areas. Wang et al. (2001) studied a total of 22 benign solid masses of the head and neck, including 3 Warthin's tumors and 10 pleomorphic adenomas. They suggested that an ADC higher than 1.22×10^{-3} mm^2/s for a mass in the parotid region indicates a benign tumor. Ikeda and coworkers (2004) compared ADC values for malignant parotid tumors and Warthin's tumors, and found average ADCs of $1.19 \pm 0.19 \times 10^{-3}$ mm^2/s and $0.96 \pm 0.39 \times 10^{-3}$ mm^2/s, respectively (Table 1). We determined a similar mean ADC for Warthin's tumors ($0.90 \pm 0.16 \times 10^{-3}$ mm^2/s) (Yerli et al., 2005).

Other Advanced Imaging Techniques

Warthin's tumors usually show increased isotope uptake on Tc-99^m scintigraphic imaging. Distinguishing Warthin's tumors from other parotid gland tumors may be possible through Tc-99^m scintigraphy (Uchida et al., 2005) because other parotid gland tumors usually show low uptake. The mechanism of Tc-99m pertechnetate uptake in Warthin's tumors is not known. However, the size of Warthin's tumors is important in the accumulation degree. Motoori et al. (2005) reported that tumors 3 cm in diameter showed relatively higher uptake than tumors of 2 cm diameter. In addition, Warthin's tumors with a large cystic component tend to have relatively lower uptake. Cystic and small Warthin's tumors show a cold scan. The sensitivity and specificity of Tc-99^m scintigraphic imaging for diagnosing Warthin's tumors are 56–63% and 94–100%, respectively (Motoori et al., 2005).

Warthin's tumors have higher Cho/Cr and Cho/water ratios than malignant tumors and pleomorphic adenomas. King et al. (2005) found that the average Cho/Cr at an echo time of 136 msec and 272 msec for the Warthin's tumors were 5.49 ± 1.86 and 6.92 ± 1.47, respectively. The mean Cho/water ratios for the Warthin's tumors at an echo time of 136 msec and 272 msec were 1.35 ± 0.89 and 3.29 ± 2.07, respectively.

Warthin's tumors show mostly high FDG accumulation (Table 2). It has been reported that epithelial cells containing

Table 1 Mean Apparent Diffusion Coefficients (ADCs) for the Parotid Gland Tumor Types

	Pleomorphic Adenoma	Warthin's Tumor	Malignant Tumor
	Mean ± SD ($\times 10^{-3}$ mm^2/s)	Mean ± SD ($\times 10^{-3}$ mm^2/s)	Mean ± SD ($\times 10^{-3}$ mm^2/s)
Motoori et al. (2004)	2.03 ± 0.32	—	1.40 ± 0.39
Ikeda et al. (2004)	—	0.96 ± 0.13	1.19 ± 0.19
Habermann et al. (2005)	2.14 ± 0.11	0.85 ± 0.1	1.04 ± 0.3
Yerli et al. (2005)	1.78 ± 0.39	0.90 ± 0.16	0.88 ± 0.27

Table 2 **Mean Standardized Uptake Values (SUVs) for the Parotid Gland Tumor Types**

	Pleomorphic Adenoma	Warthin's Tumor	Malignant Tumor
	Mean ± SD	Mean ± SD	Mean ± SD
Okamura *et al.* (1998)	4.07 ± 1.55	7.03 ± 2.49	5.92 ± 2.05
Matsuda *et al.* (1998)	4.12 ± 1.82	7.42 ± 2.37	5.20 ± 1.71
Uchida *et al.* (2005)	—	7.06 ± 3.99	5.82 ± 3.95

a large number of mitochondria may be associated with accumulation of FDG. The mean SUV of Warthin's tumors on PET-FDG is greater than that of other benign parotid tumors and overlap with that of malignant tumors (Okamura *et al.*, 1998).

Basal Cell Adenoma

Basal cell adenoma (BCA) of the parotid gland is a relatively rare benign epithelial neoplasm. This adenoma almost always affects persons over 50 years of age and is found more often in female patients. The average age of cases is 58, more than a decade older than the average age of cases with pleomorphic adenoma. The incidence of BCA is 7.5% among primary epithelial parotid gland tumors. Malignant progression of BCA of the parotid gland is rare, but when it occurs, it can develop into basal cell adenocarcinoma or adenoid carcinoma (Lee *et al.*, 2005). The recurrence rate following total excision is high for a membranous-type tumor, and treatment requires total parotidectomy for this type.

Histopathologically, these neoplasms feature relatively uniform small dark basaloid epithelial cells consisting of a monomorphic population in a stroma and are well encapsulated by fibrous connective tissue. The basaloid cells are arranged into solid, trabecular, tubular, and membranous areas. The solid type is the most common variant. The absence of myxochondroid character and myoepithelial cells differentiates BCA from pleomorphic adenomas (Jang *et al.*, 2004; Rehberg *et al.*, 1998). The typical vascular pattern in BCAs features large numbers of endothelial-lined small capillaries and venules due to neovascularization.

Basal cell adenoma may be predominantly solid or cystic. The solid component shows intense enhancement after intravenous contrast injection. Two different enhancement patterns have demonstrated the use of biphasic and multiphase dynamic CECT for BCA of the parotid gland (Lee *et al.*, 2005; Yerli *et al.*, 2005). Seven cases demonstrating dynamic CT findings of BCA are reported in the literature. Lee *et al.* (2005) reported four BCA cases showing marked contrast enhancement on the early phase and decrease in attenuation on the delayed phase (Fig. 1). These researchers also demonstrated two BCA cases with large cystic areas showing additional enhancement in the delayed phase. We determined one BCA exhibited marked enhancement at the early phase

and gradually reduced levels during the other three phases. Dynamic CECT might be helpful to differentiate BCA from pleomorphic adenoma. The strong contrast enhancement in the early phase might be related to the vascular architecture in BCA. Lee *et al.* (2005) thought the presence of myxoid change, including sparse vascularity, adjacent to the cystic space might play a role in additional enhancement in the delayed images.

Basal cell adenoma is hypointense or isointense compared to muscle on T1-weighted images and hyperintense on T2-weighted images. The tumor may contain a markedly hemorrhagic component. The capsule surrounding the tumor shows low signal intensity on T2-weighted images in BCA as in pleomorphic adenoma. The literature contains just one report of a BCA describing ADC value. In our study one BCA case was determined, and it had an ADC value of 1.40 × 10^{-3} mm^2/s (Yerli *et al.*, 2005). This tumor exhibited diffusion characteristics similar to the pleomorphic adenomas, probably because of its adenomatous nature.

Other Benign Parotid Tumors

Hemangiomas are the most common tumor type of the parotid gland in the pediatric population. They may contain signal voids reflecting dilated vessels and may have calcification in the vascular spaces (Andronikou *et al.*, 2003). Neurogenic tumors arising from facial nerve complex may be located within the parotid gland. Hemangiomas and neurogenic tumors may also show gradual enhancement in dynamic imaging (Takashima *et al.*, 1993). Lipomas of the parotid gland are uncommon, and diagnosis is straightforward. The fat densities are determined on CT, and all imaging sequences in MR exhibit signals consistent with fat. Lipomas have a flat curve in the dynamic imaging. Recurrent tumors show the same dynamic curves as the original tumor (Takashima *et al.*, 1993).

Malignant Parotid Tumors

The most common primary malignant parotid tumor is mucoepidermoid carcinoma, and it accounts for 80 to 90% of all cases. Adenoid cystic carcinoma, acinic cell carcinoma, adenocarcinoma, and squamous cell carcinoma are other forms of primary parotid malignant tumors (Howlett *et al.*, 2002). Primary lymphoma and metastatic involvement of the parotid gland are rare. Whole neck examination, from the skull base to the thoracic inlet level, is essential to rule out the possibility of lymph node metastases in evaluation of a suspected malignant parotid mass; careful examination of the cervical region for lymph nodes is needed (Suh *et al.*, 2005).

Dynamic Contrast-Enhanced Imaging

Some researchers have reported that malignant parotid tumors have irregular tumor margins, heterogeneous signal intensity, and infiltration into surrounding tissue. A group of investigators have reported that none of these MR features could reliably predict malignant tumors (Takashima *et al.*, 1993; Yabuuchi *et al.*, 2003; Motoori *et al.*, 2005). In dynamic imaging, malignant parotid tumors show mostly rapid contrast enhancement in the early phase and decreasing enhancement in late phases due to the high microvessel count similar to that in Warthin's tumor; the evaluation of peak enhancement time alone cannot help differentiate malignant tumors from Warthin's tumors. However, we determined that four of the five malignant tumors showed increasing enhancement up to 90 sec, and then decreased through the late phases and 10 of the 11 Warthin's tumors showed rapid contrast enhancement at 30 sec (first phase) and rapid reduction of enhancement from the first to the fourth phase (Fig. 1) (Yerli *et al.*, 2007). Malignant tumors also have a lower washout ratio than those of the Warthin's tumors (Yabuuchi *et al.*, 2003). It is reported that the sensitivity and specificity of the method were 91% on the basis of 30% washout ratio and early contrast enhancement to differentiate malignant from benign tumors (Yabuuchi *et al.*, 2003). Choi *et al.* (2000) reported that 11 of 20 malignant tumors showed gradual increase enhancement similar to that in pleomorphic adenoma. Takashima *et al.* (1993) reported that 4 of 10 malignant tumors showed gradually increased enhancement. The differences in the dynamic imaging for malignant tumors can be explained by various kinds of malignant parotid tumors having different histologic structures. The value of dynamic imaging in predicting malign parotid tumors appears to be controversial.

Diffusion Weighted Magnetic Resonance Imaging

The ADC value of malignant tumors in the parotid gland is lower than that of benign solid tumors (Wang *et al.*, 2001). High cellularity in the malignant tumors restricts the diffusion of the water molecules and causes the lower ADC values (Table 1). The decrease of ADC is the most prominent in the malignant lymphoma among the malignant parotid tumors (Wang *et al.*, 2001) (Fig. 3). According to our experiences, the ADC value of parotid carcinomas appears to be larger than those of malignant lymphoma ($1.17 \pm 0.03 \times 10^{-3}$ mm²/s and

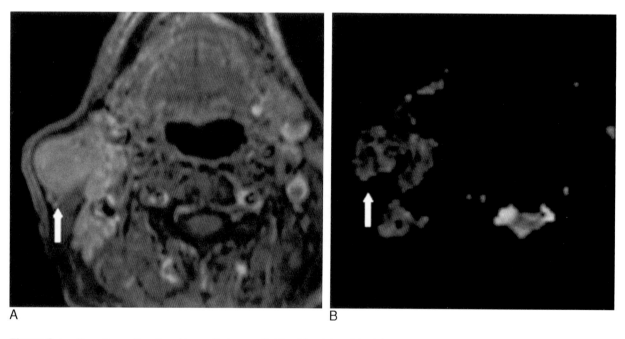

A   **B**

Figure 3 A malignant tumor (lymphoma) located in the superficial and deep lobes of the right parotid gland. (**A**) An axial fat-suppressed, postcontrast T1-weighted image (575/15, TR/TE) shows a mass lesion that is enhanced (arrow). (**B**) An ADC image shows a lesion (arrow) with a low ADC (0.63×10^{-3} mm²/s).

Table 3 Radiologic Algorithm for Diagnosis of Parotid Masses

Physical examination

Mass

US

Lymph node

Pure cyst → No further imaging

Suspected lymphadenopathy

Solid or semisolid

Cooperated patients

Impaired cooperation or + ferromagnetic device not compatible with MR

Located superficial lobe

Located deep lobe or + contrast allergy

Dynamic CT

Advantages
• Fast examination
• Cost effective
• No consideration for ferromagnetic device

Dynamic CT or MRI combined with one of the advance imaging methods (Dynamic MRI, DWMRI or ¹H-MRS)

MRI combined with one of the advance imaging methods (Dynamic MRI, DWMRI or ¹H-MRS)

Advantages
• Determination of facial nerve
• High contrast resolution
• No risk of contrast allergy
• High accuracy

Tubular signal voids

Fat density on CT, high signal on T1

• bright signal intensity on T2W MRI
• gradual enhancement
• High ADC
• low Cho/Cr ratio

• Decreasing enhancement
• High washout, 30% ↑
• Low ADC
• High Cho/Cr ratio

• Decreasing enhancement
• High ADC

• Decreasing enhancement
• Low washout, 30% ↓
• Medium ADC(Low ADC in lymphoma)
• Low Cho/Cr ratio

• Low uptake with PET
• Cold scan on Tc-99m PS

• High uptake with PET
• High uptake on Tc-99m PS

• High uptake with PET
• Cold scan on Tc-99m PS

Pleomorphic adenoma

Warthin's tumor

BCA

Malignant

Hemangioma

Lipoma

$0.68 \pm 0.05 \times 10^{-3}$ mm^2/s, respectively) and our results are consistent with those documented in a previous study. The presence of common microcystic structures and hypervascular portion in the parotid carcinomas might be the cause of higher ADC values rather than that of lymphomas. Ikeda et al. (2004) found that the mean ADC for malignant parotid tumors was higher than that for Warthin's tumors. According to our experiences, however, the ADC values of Warthin's tumor overlap those of malignant parotid tumors due to hypercellularity. The optimal threshold value for ADCs should be determined in differentiating benign and malignant tumors in the large population.

Other Advanced Imaging Techniques

Malignant tumors have lower Cho/Cr ratios than Warthin's tumors and pleomorphic adenoma associated with membrane turnover. King et al. (2005) found that the average Cho/Cr at an echo time of 136 msec and 272 msec for the malignant tumors were 1.73 ± 0.47 and 2.27 ± 0.69, respectively. Malignant parotid tumors show a cold scan on Tc-99m pertechnetate scintigraphy similar to that in pleomorphic adenoma and other benign parotid tumor except Warthin's tumor. The reported sensitivities and specificities of Tc-99m pertechnetate scintigraphy have been low (Uchida et al., 2005). However, it is reported that the sensitivity and specificity of PET with F-18 fluorodeoxyglucose used to differentiate malignant tumors from benign tumors are 75% and 67%, respectively. Uchida et al. (2005) reported a 30% false-positive rate by PET, and they pointed out that a high FDG uptake in Warthin's tumors could cause a high false-positive ratio in detecting malignant tumors. To improve the specificity and high false-positive rate, it has been suggested that Tc-99m pertechnetate parotid scintigraphy should be performed to diagnose Warthin's tumors in the first step and in cases with negative scintigraphy with Tc-99m, FDG-PET should be performed in detecting malignant tumors in the second step (Uchida et al., 2005). However, some malignant tumors with small size or low metabolism may appear as low FDG uptake and cause a false-negative ratio (Matsuda et al., 1998). Okamura et al. (1998) reported that it is not possible to differentiate malignant tumors from benign tumors with regard to SUV on FDG-PET.

In summary, the diagnosis of malignant tumors by Tc-99m pertechnetate scintigraphy is limited, and the usefulness of FDG-PET to differentiate malignant tumors from benign tumors of the parotid gland can be limited (Table 2). However, FDG-PET might have a potential role in distinguishing recurrent tumors from surgical scar formation in the gland and in monitoring (operated patients).

In conclusion, conventional CT and MRI serve as the basis of imaging to define the features of parotid gland tumors. Advanced imaging techniques provide supplementary findings as diffusivity of molecules, metabolic activity, and dynamic

enhancement features of tumor and may help in detecting tumor type in the parotid. A diagnostic radiologic algorithm that can be used in the diagnosis of parotid masses is presented in Table 3. Magnetic resonance imaging is a superior imaging technique that reflects signal, metabolite, and diffusion features and provides multiphase dynamic follow-up to evaluate parotid gland tumors. It can be possible to establish a certain diagnosis of parotid tumors on the basis of combined T1- and T2-weighted images, together with dynamic MR imaging findings and/or ADC calculation. The threshold value for ADC should be determined to differentiate benign and malignant tumors in the large population. Although dynamic CT appears to be more practical in diagnosing parotid tumors, as it is both faster and easier than MRI, it should be noted that, if there is any MRI limitation in a patient with parotid tumor, CT might be a reliable diagnostic method as an alternative versus MRI modality.

References

Andronikou, S., McHugh, K., Jadwat, S., and Linward, J. 2003. MRI features of bilateral parotid haemangiomas of infancy. Eur. Radiol. 13:711–716.

Choi, D.S., Na, D.G., Byun, H.S., Ko, Y.H., Kim, C.K., Cho, J.M., and Lee, H.K. 2000. Salivary gland tumors: evaluation with two-phase helical CT. Radiology 214:231–236.

Gritzmann, N. 1989. Sonography of the salivary glands. AJR Am. J. Roentgenol. 153:161–166.

Habermann, C.R., Gossrau, P., Graessner, J., Arndt, C., Cramer, M.C., Reitmeier, F., Jaehne, M., and Adam, G. 2005. Diffusion-weighted echo-planar MRI: a valuable tool for differentiating primary parotid gland tumors? Rofo 77:940–945.

Howlett, D.C., Kesse, K.W., Hughes, D.V., and Sallomi, D.F. 2002. The role of imaging in the evaluation of parotid disease. Clin. Radiol. 57:692–701.

Ikeda, M., Motoori, K., Hanazawa, T., Nagai, Y., Yamamoto, S., Ueda, T., Funatsu, H., and Ito, H. 2004 Warthin tumor of the parotid gland: diagnostic value of MR imaging with histopathologic correlation. AJNR Am. J. Neuroradiol. 25:1256–1262.

Jang, M., Park, D., Lee, S.R., Hahm, C.K., Kim, Y., Park, C.K., Tae, K., Park, M.H., and Park, Y.W. 2004. Basal cell adenoma in the parotid gland: CT and MR findings. AJNR Am. J. Neuroradiol. 25:631–635.

King, A.D., Yeung, D.K.W., Ahuja, A.T., Tse, G.M.K., Yuen H.Y., Wong, K.T., and Van Hasselt, A.C. 2005. Salivary gland tumors at in vivo proton MR spectroscopy. Radiology 237:563–569.

Koyuncu, M., Sesen, T., Akan, H., Ismailoglu, A.A., Tanyeri, Y., Tekat, A., Unal, R., and. Incesu, L. 2003. Comparison of computed tomography and magnetic resonance imaging in the diagnosis of parotid tumors. Otolaryngol. Head. Neck. Surg. 129:726–732.

Lee, D.K., Chung, K.W., Baek, C.H., Jeong, H.S., Ko, Y.H., and Son, Y.I. 2005. Basal cell adenoma of the parotid gland: characteristics of 2-phase helical computed tomography and magnetic resonance imaging. J. Comput. Assist. Tomogr. 9:884–888.

Martinoli, C., Derchi, L.E., Solbiati, L., Rizzatto, G., Silvestri, E., and Giannoni, M. 1994. Color Doppler sonography of salivary glands. AJR Am. J. Roentgenol. 163:933–941.

Matsuda, M., Sakamoto, H., Okamura, T., Nakai, Y., Ohashi Y., Kawabe, J., Ochi, H., and Wakasa, K. 1998. Positron emission tomographic imaging of pleomorphic adenoma in the parotid gland. Acta Otolaryngol. 538:214–220.

Motoori, K., Yamamoto, S., Ueda, T., Nakano, K., Muto, T., Nagai, Y., Ikeda, M., Funatsu, H., and Ito, H. 2004. Inter- and intratumoral variability in magnetic resonance imaging of pleomorphic adenoma: an attempt to interpret the variable magnetic resonance findings. *J. Comput. Assist. Tomogr. 28*:233–246.

Motoori, K., Ueda, T., Uchida, Y., Chazono, H., Suzuki, H., and Ito, H. 2005a. Identification of Warthin tumor: magnetic resonance imaging versus salivary scintigraphy with technetium-99m pertechnetate. *J. Comput. Assist. Tomogr. 29*:506–512.

Motoori, K., Iida, Y., Nagai, Y., Yamamoto, S., Ueda, T., Funatsu, H., Ito, H., and Yoshitaka, O. 2005b. MR imaging of salivary duct carcinoma. *AJNR Am. J. Neuroradiol. 26*:1201–1206.

Okamura, T., Kawabe, J., Koyama, K., Ochi, H., Yamada, R., Sakamato, H., Matsuda, M., Ohashi, Y., and Nakai, Y. 1998. Fluorine –18 fluorodeoxy-glucose positron emission tomography imaging of parotid mass lesions. *Acta Otolaryngol. 538*:209–213.

Rehberg, E., Schroeder, H.G., and Kleinsasser, O. 1998. Surgery in benign parotid tumors: individually adapted or standardized radical interventions? *Laryngorhinootologie 77*:283–288.

Rubin, G.D. 2003. MDCT imaging of the aorta and peripheral vessels [Suppl]. *Eur. J. Radiol. 45*:42–49.

Som, P.M, Lanzieri, C.F, Sacher, M., Lawson, W., and Biller, H.F. 1985. Extracranial tumor vascularity: determination by dynamic CT scanning. *Radiology 154*:401–405.

Stennert, E., Guntinas-Lichius, O., Klussmann, J.P., and Arnold, G. 2001. Histopathology of pleomorphic adenoma in the parotid gland: a prospective unselected series of 100 cases. *Laryngoscope 111*:2195–2200.

Suh, S., Seol, H.Y., Kim, T.K., Lee, N.J., Kim, J.H., Kim, K.A., Woo, J.S., and Lee, J.H. 2005. Acinic cell carcinoma of the head and neck: radiologic-pathologic correlation. *J. Comput. Assist. Tomogr. 29*:121–126.

Sumi, M., Takagi, Y., Uetani, M., Morikawa, M., Hayashi, K., Kabasawa, H., Aikawa, K., and Nakamura, T. 2002. Diffusion-weighted echo-planar MR imaging of the salivary glands. *AJR Am. J. Roentgenol. 178*:959–965.

Takashima, S., Noguchi, Y., Okumura, T., Aruga, H., and Kobayashi, T. 1993. Dynamic MR imaging in the head and neck. *Radiology 189*:813–821.

Uchida, Y., Minoshima, S., Kawata, T., Motoori, K., Nakano, K., Kazama, T., Uno, T., Okamoto, Y., and Ito, H. 2005. Diagnostic value of FDG PET and salivary gland scintigraphy for parotid tumors. *Clin. Nucl. Med. 30*:170–176.

Wang, J., Takashima, S., Takayama, F., Kawakami, S., Saito, A., Matsushita, T., Momose, M., and Ishiyama, T. 2001. Head and neck lesions: characterization with diffusion-weighted echo-planar MR imaging. *Radiology 220*:621–630.

Yabuuchi, H., Fukuya, T., Tajima, T., Hachitanda, Y., Tomita, K., and Koga, M. 2003. Salivary gland tumors: diagnostic value of gadolinium-enhanced dynamic MR imaging with histopathologic correlation. *Radiology 226*:345–354.

Yerli, H., Agildere, A.M., Aydin, E., Geyik, E., Haberal, N., Kaskati T., and Ozluoglu, L. 2005a. Value of apparent diffusion coefficient calculation in the differential diagnosis of parotid gland tumors. Presented in the 30th Congress of the ESNR, Annual Meeting, Barcelona, Spain.

Yerli, H., Teksam, M., Aydin, E., Coskun, M., Ozdemir, H., and Agildere, A.M. 2005b. Basal cell adenoma of the parotid gland: dynamic CT and MRI findings. *Br. J. Radiol. 78*:642–645.

Yerli, H., Aydin, E., Coskun, M., Geyik, E., Ozluoglu, L., Haberal, N., and Kaskati, T. 2007. Dynamic multi-slice computed tomography findings for parotid gland tumors. *J. Comput. Assist. Tomogr. 31*:309–316.

40

Pituitary Macroadenomas: Intraoperative Magnetic Resonance Imaging and Endonasal Endoscopy

Ilya Laufer, Vijay K. Anand, and Theodore H. Schwartz

Introduction

Pituitary macroadenomas are benign tumors of the pituitary gland, measuring > 1 cm in diameter. They may cause diffuse enlargement and destruction of the sella and frequently extend into one of the parasellar spaces (Thapar and Laws, 2004). Complete removal of these lesions is challenging because of the difficulty in visualizing and accessing the entire tumor through a long and narrow retractor. Pituitary macroadenomas have been approached via transsphenoidal and transcranial routes. In our experience, the transsphenoidal approach offers a lower risk of morbidity than the transcranial approach by minimizing retraction injury and providing a less invasive route to the sella. To further minimize the morbidity of transsphenoidal surgery, we use an exclusively endoscopic approach for resection of pituitary lesions. The exclusive use of the endoscope obviates the need for nasal retractors, provides superior visualization and illumination of the sellar contents by advancing the lens and light source intracranially, and eliminates postoperative nasal packing.

Another method for improving visualization into the parasellar spaces has been the use of intraoperative magnetic resonance imaging (IMRI) during transsphenoidal surgery. The ability to obtain intraoperative images after an initial attempt at resection permits the visualization of unseen residual tumor that can be removed with a "second look." We have used IMRI to augment the excellent visualization obtained with the endoscope. The combination of these techniques offers the surgeon maximal intraoperative visualization of the lesion and provides definitive information about the extent of the resection.

In this chapter, we describe our method for combining endonasal endoscopy with IMRI in the removal of pituitary tumors and present our experience with the combined use in a series of 15 patients. On the basis of our experience, we can compare the relative value of each technology in the effort to achieve complete resection.

Methods

Surgical Procedure

Patients are intubated and positioned supine on the operating table, and a Foley catheter is placed. Antibiotics, glucocorticoids, and antihistamines are administered. MRI-compatible EKG leads are placed and attached to an MRI-compatible anesthesia machine (Datex-Ohmeda, Madison, Wisconsin). A 10-ml aliquot of cerebrospinal fluid (CSF) obtained via lumbar puncture is mixed with 0.2 ml of 10% fluorescein (AK-Flour, AKORN, Illinois) and introduced into the CSF space via a lumbar puncture to help visualize CSF leaks. The patient's head is fixed in a neutral position and is slightly elevated with an MRI-compatible headholder (Medtronic, Minneapolis, Minnesota). A disposable surface coil is placed over the crown of the head and left in position during the surgery.

The nasal mucosa is vasoconstricted topically with cottonoids soaked in 4 ml of 4% cocaine. Using a 0° endoscope (Karl Storz, Tuttlingen, Germany), the sphenopalatine arteries and middle turbinates are injected with a mixture of 1% lidocaine and epinephrine (1:100,000). The middle and superior turbinates are retracted laterally under endoscopic visualization, and the sphenoid ostia are identified. The posterior third of the nasal septum is resected with a tissue shaver. This provides a panoramic view of the sphenoid sinus rostrum and the ostia bilaterally. Once the sphenoid sinus mucosa is retracted laterally, rongeur forceps are used to remove the intersinus sphenoid septum. This step brings the posterior wall of the sphenoid sinus into full view. At this point, image guidance is used to confirm localization and identify the location of the carotid arteries.

A 0°, 30-cm, rigid 4-mm endoscope (Karl Storz) is introduced through the left nostril and held in place with a flexible scope holder (Karl Storz). The right nostril is used for introduction of surgical instruments. The floor of the sella is opened with an osteotome or a high-speed drill, curette, or a Kerrison rongeur. If the tumor is larger than 2 cm, we often remove the tuberculum sellae and planum sphenoidal to improve the exposure. A sickle knife or microscissors is used to open the dura in a cruciate fashion, and the circular sinus is coagulated and cut if necessary. The adenoma is identified and removed using ring curettes. Starting inferiorly, then laterally, then superiorly to prevent premature herniation of the arachnoid, which can obscure laterally placed tumor fragments, a 45°, 18-cm, 4-mm endoscope is used to examine the sella and the suprasellar space for residual tumor.

After completion of tumor resection, a careful inspection for CSF leak is carried out using an endoscope. Blocking light filters are used to highlight the fluorescein. If a leak is seen, a fat graft is harvested through a small incision in the anterior abdominal wall and is used to fill the sella. If a transtuberculum or transplanum approach is required for the resection of a large tumor, a fascia lata inlay graft is placed after the fat graft. Vomeric bone is used to buttress the closure. Polymerized hydrogel (Duraseal; Confluent Surgical, Massachusetts) spray is used to provide a water-tight closure. A lumbar drain can be placed to divert CSF if the patient is at risk of CSF leak because of factors that include obesity, hydrocephalus, or visualization of fluorescein at the end of the closure.

Intraoperative Magnetic Resonance Imaging

When IMRI is implemented, a radiofrequency-shielded operating room must be used along with dedicated anesthesia equipment, including ventilator, infusion pumps, and monitoring screens. Pressure transducers must be kept outside the scanner to prevent artifacts. We use the Odin Polestar N-10 IMRI, which is positioned under the OR table. Its "home" position is beneath the head of the patient, and it may be robotically raised into the "scanning" position (Fig. 1).

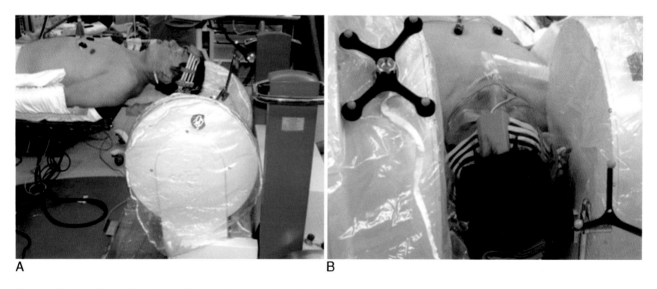

A   B

Figure 1 (**A**) A disposable surface coil is placed on the patient's head. The magnet is in the "home" position in this photograph. (**B**) Photograph of the magnet in the "scanning" position. The magnet reference frame is on the left, and the patient reference frame is on the right. Reprinted with permission from Lippincott, Williams & Wilkins; Schwartz *et al.* 2006. Endoscopic transsphenoidal pituitary surgery with intraoperative magnetic resonance imaging. *Neurosurgery 58*:44–51.

Daily quality assurance and shimming are performed on the magnet. All electronic equipment is unplugged during quality assurance and image acquisition. The magnet and patient reference frames must be placed in the line of sight of the infrared camera. The infrared camera is placed at the head of the bed to prevent having the surgeon in its line of sight (Fig. 2). Endoscope images are projected on a wall-mounted 42-inch plasma screen (Panasonic TH42PWD5; Matsushita Electronic Industrial Co., Osaka, Japan).

Pre-resection images of the sella, parasellar structures, and nasopharynx are obtained before and after administration of intravenous contrast (gadolinium, 0.6 ml/kg) and are subsequently used for stereotactic navigation. During the surgical procedure, the magnet is lowered under the bed. It is raised after the resection is complete, all electronic equipment is unplugged, and images are obtained with and without intravenous contrast. Post-resection images are compared to pre-resection images (Fig. 3). If residual tumor is noted on the post-resection scans, reexploration with the endoscope is performed to visualize and resect tumor remnants, using stereotactic navigation for localization.

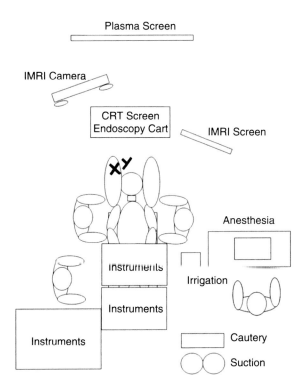

Figure 2 Schematic representation of the operating room setup. The magnet and patient reference frames are placed in the line of sight of the infrared camera. A cathode ray tube (CRT) screen is positioned at the head of the operating table in cases where IMRI is not used. IMRI causes distortion of color and image in CRT screens. Thus in cases where IMRI is used, the endoscopic image is projected on a plasma screen. Reprinted with permission from Lippincott, Williams & Wilkins; Schwartz *et al.* 2006. Endoscopic transsphenoidal pituitary surgery with intraoperative magnetic resonance imaging. *Neurosurgery 58*:44–51.

Results

We combined endoscopic endonasal surgery with IMRI to remove pituitary adenomas in a series of 15 patients (Schwartz *et al.*, 2006). There were no intraoperative complications. In three patients, residual tumor was identified on post-resection IMRI. On examination with a 45° endoscope, tumor remnants tucked behind the edge of the dura or within arachnoid folds were identified and resected. In four patients, possible residual tumor on IMRI turned out to be pooled blood or folds of the arachnoid. Residual tumor in the cavernous sinus was intentionally left in three patients and was observed on IMRI. Finally, in five patients no residual tumor was observed on IMRI. On postoperative 1.5 T MRI performed immediately after surgery and three months later, no tumor was present, except in the patients with intentionally left cavernous sinus disease.

Discussion

The first neurosurgeon to employ an endoscope while operating on the sella was Gerard Guiot in the 1960s (Guiot *et al.*, 1963). However, it was only in the 1990s that neurosurgeons began to actively use the endoscope in pituitary surgery. In 1992, Jankowski *et al.* (1992) first reported a purely endoscopic endonasal approach to the pituitary. More recently, Cappabianca, de Divitiis, and Jho, with multiple associates, have popularized this technique and published their experience (Cappabianca *et al.*, 2004; Jho and Ha, 2004). Use of an endoscope brings the light source directly into the sella, providing illumination that is superior to the illumination provided by an operating microscope. Furthermore, the use of angled endoscopes allows visualization of areas not accessible to linear sight lines afforded by the microscope. Postoperatively, patient comfort is greater after endoscopic procedures because nasal packing is not required. An endonasal retractor, which is required during microscope-assisted pituitary surgery, is not used in endoscopic surgery, thus eliminating the potential risk of skull base or nasal fractures. Sphenoid mucosa and mucociliary transport are better preserved after endoscopic surgery, further minimizing postoperative discomfort. The main shortcoming of endoscopic surgery is the lack of stereoscopic vision, which with increasing operator experience becomes less important. The ongoing development of stereoscopic endoscopes should eliminate this problem.

MRI technology has revolutionized neurosurgery by allowing us to diagnose, localize, and visualize pathologic processes in the central nervous system with unprecedented clarity. Preoperatively, it provides us with information about the location, size, and boundaries of the lesion and its relationship to adjoining structures. Postoperatively, MRI shows us the extent of the resection and the effect of the surgery

Pre-resection
−Gado   + Gado

Post-resection
−Gado   + Gado

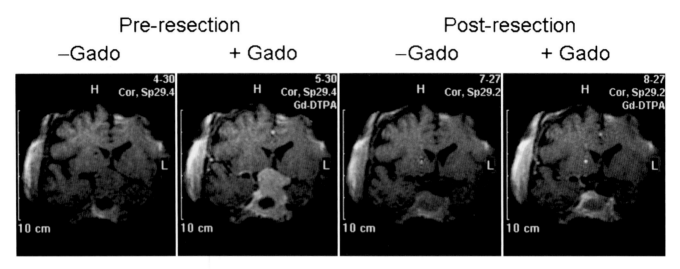

Figure 3 Example of pre- and post-resection images obtained with the 0.1-Tesla magnet with (+ Gado) and without (− Gado) gadolinium contrast. The optic nerves and the stalk can be visualized. Reprinted with permission from Lippincott, Williams & Wilkins; Schwartz *et al.* 2006. Endoscopic transsphenoidal pituitary surgery with intraoperative magnetic resonance imaging. *Neurosurgery 58*:44–51.

on surrounding structures. The goal of surgical treatment of benign or low-grade lesions in the central nervous system is gross total resection with minimal damage to adjoining parenchyma. The appearance of residual tumor on postoperative imaging and, especially, the progression of these residual lesions on follow-up imaging frequently prompt surgeons to reattempt resection. Thus, it is most logical to bring MRI technology into the operating room, in order to permit surgeons to evaluate the extent of the resection before deciding to end the surgery.

On occasion, the margin of a macroadenoma is indistinguishable from normal pituitary parenchyma to the naked eye. However, it is distinguishable on MRI. Furthermore, macroadenomas may extend outside of the normal sellar boundaries into the suprasellar space or the cavernous sinus. This extension may not be obvious on preoperative imaging or intraoperatively and would become apparent only postoperatively when residual tumor is seen on MRI. Macroadenomas may also envelop the carotid arteries. During surgery, it may not be clear how much of the tumor may safely be removed before damaging a carotid artery, and IMRI can elucidate the relation of the residual tumor to the artery. Finally, IMRI can serve as an important adjunct to intraoperative frameless navigation systems. The navigation systems rely on preoperative location of brain structures. However, because of retraction, CSF loss, and resection, brain structures may shift by as much as 1–1.5 cm. Therefore, static image-guided systems frequently become inaccurate intraoperatively, and real-time imaging is required. Hence, IMRI seems to be a useful addition to the operating room, allowing a more complete and safer resection of macroadenomas.

Several groups have reported on their experience with IMRI and transsphenoidal surgery. In 1999, Martin *et al.*

(1999) published their experience with five patients with pituitary macroadenomas who underwent IMRI-assisted transsphenoidal resection. They used a 0.5-Tesla imager and an MRI-compatible microscope and speculum during their surgeries. In three patients, IMRI revealed residual tumor that was not visualized in the microscopic field-of-view and that was subsequently safely removed, thereby providing maximal tumor resection. Furthermore, in one patient, after the fat graft was placed, an expanding intrasellar mass was identified, which turned out to be a developing clot. The clot was evacuated, and adequate hemostasis was obtained before completion of surgery. Bohinski *et al.* (2001) reported on their experience with a 0.3-Tesla IMRI. Between 1998 and 2000, 30 patients with macroadenomas underwent microscope-assisted transsphenoidal tumor resection via a sublabial-transseptal approach. In one patient, a hemorrhage was detected and the operation was converted to a craniotomy. In the remaining 29 patients, IMRI revealed optimal tumor resection in 34% of the patients. In the remaining 66%, 16 patients underwent one reexploration, and three underwent two reexplorations to achieve maximal safe tumor evacuation.

Finally, Fahlbusch's group in Erlangen, Germany, has been actively implementing and developing IMRI for use during tumor resection. In a series of 106 patients with hormonally inactive pituitary macroadenomas, they obtained intraoperative imaging with a 1.5-Tesla magnet (Fahlbusch *et al.*, 2001). They used a transsphenoidal microsurgical technique with endoscopic assistance. Surgery took place 4 meters away from the center of the scanner, allowing them to use conventional surgical instruments. Each scan added approximately 15 minutes to operative time. Although complete tumor removal was intended in 85 of the 106 patients,

IMRI revealed that residual tumor remained in 36 of the 85. The resection was extended in 29 of these patients, and complete resection was achieved in 21 patients. Thus, the rate of complete tumor removal increased from 58 (49 of 85) to 82% (70 of 85).

Our experience with the combined use of endonasal endoscopy and IMRI has allowed us to compare the relative value of each technology in extent of resection. The amount of residual tumor found with IMRI was smaller in our series than in previous reports in which the endoscope was not used. We therefore conclude that the endoscope permits a more aggressive resection than the microscope. The small number of cases in which residual tumor was identified with IMRI was balanced by the number of cases in which interpretation of the images was ambiguous and led to unnecessary reexploration of the sella and increased risk of complications. We believe that the relative increased value of IMRI with low-resolution, low-Tesla magnets is insufficient to support its routine use if endonasal endoscopy is employed. However, higher Tesla magnets will likely be sufficiently sensitive and specific for residual tumor to be of added value after an endoscopic resection.

Future Directions

Intraoperative MRI is being actively implemented and developed in several academic centers. One of the main challenges before the neurosurgical community at this time is the design and performance of high-volume outcome studies in order to determine whether this novel technology truly improves the outcome of surgical intervention. Furthermore, it is important to determine whether its high cost justifies its implementation in routine neurosurgical practice.

Neuroendoscopy has become a well-accepted adjunct to pituitary microsurgery. Several groups recommend that purely endoscopic transsphenoidal surgery should replace conventional microscope-assisted pituitary operations, citing increased patient comfort, improved visualization, and decreased risk of morbidity. However, most of this evidence is anecdotal or is based on small cohorts of patients. Studies in high-volume endoscopic academic centers are currently under way to explore these claims. Finally, the development and improvement of stereoscopic endoscopy will make this technology more accessible and safer to use.

References

Bohinski, R.J., Warnick, R.E., Gaskill-Shipley, M.F., Zuccarello, M., van Loveren, H.R., Kormos, D.W., and Tew, J.M., Jr. 2001. Intraoperative magnetic resonance imaging to determine the extent of resection of pituitary macroadenomas during transsphenoidal microsurgery. *Neurosurgery 49*:1133–1143.

Cappabianca, P., Cavallo, L.M., and de Divitiis, E. 2004. Endoscopic endonasal transsphenoidal surgery. *Neurosurgery 55*:933–940; discussion 940–941.

Fahlbusch, R., Ganslandt, O., Buchfelder, M., Schott, W., and Nimsky, C. 2001. Intraoperative magnetic resonance imaging during transsphenoidal surgery. *J. Neurosurgery 95*:381–390.

Guiot, G., Rougerie, J., Fourestier, M., Fournier, A., Comoy, C., Voulmiere, J., and Groux, R. 1963. Intracranial endoscopic explorations. *Presse Med. 71*:1225–1228.

Jankowski, R., Auque J., Simon, C., Marchal, J.C., Hepner, H., and Wayoff, M. 1992. Endoscopic pituitary tumor surgery. *Laryngoscope 102*:198–202.

Jho, H.D., and Ha, H.G. 2004. Endoscopic endonasal skull base surgery: Part 1—the midline anterior fossa skull base. *Minim. Invasive Neurosurg. 47*:1–8.

Martin, C.H., Schwartz, R., Jolesz, F., and Black, P.M. 1999. Transsphenoidal resection of pituitary adenomas in an intraoperative MRI unit. *Pituitary 2*:155–162.

Schwartz, T.H., Stieg, P.E., and Anand, V.K. 2006. Endoscopic transsphenoidal pituitary surgery with intraoperative magnetic resonance imaging. *Neurosurgery 58*:44–51.

Thapar, K., and Laws, E.R. 2004. Pituitary tumors: functioning and nonfunctioning. In: Winn, H. (Ed.), *Youmans Neurological Surgery*. Philadelphia: Saunders, 1, pp. 1169–1206.

41

Penile Cancer Staging: ^{18}F-Fluorodeoxyglucose-Positron Emission Tomography/Computed Tomography

Bernhard Scher, M. Seitz, B. Schlenker, M. Reiser, and R. Tiling

Introduction

The prevalence of penile carcinoma shows a clear geographical distribution. In industrial countries such as Europe and the United States, the incidence of penile cancer ranges from to 0.3 to 1.5, and this tumor entity makes up 0.4 to 0.65% of all malignant diseases. Prevalence of penile cancer is more than four times higher in South America, Asia, and Africa, and in some areas reaches a prevalence of up to 17%. Inadequate hygienic conditions, rarely performed therapeutic circumcisions, and lack of medical treatment for pre-cancerous lesions such as *lichen sclerosus et atrophicus* are reasons for this geographical difference. Also, chronic and untreated human papillomavirus (HPV) infections with the high-risk subtypes 16 and 18 lead to an increased prevalence of penile cancer (McCance *et al.*, 1986). When the diagnosis is established, patients are on average 57 years of age (Derakhshani *et al.*, 1999; Derrick *et al.*, 1973); however, in rare cases penile cancer also occurs in patients younger than 30 years of age.

Generally, penile carcinoma has a slow growth rate. However, when the first symptoms show up, many patients are hesitant to visit a doctor because they feel embarrassed and fear therapeutic implications. Especially in developing countries additional factors that contribute to a late diagnosis are social and cultural traditions, level of education, shame, but also ignorance. Therefore, precancerous lesions and early disease stages are rather rare at the time of first diagnosis, and in many cases metastatic spread has already taken place.

The difficulties that arise from late diagnosis are reflected by a mean 5-year survival rate of 52%. While the 5-year survival rate is 66% in patients without metastatic spread, it decreases dramatically with the presence of metastatic disease to ~ 27% (Horenblas, 2001). An infiltration of the corpora cavernosa by the primary tumor is associated with lymph node metastases in > 75% of cases. Metastatic spread takes place primarily along the lymphatic system. Generally, metastases occur at first in the superficial inguinal lymph node basins, followed by the deep inguinal basins and the pelvic basins. However, in some cases skip-lesions can be found, so that pelvic lymph node metastases can occur without involvement of inguinal lymph nodes.

Etiology, Histology, and Staging

In > 95% of cases penile carcinomas are of the squamous cell type. Adenocarcinomas, malignant melanomas, or basal cell carcinomas can also be found in rare cases. Also, metastases of other urological tumors can be located at the penis. The etiology of penile cancer seems to be based on two different pathways. On the one hand, chronic inflammations caused by phimosis or insufficient hygienical conditions are regarded as a triggering factor for the genesis of penile carcinoma. On the other hand, chronic infections with high-risk human papillomavirus subtypes seem to be responsible for precancerous lesions such as Bowen's disease, erythroplasia de Queyrat, or balantitis xerotica obliterans. In the early stages, penile carcinoma can often be demarcated as a flat rubefaction, which later gradually merges into a painless exophytic tumor that can also ulcerate. Sometimes penile cancer is mistaken in its early stages for chronic balantitis. The localization of the primary malignancy is in > 50% of cases at the penile glans. The preputium is also frequently involved.

At clinical examination, localization, size, pattern of growth, and neighboring structures should be documented. Although benign exophytic lesions such as condylomas can often be differentiated from a malignant lesion by their macroscopic aspect, all suspicious lesions should nevertheless be evaluated by means of biopsy and subsequent histopathological work-up. This approach is further corroborated by the fact that benign penile changes can often be accompanied by precancerous lesions (Jaleel et al., 1999; Pizzocaro et al., 1997). Another advantage of biopsy is the possibility of assessing the histologic grade of the primary cancer. Furthermore, an HPV classification can be carried out. In future, the HPV status may be utilized to develop new treatment strategies such as the HPV vaccination.

Therapy

Therapy of the primary malignancy strongly depends on the exact localization, grading, T-stage, patient age, and patient compliance. For precancerous lesions and tumors at stage T1 and grade G1 or G2, an organ-preserving surgical approach will be chosen most frequently. Laser therapy supplemented by photodynamic diagnostics (PDD) or a local excision and brachytherapy may be preferred in these patients. In addition, in all of these cases circumcision of the preputium will be performed to remove possible satellite lesions and to accelerate wound healing. At this stage the rate of tumor recurrence ranges from 12 to 17%, depending on tumor grade and size. In case of a tumor at grade G3 and for T-stages of T2 or greater, complete or partial amputation of the penis cannot be avoided in the majority of cases. Patients with positive lymph node status

or distant metastases may also profit from additional chemotherapy or radiation therapy. Prognosis of penile carcinoma depends heavily on tumor stage, histologic grade, and regional lymph node involvement (Chen et al., 2004; Singh and Khaitan, 2003). Despite surgical therapy and lymphadenectomy with curative intention, tumor progression will take place in ~ 40% of cases (Syed et al., 2003).

Diagnostics of the Primary Malignancy

To beware as many patients as possible from mutilating partial or total penectomy, sensitive diagnostic methods are necessary to be able to exactly assess the extent of tumor growth and involvement of surrounding structures, and to detect possible satellite lesions. For this purpose, several diagnostic procedures have been in use to evaluate the primary malignancy.

Acetic acid test. Five percent acetic acid is applied > 10 min upon a suspected lesion. Human papillomavirus infections as well as HPV-associated carcinoma *in situ* can be demarcated by showing a whitish discoloration. The sensitivity of the acetic acid test is up to 95%. However, the rate of false positives is high because areas with inflammatory changes can also show a whitish discoloration.

Photodynamic diagnostics. Photodynamic diagnostics (PDD) is an established method for the detection of precancerous lesions and malignant changes. Underutilization of PDD satellite lesions in the proximity of the primary malignancy can be detected. For this procedure 5-aminolevulinacid (5-ALA) is applied on the penis and after ~ 1 hr malignant lesions typically demarcate themselves as reddish fluorescent areas under a flashing blue light of a xenon arc lamp (Frimberger et al., 2002). Furthermore, in combination with organ-preserving laser coagulation therapy, PDD may be used to assess complete ablation of the tumor.

Radiologic imaging methods. These procedures play a minor role in the diagnostics of the primary tumor. In the past, ultrasonography (US) and magnetic resonance imaging (MRI) have been used to evaluate possible infiltration of the corpora cavernosa. However, these imaging modalities have not proven sufficiently robust in the assessment of the T-stage (Agrawal et al., 2000; Lont et al., 2003).

Lymph Node Metastases

At first diagnosis of a penile cancer, the palpation of inguinal lymph nodes is obligatory. When suspicion of lymph node spread arises, radical lymphadenectomy will be performed. However, because of the frequency and the high prognostic consequence of the presence of lymph node spread and because of the unsatisfactory diagnostic accuracy of currently available imaging techniques, this invasive procedure is routinely carried out in cases with high tumor grade and at stage T2 and higher (Chen *et al.*, 2004). In contrast to other tumor entities, lymphadenectomy is considered a curative approach with regard to penile carcinoma and can lead to a complete cure in some instances. Unfortunately, lymphadenectomy is frequently associated with serious complications, such as lymphoceles, lymphedemas of the legs, scrotal edemas, or necrosis at the resection site (Nelson *et al.*, 2004). To reduce comorbidity, operation techniques have been modified by Catalona (1988) and Cabanas (1977) and supplemented by sentinel lymph node biopsy (SLNB). However, as the lymphatic drainage has a considerable individual variation in this region of the body, both of these altered operation techniques could not gain acceptance as a gold standard.

Scintigraphic Sentinel Lymph Node Biopsy

Horenblas (2001) and Kroon *et al.* (2005) introduced scintigraphic sentinel lymph node biopsy after peritumoral and intradermal injection of radiolabeled nano-colloid particles. Contrary to the aforementioned lymphadenectomy techniques, the radiolabeled sentinel lymph node can be reliably detected intraoperatively by using a gamma probe. Only in cases with metastatic spread, verified by intraoperative frozen section, an extensive radical bilateral lymphadenectomy would be carried out. This novel approach has shown first promising results and has the potential to reduce the frequency of generally performed radical lymphadenectomy. While SLNB is known to have high accuracy particularly regarding mammary cancer, Tanis *et al.* (2002) reported a comparatively low overall sensitivity of 78% for penile cancer. This may be attributed to the highly variable lymphatic drainage in this body region. Furthermore, it is well known, that kip lesions and bilateral involvement are not uncommon in penile cancer patients (Algaba *et al.*, 2002).

Conventional Imaging Modalities for Staging of Penile Cancer

Verification of the primary penile cancer is most often obtained on the basis of histopathological work-up of biopsy specimens of the suspected area. Therefore, diagnostic imaging techniques are rarely applied for evaluation of the primary malignancy. If penile cancer is present, clinical palpation will be carried out as a first-line examination to assess the N-stage. However, Algaba *et al.* (2002) have reported that 20–96% of penile cancer patients have palpable lymph nodes at the time of first diagnosis, although metastatic infiltration is present in only 17–45% of these cases. Therefore, additional radiologic imaging modalities, such as US, computed tomography (CT),

or MRI can be performed in the majority of cases. While US is a widely available imaging procedure, it has its limitations with regard to N-staging, especially when lymph node metastases in the deeper lymphatic basins are present (Algaba *et al.*, 2002). Radiologic cross-sectional imaging techniques, such as CT and MRI, provide high anatomical detail. However, as these procedures rely mainly on a system of classification based on morphologic aspects, such as the size of a respective lymph node, Derakhshani *et al.* (1999) found them to be not sufficiently robust regarding N-staging. Furthermore, Lont *et al.* (2003) demonstrated that the rate of false-positive lymph node findings is comparably high for CT and MRI. An explanation for these findings may be that lymph nodes frequently undergo reactive changes on the basis of the underlying primary penile carcinoma (Chen *et al.*, 2004). Even under physiological conditions, lymph nodes in the inguinal region can exceed 2 cm in diameter without malignant infiltration.

PET and PET/CT for Staging of Penile Cancer

As a whole-body procedure, functional PET imaging by using ^{18}F-fluoro-deoxyglucose (^{18}F-FDG) has proven to be a valuable diagnostic tool for the assessment of metastatic spread. Recently introduced combined PET/CT scanners may further improve the diagnostic accuracy in certain scenarios by providing exact image fusion between PET and detailed anatomic CT images. To utilize PET or PET/CT for imaging penile cancer, the principal question that needs to be tackled is whether penile cancer and its metastases exhibit high enough ^{18}F-FDG-uptake to be detectable with PET. It is well known that glucose metabolism in squamous-type carcinomas is generally high. Therefore, in theory, penile carcinoma should be amenable to ^{18}F-FDG-PET imaging. Until recently, only three case reports in the international literature hint that ^{18}F-FDG-PET may be used for penile cancer imaging. In a publication that primarily investigated a novel polychemotherapy regimen in a patient with penile cancer, the authors report that an incidentally discovered metastatic lymph node showed focal ^{18}F-FDG accumulation (Joerger *et al.*, 2004). Another case report addressed a lesion with increased ^{18}F-FDG metabolism in a patient with underlying penile carcinoma (Ravizzini *et al.*, 2001). In a third publication, Langen *et al.* (2001) reported that a coincidentally discovered inguinal lymph node metastasis originating from penile cancer showed focal ^{18}F-FDG uptake. However, in none of these case reports has ^{18}F-FDG-PET imaging of penile cancer been the primary focus.

In a pilot study investigating 13 patients with suspected penile cancer, we systematically demonstrated for the first time that the primary penile cancer as well as lymph node metastases originating from penile cancer exhibit increased FDG-uptake typically for malignancy (Scher *et al.*, 2005).

The reference standard of this study based on histopathological correlation was obtained at biopsy or surgery. ^{18}F-FDG-PET/CT was carried out for whole-body staging in all patients by using a dual-slice PET/CT system; 200 MBq of ^{18}F-FDG were administered intravenously. A native low dose CT scan was used for attenuation correction. Following that, emission scanning was performed, and afterward a diagnostic contrast-enhanced CT of the thorax, abdomen, and pelvis was carried out. All studies were evaluated by readers blinded to any clinical information and to results of other imaging procedures. However, readers were aware of the patient's underlying disease. The classification of whether a lesion had to be considered benign or malignant was based predominantly on a visual image analysis of the PET scan. Computed tomography was exclusively used for anatomic allocation, and SUV_{max} values served as guidance only.

The primary penile cancer as well as regional lymph node metastases exhibited a pattern of tracer uptake typical for malignant processes (Fig. 1). In the included patient population, sensitivity in the detection of the primary malignancy was 75%, with a specificity of 75%. On a per-patient basis, sensitivity in the detection of lymphatic spread was 80% with a specificity of 100%. PET/CT missed one single lymph node micrometastasis. On a nodal-group basis, PET/CT had a sensitivity of 89% in the detection of metastases in the superficial inguinal lymph node basins and a sensitivity of 100% in the deep inguinal and obturator lymph node basins. Due to the generally intense pattern of tracer uptake of penile cancer lesions, even small lesions could be reliably detected by PET/CT. However, interpretation of lesions below 1 cm in diameter may be difficult because significant partial-volume effects must be taken into account during PET interpretation. Therefore, SUV_{max} values should serve as guidance only. Although not in the case of the limited number of 13 included patients, false-positive findings may occur because inguinal lymph nodes frequently undergo reactive changes secondary to the primary penile cancer. This could lead to increased FDG accumulation. Despite the fact that metastatic processes most often exhibit a higher ^{18}F-FDG metabolism than do reactive changes, the possibility of false-positive findings has to be taken into consideration during routine image interpretation. This is particularly true for inguinal lymph nodes.

An intrinsic advantage of PET/CT is the ability to assess the malignancy of lymph nodes based on functional information, independently from morphologic criteria, as is the case with stand-alone CT and MRI. As the primary penile cancer is generally verified at biopsy, the main indication of ^{18}F-FDG-PET/CT in penile cancer patients needs to be considered as the prognostically crucial search for lymph node metastases. In this respect, Solsona et al. (2001), in a study covering 103 patients, reported that the likelihood of the presence of occult lymph node metastases is associated with tumor grade and stage. Distant metastases originating from penile cancer are rare, occur only in high tumor stages, and are generally accompanied with regional lymph node involvement (Misra et al., 2004).

Summary

Penile cancer is a rare tumor entity in industrial countries and is frequently diagnosed late. Urologists often find themselves in a diagnostic dilemma in selecting patients for radical lymphadenectomy, a procedure associated with a high morbidity rate. Conventional radiologic imaging procedures have proven insufficiently robust in the assessment of lymphatic spread. Regarding functional PET imaging, our own findings and the limited number of three additional case reports in the international literature indicate that squamous cell-type penile carcinoma as well as its metastases are in principle amenable to PET or PET/CT imaging. Positron emission tomography is considered the gold standard for whole-body staging and the search for regional or distant metastases in a variety of malignant diseases. In our patient collective, ^{18}F-FDG-PET/CT showed promising first results

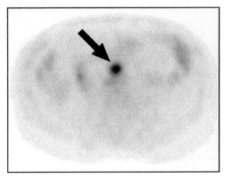 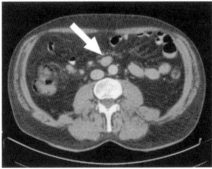 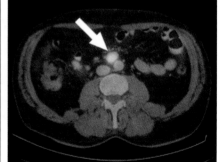

Figure 1 Patient (73 years old) with histopathologically verified penile cancer. The lymph node status in the inguinal and obturatoric region was negative. However, PET/CT revealed a para-aortal skip lesion located more cranially in the abdominal region (arrows). The lesion could be identified as a lymph node metastasis at follow-up.

in staging patients who suffer from penile cancer. However, independently of the underlying malignant disease, a known limitation of PET or PET/CT lies in the detection of micrometastases. While the resolution of modern PET and PET/CT devices is significantly below 1 cm if the lesions exhibit high FDG uptake, it is generally not possible to detect micrometastases by means of PET imaging.

Because of its different methodical approach, SLNB can be frequently used to verify micrometastatic invasion of the sentinel lymph node(s). A combination of PET and SLNB may compensate for the shortcomings of each respective procedure. While an application of SLNB parallel to PET or PET/CT may minimize the risk of undetected micrometastases, PET has the ability to detect skip lesions and to provide whole-body staging. It is speculated that a negative PET scan in combination with negative SLNB findings could provide a sufficiently high level of diagnostic security to dispense with prophylactic lymphadenectomy, particularly in cases with low tumor grade and stage. In consequence, the comorbidity rate caused by lymphadenectomy could be reduced. Eventually, PET may prove to be a valuable method to evaluate the need of lymphadenectomy or to opt for a "wait-and-see" strategy with regular follow-up examinations. A future implementation of PET and PET/CT into the diagnostic work-up of penile cancer patients may therefore help in selecting a stage for appropriate therapy and in improving follow-up.

Combined PET/CT systems may eventually be favored over stand-alone PET scanners. The possibility of allocating a focus seen in PET to a certain anatomic region or structure can lead to an increase in diagnostic assertiveness, for example, by assigning a discrete PET lesion to a lymph node in the respective CT scan. Furthermore, the additional morphologic information provided by CT and the use of exact image fusion may be particularly useful for planning surgery.

References

Agrawal, A., Pai, D., Ananthakrishnan, N., Smile, S.R., and Ratnakar, C. 2000. Clinical and sonographic findings in carcinoma of the penis. *J. Clin. Ultrasound 8*:399–406.

Algaba, F., Horenblas, S., Pizzocaro-Luigi Piva, G., Solsona, E., and Windahl, T. 2002. EAU guidelines on penile cancer. *Eur. Urol. 3*:199–203.

Cabanas, R.M. 1977. An approach for the treatment of penile carcinoma. *Cancer 2*:456–466.

Catalona, W.J. 1988. Modified inguinal lymphadenectomy for carcinoma of the penis with preservation of saphenous veins: technique and preliminary results. *J. Urol. 2*:306–310.

Chen, M.F., Chen, W.C., Wu, C.T., Chuang, C.K., Ng, K.F., and Chang, J.T. 2004. Contemporary management of penile cancer including surgery and adjuvant radiotherapy: an experience in Taiwan. *World J. Urol. 1*:60–66.

Derakhshani, P., Neubauer, S., Braun, M., Bargmann, H., Heidenreich, A., and Engelmann, U. 1999. Results and 10-year follow-up in patients with squamous cell carcinoma of the penis. *Urol. Int. 4*:238–244.

Derrick, F.C., Jr., Lynch, K.M., Jr., Kretkowski, R.C., and Yarbrough, W.J. 1973. Epidermoid carcinoma of the penis: computer analysis of 87 cases. *J. Urol. 3*:303–305.

Frimberger, D., Schneede, P., Hungerhuber, E., Sroka, R., Zaak, D., Siebels, M., and Hofstetter, A. 2002. Autofluorescence and 5-aminolevulinic acid induced fluorescence diagnosis of penile carcinoma—new techniques to monitor Nd: YAG laser therapy. *Urol. Res. 5*:295–300.

Horenblas, S. 2001. Lymphadenectomy for squamous cell carcinoma of the penis. Part 2: the role and technique of lymph node dissection. *BJU Int. 5*:473–483.

Jaleel, H., Narouz, N., Wade, A.A., and Allan, P.S. 1999. Penile intraepithelial neoplasia—a veiled lesion in genitourinary medicine. *Sex. Transm. Infect. 6*:435–436.

Joerger, M., Warzinek, T., Klaeser, B., Kluckert, J.T., Schmid, H.P., and Gillessen, S. 2004. Major tumor regression after paclitaxel and carboplatin polychemotherapy in a patient with advanced penile cancer. *Urology 4*:778–780.

Kroon, B.K., Horenblas, S., Meinhardt, W., van der Poel, H.G., Bex, A., van Tinteren, H., Valdes Olmos, R.A., and Nieweg, O.E. 2005. Dynamic sentinel node biopsy in penile carcinoma: evaluation of 10 years experience. *Eur. Urol. 5*:601–606; discussion 606.

Langen, K.J., Borner, A.R., Muller-Mattheis, V., Hamacher, K., Herzog, H., Ackermann, R., and Coenen, H.H. 2001. Uptake of cis-4-[18F]fluoro-L-proline in urologic tumors. *J. Nucl. Med. 5*:752–754.

Lont, A.P., Besnard, A.P., Gallee, M.P., van Tinteren, H., and Horenblas, S. 2003. A comparison of physical examination and imaging in determining the extent of primary penile carcinoma. *BJU Int. 6*:493–495.

McCance, D.J., Kalache, A., Ashdown, K., Andrade, L., Menezes, F., Smith, P., and Doll, R. 1986. Human papillomavirus types 16 and 18 in carcinomas of the penis from Brazil. *Int. J. Cancer. 1*:55–59.

Misra, S., Chaturvedi, A., and Misra, N.C. 2004. Penile carcinoma: a challenge for the developing world. *Lancet Oncol. 4*:240–247.

Nelson, B.A., Cookson, M.S., Smith, J.A., Jr., and Chang, S.S. 2004. Complications of inguinal and pelvic lymphadenectomy for squamous cell carcinoma of the penis: a contemporary series. *J. Urol. 2*:494–497.

Pizzocaro, G., Piva, L., Bandieramonte, G., and Tana, S. 1997. Up-to-date management of carcinoma of the penis. *Eur. Urol. 1*:5–15.

Ravizzini, G.C., Wagner, M., and Borges-Neto, S. 2001. Positron emission tomography detection of metastatic penile squamous cell carcinoma. *J. Urol. 5*:1633–1634.

Scher, B., Seitz, M., Reiser, M., Hungerhuber, E., Hahn, K., Tiling, R., Herzog, P., Reiser, M., Schneede, P., and Dresel, S. 2005. 18F-FDG PET/CT for staging of penile cancer. *J. Nucl. Med. 9*:1460–1465.

Singh, I., and Khaitan, A. 2003. Current trends in the management of carcinoma penis—a review. *Int. Urol. Nephrol. 2*:215–225.

Solsona, E., Iborra, I., Rubio, J., Casanova, J.L., Ricos, J.V., and Calabuig, C. 2001. Prospective validation of the association of local tumor stage and grade as a predictive factor for occult lymph node micrometastasis in patients with penile carcinoma and clinically negative inguinal lymph nodes. *J. Urol. 5*:1506–1509.

Syed, S., Eng, T.Y., Thomas, C.R., Thompson, I.M., and Weiss, G.R. 2003. Current issues in the management of advanced squamous cell carcinoma of the penis. *Urol. Oncol. 6*:431–438.

Tanis, P.J., Lont, A.P., Meinhardt, W., Olmos, R.A., Nieweg, O.E., and Horenblas, S. 2002. Dynamic sentinel node biopsy for penile cancer: reliability of a staging technique. *J. Urol. 1*:76–80.

42

Malignant Peripheral Nerve Sheath Tumors: [¹⁸F]Fluorodeoxyglucose-Positron Emission Tomography

Winfried Brenner and Victor F. Mautner

Introduction

Malignant peripheral nerve sheath tumor (MPNST) is a rare tumor entity within the sarcoma tumor family comprising 10% of all soft tissue sarcomas. Older terms used for this tumor are malignant schwannoma, neurogenic sarcoma, or neurofibrosarcoma. These tumors are usually large tumors of more than 5 cm in diameter at initial diagnosis located in the deep soft tissue in close proximity to a nerve trunk, most commonly the sciatic nerve, brachial, and sacral plexus. The most frequent clinical symptom is pain. In a large series of 120 patients with MPNST, about half of these tumors arose from (plexiform neurofibromas (PNF)) in patients with neurofibromatosis type-1 (NF1; von Recklinghausen's disease), 16% from preexisting metaplastic foci, and 11% in previously irradiated tissue (Ducatman *et al.*, 1986). Approximately, 20% are sporadic MPNST; that is, these tumors developed in patients with no preexisting neurofibromatosis or other pre-sarcomatous lesions.

Neurofibromatosis type-1 is an autosomal dominant disease with an incidence of 1 in 2500–3000 (Huson *et al.*, 1989; Lammert *et al.*, 2005). Most of these patients develop

multiple neurofibromas (NF) all over their body, but mainly PNF may undergo malignant sarcomatous transformation into an MPNST (Ferner and Gutmann, 2002). Plexiform neurofibromas are comprised of the same cell types as dermal neurofibromas. They may grow along the length of a nerve, involving multiple fascicles and branches and extend into surrounding structures. Plexiform neurofibromas may already be present at birth or may become apparent later in life. Their incidence in patients with NF1 is suggested to range from 15 to 30% according to population-based studies (Huson *et al.*, 1988; McGaughran *et al.*, 1999), but internal PNF are frequently undetected without radiological investigation. In contrast to NF, PNF often result in morbidity due to their continued growth. PNF in NF1 is accompanied by a 10% risk for transformation into MPNST (McGaughran *et al.*, 1999; Rasmussen *et al.*, 2001). Clinical indicators of malignancy are persistent or increasing pain, swelling and increase in size, and neurological deficits (Stark *et al.*, 2001). In NF1 patients with MPNST, overall survival rates are low due to high local recurrence rates and early onset of metastases to lungs, pleura, liver, brain, soft tissue, bone, regional lymph nodes, skin, and retroperitoneum (Ducatman *et al.*,

1986; Stark *et al.*, 2001). Time to death is often less than 2 years (Mautner *et al.*, 2003), and overall 5-year survival rates range from 34 to 52% (Woodruff, 1999). MPNSTs in NF1 patients are often large heterogeneous tumors that develop within benign plexiform neurofibromas. They are poorly differentiated and frequently necrotic but may contain varying amounts of benign tissue. Incomplete sampling at surgery or during histopathological work-up in these tumors can result in either an over- or underestimation of the higher risk cell population and, thus, of tumor grade (Fletcher, 1994). These sampling errors may be one reason for the wide range of relapse rates in each histological grade category. But even in the careful pathological work-up, histopathology and tumor grading are not strictly correlated with prognosis in MPNST patients (Ducatman *et al.*, 1986).

Sporadic MPNST is an even rarer tumor entity arising in patients of all age groups with an incidence of 1 in 100,000 in the general population (Ducatman *et al.*, 1986). In contrast to the more common NF1-associated MPNST, no risk factors or premalignant tumor lesions are known for this tumor subtype. Presently, it is not clear whether patients with sporadic MPNST and patients with NF1-associated MPNST have a different clinical course or response to treatment (Ferner and Gutmann, 2002), although it seems more and more that sporadic MPNSTs have a more favorable outcome and a lower risk of developing metastases (Hagel *et al.*, 2007; Loree *et al.*, 2000; Pollack and Mulvihill, 1997; Stark *et al.*, 2001).

Standard Diagnostic Procedures

Since MPNST is a rare disease and patients present to specialists from widely differing disciplines, no guidelines or consistent patterns of patient management exist. The first international consensus statement on this tumor entity was published as late as 2002 (Ferner and Gutmann, 2002). Most patients initially suffer from pain, or neurologic deficits or observe a tumor increasing in size. These symptoms, depending on their localization, usually prompt imaging such as X-ray, ultrasound, computer tomography (CT), or magnetic resonance imaging (MRI) to start the diagnostic work-up. For subsequent tumor staging, X-ray and/or CT of the lungs and ultrasound and/or CT of the liver and the abdomen are usually recommended with respect to frequent metastasis in liver and lungs (Ferner and Gutmann, 2002; Stark *et al.*, 2001). Positron emission tomography (PET) with [^{18}F]fluorodeoxyglucose (FDG), nowadays often performed in combination with CT on a combined PET/CT scanner, is another promising diagnostic tool that allows performing whole-body imaging in one single session (Ferner and Gutmann, 2002). The final preoperative diagnosis of MPNST is usually achieved by histopathology and immunohistochemistry based on fine needle aspiration or biopsy.

After surgery, baseline MRI of the tumor region is recommended after 2–3 months (Ferner and Gutmann, 2002). Additional imaging studies and their timing during follow-up depend on the nature and location of the initial tumor, known metastases, and clinical symptoms of the patient. Whole-body procedures such as whole-body MRI or PET and PET/CT are gaining interest because they provide information on both the local and the whole-body status of a patient in one session. This is of particular interest in the long-time follow-up in patients with NF1-associated MPNST to monitor all their lesions (Friedrich *et al.*, 2005; Kehrer-Sawatzki *et al.*, 2005).

Treatment and Outcome

The most important therapeutic intervention in MPNST is complete removal of the tumor with wide margins. Lesions should be widely resected with the margins well into normal tissue as far as possible (≥ 10 cm) (Ferner and Gutmann, 2002). Amputation may be indicated for extensive or recurrent tumors of the limbs. The paramount effect of complete resection of MPNST with negative margins is emphasized by the fact that wide and complete tumor resection as well as location of the tumor, which defines the extent of surgery, and, thus, complete resection, are significant and independent predictors for outcome (Ferner and Gutmann, 2002; Mundt *et al.*, 1995; Stark *et al.*, 2001; Wong *et al.*, 1998).

Based on the Consensus Statement, radiotherapy may help to provide local control and delay the onset of local recurrence but so far has little effect on long-term survival, which is determined by metastases. Adjuvant radiotherapy therefore is recommended only in case of intermediate and high-grade tumors as well as in low-grade tumors with marginal or incomplete resection in order to achieve local control (Ferner and Gutmann, 2002; Wong *et al.*, 1998).

Chemotherapy is usually restricted to patients with metastatic disease. Only very few drugs or drug combinations have shown to be effective at all, resulting in treatment regimens that apply doxorubicin or doxorubicin in combination with ifosfamide (Santoro *et al.*, 1995). Although it is not clear whether chemotherapy is of survival benefit for the patient, it is clearly not a curative treatment strategy (Ferner *et al.*, 2002; Sarcoma Meta-Analysis Collaboration, 1997). However, it may achieve palliation in many patients, and complete or long-lasting remissions are observed in rare cases. Chemotherapy might also be useful in the preoperative setting to downstage patients with initially unresectable tumors (Ferner and Gutmann, 2002).

Recently, the detection of mutations in the c-kit oncogene of patients with MPNST has led to potentially new forms of treatment based on receptor tyrosine kinase inhibitors such as imatinib (Glivec®). First clinical trials investigating the therapeutic benefit of receptor tyrosine kinase inhibitors in

MPNST are already underway. Despite all the above-mentioned treatment options, outcome in MPNST patients is still poor, with 5-year survival rates of 34 to 50% (Stark *et al.*, 2001; Woodruff 1999). Partial response rates to chemotherapy are even lower in the range of 25–30% (Santoro *et al.*, 1995), and the magnitude of any survival benefit of adjuvant chemotherapy was very small (approximately 4%) and thus not statistically significant (Sarcoma Meta-Analysis Collaboration, 1997).

Positron Emission Tomography Imaging in Malignant Peripheral Nerve Sheath Tumor

Because long-time survival and outcome are based on successful and complete tumor excision, early diagnosis of MPNST is of utmost importance in order to detect the primary or recurrent tumor in early stages when it is still small and resectable. Reliable diagnosis is particularly important in patients with NF1 and multiple tumorous lesions to differentiate MPNST from PNF. Both can present with similar clinical symptoms such as pain, neurologic deficits, and increase in size. Therefore, apart from conventional, well-standardized anatomic imaging procedures such as MRI and CT which use tumor size and increase in size as predominant parameters, metabolic PET imaging has become the focus of ongoing research (Brenner *et al.*, 2006b; Cardona *et al.*, 2003; Ferner *et al.*, 2000; Ferner *et al.*, 2005). The most widely used PET tracer for neurogenic tumors is [^{18}F]fluorodeoxyglucose (FDG). Other clinical PET tracers with reported utility for imaging of neurogenic tumors in patients are [^{18}F]fluorine α-methyl tyrosine (FMT) (Ahmed *et al.*, 2001) and [^{11}C]L-methyl methionine (Nyberg *et al.*, 1997). However, presently none of these tracers has been used in MPNST besides FDG.

[^{18}F]Fluorodeoxyglucose (FDG)

[^{18}F]Fluorodeoxyglucose is the most widely used PET tracer in oncology and the most commonly used tracer for sarcoma imaging. FDG-PET studies produce images that represent the rate of glycolysis in tissues: the glucose analog 2-[^{18}F]fluoro-2-deoxy-D-glucose undergoes membrane transport and phosphorylation by hexokinase to FDG-6-phosphate similar to the pathway of glucose metabolism to glucose-6-phosphate. However, while glucose-6-phophate is metabolized in the normal glycolysis pathway, FDG-6-phosphate is not a substrate for further metabolism. Because FDG is not able to diffuse back across the cell membrane after phosphorylation, nor can phosphorylation be reversed to a significant extent in most tissues, FDG is trapped in the cell in proportion to the rate of glycolysis. This metabolic pathway enables FDG to be used for quantitative metabolic imaging. Common quantitative procedures for FDG imaging in tumor are standardized uptake value (SUV), Patlak graphical analysis, and nonlinear regression analysis based on a three-compartment model for FDG. Tumor SUV is a semiquantitative parameter that represents the metabolic activity in a static image as measured by region of interest (ROI) technique and corrected for both the injected activity per kg body weight and the blood glucose level.

Two different types of SUV are known, which represent different biological information. Average tumor SUV (SUV_{mean}) is the mean of all pixel-related SUV values within an ROI as a statistical measure of tumor metabolism in general. In heterogeneous tumors such as sarcomas, however, maximum SUV (SUV_{max}), that is, the highest single SUV value within an ROI, is thought to be more reliable to describe biological features because the highest uptake areas determine tumor activity and thus tumor aggressiveness. Consequently, SUV_{max} has been shown to be a useful parameter for risk assessment in sarcomas. Eary *et al.* (2002) found that pretherapy tumor SUV obtained by FDG-PET in 209 patients with different types of sarcoma was an independent and significant predictor of survival and disease progression and had the same prognostic power as tumor histologic grade as shown by multivariate analysis. Patlak analysis and the more sophisticated nonlinear regression analysis allow true quantitative calculation of kinetic parameters, but require dynamic PET imaging for 60–90 min in combination with arterial rather than venous blood sampling. These complex techniques are often limited to research while SUV is commonly used for clinical studies and routine use in daily practice.

[^{18}F]Fluorodeoxyglucose Positron Emission Tomography Imaging

Because MPNSTs are rare tumors, many publications on FDG-PET imaging in patients with MPNST are case reports (Basu and Nair, 2006; Chander *et al.*, 2004; Otsuka *et al.*, 2005; Ruiz-Hernandez *et al.*, 2003; Santaella *et al.*, 2005; Solomon *et al.*, 2001). Only few studies deal with PET imaging in large patient subsets, and FDG has been used as a tracer in all of these studies (Brenner *et al.*, 2006b; Cardona *et al.*, 2003; Ferner *et al.*, 2000; Ferner *et al.*, 2005; Wegner *et al.*, 2005).

In all case reports MPNST was described as a tumor with high to intense FDG uptake that could be easily recognized on PET images. Local recurrences of MPNST could also be detected (Ruiz-Hernandez *et al.*, 2003; Santaella *et al.*, 2005), and FDG-PET was especially helpful in a patient after combined surgery and radiation therapy when MRI was inconclusive in differentiating between postirradiation fibrosis and recurrent tumor (Santaella *et al.*, 2005). In a patient with NF1, PET/CT imaging identified an area of clearly increased FDG uptake (SUV_{max}: 6.6) within a huge tumor lesion in the left gluteal area. As confirmed by histopathology, the area with intense FDG uptake showed signs of sarcomatous transformation within the tumor lesion and corresponded to a high-grade MPNST (Otsuka *et al.*, 2005). The ability of FDG-PET imaging to detect sarcomatous transformation in NF1 patients is addressed in two other case reports thus emphasizing the importance of an imaging modality that can differentiate NF and PNF from MPNST in NF1 patients. In these patients with a multitude of concurrent lesions all over their bodies and the intrinsic risk to develop MPNST, it would be a milestone for the follow-up to reliably detect MPNST at an early stage.

Biopsy of all growing or painful lesions is rather cumbersome for the patient, and sampling errors are common because MPNST often arises in preexisting PNF. Solomon *et al.* (2001) could nicely demonstrate that in an NF1 patient with multiple neurofibromas increased FDG uptake was observed in the periphery of a large hemipelvic mass, while the center of the lesion was devoid of radioactivity consistent with necrosis as confirmed by histopathology. The areas of increased FDG uptake correlated with focal areas of high-grade MPNST arising within a neurofibroma. The postoperative PET study revealed no residual MPNST despite a residual mass demonstrated on CT. In this patient, metabolic PET imaging was the most sensitive technique for detecting malignant tumor tissue as compared to CT and MRI.

Similar findings have been reported by Basu and Nair (2006), who concluded "that FDG-PET is the most sensitive noninvasive probe to diagnose malignant transformation in NF1 and hence likely to appear as the screening procedure of choice in their follow up to rule out malignant transformation." They reported on an NF1 patient with recurrent MPNST and numerous tumors as shown by MRI, while on PET images only three lesions revealed increased FDG uptake. All these lesions could be proven as either recurrent MPNST or metastases by histopathology. The authors emphasized that only malignant lesions showed FDG uptake, while numerous benign NF and PNF did not show enhanced FDG uptake in this patient. FDG-PET was also helpful in detecting metastatic spread of retroperitoneal MPNST in an NF1 patient as shown by Chander *et al.* (2004). Even more interesting in this case report was the fact that serial FDG-PET could be used for monitoring the effects of chemotherapy with doxorubicin and ifosfamide. Eight weeks after starting chemotherapy, the metastatic lesion with a pretherapeutic SUV of 4.0 showed no FDG uptake anymore, indicating favorable response to chemotherapy. Positron emission tomography results were confirmed by the clinical course, which revealed a relapse of the lesion only after 5 months after chemotherapy (Chander *et al.*, 2004).

Differentiation between benign and malignant lesions is the most important task in patients with NF1 because MPNST is the main reason for death in these patients. Detection of lesions and confirmation of growth can be easily achieved by morphological imaging techniques such as ultrasound, CT, or MRI. However, these methods are unreliable in char-

acterizing the nature of lesions as benign or malignant. Characteristic signs of MPNST such as large tumors increasing in size, heterogeneous signal patterns within the lesions, and invasion of adjacent structures can be observed in benign infiltrating plexiform neurofibromas as well. Attempts to overcome this diagnostic dilemma include the use of metabolic imaging, encouraged by case reports on the usefulness of FDG-PET in detecting MPNST by means of increased FDG uptake. Ferner *et al.* (2000) published the first full paper on FDG-PET imaging in 18 patients with NF1, seven of these with MPNST. In contrast to the one patient presented by Basu and Nair (2006), Ferner *et al.* (2000) observed FDG uptake not only in malignant lesions, that is, in MPNST, but also in benign neurofibroma.

Although MPNST had significantly higher SUV values than benign tumors, there was an overlap between the SUV of both subgroups. In MPNST, SUV ranged from 2.7 to 8.4 with a mean of 5.4 compared to values ranging from 0.6 to 3.3 with a mean of 1.5 in benign NF or PNF. Using a cut-off of 2.5 for SUV measured at a mean time of 111 min (range: 45–206 min) after FDG injection, no malignant tumor was classified as benign, but two benign lesions were rated as malignant (false positive). FDG-PET imaging therefore was a useful method of identifying malignant transformation in plexiform neurofibromas (Ferner *et al.*, 2000). Based on these findings, Ferner *et al.* (2005) started to systematically investigate the potential of FDG-PET as a diagnostic tool for MPNST in patients with NF1. FDG-PET was performed in 105 NF1 patients with PNF and one or more associated clinical symptoms such as persistent pain, change in texture, rapid growth, and impaired neurological function. In this patient population, 80 benign PNF and 35 MPNST were detected. FDG-PET was false positive in 4 patients and false negative in 3 patients with low-grade MPNST, resulting in a sensitivity in detecting NF1-associated MPNST of 0.83–0.90 and a specificity of 0.95–0.97. In this large study, the authors could confirm their previous promising results showing that FDG-PET is a highly sensitive and specific tool for differentiating benign PNF from MPNST.

In another study on the value of FDG-PET imaging in neurogenic tumors to detect MPNST, Cardona *et al.* (2003) analyzed PET images in 13 patients with a total of 25 tumors. Five patients had NF1, and in 8 patients the lesions were described as sporadic. Twelve lesions were classified as benign and 13 lesions as MPNST (6 primary tumors and 7 recurrent MPNSTs). Malignant peripheral nerve sheath tumor showed a 2.6-fold higher FDG uptake (range: 1.8–12.3; median: 2.9) than benign tumors (range: 0.5–1.8; median: 1.1; $p < 0.001$). Using a cut-off value of 1.8 for SUV measured after a fixed 5-min interval 55–60 min after FDG injection, FDG-PET showed a sensitivity of 100% and a specificity of 83% in distinguishing between benign neurogenic tumors and MPNST (Cardona *et al.*, 2003). In contrast to the study by Ferner *et al.* (2000), who measured tumor

SUV after varying time intervals, Cardona *et al.* (2003) used a standardized time for SUV measurement. This is a very important methodological point because in almost all tumors FDG uptake increases over time. Beaulieu *et al.* (2003), in their publication on time dependency of SUV, showed that breast cancer tumors can have a 20–25% increase in SUV in only 15 min. In future studies on tumor SUV in MPNST, therefore, standardized conditions should be considered as *conditio sine qua non* to facilitate comparison between patients and, even more important, within single patients during follow-up scans.

Another interesting point in the work by Cardona *et al.* (2003) is the fact that they investigated not only patients with NF1-associated MPNST but also patients with sporadic MPNST. According to the presented data, 6 NF1-associated MPNSTs showed SUV ranging from 1.8 to 12.3 with a median of 3.3 (mean: 4.8). Four sporadic MPNSTs had similar values ranging from 2.1 to 4.4, with a median of 2.7 (mean: 3.0). With their publication, these workers confirmed the findings of Ferner *et al.* (2000), demonstrating that FDG-PET can help to discriminate benign neurogenic tumors from MPNST. The lower cut-off of tumor SUV (1.8 versus 2.5) used by Cardona *et al.* (2003) is probably only due to an earlier time point of imaging after tracer injection (60 min versus median 111 min) (Ferner *et al.*, 2000).

In an interesting study on the general impact of PET scanning on the management of 165 pediatric oncology patients, Wegner *et al.* (2005, p. 29) reported the results of 16 scans in 13 patients with plexiform neurofibroma and suspicion of malignant transformation. Positron emission tomography changed the management in 9/16 (56%) cases. In 8 cases, the change was from biopsy/surgery to no treatment, while in one case extensive surgery and radiotherapy were performed instead of the planned biopsy. Positron emission tomography findings were confirmed either by histology or by long-time follow-up. Positron emission tomography was proven false positive in one patient, where a lesion reported as malignant was demonstrated to be benign on histology. In their discussion the authors therefore state: "PET had the greatest impact on patients with plexiform neurofibroma, altering management in 56% of cases. This is understandable, as the symptoms of MPNST, such as pain, neurological symptoms and increase in size of the lesion, are non-specific and can overlap with the features of a symptomatic benign neurofibroma. Before PET was available, biopsy or surgical excision was required to demonstrate malignancy. In this study, in seven cases PET saved the child from having an unnecessary invasive procedure. In other cases, PET was helpful by confirming the suspicion of malignant transformation and guiding the biopsy to the most metabolically active area or by changing the surgical approach."

A different aspect of metabolic tumor imaging has been presented by our group reporting on the prognostic relevance of pretherapy FDG tumor uptake in NF1-associated MPNST

(Brenner *et al.*, 2006b). Current thinking in tumor biology is that SUV in a tumor reflects the metabolic activity of the tumor; the inherent assumption in this concept is that tumor grade and the overall behavior of the tumor are predicted by this metabolic activity. In accordance with this hypothesis, SUV has been shown to be a suitable parameter for risk assessment in terms of nonhistopathological tumor grading and prediction of outcome in patients with different types of sarcoma (Brenner *et al.*, 2004, 2006a; Eary *et al.*, 2002). This idea has been transferred to patients with NF1 and MPNST. Survival rates in most patients are low, and time to death is often less than 2 years. However, there are patients with a more favorable prognosis who develop metastases rather late or not at all.

Because histopathology and tumor grading are not well correlated with prognosis in NF1-associated MPNST, we aimed to evaluate the potential of FDG-PET for prediction of outcome in 16 NF1 patients with MPNST of tumor grades II and III according to the French Federation of Cancer Centers Sarcoma Group system (Brenner *et al.*, 2006b; Coindre *et al.*, 2001). Tumor SUV did not show a significant difference between grade II (4.7 ± 3.1; range: $2.1 - 11.0$; $n = 7$) and grade III tumors (6.4 ± 2.6; $3.2 - 11.6$; $n = 9$; $p = 0.270$). Significant differences in SUV, however, were found between patients who were still alive after 36 months (SUV: 2.5 ± 0.4; $2.1 - 2.8$, $n = 3$) and patients who died (6.3 ± 2.7; $3.2 - 11.6$; $n = 12$, $p < 0.001$). Three patients with tumor grade II had SUV < 3. None of these patients developed metastases or died during a follow-up of 41–62 months; 13 patients with both tumor grades II and III had SUV > 3. Only 1 of these patients was alive after 36 months, while 12 patients passed away within 4–33 months. Using a cut-off of 3, SUV predicted long-time survival with an accuracy of 94% compared to 69% for histopathological tumor grade.

In Kaplan-Meier survival analysis, patients with SUV > 3 had a significantly shorter mean survival time of 13 months compared to 52 months in patients with SUV < 3, while tumor grading did not reveal differences in survival time (15 versus 12 months). Thus, tumor SUV allowed identification of low-risk MPNST patients with favorable outcome independently of histopathological findings. Therefore, we concluded that tumor SUV obtained by FDG-PET was a significant parameter for prediction of survival in NF1 patients with MPNST, while histopathological tumor grading did not predict outcome (Brenner *et al.*, 2006b). Consequently, FDG-PET as a new risk stratification tool might be useful for the management of NF1 patients with MPNST. Oncologic follow-up investigations are usually performed at 3-month intervals, including MRI of the whole body and MRI of the original tumor site in all tumor grades, because relapse rates are not strictly linked to grade. Standardized uptake value, however, might help to individualize follow-up regimens in MPNST. Because we did not observe metastatic disease in patients with tumor SUV < 3, in this low-risk population follow-up might be limited to tight check-ups for local recurrences while check-ups for distant metastases to lungs or other organs might be performed at longer time intervals (Brenner *et al.*, 2006b).

In a recent study, sporadic MPNST was shown to have a more favorable outcome than NF1-associated MPNST accompanied by differences in histopathological parameters (Hagel *et al.*, 2007). These findings indicate the necessity for a separate grading scheme that takes into account the genetic background in NF1 patients and the differences in histopathology, and, thus, the tumor biology of these two tumor entities. Because tumor SUV in FDG-PET is considered to reflect biological tumor aggressiveness, we started to test if sporadic MPNSTs show lower SUV values according to their suggested more favorable outcome than NF1-associated MPNST. The aim of our so far unpublished study was to compare pretherapy tumor SUV in patients with sporadic and NF1-associated MPNST and to check whether cut-off values used in NF1-associated MPNST can also be applied in sporadic MPNST. Tumor SUV ranged from 2.1 to 11.6 in 16 NF1-associated MPNSTs with a mean of 5.7 ± 2.9. In 3 sporadic MPNSTs, SUV values were 1.0, 1.8, and 3.2, and, thus, significantly lower than those in NF1-associated MPNST ($p < 0.005$). Despite the low SUV, two out of three patients with sporadic MPNST (SUV 1.0 and 3.2) died within two years after diagnosis (unpublished data). Based on these preliminary results, sporadic MPNST seems to have significantly lower tumor SUV in FDG-PET than NF1-associated MPNST, which may reflect differences in biological behavior as suggested by outcome data in patients with sporadic MPNST. If our observation is confirmed in a larger number of patients with sporadic MPNST, lower cut-off values in SUV will be necessary for definition of malignancy and prediction of outcome in these patients than currently used in NF1-associated cases.

In conclusion, the available literature on PET imaging in MPNST is small and focuses primarily on differentiation of MPNST from NF and PNF in NF1 patients. Although FDG-PET has been shown to be a very useful tool for making this differentiation, it has to be kept in mind that distinguishing MPNST from other sarcoma and even other benign tumors such as schwannoma is not feasible by PET imaging. For benign schwannoma, high FDG uptake with SUV up to 3.7 (Ahmed *et al.*, 2001) and 6.6 (Beaulieu *et al.*, 2004) has been reported showing a wide overlap with tumor SUV observed in MPNST. Differential diagnosis between MPNST and schwannoma, therefore, is not possible according to the available literature.

Summary

Although development of MPNST is a life-threatening complication in up to 10% of patients with NF1, MPNST in general is a very rare malignant tumor. This fact is the very reason for the lack of large prospective clinical studies, and there are even fewer reports on PET imaging in patients

with MPNST. It is therefore not yet possible to draw definite conclusions resulting in approved indications for PET imaging in MPNST because the number of studies and the number of enrolled patients are too small. Furthermore, the methods used for the different studies (e.g., time of PET scan after tracer injection and method of quantification) differ per study. Nevertheless, based on the available literature, in some clinical settings FDG-PET has been shown very helpful for patient management in MPNST:

- Detecting sarcomatous transformation in NF1 patients and differentiation of NF and PNF from MPNST by means of increased tumor SUV, especially in patients with clinical symptoms such as tumor growth, pain, or neurological deficits
- Predicting outcome in NF1-associated MPNST and defining patients at low risk for metastatic disease

Yet further indications are suggested by various case reports:

- Guiding biopsy in suspected MPNST withing preexisting PNF
- Whole-body imaging for detecting hematogenous spread during primary staging and follow-up
- Differentiating postoperative changes and postirradiation fibrosis from residual tumor tissue or local relapse
- Monitoring response to chemotherapy

Further research needs to be done in prospective studies in larger patient series to define the various indications that have been suggested as useful for management of patients with MPNST. Multicenter trials using well-defined diagnostic and therapeutic settings therefore seem the appropriate tool to increase the data on FDG-PET imaging in both sporadic and NF1-associated MPNST.

References

Ahmed, A.R., Watanabe, H., Aoki, J., Shinozaki, T., and Takagishi, K. 2001. Schwannoma of the extremities: the role of PET in preoperative planning. *Eur. J. Nucl. Med. 28*:1541–1551.

Basu, S., and Nair, N. 2006. Potential clinical role of FDG-PET in detecting sarcomatous transformation in von Recklinghausen's disease: a case study and review of the literature. *J. Neurooncol. 80*:91–95.

Beaulieu, S., Kinahan, P., Tseng, J., Dunnwald, L.K., Schubert, E.K., Pham, P., Lewellen, B., and Mankoff, D.A. 2003. SUV varies with time after injection in (18)F-FDG PET of breast cancer: characterization and method to adjust for time differences. *J. Nucl. Med. 44*:1044–1050.

Beaulieu, S., Rubin, B., Djang, D., Conrad, E., Turcotte, E., and Eary, J.F. 2004. Positron emission tomography of schwannomas: emphasizing its potential in preoperative planning. *Am. J. Roentgenol. 182*:971–974.

Brenner, W., Conrad, E.U., and Eary, J.F. 2004. FDG PET imaging for grading and prediction of outcome in chondrosarcoma patients. *Eur. J. Nucl. Med. Mol. Imaging 31*:189–195.

Brenner, W., Eary, J.F., Hwang, W., Vernon, C., and Conrad, E.U. 2006a. Risk assessment in liposarcoma patients based on FDG PET imaging. *Eur. J. Nucl. Med. Mol. Imaging 33*:1290–1295.

Brenner, W., Friedrich, R.E., Gawad, K.A., Hagel, C., von Deimling, A., de Wit, M., Buchert, R., Clausen, M., and Mautner, V.F. 2006b. Prognostic relevance of FDG PET in patients with neurofibromatosis type-1 and malignant peripheral nerve sheath tumours. *Eur. J. Nucl. Med. Mol. Imaging 33*:428–432.

Cardona, S., Schwarzbach, M., Hinz, U., Dimitrakopoulou-Strauss, A., Attigah, N., Mechtersheimer, G., and Lehnert, T. 2003. Evaluation of F18-deoxyglucose positron emission tomography (FDG-PET) to assess the nature of neurogenic tumours. *Eur. J. Surg. Oncol. 29*:536–541.

Chander, S., Westphal, S.M., Zak, I.T., Bloom, D.A., Zingas, A.P., Joyrich, R.N., Littrup, P.J., Taub, J.W., and Getzen, T.M. 2004. Retroperitoneal malignant peripheral nerve sheath tumor: evaluation with serial FDG-PET. *Clin. Nucl. Med. 29*:415–418.

Coindre, J.M., Terrier, P., Guillou, L., Le Doussal, V., Collin, F., Ranchere, D., Sastre, X., Vilain, M.O., Bonichon, F., and N'Guyen Bui, B. 2001. Predictive value of grade for metastasis development in the main histologic types of adult soft tissue sarcomas: a study of 1240 patients from the French Federation of Cancer Centers Sarcoma Group. *Cancer 91*:1914–1926.

Ducatman, B.S., Scheithauer, B.W., Piepgras, D.G., Reiman, H.M., and Ilstrup, D.M. 1986. Malignant peripheral nerve sheath tumors. A clinicopathologic study of 120 cases. *Cancer 57*:2006–2021.

Eary J.F., O'Sullivan, F., Powitan, Y., Chandhury, K.R., Vernon, C., Bruckner, J.D., and Conrad, E.U. 2002. Sarcoma tumor FDG uptake measured by PET and patient outcome: a retrospective analysis. *Eur. J. Nucl. Med. 29*:1149–1154.

Ferner, R.E., Lucas, J.D., O'Doherty, M.J., Hughes, R.A., Smith, M.A., Cronin, B. F., and Bingham, J. 2000. Evaluation of (18)fluorodeoxyglucose positron emission tomography ((18)FDG PET) in the detection of malignant peripheral nerve sheath tumours arising from within plexiform neurofibromas in neurofibromatosis 1. *J. Neurol. Neurosurg. Psychiatry 68*:353–357.

Ferner, R.E., and Gutmann, D.H. 2002. International consensus statement on malignant peripheral nerve sheath tumors in neurofibromatosis. *Cancer Res. 62*:1573–1577.

Ferner, R.E., O'Doherty, M., Golding, J.F., Chaundhry, I., Calonje, E., Robson, A., and Smith, M.A. 2005. Evaluation of 18-fluorodeoxyglucose positron emission tomography as a diagnostic tool for malignant peripheral nerve sheath tumors (MPNST) in neurofibromatosis 1 (NF1). *Anticancer Research 25*:4845–4846 (abstract).

Fletcher, C.D. 1994. [The histological features of local recurrences of soft tissue sarcomas]. *Pathologe 15*:196–200.

Friedrich, R.E., Kluwe, L., Funsterer, C., and Mautner, V.F. 2005. Malignant peripheral nerve sheath tumors (MPNST) in neurofibromatosis type 1 (NF1): diagnostic findings on magnetic resonance images and mutation analysis of the NF1 gene. *Anticancer Res. 25*:1699–1702.

Hagel, C., Zils, U., Peiper, M., Kluwe, L., Gotthard, S., Friedrich, R.E., Zurakowski, D., von Deimling, A., and Mautner, V.F. 2007. Histopathology and clinical outcome of NF1-associated vs. sporadic malignant peripheral nerve sheath tumors. *J. Neurooncol. 82*:187–192

Huson, S.M., Harper, P.S., and Compston, D.A. 1988. Von Recklinghausen neurofibromatosis: a clinical and population study in south-east Wales. *Brain 111*:1355–1381.

Huson, S.M., Compston, D.A., Clark, P., and Harper, P.S. 1989. A genetic study of von Recklinghausen neurofibromatosis in south east Wales. I. Prevalence, fitness, mutation rate, and effect of parental transmission on severity. *J. Med. Genet. 26*:704–711.

Kehrer-Sawatzki, H., Kluwe, L., Funsterer, C., and Mautner, V.F. 2005. Extensively high load of internal tumors determined by whole body MRI scanning in a patient with neurofibromatosis type 1 and a non-LCR-mediated 2-Mb deletion in 17q11.2. *Hum. Genet. 116*:466–475.

Lammert, M., Friedman, J.M., Kluwe, L., and Mautner, V.F. 2005. Prevalence of neurofibromatosis 1 in German children at elementary school enrollment. *Arch. Dermatol. 141*:71–74.

Loree, T.R., North, J.H., Jr., Werness, B.A., Nangia, R., Mullins, A.P., and Hicks, W.L., Jr. 2000. Malignant peripheral nerve sheath tumors of the head and neck: analysis of prognostic factors. *Otolaryngol. Head Neck Surg. 122*:667–672.

Mautner, V.F., Friedrich, R.E., von Deimling, A., Hagel, C., Korf, B., Knofel, M.T., Wenzel, R., and Funsterer, C. 2003. Malignant peripheral nerve sheath tumours in neurofibromatosis type 1: MRI supports the diagnosis of malignant plexiform neurofibroma. *Neuroradiology 45*:618–625.

McGaughran, J.M., Harris, D.I., Donnai, D., Teare, D., MacLeod, R., Westerbeek, R., Kingston, H., Super, M., Harris, R., and Evans, D.G. 1999. A clinical study of type 1 neurofibromatosis in north west England. *J. Med. Genet. 36*:197–203.

Mundt, A.J., Awan, A., Sibley, G.S., Simon, M., Rubin, S.J., Samuels, B., Wong, W., Beckett, M., Vijayakumar, S., and Weichselbaum, R.R. 1995. Conservative surgery and adjuvant radiation therapy in the management of adult soft tissue sarcoma of the extremities: clinical and radiobiological results. *Int. J. Radiat. Oncol. Biol. Phys. 32*:977–985.

Nyberg, G., Bergstrom, M., Enblad, P., Lilja, A., Muhr, C., and Langstrom, B. 1997. PET-methionine of skull base neuromas and meningiomas. *Acta Otolaryngol. 117*:482–489.

Otsuka, H., Graham, M.M., Kubo, A., and Nishitani, H. 2005. FDG-PET/CT findings of sarcomatous transformation in neurofibromatosis: a case report. *Ann. Nucl. Med. 19*:55–58.

Pollack, I.F., and Mulvihill, J.J. 1997. Neurofibromatosis 1 and 2. *Brain Pathol. 7*:823–836.

Rasmussen, S.A., Yang, Q., and Friedman, J.M. 2001. Mortality in neurofibromatosis 1: an analysis using U.S. death certificates. *Am. J. Hum. Genet. 68*:1110–1118.

Ruiz-Hernandez, G., Hornedo-Muguiro, J., Salinas-Hernandez, P., Perez-Castejon, M.J., Lapena-Guticrrez, L., Montz-Andree, R., and Carreras-Delgado, J.L. 2003. [Positron emission tomography in a patient with Von Recklinghausen disease and left dorsal neurofibrosarcoma]. *Rev. Esp. Med. Nucl. 22*:418–423.

Santaella, Y., Borrego, I., Lopez, J., Ortiz, M.J., and Vazquez, R. 2005. [18-FDG-PET in a case of recurrent malignant schwannoma]. *Rev. Esp. Med. Nucl. 24*:127–130.

Santoro, A., Tursz, T., Mouridsen, H., Verweij, J., Steward, W., Somers, R., Buesa, J., Casali, P., Spooner, D., and Rankin, E. 1995. Doxorubicin versus CYVADIC versus doxorubicin plus ifosfamide in first-line treatment of advanced soft tissue sarcomas: a randomized study of the European Organization for Research and Treatment of Cancer Soft Tissue and Bone Sarcoma Group. *J. Clin. Oncol. 13*:1537–1545.

Sarcoma Meta-Analysis Collaboration. 1997. Adjuvant chemotherapy for localised resectable soft-tissue sarcoma of adults: meta-analysis of individual data. Sarcoma Meta-analysis Collaboration. *Lancet 350*:1647–1654.

Solomon, S.B., Semih Dogan, A., Nicol, T.L., Campbell, J.N., and Pomper, M.G. 2001. Positron emission tomography in the detection and management of sarcomatous transformation in neurofibromatosis. *Clin. Nucl. Med. 26*:525–528.

Stark, A.M., Buhl, R., Hugo, H.H., and Mehdorn, H.M. 2001. Malignant peripheral nerve sheath tumours—report of 8 cases and review of the literature. *Acta Neurochir. (Wien) 143*:357–363; discussion 363–354.

Wegner, E.A., Barrington, S.F., Kingston, J.E., Robinson, R.O., Ferner, R.E., Taj, M., Smith, M.A., and O'Doherty, M.J. 2005. The impact of PET scanning on management of paediatric oncology patients. *Eur. J. Nucl. Med. Mol. Imaging 32*:23–30.

Wong, W.W., Hirose, T., Scheithauer, B.W., Schild, S.E., and Gunderson, L.L. 1998. Malignant peripheral nerve sheath tumor: analysis of treatment outcome. *Int. J. Radiat. Oncol. Biol. Phys. 42*:351–360.

Woodruff, J.M. 1999. Pathology of tumors of the peripheral nerve sheath in type 1 neurofibromatosis. *Am. J. Med. Genet. 89*:23–30.

43

Prostate Cancer: ^{11}C-Choline-Positron Emission Tomography

Mohsen Farsad and Paolo Castellucci

Introduction

Prostate cancer is the most common cancer in elderly men and is the second most common cause of cancer death in men over age 50. The incidence of prostate cancer increases dramatically with each decade after 50, but disease rates appear to vary by population. The clinical incidence of prostate cancer varies ranging from 1 in 100,000 in China, 45–65 in 100,000 in the U.S. white subjects, 55–65 in 100,000 in European countries, to 102 in 100,000 in African Americans (Hsing and Devesa, 2001). Fortunately, prostate cancer tends to be slow-growing compared to many other cancers, and the majority of prostate cancers do not spread or cause harm for decades. Survival of the patient with prostate cancer is related to the extent of the tumor; many patients, especially those with localized tumors, may die of other illnesses without ever having suffered significant disability from their cancer; patients with locally advanced cancer are not usually curable, and a substantial fraction will eventually die of their tumor. However, some patients may have prolonged survival even after the cancer has metastasized to distant sites such as bone.

The approach to treatment is influenced by age and coexisting medical problems. Usually, if prostate cancer is detected early, treatment involves either surgical removal of the prostate or radiation therapy. For more advanced cases of prostate cancer, or if cancer spreads beyond the prostate, hormone medications are the preferred treatment. If the individual is older than 70 and has only a slow-growing tumor, the best treatment strategy may be "watchful waiting" (Aus et al., 2005).

Despite the recent advances in the early detection and diagnosis of prostate carcinoma, imaging has had a minor role in the care of prostate cancer, and many challenges remain. Strictly anatomic imaging is unlikely to yield much better results in the future. The diagnostic limitations of the anatomic imaging methods led clinicians to introduce new imaging techniques able to study more accurately prostate carcinoma. Of all available imaging modalities, metabolic diagnostic methods seems to be the most promising (Sedelaar et al., 2003).

Positron emission tomography (PET) imaging using different positron-emitting radiopharmaceuticals has emerged as a promising new metabolic diagnostic tool for evaluation of a variety of malignant diseases. Most of the success gained has been achieved with positron-emitter ^{18}F-FDG, since most malignant tumor cells have an increased glucose metabolism and increased glycolysis. Although the first published studies with widely available ^{18}F-FDG showed encouraging results for detection of prostate cancer recurrence in biochemical relapse, FDG-PET has proven to be disappointing in prostate cancer (Jana and Blaufox, 2006).

In recent years, new radiopharmaceuticals have been introduced for tumor identification in PET studies (Jana and Blaufox, 2006). The PET tracers used for clinical studies of prostate cancer are ^{11}C-acetate, ^{18}F-acetate, ^{11}C-methionine, ^{11}C-choline, ^{18}F-choline, and ^{18}F-FDHT (16-^{18}F-fluoro-5-dihydrotestosterone).

^{11}C-acetate and ^{11}C-choline seem to be the most promising and clinically useful positron-labeled tracers for the study of prostate cancer. The value of these two tracers appears nearly identical, and none of them can be favored (Kotzerke et al., 2003).

Principle and Methods

^{11}C-choline is a substrate for the synthesis of phosphatidylcholine, which is a major phospholipid in the cell membrane. ^{11}C-choline is first incorporated into cells by conversion into ^{11}C-phosphorylcholine, which is trapped inside the cell and then converted to phosphatidylcholine. It has been hypothesized that uptake of ^{11}C-choline reflects proliferative activity by estimating membrane lipid synthesis. However, a recent study found that radiolabeled choline uptake does not correlate with cell proliferation in prostate cancer (Breeuwsma et al., 2005). Thus, the exact uptake mechanism has to be established. ^{11}C-choline is cleared very rapidly from the blood, and optimal tumor-to-background contrast is reached within 5–7 minutes after administration of tracer. This allows for imaging as early as 3–5 min after tracer injection and provides images of good diagnostic quality. Physiologically increased tracer uptake is noted in salivary glands, liver, kidney parenchyma, and pancreas, and faint uptake in spleen, bone marrow, and muscles. Bowel activity is variable, and occasionally urinary bladder activity can be observed. The short half-life for ^{11}C (20 min) poses a logistic challenge in many institutions, and its use is limited to facilities with an on-site cyclotron.

Most of the knowledge has been gained through dedicated PET technology, but a number of developments, especially the introduction of hybrid tomographs, will impact the use of this metabolic imaging. Recently introduced dual-modality PET/CT tomography (Townsend and Beyer, 2002) allows the acquisition of anatomical (CT) and metabolic images (PET) simultaneously with the same imaging device and without moving the patient off and on the table in between examinations. Anatomical landmarks provided by CT greatly facilitate the assignment of biological abnormalities to anatomical structures and the interpretation of pathological findings, thereby improving the specificity of the test.

^{11}C-choline PET has been proposed for early intraprostatic tumor localization, for staging of prostate cancer, for identification of nodal involvement, and for detection of tumor recurrence.

^{11}C-Choline PET for Intraprostatic Tumor Localization

Early detection of prostate cancer may lead to an increase in curable disease, amenable to curative radical prostatectomy or curative radiation therapy. Serum prostate specific antigen (PSA) measurements and digital rectal exploration (DRE) are currently considered the best diagnostic methods for prostate cancer screening. However, there is an important lack of specificity of PSA, because prevalence of prostate cancer with PSA values lower than the traditional cut-off point of 4.0 ng/ml is higher than was initially thought and, furthermore, because there is an important overlap of benign conditions and prostate cancer in subjects with PSA values between 4.1 and 10 ng/ml. On the other hand, DRE is a specific test with low sensitivity for the diagnosis and staging of prostate cancer, with a poor correlation with localization and extension of cancer.

If screening tests suggest a possible presence of prostate cancer, a transrectal ultrasound (TRUS) can be performed. TRUS is the most commonly used imaging modality for viewing the prostate; the volume of the prostate can be estimated, and the test facilitates biopsy. Unfortunately, this diagnostic modality also presents low sensitivity and specificity for prostate cancer localization. First, only 20% of hypoechoic lesions are malignant, and second up to 30% of palpable lesions are isoechoic or show little hypoechogenicity in relation to the surrounding tissue.

Because of the limited detection rate that all the above-mentioned techniques offer, in cases of highly suspected prostate cancer, random systemic TRUS-guided biopsies are usually performed. However, despite efforts to refine the indication for prostate biopsies by means of using PSA-derived indexes such as PSA free ratio, PSA density, PSA velocity, and PSA age related, the negative biopsy rate remains unacceptably high (30–40%), especially for anterior located tumors.

The low accuracy of TRUS has led urologists to perform repeated biopsies for patients at risk of prostate cancer (persistently elevated serum PSA values or abnormal histological findings in the initial biopsy specimens) in order to decrease the proportion of prostate cancer missed by initial biopsy. Although various prostate biopsy schemes and biopsy needle trajectories have been proposed, the optimal biopsy strategy still remains to be defined. Some of the diagnostic limitations of TRUS were overcome with the development of new techniques such as color-encoded Doppler US, power Doppler US, and contrast-enhanced three-dimensional power Doppler US. However to date none of these newly introduced techniques is a fully reliable method for significantly improving the detection rate of TRUS-guided biopsy (Aus *et al.*, 2005).

On the other side, patients often refuse to undergo repeated biopsy, regardless of the prior number of biopsies. In this scenario, it is reasonable to look for other imaging techniques that can visualize a suspected area in a certain sextant of gland, which could increase the cancer detection rate by performing additional guided biopsy cores.

Magnetic resonance with endorectal coil shows good accuracy in local staging of prostate cancer and is more accurate than TRUS in tumor detection. However, it lacks specificity (benign conditions like prostatitis, post-biopsy bleeding, or scarring mimic cancer). Recent studies have demonstrated that spectroscopic evaluation of citrate and choline metabolism (MRSI) improves the specificity of this diagnostic method. Promising advances are expected in this field (Rajesh and Coakley, 2004). The development of prostate cancer is associated with changes in the metabolism of tumor cells, and therefore metabolic imaging such as PET imaging is of advantage.

The first published literature regarding the value of PET imaging in early prostate cancer localization demonstrated the feasibility of ¹¹C-choline PET for visualizing prostate cancer foci and showed, on average, a lower uptake of noncancerous prostate tissue compared to cancer tissue (de Jong *et al.*, 2002).

The last two studies published on this issue correlated PET/CT findings with whole prostate histopathological analysis on a sextant basis (Farsad *et al.*, 2005; Martorana *et al.*, 2006). These two studies confirmed that ¹¹C-choline PET is able to visualize prostate cancer foci and has demonstrated a good sensitivity for intraprostatic localization of primary cancer nodules greater than 5 mm. However, considering all cancer foci (regardless of size), these studies showed a low sensitivity of ¹¹C-choline PET for prostate cancer foci localization, and accuracy values appeared similar to TRUS biopsy. This is basically due to the limited spatial resolution of PET/CT scanners (5 mm) and to the effects of partial volume.

Any of these studies found a correlation between uptake of ¹¹C-choline and Gleason's score, PSA values, tumor grade, or prostate volume. Thus, we may assume that ¹¹C-choline PET cannot serve as an indicator of biologic aggressiveness.

At the same time, these studies underlined PET's inability to distinguish between primary prostate cancer and high-grade PIN or benign prostate hyperplasia (BPH) by demonstrating a significant overlap in uptake values of ¹¹C-choline between prostate cancer and BPH. Possible explanation of this phenomenon may be the heterogeneity and mixture of cell clones in tumors and other benign conditions.

Taking all preliminary results into account, ¹¹C-choline PET cannot be recommended for a routine use as a "first-line" screening procedure in men at high risk of prostate cancer.

¹¹C-Choline PET for Staging of Prostate Cancer

The major reason for a high failure rate after intended curative therapy of prostate cancer is undiagnosed disseminated disease (undetected extracapsular growth, seminal vesicle involvement, hematogenous, or lymphogenous metastases). Currently, tables based on clinical stage, serum PSA level, and the biopsy-determined Gleason grade are being used to predict the pathologic extent of prostate cancer. Men with high-grade (Gleason grade = 8–10) or advanced-stage prostate cancer are much less likely to be cured by radical prostatectomy or radiation therapy than are men with organ-confined and a low or moderate grade of prostate cancer. However, these facts merely provide statistical information, and uncertainties remain regarding optimal therapy for a particular patient. In this context, the accurate staging of prostate cancer is becoming increasingly important, as it can affect treatment planning and help to differentiate aggressive from indolent cancer. There is much interest in new imaging techniques designed to detect preoperatively the spread of disease from the gland. If men with clinically occult advanced disease could be identified before surgery using imaging, some of them could be spared the unnecessary risks and costs of prostatectomy, and in the future could be treated with other methods that are more suited to the advanced stage of their disease (Aus *et al.*, 2005).

Neither CT nor MRI, as currently practiced, seems to be accurate enough for preoperative staging, especially for assessment of nodal involvement (Sedelaar *et al.*, 2003). ¹¹C-choline PET, when used in pretreatment staging, may detect lymph node metastases with a higher sensitivity than the conventional modalities, thereby avoiding exploratory surgical procedures. De Jong and colleagues evaluated the strength and accuracy of ¹¹C-choline PET in the preoperative staging of lymph nodes in prostate cancer. In 67 patients, lymph node metastases were detected with a sensitivity of 80%, a specificity of 96%, and an accuracy of 93% for staging metastatic lymph node disease. Of note, a significant number of solitary distant nodal metastasis were found outside the fields of standard pelvic lymphadenectomy (de Jong *et al.*, 2003a).

Existing data in literature also indicate that ¹¹C-choline PET has very poor sensitivity and accuracy for detection of extracapsular extension (Martorana *et al.*, 2006). This result can be partially attributed to the limitations of CT for detailed visualization of prostatic anatomy, in addition to the poor spatial resolution (5 mm) of PET. Similarly, ¹¹C-choline PET fails to detect nodal micrometastasis due to low spatial resolution. Modern PET/CT devices can identify lesions in the range of 5 to 8 mm.

In summary, with regard to prostate staging, ¹¹C-choline PET has not been studied in an acceptable number of patients.

However, it does not seem to be accurate enough to utilize for evaluating extracapsular extension and seminal vesicle involvement, while showing promising results for detecting nodal and bone metastases. Currently, its use in predicting stage at presentation should be limited to research studies; a routine clinical use cannot be recommended.

¹¹C-Choline PET for Detection of Prostate Cancer Recurrence

Patients with prostate cancer and treated with radical prostatectomy are routinely followed with DRE and PSA measurements for surveillance of recurrent disease. Actually, PSA measurement is the most useful tool for evaluating treatment efficacy. Biochemical recurrence is generally considered to have occurred when two separate measurements reveal a PSA of 0.2 ng/ml or greater and rising. The probability of biochemical relapse at 5 years, reported in several large series, has ranged between 20% and 31%.

The spectrum of PSA relapse disease is very wide, however, with multiple prognostic variables. The type of prior therapy (surgery, radiation, both, or hormone therapy), PSA kinetics (PSA elevation, PSA doubling time, PSA velocity), duration of prior remission, prostate cancer histology, and extent of primary cancer (margin involvement, seminal vesicle involvement, lymph node involvement) are some of the most important prognostic variables predictive of overall outcome. All these parameters are important for an appropriate further treatment strategy. Patient characteristics such as age, comorbid conditions, and life expectancy also play a role in treatment recommendation for PSA relapse disease.

In this scenario, the major objective of the imaging methods is to assess patients for the presence of distant metastatic disease. This would enable selection of patients with absence of distant metastases for local therapies. However, the precise determination of the actual site of recurrence is frequently unsuccessful. TRUS with biopsy of the anastomotic site, radionuclide bone scans, CT, and MR alone, or in combination have traditionally been associated with a low sensitivity and/or specificity. Thus, in a substantial proportion of patients, PSA recurrence will remain the only evidence of disease activity, and an increasing number of patients will receive early androgen deprivation treatment solely on the basis of a rising PSA without defining the exact site(s) of disease. An improvement of detection rate in evaluation of disease recurrence can be achieved through employment of functional imaging tools like PET.

Preliminary results published by Hara *et al.* (1998) demonstrated the successful use of ¹¹C-choline PET in identifying both local and distant metastasis in patients with prostate cancer. Although this study was limited by having no histologic reference for the metastatic sites, the likelihood of positive ¹¹C-choline findings was high for tumor tissue, and the data were encouraging. Subsequent studies confirmed the feasibility of ¹¹C-choline PET for detecting the site of

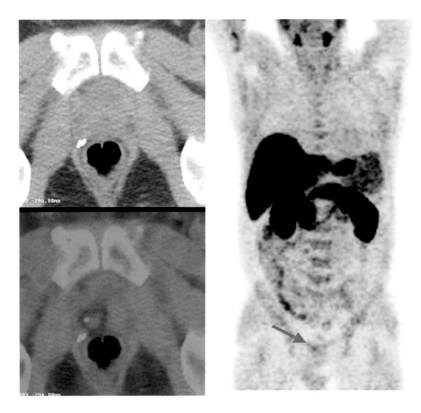

Figure 1 Patient treated with radical prostatectomy for a prostate cancer and biochemical recurrence (PSA 3.1 ng/ml). ¹¹C-choline PET/CT detected local recurrence confirmed by biopsy.

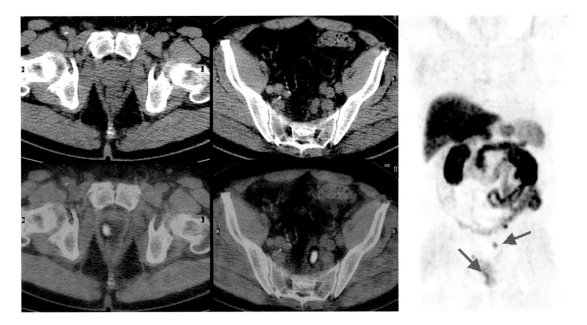

Figure 2 Patient with biopsy proved primary prostate cancer and biochemical recurrence (PSA 6.1 ng/ml). ¹¹C-choline PET/CT identified intraprostatic cancer and node metastasis.

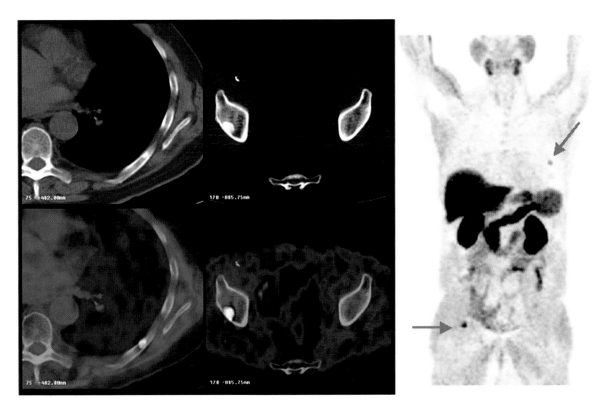

Figure 3 Patient treated with radical prostatectomy for prostate cancer; biochemical recurrence (PSA 7 ng/ml) nondetected by other imaging methods. ¹¹C-choline PET/CT identified two small bone metastases.

disease recurrence in about half of patients with rising PSA. The sensitivity of ^{11}C-choline PET for detection of disease recurrence ranges from 47 to 59% (Jana and Blaufox, 2006).

[11]C-choline PET, supplying a whole-body tomography exam, has the major advantage of detecting local and distant metastasis (lymphogenous or hematogenous) within a single session. Furthermore, the added value of ^{11}C-choline PET compared to conventional imaging seems to be the higher sensitivity for detecting of nodal metastasis (Yoshida et al., 2005). Although locating nodal recurrences only occasionally leads to surgery, identifying the source of the rising PSA level allows the patient and the surgeon to explain the rising level and to choose the best type of treatment (e.g., local radiotherapy).

[11]C-choline PET might not demonstrate more bone lesions than conventional bone scintigraphy, but it shows higher specificity and consequently higher accuracy. ^{99m}Tc-MDP, the widely used tracer for bone scan, is not tumor specific, and, therefore, it is prone to yield false-positive findings. Lower bone lesion detection is reported primarily for lesions located at the vertebral column. Therefore, taking advantage of both the favorable tumor-specific characteristics of ^{11}C-choline and the better performance of PET scanners, ^{11}C-choline PET results are more accurate for detecting metastases than bone scan (Jana and Blaufox, 2006). However, in patients with high-risk cancer, suspicious bone metastasis (elevated serum alkaline phosphatase levels and bone pain), and PSA levels higher than 10 ng/ml, the more easily available and cheaper bone scan should be performed as the first diagnostic method. In the case of skeletal spread, systemic therapy can be proposed without any further diagnostic investigation. ^{11}C-choline PET should be reserved for patients with biochemical recurrence and negative bone scan, apparently single lesions or unequivocal findings.

Available studies suggest a higher detection rate of ^{11}C-choline PET for detection of distant metastasis compared to local recurrences (Picchio et al., 2003). Local recurrence has been postulated to have a more linear increase in PSA (velocity < 0.75 ng/ml per year), while distant metastases display an exponential increase (velocity > 0.75 ng/ml per year). When local recurrence is suspected, TRUS biopsy should be preferred as a "first-line" imaging method, despite its inability to detect minimal tumor mass at very low PSA levels (< 1 ng/ml). TRUS biopsy seems to be more sensitive than ^{11}C-choline PET for detecting local recurrence, especially if PSA levels are low. The rationale for using ^{11}C-choline PET should be exclusion of distant metastasis before performing salvage radiotherapy.

Although ^{11}C-choline PET should be considered an established clinical procedure in detecting prostate cancer recurrence, patient referral criteria have still to be defined. At present, no definite data exist with regard to the thresholds of serum PSA level above which ^{11}C-choline is more likely to detect disease. More importantly, the influence of anti-androgen therapy on ^{11}C-choline uptake in patients with prostate cancer should be clarified. Preliminary results (own unpublished data) suggest that anti-androgen treatment reduces tumor metabolic activity and, consequently, ^{11}C-choline uptake in androgen-sensitive prostate cancer.

As far as the assessment of disease recurrence is concerned, ^{11}C-choline PET has to be performed only if it will influence treatment decisions. The use of ^{11}C-choline PET is considered appropriate in cases in which findings of conventional imaging are doubtful or inconclusive or where lesions are seemingly unique or susceptible to surgery and/or radiation therapy. The opportunity to screen the whole body by PET imaging is particularly important as local recurrence and distant metastasis can be detected.

Although ^{11}C-choline is not the "perfect" radiotracer for prostate cancer imaging, ^{11}C-choline PET generally shows more sites of disease compared to all conventional imaging methods together. At present, the only clinical indication for studying prostate cancer with ^{11}C-choline PET is the evaluation of suspected recurrence after first-line treatment. Further studies are warranted to evaluate the true role of ^{11}C-choline-PET for detection of intraprostatic cancer and for prostate cancer preoperative staging.

Acknowledgments

We used our own PET cases (University Hospital S. Orsola-Malpighi Bologna-Italy) with a GE Discovery PET/CT scanner. All patients provided informed consent for participation and anonymous publication of data.

References

Aus, G., Abbou, C.C., Bolla, M., Heidenreich, A., Schmid, H.P., van Poppel, H., Wolff, J., and Zattoni, F. 2005. EAU guidelines on prostate cancer. Eur Urol. 48:546–551.

Breeuwsma, A.J., Pruim, J., Jongen, M.M., Suurmeijer, A.J., Vaalburg, W., Nijman, R.J., and de Jong, I.J. 2005. In vivo uptake of [11C]choline does not correlate with cell proliferation in human prostate cancer. Eur. J. Nucl. Med. Mol. Imaging 32:668–673.

de Jong, I.J., Pruim, J., Elsinga, P.H., Vaalburg, W., and Mensink, H.J. 2003a. Preoperative staging of pelvic lymph nodes in prostate cancer by 11C-choline PET. J. Nucl. Med. 44:331–335.

de Jong, I.J., Pruim, J., Elsinga, P.H., Vaalburg, W., and Mensink, H.J. 2003b. 11C-choline positron emission tomography for the evaluation after treatment of localized prostate cancer. Eur. Urol. 44:32–38.

de Jong, I.J., Pruim, J., Elsinga, P.H., Vaalburg, W., and Mensink, H.J. 2002. Visualization of prostate cancer with 11C-choline positron emission tomography. Eur. Urol. 42:18–23

Farsad, M., Schiavina, R., Castellucci, P., Nanni, C., Corti, B., Martorana, G., Canini, R., Grigioni, W., Boschi, S., Marengo, M., Pettinato C., Salizzoni, E., Monetti, N., Franchi, R., and Fanti, S. 2005. Detection and localization of intra prostate cancer: correlation of ^{11}C-choline PET/CT with histopathologic step-section analysis. J. Nucl. Med. 46:1642–1649.

Hara, T., Kosaka, N., and Kishi, H. 1998. PET imaging of prostate cancer using carbon-11-choline. J. Nucl. Med. 39:990–995.

Hsing, A.W., and Devesa, S.S. 2001. Trends and patterns of prostate cancer: what do they suggest? *Epidemiol Rev. 23*:3–13.

Jana, S., and Blaufox, M.D. 2006. Nuclear medicine studies of the prostate, testes, and bladder. *Semin. Nucl. Med. 36*:51–72.

Kotzerke, J., Prang, J., Neumaier, B., Volkmer, B., Guhlmann, A., Kleinschmidt, K., Hautmann, R., and Reske, S.N. 2000. Experience with carbon-11 choline positron emission tomography in prostate carcinoma. *Eur. J. Nucl. Med. 27*:1415–1419.

Kotzerke, J., Volkmer, B.G., Glatting, G., Van den Hoff, J., Gschwend, J.E., Messer, P., Reske, S.N., and Neumaier, B. 2003. Intraindividual comparison of [11C]acetate and [11C]choline PET for detection of metastases of prostate cancer. *Nuklearmedizin 42*:25–30.

Martorana, G., Schiavina, R., Corti, B., Farsad, M., Salizzoni, E., Brunocilla, E., Bertaccini, A., Manferrari, F., Castellucci, P., Fanti, S., Canini, R., Grigioni, W.F., Morselli Labate, A.M., and D'Errico Grigioni, A. 2006. ¹¹C-choline PET/CT for tumor localization of primary prostate cancer in comparison with 12-core biopsy *J. Urol. 176*:954–960.

Picchio, M., Messa, C., Landoni, C., Gianolli, L., Sironi, S., Brioschi, M., Matarrese, M., Matei, D.V., De Cobelli, F., Del Maschio, A., Rocco, F., Rigatti P., and Fazio, F. 2003. Value of [11C]choline-positron emission tomography for re-staging prostate cancer: a comparison with [18F]fluorodeoxyglucose-positron emission tomography. *J. Urol. 169*:1337–1340.

Rajesh, A., and Coakley, F.V. MR imaging and MR spectroscopic imaging of prostate cancer. 2004. *Magn. Reson. Imaging Clin. N. Am. 12*:557–579.

Sedelaar, J.P., de la Rosette, J.J., and Debruyne, F.M. 2003. Progress in the imaging of the prostate gland. *Curr. Urol. Rep. 4*:1–2.

Sutinen, E., Nurmi, M., Roivainen, A., Varpula, M., Tolvanen, T., Lehikoinen, P., and Minn, H. 2004. Kinetics of [(11)C]choline uptake in prostate cancer: a PET study. *Eur. J. Nucl. Med. Mol. Imaging 31*:317–324.

Townsend, D.W., and Beyer, T. 2002. A combined PET/CT scanner: the path to true image fusion. *Br. J. Radiol. 75*:S24–S30.

Yoshida, S., Nakagomi, K., Goto, S., Futatsubashi, M., and Torizuka, T. 2005. 11C-choline positron emission tomography in prostate cancer: primary staging and recurrent site staging. *Urol. Int. 74*:214–220.

44

Metabolic Characterization of Prostate Cancer: Magnetic Resonance Spectroscopy

Kate W. Jordan and Leo L. Cheng

Introduction

From Metabolites to Metabolomics

To evaluate prospectively the clinical utility of magnetic resonance spectroscopy, one must first understand the rationale for how metabolomics in the era of genomics and proteomics offers a potentially powerful tool for disease evaluation. Simplifying the complex networks of biological metabolisms that control and regulate a human life by ignoring feedback loops and parallel processes, we can generally consider metabolites (such as those found in one's bodily fluids or tissues) as downstream products of genomic and proteomic changes. However, compared with genes and proteins, the advantage of metabolites is that they are, in many ways, the stepping-stones of cellular pathways through which the current, existing molecular processes can be probed. We define current oncological metabolomics as the study of the global variations of metabolites, and a measurement of global profiles of metabolites from various metabolic pathways under the influence of oncological developments and progressions. The intrinsic interconnectivity of the entire metabolism, both physiological and pathological, of a human body under the influence of oncological processes is reflected in the emphasized word

"global" in the above definition. Metabolomics is a science that evolved from studies of individual metabolites and their specific relationship with physiology and pathology into a discipline that now surveys the entire measurable metabolite profile for correlations with biomedicine.

Metabolomics for Prostate Cancer

The majority of prostate cancers (PCs), > 70%, are adenocarcinomas originating from the secretory epithelium of the peripheral zone; 15% arise from the transitional zone; and very few cancers derive from central zone tissue (Carroll *et al.*, 2001). Despite this seemingly straightforward analysis of the prostate, in clinical reality the disease is very heterogeneous. Prostate cancer is a pathologically multifocal disease that can be found throughout the gland. The innate heterogeneity of prostate cancer complicates disease diagnosis. While 1 in 4 men may harbor PC in their gland, only 3.6% of those diagnosed will die of the disease, and an estimated 30% of PC patients are overtreated (Carter *et al.*, 2002). Regrettably, there are currently no clinical paradigms to assess the virulent from indolent cancers. Each day > 150 radical prostatectomies are performed in the United States, resulting in impotence and/or incontinence of urine for more than 95 and 45 men, respectively (Ransohoff *et al.*, 2002).

Understandably, these are alarming statistics for both patients and clinicians. The NCI's Prostate Cancer Progress Review Group (PRG) (1998) has, therefore, outlined "crucial directions for research," which include discovering new markers to differentiate less harmful from aggressive tumors, improving prognostic markers to better guide individual therapy, and improving diagnosis to ensure that destructive PCs are not missed. Of all the various avenues that could be pursued, metabolomics offers a unique, sensitive, and specific solution to the issues raised by the PRG. In this chapter, we show that metabolomics can be evaluated with magnetic resonance spectroscopy (MRS), which has demonstrated its potential to refine the PC clinic, and may offer new paradigms that may advance diagnosis and management of the disease to a new, high level.

Malignant Changes in Prostate Metabolism

Magnetic resonance spectroscopy, also known as nuclear magnetic resonance (NMR), was discovered independently by Felix Bloch and Edward Mills Purcell in 1945 (Sohlman, 2003). Following the development of NMR, German and English researchers in the 1970s found that small changes in cellular pathways could lead to large changes in metabolic concentrations (Daviss, 2005). This crucial discovery became the foundation of metabolomics as it describes the ability of metabolites to signify otherwise undetectable biological changes in cellular processes.

A number of specific metabolites have particular importance in studying the prostate. Historically, citrate and choline have the most well-categorized biochemical role in prostate malignant transformation. In the epithelial cells of a healthy prostate, there is a high cellular accumulation of zinc (Franklin et al., 2005). High levels of zinc inhibit oxidation of citrate in the Krebs cycle, leading to high levels of citrate, which is secreted into prostatic fluid. The metabolic transformation from citric-production to citric-oxidization is the most consistent modification from normal to malignant prostate tissue. Elevated levels of choline are associated with changes in cell membrane synthesis accompanying cancerous development (Podo, 1999). In addition to citrate and choline, other common metabolites that have been evaluated as diagnostic markers for prostate cancer include creatine, the choline-containing compounds phosphocholine and glycerophosphocholine, spermine, spermadine, taurine, and myo-inositol. Integrating the polyamines allows the differentiation of cancer from healthy or benign prostatic tissue, as the polyamine levels are elevated in benign conditions but are reduced in malignant situations (Cheng et al., 2001). Polyamines stabilize the membranes of both cells and organelles, and assist the formation of disulfide crosslinks (such as those important to sperm fusion and adhesion proteins). Significant data from cell-extract studies have shown that the alterations in prostate cellular metabolism

that accompany malignant changes are in fact cancer specific and are not due to changes in cellular volume or doubling time (Ackerstaff et al., 2001).

When investigating metabolic alterations in relation to physiological and pathological conditions, the predecessors to current PC spectroscopy often focused on individual metabolites, usually choline, creatine, and citrate. As spectroscopy developed, analysis of concentrations of individual metabolites gave way to examining ratios of metabolites to one another. Current in vivo spectroscopy continues to use the ratios of choline, citrate, and creatine to one another as their litmus test. Probing the concentrations of other metabolites, such as the polyamines, in in vivo spectroscopy is not easy because at 1.5T (T for Tesla, the unit of magnetic field strength) the polyamine resonances overlap with the peaks for choline and creatine.

Ex vivo spectroscopy of biological samples, utilizing the advantages of high field strength and more achievable field homogeneity, can reveal dozens of cellular metabolites that are not distinguishable in vivo. Ex vivo studies can be performed either on intact tissue samples or on solutions of tissue extracts. These solutions or intact tissues, if analyzed effectively with appropriate methodologies, are likely to produce spectra with > 100 resonance peaks. The collections of these peaks, reflecting the MRS visible cellular metabolomics of the analyzed samples from an individual, vary according to individual biological diversity, disease status, and pathological conditions. Thus, instead of considering each individual metabolite independently, one needs to collectively and simultaneously evaluate them as an entire group. Fortunately, existing statistical models and methods can readily be used for this type of data mining and analysis (e.g., principal component analysis).

Magnetic Resonance Spectroscopy

Magnetic Resonance Spectroscopy

Innate nuclear momentum is known to have different states that become degenerated, for instance, into α and β states for protons, when the nucleus is placed in an external magnetic field (B_0). This splitting of momentum states results in an energy differential in which more atoms exist in the lower energy state (populations are now given by Boltzmann's law, $N^-/N^+ = e^{-E/kT}$, T: absolute temperature). The effective field at the nucleus is in reality not the full strength of the applied field due to electron circulation; the net magnetic field is referred to as B. The electron density at each nucleus varies, an effect referred to as chemical shift. In a given magnetic field, B_0, the energy needed to transfer between α and β states is proportional not to B_0, but to the field strength B.

Magnetic resonance occurs between the states when a second magnetic field, B_1, is applied through a coil at a radiofrequency

(RF) that matches the required energy to transition between the α and β states:

$$\Delta E = h v$$

where h is Planck constant and v is the resonance frequency that can be written as:

$$v = \gamma B/2\pi$$

In this formula, γ is the gyromagnetic ratio that relates directly to the type of the examined nucleus. The equation $v = \gamma B/2\pi$ is known as the Larmor equation; which is fundamental to MR spectroscopy, where chemical environments affect B through chemical shift α, and hence alter the Larmor frequency, v.

The samples studied by MRS are not homogeneous; the MR spectra are produced by the nuclei, for instance, protons, with different Larmor frequencies in a given molecule or a mixture of different molecules. Each nucleus in a different chemical environment will have a unique Larmor frequency, in an applied B_0 field, and resonate when the applied B_1 energy matches that frequency. A nucleus is said to be "on resonance" when it is absorbing RF energy. Magnetic resonance uses the response of the magnetic moment of a nucleus when placed in a static external magnetic field and perturbed by a second oscillating field. Because the level of the response of a particular nucleus depends on its type as well as the chemical environment in which it resides, and by measuring a range or a spectrum of the responding levels for a given sample, the identification of the contained chemical components can be determined.

Pulse and Fourier Transform Magnetic Resonance Spectroscopy

Magnetic resonance spectroscopy was initially practiced using the continuous-wave (CW) technique, meaning either: (a) the magnetic field was constant and the oscillating wave was swept to detect on resonance molecules; or, more commonly, (b) the oscillating field was fixed at a certain frequency and the magnetic field was swept. In CW MRS each Larmor frequency of interest must be probed individually. The CW modality lost favor to pulse MRS by the 1970s. Pulse MRS, as indicated by its title, instead of swiping through magnetic fields, pulses the applied RF B_1 field through the sample with a short square pulse that, according to the mathematics of Fourier transform, contains all the frequencies of interest. Therefore, all the Larmor frequencies can be excited simultaneously, and nuclear behavior can be recorded after the RF B_1 field is turned off.

The advantages of Pulse MRS over CW MRS are evident. The most obvious improvement is an increase in the S/N, resulting in the capability to do more measurements per unit of time. The signal is the measurable output of the nuclei, while noise is the appearance of outside interference

on the spectra. Signal-to-noise ratio (S/N) increases with the number of scans performed, proportional to $\sqrt{N}$. Pulse MRS allows one to take more scans in a dramatically reduced time period compared to CW MRS (seconds vs. minutes or longer); thus, pulse MRS provides a remarkably impressive S/N benefit. Besides this advantage, the most important contribution of pulse MRS is its ability to manipulate nuclei of interest and force them to yield the desired chemical information, which we will discuss later.

In pulse MRS, the B_1 field is introduced by applying a sinusoidal RF current much greater than that used in CW MRS. The frequency of the RF pulse excites the nuclei to be on resonance for a time, t, which rotates the net magnetization of the nuclei $\gamma B_1 t$. For example, a pulse that can rotate the nuclei 90° is called a 90° (or $\pi/2$) pulse. Doubling the time the RF is applied will result in doubling the degree to which the nuclei are rotated (e.g., a π pulse turns the nuclei 180°). When the pulse is turned off, the nuclei attempt to return to their ground state and require a set length of time for the nuclei to relax back to equilibrium (Fig. 1). During this time, the nuclei emit energy signals that can be registered in the time domain as a signal/time plot known as the free induction decay (FID). The FID measured from a sample is the algebraic sum of all the decaying waves for the measured nuclei. After the FID is induced and recorded, it is translated into a frequency-dependent pattern (a spectrum) using the Fourier transformation (Fig. 2). Fourier transformation is a very powerful tool because it allows us to relate the frequency and time domains to extract meaningful spectra, and also because it integrates the complex amalgam of

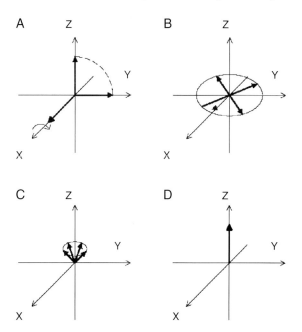

Figure 1 (Modified from Farrar, 1997) When (**A**) a 90° B_1 pulse is applied to the nuclei in the magnetic field, they (**B**) dephase from one another, (**C**) precess, and finally (**D**) the full macroscopic magnetization has returned the nuclei to the Z plane.

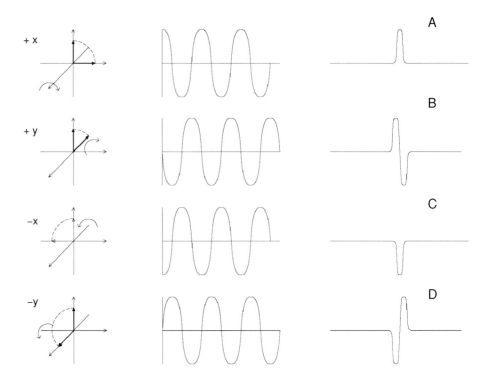

Figure 2 (Modified from Farrar, 1997) From left to right note the position of the nuclei in the rotating frame, the FID signal generated, and spectral signal after Fourier transformation for nuclei among the: (**A**) +*x*-axis, (**B**) +*y*-axis, (**C**) −*x*-axis, and (**D**) −*y*-azis.

sinusoidal patterns produced by each individual molecule as their nuclei decay to produce the spectra.

The nuclear decay to the ground state takes place in two arenas, the *z*-direction (i.e., the direction of the external magnetic field) and a plane (*x-y*) perpendicular to the field direction. The relaxation times of the nuclei with regard to the *z*-direction and the *x-y* plane can provide such useful information as chemical shifts, conformational changes in macromolecules, bond distances, spin-spin couplings (the interaction of two hydrogen nuclei on the same molecule splitting the spectral lines), molecular diffusion, and molecular correlation times. Most often, the three types of relaxation time discussed in regard to MRS are T_1, T_2, and T_2^*.

T_1 is the first-order relaxation, commonly referred to as spin-lattice relaxation time; it relates the time required for the nuclei to return to equilibrium by exchanging energy with their surroundings. The lattice is a general term for the nucleus's surroundings, which can absorb energy given off by the nuclei. In addition to nuclear effects of magnetization, MRS must also acknowledge the innate thermodynamic processes taking place. T_1 time is the relaxation order that reestablishes thermal equilibrium. After $5 \times T_1$ time, the 99.3% magnetization has been reestablished in the *z*-direction and thermo-equilibrium is restored; however, since the signals can only be detected in the *x-y* plane, one can use a second pulse to rotate the already recovered nuclear magnetizations away from the *z*-direction after a certain recovery time. Variations in the length of this recovering time allow one to measure the T_1 value.

T_2 takes into account nuclei relaxing back to equilibrium not with their external environment but instead with each other, among the like nuclei. As nuclei relax, they do not remain in phase with one another, as each experiences a slightly different local magnetic field and rotates at its own Larmor frequency. T_2 is always less than or equal to T_1.

T_2^* is the relaxation time that acknowledges both the natural line width (T_2) and the fact that a magnetic field can never, in reality, be perfectly homogeneous. Therefore, nuclei in different parts of the field experience differing net magnetism and thus have different resonances. At the moment of the initial RF pulse, all nuclei are rotated a certain degree from the *z*-direction, as they rotate (or more precisely precess), they become dephased in the *x-y* plane. Figure 1 depicts the fan-like array of dephased nuclei. As previously described, this means certain nuclei will, in essence, precess more quickly than others (the portions of the sample experiencing the greatest net magnetization precess most rapidly). Within the sample the nuclei that precess at the same speed, which have the same Larmor frequency and experience the same magnetization, are called spin isochromats. When discussing dephasing and the relaxation back to 0 in the *x-y* plane, it is these isochromats to which we are specifically referring.

Increasing field homogeneity will bring T_2^* closer to T_2. However, the mechanical and technical aspects of increasing field homogeneity have a limit. Therefore, spin-echo techniques are used to diminish the effects of field inhomogeneity.

Spin-echo techniques involve multiple pulses that reverse the order of the spin isochromats. This is accomplished in the following way: first, the sample is pulsed to a certain extent (usually 90°) after which the spin isochromats dephase. After a certain time, t, during which the spin isochromats become out of phase with each other, but *before* they have a chance to internally dephase, there is a second, 180° pulse applied along the x'-direction in the x'-y' plane (x' being the plane in the rotating frame of the coil and sample, versus the x plane of the static magnet). The net magnetization in the z'-direction is inverted and has no effect on the experiment, while the order of the spin isochromats is now reversed so that the fastest isochromats are behind the slowest. The benefit of this rearrangement is that the faster spin isochromats catch up with the slower ones, resulting in refocused magnetization along the y'-direction at time $2t$. The representation of the spin echo is an inverted FID. Several pulse techniques have been created to generate what is known as an echo-train.

An echo-train consists of the FIDs produced by a pulse sequence rephasing the isochromats at multiples of time, t. The maximal echo amplitude in the spin echo should decay at a time constant that is consistent with T_2. The Carr-Purcell echo-train combines 180° pulses with 180° phase shifts (e.g., echo one $+x$, echo two $-x$) and diminishes any pulse errors resulting from field inhomogeneity or pulse-length discrepancies; alternatively, phase shifting all echo pulses so they are 90° with respect to the initial pulse simplifies the process (e.g., all echoes are in the direction of the initial FID). This is known as the very common Meiboom-Gill modification of the Carr-Purcell sequence (CPMG).

A further importance of pulse MRS is the ability to decrease the time requisite for accumulating FIDs. In order for an FID to be complete, enough time must elapse between pulses for the magnetization to accrue along the z-direction. This is not as large a problem in liquids as it is in solids because in liquids T_1 is closer to T_2^*. To overcome the FID time requirement in samples such as nonliquid biological samples, one must force the system to return to thermal equilibrium faster than is natural. Driven equilibrium Fourier transform (DEFT) involves the initiation of a pulse-echo sequence, and at the peak of a spin echo a 90° pulse rotates the nuclei back to the z-direction, preparing the sample to start the process of gather FID again.

Magnetic Resonance Spectroscopy of Nonaqueous Solutions and Solids

In the above discussion, we categorically considered the notion that identical molecules, or nuclei in the same chemical functional group of molecules, are physically the same; that is, they are identical and have exactly the same Larmor frequency. In reality, the closest system that may mimic such an ideal condition is an aqueous solution, where molecules of interest are all surrounded by solvent molecules and are a distance away from each other. Thus, by the additional assistance of molecular tumbling,

these molecules, and hence their nuclei of the same functional group, may be considered identical. In a nonideal case, there exist differences in the chemical shift factor σ for these nuclei. This is known as an anisotropic effect, and it results in nuclei of the same type resonating at a range of Larmor frequencies. This fact is reflected in an MR spectrum, where the resonance peak corresponding to these nuclei is broadened, as a spectrum is in fact a pictorial presentation of population distributions. This phenomenon is seen everywhere from classical solids to biological samples of nonaqueous solution, to *in vivo* MRS of any physiological structures and organs.

Considerations of MRS for nonaqueous solution can be applied to the study of any biological tissues. For this reason, historically researchers have investigated solutions of tissue extracts instead of dealing with biological tissues, which are of a semisolid nature. However, although individual metabolites can be quantified within the extract solution using this method, the metabolites are altered to an unknown (unquantifiable) degree when going through the extraction processes. Furthermore, extraction methods destroy tissue pathological structures and preclude histopathological evaluation of the analyzed samples, preventing a correlation between the spectra and the pathology that produced it. This issue might not present a problem if tumors consisted of pathologically homogeneous structures. Unfortunately, when dealing with human malignancies, tissue heterogeneity must be assumed and accounted for when analyzing MR spectra. While hundreds, if not thousands, of past publications were based on extraction MRS, the ability to compare biological and metabolic process with their underlying pathology (which may be considered essential) has been forever lost.

Magnetic Resonance Spectroscopy with Magic Angle Spinning

The issues described earlier in this chapter, whereby spectra are produced with broad linewidths is the result of something that can be categorically termed *solid effects* produced by using MRS to study anything other than liquids. The quintessential example of a solid effect, the one most often referred to in MRS texts, is that of orientation-dependent interactions, such as dipolar interactions. Dipolar interactions take place between nuclei when the nuclei are susceptible to the magnetic field generated by the surrounding nuclei. The magnitude of the dipole-dipole interaction effect on spectral broadening is dependent on the distance between the nuclei, the angle between the nuclear vector, and the applied magnetic field, B_0; and is proportional to $(3\cos^2 \theta - 1)$. This condition accounts not only for dipolar interactions, but also other solid effects. Andrew *et al.* (1959) addressed the dipolar situation when they showed that dipolar interactions could be overcome if the angle θ in the above equation was 54.74° away from the applied magnetic field. Hence, 54.74° is known as the magic angle—the angle at which dipolar interactions are greatly reduced. In order to achieve such manipulation, the sample is placed in a rotor and mechanically tipped to the magic angle.

When the sample is spinning, at rates anywhere up to ~ 35 kHz (the current technical limit), the time average internuclear vector aligns at the magic angle and the spectra produced are extremely well resolved. The effective spinning rate is defined as the rate equal to or greater than the linewidth produced by solid effects. When Lowe and Andrew (1959) observed that magic angle spinning (MAS) MR spectroscopy resulted in the Lorentzian-shaped spectra previously only observed in aqueous solutions, the technique was adopted for solid-state MAS. Figure 3 exemplifies the capability of the MAS technique. The spectra in Figure 3A and 3B are produced from the same human prostate tissue sample, without and with spinning, respectively without spinning, the spectra are little more than several broad peaks and noise; 3C is an expansion of the 0.5 ppm to 3.0 ppm range of 3B, in which individual metabolites from human prostatic tissue are clear and quantifiable when the sample is spun at 600 Hz.

Although the MAS technique was well known to MRS physicists, only many years later was it adopted for studying biological tissues. During his postdoctoral work at the Massachusetts General Hospital and Harvard Medical School, one of the authors of this chapter discovered that the MAS could be used on *unaltered* biological tissue specimens (Cheng *et al.*, 1996). Proton (1H) MR spectroscopy of tissue samples, when mechanically rotated at the magic angle, produces spectra with resolution close to those measured in solution, which is sufficient for the detection and quantification of individual metabolites. For the purpose of measuring unaltered tissue specimens the procedure became known as high-resolution magic angle spinning (HRMAS).

The technique was further improved by D.C. Anthony's observation that at a restrained rotation tissue architecture was not damaged by the centrifugal force of HRMAS (Cheng *et al.*, 2000). This property is critical, for it allows histopathology to be performed on the same sample after spectroscopy is measured, permitting the methodology to address the aforementioned issue of human tumor heterogeneity. The ability to correlate spectroscopy with tissue pathology made HRMAS a premier modality for spectroscopic disease analysis. Figure 4 displays HRMAS 1HMRS spectra with metabolites of interest labeled, as well as an H&E slide of the unaltered prostate tissue that was analyzed and produced the pictured spectra. Since its advent in the mid 1990s, HRMAS 1HMRS has been adopted for a wide variety of research studies.

Current Techniques

Histopathology from biopsy cores remains the gold standard for diagnosing and determining treatment of prostate cancer. But although histopathology has served well in the past, it cannot meet the needs of the current oncology clinic in which evolving technologies have drastically increased the number of men diagnosed with early-stage, moderately differentiated PC. MR spectroscopy may present one of many modalities being examined at present to meet the demands of twenty-first-century diagnosis, prognosis, and treatment planning.

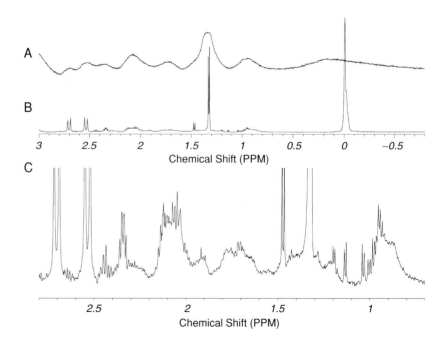

Figure 3 (A) Spectra produced by the same sample without MAS and (B) with MAS, clearly indicating that the metabolites are distinguishable and quantifiable with MAS but not conventional MRS; (C) expansion for better detail is provided of the 3.0 to 0.5 ppm range of the MAS spectra in (B).

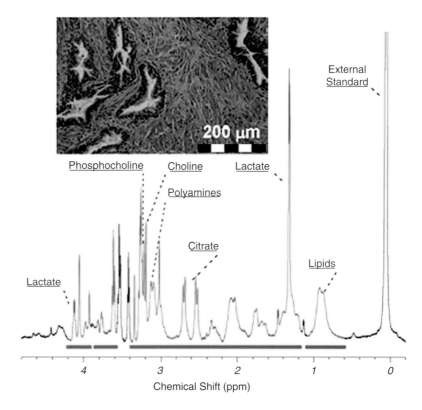

Figure 4 (Modified from Cheng *et al.*, 2005) HRMAS 1HMRS spectra of an intact, surgical prostate sample. The sample was spun at 600 and 700 Hz, which was not damaging to the tissue architecture, and histopathology on the slide shown was performed on the same sample following spectroscopic analysis.

Current *In Vivo* Prostate Cancer Spectroscopy

The origins of modern *in vivo* MR spectroscopy for the human prostate date back to ~ 1980; like many applications of spectroscopy, MRS advanced with the rate of technological improvements in coils, field strength, pulse sequences, and so on. Most commonly current *in vivo* MRS data are collected at the clinical field strength of 1.5 T, with an increasing trend toward utilization of 3 T, using phased-array and endorectal coils. The advantage of the increase to 3 T is the doubling of the S/N, and theoretically a drastic improvement in spectral resolution. However, prostate spectroscopy and/ or imaging at 3 T is still being evaluated, and, in many ways, it is still in its infancy. Toward the same end of increased S/N, the endorectal coil produces spectra with ~ 10-fold increase in S/N versus a pelvic phased coil (Kurhanewicz *et al.*, 2002). Normally, cancer is differentiated from healthy prostatic tissue by an increased ratio of choline (Cho) plus creatine (Cr) to citrate (Cit), as in [Cho + Cr]/Cit. Current *in vivo* MR spectroscopy has a reported sensitivity, specificity, and accuracy in detecting prostate cancer of up to 89%, 77%, and 83%, respectively (Squillaci *et al.*, 2005). This means that MR spectroscopy is more sensitive than MR imaging, biopsy, and digital rectal exams. More crucially, when MRS was combined with magnetic resonance spectroscopic imaging (MRSI), it increased the latter's specificity and accuracy in detecting cancer by 14 to 15% (Squillaci *et al.*, 2005).

These data clearly illustrate the additional benefit patients might have if they undergo MRS in conjunction with MRSI. However, *in vivo* MRS is often excluded at the time of diagnosis because it is considered time consuming and is not cost effective as a screening tool.

In the last five years, as clinical interest in prostate *in vivo* MRSI has increased, MR spectroscopic studies have become an adjunct to MRSI. Briefly, MRSI is a metabolic imaging modality that combines the imaging capability of MRI with a very limited amount of spectroscopic information provided by MRS. The metabolite distributions of a single metabolite (or the ratio of two metabolites) are recorded for the voxels of interest (in three dimensions) and surrounding tissue, then overlaid onto the MRI image to examine metabolites within the anatomy. Interpretation of MRSI is a complicated procedure for the prostate owing to the potential of several histological tissue types being present in a single voxel. Thus, there can exist an inability to correlate the single metabolite (or ratio) with specific pathology. Despite the ability of MRS to indicate abnormal regions, it is normally used secondarily to MRI/MRSI to study the metabolism of areas that are already believed to be anomalous. Only time will reveal whether the experimental research that supports the use of MRS will be enough to vault *in vivo* MR spectroscopy out of its current backseat clinical role.

Ex Vivo Prostate Cancer Magnetic Resonance Spectroscopy

The history of *ex vivo* prostate spectroscopy is almost 20 years long and has been improved drastically by the implementation of HRMAS techniques. The original aims of *ex vivo* PC spectroscopy were to gain a better insight into the underlying tumor biology accompanying metabolic changes; to correlate tumor pathology with spectroscopic results; and to improve techniques for *in vivo* application. Unlike *in vivo* spectroscopy, *ex vivo* is rarely used in conjunction with imaging.

Ex Vivo Fluid Studies

Seminal fluid studies linking changes in citrate concentrations to prostate tumorigenesis started after citrate was discovered in human semen by Bertil in 1929 (Averna *et al.*, 2005). Prostatic fluid makes up 50% of the volume of seminal fluid, and it is, therefore, logical to assume that changes in prostate metabolism may be indicated in changes in seminal fluid metabolite concentrations.

In 1997, one of the first published studies linking seminal fluid to disease status using MRS focused on correlating several metabolites with one another and with the malignant condition (Lynch and Nicholson, 1997). In the words of the authors, "High resolution proton (1 H) NMR spectroscopy is an ideal analytical probe where a range of structurally dissimilar metabolites are being measured in a complex matrix such as a biofluid. In addition to analytical information forthcoming from NMR measurements, dynamic molecular interactions of metabolites can also be studied in whole biofluids such as binding phenomena, metal complexation reactions, and enzymatic conversions" (Lynch *et al.*, 1997). It was found in the study (with 38 subjects) that the concentrations of citrate and spermine are linearly correlated ($p < 0.05 \times 10^{-10}$), and that there is a significant difference between the ratio of citrate to spermine in PC patients versus normal controls ($p < 0.02$). It was also found that no significant differences existed between samples collected by prostatic massage and those from ejaculation. This study was followed by a more recent and more striking study of the relationship between citrate concentration in seminal fluid and the presence of prostate cancer.

Averna *et al.* (2005) indicated that 1 H NMR measurement of citrate in seminal fluid could provide a new, rapid, noninvasive screening method. While this claim could be very relevant, the study could not report sensitivity or specificity, presumably due to a small sample pool ($n = 7$). Not only were the authors able to distinguish differences in citrate concentrations between PC patients, healthy controls, and men with BPH, but they also developed spectral editing techniques to identify citrate in clinical *in vivo* MRS. The authors noted that seminal MRS could take as little as 5 min, rendering it more useful as a screening tool than currently lengthy and non–cost-effective clinical MRS. Furthermore, they suggest that combining measurements of citrate and

other metabolites could lead to the development of computer-aided pattern recognition techniques. Studies by Lynch and Nicholson (1997) and Averna *et al.* (2005) demonstrate the novelty, benefits, and deficits of using *ex vivo* MRS to study biofluids.

The most evident advantage of studying seminal fluid is its noninvasive nature. Collecting seminal fluid, either voluntarily or by prostate massage, is as straightforward as obtaining blood samples and less invasive than a core needle biopsy. Unfortunately, the published studies on MRS of seminal fluid are marred by meager participation ($n < 50$ from < 30 subjects in all studies). It is very plausible that most men have a conceptual issue with volunteering their seminal fluid, feeling that such specimen collection is embarrassing and crosses the boundary of personal space. While the seminal fluid studies presented here are promising, more conclusive evidence will likely be needed before such measures are clinically implemented. Moreover, advanced prostate cancer is known to mutate the acini, prohibiting the excretion of prostatic fluid. Thus, such fluid examination is only possible for a select group of patients. Finally, threshold values for what citrate concentration is conclusively indicative of each clinical status need to be established if seminal fluid MRS is to be of any utility. Nevertheless, the results of the aforementioned studies are very encouraging and may help refine *in vivo* prostate MRS and establish more accurate screening methods.

Pre-Clinical Drug Studies

Studies discussed in this section are classified, for the purpose of this chapter, as *ex vivo* because they examine either cell lines or animal models. The authors acknowledge, however, that incorporation of MRS for drug studies clinically would most likely involve *in vivo* MRS.

A very different, but equally intriguing, application of MRS is in toxicology studies, monitoring the metabolic effects of certain drugs on prostate cells and/or tumors. Presently, differentiating agents to treat prostate cancer are being explored in clinical trials. Such chemicals promote cell differentiation and apoptosis, often through poorly understood mechanisms of actions. Phenylacetate (PA) and phenylbutyrate (PB) are two such aromatic acids being investigated as differentiation inducers. Milkewitch *et al.* (2005) described the behavior of these compounds by treating DU145 human prostate carcinoma cells with PA and PB, then monitoring the metabolic changes induced with 1 H and 31 P diffusion-weighted MRS. DU145 cells (originally established from a metastatic brain lesion of prostate carcinoma) are a model of androgen-independent prostate cancer. In the study the cells were cultured and then treated with 10 mM PA or PB while being continually monitored via MRS for 16 hr. The single-pulse, water-suppressed spectra gathered on the 9.4 T spectrometer revealed significant metabolic changes in the signals from lactate, mobile lipids and neutral amino acids, fatty acids, total choline, and glycerophosphorylcholine (GPC).

The results were compared with electron and light micros-copy to associate metabolic changes with morphological vari-ations. Further analysis of the spectroscopy and microscopy data indicates that PB treatment causes an arrest in the G1 phase of the cell cycle leading to induction of apoptosis. Phen-ylacetate treatment, on the other hand, leads to an accumula-tion of G2/M cells and did not induce apoptosis (Milkevitch *et al.*, 2005). Thus, the two differentiating agents, though structurally similar, affect different stages of the cell cycle. Not only did this study elucidate the cellular effects of PB and PA, but it also demonstrated the feasibility of using MRS to monitor metabolic changes and analyze toxicologi-cal effects of potential chemotherapeutic agents.

The capacity of MRS to be used as a noninvasive monitor of drug efficacy is also supported by a study utilizing 1 H and 31 P spectroscopy to discriminate if genetic pro-drug activa-tion therapy (GPAT) could be used to treat hormone refrac-tory prostate cancer (Eaton *et al.*, 2001). Hormone refractory prostate cancer is an advanced disease with poor prognosis. Novel therapies being explored include gene therapy, often in combination with immunotherapy. Disease manage-ment of this type has demonstrated tumor-specific immune response, and GPAT functions by inserting "suicide" genes (usually the herpes simplex virus thymadine kinase enzyme/ ganciclovir pro-drug system) into tumor cells. Cells treated with GPAT not only die during the cell cycle, but also initi-ate an immune response important for the "bystander effect" and, potentially, distant metastasis. Clinical trials, as of the early 2000s, produced limited clinical response, and MRS was proposed as a means to directly monitor cellular effects of the GPAT system. Serial monitoring similar to the previ-ously described PA/PB study was undertaken. However, in the GPAT study MRS was done *in vivo* on animals from two mouse models. Significant changes were observed in tumor ATP/Pi and phosphomonoester (PME)/phosphate ratios. In tumors of treated animals the ATP/Pi ratio increased, while the PME/phosphate ratio decreased; in contrast, tumors of the control animals had a decrease in the ATP/Pi ratio and no change over time of the PME/phosphate ratio (Eaton *et al.*, 2001). Changes to the PME/phosphate ratio are commonly observed in human prostate tumors and are associated with an increased response to treatment. Further data from this study showed that the metabolic changes associated with the GPAT system are similar to those produced by other, more widely used, chemotherapies. It was also reported that these metabolic effects, established by the MR spectra, were also present in cells subject to the "bystander effect." These data support the use of MRS to observe the effects of drugs *in vivo*.

The above-discussed studies expressly recommend the use of MRS for examining the toxicological effects of drugs ear-marked as potential prostate cancer therapies. Although we are encouraged by these studies, there remains a lack of clini-cal interest in utilizing this methodology. One explanation for this lack of interest may be the slow pace at which clinical paradigms for treatment change. As previously mentioned, radical prostatectomy remains the gold standard of treatment. Understandably, without reliable *in vivo* disease indicators that suggest the rate of tumor growth, many patients may not feel comfortable taking novel drugs to treat their disease when an alterative to remove the tumor entirely exists. One would hope that as early diagnosis and drug discovery increase, there may be more of a clinical demand to study new drug treatments, at which point *in vivo* MRS alone (or in conjunc-tion with MRI) may be the best way to monitor treatment.

High-Resolution Magic Angle Spinning Proton Magnetic Resonance Spectroscopy

Ex vivo prostate HRMAS 1HMRS has advanced rapidly and is currently being tested in our lab as a potential new diagnostic modality. In 2001 we first reported the use of the HRMAS 1HMRS methodology for investigating prostate cancer. The pivotal aspects of the study were the ability to successfully analyze delicate prostate tissues with HRMAS 1HMRS and the capacity to quantify the heterogeneous sample pathology following spectroscopic measurement. The demonstration that both MRS and pathology data could be collected from the same sample indicated the potential for HRMAS 1HMRS to become a critical tool in PC research. The study found that spermine concentration (measured by MRS) correlated with volume percentage (vol%) normal prostatic epithelial cells (Cheng *et al.*, 2001). This study not only verified the capacity of HRMAS 1HMRS to probe the metabolic characteristics of prostate cancer, it also exempli-fied the importance of methodologies that preserve tissue architecture.

A report from Swanson *et al.* (2003) on the diagnostic ability of *ex vivo* prostate HRMAS 1HMRS examined the ability of MRI/3D-MRSI to target samples for *ex vivo* anal-ysis, and the capacity of HRMAS 1HMRS to predict can-cer. The authors found that HRMAS 1HMRS was able to significantly distinguish normal from malignant tissue on the basis of higher levels of citrate and the polyamines in normal gland, and increased choline compounds (choline, GPC, and phosphocholine) in cancer. The samples analyzed were chosen based on *in vivo* MRI/3D-MRSI analysis, and it was found that the *in vivo* techniques targeted healthy tissue with 90% accuracy and cancerous gland with 71% accuracy. They were able to confirm that *ex vivo* analysis yields simi-lar findings to *in vivo* analysis, mainly that choline is greatly increased in the malignant condition. They also studied sev-eral metabolites (including the polyamines) that were not quantifiable with *in vivo* methods.

The ability to analyze a wider array of metabolites could lead to the elucidation of the underlying biology of prostate tumorigenesis, and the improvement of *in vivo* MRS/MRSI. While the study can be viewed as highly successful, the authors acknowledge the difficulties arising in their study from prostate heterogeneity. While generalizations could be made regarding "increased" or "decreased" metabolite levels, there was a large amount of variegation between metabolite profiles due to the heterogeneity of the samples. The spectral profiles were most reflective of the sample's disease status when 20% of the sample was cancer; unfortunately, this is a condition that could not be guaranteed as the 3D-MRSI had an accuracy of 71% when targeting tumor tissue. The authors acknowledged that a more comprehensive study needed to be undertaken, specifically one which overcomes issues of heterogeneity, and find a way to classify metabolites so they reflect tissue pathology regardless of the percentage of each feature present.

Our group (Cheng et al., 2005) reported the first preclinical study of HRMAS 1HMRS on 199 ex vivo human prostate samples from prostatectomies of 82 PC cancer patients. Prior to this large-scale investigation of prostate cancer metabolic profiles, several technical developments have been necessary for prostate HRMAS to reach an optimal level. First, it must be acknowledged that prostatic tissues are fragile. While tissue architecture of breast samples may not be damaged at spinning rates up to 3.6 kHz, accurate prostate tissue histopathology is only possible if the tissue is spun at a rate < 1 kHz. For the purpose of most studies a speed of 600 or 700 Hz is sufficient. Unfortunately, at these relatively slow rates, spinning side bands (SSBs) appear in the spectra and overlap with regions of interest. Two SSB reduction schemes can be utilized to procure the entire prostate tissue spectra. First, rotor-synchronized delays alternating with nutation for tailored excitation (DANTE) sequence is effective if the spectral SSBs are primarily from water and not from other metabolites (Taylor et al., 2003). If, however, the sample is contaminated by alcohol (a frequent occurrence in surgical samples) or SSBs are produced by metabolites, an editing procedure known as Min(A,B) is most useful (Burns et al., 2005). Min(A,B) is a mathematical model which edits two spectra (A,B) acquired at different spinning rates, such as 600 and 700 Hz, by the formula: $(A + B - |A - B|/2)$ (Burns et al., 2005).

Following the establishment of spectral editing protocols, we were able to test the efficacy of using prostate metabolic profiles (measured with HRMAS 1HMRS) to predict disease status (Cheng et al., 2005). The study found that tissue metabolite profiles can: (1) differentiate malignant from benign samples (collected from the same patient); (2) correlate with patient PSA levels; (3) differentiate between aggressive and indolent tumors; and (4) predict tumor perineural invasion. All of these results were found to be significant with $p < 0.03$. Receiver operating characteristic curves (ROC) revealed the overall accuracy of using metabolic profiles to determine cancerous status was 98.2% based on evaluating paired metabolic profiles and histopathological analysis of samples from 13 patients.

Equally important, histopathology not only allows the correlation of the metabolic profile and tissue components, but also shows that no coincidental correlation exists between patient status information and percent volume of each cell type; this shows that the metabolic profiles are independent of cell volume, doubling time, etc. Additionally, though AJCC/TMN staging does not currently include tumor perineural invasion, the perineural invasion status does indicate prostate tumor aggressiveness and is thus incorporated into treatment planning. The ability of metabolic profiles generated by HRMAS 1HMRS to indicate cancer or benign status, identify tumor aggressiveness, and correlate with other clinical status features indicates the potential for said profiles to provide a "second opinion" for biopsy evaluation. More fascinatingly, the data support the analysis of a biopsy core to predict tumor stage, even if the core itself contains no cancerous glands. Our findings indicate that HRMAS 1HMRS has the ability to generate profiles indicative of processes actively taking place, which has great implications in patient prognosis and treatment but has not yet manifested itself in morphological changes identifiable histopathologically.

We value the potential impact this research may have on the prostate clinic, but we also acknowledge the unanswered questions that remain following our investigations. First, our data indicate the existence of a metabolic field effect (i.e., malignant metabolic profiles are delocalized from cancer cells). However, at present we do not know if these cancer metabolic profiles are only local near cancer-containing glands or global throughout the organ. We do not have data regarding the proximity of the histo-benign tissue sample we analyzed to the cancer in the gland. Second, it is almost impossible to identify "normal" controls due to the possibility that many men over the age of 39 harbor a certain amount of PC in their prostate gland, which questions even the use of human autopsy if the entire prostate has not been thoroughly examined for complete pathological composition.

Future Directions

Magnetic resonance spectroscopy, both in vivo and ex vivo, has advanced in a remarkable way in a relatively short period of time. The biomedical uses for the modality, combined with the potential for further clinical integration, may present it as an extremely powerful tool for the management of human prostate cancer. The diversity of the studies presented here is an illustration of the wide scope of MRS and its implementation in the diagnosis, prognosis, and treatment planning for PC. We appreciate that histopathology remains the gold standard by which all techniques will be evaluated, but we also understand the limitations of this extremely subjective field. The objectivity of MRS combined with its ability to be noninvasive, sensitive, and specific will, we believe, continue to assert MRS as a premier technique of the twenty-first century.

In the coming months and years we look forward to further refinement of MRS, which will come in two major waves: first, the improvement of *in vivo* MRS and second, the clinical acceptance of using *ex vivo* MRS. With regard to *in vivo* MRS, as technology improves (resulting in higher clinical field strength and better resolution of individual metabolites), the cost of MRS will decrease, which means that patients will have the benefit of utilizing MRS in conjunction with MRSI. This will be especially imperative if treatment moves away from radical prostatectomy and MRS becomes necessary to monitor tumor reaction to novel therapies. *Ex vivo* MRS, on the other hand, must bridge the gap between phenomenal research work and clinical inclusion. For this purpose we consider HRMAS 1HMRS to have the most relevance and potential.

As acceptance grows and we can move away from the "seeing is believing" method of diagnosis, new clinical paradigms will emerge in which MRS is an integral part. An essential part of improving MRS will come in the form of full automation, such that an entire metabolic profile can be constructed from spectra, compared to literature values, and assigned a disease status. The ability of metabolic profiles to designate benign from malignant, and the aggressiveness of a tumor if present, would make spectroscopy a clinical necessity. One proposed combination of *in vivo* and *ex vivo* work would be to use *ex vivo* HRMAS 1HMRS to define the predictive metabolic signatures; these signatures could then be searched for *in vivo* to provide more accurate diagnosis or preventative screening. In this way, spectroscopy will provide a truly "systems biology" approach to PC management, one in which *in vivo* and *ex vivo* modalities are used in combination to provide maximal benefit to the patient. In closing, we hope this chapter has provided an introductory account of the theory of MRS and the rationale behind applying MRS to prostate cancer, as well as the current and future prospects for spectroscopy in the field of medical oncology as it relates to prostate cancer.

Acknowledgement

Authors acknowledge support from NIH grants CA211478, CA095624, and DOD grant W81XWH-04-1-0190.

References

Ackerstaff, E., Pflug, B.R., Nelson, J.B., and Bhujwalla, Z.M. 2001. Detection of increased choline compounds with proton nuclear magnetic resonance spectroscopy subsequent to malignant transformation of human prostatic epithelial cells. *Cancer Res. 61*:3599–3603.

Andrew, E.R., Bradbury, A., and Eades, R.G. 1959. Removal of dipolar broadening of nuclear magnetic resonance spectra of solids by specimen rotation. *Nature 183*:1802–1803.

Averna, T.A., Kline, E.E., Smith, A.Y., and Sillerud, L.O. 2005. A decrease in 1H nuclear magnetic resonance spectroscopically determined citrate in human seminal fluid accompanies the development of prostate adenocarcinoma. *J. Urol. 173*:433–438.

Burns, M.A., Taylor, J.L., Wu, C.L., Zepeda, A.G., Bielecki, A., Cory, D., and Cheng, L. L. 2005. Reduction of spinning sidebands in proton NMR of human prostate tissue with slow high-resolution magic angle spinning. *Magn. Reson. Med. 54*:34–42.

Carroll, P.R., Lee, K.L., Fuks, Z.Y., and Kantoff, P. W. 2001. Cancer of the prostate. In: DeVito, V.T., Hellman, S., and Rosenberg, S.A. (Eds.) *Cancer: Principles and Practice of Oncology, Sixth Edition*, pp. 1418–1479. Philadelphia: Lippincott Williams and Wilkins.

Carter, H.B., Walsh, P.C., Landis, P., and Epstein, J.I. 2002. Expectant management of nonpalpable prostate cancer with curative intent: preliminary results. *J. Urol. 167*:1231–1234.

Cheng, L.L., Burns, M.A., Taylor, J.L., He, W., Halpern, E.F., McDougal, W. S., and Wu, C.L. 2005. Metabolic characterization of human prostate cancer with tissue magnetic resonance spectroscopy. *Cancer Res. 65*:3030–3034.

Cheng, L.L., Lean, C.L., Bogdanova, A., Wright, S.D., Jr., Ackerman, J.L., Brady, T.J., and Garrido, L. 1996. Enhanced resolution of proton NMR spectra of malignant lymph nodes using magic-angle spinning. *Magn. Reson. Med. 35*:653–658.

Cheng, L.L., Anthony, D.C., Comite, A.R., Black, P.M., Tzika, A.A., and Gonzalez, R.G. 2000 Quantification of microheterogeneity in glioblastoma multiforme with *ex vivo* high-resolution magic-angle spinning (HRMAS) proton magnetic resonance spectroscopy. *Neuro-oncolog. 2*:87–95.

Cheng, L.L., Wu, C., Smith, M.R., and Gonzalez, R.G. 2001. Non-destructive quantitation of spermine in human prostate tissue samples using HRMAS 1 H NMR spectroscopy at 9.4 T. *FEBS Lett. 494*:112–116.

Daviss, B. 2005. Growing pains for metabolomics. *The Scientist 19*:25–28.

Eaton, J.D., Perry, M.J., Todryk, S.M., Mazucco, R.A., Kirby, R.S., Griffiths, J.R., and Dalgleish, A.G. 2001. Genetic prodrug activation therapy (GPAT) in two rat prostate models generates an immune bystander effect and can be monitored by magnetic resonance techniques. *Gene Ther. 8*:557–567.

Farrar, T.C. 1997. *Introduction to Pulse NMR Spectroscopy*. Madison, WI: Farragut Press.

Franklin, R.B., Milon, B., Feng, P., and Costello, L.C. 2005. Zinc and zinc transporters in normal prostate and the pathogenesis of prostate cancer. *Front. Biosci. 10*:2230–2239.

Kurhanewicz, J., Swanson, M.G., Nelson, S.J., and Vigneron, D.B. 2002. Combined magnetic resonance imaging and spectroscopic imaging approach to molecular imaging of prostate cancer. *J. Magn. Reson. Imag. 16*:451–463.

Lynch, M.J., and Nicholson, J.K. 1997. Proton MRS of human prostatic fluid: correlations between citrate, spermine, and myo-inositol levels and changes with disease. *Prostate 30*:248–255.

Milkevitch, M., Shim, H., Pilatus, U., Pickup, S., Wehrle, J. P., Samid, D., Poptani, H., Glickson, J.D., and Delikatny, E.J. 2005. Increases in NMR-visible lipid and glycerophosphocholine during phenylbutyrate-induced apoptosis in human prostate cancer cells. *Bioch. Biophys. Acta 1734*:1–12.

Podo, F. 1999. Tumour phospholipid metabolism. *NMR Biomed. 12*:413–439.

Ransohoff, D.F., McNaughton Collins, M., and Fowler, F.J. 2002. Why is prostate cancer screening so common when the evidence is so uncertain? A system without negative feedback. *Am. J. Med. 113*:663–667.

Sohlman, M.E. 2003. *Nobel Foundation Directory 2003*. Vastervik, Sweden: AB CO Ekblad.

Squillaci, E., Manenti, G., Mancino, S., Carlani, M., Di Roma, M., Colangelo, V., and Simonetti, G. 2005. MR spectroscopy of prostate cancer: initial clinical experience. *J. Exp. Clin. Cancer Res. 24*:523–530.

Swanson, M.G., Vigneron, D.B., Tabatabai, Z.L., Males, R.G., Schmitt, L., Carroll, P.R., James, J.K., Hurd, R.E., and Kurhanewicz, J. 2003. Proton HRMAS spectroscopy and quantitative pathologic analysis of MRI/3D-MRSI-targeted postsurgical prostate tissues. *Magn. Reson. Med. 50*:944–954.

Taylor, J. L., Wu, C. L., Cory, D., Gonzalez, R. G., Bielecki, A., and Cheng, L. L. 2003. High-resolution magic angle spinning proton NMR analysis of human prostate tissue with slow spinning rates. *Magn. Reson. Med. 50*:627–632.

45

Prostate Cancer: Diffusion-Weighted Imaging

Ryota Shimofusa

Introduction

Diffusion-weighted (DW) magnetic resonance (MR) imaging provides potentially unique information on prostatic tissue. DW MR imaging reflects the molecular diffusion of water caused by the random, microscopic translational motion of molecules known as Brownian motion. This imaging technique can provide image contrast that is independent of conventional MR imaging. Although every system has several limitations, DW imaging is easily performed in a short time span on recent MR scanners without additional hardware or software. In the evaluation of prostate cancer, DW MR imaging is a new functional imaging technique that will soon become more universally available to clinicians.

Basics and Recent Advances of Diffusion-Weighted Imaging

The primary application of DW MR imaging has been in brain imaging, mainly for the evaluation of acute ischemic stroke, intracranial tumors, and demyelinating disease. Because DW MR imaging is highly sensitive to gross physiological motion, this technique used to be difficult to apply to abdominal and pelvic organs. However, with the recent advent of the fast imaging technique, DW MR imaging of pelvic organs has become a reality. One of these rapid imaging methods is echo-planar imaging. The use of echo-planar imaging with a preparation pulse sensitive to diffusion allows DW images to be obtained in a subsecond time interval with greatly reduced motion artifacts. On the other hand, the image quality of echo-planar imaging can be influenced by susceptibility artifacts. Susceptibility artifacts occur at the interface of substances with large magnetic susceptibility differences and are prevalent at the boundary of air-containing organs such as the intestines. This is the major problem when obtaining DW images of the prostate, which is located adjacent to gas in the rectum. Most recently, another fast imaging technique, parallel imaging, has become available. By parallel imaging, the accumulating phase that causes susceptibility artifacts is decreased because of a reduction in the train of gradient echoes and sampling time. With these recent technical evolutions, DW imaging of the prostate is now clinically applicable.

The most commonly used sequences of DW imaging are the echo-planar sequences with supplementary gradients, called motion proving gradients, sensitized to the diffusion phenomenon in at least three main axes in space. The intensity and duration of the motion proving gradients are generally denoted as the b-value (sec/mm^2). A b-value of 1000 sec/mm^2 is widely used for brain diffusion studies. As the b-value increases, the degree of diffusion-weighting also increases. However, maximum b-values are usually in the range of 800–2000 sec/mm^2 because of the limits of each MR gradient performance. Higher *b*-values also negatively affect the image quality of DW imaging owing to the prolonged echo time. Because of these limitations, *b*-values less than $800 \, \text{sec/mm}^2$ were used in the preliminary studies of diffusion-weighted imaging of the prostate. The more recent MR gradient technology and parallel imaging technique have permitted the use of higher *b*-values ($b = 1000 - 2000 \, \text{sec/mm}^2$) and greater diffusion sensitivity in prostatic DW imaging.

In a narrow sense, DW MR images are the source images acquired with the motion proving gradients in the three planes. Because DW images are inherently T2-weighted (T2W), changes in tissue T2 can influence the signal intensities of the DW images independent of tissue diffusibility. The effect of prolonged T2 in DW images is known as T2 shine-through. To remove the T2W contrast, an apparent diffusion coefficient (ADC) value is calculated. Decreased ADC value means restricted diffusion. At least two image sets with different *b*-values are needed to determine ADC. Thus, ADC is usually calculated by images with $b = 0 \, \text{sec/mm}^2$ and $b = 1000 \, \text{sec/mm}^2$. It is possible to determine ADC graphically instead. This is accomplished by obtaining more than two image sets. By plotting the natural logarithm of signal intensity versus *b* for these *b* values, ADC can be determined from the slope of the line. An ADC map, which is an image with a signal intensity equal to the magnitude of ADC, allows a quantitative and reproducible assessment of the diffusion changes of the tissue.

Diffusion-Weighted Imaging of Prostate Cancer

MR imaging is widely used for determination of prostatic disease. On conventional T2W imaging, regions of prostate cancer show decreased signal intensity relative to normal peripheral zone tissue because of increased cell density and loss of prostatic ducts. Because of the similarity in signal intensity between prostate cancer and other benign lesions such as benign prostatic hyperplasia on T2W imaging, however, conventional MR imaging has good sensitivity (78–83%) but low specificity (50–55%) in detecting and localizing prostate cancer (Shimofusa *et al.*, 2005). Conventional MR lacks histological specificity, resulting in benign and normal prostatic tissues being interpreted as cancer.

Recent studies (Issa, 2002; Hosseinzadeh and Schwarz, 2004; Sato *et al.*, 2005; Pickles *et al.*, 2006) demonstrated that the ADC values of prostate cancer were significantly lower than those of nonmalignant prostatic tissue. These studies reported that the mean ADC values of prostate cancer ranged from 1.11×10^{-3} to $1.38 \times 10^{-3} \, \text{mm}^2/\text{sec}$, whereas the values of noncancerous tissue were in a range of 1.58×10^{-3} to $1.95 \times 10^{-3} \, \text{mm}^2/\text{sec}$. Although the exact mechanism responsible for the decreasing ADC value is still unknown, the difference may be explained by certain anatomical changes caused by the replacement of normal tissue with cancer. The normal prostate consists of a glandular component of the prostate consisting of water-rich ducts. In prostate cancer, the normal architecture of the gland is replaced by adenocarcinoma. The tumor has numerous small, closely packed glands with little stroma between them, and this tight glandular packing presents increased restriction or hindrance on water displacement.

Reflecting lower ADC, prostate cancer was depicted as a hyperintense focal lesion on DW imaging with markedly enhanced contrast compared with T2W imaging (Fig. 1). Although the most appropriate *b*-value for DW imaging of the prostate is still to be established, a *b*-value higher than the commonly applied value for other abdominal organs ($b = 300 - 800 \, \text{sec/mm}^2$) may be needed to clearly depict prostate cancer. When using a lower *b*-value, the effects of coherent motion (perfusion) and of T2 shine-through become more dominant. The increased effect of coherent motion makes it difficult to assess microscopic diffusibility of cancerous tissue, and the increased T2 shine-through effect may cause decreased contrast enhancement between normal and malignant tissue on DW imaging, as regions of prostate cancer usually show decreased signal intensity relative to normal prostatic tissue on T2W imaging.

There are few reports about DW imaging of prostate cancer with a high *b*-value ($b > 800 \, \text{sec/mm}^2$). This is presumably because the decreased signal-to-noise ratio due to the increased *b*-value makes an adequate evaluation of images difficult. Recent advances in MR gradient technology, however, have enabled us to obtain assessable images with higher *b*-values. We have evaluated the detectability of prostate cancer by combined T2W and DW imaging with a high *b*-value ($b = 1000 \, \text{sec/mm}^2$) and with parallel imaging (Shimofusa *et al.*, 2005). Receiver operating characteristic analysis revealed that the addition of DW imaging to conventional T2W imaging provides better detection of prostate cancer. Another report (Hosseinzadeh and Schwarz, 2004) demonstrated that DW imaging and an ADC map of the prostate with $b = 1000 \, \text{sec/mm}^2$ was possible with an endorectal coil.

Some reports have suggested that DW images, including an ADC map, may also be useful in detecting and discriminating bone and lymph node metastases (Sumi *et al.*, 2003; Park *et al.*, 2004). On DW imaging with a high *b*-value ($b > 800 \, \text{sec/mm}^2$), metastatic bone tumors tend to be depicted as hyperintense (Fig. 2). Although the clinical efficacy is still to be established, DW imaging has the potential to help in the detection of the metastatic focus originating from prostate cancer.

Current Problems and Future Directions of Diffusion-Weighted Imaging

The apparent diffusion coefficient for prostate cancer is significantly less than that for nonmalignant tissue, but some studies (Issa, 2002; Hosseinzadeh and Schwarz, 2004; Pickles

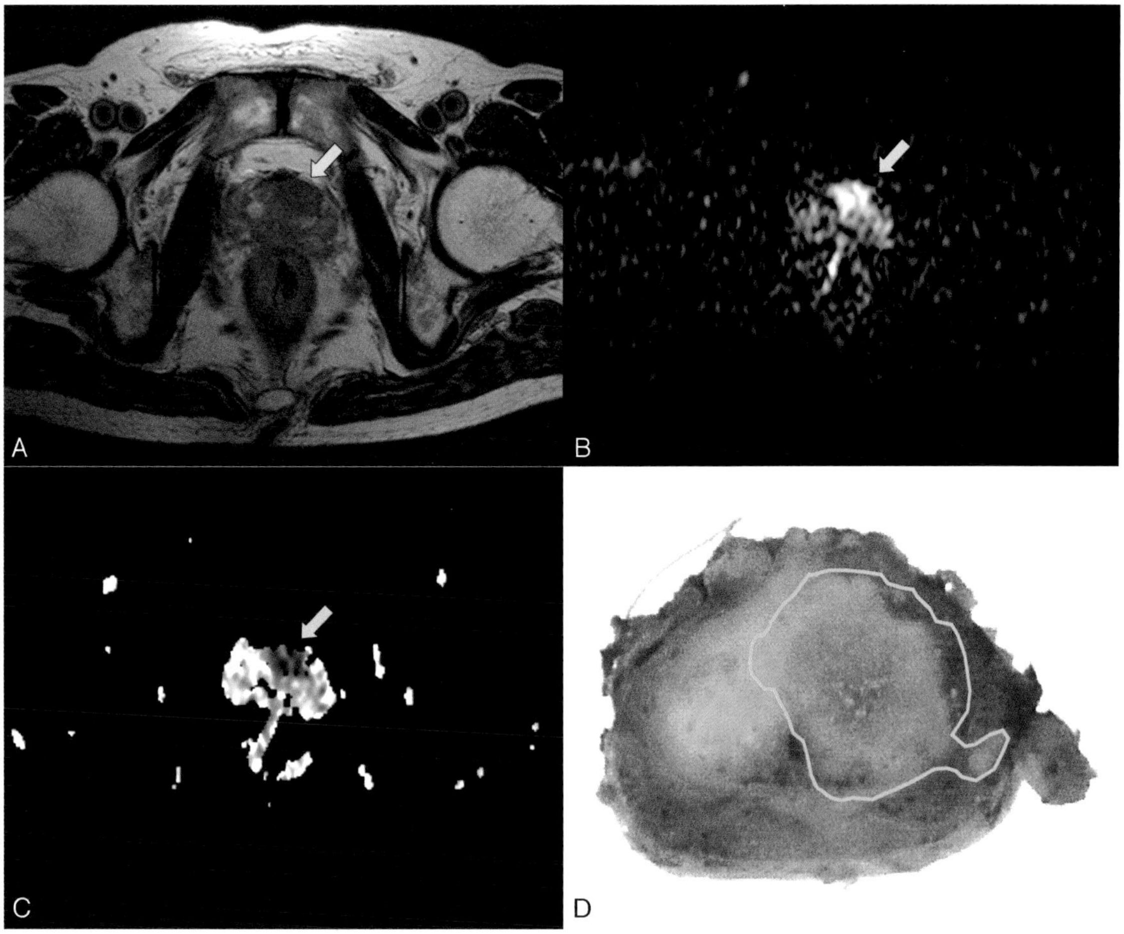

Figure 1 Prostate cancer in a 72-year-old man. (**A**) Axial T2W image (3880 ms/120 ms [repetition time/echo time]) shows a 20-mm diameter hypointense area in the left central gland (arrow). Discrimination of prostate cancer from other benign lesions, such as a benign prostatic hyperplastic nodule, is difficult. (**B**) Axial DW image (2500 ms/90 ms [repetition time/echo time], $b = 1000 \, \text{sec/mm}^2$, with parallel imaging technique) of the same plane clearly demonstrates a focal hyperintense lesion (arrow). (**C**) ADC map image shows decreased signal intensity (arrow), indicating decreased ADC. (**D**) Radical prostatectomy specimen revealed moderately differentiated adenocarcinoma (outlined).

et al., 2006) have also reported an overlap in individual values. The reason for this overlap, presumably, is that tissue structure that can affect the properties of water diffusion is altered due to age-related anatomic changes within the prostate gland. In addition, diffusion properties may also be changed as a result of morphological changes caused by benign disease such as prostatic hyperplasia or hemorrhage. Because of these considerable intersubject variations, a quantitative ADC threshold value presently does not permit distinguishing malignant from nonmalignant prostatic tissue. DW imaging including an ADC map should be used in conjunction with a morphological study with conventional MR imaging as well as together with complementary functional studies, such as dynamic contrast-enhanced study and/or proton MR spectroscopy. Dynamic contrast-enhanced study is believed to provide insights into tissue vasculature. Since angiogenesis is uncontrolled in tumors, their vasculature can be highly permeable, resulting in significantly different pharmacokinetics compared to surrounding

normal tissue. Proton MR spectroscopy allows metabolites within tissues to be examined. The healthy peripheral zone is known to have a high citrate content, whereas in areas of prostate tumor the resonance signal from citrate is reduced or even absent.

Echo-planar imaging-based DW imaging is a technique with an inherently low signal-to-noise ratio and low resolution. As a result, a small cancer focus or a small extracapsular extension can be missed or misdiagnosed. Multiple averaging should be performed to increase the signal-to-noise ratio, which would result in a relatively long scan time. 3.0 Tesla-MR (Pickles *et al.*, 2006) or an endorectal coil (Hosseinzadeh and Schwarz, 2004) may be alternative solutions for increasing the signal-to-noise ratio and resolution. Applying these techniques, DW imaging may have the potential to assess extracapsular extensions of prostate cancer with high spatial resolution, and it may contribute to improving staging accuracy.

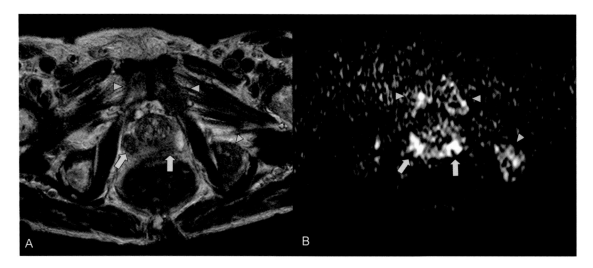

Figure 2 Prostate cancer in an 82-year-old man, with multiple bone metastases. (**A**) Axial T2W image (3900 ms/120 ms [repetition time/echo time]) revealed prostate cancer as multiple hypointense foci in the peripheral zone (arrows). Multiple hypointense lesions, suggesting bone metastases, are also shown in the pelvic bone (arrowheads). (**B**) Axial DW image (2500 ms/90 ms [repetition time/echo time], $b = 1000$ sec/mm², with parallel imaging technique) of the same plane clearly demonstrates prostate and pelvic bone lesions as focal hyperintense areas with markedly enhanced contrast compared with T2W imaging (arrows and arrowheads).

Diffusion anisotropy of prostatic tissue can also be measured by DW imaging. Diffusion tensor imaging, which can be obtained by six or more directions of the motion-proving gradients, provides information regarding diffusion anisotropy and fiber orientation. Reportedly, the diffusion properties in prostate tissue are anisotropic, and the prostate fiber orientations are predominantly in the superior-inferior direction for both the peripheral zone and central gland, consistent with the tissue architecture (Sinha and Sinha, 2004). By measuring diffusion anisotropy and orientation, early changes in the structural organization of prostate tissue can be detected before any gross morphological changes take place. It is hoped that the diffusion tensor imaging technique will contribute to earlier and more specific diagnosis of prostate cancer.

In conclusion, DW imaging is a relatively new functional imaging technique complementary to conventional MR imaging in the evaluation of prostate cancer. Diffusion-weighted imaging is certain to become an important option for prostate cancer detection and characterization.

References

Hosseinzadeh, K., and Schwarz, S.D. 2004. Endorectal diffusion-weighted imaging in prostate cancer to differentiate malignant and benign peripheral zone tissue. *J. Magn. Reson. Imaging 20*:654–661.

Issa, B. 2002. *In vivo* measurement of the apparent diffusion coefficient in normal and malignant prostatic tissues using echo-planar imaging. *J. Magn. Reson. Imaging 16*:196–200.

Park, S.W., Lee, J.H., Ehara, S., Park, Y.B., Sung, S.O., Choi, J.A., and Joo, Y.E. 2004. Single shot fast spin echo diffusion-weighted MR imaging of the spine; is it useful in differentiating malignant metastatic tumor infiltration from benign fracture edema? *Clin. Imaging 28*:102–108.

Pickles, M.D., Gibbs, P., Sreenivas, M., and Turnbull, L.W. 2006. Diffusion-weighted imaging of normal and malignant prostate tissue at 3.0T. *J. Magn. Reson. Imaging 23*:130–134.

Sato, C., Naganawa, S., Nakamura, T., Kumada, H., Miura, S., Takizawa, O., and Ishigaki, T. 2005. Differentiation of noncancerous tissue and cancer lesions by apparent diffusion coefficient values in transition and peripheral zones of the prostate. *J. Magn. Reson. Imaging 21*:258–262.

Shimofusa, R., Fujimoto, H., Akamata, H., Motoori, K., Yamamoto, S., Ueda, T., and Ito, H. 2005. Diffusion-weighted imaging of prostate cancer. *J. Comput. Assist. Tomogr. 29*:149–153.

Sinha, S., and Sinha, U. 2004. In vivo diffusion tensor imaging of the human prostate. *Magn. Reson. Med. 52*:530–537.

Sumi, M., Sakihama, N., Sumi, T., Morikawa, M., Uetani, M., Kabasawa, H., Shigeno, K., Hayashi, K., Takahashi, H., and Nakamura, T. 2003. Discrimination of metastatic cervical lymph nodes with diffusion-weighted MR imaging in patients with head and neck cancer. *AJNR Am. J. Neuroradiol. 24*:1627–1634.

46

Prostatic Secretory Protein of 94 Amino Acids Gene-Directed Transgenic Prostate Cancer: Three-Dimensional Ultrasound Microimaging

Jim W. Xuan, James C. Lacefield, Lauren A. Wirtzfeld,
Michael Bygrave, Hongyi Jiang, Jonathan I. Izawa, Madeleine Moussa,
Joseph L. Chin, and Aaron Fenster

Introduction

Prostate cancer (PC) is the most common cancer in adult men in North America. Mice have been the most prominent model organisms for preclinical cancer research. However, PC does not occur naturally in rodents, so preclinical studies frequently employ genetically engineered (GE) mouse models for basic research and preclinical studies. These GE mouse PC models normally employ promoters from prostate specific genes. In this chapter, we review the utilization of a prostate tissue specific gene, PSP94 (prostate secretory protein of 94 amino acids) to specifically target expression of the oncogene, SV40 T antigen (T and/or1), in the prostate gland. We established two PSP94 gene-directed mouse PC models: the TGMAP (Trans-Genic Mouse Adenocarcinoma Prostate) and KIMAP (Knock-In Mouse Adenocarcinoma Prostate). The TGMAP model exhibits the features of highly precise prostate-tissue specific

targeting and mimics the widely used TRAMP model in terms of tumorigenesis and rapid tumor growth kinetics. We have demonstrated that three-dimensional ultrasound microimaging of the TGMAP model enables longitudinal measurements of tumor volume and growth kinetics, and that correspondence of tumor histology and ultrasound image texture aids interpretation of the ultrasonic appearance of TGMAP tumors. The utility of ultrasound microimaging for assessing tumor progression and treatment response in GE models of PC will improves as technology for imaging tumor blood flow becomes available.

Genetically Engineered Mouse Prostate Cancer Models

Transgenic models of PC were first generated in the mid-1990s and now are fast becoming the models of choice

(Greenberg *et al.*, 1995). In general, transgenic models feature higher penetrance, faster progression, and greater overall reproducibility of metastatic properties compared to other spontaneous, steroid, or hormone-induced PC models (reviewed by Winter *et al.*, 2003).

The transgenic adenocarcinoma of the mouse prostate (TRAMP) model developed by Greenberg *et al.* (1995) is the most widely used model in the world in both basic and preclinical studies. The TRAMP model is based on a minimal rat probasin promoter (rat PB, −426/+28) directing expression of the heterologous simian virus 40 (SV40) early genes (T/t, large T and small t; Tag) specifically to the mouse prostatic epithelium. Consistent with the spatial and temporal expression pattern of the rat PB gene, PB-Tag expression begins between 4 and 6 weeks of age, and TRAMP mice consequently develop mild to severe prostatic hyperplasia by 12 weeks of age. At 24 weeks of age, virtually 100% of male mice have poorly differentiated and invasive PC. Lymph node and lung metastases are common in these mice, while osseous, renal, and adrenal metastases are also observed. Castration of TRAMP mice at 12 weeks of age causes an initial regression of the prostate, indicating that tumors are initially androgen sensitive. Castration at 12 weeks is curative in 20% of TRAMP mice, but the remainder eventually progress to poorly differentiated, androgen-insensitive PC with frequent metastases by 24 weeks of age.

The LADY model (reviewed by Abate-Shen and Shen, 2002) is based on a large rat PB promoter (11.5 kb/+28) driving the expression of only the SV40 large T antigen to the prostate epithelium. Seven transgenic lines have been generated and are collectively called the "LADY" system. Six of the seven lines develop androgen-dependent (AD) PC that rarely metastasizes. However, one line, 12T-10, exhibits reproducible metastases with both glandular and neuroendocrine (NE) characteristics. At least 14 different kinds of vector genes have been tested for prostate targeting in GE-PC modeling (Winter *et al.*, 2003). However, the majority of genes are not prostate-tissue specific (Abate-Shen and Shen, 2002).

Brief Review of PSP94

PSP94 (Prostatic Secretory Protein of 94 Amino Acids), also known as β-Microseminoprotein (β-MSP), is one of the three most abundant secretory proteins (the other two are PSA—prostate specific antigen—and PAP—prostatic acid phosphatase) of the prostate gland. Although PSP94 is abundantly (at a concentration of mg/ml) secreted in the semen, its real biological function is still unknown. A variety of functions have been hypothesized (for a mini-review see Xuan *et al.*, 1999). The function of PSP94 in the female pig is also reported by its preferential expression at the functional stage of the corpus luteum. We hypothesized that PSP94 may serve as a barrier for interspecies fertilization (Xuan *et al.*, 1999).

PSP94 was proposed to be a prostatic inhibin protein (PSP) or β-inhibin, which refers to its possible function as a tumor suppressor, an inhibitory factor for the secretion of β-follicle stimulating hormone (FSH) from the pituitary gland. Recently, its inhibitory function, or tumor suppressor function, has been reported (Shukeir *et al.*, 2003). However, this function was not confirmed, as the real β-inhibin/activin from the prostate was widely recognized as a 60-kDa protein from the prostate (Risbridger *et al.*, 2001).

Studies in human, primate, porcine, and rodent (Fernlund *et al.*, 1996) PSP94 have shown that PSP94 is a conserved, but also a rapidly evolving, protein (Xuan *et al.*, 1999). PSP94 or PSP94-like molecules have been identified in birds (ratite), bovids, batracians, and fish (Lazure *et al.*, 2001). This is in contrast to rPB and PSA, where neither human probasin nor mouse PSA homologues have been identified. However, the only structural connection among these species is with the conserved cysteine-rich sites, and no definitive biological functions have been identified. Promoter region of PSP94 gene and isoforms of PSP94 protein have been studied in various species. The promoter region of PSP94/β-MSP has been cloned and sequenced from human, primates, and rodents (Xuan *et al.*, 1999).

As with PSA and PAP, PSP94 has been localized in the prostate epithelial cells by immunohistochemistry (IHC) and *in situ* hybridization (ISH). PSP94 expression in PC tissue by IHC and ISH showed decreased levels as compared to benign prostate tissue, and more intense staining in prostate tissue was associated with a better prognosis. As with PSA (prostatic specific antigen), the decreased level of PSP94 expression in PC tissue can account for the decreased free form of PSP94 in serum, which normally represents the level of secreted proteins (e.g., PSP94 and PSA) leaking into the systemic circulation. In contrast, levels of serum bound and total PSP94 determined by enzyme-linked immunosorbent assay (ELISA) were elevated in PC patients. As with differential testing of PSA (ratio of free-to-total serum PSA), PSP94 has been shown to exist in serum in both free and bound forms (Reeves *et al.*, 2005). Preliminary clinical results demonstrate the potential of PSP94 as a serum prognostic marker for PC patients (Reeves *et al.*, 2005).

As with PSA (prostatic specific antigen), PSP94 is a prostate tissue-specific protein. PSA and PSP94 are predominant secretory proteins of the prostate. We have found prostate-tissue-specific gene expression in human tissues, in both rat and mouse PSP94 (Xuan *et al.*, 1999). PSP94 is specific to the peripheral zone (where most human PC occurs) in the human prostate. Both PSA and PSP94 were initially believed to be prostate tissue specific; however, both were later found to be present in a number of secretory tissues and fluids: lung, paraurethral and perianal glands, bronchi, trachea, gastric juice, milk, amniotic fluid, and saliva. The pattern of tissue distribution in humans and other primates indicates that PSP94 is possibly a mucous secretory protein

(Fernlund *et al.*, 1996). However, these observations have not been confirmed in rodents (Xuan *et al.*, 1999) and porcine subjects. Moreover, in humans, these observations were made mostly in clinical and pathological samples. Nonprostate tissue PSP94 (ng/ml) has been detected in much lower magnitudes than prostatic PSP94 (mg/ml). As demonstrated in our transgenic and knock-out mouse experiments testing the temporal and spatial specificity of the mouse PSP94 promoter, the PSP94 gene appears to be a prostate tissue-specific gene, because we have never observed any tumor formation in extraprostatic tissues secretions, including gastric, bronchial, and tracheal tissues.

A number of reports (Fernlund *et al.*, 1996; Imasato *et al.*, 2001) indicated that rat PSP94 was found specifically in the dorsal lateral prostate (DLP). The lateral prostate lobe (LP) expressed the highest level of PSP94 mRNA and protein, respectively. The differential distribution pattern of PSP94 has been examined differential distribution pattern of PSP94 expression specifically in the peripheral zone in fetal, pubertal, and adult human prostates by ISH and IHC.

PSP94 Gene-Directed Genetically Engineered Mouse Prostate Cancer Models

The promoter/enhancer region of the mouse PSP94 gene has been utilized to establish two mouse GE-PC models: the PSP-TGMAP model (PSP94-directed transgenic mouse adenocarcinoma of the prostate) (Gabril *et al.*, 2002) and the PSP-KIMAP model (PSP94 gene-directed knock-in of adenocarcinoma of the prostate) (Duan *et al.*, 2005). Both of these genetically engineered models are based on mouse prostate tissue-specific targeting and expression of an SV40 Tag (T/t) oncogene.

To determine whether the PSP94 promoter/enhancer region is capable of directing the prostate tissue-specific transgene expression, a series of progressive deletions of the promoter/enhancer region fused with a reporter gene (Lac Z) were constructed for *in vitro* cell culture studies. Two transgenes (183 and 186) were constructed using both SV40T/t antigens. Transgene 183 contains exon 1 and 186 contains part of intron 1 sequences, in addition to the promoter/enhancer, in order to enhance the transgene expression. Transgenic mice were identified by a quick PCR test of toe/tail samples, followed by Southern blotting experiments (Gabril *et al.*, 2002).

After breeding with wild-type [C57BL/6 × CBA] F1 hybrids, out of 18 transgenic mice, 3 transgenic founder breeding lines (F0 of A, B, C) were characterized and successfully established: line A from transgene 183 (183–2) and lines B and C from 186. In this study, most of the TGMAP mice are from the 183A line (Fig. 1), because of its stable phenotype and rapid tumor growth. Targeting of transgene

expression in three transgenic breeding lines specifically to the prostate was first demonstrated. The PSP-TGMAP model was further characterized and demonstrated in three breeding lines by correlating tumor grades with age (10–32 weeks), and IHC staining of SV40 Tag protein expression in the prostate with tumor grading (Fig. 1D–G) (Gabril *et al.*, 2002). According to the diagnostic criteria set up in human PC and the basic conceptual similarity, the neoplastic changes were classified using the following five grading categories: low and high mouse PIN, well-differentiated PC, moderately differentiated PC, and poorly differentiated PC. Tumor progression and metastasis at 20 weeks of age in one PSP-TGMAP line (A) were found. Metastatic deposits were observed primarily in lymph nodes (Fig. 1A and 1B), as well as in the lung, liver, and kidney. Since androgen responsiveness is a physiologic characteristic of the prostate, two groups (A and C) of mice at 20–26 weeks of age were selected by responsiveness to castration. The responsiveness of the PSP94-TGMAP model to androgen deprivation was demonstrated by involution of the prostate and elimination of SV40 Tag expression as early as two weeks until one month after castration. Castrated A line mice refractory to androgen deprivation were identified. The PSP94-TGMAP model demonstrated similarities to the most commonly used transgenic mouse prostate cancer model, the TRAMP model (Greenberg *et al.*, 1995). These features include spatial (prostate tissue) and temporal (postpuberty) specificity of tumor induction, rapidity of tumor growth, histopathology, androgen dependence, and responsiveness and refractoriness to androgen deprivation therapy (Gabril *et al.*, 2002).

The knock-in technology with this KIMAP model demonstrates highly predictive cancer development and has some advantages over the traditional transgenic technique-derived PC models (Duan *et al.*, 2005). These advantages include the stability of both the phenotype and genotype, the synchronicity of prostate cancer development, the precision of prostate tissue targeting, and the absence of founder-line variability. As a mouse preclinical model, fast-growing PC is preferable for short-term studies. Since most tumors in the KIMAP model were very small and slowly growing, in this regard, the PSP-KIMAP model is less suitable than the PSP-TGMAP model for noninvasive microimaging studies. However, since the majority of men in North America who are diagnosed with prostate cancer are at low to intermediate risk for disease-specific mortality, the KIMAP models may have other utility for preclinical studies.

The terms *microscopic* and *macroscopic* cancer were introduced in this microimaging study to distinguish tumors of sizes that could be expected to be detectable with ultrasound microimaging from cancer on scales relevant to histopathology. Macroscopic tumors, meaning PC larger than 1 mm in diameter, were the focus of the imaging studies. However, it should be noted that mice from both the PSP-TGMAP and PSP-KIMAP models that are classified as

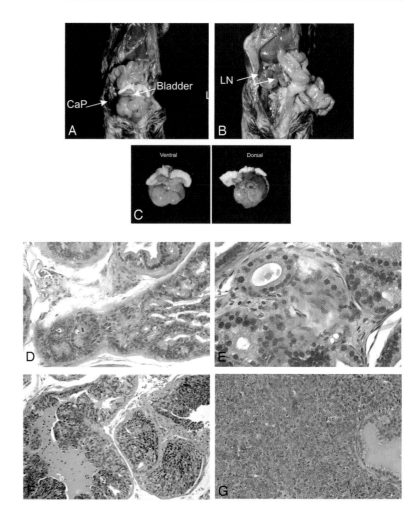

Figure 1 (**A**) Gross pathological dissection of a transgenic mouse at 16 weeks of age. Arrows show locations of the bladder and a large-sized (2.5 cm in diameter) prostate cancer. (**B**) The same mouse showing enlarged renal lymph nodes after removal of the large prostate cancer mass. (**C**) Dissected transgenic prostate tumor viewed from dorsal and ventral sides separately. (**D–G**) Histopathological determination of genetically engineered CaP for mPIN (mouse prostatic intraepithelial neoplasia, (**D**), well (**E**), moderately (**F**), and poorly differentiated (**G**) CaP.

tumor negative by ultrasound still possess microscopic foci of various degrees of mouse PC that have not formed large, fast-growing masses.

Microimaging of GE-PC Mouse Models: Importance of Noninvasive Techniques

Tumor initiation in transgenic models varies over a significant period of time, so it is difficult to evaluate the early stages of tumor progression using conventional biological methods. Prostate tumor development in transgenic models cannot be detected by palpation until the tumor reaches 0.5 to 1 cm in diameter. At this size, the tumors may already have passed clinically relevant stages for diagnosis and treatment. Therefore, noninvasive imaging techniques are required to monitor tumor initiation and development in mouse PC models. The ability to noninvasively quantify tumor burden in live mouse models will ultimately lead to the development

of more accurate models of human cancer that are better suited for preclinical evaluation and optimization of cancer therapy.

Microimaging systems, by definition, provide *in vivo* spatial resolution finer than 200 μm, which yields anatomical detail in mice comparable to that obtained in clinical imaging of humans. Microimaging of mouse cancer models can be performed using instruments analogous to any of the prominent medical imaging modalities, including X-ray computed tomography (CT), magnetic resonance imaging (MRI) and spectroscopy, radionuclide imaging, and ultrasound, as well as optical techniques such as bioluminescence imaging and optical coherence tomography (Weissleder, 2002). Selection of a microimaging modality involves balancing trade-offs between equipment costs, spatial resolution, image acquisition time, the technical feasibility of imaging specific regions of the body, and the sensitivity and specificity of anatomic, functional, and molecular information required for a particular application.

Preclinical imaging studies of prostate cancer models have been reported using several modalities. For example, micro-positron emission tomography (microPET) has been used to monitor the growth of xenograft tumors in immunodeficient mice (Yang *et al.*, 2003). The LNCaP tumors cells that are frequently used in preclinical models were transfected with a PET reporter gene, which allowed the tumors to be monitored with microPET imaging and the PET image to be confirmed postmortem with autoradiographic images. Hsu *et al.* (1998) employed MRI to longitudinally monitor the growth of tumors in their TRAMP model. Differences in tumor growth were measured in castrated versus normal TRAMP mice in that study. The development of prostate-specific promoters has also made *in vivo* monitoring of transgenic expression possible using bioluminescence imaging of luciferase reporter genes. This technique was first demonstrated by manipulation of human PSA promoter-directed luciferase in recombinant adenovirus in a xenograft-based model (Adams *et al.*, 2002).

Ultrasound is another modality that can be used for preclinical imaging of mouse PC models. Ultrasound is the most frequently used clinical diagnostic imaging modality, accounting for ~ 25% of all imaging exams worldwide. Most clinical ultrasound systems employ frequencies in the range of 5 to 12 MHz, which provide in-plane spatial resolution on the order of 0.5 to 1.0 mm. In contrast, ultrasound microimaging systems use frequencies > 20 MHz to produce high-resolution images, e.g., ~ 100 µm when imaging at 30 MHz. The depth of penetration of high-frequency ultrasound into tissue is limited to ~ 5 to 15 mm by frequency-dependent attenuation, which restricts clinical applications of high-frequency ultrasound to dermatology, ophthalmology, and intravascular imaging, but has sufficient penetration depth for most mouse imaging tasks.

The primary goals of preclinical imaging of small-animal cancer models are usually to detect tumors as early as possible after initiation and to follow the progression or regression of tumors over time. It is therefore desirable for a preclinical imaging system to be able to acquire and display images rapidly to facilitate monitoring of a large number of mice, while minimizing the risks to the animals created by repeated imaging. Ultrasound microimaging systems produce images in real time, implying at least 30 two-dimensional frames are acquired and displayed each second. Repeated ultrasound exposure is not hazardous to the animal, and anatomical imaging does not require injection of exogenous contrast agents or genetic manipulation of reporter cell lines. These characteristics are especially attractive for longitudinal studies.

Two-dimensional (2D) imaging is often sufficient for lesion detection. However, three-dimensional (3D) imaging provides more accurate tumor volume measurements than volumes estimated from 2D images, because volume estimation from 2D images requires an assumption that the image plane contains the maximum tumor diameter and the tumor has a smooth spherical or ellipsoidal shape.

In addition, 3D imaging depicts more landmarks in the anatomy surrounding a tumor, which is valuable for identifying individual tumors during longitudinal studies of models that exhibit multifocal cancers. For the reasons outlined in the preceding paragraphs, our laboratory employs 3D ultrasound microimaging for longitudinal studies of the PSP-TGMAP model.

PSP-TGMAP Microimaging Methods

Image Acquisition

During an ultrasound examination, mice are anesthetized by inhalation of isoflurane and are positioned on a heated stage to maintain body temperature. The abdomen is depilated with a consumer hair removal cream and ultrasound contact gel is applied over the area of interest to enhance transmission of ultrasound into the animal.

Ultrasound images are acquired using a Vevo 660 microimaging system (VisualSonics Inc., Toronto, Ontario, Canada) similar in design to the instrument described by Foster *et al.* (2002). This system includes on-board three-dimensional image reconstruction and visualization software developed by our laboratory (Fenster *et al.*, 2001). All images of the PSP-TGMAP model are acquired using a mechanically scanned 30 MHz probe that produces a 55 × 115 × 115 µm³ resolution volume at the 12.7 mm focal depth.

To acquire 3D images, the ultrasound probe is translated by a stepper motor, and parallel planes are acquired at a spacing of 30 µm. Three-dimensional images of the region of interest are acquired, including the tumor, prostate, bladder, and seminal vesicles. Images showing a volume 12 × 12 × 9 mm³ are acquired and displayed in approximately 30 seconds. The total time to prepare a mouse and acquire a complete set of 3D images is about 30 min. Tumor volumes can be measured in the 3D images by manually outlining the tumor in closely spaced parallel planes, summing the cross-sectional areas of the outlines, and multiplying by the slice thickness (Fenster *et al.*, 2001).

Initial Imaging Studies

Initial cross-sectional and longitudinal imaging studies were performed to determine the sensitivity and specificity of 3D ultrasound microimaging for detecting PSP-TGMAP prostate tumors and demonstrate the use of 3D ultrasound to measure the growth of the tumors *in situ*. In addition, qualitative comparison of ultrasound images with hemotoxylin and eosin (H&E)-stained histology slides suggested some histologic features of PSP-TGMAP tumors that may contribute to tumor detection in the ultrasound images. The methods employed in these studies are summarized in the following paragraphs and were described in detail by Wirtzfeld *et al.* (2005).

After mice were euthanized, the prostate tissue including the VP, DLP, and AP, the male accessory gland (seminal vesicles), and the entire urinary tract were removed for gross examination and serial sectioning. The excised tissues were fixed, embedded in paraffin, sliced into 5-μm thick slides, and H&E-stained. Every tenth slide (i.e., slides at 50-μm spacing) was digitized at 10× magnification using a video microscopy system. Three-dimensional serial histology images were constructed from the digitized slides.

Visual correlation of ultrasound and histology images was achieved by slicing through a 3D ultrasound image in different orientations to search for ultrasound views that matched the planes of the histology slides from that tumor. Corresponding planes were identified by comparing the shape of the prostate and the appearance of regions of the most poorly differentiated high-grade tumor in the ultrasound and histology images, and by using the points where the seminal vesicles joined the prostate as anatomical landmarks for aligning the two sets of images.

Tumors were identified prospectively in the 3D ultrasound images by consensus of the ultrasound system operators and retrospectively by a blinded radiologist experienced in human prostate ultrasound imaging. The accuracy of each diagnosis was determined based on the presence or absence of macroscopic tumors larger than 1 mm diameter that were identified at autopsy and confirmed to be cancerous by histopathology. These data were used to compute tumor detection sensitivities and specificities for the ultrasound microimaging system.

To verify ultrasound tumor size measurements, maximum sagittal diameters of macroscopic tumors were measured using a ruler and compared to diameters measured using the 3D ultrasound image analysis software. Pearson's correlation coefficient, r, was computed for the paired ultrasound and gross pathology diameter estimates. A p-value of less than 0.05 from a t-test was considered evidence of statistically significant correlation.

Diameter growth curves were constructed for tumors that remained small enough to fit within the 12×12-mm^2 two-dimensional field-of-view of the ultrasound system in at least three imaging sessions, and volume growth curves were constructed for tumors that were contained by the $12 \times 12 \times 9$-mm^3 three-dimensional ultrasound field-of-view in at least three imaging sessions. For each tumor, the measured diameters (or volumes) were plotted as functions of time elapsed since initial detection, separate exponential growth curves were fit by linear regression, and doubling times were estimated from the fitted curves. Agreement between the experimental data and the fitted exponentials was assessed by computing coefficients of determination, r^2, for the fitted curves.

Results of PSP-TGMAP Imaging Studies

Three-dimensional ultrasound images were compared with reconstructed serial histology sections to show the fidelity of the ultrasound images of PSP-TGMAP tumors. Figure 2A shows three orthogonal planes through a 3D ultrasound image of a VP tumor and Figure 2B shows orthogonal planes through a 3D reconstruction of 70 H&E-stained serial histology slides obtained from the same tumor. Figure 2C shows a transverse two-dimensional ultrasound image of this tumor, and Figure 2D shows the corresponding 4× magnification histology slide.

Figure 2 illustrates several characteristics of the PSP-TGMAP tumor model that can be observed using 3D ultrasound microimaging. First, the size and shape of the tumor can be determined by slicing through the image volume. Second, the ultrasound image plane in Figure 2C shows a hypoechoic ring (i.e., the outer tumor area scatters ultrasound weakly and therefore appears dark in the image) surrounding a central region of heterogeneous image texture. High-magnification histologic examination indicates that the outer hypoechoic area consisted of a high density of sheets of poorly differentiated PC cells, including small cell carcinoma, with few blood vessels. The high-power view of the H&E-stained slides also reveals that the central core, where the tumor appears brighter in the ultrasound images, contains a lower density of poorly differentiated PC cells surrounded by vascular and hemorrhaged regions. The histology slides show that the peripheral dark ring and the brighter central area are separated by a thin layer of ill-defined fibrous stroma tissues. The appearance of a hypoechoic outer ring appears to be the primary factor that allows these murine prostate tumors to be detected in ultrasound images.

Prospective diagnoses of tumor development were determined from ultrasound images acquired from 33 mice, including 14 with macroscopic prostate tumors subsequently confirmed by pathology and 19 without macroscopic tumors. Tumor detection sensitivity and specificity were 95% and 100%, respectively, which demonstrates that ultrasound microimaging is a reliable means of assessing tumor development in PSP-TGMAP mice.

Paired sagittal diameter measurements obtained from 3D ultrasound images and gross pathology specimens of 11 tumors showed good agreement. Pearson's correlation coefficient indicated significant correlation ($r = 0.998$, $p < 0.001$) between the ultrasound and gross pathology diameter measurements. This result demonstrates that the regions of the prostate identified as cancerous by ultrasound are consistent with the cancerous regions identified by gross pathology.

Exponential growth curves closely fit longitudinal measurements of sagittal tumor diameter. The coefficients of determination, r^2, for the four diameter growth curves ranged from 0.943 to 0.996. Diameter doubling times estimated

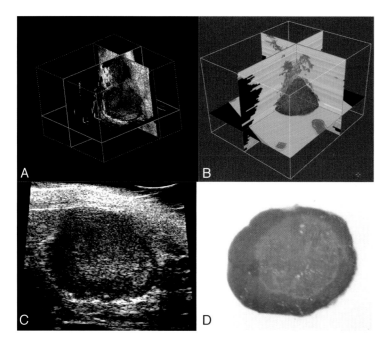

Figure 2 Corresponding ultrasound and histology images of a 7-mm diameter PSP-TGMAP tumor. (**A**) 3D ultrasound image displayed in three orthogonal planes through the tumor. (**B**) Corresponding view of a 3D serial H&E-histology reconstruction of the same tumor. (**C**) A 2D slice through the 3D ultrasound volume. (**D**) An H&E-histology slide corresponding to the ultrasound image in (c), displayed at 4× magnification. Reprinted with permission from Wirtzfeld *et al.* (2005).

from the exponential curve fits were between 10.3 and 42.8 days for these tumors. Exponential functions also fit the volume growth data well ($r^2 = 0.939$ and 0.986) in the two tumors from which at least three volume measurements were obtained. Volume doubling times estimated from the exponential curve fits were 4.9 and 12.9 days. These results indicate that the exponential function accurately describes PSP-TGMAP tumor development during the rapid phase of growth observed in this study.

Since ultrasound microimaging can be used to both detect murine prostate tumors as small as 2 to 3 mm diameter and document tumor growth in longitudinal studies, ultrasound imaging is expected to be effective for evaluating treatment responses in transgenic PC models. For example, ultrasound microimaging has been used to measure a delay in PSP-TGMAP tumor growth following castration (Van Huizen *et al.*, 2005). Measurements of growth delays following treatments are a commonly used preclinical outcome measure because the duration of growth delay is considered an indication of the proportion of the tumor cells killed by a treatment.

Future Directions: Imaging of Prostate Tumor Vascularity

The 2D and 3D ultrasound imaging techniques described in this chapter are limited to providing morphological information about tumor size, growth rate, shape, and possibly changes in internal microstructure. However, functional information relevant to preclinical PC research can be obtained from ultrasound Doppler imaging, which can be used to detect blood flow and measure flow velocity. Blood flow can be measured directly from ultrasound echoes produced by moving red blood cells, so Doppler flow images have the attractive characteristic of being acquired without the use of injected contrast agents.

The development of noninvasive blood flow measurement technologies will be particularly valuable for cancer research because angiogenesis, the formation of new blood vessels, is an essential aspect of disease progression. The extent of tumor vascularization and the organization of the vascularity may provide important clues about the biological processes involved in tumor initiation and growth. In addition, angiogenesis is considered a promising therapeutic target, and the ability to measure tumor vascularity in mice would allow prospective anti-angiogenic agents to be tested in preclinical models.

Two approaches to displaying Doppler ultrasound flow data are in widespread use. One method is *color Doppler* imaging, in which image pixels are color-coded, usually using red for flow directed toward the ultrasound probe and blue for flow away from the probe, to represent the mean blood velocity at each location in the image. Color Doppler images display 2D or 3D maps of the vasculature that enable discrimination between regions of slow and fast flow. However, accurate estimation of flow velocities requires the angle between the blood flow direction and the axis of the ultrasound beam to be determined everywhere in the field-of-view, which can be a difficult task in the tortuous vessels frequently associated with tumors. This Doppler angle artifact can complicate interpretation of color Doppler images of tumors.

The second prominent approach to ultrasound blood flow imaging, *power Doppler*, is named for the fact that the images are colored to depict the total ultrasound power reflected from moving blood cells. Power Doppler images display a quantity proportional to the number of moving blood cells, rather than their velocity, at each point in the image, typically using an orange-to-yellow color scale with more saturated colors corresponding to higher concentrations of moving cells. This approach eliminates the angle dependence of the flow measurement and also serves to reduce the level of noise in the image, which can be beneficial for detecting flow in circumstances where the ultrasound signal received from the blood is relatively weak. The latter characteristic of power Doppler implies an improved ability to detect low concentrations of moving blood cells compared to color Doppler, but it does not imply an improved ability to detect very slow flow (Ferrara *et al.*, 2000). Both color and power Doppler systems ignore echoes suggesting flow at velocities slower than a few millimeters per second to prevent the images from being overwhelmed by artifacts arising from soft tissue motion.

Recent progress in ultrasound technology has enabled development of high-frequency color (Kruse *et al.*, 1998) and power (Goertz *et al.*, 2002) Doppler systems suitable for preclinical applications. Frequency-dependent ultrasound attenuation limits the maximum depth of Doppler measurements to the same 5 to 15 mm cut-off observed in anatomical imaging. However, the primary advantage of high-frequency Doppler compared to clinical Doppler systems is that the high-frequency systems provide sufficient spatial resolution to potentially distinguish adjacent vessels separated by 100 to 200 μm, which is the spatial scale needed to depict tumor microvasculature (Ferrara *et al.*, 2000). Realization of this potential will depend in part on future improvements in the sensitivity of Doppler ultrasound to the slow velocities typical of capillary flow, which is a topic of active research.

As an example of the current state of the art in preclinical Doppler imaging, Figure 3 shows 2D and 3D power Doppler images of a 7.3-mm diameter PSP-TGMAP tumor acquired in our laboratory. The 3D power Doppler image was reconstructed and displayed using flow imaging software developed by our research team (Fenster *et al.*, 2001). The 3D image effectively depicts the three-dimensional nature of the tumor's blood supply (Xuan *et al.*, 2007), including the tortuosity and complex bifurcations of the vascular tree. Capsular vessels appearing as branching structures around the outside of the tumor are commonly seen in power Doppler images of the PSP-TGMAP model. In our preliminary studies, intratumor vessels have been more readily detected in larger tumors at later stages of development.

Recent reports have demonstrated the ability of high-frequency 3D color and power (Goertz *et al.*, 2002) Doppler to measure the responses of an orthotopic melanoma model to an antivascular agent. Doppler images acquired immediately before, 4 hr after, and 24 hr after injection of the antivascular

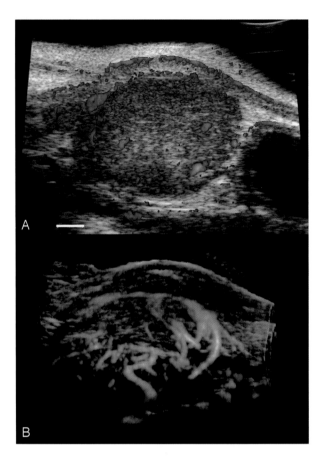

Figure 3 Vascular images of a 7.2-mm diameter (140 mm³ volume) PSP-TGMAP tumor. (**A**) In a 2D slice through the 3D gray-scale and power Doppler image, blood flow is depicted in the skin, around the tumor (capsular vessels), and within the tumor (intratumoral). (**B**) In a 3D-rendered power Doppler image of the same tumor, vessels are depicted surrounding the tumor, and some smaller vessels are apparent within the tumor. The scale bar in (A) is 1 mm.

agent demonstrated a significant reduction in the first four hours of the total Doppler power measured from blood flow within the tumors, followed by recovery of Doppler-detected flow between 4 and 24 hr. The flow levels measured by Doppler ultrasound were correlated with Hoechst perfusion staining results.

The literature addressing clinical color and power Doppler imaging of prostate cancer indicates some potential contributions of high-frequency Doppler to studies of preclinical PC models. For example, the use of power Doppler imaging has been shown to improve the positive predictive value of ultrasound for discriminating benign from malignant prostate lesions compared to diagnoses based on anatomical ultrasound imaging alone (Inahara *et al.*, 2004). This result suggests that power Doppler may improve the ability of ultrasound microimaging to detect small (i.e., < 3 mm diameter) prostate tumors, which typically yield lower contrast images than larger tumors in the PSP-TGMAP model. Prostate tumor vascularity depicted by clinical power Doppler also appears to be qualitatively correlated with histological estimates of microvessel density in pathology samples (Wilson *et al.*, 2004; Xuan *et al.*, 2007). Microvessel density is correlated with the pathological stages of prostate cancer (Brawer, 1996), suggesting that Doppler vascularity data could supplement tumor volume measured by 3D imaging as a means of assessing tumor progression and may also support comparisons of the role of angiogenesis in tumor progression in different transgenic PC models. A third clinical study demonstrated a correlation of pretreatment power Doppler vessel density and the reduction in PSA produced by radiation therapy (Sehgal *et al.*, 2003), which suggests that Doppler imaging may be useful for identifying times at which treatments are most likely to be effective in preclinical studies.

Further progress toward establishing correlations such as those presented in the preceding paragraph may depend on the development of more sophisticated methods for quantifying vascularity in Doppler images. The approaches most commonly investigated for clinical PC imaging estimate total vascularity or vascular density (Arger *et al.*, 2004). *Total vascularity* as determined by Doppler imaging is simply the number of pixels in which flow is detected. This approach was employed by Goertz *et al.* (2002) in the high-frequency studies of antivascular treatment response that were reviewed above. *Vascular density* is defined as the number of pixels exhibiting detectable flow divided by the total number of pixels in a region of interest. It seems reasonable to expect vascular density to be more closely related to histological microvessel density, but accurate interpretation of Doppler vascular density estimates will also require consideration of physical and instrumentation factors influencing Doppler measurement variability.

The uncertainty of quantitative vascularity estimates might be reduced by the use of metrics weighted by the velocity or Doppler power measured (in the color and power imaging modes, respectively) at each pixel and metrics normalized by Doppler data acquired from vessels distant from the tumor. These methods can be used for clinical and preclinical PC imaging if appropriate measurement sites within and external to prostate tumors can be identified.

The ability to image blood flow without using injected contrast agents maintains two important advantages of ultrasound relative to other preclinical imaging modalities: rapid examinations and minimal risk to the animal from repeated imaging. However, the preclinical cancer researcher should bear in mind that the use of contrast agents may nevertheless be advisable if the agents prove to significantly improve the sensitivity of ultrasound to microvascular flow.

Ultrasound contrast agents are micron-sized bubbles of inert perfluorocarbon gas encapsulated in an albumin or phospholipid shell. A single microbubble produces ultrasound echoes several orders of magnitude more powerful than an echo from a single red blood cell, so microbubble contrast agents should significantly improve the sensitivity of ultrasound to capillary flow, where the red blood cell concentration is particularly sparse. Furthermore, the scattering of ultrasound from microbubbles includes significant harmonic components that permit microbubble echoes to be distinguished from tissue echoes using specialized signal processing. This feature of contrast agent imaging should improve the ability of ultrasound to depict very slow flow because contrast-enhanced images are less susceptible to tissue motion artifacts than conventional Doppler flow images. However, microbubble contrast agents are best suited for imaging at clinical frequencies, so further technical development is needed to permit the agents to be employed routinely for preclinical vascular imaging. Graham *et al.* present further discussion of potential roles of ultrasound contrast agents in preclinical cancer research in the companion volume of *Cancer Imaging*.

In summary, transgenic mouse models such as the PSP-TGMAP are expected to provide insight into the processes underlying prostate cancer initiation and progression and to provide clinically relevant models for preclinical evaluation of prospective therapies. Three-dimensional ultrasound microimaging is an effective and efficient means of measuring murine PC tumor growth and changes in growth in response to treatment. The strengths of ultrasound include relatively low equipment costs, rapid image acquisition, and little or no risk to the animals from repeated imaging. Quantitative vascular imaging is a promising, rapidly developing capability of ultrasound microimaging that is relevant to preclinical PC research. Initial results indicate that 3D power Doppler ultrasound can depict the distribution of blood flow to and within murine PC tumors. Power Doppler is expected to be capable of measuring changes in tumor vascularity produced by anti-angiogenic agents. The role of ultrasound microimaging in preclinical PC research will continue to increase in prominence as the technology advances.

References

Abate-Shen, C., and Shen, M.M. 2002. Mouse models of prostate carcinogenesis. *Trends Genet. 18*:S1–S5.

Adams, J.Y., Johnson, M., Sato, M., Berger, F., Gambhir, S.S., Carey, M., Iruela-Arispe, M.L., and Wu, L. 2002. Visualization of advanced human prostate cancer lesions in living mice by a targeted gene transfer vector and optical imaging. *Nat. Med. 8*:891–897.

Arger, P.H., Malkowicz, S.B., Vanarsdalen, K.N., Sehgal, C.M., Holzer, A., and Schultz, S.M. 2004. Color and power Doppler sonography in the diagnosis of prostate cancer: comparison between vascular density and total vascularity. *J. Ultrasound Med. 23*:623–630.

Brawer, M.K. 1996. Quantitative microvessel density: a staging and prognostic marker for human prostatic carcinoma. *Cancer 78*:345–349.

Duan, W., Gabril, M.Y., Moussa, M., Chan, F.L., Sakai, H., Fong, G., and Xuan, J.W. 2005. Knockin of SV40 Tag oncogene in a mouse adenocarcinoma of the prostate model demonstrates advantageous features over the transgenic model. *Oncogene 24*:1510–1524.

Fenster, A., Downey, D.B., and Cardinal, H.N. 2001. Three-dimensional ultrasound imaging. *Phys. Med. Biol. 46*:R67–R99.

Fernlund, P., Granberg, L.B., and Larsson, I. 1996. Cloning of beta-microseminoprotein of the rat: a rapidly evolving mucosal surface protein. *Arch. Biochem. Biophys. 334*:73–82.

Ferrara, K.W., Merritt, C.R.B., Burns, P.N., Stuart Foster, F., Mattrey, R.F., and Wickline, S.A. 2000. Evaluation of tumor angiogenesis with US: imaging, Doppler, and contrast agents. *Acad. Radiol. 7*:824–839.

Foster, F.S., Zhang, M.Y., Yq, Y.Q.Z., G. Liu, J. Mehi, E. Cherin, Harasiewicz, K.A., Starkoski, B.G., Zan, L., Knapik, D.A., and Adamson, S.L. 2002. A new ultrasound instrument for *in vivo* microimaging of mice. *Ultrasound Med. Biol. 28*:1165–1172.

Gabril, M.Y., Onita, T., Ji, P.G., Sakai, H., Chan, F.L., Koropatnick, J., Chin, J.L., Moussa, M., and Xuan, J.W. 2002. Prostate targeting: PSP94 gene promoter/enhancer region directed prostate tissue-specific expression in a transgenic mouse prostate cancer model. *Gene Ther. 9*:1589–1599.

Goertz, D.E., Yu, J.L., Kerbel, R.S., Burns, P.N., and Foster, F.S. 2002. High-frequency Doppler ultrasound monitors the effects of antivascular therapy on tumor blood flow. *Cancer Res. 62*:6371–6375.

Greenberg, N.M., Demayo, F., Finegold, M.J., Medina, D., Tilley, W.D., Aspinall, J.O., Cunha, G.R., Donjacour, A.A., Matusik, R.J., and Rosen, J.M. 1995. Prostate cancer in a transgenic mouse. *Proc. Natl. Acad. Sci. U S A 92*:3439–3443.

Hsu, C.X., Ross, B.D., Chrisp, C.E., Derrow, S.Z., Charles, L.G., Pienta, K.M., Greenberg, M.M., Zeng, M., and Sanda, M.M. 1998. Longitudinal cohort analysis of lethal prostate cancer progression in transgenic mice. *J. Urol. 160*:1500–1505.

Imasato, Y., Onita, T., Moussa, M., Sakai, H., Chan, F.L., Koropatnick, J., Chin, J.L., and Xuan, J.W. 2001. Rodent PSP94 gene expression is more specific to the dorsolateral prostate and less sensitive to androgen ablation than probasin. *Endocrinology 142*:2138–2146.

Inahara, M., Suzuki, H., Nakamachi, H., Kamiya, N., Shimbo, M., Komiya, A., Ueda, T., Ichikawa, T., Akakura, K., and Ito, H. 2004. Clinical evaluation of transrectal power Doppler imaging in the detection of prostate cancer. *Int. Urol. Nephrol. 36*:175–180.

Kruse, D.E., Silverman, R.H., Fornaris, R.J., Coleman, D.J., and Ferrara, K.W. 1998. Swept-scanning mode for estimation of blood velocity in the microvasculature. *IEEE Trans. Ultrason. Ferroelect. Freq. Contr. 45*:1437–1440.

Lazure, C., Villemure, M., Gauthier, D., Naude, R.J., and Mbikay, M. 2001. Characterization of ostrich (Struthio camelus) beta-microseminoprotein (MSP): identification of homologous sequences in EST databases and analysis of their evolution during speciation. *Protein Sci. 10*:2207–2218.

Reeves, J.R., Xuan, J.W., Arfanis, K., Morin, C., Garde, S.V., Ruiz, M.T., Wisniewski, J., Panchal, C., and Tanner, J.E. 2005. Identification, purification and characterization of a novel human blood protein with binding affinity for prostate secretory protein of 94 amino acids. *Biochem. J. 385*:105–114.

Risbridger, G.P., Schmitt, J.F., and Robertson, D.M. 2001. Activins and inhibins in endocrine and other tumors. *Endocr. Rev. 22*:836–858.

Sehgal, C.M., Arger, P.H., Holzer, A.C., and Krisch, R.E. 2003. Correlation between Doppler vascular density and PSA response to radiation therapy in patients with localized prostate carcinoma. *Acad. Radiol. 10*:366–372.

Shukeir, N., Arakelian, A., Kadhim, S., Garde, S., and Rabbani, S.A. 2003. Prostate secretory protein PSP-94 decreases tumor growth and hypercalcemia of malignancy in a syngenic *in vivo* model of prostate cancer. *Cancer Res. 63*:2072–2078.

Van Huizen, I., Wu, G., Moussa, M., Chin, J.L., Fenster, A., Lacefield, J.C., Sakai, H., Greenberg, N.M., and Xuan, J.W. 2005. Establishment of a serum tumor marker for pre-clinical trials of mouse prostate cancer models. *Clinic. Can. Res. 11*:7911–7919.

Weissleder, R. 2002. Scaling down imaging: molecular mapping of cancer in mice. *Nat. Rev. Cancer 2*:11–18.

Wilson, N.M., Masoud, A.M., Barsoum, H.B., Refaat, M.M., Moustafa, M.I., and Kamal, T.A. 2004. Correlation of power Doppler with microvessel density in assessing prostate needle biopsy. *Clin. Radiol. 59*:946–950.

Winter, S.F., Cooper, A.B., and Greenberg, N.M. 2003. Models of metastatic prostate cancer: a transgenic perspective. *Prostate Cancer Prostatic Dis. 6*:204–211.

Wirtzfeld, L.A., Wu, G., Bygrave, M., Yamasaki, Y., Sakai, H., Moussa, M., Izawa, J.I., Downey, D.B., Greenberg, N.M., Fenster, A., Xuan, J.W., and Lacefield, J.C. 2005. A new three-dimensional ultrasound microimaging technology for preclinical studies using a transgenic prostate cancer mouse model. *Cancer Res. 65*:6337–6345.

Xuan, J.W., Kwong, J., Chan, F.L., Ricci, M., Imasato, Y., Sakai, H., Fong, G.H., Panchal, C., and Chin, J.L. 1999. cDNA, genomic cloning, and gene expression analysis of mouse PSP94 (prostate secretory protein of 94 amino acids). *DNA Cell. Biol. 18*:11–26.

Xuan, J.W., Bygrave, M., Jiang, H., Valiyeva, F., Dunmore-Buyze, J., Holdsworth, D.W., Izawa, J.I., Bauman, G., Moussa, M., Winter, S., Greenberg, N.M., Chin, J.L., Drangova, M., Fenster, A., and Lacefield, J.C. 2007. Functional neo-angiogenesis imaging of transgeneic mouse prostate cancer by three dimensional power Doppler ultrasound. *Cancer Res. 67*:2830–2839.

Yang, H., Berger, F., Tran, C., Gambhir, S.S., and Sawyers, C.L. 2003. MicroPET imaging of prostate cancer in LNPC-SR39TK-GFP mouse xenografts. *Prostate 55*:39–47.

47

Prostate Cancer within the Transition Zone: Gadolinium-Enhanced Magnetic Resonance Imaging

Hong Li, Ryo Sugihara, and Kazuro Sugimura

Introduction

Prostate carcinoma is the most common cancer in males over 50 years of age and remains a leading cause of cancer death (Dennis and Resnick, 2000; Dijkman and Debruyne, 1996). Accurate preoperative staging and early detection are very important in selecting the therapeutic strategies for prostate cancer (Quinn and Babb, 2002; Franceschi and La Veachia, 2001). Magnetic resonance (MR) imaging has been gaining acceptance as an important tool in the evaluation of prostate cancer—mainly that which occurs in the peripheral zone (Claus et al., 2004; Engelhard et al., 2000). Although most prostate cancers originate in the peripheral zone, up to ~ 30% of prostate cancers occur within the transition zone (TZ) (McNeal et al., 1988). Transition zone cancer has made substantial contributions to the morbidity and mortality of prostate cancer. Recently reports have shown that evaluating prostate cancer using MR imaging has focused on transition zone cancer (Li et al., 2006; Akin et al., 2006).

The zonal description of the prostate by McNeal (1968) has led to a better understanding of the anatomy of the transition zone as visualized by MR imaging (Schnall et al., 1990; Schiebler et al., 1993). On T2-weighted images, the transition zone has lower signal intensity than the peripheral zone. With advancing age, the transition zone gradually increases and produces hyperplasia. Hyperplasia can be diffuse and homogeneous, but in general hyperplastic tissue appears to be multinodular. Depending on the ratio of stromal-to-glandular hyperplasia, nodules with a mixed-tissue composition display different heterogeneous intensity appearance on T2-weighted imaging. High-signal areas are due to cystic involution of areas of hyperplasia. Low-signal areas are explained by predominant stromal hyperplasia. Purely stromal hyperplasia is usually homogeneous and low intensity, while pure glandular hyperplasia tends from low to iso-homogeneous intensity on T2-weighted imaging.

Transition zone cancer tends to have uniform low intensity on T2-weighted imaging with a lenticular shape (Li et al., 2006; Akin et al., 2006). However, MR imaging is generally considered inadequate for detection of transition zone cancer because the uniform low intensities of transition zone cancers are too uncertain to assist with the diagnosis of transition zone cancer in the presence of a coexisting benign disease (Akin *et al.*, 2006). However, some transition zone cancers may not show uniform low intensities (Li *et al.*, 2006).

Criteria for MR imaging in detecting prostate cancers in the peripheral zone have been published (Engelhard *et al.*, 2000). However, criteria for MR imaging for cancers in the transition zone have not been studied. It is important to establish the diagnostic criteria for detecting transition zone cancers and for differentiating transition zone cancers from coexisting benign lesions because a considerable number of cancers originate in the transition zone, and research is needed in this part of the prostate.

The limited value of enhanced MR imaging in patients with a transition zone cancer has been reported before (Brown *et al.*, 1995). We have suggested that MR imaging using gadolinium-enhancement can be useful in the detection and differentiation of transition zone cancer from other benign lesions such as BPH nodules (Li *et al.*, 2006). With gadopentetate dimeglumine administration, the transition zone showed markedly inhomogeneous signal intensity in advancing age. However, the configuration and the homogeneous enhancement pattern of the transition zone cancer could be depicted better than the appearance on T2-weighted imaging alone (Li *et al.*, 2006).

Methods

Patients

A total of 121 patients with untreated prostate cancer underwent conventional MRI followed by radical prostatectomy. After eliminating patients with unenhanced MRI because of a history of drug allergies ($n = 3$) or serious obstructive voiding symptoms ($n = 2$), medical records, MRI, and histopathologic data of 116 patients were studied. The patients ranged from 52 to 76 years of age (mean, 65 years). In all, 108 out of 116 patients were referred for MRI before the sextant biopsy; the remaining eight patients received MRI after the sextant biopsy with a mean interval of 4 weeks (range, 3–6 weeks). For all patients, the period from MRI to radical prostatectomy surgery ranged from 1 to 7 weeks (mean interval, 4 weeks).

Magnetic Resonance Imaging Techniques

Magnetic resonance imaging studies were performed with a 1.5–T MRI system (Signa, GE Healthcare) using a pelvic phased-array coil. Hyoscine-N-butylbromide (Buscopan, Boehringer Ingelheim) was injected IV in all patients to minimize peristaltic artifacts. Contrast enhancement has been used in routine clinical examinations in our hospital when prostate cancer is suspected since 1999. Informed consent was obtained from all patients according to a protocol that has been approved by our institutional review board.

T1-weighted (TR/TE, 500-685/9-20) and T2-weighted turbo spin-echo (3500–5500/100–155; echo-train length, 8–16) sequences were performed in the axial, sagittal, and coronal planes for all patients using a multisection technique. Slice thickness was 4 mm with a 1-mm interslice gap, matrix size was 512 × 512, and field-of-view was 220 × 220 mm.

After these initial sequences, the enhanced fat-saturated axial T1-weighted imaging was repeated immediately after a bolus injection of IV gadolinium (Magnevist, 0.2 ml/kg, Schering). This set of images was obtained at ~ 2 min 30 sec. Enhanced images through the prostate from the apex to the base of the prostate were obtained within a time of ~ 60 sec variable to the number of slices. The mean number in each sequence of MRI slices of the prostate was six slices (range, 4–9 slices).

Histopathologic Examination

All specimens were coated with India blue or red ink to allow the microscopic evaluation of surgical resection margins and fixed in 5% buffered formalin for 24 hr. After dehydration, the prostate glands were serially blocked into 4-mm-thick sections from the apex to the base in transverse planes corresponding to MRI carried out by two doctors. Next, 719 step-sectioned pathologic specimens were obtained (mean, 6.2 slices for each gland). Each section was copied on paper and then the mounted prostate specimens were embedded in paraffin. A 7-μm-thick slice was obtained from the superior surface of each section and stained with hem-eos. The contour and size of each lesion were drawn on copying paper, and the diagnosis was reported on a separate paper by a pathologist who used the following classification: prostatic adenocarcinoma, benign prostatic hyperplasia subdivided into glandular (> 5% glandular elements), stroma (< 5% glandular elements), mixed glandular and stroma, prostatitis, bleeding, scar, necrosis, and normal stromal and glandular elements.

Based on microscopic examination, the pathologist diagnosed 196 discrete prostate cancers, including 53 in the transition zone (27%), 134 in the peripheral zone (68%), and nine (5%) for which the origin could not be identified.

Magnetic Resonance Imaging Analysis

Magnetic resonance images of each patient were downloaded individually and were separately transferred to a computer from the DICOM server in the PACS system of our hospital. The names, ages, and identification numbers recorded on each image were erased by members of this study group. Two reviewers (with 9 and 15 years of experience, respectively, in prostate images) who were not given the histopathologic results independently analyzed all images. Both reviewers knew that all the patients had prostatectomy-proven prostate cancer.

One reviewer traced each prostate onto paper according to each axial T2-weighted slice for correlation with the pathologic maps. Lesions of the transition zone in which signal intensity was abnormally low compared with the transition zone area or which the reviewer thought were possibly prostatic lesions were drawn on each of the traced prostate images.

Lesions were subsequently recorded and rated by the two reviewers. They were restricted to the sites identified by one of the reviewers to ensure they were both rating the same areas. Cancer was considered present on MR image analysis when there was uniform low signal intensity on T2-weighted images, homogeneous gadolinium enhancement, or where the interface between the lesion and the inner gland was irregular on gadolinium-enhanced and T2-weighted images (irregular margin was considered according to gadolinium enhancement and T2-weighted images because the interface between cancer and the area of the inner gland was sometimes not easy to identify on T2-weighted images). However, all other nodules showing heterogeneous low intensity with regular margins and heterogeneous gadolinium enhancement were considered benign lesions. The diagnostic base criteria of the MR images were determined for detecting transition zone cancer as follows: lesions with A, uniform low intensity on T2-weighted images; B, homogeneous gadolinium enhancement; and C, irregular margins both on gadolinium-enhanced and T2-weighted images.

The criteria for each area was rated by the two reviewers on a five-point scale: (1) definitely cancer; (2) probably cancer; (3) possibly cancer; (4) probably benign; or (5) definitely benign. When a lesion was difficult to rate or when lesions were rated significantly differently, consensus readings were performed until the lesion could be rated.

The reviewers also noted that the images did not have large or extensive motion artifacts with the exception of those in two patients, where artifacts on gadolinium-enhanced imaging arose from hip prostheses. No bleeding was seen within the transition zone areas in any of the MR imaging, with the exception of those in one patient who had no history of biopsy before MRI was performed.

Statistical Analysis

The units of analysis were the cancers and benign diseases in the transition zone. Cancer within the transition zone detected with MRI was considered a true positive (rated 1–3, cancer present) when cancer was present on the histopathologic copying papers on which each transition zone cancer was drawn within the same region. False-positive results (rated 1–3, cancer absent) were considered if the cancer in the transition zone was diagnosed using MRI but a benign lesion was reported on the histopathologic copying papers. True-negative results (rated 4–5, cancer absent) were considered when benign lesions detected with MRI were compared with histopathologic copying papers with benign lesions.

If the MRI was considered negative but the histopathologic copying papers showed cancers, then the results were false negative (rated 4–5, cancer present).

The sensitivity of each criterion was determined by confidence ratings of 1–3. Similarly, specificity was determined by confidence ratings of 4–5 (Obuchowski, 2003). The sensitivity, specificity, and correct characterization rates were determined with each diagnostic criterion, which was rated on the five-point scale by each reviewer. Statistical differences, receiver operating characteristic curve analysis, and 95% confidence intervals were calculated using StatMate III software (ATMS Co. Ltd.). Interobserver agreement was assessed with kappa statistics. Kappa analysis was performed using formulas described by Kundel and Polansky (2003). A kappa value of up to 0.20 stood for slight agreement; a value of 0.21–0.40, fair agreement; 0.41–0.60, moderate agreement; 0.61–0.80, substantial agreement; and 0.81 or greater, almost perfect agreement. In all statistical analyses, a p value of < 0.05 was considered to indicate a statistically significant difference.

Results

The serum prostate-specific antigen (PSA) level was reduced in 116 patients, ranging from 2.2 to 71.4 ng/ml before operation (mean, 16.9 ng/ml). All 116 prostatectomy specimens evaluated in this study had a histopathologic diagnosis of cancer, and the histologic grades were further defined using the Gleason score. A total of 53 transition zone cancers were identified on histopathologic evaluation by a pathologist. According to criterion A of the uniform low intensity on T2-weighted imaging, the sensitivity, specificity, and accuracy were 50%, 51%, and 51%, respectively.

In comparison with schematic prostate MRI diagrams, criterion A of the uniform low intensity on T2-weighted imaging was seen in 27 (51%) of the 53 transition zone cancers (Fig. 1A, 1B). The remaining 26 (49%) false-negative MRI results were reviewed with histopathologic copying papers as follows: A, mixed with benign prostatic hyperplasia ($n = 3$) (Fig. 1A, 1B); B, hypernephroid pattern ($n = 2$, of two revealed on histopathologic copying papers); C, well-differentiated adenocarcinoma ($n = 3$ of 7); D, ordinary pattern in histopathology ($n = 4$); E, mixed with the edema fibrosis tissue secondary to prostatitis ($n = 1$); F, arising within benign prostatic hyperplasia nodules ($n = 2$); G, arising from residual tissue of the transition zone after a transurethral resection of the prostate ($n = 1$); H, multiple cancer foci sporadically distributed among the normal gland of the prostate ($n = 1$); and I, nine cancers that could not be visualized using MRI, including six cancers smaller than 5 mm^2 in size.

A total of 33 low-intensity lesions on T2-weighted images were identified as benign lesions when a schematic prostate diagram of imaging papers was compared with the

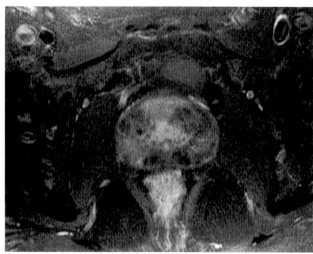

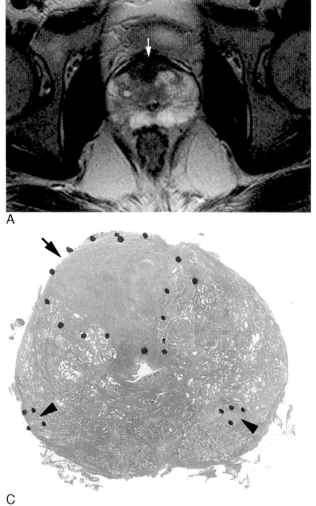

Figure 1 Prostatic cancer in 68-year-old man with prostate-specific antigen level of 19.3 ng/ml and negative findings on endorectal sonography-guided biopsy. Stage is T2b. No suspicious findings were seen on digital rectal examination or endorectal sonography. (**A**) Axial T2-weighted images (TR/TE, 5000/155, and 4700/119; echo-train length, 8) show uniform hypointense area with irregular margin in anterior location of inner gland, which extends toward anterior fibromuscular stroma (*arrows*). Heterogeneous decreased intensity area is seen in right peripheral zone. (**B**) Contrast-enhanced T1-weighted image (600/20) with fat suppression shows homogeneous enhancement of lesion at inner gland and enhancement of both peripheral zones. (**C**) Histopathologic specimen obtained at corresponding level reveals moderately differentiated adenocarcinoma in anterior position of inner gland (*arrow*). Tumor size is 35 × 15 mm. Two small tumor foci indicating prostatic intraepithelial neoplasia are seen in background of both peripheral zones (*arrowheads*) (original magnification, H and E staining).

pathologic copying papers. Among them, 17 (51%) lesions showed inhomogeneous low intensity on T2-weighted imaging. Sixteen (48%) false-positive MRI results were attributed to the fact that histopathologic examination revealed benign prostatic hyperplasia ($n = 11$), bleeding ($n = 1$), prostatitis ($n = 1$), inflammation in the periurethral duct ($n = 1$), inflammation in the anterior fibromuscular stroma ($n = 1$), and stromal tissue ($n = 1$).

Based on criterion B of the homogeneous gadolinium enhancement, the sensitivity, specificity, and accuracy were 66%, 75%, and 70%, respectively. Thirty-five (66%) of 53 transition zone cancers showed homogeneous enhancement identified by histopathologic copying reports (Fig. 1B). The remaining 18 (34%) false-negative MRI results were reviewed as cancer blended with benign prostatic hyperplasia ($n = 3$), fibrosis tissue with edema ($n = 1$), multiple cancer foci sporadically distributed among a normal prostate gland ($n = 1$), unenhanced ($n = 4$), a hypernephroid

pattern of adenocarcinoma ($n = 1$), pseudohyperplastic adenocarcinoma ($n = 2$ of two revealed on histopathologic copying papers) (Arista-Nasr *et al.*, 2003), and well-differentiated adenocarcinoma ($n = 1$). The remaining five cancers smaller than 5 mm² in size were not visualized on the MRI. Twenty-five (76%) of 33 benign lesions showed inhomogeneous enhancement. Eight (24%) false-positive MRI results were due to stroma benign prostatic hyperplasia ($n = 2$), glandular benign prostatic hyperplasia without degeneration ($n = 4$), inflammation in the anterior fibromuscular stroma ($n = 1$), and inflammation in the periurethral duct ($n = 1$).

According to criterion C of the irregular margin analysis, the sensitivity, specificity, and accuracy were 60, 72, and 65, respectively. Based on histopathologic examination, 21 (39%) false-negative MRI results showed some cancers were globular surrounded by a pseudo-well-circumscribed margin mimicking benign prostatic hyperplasia; others were in contact with the benign prostatic hyperplasia nodule or could not be identified. In the 33 benign lessons, 9 (27%) false-positive MRI results showed benign prostatic hyperplasia ($n = 6$), prostatitis ($n = 2$), and periurethral duct inflammation ($n = 1$).

According to the analysis of base criteria A, B, and C, the following two steps were performed for further analysis. First, the base criteria were combined into three groups of A-B, A-C, and B-C. Sensitivities, specificities, and accuracy of three groups were 43%, 88%, and 60% in group A-B; 42%, 88%, and 59% in group A-C; and 52%, 79%, and 63% in group B-C, respectively. They were then compared with each other. Sensitivities, specificities, and accuracy for each comparison were not found to differ significantly. When groups A-B, A-C, and B-C were compared with the individual criteria A, B, and C, their sensitivities were lower and their specificities were higher. Then, the three subgroups (subgroup G, H, and I) were further divided according to base criteria A, B, and C. Subgroup G is that cancer was considered present if the lesion satisfied any one criterion among base criteria A, B, and C; subgroup H is that any two criteria among base criteria A, B, C; subgroup I is that all three criteria were among base criteria A, B, C. Sensitivities, specificities, and accuracy were 79%, 27%, and 50%, respectively, in subgroup G; 68%, 82%, and 73% in subgroup H; and 34%, 91%, and 56% in subgroup I.

To obtain better accuracy, the second subgroup H was considered the best of the three subgroups according to results. This was not the case when criteria A, B, and C were analyzed independently, or when they were analyzed in combination (A-B, A-C, and B-C). The 95% confidence interval of each criterion and the kappa statistics acted to measure the agreement between two reviewers. There was a very good to excellent agreement between the two reviewers for detecting transition zone cancer when using our three criteria.

Discussion

Although most prostate cancers originate from the peripheral zone, up to ~ 30% of prostate cancers occur within the transition zone (TZ) (McNeal et al., 1988). The latter cancer has substantial contributors to the morbidity and mortality of prostate cancer. Patients with transition zone cancers show clinical features that are different from those shown by cancers in the peripheral zone. It is more difficult to detect transition zone cancers located anterior of the prostate and far from the rectum when using digital rectal examination and transrectal needle biopsy (Noguchi et al., 2000; Lui et al., 1995). They are most frequently diagnosed incidentally in transurethral resection specimens (TURP) and prostatectomy specimens (McNeal et al., 1988).

Although transition zone cancers often have markedly higher mean prostate specific antigen levels (Noguchi et al., 2000) and higher tumor volumes (Stamey et al., 1993), transition zone cancers more frequently show organ-confined disease (Augustin et al., 2003) and lower Gleason scores (Stamey and Yemoto, 1995) than patients with peripheral zone cancers. Furthermore, patients with transition zone cancers have more favorable prognoses than patients with peripheral zone cancers (Noguchi et al., 2000), although some controversy remains (Augustin et al., 2003).

Transition zone cancers and peripheral zone cancers differ not only in their clinical and pathologic characteristics but also in the MR imaging features they display (Akin et al., 2006). Peripheral zone cancers are depicted as areas of low T2 signal intensity within the relatively homogeneous high T2 intensity peripheral zone. However, transition zone cancer is the site of origin of benign prostatic hyperplasia, which can be hampered in the evaluation of transition zone cancers by heterogeneous signal intensity on T2-weighted intensity (Muramoto et al., 2002). Evaluation of transition zone cancer with MR imaging is more difficult than with peripheral zone cancer.

It has been suggested that patients with multiple negative biopsy results and an elevated PSA level should undergo biopsies in which the transition zone is specifically targeted (Liu et al., 2001). Even when the transition zone is specifically targeted, small tumors (< 2 cm^3) may be missed (McNeal and Noldus, 1996). Magnetic resonance imaging guidance may improve the accuracy of biopsy results. Recently, reports have shown that evaluating prostate cancer by MR imaging has focused on transition zone cancers (Li et al., 2006; Akin et al., 2006). Variable MR imaging techniques have been used for detecting transition zone cancers. These include conventional MR imaging with (Li et al., 2006) or without gadopentetate dimeglumine administration (Kitamura et al., 2002), endorectal MR imaging (Akin et al., 2006), dynamic subtraction contrast-enhanced MR imaging (Ogura et al., 2001), proton MR spectroscopic imaging (Zakian et al., 2003), and diffusion-weighted images (Sato et al., 2005).

On conventional spin-echo T2-weighted MR imaging, the transition zone shows a heterogeneously variable signal intensity appearance in older people with benign prostatic hyperplasia, while transition zone cancer tends to have uniform low intensity (Kitamura et al., 2002). However, diagnosis is limited by false-negative findings. The uniform low intensities of transition zone cancers are too uncertain to assist with the diagnosis of transition zone cancers in the presence of a coexisting benign disease. On the other hand, some transition zone cancers do not show uniform low intensity, instead showing heterogeneous low intensity on T2-weighted imaging.

Endorectal surface coil MR imaging can detect and stage the prostate cancer, mainly in the peripheral zone. However, the endorectal coil has limitations in detecting the transition zone cancers because transition zone cancers are located anteriorly in the prostate and far from the rectum. Outwater et al. (1994) did not identify any of 29 central gland tumors and 41 of 56 (73%) peripheral tumors on MR imaging that used an ERC technique. Recently, Akin *et al.* (2006) reported that MR imaging with an endorectal coil was useful in detecting transition zone cancers. The sensitivity and specificity of detecting transition zones were 75% and 87% in reader 1, and 80% and 78% in reader 2, respectively. In addition, they show that local staging of transition zone cancers is possible with MR imaging using an endorectal coil.

Dynamic subtraction contrast-enhanced MR imaging could detect an early cancer in peripheral zone cancer (Namimoto *et al.*, 1998). In a normal prostate, enhancement occurs initially at the inner portion, with a slight, gradual enhancement of the peripheral zone. Therefore, cancers in the peripheral zone can demonstrate an enhancement earlier and more intensely than those in the peripheral zone. However, it is difficult to demonstrate transition zone cancers because the period of enhancement of the transition zone is similar to that in the transition zone cancers (Namimoto *et al.*, 1998). Using endorectal coil MR imaging with the contrast enhanced, the detection rate of tumor localization was higher in the peripheral zone (81%) and lower in the transition zone (37%) (Ogura *et al.*, 2001). In addition, findings from previous dynamic studies were insufficient for purposes of differentiating between transition zone cancers and BPH (Jager *et al.*, 1997; Padhani *et al.*, 2000).

Proton MR spectroscopic imaging has been successfully applied to the diagnosis of cancer in the peripheral zone on the basis of the elevation of choline and the reduction of citrate in cancerous tissue (Dhingsa *et al.*, 2004; Swindle *et al.*, 2003). However, the broad range of metabolite ratios observed in transition zone cancer precludes the use of a single ratio to differentiate transition zone cancer from benign transition zone lesions (Zakian *et al.*, 2003; Shukla-Dave *et al.*, 2004). In conventional MR imaging with gadopentetate dimeglumine administration, no relevant increase was found for detecting peripheral zone cancer (Brown *et al.*, 1995; Mirowitz *et al.*, 1993). However, the transition zone shows markedly inhomogeneous signal intensity after gadopentetate dimeglumine administration, while the configuration and homogeneous enhancement pattern of the transition zone cancer could be depicted better than the appearance on T2-weighted imaging alone (Li *et al.*, 2006).

The importance of recognizing the presence of transition zone cancer was described by Padhani and Nutting (Padhani *et al.*, 2000; Padhani and Nutting, 2003). In a previous study aimed at detecting transition zone cancer, Outwater *et al.* (1994) identified none of the 29 central gland tumors in their study. Carter *et al.* (1991) reported 15% sensitivity, and Ikonen *et al.* (1998) reported 55% sensitivity. Our data of overall sensitivity, specificity, and accuracy were 68%, 82%, and 73%, respectively, and thus similar to data from Ito *et al.* (2003), who lacked pathologic correlation with radical prostatectomy specimen examinations (invisible cancers smaller than 5 mm^2 in size were not included). The improved accuracy of identification in our study was probably due to the use of our three criteria for detecting transition zone cancer.

Not all transition zone cancers show uniform low-intensity appearances (so-called T2-isointense prostate cancer [PCa]) (Oyen, 2003). By excluding six nonvisualized transition zone cancers < 5 mm^2 in size (Ikonen *et al.*, 1998; Stamey *et al.*, 1993), our histopathologic data revealed that 20 of 53 transition zone cancers did not show uniform low intensity. False-negative imaging results were obtained: adenocarcinomas with low grade (well-differentiated and pseudohyperplasic pattern) or hypernephroid components (Turnbull *et al.*, 1999; Rouviere *et al.*, 2003; Dhingsa *et al.*, 2004); or adenocarcinomas blending with benign prostatic hyperplasia, edema tissue or normal tissue, and so on (Engelhard *et al.*, 2000). However, by using the criteria of homogeneous enhancement and irregular margins, 38% of false-negative cases could be correctly diagnosed as transition zone cancer in our study.

The specificity was low when transition zone cancers were detected using only sequential T2-weighted imaging. T2 hypointense foci in the inner gland can be caused by numerous other conditions such as prostatitis, granulomatous disease, smooth muscle hyperplasia, fibromuscular hyperplasia, atypical adenomatous hyperplasia, scar, infarction, and bleeding that contribute to the poor specificity (Engelhard *et al.*, 2000; Schiebler *et al.*, 1993; Rouviere, 2003; Padhani *et al.*, 2000; Ikonen 1998; Dhingsa *et al.*, 2004; Swindle *et al.*, 2003; Zakian *et al.*, 2003). However, if the criteria of homogeneous enhancement and irregular margins were used, the specificity rates could be increased from 51 to 82% in this study.

Inflammation in the anterior fibromuscular stroma (AFS) or periurethral duct may result from false-positive imaging results in our study. Normally, both the anterior fibromuscular stroma and the periurethral duct show low intensity on T2-weighted imaging without enhancement (Schiebler *et al.*, 1993). However, when inflammation occurs, both of these show enhancement similar to transition zone cancer. Our study showed that the addition of gadolinium-enhanced MRI to T2-weighted imaging provides better accuracy for detecting transition zone cancers than the use of T2-weighted imaging alone. We also revealed that one-third of cancers in the transition zone do not show uniform low intensity on T2-weighted imaging, and that when transition zone cancer is suspected, a gadolinium-enhanced imaging study should be used. The most promising clinical application of this technique could be to study patients with a previous negative endorectal sonography-guided biopsy, persistently elevated PSA, and abnormal low intensity in the transition zone on T2-weighted imaging.

References

Akin, O., Sala, E., Moskowitz, C.S., Kuroiwa, K., Ishill, N.M., Pucar, D., Scardino, P.T., Hricak, H. 2006. Transition zone prostate cancers: features, detection, localization, and staging at endorectal MR imaging. *Radiology* 239:784–792.

Arista-Nasr, J., Martinez-Benitez, B., Valdes, S., Hernandez, M., and Bornstein-Quevedo, L. 2003. Pseudohyperplastic prostatic adenocarcinoma in transurethral resections of the prostate. *Pathol. Oncol. Res. 9*:232–235.

Augustin, H., Erbersdobler, A., Graefen, M., Fernandez, S., Palisaar, J., Huland and H., Hammerer, P. 2003. Biochemical recurrence following radical prostatectomy: a comparison between prostate cancers located in different anatomical zones. *Prostate 55*:48–54.

Brown, G., Macvicar, D.A., Ayton, V., and Husband, J.E. 1995. The role of intravenous contrast enhancement in magnetic resonance imaging of prostatic carcinoma. *Clin Radiol. 50*:601–606.

Carter, H.B., Brem, R.F., Tempany, C.M., Yang, A., Epstein, J.I., Walsh, P.C., and Zerhouni, E.A. 1991. Nonpalpable prostate cancer: detection with MR imaging. *Radiology 178*:523–525.

Claus, F.G., Hricak, H., and Hattery, R.R. 2004. Pretreatment evaluation of prostate cancer: role of MR imaging and 1H MR spectroscopy. *Radiographics 24*:167–180.

Dennis, L.K., and Resnick, M.I. 2000. Analysis of recent trends in prostate cancer incidence and mortality. *Prostate 42*:247–252.

Dhingsa, R., Qayyum, A., Coakley, F.V., Lu, Y., Jones, K.D., Swanson, M.G., Carroll, P.R., Hricak, H., and Kurhanewicz, J. 2004. Prostate cancer localization with endorectal MR imaging and MR spectroscopic imaging: effect of clinical data on reader accuracy. *Radiology 230*:215–220.

Dijkman, G.A., and Debruyne, F.M.J. 1996. Epidemiology of prostate cancer. *Eur Urol. 30*:281–295.

Engelhard, K., Hollenbach, H.P., Deimling, M., Kreckel, M., and Riedl, C. 2000. Combination of signal intensity measurements of lesions in the peripheral zone of prostate with MRI and serum PSA level for differentiating benign disease from prostate cancer. *Eur Radiol. 10*:1947–1953.

Franceschi, S., and La Vecchia, C. 2001. Cancer epidemiology in the elderly. *Crit. Rev. Oncol. Hematol. 39*:219–226.

Ikonen, S., Karkkainen, P., Kivisaari, L., Salo, J.O., Taari, K., Vehmas, T., Tervahartiala, P., Rannikko, S. 1998. Magnetic resonance imaging of clinically localized prostatic cancer. *J. Urol. 159*:915–919.

Ito, H., Kamoi, K., Yokoyama, K., Yamada, K., and Nishimura, T. 2003. Visualization of prostate cancer using dynamic contrast-enhanced MRI: comparison with transrectal power Doppler ultrasound. *Brit. J. Radiol. 76*:617–624.

Jager, G.J., Ruijter, E.T., van de Kaa, CA., de la Rosette, J.J., Oosterhof, G.O., Thornbury, J.R., Ruijs, S.H., and Barentsz, J.O. 1997. Dynamic turbo FLASH subtraction technique for contrast-enhanced MR imaging of the prostate: correlation with histopathologic results. *Radiology 203*:645–652.

Kitamura, Y., Kaji, Y., Li, H., Manabe, T., Sugimura, K., and Tachibana, M. 2002. Prostate cancer derived from transition zone specific findings on MR imaging. Presented at the 9th annual symposium on urogenital radiology of the European Society of Urogenital Radiology, Genoa, Italy, June 15–20.

Kundel, H.I.., and Polansky, M. 2003. Measurement of observer agreement. *Radiology 228*:303–308.

Li, H., Sugimura, K., Kaji, Y., Kitamura, Y., Fujii, M., Hara, I., and Tachibana, M. 2006. Conventional MRI capabilities in the diagnosis of prostate cancer in the transition zone. *Am. J. Roentgenol. 186*:729–742.

Liu, I.J., Macy, M., Lai, Y.H., and Terris, M.K. 2001. Critical evaluation of the current indications for transition zone biopsies. *Urology 57*:1117–1120.

Lui, P.D., Terris, M.K., McNeal, J.E., and Stamey, T.A. 1995. Indications for ultrasound guided transition zone biopsies in the detection of prostate cancer. *J. Urol. 153*:1000–1003.

McNeal, J.E. 1968. Regional morphology and pathology of the prostate. *Am. J. Clin. Pathol. 49*:347–357.

McNeal, J.E., and Noldus, J. 1996. Limitations of transition zone needle biopsy findings in the prediction of transition zone cancer and tissue composition of benign nodular hyperplasia. *Urology 48*:751–756.

McNeal, J.E., Redwine, E.A., Freiha, F.S., and Stamey, T.A. 1988. Zonal distribution of prostatic adenocarcinoma. Correlation with histologic pattern and direction of spread. *Am. J. Surg. Pathol. 12*:897–906.

Mirowitz, S.A., Brown, J.J., and Heiken, J.P. 1993. Evaluation of the prostate and prostatic carcinoma with gadolinium-enhanced endorectal coil MR imaging. *Radiology 186*:153–157.

Muramoto, S., Uematsu, H., Kimura, H., Ishimori, Y., Sadato, N., Oyama, N., Matsuda, T., Kawamura, Y., Yonekura, Y., Okada, K., and Itoh, H. 2002. Differentiation of prostate cancer from benign prostate hypertrophy using dual-echo dynamic contrast MR imaging. *Eur. J. Radiol. 44*:52–58.

Namimoto, T., Morishita, S., Saitoh, R., Kudoh, J., Yamashita, Y., and Takahashi, M. 1998. The value of dynamic MR imaging for hypointensity lesions of the peripheral zone of the prostate. *Comput. Med. Imaging Graph. 22*:239–245.

Noguchi, M., Stamey, T.A., Neal, J.E., and Yemoto, C.E. 2000. An analysis of 148 consecutive transition zone cancers: clinical and histological characteristics. *J. Urol. 163*:1751–1755.

Obuchowski, N.A. 2003. Receiver operating characteristic curves and their use in radiology. *Radiology 229*:3–8.

Ogura, K., Maekawa, S., Okubo, K., Aoki, Y., Okada, T., Oda, K., Watanabe, Y., Tsukayama, C., and Arai, Y. 2001. Dynamic endorectal magnetic resonance imaging for local staging and detection of neurovascular bundle involvement of prostate cancer: correlation with histopathologic results. *Urology 57*:721–726.

Outwater, E.K., Petersen, R.O., Siegelman, E.S., Gomella, L.G., Chernesky, C.E., and Mitchell, D.G. 1994. Prostate carcinoma: assessment of diagnostic criteria for capsular penetration on endorectal coil MR images. *Radiology 193*:333–339.

Oyen, R.H. 2003. Dynamic contrast-enhanced MRI of the prostate: is this the way to proceed for characterization of prostatic carcinoma? *Eur. Radiol. 13*:921–924.

Padhani, A.R., Gapinski, C.J., Macvicar, D.A., Parker, G.J., Suckling, J., Revell, P.B., Leach, M.O., Dearnaley, D.P., and Husband, J.E. 2000. Dynamic contrast enhanced MRI of prostate cancer: correlation with morphology and tumour stage, histological grade and PSA. *Clin. Radiol. 55*:99–109.

Padhani, A.R., and Nutting, C.M. 2003. Why do we need more accurate intraprostatic localization of cancer? *Br. J. Radiol. 76*:585–586.

Quinn, M., and Babb, P. 2002. Patterns and trends in prostate cancer incidence, survival, prevalence and mortality. Part I: international comparisons. *BJU Int. 90*:162–173.

Rouviere, O., Raudrant, A., Ecochard, R., Colin-Pangaud, C., Pasquiou, C., Bouvier, R., Marechal, J.M., and Lyonnet, D. 2003. Characterization of time-enhancement curves of benign and malignant prostate tissue at dynamic MR imaging. *Eur. Radiol. 13*:931–942.

Sato, C., Naganawa, S., Nakamura, T., Kumada, H., Miura, S., Takizawa, O., and Ishigaki, T. 2005. Differentiation of noncancerous tissue and cancer lesions by apparent diffusion coefficient values in transition and peripheral zones of the prostate. *J. Magn. Reson. Imaging 21*:258–262.

Schiebler, M.L., Schnall, M.D., Pollack, H.M., Lenkinski, R.E., Tomaszewski, J.E., Wein, A.J., Whittington, R., Rauschning, W., and Kressel, H.Y. 1993. Current role of MR imaging in the staging of adenocarcinoma of the prostate. *Radiology 189*:339–352.

Schnall, M.D., Bezzi, M., Pollack, H.M., and Kressel, H.Y. 1990. Magnetic resonance imaging of the prostate. *Magn. Reson. Q. 6*:1–16

Shukla-Dave, A., Hricak, H., Eberhardt, S.C., Olgac, S., Muruganandham, M., Scardino, P.T., Reuter, V.E., Koutcher, J.A., and Zakian, K.L. 2004. Chronic prostatitis: MR imaging and 1H MR spectroscopic imaging findings–initial observations. *Radiology 231*:717–724.

Stamey, T.A., Freiha, F.S., McNeal, J.E., Redwine, E.A., Whittemore, A.S., and Schmid, H.P. 1993. Localized prostate cancer: relationship of tumor volume to clinical significance for treatment of prostate cancer. *Cancer 71*:933–938.

Stamey, T.A., and Yemoto, C.E. 1995. The clinical importance of separating transition zone (TZ) from peripheral zone (PZ) cancers (abstract). *J. Urol. 159*:22.

Swindle, P., McCredie, S., Russell, P., Himmelreich, U., Khadra, M., Lean, C., and Mountford, C. 2003. Pathologic characterization of human prostate tissue with proton MR spectroscopy. *Radiology 228*:144–151.

Turnbull, L.W., Buckley, D.L., Turnbull, L.S., Liney, G.P., and Knowles, A.J. 1999. Differentiation of prostatic carcinoma and benign prostatic hyper-

plasia: correlation between dynamic Gd-DTPA-enhanced MR imaging and histopathology. *J. Magn. Reson. Imaging 9*:311–316.

Zakian, K.L., Eberhardt, S., Hricak, H., Shukla-Dave, A., Kleinman, S., Muruganandham, M., Sircar, K., Kattan, M.W., Reuter, V.E., Scardino, P.T., and Koutcher, J.A. 2003. Transition zone prostate cancer: metabolic characteristics at 1 H MR spectroscopic imaging—initial results. *Radiology 229*:241–247.

48

Rectal Wall Invasion of Locally Advanced Prostate Cancer: Comparison of Magnetic Resonance Imaging with Transrectal Ultrasound

Dan Leibovici, Philippe E. Spiess, and Louis L. Pisters

Introduction

Because of the major contributions by Walsh and Jewett (1980), radical retropubic prostatectomy has become central in the treatment of localized prostate cancer. When the tumor is confined to the prostate, radical surgery is curative in the majority of cases; however, if the cancer extends beyond the prostatic capsule or invades any structures nearby, cure is unlikely with surgery or radiation therapy alone. Locally advanced prostate cancer (LAPC) is a complex clinical problem, even in the absence of distant metastasis. Such cancer may present as a late event of local cancer recurrence after primary curative treatment, or it may be present at the time of diagnosis of a primary aggressive tumor that has invaded surrounding structures before becoming clinically evident. Locally advanced prostate cancer generally consists of a bulky tumor invading pelvic organs, such as the seminal vesicles, bladder, ureters, rectum, and pelvic side wall. These tumors may be associated with substantial morbidity

and even mortality, and can significantly affect the patient's quality of life.

The most common symptoms of LAPC are those associated with bladder outlet obstruction (e.g., weak urinary stream, urinary frequency, incomplete bladder emptying, and frank retention). Other symptoms include severe pelvic pain, dysuria, refractory hematuria, urinary and fecal incontinence, rectal pain, tenesmus, and renal failure. The syndrome of symptomatic LAPC is associated with decreased performance status and specific morbidity from obstructive renal failure and bleeding. The majority of patients with these symptoms will require urinary tract drainage via nephrostomy tube, ureteral stent, or urethral catheter. These devices are subject to dislodgement, functional failure, and infection and all of these conditions increase the patient's risk for morbidity and the potential need for additional ancillary procedures.

In addition to the risks associated with urinary tract drainage, the large cancerous pelvic mass is an ongoing source of metastasis seeding and may eventually cause disease progression and death. In the absence of widespread metastatic disease, the life expectancy of patients with LAPC may be several years; therefore, palliation of the symptoms associated with this disease and achievement of adequate local control become primary clinical end points independent of disease-specific survival (Leibovici *et al.*, 2005).

Traditional treatment modalities used in this setting have included radiation therapy, androgen ablation, transurethral prostatectomy (channeling), and chemotherapy. Unfortunately, none of these treatments provides effective palliation because they fail to eliminate tumor bulk in the pelvis (Fowler *et al.*, 2002; Senzer, 2001). At M. D. Anderson Cancer Center, we recently showed that radical surgery offers effective and durable palliation for patients with symptomatic LAPC (Kamat *et al.*, 2003; Mazur and Thompson, 1991). In 85% of well-selected patients, radical pelvic surgery eliminated local symptoms indefinitely. On an average, the patients gained two years of improved quality of life before the onset of symptoms related to metastatic disease.

The apparent advantage of radical surgery over other treatment modalities in achieving effective palliation is that in the surgical approach, the bulk of tumor is removed from the pelvis, and the lower urinary tract is reconstructed in all areas not affected by cancer. In theory, this outcome can be accomplished in some cases by radical prostatectomy alone; however, the majority of patients need more extensive surgery, for example, radical cystoprostatectomy or total pelvic exenteration (TPE). The extent of surgery depends largely on the organs and anatomic structures invaded by cancer; the functional implications of the diversion to be performed must also be considered. Although radical surgery is an effective means of palliation for the patient with LAPC, due to the extent of surgery and the potential morbidity associated with this approach, careful patient and procedure selection are crucial to optimizing outcome.

Selection of Patients for Radical Surgery

The best surgery results are achieved in patients with true LAPC, that is, those with no metastasis, an adequate performance status, and no significant comorbidities. Because the purpose of the surgery is palliation, operating on patients with metastatic disease is not absolutely contraindicated; however, the patient should be expected to live long enough to benefit from symptomatic relief and thus justify the risks associated with surgery. Distinguishing between isolated LAPC and LAPC with concomitant metastasis is not easy. Unfortunately, imaging studies such as bone scintigraphy computerized axial tomography (CAT) often lack sensitivity and fail to show metastasis in its early phase (Lee *et al.*, 1999, 2000). Monoclonal antibody-based radioisotope scans were developed for the purpose of locating the site of recurrent tumor. However, in a study by Lange (2001), this

modality did not demonstrate expected accuracy in ruling out metastatic disease, although it did demonstrate a high predictive value of a positive extrapelvic scan. Measuring the rate with which the serum prostate specific antigen (PSA) level increases, specifically the serum PSA doubling time, is helpful in distinguishing between localized and systemic disease. D'Amico *et al.* (2003) showed that a short serum PSA doubling time is characteristic of metastatic disease, whereas a long doubling time is characteristic of localized prostate cancer. Serum PSA doubling time is more sensitive than most imaging studies in detecting metastasis in its early phase.

Determining the Appropriate Surgical Procedure

The type of surgical procedure to be performed depends on the extent of cancer involvement. When the cancer is limited to the prostate or when its extension beyond the prostate is considered minimal, radical prostatectomy may be appropriate. Invasion of cancer into the bladder necessitates cystoprostatectomy, and when the rectal wall is invaded by cancer or cannot be surgically separated off the prostate, TPE is indicated. The extent of cancer involvement into pelvic organs must be determined preoperatively by imaging analysis, facilitating preoperative planning of the most appropriate surgical procedure on a patient-by-patient basis. Preoperative planning should include a discussion with the patient about the specific surgical procedure to be used and coordination with other clinicians, for example, general surgeons and plastic reconstructive surgeons, when their assistance is anticipated.

In its early phase, invasion of prostate cancer into the bladder area typically occurs at the bladder neck, and the tumors tend to spread into the bladder wall underneath the mucosa (Figs. 1A and 1B). The tumor eventually grows and erodes through the mucosa, creating the typical appearance of a solid friable fungating mass that may be difficult to distinguish from an invasive primary bladder cancer. Although CAT and magnetic resonance imaging (MRI) scans may suggest bladder invasion by prostate cancer, cystoscopy is the most useful diagnostic modality. Cystoscopy permits assessment of the extent of invasion with confirmation by biopsy and examination under anesthesia. The latter modality is of paramount importance and is useful in the detection of advanced-stage tumors, such as tumors fixed to the pelvic side wall, which are generally considered inoperable.

Although cystoprostatectomy is required for treatment of bladder invasion by prostate cancer, removal of the bladder *en bloc* with the prostate is justified in the occasional patient who has a dysfunctional bladder or refractory radiation-induced cystitis. Furthermore, because urinary incontinence occurs in virtually 50% of patients undergoing salvage radical prostatectomy

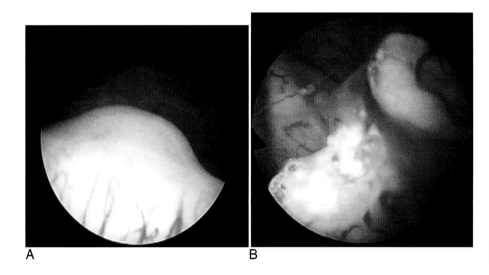

Figure 1 Cystoscopic view of early (**A**) and late (**B**) bladder invasion by prostate cancer.

after previous radiation therapy, performing cystoprostatectomy rather than radical prostatectomy in this setting may reduce the frequency of this complication and render salvage radical surgery more acceptable to the patient.

When cystoprostatectomy is considered, ileal conduit is probably the safest type of urinary diversion for patients with LAPC. Ileal conduits can be performed faster than orthotopic urinary diversions, thus allowing for more rapid recovery. This procedure also removes the entire urinary tract from the area inflicted with cancer and decreases the risk of cancer-related urinary symptoms and morbidity. However, creation of an orthotopic neobladder has been described in this setting and is an acceptable alternative in appropriately selected patients (Bochner *et al.*, 1998).

Preoperative detection of cancer invasion into the rectal wall is crucial in deciding whether to proceed with TPE or to attempt to spare the rectum. Digital rectal examination alone may produce misleading results, especially in patients who have previously undergone radiation therapy and in whom the distinction between perirectal scarring and tumor is difficult on the basis of palpation alone. Both transrectal ultrasound (TRUS) and MRI can be useful in

examining the rectal wall. We compared the accuracy of these two modalities in a series of 16 patients who underwent TPE and 24 who underwent cystoprostatectomy for palliation of symptomatic LAPC (Leibovici *et al.*, 2005). Cancer invasion into the rectum was confirmed by histology in 15 (94%) of the patients who underwent TPE. Among the patients who underwent cystoprostatectomy, rectal wall invasion was ruled out by achieving negative surgical margins on the posterior aspects of the specimen and by close follow-up, during which no clinical evidence of local cancer recurrence was observed. In one patient who had undergone cystoprostatectomy, rectal and perineal recurrences were clinically evident 10 months after surgery. We found that TRUS was highly specific and sensitive in detecting rectal wall invasion by LAPC, whereas MRI demonstrated 100% specificity but poor sensitivity (Leibovici *et al.*, 2005) (Table 1).

Although our results imply that MRI can reliably rule out rectal wall invasion, when the two imaging examinations are performed preoperatively, MRI cannot reliably rule out rectal wall invasion if the TRUS is positive. Conversely, when the TRUS is negative and the MRI is positive, the likelihood

Table 1 Comparison of TRUS and MRI Performances in the Detection of Rectal Wall Invasion by Prostate Cancer (Leibovici *et al.*, 2005)

	Sensitivity	Specificity	Overall Accuracy	PPV	NPV
TRUS	92.9 (66.1–99.8)	87.0 (66.4–97.2)	89.2 (74.6–97.0)	81.3 (54.4–96.0)	95.2 (76.2–99.9)
MRI	54.6 (23.4–83.3)	100 (76.8–100)	80 (59.3–93.2)	100 (54.1–100.0)	73.7 (48.8–90.9)

TRUS: transrectal ultrasound; MRI: magnetic resonance imaging; PPV: positive-predictive value; NPV: negative-predictive value
Probabilities are given in percentages. The numbers in parentheses are 95% confidence intervals.

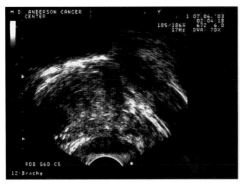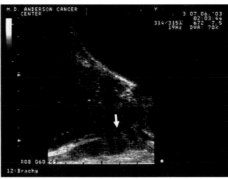

Figure 2 TRUS image showing the invasion of prostate cancer (observed as a hypoechoic lesion) into the rectal wall. Note the loss of continuity of the perirectal fascia (indicated by arrow) with transmural invasion of the rectum by prostate cancer.

of actual rectal wall invasion is ~ 5%. We concluded that in experienced hands, TRUS is the modality of choice for examining the rectal wall for evidence of tumor invasion, and, in most cases, MRI is noncontributory (Fig. 2).

Pelvic MRI using an endorectal coil may provide better resolution and may be more sensitive than conventional MRI. The role of endorectal MRI in the preoperative evaluation of patients with LAPC is yet to be determined (Futterer *et al.*, 2004).

To date, no imaging modality has been shown to be accurate and reliable in diagnosing cancer foci within the prostate. Despite early promise, TRUS has been inaccurate in detecting malignant foci within the prostate, and it is used merely as an aiming mechanism for random biopsies. Conversely, endorectal MRI with spectroscopy was recently shown to detect cancer foci within the prostate following a previous negative prostate biopsy (Prando *et al.*, 2005). However, TRUS of the rectal wall is very accurate in showing invasion by prostate cancer owing to the tangency of the rectal wall with the probe and the homogeneous echo pattern of that structure. Indeed, TRUS has been successfully used to stage primary rectal cancer (Kyu *et al.*, 1999).

In conclusion, radical surgery may be offered to carefully selected patients with LAPC; however, preoperative staging to determine the extent of local invasion and the affected pelvic structures is mandatory. Cystoscopy with biopsy and examination under anesthesia are useful in assessing the extent of bladder involvement and resectability, and TRUS is an accurate means of detecting invasion of the cancer into the rectal wall. Magnetic resonance imaging adds little to the accuracy of TRUS; thus the advantages of MRI spectroscopy and the use of an endorectal coil are yet to be determined.

References

Bochner, B.H., Figueroa, A.J., Skinner E.C., Lieskovsky, G., Petrovich, Z., Boyd, S.D., and Skinner, D.G. 1998. Salvage cystoprostatectomy and orthotopic urinary diversion following radiation failure. *J. Urol. 160*:29–33.

D'Amico, A.V., Moul, J.W., Carroll, P.R., Sun, L., Lubeck, D., and Chen, M.H. 2003. Surrogate endpoint for prostate cancer-specific mortality after radical prostatectomy or radiation therapy. *J. Natl. Cancer Inst. 95*:1376–1383.

Fowler, J.E., Jr., Bigler, S.A., White, P.C., and Duncan, W.L. 2002. Hormone therapy for locally advanced prostate cancer. *J. Urol. 168*:546–549.

Futterer, J.J., Scheenen, T.W., Huisman, H.J., Klomp, D.W., van Dorsten, F.A., Hulsbergen-van de Kaa, C.A., Wijtes, J.A., Heerschap, A., and Barentsz, J.O. 2004. Initial experience of 3 Tesla endorectal coil magnetic resonance imaging and 1H-spectroscopic imaging of the prostate. *Invest. Radiol. 39*:671–680.

Kamat, A.M., Huang, S.F., Bermejo, C.E., Rosser, C.J., Pettaway, C.A., Pisters, P.W., Guitreau, D.P., and Pisters, L.L. 2003. Total pelvic exenteration: effective palliation of perineal pain in patients with locally recurrent prostate cancer. *J. Urol. 170*:1868–1871.

Kyu, K.N., Kim, M.Z., Seong, H.Y., Kook, S.S., and Sik, M.J. 1999. Comparative study of transrectal ultrasonography, pelvic computerized tomography, and magnetic resonance imaging in preoperative staging of rectal cancer. *Dis. Colon Rectum 42*:770–775.

Lange, P.H. 2001. Prostascint scan for staging of prostate cancer. *Urology 57*:402–406.

Lee, N., Fawaaz, R., Olsson, C.A., Benson, M.C., Petrylak, D.P., Schiff, P.B., Bagiella, E., Singh, A., and Ennis, R.D. 2000. Which patients with newly diagnosed prostate cancer need a radionuclide bone scan? An analysis based on 631 patients. *Int. J. Radiat. Oncol. Biol. Phys. 48*:1443–1446.

Lee, N., Newhouse, J.H., Olsson, C.A., Benson, M.C., Petrylak, D.P., Schiff, P.B., Bagiella, E., Malyszlto, B., and Ennis, R.D. 1999. Which patients with newly diagnosed prostate cancer need a computed tomography of the abdomen and pelvis? An analysis based on 588 patients. *Urology 54*:490–494.

Leibovici, D., Kamat, A.M., Do, K.A., Pettaway, C.A., Ng, C.S., Evans, R.B., Rodriguez-Bigas, M., Skibber, J., Wang, X., and Pisters, L.L. 2005a. Transrectal ultrasound versus magnetic resonance imaging for detection of rectal wall invasion by prostate cancer. *The Prostate 62*:101–104.

Leibovici, D., Kamat, A.M., Pettaway, C.A., Pagliaro, L., Rosser, C.J., Logothetis, C.J., and Pisters, L.L. 2005b. Cystoprostatectomy for effective palliation of symptomatic bladder invasion by prostate cancer. *J. Urol. 174*:2186–2190.

Leibovici, D., Lee, A.K., Cheung, R.M., Spiess, P.E., Kuban, D.A., Rosser, C.J., Shen, Y., Yang, Y., Chichakli, R., and Pisters, L.L. 2005c. Symptomatic local recurrence of prostate carcinoma after radiation therapy. *Cancer 103*:2060–2066.

Mazur, A.W., and Thompson, I.M. 1991. Efficacy and morbidity of "channel" TURP. *Urology 38*:526–528.

Prando, A., Kurhanewicz, J., Borges, A.P., Oliveira, E.M., Jr., and Figuereido, E. 2005. Prostatic biopsy directed with endorectal MR spectroscopic imaging findings in patients with elevated prostate specific antigen levels and prior negative biopsy findings: early experience. *Radiology 236*:903–910.

Senzer, N.N. 2001. Prostate cancer: multimodality approaches with docetaxel. *Semin. Oncol. 4*:77–85.

Walsh, P.C., and Jewett, H.J. 1980. Radical surgery for prostate cancer. *Cancer 45*:1906–1916.

49

Local Staging of Prostate Cancer Using Endorectal Coil Magnetic Resonance Imaging

Thomas Hambrock, Jelle O. Barentsz, and Jurgen J. Fütterer

Introduction

Prostate cancer is the second most common cause of cancer-related death in men in most Western countries and poses a growing health problem. In 2007, approximately 218,000 men will be diagnosed with prostate cancer in the United States. Presently, more than one out of every three new cancers among males in the United States is prostate cancer (Jemal *et al.*, 2007). The wider use of serum prostate-specific antigen (PSA) tests and ever-lower PSA thresholds for performing biopsies will further increase the incidence of this disease. Like many cancers, prostate cancer is treated most effectively when detected early. Two of the most important tests for the early detection of prostate cancer are the digital rectal examination (DRE) and PSA blood test. Common diagnostic imaging methods such as (transrectal) ultrasound are often inadequate for staging and localization of prostate cancer (Sauvain *et al.*, 2003). This is a serious challenge, because accurate tumor staging and localization will critically influence patient management. To date, the histopathological examination of transrectal ultrasound-guided biopsy-obtained tissue remains the gold standard for diagnosis of prostate cancer. Such examination is still being used despite its inherent limitations that prostate malignancies are easily overlooked and tumor aggressiveness underestimated

because of their multifocal and heterogeneous nature (Hodge *et al.*, 1989).

Tumor Characteristics

Knowledge of the natural progression of prostate cancer is needed to give an indication of the prognosis once the disease is diagnosed. Relevant information on the expected course of the disease should be available before making treatment decisions. Several treatment options are available for patients with prostate cancer confined to the prostate. Radical prostatectomy or radiation therapy is advocated for local treatment with curative intention. Each of these treatment modalities has its own set of side effects that can influence patient decision on choice.

The available statistics on the rising morbidity and mortality associated with prostate cancer must be balanced against the fact that the histological incidence of prostate cancer far exceeds the prevalence of clinically manifest disease. It is known that > 30% of men older than 50 years have microscopic prostatic carcinoma at autopsy, yet fewer than 10% of men develop clinical prostate cancer in their lifetime. These data suggest that the majority of prostate cancers remain dormant and do not progress to a clinically relevant stage. The observation that many men die with prostate cancer but do not die from prostate cancer has been the basis of debate with regard to the most optimal treatment modalities for patients with tumors confined to the prostate, with the least mortality and morbidity.

The increasing use of early screening programs has created what appears to be a "stage migration." This means that more men are currently diagnosed with prostate cancer that is confined to the prostate and are thus more likely to be permanently cured with conventional therapy. Furthermore, a dilemma in the management of prostate cancer is that nonaggressive cancers (which do not require aggressive treatment) cannot easily be distinguished from cancers with a highly malignant potential. Thus, accurate methods are needed to define the aggressive malignant potential of an individual prostate tumor.

Grading and Partin Tables

As is true in many other organ systems, the grade of a malignancy or its degree of departure from normal has been established as an important prognostic marker in the prostate. A number of grading systems have been advocated, but currently the most widely used is that of Gleason. The Gleason grading system uses low-power microscopy to identify the architectural patterns of the tumor. The Gleason system has been shown not only to offer the most significant prognostic information but also to have a high reproducibility between pathologists (Kirby et al., 1996; Hayat et al., 2002).

Presently, DRE has been shown to have a fair reproducibility between experienced urologists. However, DRE misses a substantial proportion of cancers, especially tumors in the transition and the central zone, yet it identifies most large palpable peripheral zone tumors, with a more advanced pathological stage. Partin et al. (1993) demonstrated a sensitivity and specificity of 52% and 81%, respectively, for the prediction of organ-confined disease by DRE alone.

Currently, PSA is still recognized as the most useful hematological tumor marker available in clinical practice for the diagnosis, staging, and monitoring of prostate cancer. However, although studies have shown that serum PSA correlates directly with advancing clinical and pathological stages in most cases serum PSA level alone is not sufficiently accurate to stage individual patients due to the large overlap between different tumor stages. Furthermore, other disease processes, such as benign prostatic hyperplasia and prostatitis, can also influence serum PSA levels.

The Gleason score determined from ultrasound guided biopsy specimens has been shown to correlate most closely with the actual pathological stage for patients at either extreme of the score (i.e., 2–4 and 8–10) (Partin et al., 1990). Unfortunately, most men present with Gleason scores of 5–7, where the prediction of true pathological stage is less accurate.

Because of the multifocal and heterogeneous nature of prostate cancer, biopsy might not always represent the area within the prostate that has the highest Gleason score. This will result in an underestimation of the actual disease grade.

Nomograms, that is, Partin tables, which use three variables of serum PSA, biopsy Gleason score as well as clinical tumor stage determined with DRE, were initially developed in the early 1990s to assist urologists in the preoperative prediction of true pathological stage for patients who had clinically localized prostate cancer. Wider application and acceptance of these nomograms were subsequently validated in a multi-institutional study (Partin et al., 1997) as well as by other investigators. However, these three individual preoperative variables resulted in a large discrepancy between clinical prediction of organ-confined disease and actual pathological staging. The older Partin tables were therefore modified (Partin et al., 1997), using logistic regression analysis, with the probability of organ-confined disease improving across groups.

Partin tables have been validated as a predictive tool and are widely used for patient counselling. However, as a treatment-planning tool they are limited because they do not incorporate anatomic information that could guide interventions to control local disease. If cancer extends through the prostate capsule, the chances of cure are substantially diminished, and the surgical or radiation treatment planning must be adapted to ensure complete eradication of the cancer. Despite the strong predictive ability and the cost-effectiveness of the staging nomograms, there is room for improvement in staging accuracy, particularly because clinical staging in the staging nomograms is based only on digital rectal examination. Moreover, the staging nomograms cannot assist in the localization of extracapsular extension, which may be critical for optimal treatment planning.

Prognostic Factors

To determine the most effective treatment method with the least morbidity/mortality and best chance of cure, numerous prognostic variables could be taken into consideration. Partin tables were developed to incorporate some of these variables. A vast array of additional prognostic indicators is available which could guide the urologist. Unfortunately, due to the complexity of identifying many of these factors, urologists are not yet able to include these variables in decision making. Tumor aggressiveness, and thus the potential to metastasize, depends on a number of factors, of which pathological stage, histological grading, microvessel density (MVD), tumor volume, PSA levels, and vascular endothelial growth factor (VEGF) are the most important. Although the primary histological grade of the tumor best predicts aggressiveness and thus metastatic potential, some aggressive tumor areas within the prostate are often missed on biopsy, restricting its usefulness (Chodak *et al.*, 1994). Noninvasive techniques for accurate grading of prostatic tumors, therefore, will be of great benefit and might reduce the need for invasive procedures.

Recently, MVD and VEGF expressions have been found to have significant prognostic values. In prostate cancer, high MVD has been linked to aggressive behavior and thus correlated with histological grade, tumor stage, preoperative serum PSA, and time to recurrence (Gravdal *et al.*, 2006). There is strong evidence that angiogenesis in prostate cancer significantly correlates with the incidence of systemic metastases. Furthermore, it has been stated that MVD is a better predictor for extracapsular invasion of prostate cancer than PSA (Strohmeyer *et al.*, 2000). Increased expressions of VEGF and VEGF-C are closely associated with progression of prostate cancer through their role in maintaining angiogenesis and stimulating lymphangiogenesis (Yang *et al.*, 2006).

It has been reported that tumor volume and Gleason grade are closely correlated. Results indicate that extraprostatic extension only begins when tumors have reached a volume of $0.5\,cm^3$ or more and is found most often when tumor volume is greater than $1.4\,cm^3$ (McNeal, 1992). Because tumor volume has emerged as an important factor in predicting pathologic stage and tumor recurrence, the percentage of positive biopsy cores has been used to predict pathological stage, as there is a linear relationship between percentage positive biopsy cores and tumor volume.

Staging of Prostate Cancer

Clinical staging of prostate cancer currently entails the use of DRE, PSA, and transrectal US. The clinical stage is identified using these variables and is expressed in the Tumor Node Metastases (TNM) staging classification (Table 1).

Stages T1a–T1c

Stages T1a and T1b are not identified by digital rectal examination of the prostate. They are found incidentally in the prostatic tissue removed during transurethral resection or during prostatectomy performed for benign prostate hyperplasia (BPH). Tumors of these stages are generally referred to as incidental carcinomas. These tumors are found in 8 to 12% of the patients undergoing surgery for benign disease. Patients

Table 1   TNM Staging System for Prostate Cancer (Greene F.L. 2002)

TNM Staging System for Prostate Cancer	
Stage	Definition
Primary tumor	
TX	Primary tumor cannot be assessed
T0	No evidence of primary tumor
T1	Clinically the tumor is neither palpable nor visible with imaging
T1a	Tumor is an incidental histologic finding in 5% or less of tissue resected
T1b	Tumor is an incidental histologic finding in > 5% of tissue resected
T1c	Tumor identified with needle biopsy (e.g., because of an elevated PSA)
T2	Tumor confined within the prostate
T2a	Tumor involves one-half of one lobe or less
T2b	Tumor involves more than one-half of one lobe but not both lobes
T2c	Tumor involves both lobes
T3	Tumor extends through the prostate capsule
T3a	Extracapsular extension (unilateral or bilateral)
T3b	Tumor invades seminal vesicle(s)
T4	Tumor is fixed or invades adjacent structures other than seminal vesicles: bladder neck, external sphincter, rectum, levator muscles, and/or pelvic wall
Regional lymph nodes	
NX	Regional lymph nodes were not assessed
N0	No regional lymph node metastasis
N1	Metastasis in regional lymph node(s)
Distant metastasis	
MX	Distant metastasis cannot be assessed (not evaluated with any modality)
M0	No distant metastasis
M1	Distant metastasis
M1a	Non-regional lymph node(s)
M1b	Bone(s)
M1c	Other site(s) with or without bone disease

rarely die from T1a or T1b disease but rather from age-related problems. Prostate cancer diagnosed by needle biopsy after an elevated PSA was found and is termed stage T1c disease if both DRE are normal and no lesions are visible on TRUS.

Stages T2a–T2c

In stages T2a to T2c disease, there is either an organ-confined palpable nodule on DRE or evidence of one or multiple tumors on imaging. This category of prostate cancers is considered potentially curable. In stage T2, lymph node dissection in patients reveals lymph node metastasis in 10–25% of cases. The natural history of T2 prostate cancer has been shown to be associated with a 10-year local progression of 66% and progression to metastatic disease in 33%.

Stage T3 Prostate Cancer

T3 prostate cancers have extracapsular extension and a much poorer prognosis. These tumors are at the limit of potential surgical curability, with microscopic invasive tumors having a more favorable outcome. Lymph node metastases occur in 50% of these cases. In the event of lymph node involvement, prognosis is determined by the N status rather than by the T category. It has been shown that cure rates with surgery alone are not to be expected to exceed 30%.

N+ and M+ Disease

During pelvic lymphadenectomy, metastatic lymph nodes are found to various degrees. Median time progression in this group is in the order of 11–24 months. In terms of survival, it seems to be of little importance whether hormonal treatment is deferred or started immediately. The reported median time to progression can be prolonged up to 5 years with early hormonal treatment; this is achieved at the cost of side effects.

Imaging Techniques In Staging

Because DRE and/or PSA has been shown to be of limited value in the prediction of stage T3 tumors, numerous imaging modalities have been incorporated to improve the accuracy of staging. The most common imaging modalities, albeit with different accuracy, are power Doppler and contrast-enhanced transrectal ultrasound (TRUS), CT, glucose/choline positron emission tomography (PET) as well as MRI.

Transrectal Ultrasound, Power Doppler Ultrasound, and Contrast-Enhanced Ultrasound

Since its clinical introduction in 1971, TRUS has become the cheapest and most frequently used imaging technique in the evaluation of the prostate. Its value in assessing prostate volume and guiding biopsy is well known. The role of transrectal ultrasound in detecting and staging prostate cancer is more controversial. Transrectal ultrasound can be used to examine the prostate for hypoechoic lesions, as these have an increased probability of being malignant, especially when they are present in the peripheral zone with a 17–57% chance of malignancy. Unfortunately, prostate tumors can present as isoechoic (12–30%) or even hyperechoic lesions. When staging prostate cancer by TRUS, any change in the prostatic capsule, such as bulging or irregularity, adjacent to the hypoechoic lesion is suspicious of extracapsular extension. Invasion of tumor into the seminal vesicles may also be identified on TRUS. Transrectal ultrasound has a limited value in tumor staging, with positive predictive values of 50–63% for detecting extracapsular extension. Therefore, the merit of TRUS lies in guiding biopsies to provide a histopathological diagnosis (Giesen et al., 1995). Duplex Doppler studies with TRUS, as well as microbubble ultrasonographic contrast agents to enhance the visibility of blood flow, are new methods to study tumor vascularity. These blood flow-enhancing TRUS methods have the potential to improve the detection and staging of prostate cancer (Pelzer et al., 2005). Future research will indicate their exact role.

Computed Tomography

In the 1980s and early 1990s, the value of CT in prostate staging was assessed. While CT may be useful to define locally advanced cancers (T4), by showing the involvement of pelvic structures and lymph nodes, it has no use in assessing clinically confined lesions (local stage T2 or T3 disease) (Huncharek and Muscat, 1996).

Positron Emission Tomography

Positron emission tomography is an imaging technique that provides noninvasive, three-dimensional (3D), whole-body, quantitative images of radioactivity from radioisotopes undergoing positron emission decay. FDG-PET imaging in prostate cancer has been difficult because of the low glucose utilization of these tumors and the anatomical close connection to the bladder, where intense accumulation of FDG in the urinary pool makes assessment of the prostate difficult. Fibrosis, inflammation, BPH, and androgen ablation therapy restrict uptake of FDG and reduce delineation of tumor. Newer molecular imaging techniques with radiotracers have emerged as powerful methods in guiding the management of patients with prostate cancer. Positron emission tomography, however, has a role only in the staging of metastatic disease and biological characterization of prostate cancer. New PET tracers, including C^{11}-choline and C^{11}-acetate, show potential for identifying nodal disease. Although FDG-PET has a role in the staging of metastatic prostate cancer and detection of recurrence, its role in local prostate staging to differentiate T2 from T3 disease is very limited owing to the very low spatial resolution of this technique as well as the low uptake of the tracer within the primary tumor as mentioned above (Lawrentschuk, 2006).

Endorectal Magnetic Resonance Imaging in Local Staging of Prostate Cancer

Magnetic resonance imaging is currently the most accurate modality for the preoperative staging of prostate cancer. It has a higher accuracy in the assessment of intraprostatic disease (stage T2), extracapsular extension, and seminal vesicle invasion (stage T3), as well as invasion of periprostatic structures (stage T4), compared to CT, TRUS, or FDG-PET. Magnetic resonance imaging performed at low field strengths with the conventional body coil or phased-array surface coils lacks sufficient resolution and signal-to-noise ratio (SNR) to identify fine anatomic details of the prostate gland and periprostatic tissues necessary for accurate staging. Hence, small extracapsular extension of tumor or infiltration into the seminal vesicles is usually not visible, and the accuracy in defining local tumor stage is as low as 57% in clinically confined tumors (Rifkin *et al.*, 1990). The introduction of balloon-type endorectal coils was shown to drastically increase the spatial resolution and SNR of prostate MR imaging. Consequently, the ability of MR imaging to correctly stage local tumor cancer was significantly increased. Despite this, a large heterogeneity of staging accuracy with endorectal 1.5T MR imaging has been reported (Bartolozzi *et al.*, 2001).

Despite its high specificity in the identification of extracapsular extension, increased experience in interpretation and a better understanding of anatomical criteria used to diagnose T3 disease are the key to further improving the accuracy of MR imaging in staging. Apart from extracapsular extension, seminal vesicle invasion is an important prognostic factor because it is associated with the highest rates of recurrence, second only to lymph node metastases (Blute *et al.*, 2001). Magnetic resonance imaging is also helpful in identifying the invasion of adjacent organs (e.g., the bladder, pelvic floor muscles, and rectum).

The most cost-effective group of patients to undergo local staging with endorectal MR imaging are those considered to have an intermediate risk of T3 prostate cancer, based on a PSA level between 4 and 20 ng/ml and a Gleason score between 5 and 7 (Engelbrecht *et al.*, 2001). In this group of patients, endorectal MR imaging is useful because the decision on selection of treatment (prostatectomy or local radiotherapy and/or hormonal treatment) depends on the imaging results. Inclusion of MR imaging results in clinical nomograms helps improve the prediction of cancer extent, thereby improving patient selection for local therapy.

These findings and a recent report (Saito *et al.*, 2006) indicating a 5-year survival benefit for men with locally advanced prostate cancer treated with external beam radiation therapy (RT) and adjuvant androgen suppression as opposed to external beam RT alone provide weight for consideration of combined modality therapy (i.e., RT + androgen suppression) for the subset of patients identified on MR imaging to have T3 disease. Thus, in this select patient subgroup, the endorectal MR imaging stage provided an identification of patients at very high risk for PSA failure postoperatively. Therefore, this radiologic tool could influence the decision on management and potentially improve clinical outcome for the individual patient.

Ideally, endorectal MR imaging of the prostate should have a low percentage of false positives for extracapsular extension and seminal vesicle invasion to ensure that few, if any, patients will be deprived of potentially curative treatment. Sensitivity for periprostatic extension is less important because even a low sensitivity is an improvement on clinical staging.

Imaging Protocol

Endorectal MR imaging should be obtained at least 4 weeks after TRUS-guided biopsy as hemorrhage decreases the localization accuracy and thus staging (White *et al.*, 1995). Prostate MR imaging is performed using radiofrequency (RF) coils, which can transmit radiofrequencies and receive MR signals. Three types of coils can be used for prostatic MRI. Initially, the body coil was used, which is a built-in coil present in most MRI scanners. Surface coils, which are placed on the surface of the patient at the anatomic region of interest, have become the preferred method of imaging. In prostate MR imaging, the pelvic phased-array coil and the endorectal coil are used at 1.5 Tesla, while either the pelvic phased array or endorectal coil is used at 3 Tesla. Given these different techniques, use of an endorectal coil is considered to be a significant improvement over the body or pelvic phased-array coils. Patients tolerate the endorectal coil well, although the insertion remains uncomfortable. For the endorectal coil, the only reported adverse effect on imaging is an increase in the incidence of movement artifacts, which causes image quality to deteriorate (Heijmink *et al.*, 2007).

A typical imaging sequence for integrated endorectal-pelvic phased-array coil imaging at 1.5T for staging of prostate cancer includes: turbo spin-echo sequence with repetition time (TR) of 4000 ms, echo time (TE) of 128 ms, echo-train length of 15, averages 2, field-of-view 280 mm, matrix size 240×512, and a slice thickness of 4 mm. There is no evidence for the usefulness of fat suppression in T2-weighted sequences. Use of frequency-selective fat suppression does not significantly improve the diagnosis of extraprostatic disease and decreases the SNR, which may limit visualization of anatomic details and reduce the definition of the prostatic capsule. Moreover, suppression of fat signal intensity leads to reduced definition of periprostatic anatomic planes and degrades visualization of structures within the prostatic fat, such as the neurovascular bundles. Contrast between extra-prostatic tumor and peri-prostatic fat may also be reduced (Tsuda *et al.*, 1999).

T2-Weighted Magnetic Resonance Imaging Features

It has been established that 70% of prostate cancers originate in the peripheral zone, ~ 25% arise in the transition zone, and the remaining 5% are located in the central zone (Sakai *et al.*, 2005). Prostate cancer usually appears as an area of low signal intensity within the high signal intensity of the normal peripheral zone on T2-weighted images (Fig. 1). These differences in signal intensity make it possible to identify tumors in the peripheral zone. Focal areas of low signal intensity within the peripheral zone, however, do not always represent cancer because chronic prostatitis (especially granulomatous prostatitis), atrophy, and postbiopsy hemorrhage with blood in the methemoglobin state may mimic tumor (White *et al.*, 1995). The latter can be differentiated from the other causes by visualizing a high signal intensity area on T1-weighted images (methemoglobin is diamagnetic), in which prostate cancer is usually undetectable. To prevent false interpretation of T2-weighted images (especially when assessing tumor stage), MR imaging should be performed at least four weeks after prostatic biopsy. A rare subtype of prostate carcinoma, termed mucinous carcinoma, can appear as a hyperintense lesion on T2-weighted images because of its rich mucinous content. The detection of tumors located within the central portion of the gland is much more difficult, especially because of the coexisting benign prostatic hyperplasia with nodular appearance. Nevertheless, endorectal MR imaging can sometimes depict centrally located tumors that are usually undetectable by DRE or TRUS.

The TNM staging system today includes information obtained from imaging modalities to define the presence and extent of the neoplasm. Among locally invading tumors, however, the distinction between those penetrating the prostate capsule but sparing the seminal vesicles (T3a) and those invading the seminal vesicles (T3b) is important in both therapeutic planning and patient prognosis. It is important to remember that according to the TNM staging system, tumors invading but not penetrating the capsule are classified as T2 and not as T3. Magnetic resonance imaging with the endorectal coil allows evaluation of the tumor location, tumor volume, capsular penetration, invasion of neurovascular bundle, and seminal vesicle involvement (Jager *et al.*, 2000). Precise analysis of all these MR features is crucial for accurate treatment planning.

Location of the tumor within the prostate has important prognostic and therapeutic consequences. Some areas have a higher risk for extraglandular invasion. These areas include the implant of the seminal vesicles where the capsule insinuates itself, and the apex where the anatomic fibromuscular capsule no longer exists. The latter location could be considered extra-capsular. Apical tumors, moreover, increase the difficulties of performing radical surgical removal of the malignancy. When the apex is involved, the percentage of positive surgical margins is substantial. In addition, urinary continence is seldom preserved after surgical removal of apical tumors.

The appearance of the prostatic capsule is that of a thin low signal intensity rim located between the hyperintensity

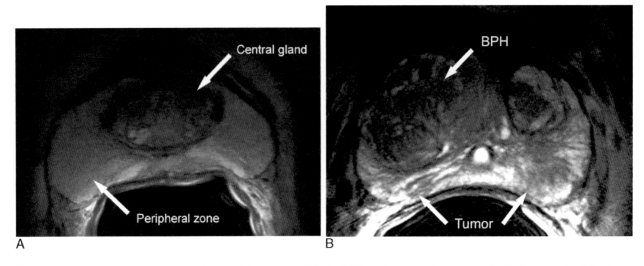

Figure 1 T2-weighted endorectal coil MR images of the prostate at 3 Tesla. (**A**) Normal prostate—bottom arrow indicating normal peripheral zone and top arrow showing normal central gland (**B**) Prostate with two peripheral zone tumors (bottom arrows) and area of BPH (top arrow).

of the peripheral zone and that of the periprostatic fat on T2-weighted imaging. Chemical shift adds to improving delineating the prostate capsule. Prostate cancer can be regarded as intracapsular when normal appearing hyperintense prostatic tissue is visible between the tumor and the capsule or when the capsule is clearly delineated, despite bordering on the tumor. In contrast, bulging or irregularity of the border of the prostate, low signal intensity focal thickening of the capsule at the capsular margin of the tumor or at the edges of the tumor, and retraction of the capsule adjacent to the tumor should be regarded with great suspicion as most likely signs of extracapsular extension. Low signal intensity lesions within the periprostatic fat, adjacent to the lesion, and evidence of obvious extracapsular tumor provide evidence of extraprostatic infiltration (Fig. 2). It is important to know that the prostate capsule can show irregularity at any time after biopsy and is independent of the degree of hemorrhage. Thus, capsular irregularity should be interpreted with caution when evaluated after biopsy. With increased experience, subtle findings of extracapsular spread can also be correctly interpreted in many instances.

At the site where the neurovascular bundle enters the capsule, the capsule is less well developed, particularly at the apex of the gland. These capsular weaknesses are preferential paths for spread of the tumor. The neurovascular bundles are best visualized on transverse T1-weighted images and appear as hypointense structures, located at the postero-lateral areas of the prostate, within the hyperintense periprostatic fat. Tracing the neurovascular bundle along its whole path is quite difficult, especially in the area of the apex (Bartolozzi *et al.*, 2001).

Seminal vesicles on T2-weighted images appear as irregular structures with thin hypointense walls and filled with hyperintense fluid. The diagnosis of seminal vesicle invasion is made when focal or diffuse thickening (hypointense) of the tubular walls, associated with focal hypointense luminal lesions, is present (Fig. 3). It can also be diagnosed when diffuse anatomical or morphologic changes of the seminal vesicles occur as a result of advanced tumor infiltration. When the tumor has reached and infiltrated the ejaculatory ducts, the seminal vesicles can be considered affected. False-positive findings of seminal vesicle infiltration can occur when hemorrhage (post-biopsy), occurs or due to inflammatory processes within the prostate. In the presence of post-biopsy hemorrhage, low-intensity lesions tend to be diffuse, and as in the prostate gland itself, the presence of blood in the methemoglobin state can be confirmed by high signal intensity on T1-weighted images (Bartolozzi *et al.*, 2001).

Accuracy of T2-Weighted Magnetic Resonance Imaging in Staging of Prostate Cancer

A large number of studies have been performed over the last years to show the accuracy of MRI in staging prostate. Engelbrecht (Engelbrecht *et al.*, 2002) showed in a meta-analysis that it is not yet possible to state the "overall" accuracy of MR imaging for staging prostate cancer because of a wide divergence in the literature. For example, the accuracy of assessing extracapsular extension with the endorectal coil varied widely between 58% and 90%. There were several possible explanations: the use of different imaging protocols, differences in reader experience, patient selection, and use of

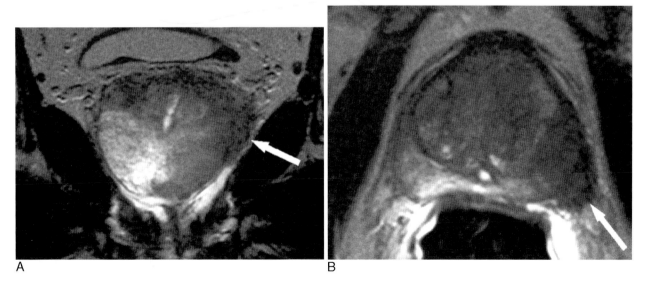

Figure 2 (**A**) Coronal and (**B**) transverse, T2-weighted MR images showing a low signal intensity lesion (arrow), indicative of extracapsular extension in the area of the left neurovascular bundle.

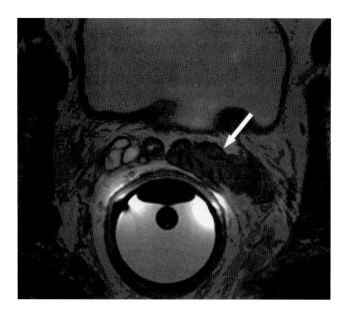

Figure 3 Transverse T2-weighted MR image showing low-intensity lesions with vascular wall thickening (arrow) due to prostate cancer invasion of the seminal vesicles.

different criteria for extracapsular extension. A limitation of endorectal MR imaging on which there was consensus is that it is still not possible to detect microscopic extracapsular extension. Their meta-analysis showed that the detection of seminal vesicle invasion was generally good using the endorectal coil, with accuracies ranging between 81% and 96%. However, it appeared that the most specific criterion for extracapsular extension is asymmetry of the neurovascular bundle (sensitivity 38%, specificity 95%). The most sensitive criterion is overall impression of the tumor (sensitivity 68%, specificity 72%) (subjective combination of all available criteria). Other reliable criteria are obliteration of the rectoprostatic angle, bulging, and extracapsular tumor extension. However, in the meta-analysis they could not determine the effect that the criteria for extracapsular extension have on staging performance.

Engelbrecht's summary receiver operating characteristic (ROC) curve for MR imaging in prostate cancer staging (T2 vs. T3) had a joint maximum sensitivity and specificity of 71%. At a specificity of 80% on that curve, sensitivity was 62%, and at a specificity of 95%, sensitivity was 29%. The summary ROC curve for detection of seminal vesicle invasion had a joint maximum sensitivity and specificity of 82%. At a specificity of 95%, sensitivity was 27%. Similarly, for detection of extracapsular extension a joint maximum sensitivity and specificity of 64% was found; with a specificity of 95%, the sensitivity was 23%. Their joint sensitivity and specificity numbers for detecting stage cT3 (71%) were similar to the numbers reported by Sonnad *et al.* (2001) in their meta-analysis (74%). A limitation of these estimates is that, due to the heterogeneity in staging performance, it is difficult to discuss the average local staging performance of MR imaging. Because of poor reporting, they were not

able to fully explain the heterogeneity of performance presented in the literature. It was suggested that turbo spin echo, endorectal coil, and multiple imaging planes improved staging performance (Engelbrecht *et al.*, 2002).

Comparative studies evaluating the benefit of using a combined integrated endorectal-pelvic phased-array coil versus pelvic phased-array coil only at 1.5T have also appeared. Anatomical detail of the overall prostate is significantly better evaluated using the endorectal-pelvic phased-array coil (Fütterer *et al.*, 2007). It has been reported that, for the experienced reader, local staging accuracy increased significantly from 59% (pelvic phased-array coil) to 83% (endorectal-pelvic phased-array coil). This was mostly due to the increase in specificity, which is crucially important for staging. Use of an endorectal-pelvic phased-array coil resulted in significant improvement of anatomic details, staging accuracy, and specificity. When using an endorectal-pelvic phased-array coil, overstaging is reduced significantly with equal sensitivity. Jager *et al.* (2000) developed a decision analytic model that supported the opinion that MR staging in preoperative work-up of prostate cancer is cost-effective and should be performed with a high specificity. Langlotz *et al.* (1995) also emphasized this need for high specificity in prostate MR imaging to ensure that as few patients as possible will be unnecessarily turned away from potentially curative therapy on the basis of false-positive MR imaging results.

In patients in whom prostate cancer was diagnosed, the existence of seminal vesicle invasion is associated with high rates of tumor recurrence and therapy failure. Reported progression rates in these patients range from 40 to 95%. High PSA, a high Gleason score, the presence of tumor at the base of the prostate, and coexistent lymph node metastasis are all associated with an increased incidence of seminal vesicle invasion (Villers *et al.*, 1990). In patients with prostate cancer, the preoperative diagnosis of seminal vesicle invasion is an important factor in staging and prognosis and affects treatment decisions and planning. Routinely performing seminal vesicle biopsy during preoperative staging has been limited by the low prevalence of seminal vesicle invasion in patients with prostate cancer, the low sensitivity of this procedure, and the high rate of false-positive results (Guillonneau *et al.*, 1997).

In recent studies, MR imaging identified seminal vesicle invasion with a sensitivity of 71–80% and a specificity of 83–93% (Bartolozzi *et al.*, 1996; Rorvik *et al.*, 1999). An advantage of endorectal MR imaging is its ability to diagnose seminal vesicle invasion with good sensitivity and specificity; it therefore adds valuable information to patient management. This information can seldom be obtained by using digital rectal examination or TRUS.

Sala *et al.* (2006) reported on the accuracy of endorectal MR imaging in demonstrating seminal vesicle invasion and investigated the MR features that can predict these invasions. They showed that seminal vesicle invasion can be detected with an area-under-curve of between 0.81 and 0.93 for two readers. For both readers, the features that had the highest sensitivity and specificity were low signal intensity within the seminal vesicle and lack of preservation of seminal vesicle architecture. Tumor at the prostate base that extended beyond the capsule, as well as low signal intensity within a seminal vesicle that has lost its normal architecture, were highly predictive of seminal vesicle invasion. For both readers, dilatation of the ejaculatory ducts and obliteration of the angle between the prostate and the seminal vesicle had the lowest sensitivities but were highly specific for seminal vesicle invasion. It was also shown that at pathological examination, all patients with seminal vesicle invasion had tumor at the base of the prostate. Seminal vesicle invasion was also associated with extracapsular extension in 92% of the cases. It appeared that the combination of tumor at the base of the prostate gland and extracapsular extension with seminal vesicle invasion features is more helpful than any seminal vesicle invasion feature alone in predicting seminal vesicle invasion. The combinations of features that are predictive of seminal vesicle invasion, however, will vary for different readers.

Accidental damage or purposeful removal of the neurovascular bundle during prostatectomy can have significant detrimental consequences for the patient. Urinary incontinence and impotence can reduce the quality of life. Preoperative confirmation of absent neurovascular bundle infiltration by tumor can dictate a nerve-sparing surgery, reducing patient morbidity. Reliable selection criteria, however, are required for adequate and safe use of a nerve-sparing surgical approach without compromising cancer removal. However, presently, no objective and accepted selection criteria exist for a nerve-sparing surgery. Most reported studies addressing the results of nerve-sparing modification are for patients selected by DRE, PSA, or intraoperative findings.

The staging accuracy and detection of neurovascular bundle involvement by dynamic subtraction contrast-enhanced endorectal MRI in patients with localized prostate cancer has been assessed (Ogura et al., 2001). An accuracy rate of 84% and 97% for the detection of capsular penetration and seminal vesicle invasion, respectively, was reached, while a 97% accuracy was obtained for the assessment of neurovascular bundle involvement. It appears that this technique may be useful for the selection of patients for radical prostatectomy and particularly for identifying candidates for nerve-sparing surgery from those with clinically localized prostate cancer.

It has been shown that 25% of the cancers involve the transition zone of radical prostatectomy specimens (McNeal et al., 1988). Transition zone cancers have pathological and clinical features that differ from those portrayed by peripheral zone cancers. The importance of accurately detecting transition zone cancers is to guide biopsy, support therapy planning, and to help the surgeon to avoid positive anterior surgical margins at radical prostatectomy. Compared to peripheral zone cancers, patients with transition zone cancers have significantly higher mean PSA levels (11 ng/ml

and 31 ng/ml, respectively) (Stamey et al., 1993). Tumor volumes in patients with transition zone cancer (11.2 ml) are also larger than in peripheral zone cancers (5.0 ml). Transition zone cancers, however, have lower mean Gleason scores than patients with peripheral zone cancers (6.2 and 7.4, respectively). In addition, transition zone cancers are more often confined intraprostatically (67–89%) than peripheral zone cancers (41–56%) (Stamey and Yemoto, 1998). Furthermore, extraprostatic extension of these tumors occurs at a larger average tumor volume in transition zone cancers than in peripheral zone cancers (4.98 ml vs. 3.86 ml, respectively) (Greene et al., 1991). When tumor volumes are the same, a higher rate of organ-confined disease is thus seen in transition zone cancers as compared to peripheral zone cancers (79% and 27%, respectively) (McNeal, 1992).

Studies performed previously with older scanners and with the use of surface coils only indicated that MR imaging had limited ability in the identification of transition zone cancers. The presence of fibromuscular (stromal) benign prostatic hyperplasia makes identification of transition zone cancers particularly difficult because these have low-intensity features on T2-weighted MR images. However, preliminary reports have shown that homogeneous low T2 signal intensity, poorly defined margins, and absence of the capsule on MR images can be used to identify transition zone cancers.

Transition zone cancers and peripheral zone cancers have separate clinical, pathological, and imaging characteristics. Peripheral zone cancers receive the most focus in the current prostate MR imaging literature. The role of MR imaging in the assessment of transition zone cancers has been studied only rarely. The lower incidence of transition zone cancers may be one reason for this scarcity. In addition, the evaluation of transition zone cancer on MR imaging is hampered by the heterogeneous T2 signal intensity in the normal transition zone.

One study specifically addressed the problem of identifying and staging transition zone cancers with endorectal MR imaging. Sensitivities of 75–80% as well as specificities of 78–87% were reached. Increasing volume of tumors increased the localization rate significantly. Similar to peripheral zone cancers, low sensitivities (28–56%) but high specificities (93–94%) were reached for staging. It was found that homogeneous low T2 signal intensity and lenticular shape were significantly associated with the presence of transition zone cancer. For experienced readers it was possible to stage transition zone cancers with MR imaging (Akin et al., 2006).

Dynamic Contrast-Enhanced Magnetic Resonance Imaging

Although the literature is still sparse on the added value of dynamic contrast-enhanced MR imaging (DCE-MRI) to improve staging performance, it does appear to improve local staging performance when used in combination with T2-weighted imaging in patients with equivocal capsular penetration, seminal vesicle invasion, and neurovascular bundle involvement. Recently, Fütterer (Fütterer *et al.*, 2005) specifically investigated the ability of DCE-MRI to improve the staging of prostate cancer. They found that, for experienced radiologists, the addition of DCE-MRI to high-resolution T2-weighted imaging had little additional benefit except in equivocal cases. Reader experience is important in the staging of prostate cancer, and less experienced radiologists improved their results significantly (the area under the ROC curve improved from 0.66 to 0.82) by using DCE-MRI imaging. They noted that parametric maps helped draw the attention of less experienced readers to areas of prostate cancer, thereby allowing better staging. This suggests that DCE-MRI should be used by less experienced radiologists as an additional tool to improve the local staging performance of prostate cancer, particularly when equivocal finding is present.

Proton Spectroscopic Magnetic Resonance Imaging in the Staging of Prostate Cancer

Since the development of the endorectal coil, it has been possible to perform localized three-dimensional (3D) proton MR spectroscopy of the prostate with a spatial resolution of up to $0.22\,cm^3$. The ratio of two metabolites in the spectrum is of great importance in the prostate. Choline and citrate ratios are significantly elevated in areas of prostate cancer and do not show significant overlap with normal peripheral zone metabolite ratios (Fig. 4). The latter makes MR spectroscopy a useful method for the detection of tumor as well as estimation of tumor volume. This is particularly helpful in patients with post-biopsy hemorrhage and for those who have received previous hormonal treatment (Kurhanewicz *et al.*, 1996).

Previous studies have shown a strong association between the volume of prostate cancer determined on histopathological analysis and the presence of extracapsular extension (Bostwick *et al.*, 1993). This suggests that 3D MR spectroscopic assessment of tumor volume can predict extracapsular extension in a similar way that PSA levels predict extracapsular extension. It was noted (Stamey *et al.*, 1988) that the prevalence of extracapsular extension was only 18% in tumors with volume $< 3\,cm^3$ as compared to 79% in tumors with volume $> 3\,cm^3$. Due to the heterogeneous nature of tumors on anatomic images, TRUS and endorectal MR imaging have been disappointing in estimating tumor volume. Three-dimensional proton spectroscopic MR imaging may provide more accurate tumor volume estimation by allowing detection of significant alterations in metabolite levels of choline and citrate in the peripheral zone of the prostate in a number of voxels. The number of voxels found

positive for tumor is an indirect estimation of the tumor volume (Kurhanewicz *et al.*, 1996).

Presently, a few studies are available showing that 3D MR spectroscopic imaging has a potential in predicting extracapsular extension. Yu *et al.* (1999) have shown that patients with the least extensive tumor on 3D MR spectroscopic imaging (< 1 cancer voxel per section) were found to have only a 6% risk of extracapsular extension, whereas patients with the most extensive tumor (> 4 cancer voxels per section) had an 80% risk of extracapsular extension. These results support the use of 3D MR spectroscopic imaging as a predictor of extracapsular extension. Compared with MR imaging, 3D MR spectroscopic imaging demonstrated diagnostic accuracies comparable to those of the more experienced reader and significantly better than those for the less experienced reader. The addition of 3D MR spectroscopic imaging to MR imaging therefore improves accuracy for less experienced readers and reduces interobserver variability in the diagnosis of extracapsular extension of prostate cancer.

Staging at 3 Tesla

The increased SNR inherent in 3 Tesla (3T) as compared to 1.5T offers options for clinical MR imaging such as faster imaging, increased spatial resolution, or a combination of these. The doubling of SNR when the 3T field strength is used instead of 1.5T is similar to that achieved when localized surface coils are used for reception instead of whole-body coils at 1.5T. However, the challenges of clinical application at 3T imaging include a quadrupling of RF power deposition compared with 1.5T, signal heterogeneity from larger B1 field variations as compared with 1.5T (Greenman *et al.*, 2003), and greater susceptibility effects at the higher field strength. Changes in T1 and T2 relaxation times also need to be incorporated into sequence optimization. In addition, adjustments to dynamic contrast-enhanced sequences for kinetic analysis will be necessary. In a recent study, it has been suggested that for prostate imaging, use of an external phased-array coil at 3T yields an image quality that is equivalent to that of an endorectal coil image at 1.5T (Sosna *et al.*, 2003). Indeed, the increased SNR that has been achieved through an integrated endorectal-pelvic phased-array coil at 1.5T has facilitated MR imaging of the prostate in the detection and staging of prostate adenocarcinoma (Engelbrecht *et al.*, 2002).

It is a natural conclusion that the combined use of endorectal with external phased-array coils at 3T can further improve spatial resolution and will likely yield superior image quality compared with either an external phased-array coil alone at 3T or the combined external/endorectal coil at 1.5T. The value of T2-weighted MR imaging of the prostate depends on visualization of the tumor and prostate capsule, and ability to assess their spatial relationships. This in turn is greatly influenced by the achievable spatial resolution and tissue contrast, leading some investigators to conclude that a higher spatial

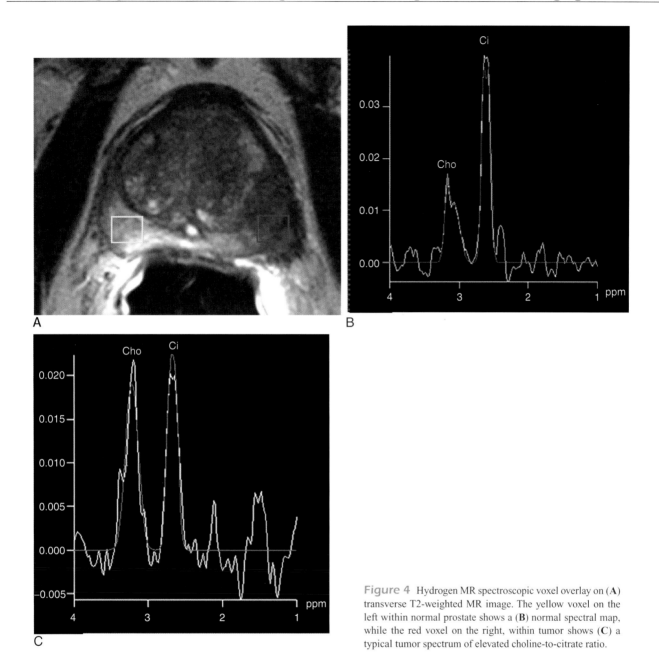

Figure 4 Hydrogen MR spectroscopic voxel overlay on (**A**) transverse T2-weighted MR image. The yellow voxel on the left within normal prostate shows a (**B**) normal spectral map, while the red voxel on the right, within tumor shows (**C**) a typical tumor spectrum of elevated choline-to-citrate ratio.

resolution facilitates better clinical performance of MR imaging of the prostate (Engelbrecht *et al.*, 2002).

In a recent study by Fütterer (Fütterer *et al.*, 2004), patients with prostate cancer were examined by using an endorectal coil at 3T MR imaging. It was shown that the increased SNR with an endorectal coil at 3T has great potential to improve the spatial resolution of T2-weighted and spectroscopic images, and either the spatial or temporal resolution of dynamic T1-weighted sequences for contrast-enhanced imaging. For the experienced radiologists, in the localization of prostate cancer, accuracies of 94% have been achieved,

which are higher than those reported for 1.5 T. Equally high sensitivities (88%) and specificities (96%) were reported. The added benefit of 3T was also noticeable for the less experienced reader (sensitivity 50%, specificity 92%). The increased resolution and SNR also seemed to increase agreement between both experienced readers. In addition, minimal capsular invasion could be detected (Fig. 5). With the demonstrated ability to detect minimal capsular penetration, the question arises whether the progression from stage T2 disease to stage T3 disease should be used as the basis on which clinicians should choose between surgical resection of

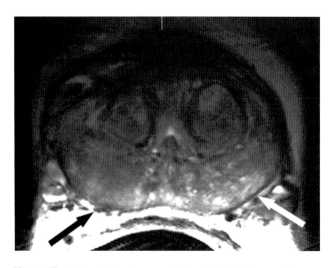

Figure 5 High-resolution transverse T2-weighted MR image of the prostate at 3T. A well-delineated, smooth, low-intensity capsule is seen on the right (white arrow). Extracapsular extension is seen on the left with loss of the capsule and low signal intensity lesions infiltrating the high-intensity periprostatic fat (black arrow).

the prostate or a combination of radiation therapy and hormonal therapy for treatment.

In another study (Fütterer *et al.*, 2006), it was confirmed that 3T endorectal coil imaging was superior in staging performances. They presented results with a high accuracy of 94% and a specificity of 96%. This has shown significant improvement over previous published results at lower field strengths. Irregular bulging of the prostatic capsule appeared to be the most sensitive indicator of extracapsular extension.

At higher field strength, the need for using an endorectal coil has been questioned. Heijmink *et al.* (2007) compared image quality and the accuracy of prostate cancer localization and staging of body array coil versus endorectal coil T2-weighted MR imaging at 3T. Significantly more motion artifacts were present when the endorectal coil was used. However, all other image quality characteristics improved significantly ($P < .001$) with endorectal coil imaging. Use of the endorectal coil significantly increased the area under the ROC curve for localizing prostate cancer from 0.62 to 0.68. Endorectal MR imaging significantly increased the staging area under the ROC curve and the sensitivity of detecting locally advanced disease in experienced readers from 7 to 73–80%, while maintaining high specificity of 97–100%. Extracapsular extension as small as 0.5 mm at histopathology could be accurately detected only with endorectal MR imaging. The significant increase in capsular delineation, visualization of the neurovascular bundle and rectoprostatic angle, and lesion visibility with endorectal MR imaging improved the staging performance. It explains the increase in sensitivity of detecting locally advanced disease for all readers. Results of their study showed that endorectal coil

MR imaging at 3T significantly improved image quality and, combined with the higher spatial resolution, significantly increased the localization and staging performance for the experienced radiologists and the less experienced radiologist (Heijmink *et al.*, 2007).

Conclusion

The increasing use of early screening programs has resulted in an ever increasing prevalence of prostate cancer and what appears to be a stage migration. In other words, more men are currently identified with prostate cancers that are confined to the prostate and are thus more likely permanently cured with conventional therapy. It has, therefore, become critically important to accurately stage prostate cancer to decide on optimal treatment techniques with the least morbidity and mortality with the best chance of permanent cure. Up until now clinical DRE examinations and imaging techniques such as TRUS and CT have been inaccurate in staging prostate cancer patients. With the introduction of endorectal coil MR imaging at 1.5 Tesla, an accurate imaging modality has become available that is also cost-effective in a subset of patients.

With increasing technological developments and higher field strengths with improved SNR and spatial resolution, these initial good results at 1.5T are likely to improve even further and will possibly reduce the variability of experienced and less experienced readers. Additional MR imaging modalities that appear to improve staging accuracies include dynamic contrast-enhanced imaging and proton spectroscopy. It can be concluded that MR imaging in prostate cancers will form the backbone of patient-oriented decision making in the diagnosing and management of prostate cancer in the years to come.

References

Akin, O., Sala, E., Moskowitz, C.S., Kuroiwa, K., Ishill, N.M., Pucar, D., Scardino, P.T., and Hricak, H. 2006. Transition zone prostate cancers: features, detection, localization, and staging at endorectal MR imaging. *Radiology 239*:784–792.

Bartolozzi, C., Crocetti, L., Menchi, I., Ortori, S., and Lencioni, R. 2001. Endorectal magnetic resonance imaging in local staging of prostate carcinoma. *Abdom. Imaging 26*:111–122.

Bartolozzi, C., Menchi, I., Lencioni, R., Serni, S., Lapini, A., Barbanti, G., Bozza, A., Amorosi, A., Manganelli, A., and Carini, M. 1996. Local staging of prostate carcinoma with endorectal coil MRI: correlation with whole-mount radical prostatectomy specimens. *Eur. Radiol. 6*:339–345.

Blute, M.L., Bergstralh, E.J., Iocca, A., Scherer, B., and Zincke, H. 2001. Use of Gleason score, prostate specific antigen, seminal vesicle and margin status to predict biochemical failure after radical prostatectomy. *J. Urol. 165*:119–125.

Bostwick, D.G., Graham, S.D., Jr., Napalkov, P., Abrahamsson, P.A., di Sant'agnese, P.A., Algaba, F., Hoisaeter, P.A., Lee, F., Littrup, P., and Mostofi, F.K. 1993. Staging of early prostate cancer: a proposed tumor volume-based prognostic index. *Urology 41*:403–411.

Chodak, G.W., Thisted, R.A., Gerber, G.S., Johansson, J.E., Adolfsson, J., Jones, G.W., Chisholm, G.D., Moskovitz, B., Livne, P.M., and Warner, J. 1994. Results of conservative management of clinically localized prostate cancer. *N. Engl. J. Med. 330*:242–248.

Engelbrecht, M.R., Jager, G.J., Laheij, R.J., Verbeek, A.L., van Lier, H.J., and Barentsz, J.O. 2002. Local staging of prostate cancer using magnetic resonance imaging: a meta-analysis. *Eur. Radiol. 12*:2294–2302.

Engelbrecht, M.R., Jager, G.J., and Severens, J.L. 2001. Patient selection for magnetic resonance imaging of prostate cancer. *Eur. Urol. 40*:300–307.

Fütterer, J.J., Engelbrecht, M.R., Jager, G.J., Hartman, R.P., King, F.B., Hulsbergen-van De Kaa, C.A., Witjes, J.A., and Barentsz, J.O. 2007. Prostate cancer: comparison of local staging accuracy of pelvic phased array coil alone versus integrated endorectal pelvic phased array coils. *Eur. Radiol. 17*:1055–1065.

Fütterer, J.J., Engelbrecht, M.R., Huisman, H.J., Jager, G.J., Hulsbergen-van De Kaa, C.A., Witjes, J.A., and Barentsz, J.O. 2005. Staging prostate cancer with dynamic contrast-enhanced endorectal MR imaging prior to radical prostatectomy: experienced versus less experienced readers. *Radiology 237*:541–549.

Fütterer, J.J., Heijmink, S.W., Scheenen, T.W., Jager, G.J., Hulsbergen-van De Kaa, C.A., Witjes, J.A., and Barentsz, J.O. 2006. Prostate cancer: local staging at 3-T endorectal MR imaging—early experience. *Radiology 238*:184–191.

Fütterer, J.J., Scheenen, T.W., Huisman, H.J., Klomp, D.W., van Dorsten, F.A., Hulsbergen-van De Kaa, C.A., Witjes, J.A., Heerschap, A., and Barentsz, J.O. 2004. Initial experience of 3 Tesla endorectal coil magnetic resonance imaging and 1H-spectroscopic imaging of the prostate. *Invest. Radiol. 39*:671–680.

Giesen, R.J., Huynen, A.L., Aarnink, R.G., de la Rosette, J.J., Hulsbergen-van De Kaa, C., Oosterhof, G.O., Debruyne, F.M., and Wijkstra, H. 1995. Computer analysis of transrectal ultrasound images of the prostate for the detection of carcinoma: a prospective study in radical prostatectomy specimens. *J. Urol. 154*:1397–1400.

Gravdal, K., Halvorsen, O.J., Haukaas, S.A., and Akslen, L.A. 2006. Expression of bFGF/FGFR-1 and vascular proliferation related to clinicopathologic features and tumor progress in localized prostate cancer. *Virchows Arch. 448*:68–74.

Greene, F.L. 2002. *AJCC Cancer Staging Manual.* (6th ed.). New York: Springer-Verlag.

Greene, D.R., Wheeler, T.M., Egawa, S., Dunn, J.K., and Scardino, P.T. 1991. A comparison of the morphological features of cancer arising in the transition zone and in the peripheral zone of the prostate. *J. Urol. 146*:1069–1076.

Greenman, R.L., Shirosky, J.E., Mulkern, R.V., and Rofsky, N.M. 2003. Double inversion black-blood fast spin-echo imaging of the human heart: a comparison between 1.5T and 3.0T. *J. Magn. Reson. Imaging 17*:648–655.

Guillonneau, B., Debras, B., Veillon, B., Bougaran, J., Chambon, E., and Vallancien, G. 1997. Indications for preoperative seminal vesicle biopsies in staging of clinically localized prostatic cancer. *Eur. Urol. 32*:160–165.

Hayat, M.A. 2002. *Microscopy, Immunohistochemistry and Antigen Retrieval Methods* New York: Kluwer Academic/Plenum Publishers.

Heijmink, S.W., Fütterer, J.J., Hambrock, T., Scheenen, T.W., Hulsbergen-van De Kaa, C.A., Huisman, H.J., and Barentsz, J.O. 2007. Body array versus endorectal coil MR imaging of prostate cancer at 3 Tesla: comparison of image quality, localization, and staging performance with whole-mount section histopathology. *Radiology 244*:184–195.

Hodge, K.K., McNeal, J.E., Terris, M.K., and Stamey, T.A. 1989. Random systematic versus directed ultrasound guided transrectal core biopsies of the prostate. *J. Urol. 142*:71–74.

Huncharek, M., and Muscat, J. 1996. Serum prostate-specific antigen as a predictor of staging abdominal/pelvic computed tomography in newly diagnosed prostate cancer. *Abdom. Imaging 21*:364–367.

Jager, G.J., Severens, J.L., Thornbury, J.R., de la Rosette, J.J., Ruijs, S.H., and Barentsz, J.O. 2000. Prostate cancer staging: should MR imaging be used?—A decision analytic approach. *Radiology 215*:445–451.

Jemal, A., Siegel, R., Ward, E., Murray, T., Xu, J., and Thun, M.J. 2007. Cancer Statistics 2007. *CA Cancer J. Clin. 57*:43–66.

Kirby, S. 1996. *Prostate Cancer*, (1st ed.). London: Mosby.

Kurhanewicz, J., Vigneron, D.B., Hricak, H., Narayan, P., Carroll, P., and Nelson, S.J. 1996. Three-dimensional H-1 MR spectroscopic imaging of the *in situ* human prostate with high (0.24–0.7-cm3) spatial resolution. *Radiology 198*:795–805.

Langlotz, C., Schnall, M., and Pollack, H. 1995. Staging of prostatic cancer: accuracy of MR imaging. *Radiology 194*:645–646.

Lawrentschuk, N. 2006. Positron emission tomography and molecular imaging of the prostate: an update. *BJU Int. 97*:923–931.

McNeal, J.E. 1992. Cancer volume and site of origin of adenocarcinoma in the prostate: relationship to local and distant spread. *Hum. Pathol. 23*:258–266.

McNeal, J.E., Redwine, E.A., Freiha, F.S., and Stamey, T.A. 1988. Zonal distribution of prostatic adenocarcinoma. Correlation with histologic pattern and direction of spread. *Am. J. Surg. Pathol. 12*:897–906.

Ogura, K., Maekawa, S., Okubo, K., Aoki, Y., Okada, T., Oda, K., Watanabe, Y., Tsukayama, C., and Arai, Y. 2001. Dynamic endorectal magnetic resonance imaging for local staging and detection of neurovascular bundle involvement of prostate cancer: correlation with histopathologic results. *Urology 57*:721–726.

Partin, A.W., Carter, H.B., Chan, D.W., Epstein, J.I., Oesterling, J.E., Rock, R.C., Weber, J.P., and Walsh, P.C. 1990. Prostate specific antigen in the staging of localized prostate cancer: influence of tumor differentiation, tumor volume and benign hyperplasia. *J. Urol. 143*:747–752.

Partin, A.W., Kattan, M.W., Subong, E.N., Walsh, P.C., Wojno, K.J., Oesterling, J.E., Scardino, P.T., and Pearson, J.D. 1997. Combination of prostate-specific antigen, clinical stage, and Gleason score to predict pathological stage of localized prostate cancer. A multi-institutional update. *JAMA 277*:1445–1451.

Partin, A.W., Yoo, J., Carter, H.B., Pearson, J.D., Chan, D.W., Epstein, J.I., and Walsh, P.C. 1993. The use of prostate specific antigen, clinical stage and Gleason score to predict pathological stage in men with localized prostate cancer. *J. Urol. 150*:110–114.

Pelzer, A., Bektic, J., Berger, A.P., Pallwein, L., Halpern, E.J., Horninger, W., Bartsch, G., and Frauscher, F. 2005. Prostate cancer detection in men with prostate specific antigen 4 to 10 ng/ml using a combined approach of contrast enhanced color Doppler targeted and systematic biopsy. *J. Urol. 173*:1926–1929.

Rifkin, M.D., Zerhouni, E.A., Gatsonis, C.A., Quint, L.E., Paushter, D.M., Epstein, J.I., Hamper, U., Walsh, P.C., and McNeil, B.J. 1990. Comparison of magnetic resonance imaging and ultrasonography in staging early prostate cancer. Results of a multi-institutional cooperative trial. *N. Engl. J. Med. 323*:621–626.

Rorvik, J., Halvorsen, O.J., Albrektsen, G., Ersland, L., Daehlin, L., and Haukaas, S. 1999. MRI with an endorectal coil for staging of clinically localised prostate cancer prior to radical prostatectomy. *Eur. Radiol. 9*:29–34.

Saito, T., Kitamura, Y., Komatsubara, S., Matsumoto, Y., Sugita, T., and Hara, N. 2006. Outcomes of locally advanced prostate cancer: a single institution study of 209 patients in Japan. *Asian J. Androl. 8*:555–561.

Sakai, I., Harada, K., Hara, I., Eto, H., and Miyake, H. 2005. A comparison of the biological features between prostate cancers arising in the transition and peripheral zones. *BJU Int. 96*:528–532.

Sala, E., Akin, O., Moskowitz, C.S., Eisenberg, H.F., Kuroiwa, K., Ishill, N.M., Rajashanker, B., Scardino, P.T., and Hricak, H. 2006. Endorectal MR imaging in the evaluation of seminal vesicle invasion: diagnostic accuracy and multivariate feature analysis. *Radiology 238*:929–937.

Sauvain, J.L., Palascak, P., Bourscheid, D., Chabi, C., Atassi, A., Bremon, J.M. and Palascak, R. 2003. Value of power Doppler and 3D vascular sonography as a method for diagnosis and staging prostate cancer. *Eur. Urol. 44*:21–30.

Sonnad, S.S., Langlotz, C.P., and Schwartz, J.S. 2001. Accuracy of MR imaging for staging prostate cancer: a meta-analysis to examine the effect of technologic change. *Acad. Radiol. 8*:149–157.

Sosna, J., Rofsky, N.M., Gaston, S.M., Dewolf, W.C., and Lenkinski, R.E. 2003. Determinations of prostate volume at 3-Tesla using an external phased array coil: comparison to pathologic specimens. *Acad. Radiol. 10*:846–853.

Stamey, T.A., and Yemoto, C.E. 1998. The clinical importance of separating transition zone (TZ) from peripheral zone (PZ) cancers [abstract]. *J. Urol. 159* (Suppl.):221.

Stamey, T.A., Dietrick, D.D., and Issa, M.M. 1993. Large, organ confined, impalpable transition zone prostate cancer: association with metastatic levels of prostate specific antigen. *J. Urol. 149*:510–515.

Stamey, T.A., McNeal, J.E., Freiha, F.S., and Redwine, E. 1988. Morphometric and clinical studies on 68 consecutive radical prostatectomies. *J. Urol. 139*:1235–1241.

Strohmeyer, D., Rossing, C., Strauss, F., Bauerfeind, A., Kaufmann, O., and Loening, S. 2000. Tumor angiogenesis is associated with progression after radical prostatectomy in pT2/pT3 prostate cancer. *Prostate 42*:26–33.

Tsuda, K., Yu, K.K., Coakley, F.V., Srivastav, S.K., Scheidler, J.E., and Hricak, H. 1999. Detection of extracapsular extension of prostate cancer: role of fat suppression endorectal MRI. *J. Comput. Assist. Tomogr. 23*:74–78.

Villers, A.A., McNeal, J.E., Redwine, E.A., Freiha, F.S., and Stamey, T.A. 1990. Pathogenesis and biological significance of seminal vesicle invasion in prostatic adenocarcinoma. *J. Urol. 143*:1183–1187.

White, S., Hricak, H., Forstner, R., Kurhanewicz, J., Vigneron, D.B., Zaloudek, C.J., Weiss, J.M., Narayan, P., and Carroll, P.R. 1995. Prostate cancer: effect of postbiopsy hemorrhage on interpretation of MR images. *Radiology 195*:385–390.

Yang, J., Wu, H.F., Qian, L.X., Zhang, W., Hua, L.X., Yu, M.L., Wang, Z., Xu, Z.Q., Sui, Y.G., and Wang, X.R. 2006. Increased expressions of vascular endothelial growth factor (VEGF), VEGF-C and VEGF receptor-3 in prostate cancer tissue are associated with tumor progression. *Asian J. Androl. 8*:169–175.

Yu, K.K., Scheidler, J., Hricak, H., Vigneron, D.B., Zaloudek, C.J., Males, R.G., Nelson, S.J., Carroll, P.R., and Kurhanewicz, J. 1999. Prostate cancer: prediction of extracapsular extension with endorectal MR imaging and three-dimensional proton MR spectroscopic imaging. *Radiology 213*:481–488.

50

Extremity Sarcoma: Positron Emission Tomography

Gazala N. Khan and Scott M. Schuetze

Introduction

Sarcomas are rare, mesenchymal malignant tumors accounting for 1% of adult and 8% of pediatric cancers. In 2005, ~ 9400 and 2500 patients were diagnosed with sarcoma of soft tissue and bone, respectively, and 4700 died from disease. More than 50% of sarcomas arise in extremities. Lung is the principal site of metastasis. The World Health Organization recognizes > 50 types of malignant bone and soft tissue tumors. Many of the sarcoma subtypes are characterized by histologic heterogeneity and may contain considerable morphological variation including cystic changes, hemorrhage, and necrosis. Imaging modalities frequently used in sarcoma management include roentgenography, computed tomography (CT), magnetic resonance imaging (MRI), bone scintigraphy, and positron emission tomography (PET).

Primary bone tumors have characteristic findings on radiography that render plain film X-ray essential in the diagnostic work-up of bone lesions. The parameters used to describe bone tumors include anatomic site, nature of the tumor border and presence of bone destruction, matrix formation, and periosteal reaction. The radiographic appearance of benign and malignant tumors is usually very different. Radiography is also useful in detecting pathologic fractures. Radiography, however, is typically not helpful in the evaluation of soft tissue tumors of the extremity because soft tissue sarcomas infrequently are ossifying or affect adjacent bone.

Computed tomography is used to determine the size and anatomic location of sarcomas; evaluate muscle, fat, and bone involvement; detect metastases to lung and the abdomen; and evaluate tumor response to chemotherapy. Computed tomography is not inferior to MRI in the evaluation of soft tissue tumors and provides complementary information regarding bone sarcomas (Panicek *et al.*, 1997). However, standard MRI provides excellent delineation of extremity sarcomas in relation to muscle and neurovascular structures, and can identify sarcoma involvement in marrow, cystic changes, and intratumoral hemorrhage. Moreover, it is important to recognize that the ability of these two methods to differentiate between benign and malignant connective tissue tumors is limited, and CT and MRI do not provide adequate insight into important biologic properties of tumor such as viability and pathologic grade.

The currently accepted convention for determining tumor response to treatment in clinical trials is the Response Evaluation Criteria in Solid Tumors (RECIST). This protocol is based on serial determination of the largest one-dimensional measurement of tumors, usually using axial images, and assumes that the bulk of the mass is composed of neoplastic cells (Therasse *et al.*, 2000). The protocol has not been validated as a surrogate measure of therapeutic benefit of chemotherapy or radiotherapy in extremity sarcomas. There are many reasons why anatomic imaging may fail to detect sarcoma response to treatment. For example, intratumoral

Cancer Imaging: Instrumentation and Applications

655

hemorrhage, myxoid degeneration, hyalinization, and/or inflammation could contribute to the make-up of a tumor mass and significantly affect tumor size. Malignant osteoid and chondroid matrices do not resorb readily after treatment of primary bone sarcomas with chemotherapy, even after complete histologic response, and bone does not rapidly reossify after elimination of tumor. The available data suggest that change in tumor size does not correlate with histologic response or outcome (Murphy, 1991; Schuetze, 2005). RECIST generally underestimates tumor response in sarcomas.

The limitations of anatomic imaging have stimulated the search for functional imaging methods that evaluate important aspects of tumor biology, such as tissue perfusion, carbohydrate metabolism, and cell proliferation, as a means to better characterize extremity masses and response to preoperative therapy. Dynamic contrast-enhanced MRI is an emerging technology that has been explored as a method to assess relative capillary density, diffusion, tumor viability, and response to preoperative therapy in sarcomas of bone and soft tissue (Reddick et al., 2001; Shapeero et al., 2002). Use of radiotracers that are incorporated into cells by DNA synthesis, protein synthesis, and cell membrane biosynthesis to infer tumor proliferation rates and cell viability in sarcomas has been reported and is discussed in other chapters (van Ginkel et al., 1999). The utility of 18-fluorodeoxyglucose (FDG)-PET in the clinical management of patients with extremity bone and soft tissue tumors, with a focus on high-grade sarcomas, is discussed below.

Evolution of FDG-PET in Etremity Sarcoma

Since the 1930s, it has been recognized that increased carbohydrate, specifically glucose, metabolism is an inherent feature common to malignant cells compared to nonmalignant counterparts. The introduction of gamma-cameras in the 1970s led to the use of various radiopharmaceuticals in the characterization of malignant tumors. Fluoro-2-deoxy-D-glucose labeled with radioactive 18-fluorine is a glucose analog that has been employed in tumor imaging since the 1980s. FDG is actively transported into cells by membrane-bound glucose transporters. Intracellularly, FDG is phosphorylated by hexokinase but is not further metabolized and becomes trapped within the cell. The trapped tracer can be quantified and spatially resolved by PET.

The earliest published description of enhanced accumulation of FDG in a sarcoma compared with normal tissue was in 1984 (Paul et al., 1984) who used PET to image an osteosarcoma in a dog. The authors proposed that FDG would be suitable for imaging tumors in man. Kern et al. (1988) reported a correlation between increased FDG uptake and the grade of sarcoma in 5 patients with extremity musculoskeletal

tumors. Within the past decade, advances in FDG-PET have made the technology more accessible and clinically feasible.

Many of the early studies of FDG-PET in sarcomas employed dynamic imaging, time-dependent arterial and/or venous blood sampling of the radiotracer, and sophisticated computations to quantify the glucose (FDG) metabolic rates of tumors (Eary et al., 1998b; Kern et al., 1988; Nieweg et al., 1996). The rate of uptake of FDG was usually expressed as micromoles or milligrams/100 grams of tissue/min. On average, high-grade sarcomas accumulated FDG at faster rates than lower-grade sarcomas or benign lesions, but there was overlap between high-, intermediate-, and low-grade sarcomas, and between low-grade tumors and benign conditions (Dimitrakopoulou-Strauss et al., 2001; Eary et al., 1998b; Nieweg et al., 1996). FDG activity plateaus after 30 min in normal tissues but may take 4 hr or more in sarcomas (Lodge et al., 1999). The rate of FDG metabolism does not correlate with percentage of cells in S-phase of the cell cycle, suggesting that FDG-PET is not an indirect measure of cell proliferation (Eary et al., 1998b). However, FDG uptake in sarcomas has been shown to correlate with histopathologic features of higher grade lesions such as increased cellularity and mitotic index (Folpe et al., 2000).

The methods used to quantitatively measure FDG uptake are not practical for clinical facilities because they are labor and time-intensive. Methods to semiquantitatively measure FDG uptake in sarcomas are simpler and more amenable to use in a busy clinical nuclear medicine facility. The standardized uptake value (SUV) is a unit less number that represents the amount of FDG accumulated at a fixed point in time. The SUV is calculated using the formula: $SUV = (C/D)/w$, where C is the tissue concentration of tracer (FDG) activity (in mCi/g) measured by PET, D is the injected dose of the tracer (in mCi), and w is the patient weight (in kg). Images are usually acquired starting 45–60 min after injection of the radiotracer to allow for FDG diffusion through the extracellular fluid and tumor uptake. The activity within a region of interest (ROI) is normalized by the amount of tracer injected and the weight of the patient. The SUV can be further adjusted by the patient's serum glucose level and corrected for signal attenuation through tissue using a transmission scan from a rotating external radiation source. Tumor SUV correlates with metabolic rate of FDG uptake (Eary et al., 1998a; Lodge et al., 1999). The average SUV (SUVave) of a sarcoma is the mean of activity throughout the ROI, whereas the maximum SUV (SUVmax) is the highest activity within a ROI. The SUVave and SUVmax are likely to be significantly different in heterogeneous masses in contrast to homogeneous tumors. The regions of sarcoma with high FDG uptake have correlated with higher grade tissue within a heterogeneous mass (Vernon et al., 2003). The SUV is a reproducible parameter of glucose utilization, but comparisons between studies require accurate accounting of the injected dose of FDG and acquisition of the signal from the region of interest at exactly the same length of time after administration of the tracer (Weber *et al.*, 1999).

Nonquantitative measures of FDG uptake in studies of sarcomas have also been used. Qualitative visual assessment of activity is subject to interobserver variation and lacks standardization. In addition, to our knowledge, the reproducibility of qualitative visual assessment across clinical sites has not been reported. Investigators have used the ratio of tumor uptake-to-normal tissue uptake of FDG (known as tumor-to-background ratio) in studies of PET in extremity sarcomas. Calculation of tumor-to-background ratios (TBR) does not require accurate accounting of the injected dose of FDG; thus, it is not quantitative. Tumor-to-background ratios may be influenced by variation in the time after injection of tracer that images are acquired because of different rates of FDG uptake in neoplastic and normal tissues. TBR may also be affected by variation in FDG uptake in the normal tissue, for example, muscle caused by physical activity. The metabolic rates of FDG, tumor SUV, and TBR have frequently been used in research of PET in sarcoma evaluation. To some extent, analysis of results across different studies of FDG-PET in extremity sarcoma is hampered by nonstandardization of imaging protocols and results reported and by evolving technology.

Role of FDG-PET in the Differential Diagnosis of Connective Tissue Lesions

Standard radiography is very helpful in the diagnosis of primary bone lesions and can often distinguish benign from malignant processes. Computed tomography and MRI, while providing excellent anatomic definition, are not able to clearly differentiate benign from malignant soft tissue masses—for example, lipoma from well-differentiated liposarcoma. FDG-PET indirectly provides data regarding cellularity, mitotic rate, and carbohydrate metabolism. Thus, it can be of value in the work-up of connective tissue lesions. FDG-PET has been studied as an adjunct to conventional radiography in the diagnosis of malignancy, as a method to predict tumor grade, and as an aid to direct biopsy.

FDG-PET has been studied as a method to noninvasively diagnose malignancy of musculoskeletal neoplasms. Adler *et al.* (1991) reported on results of FDG activity of musculoskeletal tumors > 2 cm in size in 25 patients. There was a stronger correlation between the tumor average uptake value (SUVave) and tumor grade than between TBR and tumor grade. In the series, 6 out of 6 benign lesions and 3 out of 3 low-grade liposarcomas had an average FDG uptake value of < 1.6, whereas, all 15 high-grade sarcomas had an average uptake value of > 1.6. Two of the high-grade sarcomas (an angiosarcoma and a synovial sarcoma) had an uptake value < 2.0. The low-grade liposarcomas could not be separated

from the benign lesions by FDG-PET. In a series of 45 patients presenting with connective tissue masses reported by Feldman *et al.* (2003), overall sensitivity of FDG-PET using an SUVmax > 2.0 for differentiating malignant from benign lesions was 91.7% and specificity approached 100%. Twelve benign bone lesions, 12 malignant bone lesions, 2 benign soft tissue lesions, and 17 malignant soft tissue tumors were imaged. Pathologic diagnosis was the reference standard. The series included an inadequate number of benign soft tissue tumors to generalize the findings. Aggressive benign conditions such as fibromatosis (desmoid tumors), fibrous dysplasia, osteoblastoma, and giant cell tumors (GCT) exhibited an SUVmax > 2.0. The largest reported series evaluating preoperative assessment of soft tissue masses by FDG-PET involved 114 patients presenting prior to tissue diagnosis (Aoki *et al.*, 2003). The SUVave of lesions was determined for the analysis. There was a statistically significant ($P < 0.0001$) difference in SUVave between benign (1.8 ± 1.42) and malignant (4.2 ± 3.16) lesions. However, on average, FDG uptake in liposarcomas (2.16 ± 1.72) and synovial sarcomas (1.6 ± 0.43) was not greater than that in benign lesions. Desmoid tumors (2.77 ± 1.32), sarcoidosis (3.62 ± 1.53), and GCT of tendon sheath (5.06 ± 1.63) were associated with high SUVave despite being benign.

The results from two meta-analyses of the value of FDG-PET in the diagnosis and grading of sarcomas have been reported (Bastiaannet *et al.*, 2004; Ioannidis and Lau, 2003). The latter authors extracted data from 15 reports, including 227 subjects with soft tissue sarcoma and 214 with benign lesions that had been studied with FDG-PET. The reference standard was pathologic diagnosis, but benign-appearing lesions were not biopsied in 3 of the studies. The methods used to differentiate benign from malignant lesions varied by study and included qualitative visualization, TBR, SUV, and the metabolic rate of glucose. The semiquantitative methods appeared to be more specific but less sensitive than qualitative visualization for discriminating malignant from benign lesions. An SUV ≥ 2.0 had a sensitivity of 79% and specificity of 77% for detecting sarcomas and gave false-positive results in 13 of 68 benign cases, of which many were inflammatory. Seven of 66 intermediate/high-grade sarcomas and 16 of 24 low-grade sarcomas had an SUV below 2.0. An analysis by Bastiaannet *et al.* (2004) reviewed data from 14 studies reporting on FDG-PET in the detection and/or grading of soft tissue and bone sarcomas. The reference standard was pathologic diagnosis, but different definitions of a positive PET were used. Data from studies using SUVave of lesions were pooled with data from studies using SUVmax. The sensitivity and specificity for detection of sarcoma were 91% and 85%, respectively.

FDG-PET may be more discriminating in selected histologic subtypes of sarcoma. Using an SUVmax > 2 to differentiate malignant from benign cartilaginous lesions in 26 cases, Feldman *et al.* (2005) were able to correctly identify

10 of 11 malignant and 18 of 18 benign cases by FDG-PET. One case of a Grade 1 chondrosarcoma had an SUVmax < 2. However, other investigators have demonstrated that tumor SUVave and SUVmax are not able to discriminate malignant peripheral nerve sheath tumors from benign schwannomas because both entities have elevated FDG uptake (Beaulieu *et al.*, 2004). Clearly, results of FDG-PET in one subtype of sarcoma are not necessarily applicable across other subtypes.

Inflammatory lesions with histiocytic infiltration, lesions with a predominant fibroblastic response, and neurogenic lesions are associated with high SUVs using FDG. On the other hand, low-grade sarcomas can be associated with spuriously low SUVs. Thus, FDG-PET is not an effective screening method for the differential diagnosis of benign and malignant soft tissue tumors and should not replace histologic evaluation in the work-up of suspected malignancy. Pathology remains the gold standard in the diagnosis of sarcomas.

Role of FDG-PET in Grading Soft Tissue Sarcoma

Soft tissue sarcoma grade is assessed histologically by an experienced pathologist examining the tumor type, cellular differentiation, nuclear pleomorphism, mitotic activity, and extent of necrosis. Tumor grade is a principal component in the American Joint Commission on Cancer staging system for sarcomas and independently impacts prognosis. FDG-PET has been studied as a tool to indirectly assess the histologic grade of sarcomas of bone and soft tissue.

Preoperative determination of sarcoma grade may be useful in the clinical management of extremity soft tissue tumors. Low-grade sarcomas are usually treated with complete resection with or without adjuvant radiotherapy. Intermediate- to high-grade sarcomas, especially of large size, are often treated with neoadjuvant chemotherapy, to reduce the risk of tumor metastasis, followed by complete resection and radiotherapy. Unequivocal determination that an extremity sarcoma is high grade is often required by medical oncologists prior to proceeding with chemotherapy. Histopathology has been the accepted standard method for determination of tumor grade.

Reports involving a small number of patients with sarcomas suggested that high-grade tumors are more metabolically active than low-grade sarcomas determined by the metabolic rate of FDG uptake or SUV (Adler *et al.*, 1991; Nieweg *et al.*, 1996). Subsequently, the SUVmax of bone and soft tissue sarcomas was reported to correlate with tumor cellularity and mitotic activity (Folpe *et al.*, 2000). A larger study of 70 patients supported the findings of earlier reports of a correlation between FDG uptake and sarcoma grade (Eary *et al.*, 1998b). Tumor maximum uptake values and meta-

bolic rate of FDG were compared with histologic grade. The differences in mean SUVmax and metabolic rate of FDG between the low-grade, intermediate-grade, and high-grade sarcomas were significant, but considerable overlap in the range of SUVmax between the groups occurred. In another report, the tumor SUVmax of low-grade, intermediate-grade, and high-grade soft tissue sarcomas ranged from 0.37–1.9 to 1.2–6 and to 1.4–9.1, respectively (Schwarzbach *et al.*, 2000). Lucas *et al.* (1999) reported that the SUVave for low-grade soft tissue sarcomas ranged from 1.04 to 4.63, whereas SUVave for high-grade soft tissue sarcomas varied from 2.51 to 31.91. Using a SUVave cut-off of 2.0, all of the patients with high-grade sarcomas were correctly identified, but some of the patients with low-grade tumors were incorrectly classified as being high grade. In addition, a study of chondrosarcomas demonstrated significant overlap in the range of SUVmax between Grade I, II, and III lesions (Brenner *et al.*, 2004). Clinical decisions regarding the indication for neoadjuvant chemotherapy in a patient with extremity sarcoma should not be based on FDG-PET results in the absence of pathologic confirmation of tumor grade.

Role of FDG-PET in Directing Biopsy

Biopsy is considered an essential step in the diagnostic evaluation of sarcoma. In addition to providing an accurate diagnosis, it establishes tumor grade, which in turn impacts staging, prognosis, and treatment. Owing to often large tumor size and tissue heterogeneity within a sarcoma, inherent sampling bias may provide an inaccurate assessment of tumor grade. Biopsy results may be nondiagnostic if necrotic regions are sampled or underestimate the pathologic grade. The diagnostic accuracy of core needle biopsy has been reported to be ~ 85%, but to our knowledge, the accuracy of needle biopsy in establishing tumor grade has not been described (Mankin *et al.*, 1996; Skrzynski *et al.*, 1996). FDG-PET can identify areas of high metabolic activity within a heterogeneous mass, thereby potentially reducing the sampling error of a suspected high-grade lesion.

Hain *et al.* (2003) have demonstrated that FDG-PET has a role in directing needle biopsy of extremity soft tissue masses suspected of being sarcoma. The investigators evaluated 20 patients presenting consecutively with large, deep, growing masses with MRI and FDG-PET. Radiologists blinded to the PET results recommended the most appropriate site of biopsy on MRI for comparison. Biopsies were performed in the region of tumor with the highest uptake of FDG. All of the patients subsequently underwent surgery. In all of the cases of high-grade sarcoma, the FDG-PET correctly identified the region of the tumor with high-grade histologic features, and biopsy results presumably correlated with the final diagnosis. In 3 of the 8 cases of high-grade sarcoma, the recommended location for biopsy by MRI differed from

PET, but it was not reported whether biopsy directed by MRI would have changed the presumptive diagnosis or grade of tumor. If diagnosis of a heterogeneous mass as a high-grade sarcoma is required for neoadjuvant therapy, FDG-PET directed biopsy of the most active region may improve the diagnostic accuracy.

Role of FDG-PET in Predicting Sarcoma-Specific Death

The clinical stage of extremity sarcoma provides crude prognostic information about risks of tumor recurrence and sarcoma-specific death. Patients with large, high-grade tumors are at greater risk of mortality from sarcoma than patients with low-grade disease. Additional factors including patient age, site of disease, and location relative to fascia and subtype of sarcoma have recently been incorporated into nomograms to refine estimates of prognosis (Kattan et al., 2002). In patients with high-grade sarcoma treated with neoadjuvant therapy, the histologic response of tumor has predicted risk of tumor recurrence and mortality in some, but not all, studies (Davis et al., 1994; Eilber et al., 2001; Wunder et al., 1998). FDG-PET has been studied as an adjunctive tool in the preoperative prognostic assessment of soft tissue sarcoma.

Eary et al. (2002) reported on a retrospective analysis of patients with sarcomas of soft tissue (135 patients), bone (52 patients), and cartilage (22 patients) imaged with FDG-PET at diagnosis and followed for survival. The mean length of follow-up was relatively short at 19 months. Baseline tumor SUVmax, 45–60 min after injection of tracer ranged from 1.4 to 60, and the median value for the group was 6.0. The tumor grade was high, intermediate, and low in 96, 69, and 35 of the cases, respectively. Tumors with a high SUVmax (> 6) were associated with a worse disease-free survival (P = 0.001) and overall survival (P = 0.003) than less active tumors regardless of histology. Multivariate analysis found a significant independent association between the tumor SUVmax at diagnosis and death (Eary et al., 2002). A doubling of the tumor SUVmax was associated with a 60% increase in the adjusted risk of death. Tumor grade was also strongly associated with disease relapse and survival in univariate and multivariate analyses.

A more recently reported study by Schwarzbach et al. (2005) analyzed soft tissue sarcoma SUVave in 74 adult patients at diagnosis. Hypometabolic areas on PET corresponding to necrosis within tumor were excluded from the ROI. Outcomes were analyzed in 55 patients who underwent complete resection of sarcoma, and median length of follow-up was 40 months. Tumor was located in an extremity in 67% and was high grade in 70% of the cases. Tumor resection margins were microscopically negative in 57% of patients. In univariate analysis, a higher baseline tumor SUVave,

higher tumor grade, and microscopically positive margins were associated with an increased risk of recurrence. The estimated 5-year recurrence-free survival of patients with a sarcoma SUVave < 1.59, 1.59 to < 3.6, and ≥ 3.6 was 66%, 24%, and 11%, respectively. Prognosis was significantly better in patients with SUVave < 1.59. The 5-year overall survival of patients with tumor SUVave < 1.59 was 84%, compared to 38% for patients with SUVave ≥ 3.6. In multivariate analysis, the SUV lost statistical significance, and tumor grade was the strongest predictor of patient outcome. Seventy percent of the tumors with an SUVave < 1.59 were low grade, whereas 38 of 41 (93%) tumors with SUVave ≥ 1.59 were intermediate or high grade.

FDG-PET may be more useful as a tool to predict the risk of aggressive biologic behavior (e.g., metastatic potential) in the subset of patients with high-grade sarcomas than as a tool to predict tumor recurrence in sarcomas in general. The results of a relatively homogeneous population of patients with primary high-grade extremity soft tissue sarcoma studied with FDG-PET at diagnosis have been reported (Schuetze et al., 2005). The tumor SUVmax was recorded and used in analyses. All 46 of the patients received chemotherapy and had complete gross resection of tumor. Adjuvant radiation was given to 80% of the patients. In multivariate analysis, sarcoma SUVmax ≥ 6 was associated with an increased risk of disease recurrence and development of metastasis. The increased risks were independent of tumor grade. With a median length of follow-up of 46 months, the estimated 5-year metastasis-free survival of patients with a sarcoma SUVmax < 6 was 75% compared to 40% with an SUVmax ≥ 6. In patients with baseline sarcoma SUVmax ≥ 6, the relative risk for disease recurrence and development of metastasis was 3.2 and 3.7, respectively. The reason for the difference in the rate of recurrence of high-grade sarcomas between the studies by Schwartzbach et al. (2005) and Schuetze et al. (2005), to our knowledge, is not known but may be due, in part, to the use of chemotherapy in the later study. Overall, tumor grade appears to correlate the strongest with biologic behavior, but within the subset of high-grade soft tissue sarcomas, FDG-PET at diagnosis may provide additional prognostic information to help refine estimates of survival supplied by available nomograms.

The baseline SUV of pediatric bone sarcomas at diagnosis may not be prognostically useful. A study of FDG-PET in Ewing's sarcoma family of tumors does not support the earlier findings of a univariate subset analysis of bone sarcomas by Eary et al. (2002). Tumor SUVmax at baseline was not associated with survival in a study of 34 patients with Ewing's sarcoma (Hawkins et al., 2005). Prechemotherapy SUVmax ranged from 2.3 to 32.8 and the mean was 7.9 for the group. Progression-free survival at 4 years from diagnosis was 62% for patients with an SUVmax < 6 and 52% for patients with an SUVmax ≥ 6 (P = 0.47). The lack of a significant difference in outcome between the groups with higher and lower tumor

SUVmax at diagnosis may have been caused by an underpowered study. Alternatively, baseline FDG metabolism in Ewing's (and osteosarcoma) may be unrelated to tumor sensitivity to chemotherapy, and therefore does not correlate with outcome.

Role of FDG-PET in Monitoring Response to Therapy

As discussed previously, the radiographic assessment of soft tissue sarcoma response to chemotherapy using the RECIST criteria is challenging due to tumor heterogeneity, necrosis, and hemorrhage. Cases of enlarging masses during neoadjuvant treatment exhibiting near complete histologic response have been reported (DeLaney et al., 2003). Standard radiographic response of extremity osteosarcoma has not been shown to correlate with histologic response or with disease-free or overall survival (Lawrence et al., 1993). A practical method with which to accurately determine high-grade soft tissue sarcoma, Ewing's and osteosarcoma response to neoadjuvant therapy would be clinically useful to oncologists. Functional imaging of tumor glucose utilization has been studied as a method to depict important biologic changes, such as cell viability, in sarcomas due to preoperative radiation, isolated limb perfusion, and chemotherapy.

Hyperthermia with or without Isolated Limb Perfusion

Reports exploring the correlation of changes in FDG uptake in extremity soft tissue sarcomas treated with isolated limb perfusion (ILP) or radiation were published in 1996 (Jones et al., 1996; van Ginkel et al., 1996). van Ginkel et al. studied 20 patients with locally advanced sarcomas treated with limb infusions of tumor necrosis factor and melphalan under mildly hyperthermic conditions before surgery. FDG-PET scans were done before, 2 weeks after, and 8 weeks following ILP, and the PET results were compared with histologic findings after careful examination of macroscopic and microscopic changes in tumor (van Ginkel et al., 1996). Patients had fasted for at least 6 hr prior to the test, and blood glucose levels were normal at the time of PET scanning. The metabolic rate of FDG uptake was measured and was recorded for the most active portion, the rim and the core of the tumor. Seven and 12 patients had complete and partial pathologic responses, respectively. Tumor was not excised in 1 patient because of rapid progression of disease in distant sites. The rate of FDG uptake in tumor declined > 75% from baseline within 2 weeks after ILP in 5 of the 7 patients and within 8 weeks after ILP in 6 of the 7 patients with a complete histologic response. The greatest declines in the rate of FDG uptake occurred within 2 weeks after ILP, and additional reduction in glucose uptake between weeks 2 and 8 were minor. Even though the patients with complete

responses had dramatic declines in glucose uptake within the tumor mass, the rate of FDG accumulation remained above background levels in the pseudo-capsules because of infiltration of inflammatory cells.

In one patient with a complete pathologic response of a low-grade myxoid liposarcoma, there was little change in the low rate of FDG accumulation after ILP. FDG uptake increased in 1 patient, declined < 50% in 6 patients, and declined < 75% but > 50% in 4 patients with partial pathologic responses. In seven of the patients with partial pathologic responses, viable tumor remained in the pseudo-capsules, but increased FDG activity in the pseudo-capsules was frequently caused by an inflammatory infiltrate coexisting with viable tumor. In other patients with partial responses, regions throughout the tumor mass contained viable tumor and remained FDG avid. The authors concluded that significant declines in sarcoma glucose metabolism occur within 2 weeks of ILP, but FDG PET cannot distinguish a complete from partial histologic response based on the absolute rate of FDG uptake. A clear threshold for the metabolic rate of FDG (in micromoles/100 grams of tissue/min) to separate viable from nonviable treated sarcomas does not appear to exist. The authors did not address the issue of whether the relative degree of decline in glucose metabolism, rather than the absolute value, may be more predictive of a complete pathologic response. Substitution of L-1-11C-tyrosine for FDG to monitor changes in protein synthesis in sarcomas treated with ILP using PET has discriminated between residual viable tumor and inflammation within a pseudo-capsule and may be a better radiotracer than FDG to monitor sarcoma response to ILP (van Ginkel et al., 1999). However, experience with this agent in sarcomas is very limited.

Jones et al. (1996) studied changes in FDG uptake in a small set of 4 patients, with soft tissue sarcoma treated using radiation and hyperthermia. Patients fasted 4 hr prior to the PET studies, and blood glucose values were normal at the time of FDG injection. Positron emission tomography scans were performed prior to and at the completion of therapy in 3 of the patients. Tumor maximum SUVs were calculated from the pretreatment scans and ranged from 2.6 to 12. Moderate enlargement in the central area of tumor showing absence of FDG uptake was seen in 2 of the patients, and a minor change in FDG uptake was seen in 1 of the patients. Changes in SUVmax were not reported. Absent or diminished uptake on PET correlated with regions of pathologic necrosis in the tumor. The study was too small to draw conclusions about the correlation between changes in FDG uptake and tumor response. Neither Jones et al. (1996) nor van Ginkel et al. (1999) reported on disease recurrence.

Soft Tissue Sarcoma

Changes in tumor FDG-SUVmax in a series of 38 patients with soft tissue sarcoma treated with doxorubicin-based chemotherapy have been reported by Conrad *et al.* (2004). Patients with high-grade sarcoma involving extremities, abdomen/retroperitoneum, chest wall, and head/neck were included in the analysis. FDG-PET scans with SUVmax measurements were obtained at diagnosis prior to chemotherapy and were repeated after neoadjuvant chemotherapy prior to surgical resection. The majority of patients had 3 cycles of preoperative chemotherapy. Baseline SUVmax ranged from 2.0 to 40.3 with a median of 7.65, and SUVmax of chemotherapy-treated sarcomas ranged from 1.4 to 17.2 with a median of 4.4. The median change in SUVmax was a reduction of 36.3%. A weak inverse correlation was found between the change in SUVmax and residual viable tumor on histopathology. With a median follow-up of 140 weeks for patients without recurrence of disease, a reduction in tumor SUV max of more than 40% was associated with a significantly ($P = 0.01$) lower relapse rate and an improvement in overall survival that approached statistical significance.

A report by Schuetze *et al.* (2005) updated and expanded the analysis of Conrad *et al.* (2004) in patients with high-grade, localized soft tissue sarcoma confined to an extremity. Forty-six patients were imaged prior to and after treatment with multiple cycles of doxorubicin-based, multi-agent chemotherapy. Most of the patients received additional chemotherapy and radiation adjuvantly. Patients were followed for disease recurrence and survival. Prior to PET scanning, patients fasted for at least 6 hr, and measured blood glucose levels were < 120 mg/dl. Radiographic response using RECIST was not recorded or correlated with changes in tumor SUV or patient outcomes. An FDG-PET response was defined as a reduction in tumor SUVmax of 40% or more from the pretreatment value. Patients with evidence of an FDG-PET response to neoadjuvant chemotherapy had a significantly lower risk of disease recurrence and death from disease. Four of the 17 patients (24%) with response compared to 18 of 29 patients (62%) without response experienced relapse of disease. On multivariate analysis, the pretreatment tumor SUVmax and FDG-PET response after neoadjuvant chemotherapy correlated independently with disease-free and metastasis-free survival. A 75% disease-free survival and 80% overall survival rate at 5 years from diagnosis was estimated for 12 patients with a baseline maximum SUV ≥ 6 and a PET response. In comparison, patients with a baseline maximum SUV ≥ 6 and no PET response had an estimated 5-year disease-free and overall survival of 15% and 35%, respectively. FDG-PET may be able to predict the patients with high-grade, extremity soft tissue sarcomas who are more likely to derive benefit from chemotherapy. The findings of Schuetze *et al.* (2005) need to be confirmed by larger, multi-institutional studies before FDG PET should be used routinely to guide chemotherapeutic decisions.

Bone Sarcoma

Changes in FDG uptake in osteosarcoma and Ewing's tumors to neoadjuvant chemotherapy have correlated with histologic response and outcome. Tumor-to-background ratio was used to measure metabolic response in exploratory analyses (Franzius *et al.*, 2000; Nair *et al.*, 2000; Schulte *et al.*, 1999). The average tumor uptake of FDG was normalized to uptake in nonneoplastic tissue, for example, the analogous site in the unaffected contralateral extremity. The reference standard for tumor response was histologically determined at < 10% residual viable tumor. Accounting for both studies, 38 patients with osteosarcoma were imaged before and after chemotherapy with doxorubicin, cisplatin, methotrexate, and ifosfamide in the reports by Schulte *et al.* (1999) and Franzius *et al.* (2000). Nair *et al.* (2000) imaged 16 patients with FDG-PET before and after treatment with three cycles of carboplatin and etoposide. With response defined as a decrease in TBR of 40% or more (the threshold used by Schulte *et al.*, 1999), the sensitivity, specificity, positive, and negative predictive values of FDG-PET predicting histologic response were 88%, 75%, 85%, and 79%, respectively. With response defined as a decrease in TBR of 30% or more (the threshold used by Franzius *et al.*, 2000), the sensitivity and negative predictive values improved to 100% but the specificity and positive predictive value declined to 50% and 77%, respectively. In these three small series of patients, lowering the threshold of metabolic response of osteosarcoma to a decrease in TBR of 30% or more reduces the number of patients falsely determined to be nonresponders, but increases the number falsely determined to be responding to treatment. Because of the clear clinical benefit of chemotherapy in patients with localized osteosarcoma, the greater error would be erroneously stopping therapy that was inducing histologic response than continuing therapy of questionable antitumor activity. Thus a test with a high sensitivity is more desirable.

Nair *et al.* (2000) proposed that a threshold for TBR after chemotherapy based on the absolute number would be more useful than a change in the ratio to predict histologic response in osteosarcoma. The authors argued that TBRs at near normal values (0.8–1.4) correlated well with a good histologic response (< 10% residual viable tumor). Indeed, 6 of 7 patients with a good histologic response had a TBR < 1.5, whereas 8 of 8 patients with a poor histologic response had a post-chemotherapy TBR > 1.5 (Nair *et al.*, 2000). If the same criterion is applied to the studies by Schulte *et al.* (1999) and Franzius *et al.* (2000), only 5 of 26 patients were correctly identified by FDG-PET as having had a good histologic response, and 12 out of 12 were correctly identified as having had a poor histologic response. The negative-predictive value, however, is a poor 36%; therefore, a post-treatment TBR > 1.5 cannot be used to reliably predict poor histologic response to chemotherapy.

The median post-chemotherapy TBR of responders in the previous studies was 1.5 and 2.27, respectively. The reasons for the difference in median post-treatment TBR between the studies is not known to our knowledge, but Franzius *et al.* (2000) used an acquisition time of 5 min per bed position starting 60 min after injection of FDG and Schulte *et al.* (1999) used an acquisition time of 10 min per bed position starting 45 min after tracer infusion. Increasing the post-treatment TBR threshold to 2.0 to identify nonresponders does not significantly help; the negative-predictive value is approximately 55%. FDG-PET criteria for reliably predicting osteosarcoma response (or lack thereof) to neoadjuvant chemotherapy have not been established, but the published data suggest that the change in TBR rather than the absolute post-therapy TBR may be more informative.

Franzius *et al.* (2000) studied 6 patients with primary Ewing's using FDG-PET at diagnosis and after neoadjuvant chemotherapy. All 6 of the patients had a good histologic response to therapy and a 30% or more decline in TBR to treatment. Hawkins *et al.* (2002) measured changes in tumor SUVmax and found a correlation with histologic response in 31 patients treated with neoadjuvant chemotherapy for osteosarcoma or Ewing's. A post-therapy SUVmax < 2 or a decline in SUVmax of more than 50% was scored as response. Histologic response determined by standard methods was the reference. Analyzed separately, the sensitivity, specificity, positive-, and negative-predictive values of post-therapy SUV < 2 predicting histologic response were 78%, 97%, 93%, and 80%, respectively. Post-treatment SUVmax < 2 was more accurate than a decline in SUVmax > 50% in this mixed group of osteosarcoma and Ewing's.

Hawkins *et al.* (2005) updated and expanded the results of FDG PET in Ewing's. Thirty-six patients underwent PET before and after neoadjuvant chemotherapy and were followed for survival. Tumor SUVmax was used in the analysis and histologic response to chemotherapy was defined as < 10% residual viable neoplasia. Metastasis, a known poor prognostic factor, was present at diagnosis in one-third of the patients. The baseline SUVmax ranged from 2.3 to 32.8, with a mean of 7.9. The post-therapy SUVmax ranged from 0–4.3, and the mean reduction in SUVmax to therapy was 63%. Neither the tumor baseline SUVmax nor relative reduction in SUVmax to chemotherapy was predictive of patient outcome. However, an SUVmax of < 2.5 after neoadjuvant chemotherapy predicted progression-free survival for all patients and patients with localized disease at diagnosis. The 4-year progression-free survival was 80% and 33% for patients with localized disease having a post-treatment tumor SUVmax < 2.5 and > 2.5, respectively. Favorable histologic response (< 10% residual viable tumor) was also associated with improved progression-free survival in patients with localized disease. The sensitivity and negative-predictive value of a tumor SUVmax < 2.5 predicting favorable histologic response was 76% and 40%, respectively.

The reasons for discordance between the PET and histologic responses in the study by Hawkins *et al.* (2005) were postulated to be related to the use of SUVmax and standard methodology for assessing response by pathology. Inflammatory infiltrates and reactive fibrosis within tumor may result in an underestimation of tumor response when the SUVmax is used. It is possible that the effect of inflammation and reparative changes confounding metabolic response of tumor could be minimized by using SUVave rather than SUVmax. In additional, histologic response averages findings across the entire tumor mass, whereas measurement of the SUVmax does not. Again, the use of SUVave, by averaging metabolic activity across the tumor, may correlate better with histologic response than SUVmax. To our knowledge, correlation of changes in SUVave with histologic response in Ewing's has not been reported. A sensitivity and/or negative-predictive value approaching 100% would be necessary if PET is to be used as an early indication that a change in chemotherapy for Ewing's is warranted. Collaborations to standardize imaging methods and results reporting would be helpful for implementing routine use of FDG-PET in the management of bone sarcomas.

Role of FDG-PET in Evaluating Sarcoma Recurrence

The primary treatment modalities for soft tissue sarcoma are surgical resection, chemotherapy, and radiation. Approximately, 30 to 50% of patients with high-grade disease develop local or distant recurrences after the initial therapy. Of these patients, 15 to 47% develop local recurrences, 38 to 64% develop lung metastases, and 28 to 34% develop metastases at multiple sites. The optimal management of disease recurrence is dictated primarily by site, size, and number of lesions. Conventionally, MRI with gadolinium has been employed to detect local recurrence, and chest X-ray and/or CT has been employed to detect pulmonary metastases. Bone scans are used in selected cases, for example, in situations where patients present with bone pain and/or elevated serum alkaline phosphatase.

Local Recurrence of Sarcoma

Following primary therapy for sarcoma, a number of local changes occur within the tumor bed. A considerable amount of fibrosis and edema can result following radiation. Sarcoma surgery often results in postoperative seroma, scar tissue, and alteration of fascial planes. These changes and image artifacts from metallic prostheses limit the ability of standard imaging techniques such as CT and MRI to detect local recurrences. Scar tissue or seroma may mimic mass effect from recurrent tumor. Image artifact from metallic prosthesis on MRI may interfere with the detection of subtle tissue enhancement. Results from studies performed in the late 1980s and early 1990s suggest that the sensitivity of CT in the detection of local recurrence in musculoskeletal tumors in all sites is ~ 57 to 70% (Reuther *et al.*, 1990). The sensitivity of MRI in the detection of local recurrence is ~ 80 to 85% for extremity sarcoma, but is lower following radiation (Reuther *et al.*, 1990; Vanel *et al.*, 1987). With the availability of newer technology, subsequent studies evaluated the ability of FDG-PET to detect sarcoma recurrence. Bredella *et al.* (2002) imaged 12 patients with soft tissue sarcoma, who had undergone therapy (radiation, chemotherapy, and surgery) and were suspected of having local recurrence of disease, using gadolinium-enhanced MRI and FDG-PET. In 9 patients, MRI findings were equivocal in differentiating post-therapeutic changes from tumor recurrence. FDG-PET showed increased uptake with SUVmax ranging from 2.6 to 4.6, suggestive of recurrent tumor in five of the patients. Tumor recurrence was confirmed by biopsy. SUVmax ranging from 1.0 to 1.6 in the region of the treated tumor was reported for 4 of the cases without recurrence confirmed by long-term follow-up. FDG uptake in the region of the treated tumor was attributed to changes caused by chronic inflammation. Using an SUVmax of 2.0 and above, FDG-PET was shown to be helpful in distinguishing post-therapeutic changes from tumor recurrence in patients with equivocal MR imaging findings. Two patients with extensive metallic artifact on MRI had cold defects by PET in the region of the treated sarcoma and no evidence of recurrence on follow-up. Significant limitations of the study were its selection bias, small sample size, and the heterogeneity of the patient population. Schwarzbach *et al.* (2000) reported on the ability of FDG-PET to detect local recurrence in a series of 50 patients with soft tissue sarcoma. SUVmax was calculated in the tumor bed and normal tissue (e.g., muscle).

Histopathology of suspect lesions and clinical follow-up were used as reference standards. Local recurrence was detected by FDG-PET, with a sensitivity of 88% and a specificity of 92%. The SUVmax correlated with tumor grade but not with size or histologic type. False-positive cases were related to coexistent inflammation (colonic inflammation from diverticulitis in one instance). Benign noninflammatory tissue alterations had a lower SUVmax than local recurrence of high-grade sarcoma (median SUVmax for scar 1.2, range 0.5–2.1; median SUVmax for local recurrence 2.7, range 0.6–9.1; $P = 0.0015$). No clear difference in SUVmax was seen in scar versus recurrence of low-grade sarcoma. Inflammation was associated with a high SUVmax (median 8.5, range 8–8.9). Lucas *et al.* (1998) evaluated the ability of FDG-PET and MRI as surveillance studies to detect local recurrence in 62 patients. Biopsies were performed to confirm recurrence. The sensitivity and specificity of FDG-PET were 73.7% and 94.3%, respectively, whereas, MRI had a superior sensitivity and specificity of 88.2% and 96.0%, respectively. However, other investigators have reported a sensitivity as high as 96%

for FDG-PET in the detection of local recurrence of bone sarcomas (Franzius *et al.*, 2002). The studies discussed above provide evidence supporting FDG-PET as a useful adjunct to MRI in the detection of local recurrence when MRI findings are equivocal but not in routine surveillance.

Pulmonary Recurrence of Sarcoma

Following initial therapy for localized, high-grade sarcoma, about 38 to 64% of metastases occur in the lung, and 28 to 34% of metastases occur at multiple sites such as liver and bone. Conventionally, lung metastases are detected by CT and/or chest X-ray. Chest X-ray appears to be equivalent to chest CT as a surveillance strategy. Whooley *et al.* (2000) retrospectively analyzed data on 141 patients with extremity soft tissue sarcoma assessed every 3 months, for 2 years, by physical examination, chest X-ray, blood chemistry panel, and a complete blood count. Chest X-ray abnormalities were confirmed by chest CT and subsequently by biopsy. The positive- and negative-predictive value of chest X-ray in the detection of pulmonary metastases was 92% and 97%, respectively.

The utility of FDG-PET in detecting distant recurrence has also been the subject of several studies in sarcoma following the success of FDG-PET in detecting asymptomatic metastatic disease in breast cancer, lung cancer, colon cancer, and lymphoma. A retrospective study performed by Lucas *et al.* (1998) evaluated the ability of FDG-PET to detect metastatic recurrence in patients with sarcoma. Sixty-two patients, collectively with 15 different subtypes of soft tissue sarcoma, were included in the analysis. All of the patients underwent imaging with CT to detect pulmonary metastasis followed by a whole-body FDG-PET scan. The mean follow-up period from the time of the initial diagnosis of disease was 3 years and 2 months. Biopsies were performed when changes on the imaging studies suggested recurrence. For detection of lung metastasis, FDG-PET had a sensitivity and specificity of 86.7% and 100%, respectively. In contrast, chest CT had a sensitivity and specificity of 100% and 96.4%, respectively. There was no FDG uptake noted in two cases in which CT detected multiple pulmonary metastases ranging from 5 to 9 mm in size. The investigators hypothesized that the lung metastases may have been missed by PET because emission images were acquired too soon after injection of the tracer, photon attenuation through soft tissue in the chest reduced the signal, and/or decreased vascularity of the metastases resulted in decreased delivery of FDG. In the same study, FDG-PET identified 13 nonpulmonary sites involved by metastases, of which only 5 were clinically evident. FDG-PET has limited utility in surveillance for pulmonary metastases. Abnormalities detected by chest X-ray should be evaluated with chest CT.

Nonpulmonary Recurrence of Sarcoma

FDG-PET appears to have some utility in the detection of extrapulmonary visceral disease and may serve as an adjunct to CT or MRI, although, to our knowledge, early detection of extra-pulmonary visceral disease has not been shown to impact survival. In a retrospective analysis reported by Johnson *et al.* (2003), FDG-PET correctly identified sarcoma recurrence in 2 cases in which CT was falsely negative and did not detect recurrence in 3 cases in which CT or MRI was falsely positive. Findings on radiographic images were compared with surgical biopsy or clinical follow-up for a period of six months, but pathology was obtained in only 1 of the cases with discrepant findings between CT/MRI and PET. Five of the 6 cases involved the abdomen or retroperitoneum.

Results from published studies support the conclusion that FDG-PET is not superior to anatomic imaging methods in evaluating recurrent soft tissue sarcoma. FDG-PET is inferior to thoracic CT in detecting pulmonary metastases. However, FDG-PET may have a role in early detection of nonpulmonary visceral disease (with the caveat that early diagnosis of a nonpulmonary visceral recurrence has not been shown to impact survival) and as a useful adjunct to MRI in the evaluation of local recurrence of high-grade sarcomas in a minority of cases. At present, because of the expense and radiation exposure from PET, surveillance FDG-PET scans at regular intervals after the definitive treatment of high-grade sarcomas is not indicated nor is it supported by evidence.

Future Directions

Despite its widespread application in the staging of malignancy and monitoring response to therapy in a variety of tumor types, FDG-PET has not been universally adopted by the medical community specializing in sarcoma treatment. One reason is the relative paucity of prospective clinical studies of FDG-PET in sarcomas. Another reason is the use of different methodologies and measures of response that have made comparisons between studies and meta-analyses difficult to interpret. A standardized application of FDG-PET in prospective studies evaluating a number of response parameters such as SUVmax, SUVave, and TBR may help clarify the utility of FDG-PET in sarcoma management. At the moment, FDG-PET appears to be a useful method for predicting aggressive behavior in soft tissue sarcomas and possibly in non-Ewing's bone tumors, and for predicting response to chemotherapy in Ewing's, osteosarcoma, and soft tissue sarcoma. However, criteria for metabolic response have not been definitively established, and caution should be used in interpreting results of FDG-PET in the clinical management of sarcomas in which the benefit of chemotherapy has been clearly demonstrated (e.g., osteosarcoma and Ewing's).

Other radioactive isotopes, such as C-11 methionine (Zhang *et al.*, 2004), C-11 tyrosine (van Ginkel *et al.*, 1999),

C-11 choline (Zhang *et al.*, 2003), F-18 fluorodeoxythymidine (Cobben *et al.*, 2004), and F-18 fluoromisonidazole (Rajendran *et al.*, 2003), have been employed in conjunction with PET to study aspects of tumor metabolism, proliferation, and hypoxia in exploratory analyses. Use of C-11 methionine or C-11 tyrosine may allow for better discrimination than FDG between sarcoma recurrence and postradiation inflammatory reaction. Radiolabeled Annexin V (Yagle *et al.*, 2005) and F-18 fluorodeoxythymidine (Cobben *et al.*, 2004) may allow for direct noninvasive detection of the effect of chemotherapy on tumor apoptosis and proliferation, respectively. Advances in radiochemistry and wider availability of PET tracers will likely improve our ability to diagnose and manage sarcomas. Metabolic imaging reporting must leap from qualitative, descriptive interpretations of the rather ubiquitous process of intracellular uptake of glucose to standardized, quantitative reporting of changes in specific cellular processes intimately associated with the malignant phenotype. Recent advances in FDG-PET of sarcomas regarding standardization of the methodology and reporting of results should help to speed up the introduction of novel, potentially more useful, radiopharmaceutics.

References

Adler, L.P., Blair, H.F., Makley, J.T., Williams, R.P., Joyce, M.J., Leisure, G., al-Kaisi, N., and Miraldi, F. 1991. Noninvasive grading of musculoskeletal tumors using PET. *J. Nucl. Med. 32*:1508–1512.

Aoki, J., Watanabe, H., Shinozaki, T., Takagishi, K., Tokunaga, M., Koyama, Y., Sato, N., and Endo, K. 2003. FDG-PET for preoperative differential diagnosis between benign and malignant soft tissue masses. *Skeletal Radiol. 32*:133–138.

Bastiaannet, E., Groen, H., Jager, P.L., Cobben, D.C., van der Graaf, W.T., Vaalburg, W., and Hoekstra, H.J. 2004. The value of FDG-PET in the detection, grading and response to therapy of soft tissue and bone sarcomas; a systematic review and meta-analysis. *Cancer Treat. Rev. 30*: 83–101.

Beaulieu, S., Rubin, B., Djang, D., Conrad, E., Turcotte, E., and Eary, J.F. 2004. Positron emission tomography of schwannomas: emphasizing its potential in preoperative planning. *AJR Am. J. Roentgenol. 182*:971–974.

Brenner, W., Conrad, E.U., and Eary, J.F. 2004. FDG PET imaging for grading and prediction of outcome in chondrosarcoma patients. *Eur. J. Nucl. Med. Mol. Imaging 31*:189–195.

Cobben, D.C., Elsinga, P.H., Suurmeijer, A.J., Vaalburg, W., Maas, B., Jager, P.L., and Hoekstra, H.J. 2004. Detection and grading of soft tissue sarcomas of the extremities with (18)F-3′-fluoro-3′-deoxy-L-thymidine. *Clin. Cancer Res. 10*:1685–1690.

Davis, A.M., Bell, R.S., and Goodwin, P.J. 1994. Prognostic factors in osteosarcoma: a critical review. *J. Clin. Oncol. 12*:423–431.

DeLaney, T.F., Spiro, I.J., Suit, H.D., Gebhardt, M.C., Hornicek, F.J., Mankin, H.J., Rosenberg, A.L., Rosenthal, D.I., Miryousefi, F., Ancukiewicz, M., and Harmon, D.C. 2003. Neoadjuvant chemotherapy and radiotherapy for large extremity soft-tissue sarcomas. *Int. J. Radiat. Oncol. Biol. Phys. 56*:1117–1127.

Dimitrakopoulou-Strauss, A., Strauss, L.G., Schwarzbach, M., Burger, C., Heichel, T., Willeke, F., Mechtersheimer, G., and Lehnert, T. 2001. Dynamic PET 18F-FDG studies in patients with primary and recurrent soft-tissue sarcomas: impact on diagnosis and correlation with grading. *J. Nucl. Med. 42*:713–720.

Eary, J.F., and Mankoff, D.A. 1998a. Tumor metabolic rates in sarcoma using FDG PET. *J. Nucl. Med. 39:*250–254.

Eary, J.F., Conrad, E.U., Bruckner, J.D., Folpe, A., Hunt, K.J., Mankoff, D.A., and Howlett, A.T. 1998b. Quantitative [F-18]fluorodeoxyglucose positron emission tomography in pretreatment and grading of sarcoma. *Clin. Cancer Res. 4:*1215–1220.

Eary, J.F., O'Sullivan, F., Powitan, Y., Chandhury, K.R., Vernon, C., Bruckner, J.D., and Conrad, E.U. 2002. Sarcoma tumor FDG uptake measured by PET and patient outcome: a retrospective analysis. *Eur. J. Nucl. Med. Mol. Imaging 29:*1149–1154.

Eilber, F.C., Rosen, G., Eckardt, J., Forscher, C., Nelson, S.D., Selch, M., Dorey, F., and Eilber, F.R. 2001. Treatment-induced pathologic necrosis: a predictor of local recurrence and survival in patients receiving neoadjuvant therapy for high-grade extremity soft tissue sarcomas. *J. Clin. Oncol. 19:*3203–3209.

Folpe, A.L., Lyles, R.H., Sprouse, J.T., Conrad, E.U., III, and Eary, J.F. 2000. (F-18) fluorodeoxyglucose positron emission tomography as a predictor of pathologic grade and other prognostic variables in bone and soft tissue sarcoma. *Clin. Cancer Res. 6:*1279–1287.

Franzius, C., Sciuk, J., Brinkschmidt, C., Jurgens, H., and Schober, O. 2000. Evaluation of chemotherapy response in primary bone tumors with F-18 FDG positron emission tomography compared with histologically assessed tumor necrosis. *Clin. Nucl. Med. 25:*874–881.

Franzius, C., Daldrup-Link, H.E., Wagner-Bohn, A., Sciuk, J., Heindel, W.L., Jurgens, H., and Schober, O. 2002. FDG-PET for detection of recurrences from malignant primary bone tumors: comparison with conventional imaging. *Ann. Oncol. 13:*157–160.

Hawkins, D.S., Schuetze, S.M., Butrynski, J.E., Rajendran, J.G., Vernon, C.B., Conrad, E.U., III, and Eary, J.F. 2005. [18F]Fluorodeoxyglucose positron emission tomography predicts outcome for Ewing sarcoma family of tumors. *J. Clin. Oncol. 23:*8828–8834.

Ioannidis, J.P., and Lau, J. 2003. 18F-FDG PET for the diagnosis and grading of soft-tissue sarcoma: a meta-analysis. *J. Nucl. Med. 44:*717–724.

Jones, D.N., McCowage, G.B., Sostman, H.D., Brizel, D.M., Layfield, L., Charles, H.C., Dewhirst, M.W., Prescott, D.M., Friedman, H.S., Harrelson, J.M., Scully, S.P., and Coleman, R.E. 1996. Monitoring of neoadjuvant therapy response of soft-tissue and musculoskeletal sarcoma using fluorine-18-FDG PET. *J. Nucl. Med. 37:*1438–1444.

Kattan, M.W., Leung, D.H., and Brennan, M.F. 2002. Postoperative nomogram for 12-year sarcoma-specific death. *J. Clin. Oncol. 20:*791–796.

Kern, K.A., Brunetti, A., Norton, J.A., Chang, A.E., Malawer, M., Lack, E., Finn, R.D., Rosenberg, S.A., and Larson, S.M. 1988. Metabolic imaging of human extremity musculoskeletal tumors by PET. *J. Nucl. Med. 29:*181–186.

Lawrence, J.A., Babyn, P.S., Chan, H.S., Thorner, P.S., Pron, G.E., and Krajbich, I.J. 1993. Extremity osteosarcoma in childhood: prognostic value of radiologic imaging. *Radiology 189:*43–47.

Lodge, M.A., Lucas, J.D., Marsden, P.K., Cronin, B.F., O'Doherty, M.J., and Smith, M.A. 1999. A PET study of 18FDG uptake in soft tissue masses. *Eur. J. Nucl. Med. 26:*22–30.

Mankin, H.J., Mankin, C.J., and Simon, M.A. 1996. The hazards of the biopsy, revisited. Members of the Musculoskeletal Tumor Society. *J. Bone Joint Surg. Am. 78:*656–663.

Murphy, W.A., Jr. 1991. Imaging bone tumors in the 1990s. *Cancer 67:*1169–1176.

Nair, N., Ali, A., Green, A.A., Lamonica, G., Alibazoglu, H., Alibazoglu, B., Hollinger, E.F., and Ahmed, K. 2000. Response of osteosarcoma to chemotherapy: evaluation with F-18 FDG-PET scans. *Clin. Positron Imaging 3:*79–83.

Nieweg, O.E., Pruim, J., van Ginkel, R.J., Hoekstra, H.J., Paans, A.M., Molenaar, W.M., Koops, H.S., and Vaalburg, W. 1996. Fluorine-18-fluorodeoxyglucose PET imaging of soft-tissue sarcoma. *J. Nucl. Med. 37:*257–261.

Panicek, D.M., Gatsonis, C., Rosenthal, D.I., Seeger, L.L., Huvos, A.G., Moore, S.G., Caudry, D.J., Palmer, W.E., and McNeil, B.J. 1997. CT and MR imaging in the local staging of primary malignant musculoskeletal neoplasms: report of the Radiology Diagnostic Oncology Group. *Radiology 202:*237–246.

Paul, R., Johansson, R., Kiuru, A., Illukka, T., Talvio, T., Roeda, D., Solin, O., Soderstrom, K.O., Nordman, E., and Ahonen, A. 1984. Imaging of canine cancers with 18F-2-fluoro-2-deoxy-D-glucose (FDG) suggests further applications for cancer imaging in man. *Nucl. Med. Commun. 5:*641–646.

Rajendran, J.G., Wilson, D.C., Conrad, E.U., Peterson, L.M., Bruckner, J.D., Rasey, J.S., Chin, L.K., Hofstrand, P.D., Grierson, J.R., Eary, J.F., and Krohn, K.A. 2003. [(18)F]FMISO and [(18)F]FDG PET imaging in soft tissue sarcomas: correlation of hypoxia, metabolism and VEGF expression. *Eur. J. Nucl. Med. Mol. Imaging 30:*695–704.

Reddick, W.E., Wang, S., Xiong, X., Glass, J.O., Wu, S., Kaste, S.C., Pratt, C.B., Meyer, W.H., and Fletcher, B.D. 2001. Dynamic magnetic resonance imaging of regional contrast access as an additional prognostic factor in pediatric osteosarcoma. *Cancer 91:*2230–2237.

Reuther, G., and Mutschler, W. 1990. Detection of local recurrent disease in musculoskeletal tumors: magnetic resonance imaging versus computed tomography. *Skeletal Radiol. 19:*85–90.

Schuetze, S.M. 2005. Imaging and response in soft tissue sarcomas. *Hematol. Oncol. Clin. North. Am. 19:*471–487, vi.

Schuetze, S.M., Rubin, B.P., Vernon, C., Hawkins, D.S., Bruckner, J.D., Conrad, E.U., and Eary, J. 2005. Use of positron emission tomography in localized extremity soft tissue sarcoma treated with neoadjuvant chemotherapy. *Cancer 103:*339–348.

Schulte, M., Brecht-Krauss, D., Werner, M., Hartwig, E., Sarkar, M.R., Keppler, P., Kotzerke, J., Guhlmann, A., Delling, G., and Reske, S.N. 1999. Evaluation of neoadjuvant therapy response of osteogenic sarcoma using FDG PET. *J. Nucl. Med. 40:*1637–1643.

Schwarzbach, M.H., Dimitrakopoulou-Strauss, A., Willeke, F., Hinz, U., Strauss, L.G., Zhang, Y.M., Mechtersheimer, G., Attigah, N., Lehnert, T., and Herfarth, C. 2000. Clinical value of [18-F]] fluorodeoxyglucose positron emission tomography imaging in soft tissue sarcomas. *Ann. Surg. 231:*380–386.

Shapeero, L.G., Vanel, D., Verstraete, K.L., and Bloem, J.L. 2002. Fast magnetic resonance imaging with contrast for soft tissue sarcoma viability. *Clin. Orthop. 397:*212–227.

Skrzynski, M.C., Biermann, J.S., Montag, A., and Simon, M.A. 1996. Diagnostic accuracy and charge-savings of outpatient core needle biopsy compared with open biopsy of musculoskeletal tumors. *J. Bone Joint Surg. Am. 78:*644–649.

Therasse, P., Arbuck, S.G., Eisenhauer, E.A., Wanders, J., Kaplan, R.S., Rubinstein, L., Verweij, J., Van Glabbeke, M., van Oosterom, A.T., Christian, M.C., and Gwyther, S.G. 2000. New guidelines to evaluate the response to treatment in solid tumors. European Organization for Research and Treatment of Cancer, National Cancer Institute of the United States, National Cancer Institute of Canada. *J. Natl. Cancer Inst. 92:*205–216.

van Ginkel, R.J., Kole, A.C., Nieweg, O.E., Molenaar, W.M., Pruim, J., Koops, H.S., Vaalburg, W., and Hoekstra, H.J. 1999. L-[1-11C]-tyrosine PET to evaluate response to hyperthermic isolated limb perfusion for locally advanced soft-tissue sarcoma and skin cancer. *J. Nucl. Med. 40:*262–267.

van Ginkel, R.J., Hoekstra, H.J., Pruim, J., Nieweg, O.E., Molenaar, W.M., Paans, A.M., Willemsen, A.T., Vaalburg, W., and Koops, H.S. 1996. FDG-PET to evaluate response to hyperthermic isolated limb perfusion for locally advanced soft-tissue sarcoma. *J. Nucl. Med. 37:*984–990.

Vanel, D., Lacombe, M.J., Couanet, D., Kalifa, C., Spielmann, M., and Genin, J. 1987. Musculoskeletal tumors: follow-up with MR imaging after treatment with surgery and radiation therapy. *Radiology 164:*243–245.

Vernon, C.B., Eary, J.F., Rubin, B.P., Conrad, E.U., III, and Schuetze, S. 2003. FDG PET imaging guided re-evaluation of histopathologic response in a patient with high-grade sarcoma. *Skeletal Radiol. 32*:139–142.

Weber, W.A., Ziegler, S.I., Thodtmann, R., Hanauske, A.R., and Schwaiger, M. 1999. Reproducibility of metabolic measurements in malignant tumors using FDG PET. *J. Nucl. Med. 40*:1771–1777.

Wunder, J.S., Paulian, G., Huvos, A.G., Heller, G., Meyers, P.A., and Healey, J.H. 1998. The histological response to chemotherapy as a predictor of the oncological outcome of operative treatment of Ewing sarcoma. *J. Bone Joint Surg. Am. 80*:1020–1033.

Yagle, K.J., Eary, J.F., Tait, J.F., Grierson, J.R., Link, J.M., Lewellen, B., Gibson, D.F., and Krohn, K.A. 2005. Evaluation of 18F-Annexin V as a PET imaging agent in an animal model of apoptosis. *J. Nucl. Med. 46*:658–666.

Zhang, H., Tian, M., Oriuchi, N., Higuchi, T., Watanabe, H., Aoki, J., Tanada, S., and Endo, K. 2003. 11C-choline PET for the detection of bone and soft tissue tumours in comparison with FDG PET. *Nucl. Med. Commun. 24*:273–279.

Zhang, H., Yoshikawa, K., Tamura, K., Tomemori, T., Sagou, K., Tian, M., Kandatsu, S., Kamada, T., Tsuji, H., Suhara, T., Suzuki, K., Tanada, S., and Tsujii, H. 2004. [(11)C]methionine positron emission tomography and survival in patients with bone and soft tissue sarcomas treated by carbon ion radiotherapy. *Clin. Cancer Res. 10*:1764–1772.

51

Retroperitoneal Synovial Sarcoma: Color Doppler Ultrasound, Computed Tomography, and Magnetic Resonance Imaging

Serife Ulusan

Introduction

Synovial sarcoma is a clinically and morphologically well-defined soft tissue tumor that occurs predominantly in the extremities of adolescents and young adults. It tends to arise in the vicinity of large joints, especially the knee, bursae, and tendon sheaths, but can occur anywhere in the body in locations distant from joint spaces, such as the head and neck region, abdominal wall, and retroperitoneum.

Synovial sarcoma is a relatively common primary soft tissue sarcoma and accounts for ~ 5 to 10% of all malignant mesenchymal neoplasms. It is the most common malignancy of the foot and ankle in patients between 6 and 45 years old, and the most common malignancy of the lower extremity between the ages of 6 years and 35 years (Tateishi *et al.*, 2004).

On microscopic examination, the tumor was well demarcated. The tumor cells were large, oval, with large round hyperchromatic nuclei and eosinophilic cytoplasm, and marked nuclear pleomorphism. Bizarre and multinuclear giant cells and stromal lymphocytes were seen.

Although the immunohistochemical profile of synovial sarcoma varies, most synovial sarcomas are at least focally positive for cytokeratin and epithelial membrane antigen (EMA). It has recently been suggested that EMA, cytokeratin AE1, AE3, and E-cadherin, in combination with CD34 negativity, are the most useful and sensitive markers for diagnosing monophasic fibrous and poorly differentiated synovial sarcoma. Over 80% of reported synovial sarcomas have specific reciprocal chromosomal translocation t(x; 18) (p11.2; q11.2) (Fisher *et al.*, 2004).

Synovial sarcomas can be classified into four histopathological types: (1) biphasic; (2) monophasic fibrous; (3) monophasic epithelial; and (4) poorly differentiated. Primary retroperitoneal sarcomas may be biphasic as well as monophasic. Monophasic synovial sarcomas behave more aggressively and metastasize earlier than do biphasic tumors. No imaging differences have been reported between the monophasic and biphasic variants (Kransdorf, 1995).

Primary retroperitoneal soft tissue sarcomas are rare, and the radiological differential diagnosis is often difficult. The most frequent retroperitoneal sarcomas are malignant fibrous histiocytoma, liposarcoma, fibrosarcoma, and malignant germ cell tumor (Ziran *et al.*, 1996). The retroperitoneal region is the most uncommon site of the synovial sarcoma.

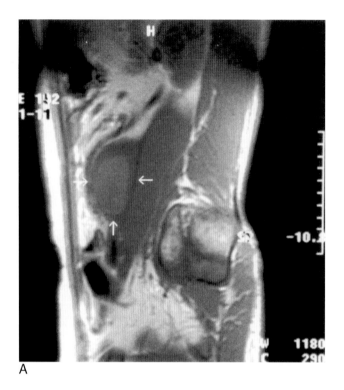

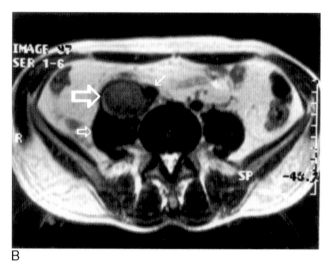

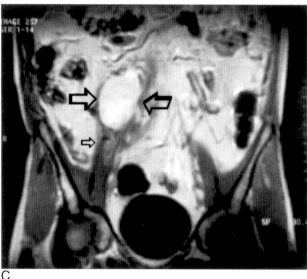

Figure 1 (A) Precontrast T1-weighted sagittal MR image shows the retroperitoneal mass, which is slightly hyperintense to adjacent muscle (arrows). (B) Axial T2-weighted MR image demonstrates slight hyperintensity of the mass (large open arrow). (C) Post-gadolinium T1-weighted image shows homogeneous enhancement of the lesion (large open arrows) compared with psoas muscle adjacent to the mass (small open arrow).

It was reported as the first retroperitoneal synovial sarcoma by Pack and Tabah (1954). Since then, 29 cases have been described (Fisher *et al.*, 2004; Ulusan *et al.*, 2005).

Approximately 50% of all synovial sarcomas recur locally, usually within 2 years, but sometimes many years later. Metastases occur mainly in lungs, and less commonly in lymph nodes and bone. All of the previously reported patients of primary retroperitoneal synovial sarcoma died (at intervals of 7 24 months) with local recurrence or extension,

but none metastasized outside the retroperiton. The mortality for these tumors is high, however, due to the local extension of disease (de Silva *et al.*, 2004; Fisher *et al.*, 2004).

Radiologic Findings

If the patient is not overweight, ultrasound will be useful in evaluating the retroperitoneal region. Retroperitoneal synovial sarcoma can be compressed or invade contiguous organs. For example, compressed ureter causes hydroureterorenephrosis, and compressed or invaded vena cava inferior may develop lower extremity venous thrombosis. These secondary findings are demonstrated with ultrasound (US) and color Doppler US. Retroperitoneal synovial sarcomas of US findings are a well-defined hypoechoic solid mass. Color Doppler US of this solid mass showed uniform hypovascularity. The mass was encircled by the vessels and extended into centripetal branches that passed into the parenchyma of the lesion (Ulusan *et al.*, 2005).

Retroperitoneal computed tomography (CT) studies should be performed with noncontrast and intravenous contrast material. Precontrast CT scan is helpful to show calcifications and, postcontrast CT scan images are helpful in allowing a distinction between vascular and nonvascular structures, determining the vascularity of a retroperitoneal mass and its effect on the urinary tract, and maximizing the detection of focal lesions in solid abdominal organs. Computed tomography is particularly useful to identify soft tissue calcifications. Such scanning may also identify areas of hemorrhage, necrosis, or cyst formation within the tumor. Postcontrast CT scans are helpful in differentiating the mass from adjacent organs and vascular structure. Thus, CT defines the mass and readily confirms contiguous organ invasion.

Retroperitoneal synovial sarcomas of CT findings are a large (5–20 cm), spherical, well-defined soft tissue mass that rarely contains calcification in the retroperitoneal region. There was marked homogeneous enhancement of the mass in the post-intravenous contrast material. The synovial sarcoma compressed or invaded the psoas muscle, inferior vena cava, and ureter, resulting in venous thrombosis or hydroureteronephrosis (Ulusan *et al.*, 2005). These compressions and invasions are more clearly seen when compared with those with US or color Doppler US.

The retroperitoneum can successfully be carried out through magnetic resonance imaging (MRI). Transverse images are obtained in all patients. In addition, coronal and sagittal images often are performed to better define invasion or compression of the aorta, inferior vena cava, and psoas muscle. Both T1- and T2-weighted sequences are required for lesion detection and characterization. Post-gadolinium T1-weighted images (WI) must be obtained in at least two different planes. On MRI, the findings of the retroperitoneal synovial sarcoma are usually nonspecific. It was defined that the intensity of this mass on T1-WI was approximately equal to that of skeletal muscle and, on T2-WI MR images, was higher than that of subcutaneous fat.

Signal intensity changes are compatible with previous hemorrhage, and fluid-fluid levels have been reported. The soft tissue calcifications frequently seen on radiographs and CT may not be detected on MRI, although larger calcifications are identified as areas of decreased signal intensity on all pulse sequences (Ulusan *et al.*, 2005).

The MRI findings of retroperitoneal synovial sarcoma are of higher signal intensity than those of skeletal muscle on spin-echo T1-WI, a moderately higher signal than those of skeletal muscle on turbo-spin-echo T2-WI, and, after administration of gadolinium contrast medium shown as T1-WI, is given marked, homogeneous enhancement (Fig. 1) (Ulusan *et al.*, 2005).

Conclusion

Early diagnosis of the retroperitoneal synovial sarcoma is impossible due to the extreme expandability of this space and deeply hidden location, which is particularly common in overweight patients (Fisher *et al.*, 2004). In the preoperative period, CT and MRI provide valuable information for management of surgery. In the postoperative period, these imaging procedures for this tumor are available for determining local recurrence and metastasis.

References

de Silva, M.V., McMahon, A.D., and Reid, R. 2004. Prognostic factors associated with local recurrence, metastases, and tumor-related death in patients with synovial sarcoma. *Am. J. Clin. Oncol. 27*:113–121.

Fisher, C., Folpe, A.L., Hashimoto, H., and Weiss, W.S. 2004. Intra-abdominal synovial sarcoma: a clinicopathological study. *Histopathology 45*:245–253.

Kransdorf, M.J. 1995. Malignant soft-tissue tumors in a large referral population: distribution of diagnoses by age, sex, and location. *Am. J. Roentgenol. 164*:129–134.

Pack G.T., and Tabah, E.J. 1954. Primary retroperitoneal tumors: a study of 120 cases. *Int. Abstr. Surg. 99*:313–341.

Tateishi, U., Hasegawa, T., Beppu, Y., Satake, M., and Moriyama, N. 2004. Synovial sarcoma of the soft tissues: prognostic significance of imaging features. *J. Comput. Assist. Tomogr. 28*:140–148.

Ulusan, S., Kizilkilic, O., Yildirim, T., Hurcan, C., Bal. N., and Nursal, T.Z. 2005. Radiological findings of primary retroperitoneal synovial sarcoma. *Br. J. Radiol. 78*:166–169.

Ziran, B.H., Makley, J.T., and Carter, J.R.1996. Primary retroperitoneal sarcomas: common symptoms, common diagnosis, uncommon disease. *Clin. Orthop. Relat. Res. 331*:277–282.

52

Thymoma: Computed Tomography

Marcello Tiseo and Francesco Monetti

Introduction

General Features

Thymic neoplasms, mostly thymomas, constitute 30% of anterior mediastinal masses in adults but only 15% of anterior mediastinal masses in children (Duwe *et al.*, 2005). A review of Surveillance, Epidemiology and End Results program (SEER) data suggests that thymomas have an incidence of 0.15 cases per 100,000 (Engels and Pfeiffer, 2003). Thymomas usually present in the fourth and fifth decades of life, although cases have been reported within the first year and into the ninth decade. There is no clear sex predisposition (Thomas *et al.*, 1999; Detterbeck and Parsons, 2004).

One-third of patients present with asymptomatic anterior mediastinal mass on chest radiograph, one-third present with local symptoms (cough, chest pain, superior vena cava syndrome, or dysphagia) and one-third of cases are detected during evaluation of myasthenia gravis (Thomas *et al.*, 1999). Approximately 30 to 50% of patients with thymoma have myasthenia gravis, compared to 10 to 15% of patients with myasthenia gravis who have a thymoma. Most patients with myasthenia gravis have a thymic hyperplasia without thymoma (Drachman, 1994). In addition to myasthenia, a host of paraneoplastic syndromes have been seen in association with thymoma, as pure red cell aplasia, hypogammaglobulinemia, and a variety of other autoimmune disorders (Thomas *et al.*, 1999).

Thymoma is an epithelial tumor generally considered to have an indolent growth pattern but malignant nonetheless because of potential for local invasion, pleural dissemination, and even systemic metastases. Distant metastases are distinctly uncommon at initial presentation; however, when present, the most common metastatic site is the pleura, with involvement of the kidney, bone, liver, and brain metastases infrequently seen (Thomas *et al.*, 1999).

Pathology and Classification

Ninety percent of thymomas occur in the anterior mediastinum, and the remainder arise in the neck or other areas of the mediastinum. Grossly, they are lobulated, firm, tan-pink to gray tumors that may contain cystic spaces, calcification, or hemorrhage. They may be encapsulated, adherent to surrounding structures, or frankly invasive. Microscopically, thymomas arise from thymic epithelial cells, although thymocytes/lymphocytes may predominate histologically. True thymomas contain cytologically bland cells and should be distinguished from thymic carcinomas, which have malignant cytologic characteristics. Confusion exists because of previous "benign" or "malignant" designations. Currently, the terms *noninvasive* and *invasive* are preferred. Noninvasive thymomas have an intact capsule, are movable, and easily resected, although they can be adherent to adjacent organs. In contrast, invasive thymomas involve surrounding structures and can be difficult to remove without *en bloc* resection of adjacent structures, despite their cytologic benign appearance (Hasserjian *et al.*, 2005).

The pathology of thymomas has undergone a sea change in the last years, culminating in the relatively new WHO histological classification. The first widely used classification proposed by Bernatz *et al.* (1961) was descriptive, distinguishing *predominantly lymphocytic*, *predominantly epithelial*, *predominantly mixed*, and *predominantly spindle-cell-type* thymoma. However, this classification was of limited clinical value. To overcome this flaw, in 1978 Levine and Rosai (1978) proposed a classification that divided into *benign* (*noninvasive*) from *malignant* (*invasive*) thymomas. Malignant thymomas were further subdivided into *category I* (with no or minimal atypia) and *category II* (with moderate to marked atypia), equivalent to thymic carcinoma. However, this classification was clinico-pathological rather than histogical, and it had little direct correlation with prognosis. In 1985, Marino and Muller-Hermelink (1985) proposed a histologic classification system determined by the thymic site of origin. Tumors arising from epithelial cells of the cortex are termed *cortical thymomas*, corresponding to traditional epithelial thymomas; those arising from spindle cells of the medullary areas are called *medullary thymomas*, corresponding to traditional spindle cell thymomas. *Mixed thymomas* have features of both. The Muller-Hermelink classification was later further divided into medullary, mixed, predominantly cortical, cortical thymomas, and well-differentiated and high-grade thymic carcinomas. Medullary and mixed thymomas were considered benign with no risk of recurrence, even with capsular invasion. Predominantly cortical and cortical thymomas exhibited intermediate invasiveness and a low but definite risk of late relapse, regardless of their invasiveness. Well-differentiated thymic carcinomas were always invasive, with a high risk of relapse and death.

Controversy about the pathology of thymic neoplasms led the World Health Organization (WHO) committee to adopt a new classification system for thymic tumors in 1999 based on prognostic significance and on cytologic similarities between normal thymic epithelial cells and neoplastic cells (Rosai and Sobin, 1999). The terminology chosen by the WHO committee is based on a combination of letters and numbers (Table 1). In particular, there are two major type of thymoma depending on whether the neoplastic epithelial cells have a spindle/oval shape (type A) or whether they have a dendritic or epithelioid appearance (type B). The type B thymomas are further subdivided into subcategories B1, B2, and B3 on the basis of an increasing epithelial-lymphocyte ratio and emergence of atypia. Thymic carcinomas (type C) are named according to their differentiation. This classification was largely confirmed and supplemented in the 2004 edition. This last edition, in particular, encompasses neuroendocrine carcinomas (including carcinoids) among the thymic carcinomas. The predominant histological subtypes in

most published series are type B2 and AB thymomas (each 20 to 35% of all cases). Types B1 and A count among the rare types (5 to 10%), while type C counts from 10 to 25% (Hasserjian *et al.*, 2005).

Diagnosis, Staging, and Prognosis

The diagnosis of thymoma is usually made clinically. Typically, a thymoma is an incidental finding on a chest radiograph or on chest computed tomography (CT), which appears as a well-defined lobulated mass in the antero-superior mediastinum (Duwe *et al.*, 2005). Further evaluation with contrast-enhanced thoracic CT scanning usually reveals an encapsulated, well-defined, soft tissue, often with hemorrhage, necrosis, or cyst formation (Maher and Shepard, 2005) (see the section Computed Tomography). Patient presenting with commonly associated diseases such as myasthenia gravis, pure red cell aplasia, or hypogammaglobulinemia should prompt investigation with a chest CT scan to rule out the presence of an asymptomatic thymoma.

Following initial clinical and CT scan evaluation, for typical small encapsulated thymomas an excisional approach for diagnosis and treatment seems reasonable, while biopsy of the anterior compartment mass may be indicated when lymphoma or locally advanced thymoma is suspected (Thomas *et al.*, 1999; Wright and Kessler, 2005). The least invasive technique is fine needle aspiration (CT-guided FNA). It must be emphasized, however, that cytology not only lacks sensitivity, but also can be misleading with respect to differentiating thymomas and lymphomas (Morrissey *et al.*, 1993). Core needle biopsies allow histological examination and, therefore, immunohistochemical staining can be performed, improving the diagnostic accuracy. If core needle biopsy is not possible, two surgical options exist for diagnostic evaluation: anterior ("Chamberlain") mediastinotomy and VATS (video-associated thoracic surgery). Standard cervical mediastinoscopy does not provide access to the anterior compartment and, therefore, should be avoided (unless significant paratracheal lymhadenopathy suspicious of metastatic disease is present) (Thomas *et al.*, 1999; Wright and Kessler, 2005).

Masaoka *et al.* (1981) developed a staging system in four stages that was widely adopted (Table 2). Staging of thymoma is based on the presence or absence of an intact tumor capsule. The Masaoka system is postsurgical because invasion of the capsule is reliably diagnosed only by pathologic examination. In this staging system, stage I thymomas do not demonstrate capsular invasion. Stage II lesions show microscopic invasion of the capsule, mediastinal fat, or surrounding pleura. Stage III tumors invade surrounding organs and structures such as the lung, pericardium, superior vena cava, and aorta. Stage IVa involves pleural or pericardial dissemination, while stage IVb involves lymphogenous or hematogenous metastases. This scheme has been incorporated with

Table 1   Comparison of the WHO Classification of Thymic Epithelial Tumors with the Clinico-Pathological Classification (Levine and Rosai, 1978) and Histogenetic Classification (Marino and Muller-Hermelink, 1985)

Tumor Type	Cells	Clinico-Pathological Classification	Histogenetic Classification
A	Spindle or oval	Benign thymoma	Medullary
B	Epithelioid or dendritic	Category I malignant thymoma	Cortical; organoid
B1			Lymphocyte-rich; predominately cortical
B2			Cortical
B3			Well-differentiated thymic carcinoma
AB		Benign thymoma	Mixed
C		Category II malignant thymoma	Nonorganotypic; thymic carcinoma, epidermoid keratinizing and nonkeratinizing carcinoma, lymphoepithelioma-like carcinoma, sarcomatoid carcinoma, clear-cell carcinoma, basaloid carcinoma, mucoepidermoid carcinoma, undifferentiated carcinoma

some modification into the TNM staging system proposed by Yamakawa (Yamakawa *et al.*, 1991).

The prognosis of thymoma is dependent on the following factors: (a) stage; (b) microscopic type; (c) completeness of excision; and (d) myasthenia gravis (Blumberg *et al.*, 1995; Strobel *et al.*, 2004; Hasserjian *et al.*, 2005). The stage remains the single most important prognostic determinant. The 5-year survival rate is of 96% for stage I, 86% for stage II, 69% for stage III, and 50% for stage IV (Masaoka *et al.*, 1981). The microscopic type of thymoma shows a close correlation with prognosis, according to this scheme of increasing aggressiveness: A < AB < B1 <B2 <B3 < C (Okumura *et al.*, 2002). Thus, types A and AB in stages I and II almost always follow a benign clinical course. Type B1 thymoma has a low malignant potential, although local recurrences or metastases may occur. Type B2, B3, and C thymomas are clear-cut malignant tumors, with well-differentiated squamous, basaloid, and mucoepidermoid carcinomas following a more favorable course than their poorly differentiated counterparts (Hasserjian *et al.*, 2005). An important prognostic parameter is completeness of excision; in fact, incomplete tumor resection was associated with a high recurrence rate and a poor prognosis (Strobel *et al.*, 2004). Previous reports have cited myasthenia gravis as a negative prognostic factor; however, more recent trials have found no adverse or even a positive effect, probably due to earlier thymoma detection (Wright and Kessler, 2005; Hasserjian *et al.*, 2005).

Computed Tomography

Computed tomography (CT) plays an important role in the management of patients with thymoma. It is often used when thymoma is suspected clinically but not detected on radiography (25% of thymomas are not seen on chest radiographs). It provides information on differential diagnosis and on the precise anatomic location of the lesion and its relationship to surrounding structures. Moreover, CT can be used in the presurgical planning providing information on the presence and degree of invasion (Wright and Kessler, 2005). Lastly, it can be used to monitor tumor behavior during chemo- and/or radiation therapy and to detect recurrent or metastatic neoplasm after the treatment has been completed (Maher and Shepard, 2005).

Diagnosis and Staging

The most frequent CT appearance of thymoma is a soft tissue mass in the anterior mediastinum, ranging from small to large and resulting in smoothly marginated, often lobulated borders against the adjacent lung (Fig. 1). Approximately, 80% of thymomas occur adjacent to the junction of the great vessels and the pericardium; other less common locations are in the cardiophrenic angle or in the adjacent cardiac border and rarely in the neck or other mediastinal compartments. After intravenous administration of contrast material, the tumor enhances homogeneously; however, areas of decreased attenuation may be present and correspond to cystic changes

Table 2   Thymoma Staging System of Masaoka

Stage	Description
I	Macroscopically completely encapsulated and microscopically no capsular invasion
II	Macroscopic invasion into surrounding fatty tissue or mediastinal pleura
	Microscopic invasion into capsule
III	Macroscopic invasion into neighboring organs (pericardium, great vessels, lung)
IVa	Pleural or pericardial dissemination
IVb	Lymphogenous or hematogenous metastasis

or foci of hemorrhage and necrosis. Calcification, even if subtle, can be easily detected with CT; the pattern of calcification is commonly linear, thin, and peripheral, corresponding to calcium deposits in the tumor capsule. Rarely, thymoma may manifest as a predominantly pleural disease, which is

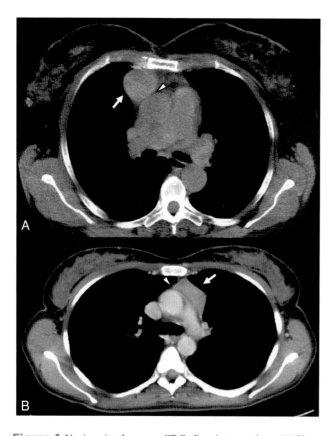

Figure 1 Noninvasive thymoma, CT findings in two patients. (**A**) Unenhanced CT section at the level of the right main pulmonary artery. A well-defined rounded mass of soft tissue attenuation is present on the right side of the anterior mediastinum (arrow); it is separated from the ascending aorta by a well-defined fat plane (arrowhead), suggesting that it is noninvasive. (**B**) Contrast-enhanced CT scan shows a heterogeneous mediastinal mass located at the level of the left pulmonary artery (arrow); it is separated from mediastinal vessels by a well-defined fat plane, suggesting that it is noninvasive (arrowhead).

usually unilateral and demonstrates nonspecific radiographic patterns such as pleural masses or diffuse, nodular, or circumferential pleural thickening that encases the ipsilateral lung. The latter presentation may mimic the appearance of diffuse malignant mesothelioma or metastatic adenocarcinoma (Naidich *et al.*, 1999).

Thymoma can be staged at the time of surgery on the presence or absence of intact tumor capsule (see the section Diagnosis, Staging, and Prognosis). As with other tumors, CT cannot be used to predict capsule invasion or resect ability with accuracy. In fact, absence of cleavage planes between tumor and mediastinal structures is not a strictly reliable criterion for predicting invasion because fibrous adhesion, without actual invasion, presents the same CT features. The only CT findings that allow a reliable diagnosis of local invasion are complete encasement or interdigitation of tumor with the mediastinal structure and bone destruction (Fig. 2). On the other hand, clear definition of fatty planes surrounding thymoma on CT should be interpreted as indicating an absence of local invasion (Fig. 1). Infiltration of the adjacent lungs or the chest wall is also possible and well demonstrated by CT (Hung *et al.*, 1999).

Thymoma can also spread by contiguity along the pleural surface potentially seeding even the diaphragmatic surface with consequent direct invasion of the abdominal organs. Transpleural spread may occur as a sheet of neoplastic tissue extending outward from the primary thymic tumor, or it may manifest as a discrete "drop metastasis" at a distance from the primary lesion. Pleural implants, when present, are often unilateral and, unlike other tumors resulting in pleural metastases, are usually unassociated with pleural effusion. Thus, CT can easily show focal, well-defined pleural masses not obscured by pleural fluid (Fig. 2). Blood-borne metastases are rare, even with extensive disease (Naidich *et al.*, 1999).

Computed tomography can be used to differentiate normal thymus and thymoma or other thymic neoplasms. Normal thymus is usually identifiable on CT in patients under the age of 25 years. It has a triangular or bilobated shape, while in such a case the left lobe is normally bigger than the right. It is usually outlined by mediastinal fat, and its margins are flat

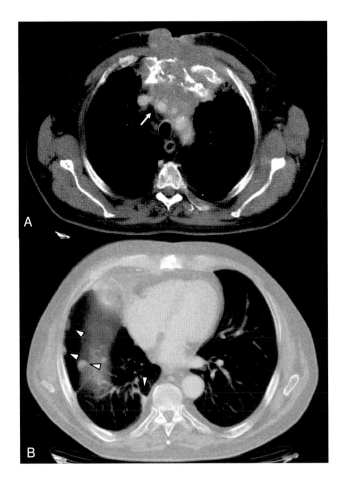

Figure 2 Invasive thymoma, CT findings. (**A**) Contrast-enhanced CT scan at the level of upper limit of the aortic arch shows a bulky homogeneous soft tissue mass in the prevascular space with encasement of brachiocephalic artery (arrow), erosion of the sternum, and deep invasion of the chest wall. (**B**) Contrast-enhanced CT scan at the level of right hemi-diaphragm shows pleural implants consistent with diffuse pleural metastatic disease (arrowheads).

or concave laterally. Normal thymus can have also a "mass" appearance, but in such a case its length is greater than its width. Its attenuation is less than that of chest wall muscle because of fatty replacement that seems to "infiltrate" the thymus, and, during its normal involution, no calcifications are usually seen. If enlargement of the thymus is encountered in patients over 30 years of age and if it is grossly asymmetric, with lobular margins, calcifications, and attenuation greater than that of chest wall muscle, a thymic mass should be suspected (Naidich *et al.*, 1999; Bogot and Quint, 2005).

Differential Diagnosis

The differential diagnosis of patients presenting with a mass in the anterior mediastinal compartment can be initially guided by patient's age, gender, association with symptoms, and other clinical findings (Duwe *et al.*, 2005; Maher and Shepard, 2005).

Germ cell tumors account for 15% of anterior mediastinal masses found in adults (Strollo and Rosado-de-Christenson, 2002). These tumors, more common in men, are classified into the following three groups based on cell type: seminomas, nonseminomas, and benign teratomas. Seminoma appears as a large mass with areas of necrosis and hemorrhage usually located in the anterior mediastinum; infiltration of mediastinal structures is infrequent, but these tumors can metastasize to local lymph nodes. On CT scan, seminomas are generally indistinguishable from thymoma or solitary lymphoma (Strollo and Rosado-de-Christenson, 2002). Teratomas are the most common mediastinal germ tumors, accounting for 60 to 75% (Bokemeyer *et al.*, 2002). On CT, teratomas typically appear as multiloculated cystic tumors protruding to one side of the midline of the anterior mediastinum; coexistence of fluid, soft tissue, calcification, and fat in an anterior mediastinal mass is highly suggestive of teratoma and is helpful in distinguishing this tumor from thymoma or lymphoma. Nonseminomatous tumors can essentially be ruled out by measuring the serum tumor marker levels of alpha fetoprotein (α-FP) and the beta subunit of chorionic gonadotropin (β-HCG) (Duwe *et al.*, 2005).

Because both the thymus and the inferior parathyroid glands arise from the third branchial complex and descend together, ectopic inferior glands can be found in the anterior mediastinum. Normal gland cannot be identified on CT; ectopic parathyroid adenomas may vary in size from 0.3 to 3 cm, and, when located in the anterior mediastinum, they may be indistinguishable from small thymic remnants or small thymomas. Their diagnosis can be aided by nuclear scans with ^{99m}Tc and ^{201}Ti (Clark *et al.*, 2005). Substernal goiter is readily identified on CT scan that shows continuity between the cervical and the mediastinal components and strong enhancement following intravenous contrast administration. Iodine nuclear medicine scans can be used to confirm a thyroid origin in rare cases when CT is equivocal (Duwe *et al.*, 2005).

Thymic involvement in lymphoma is usually indistinguishable from thymoma or other causes of anterior mediastinal mass. Ancillary findings should be searched to avoid surgical biopsy. Generally, thymoma occurs in older patients as compared with patients with lymphoma. Constitutional symptoms such as night sweats, fever, weight loss, and malaise are more consistent with lymphoma. A clinical history of immune disorder, such as myasthenia gravis, is more frequently associated with thymoma. Hilar, mediastinal, or peripheral lymphadenopathy are important findings for their association with lymphoma, often amenable to excisional biopsy, which might establish a diagnosis (Wright and Kessler, 2005). A large thymic mass showing invasion of the great vessels, mediastinal or hilar lymph node enlargement, phrenic nerve palsy, and distant metastases suggests thymic carcinoma (Jung *et al.*, 2001).

A difficult challenge for radiologists is to differentiate between thymoma and thymic hyperplasia. True thymic hyperplasia (TTH) or thymic "rebound" is an uncommon condition, consisting of enlargement of the thymus gland beyond the upper limits for the corresponding age. It can be related to "stressing" events, such as surgery, thermal burns, chemotherapy, and hyperthyroidism, or it can represent an idiopathic condition (Fig. 3). In particular, it has been regarded as a rebound immunologic phenomenon, usually regressing in a few months either spontaneously or after steroid therapy. Lymphoid follicular hyperplasia is an expression used by pathologists to describe the presence of hyperplastic lymphoid germinal centers in the thymic medulla, associated with a lymphocytic and plasmacell infiltrate. Usually, it does not produce expansion of the thymic gland, but it may also manifest as a diffuse enlargement or a focal mass up to 5 cm in diameter at CT, which does not permit radiographic differentiation from thymoma. In younger patients (< 25 years of age) who may have residual thymic tissue, biopsy is required. With increasing age, the thymus undergoes fatty involution, which makes diagnosis of thymoma easier in patients over 40 years of age (Bogot and Quint, 2005).

Thymolipoma has some important imaging features that distinguish this tumor from the others: its "habit" of conforming to adjacent structures and its classic combination of fat and soft tissue elements. Thymic cysts appear on CT as well-bounded masses located in the anterior/superior mediastinum. Some may present loculation or multiloculations with occasional visualization of septa and linear calcifications; their typical finding is the low attenuation content. Unfortunately, CT frequently fails to demonstrate internal architecture, and, occasionally, high-density material or hemorrhagic material within the cyst can make difficult a distinction from malignant tumors with cystic degeneration (Maher and Shepard, 2005).

Correlation with Histology

Several attempts have been made to correlate CT findings with various subtypes of thymic epithelial neoplasms on the basis of the 1999 World Health Organization classification (see Pathology and Classification earlier in this chapter). A retrospective study involving 53 patients who had undergone thymectomy for thymic epithelial tumors indicates that smooth contours and a round shape on CT are most suggestive of type A thymomas, whereas irregular contours are most suggestive of thymic carcinomas. In this study calcification is suggestive of type B thymomas. CT demonstrates, however, limited value in differentiating types A, B1, B2, and B3 tumors (Tomiyama *et al.*, 2002). Another retrospective study analyzed CT features of thymic epithelial tumors in 91 patients who had undergone surgery and tried to correlate these findings with the histopathologic subtypes and prognosis (Jeong *et al.*, 2004). In this study, lobulated contour was more often seen in high-risk thymomas (types B2 and B3) and thymic carcinomas (type C) than in low-risk thymomas (type A, AB, and B1 tumors). Mediastinal fat invasion was more often seen in thymic carcinomas than in low-risk thymomas, and great vessel invasion was seen only in thymic carcinomas. Tumors with a lobulated or an irregular contour, an oval shape, mediastinal fat, or great vessel invasion and pleural seeding showed significantly more frequent recurrence and metastasis. Although CT is of limited value in differentiating histological subtypes according to the WHO classification, CT findings may serve as predictors of postoperative recurrence or metastasis for the thymic epithelial tumors.

Recurrence of Disease and Response Evaluation

Computed tomography plays the major role in monitoring thymoma response during chemotherapy and/or radiotherapy treatment. In this type of neoplasia, as in other solid tumors, evaluation of therapy efficacy is normally made using Response Evaluation Criteria in Solid Tumors (RECIST) or World Health Organization (WHO) criteria (Therasse *et al.*, 2000). Moreover, CT is of great value in the detection of recurrent or metastatic disease after the treatment conclusion,

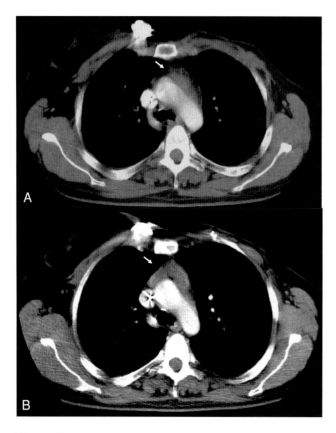

Figure 3 Thymic rebound in breast cancer, CT findings. (**A**) 33-year-old woman with thymic involution (arrow) following chemotherapy for breast cancer. (**B**) Follow-up CT obtained 6 months later shows enlargement of both lobes of the thymus (arrow).

during the follow-up. Computed tomography monitoring is particularly important because of the thymoma patients' apparent propensity to develop second primary cancer as well as the tendency for thymoma to recur after more than 5 years following treatment (Wright and Kessler, 2005).

Therapy

Thymomas are slow-growing neoplasms that should be considered potentially malignant. Surgery, radiation, and chemotherapy all may play a role in their management.

Surgery

Complete surgical resection is the mainstay of therapy for thymomas and is the most important predictor of long-term survival. Although median sternotomy is most commonly used, bilateral anterolateral thoracotomies with transverse sternotomy is preferred with advanced or laterally displaced tumors. Video-assisted thoracoscopy also has been reported, but long-term results remain unproven (Wright and Kessler, 2005).

During surgery, the surgeon should make a careful assessment of areas of possible invasion and adherence. The operation should be conducted with the goal of achieving a complete resection with *en bloc* removal of all surrounding structures that are readily removable. Certainly, surrounding mediastinal fat and pleura can be removed with no ill effects, which enhances the chance of achieving negative microscopic margins. Capsular invasion can be subtle and not detectable by the surgeon; hence, the tumor should not be shelled out but should be removed with surrounding tissue intact. Complete surgical resection is associated with an 82% overall 7-year survival rate, whereas survival with incomplete resection is 71% and with biopsy it is only 26% (Maggi *et al.*, 1991).

The role of debulking or subtotal resection in stages III and IV disease remains controversial. Several studies have documented 5-year survival rates from 60 to 75% after subtotal resection and 24 to 40% after biopsy alone (Kohman, 1997). More recent studies, however, suggest no survival advantage to debulking followed by radiation when compared to radiation alone (Ciernik *et al.*, 1994).

Since thymomas are notably indolent tumors, isolated recurrences can be surgically resected. However, the use of surgery in recurrent disease remains to be clearly defined, even though there is evidence that histology can change from primary tumor to recurrence in the direction of increased malignancy (Ciccone and Rendina, 2005).

Radiotherapy

Thymomas are radiosensitive tumors, and, consequently, radiation has been used to treat all tumor stages as well as recurrent disease (Eng and Thomas, 2005). In stage I thymomas, adjuvant radiotherapy has been administered but has not improved on the excellent results with surgery alone because recurrence is very low. In stages II and III, invasive disease adjuvant radiation can decrease recurrence rates after complete surgical resection from 28 to 5% (Koh *et al.*, 1995). Although there is general consensus regarding the use of adjuvant radiotherapy in fully resected stage III disease, its role in invasive stage II thymoma is widely debated. Despite the varying opinions expressed by different investigators, further validations of several clinical factors (cortical subtypes, fibrous adhesions, and microscopic invasions to the mediastinal pleura or pericardium) are necessary (Mangi *et al.*, 2002). Postoperative radiotherapy should be considered in all patients with completely resected stage II patients when tumor extension beyond the capsule is documented pathologically (Koh *et al.*, 1995; Thomas *et al.*, 1999).

Radiation therapy has proved beneficial in the treatment of extensive disease. Radiotherapy after incomplete surgical resection produces local control rates of 35 to 74% and 5-year survival rates ranging from 50 to 70% for stage III and 20 to 50% for stage IVa tumors (Eng and Thomas, 2005). In addition, Ciernik and collaborators have reported similar survival rates (87% 5-year and 70% 7-year) in patients treated with radiation alone compared with partial surgical resection and adjuvant radiation in small numbers of stage III and IV patients and patients with intrathoracic recurrences (Ciernik *et al.*, 1994).

Medical Treatment

Chemotherapy has been used with increasing frequency in the treatment of invasive thymomas. Single-agent and combination therapy have both demonstrated activity, and doxorubicin, cisplatin, and ifosfamide are the most active single agents (Evans and Lynch, 2005). Combination chemotherapy regimens have shown higher response rates than single agents and, in a retrospective analysis, improved overall survival (Loehrer *et al.*, 2004a). The combination regimens have been used in adjuvant and neoadjuvant settings and particularly in the treatment of advanced or recurrent disease. Cisplatin-containing regimens appear to be the most active. The best results in reasonably large Phase II studies have been obtained with the ADOC (cisplatin, doxorubicin, vincristine, and cyclophosphamide) regimen (Fornasiero *et al.*, 1991) and with the PAC (cisplatin, doxorubicin, and cyclophosphamide) regimen (Loehrer *et al.*, 1994). More recently, the European Organization for Research and Treatment of Cancer noted 31% complete and 56% overall response rates, with a median survival of 4.3 years in a small study of 16 patients with advanced thymoma treated with cisplatin and etoposide (Giaccone *et al.*, 1996).

Patients with progressive disease following first-line chemotherapy may respond to retreatment with the same chemotherapy regimen, particularly if the disease-free interval was more than 12 months (Lara *et al.*, 1996). Salvage strategies, including high-dose chemotherapy regimens with stem-cell support, corticosteroids, and somatostatin, have also been attempted (Evans and Lynch, 2005). Varying regimens of corticosteroids have shown effectiveness in the treatment of all histologic subtypes of thymoma (with and without myasthenia) (Kirkove *et al.*, 1992; Termeer *et al.*, 2001). Thymic tumors have been shown to possess receptor for somatostatin. Palmieri *et al.* (1997) reported the first case of complete response to a combination of octreotide, a synthetic somatostatin analog, and prednisone in a patient with thymoma and pure red-cell aplasia. The Eastern Cooperative Oncology Group (ECOG) reported the interesting results of Phase II trial where patients affected by advanced thymoma or thymic carcinoma were treated with octreotide, either alone or in combination with prednisone (Loherer *et al.*, 2004b). We have recently observed a dramatic complete remission by adding prednisone to octreotide in an octreotide-refractory epithelial thymoma (Tiseo *et al.*, 2005).

Combined Modality Approaches

If chemotherapy can lead to responses in the advanced disease, it is therefore possible that it may improve long-term disease-free survival for patients who are surgical candidates and, moreover, may also convert patients with unresectable thymoma into patients with operable disease. While randomized controlled trials are lacking because of the rarity of disease, there is evidence supporting the ability of chemotherapy to accomplish both of these goals (Evans and Lynch, 2005). Three prospective evaluations of neoadjuvant chemotherapy have demonstrated that this approach appears promising since the complete resection and long-term survival rates were obtained. This approach was studied with cisplatin, epirubicin, and etoposide (Macchiarini *et al.*, 1991), with ADOC regimen (Rea *et al.*, 1993) and with cisplatin, doxorubicin, cyclophosphamide, and prednisone (Shin *et al.*, 1998; Kim *et al.*, 2004), respectively. How can we be certain that this approach improves outcomes without a control group? Given the difficulty of performing randomized trials, an Italian series in which the prospective results of multimodality approach were compared with their own historical control may answer this question (Venuta *et al.*, 2003). Sixty-five patients were enrolled in the prospective phase of the study after 1989 and compared with 83 patients treated between 1965 and 1988 with surgery alone. Complete resection rates and, in particular, overall survival were significantly improved in the multimodality group.

A multi-institutional prospective trial in 23 patients with stages III–IV unresectable thymic tumors treated with two to four cycles of PAC regimen and sequential radiation therapy demonstrated results similar to those obtained with neoadjuvant chemotherapy followed by surgical resection and radiation (Loehrer *et al.*, 1997). Therefore, for the chemoradiation

definitive approach, further confirmations are needed, as for the chemoradiation induction strategy, the experience is at the anecdotal level (Evans and Lynch, 2005).

Conclusions

Thymomas are the most common primary mediastinal tumors; in most cases of thymoma, the initial diagnosis of mediastinal mass is made by CT. This method can aid in characterization of these neoplasms and plays an important role in the management of patients with thymoma. Computed tomography can provide important information on differential diagnosis and on the precise anatomic location of the lesion and its relationship to surrounding structures. Lastly, it can be used to monitor tumor behavior during chemo- and/or radiation therapy and to detect recurrent or metastatic neoplasm after the treatment has been completed. For the majority of patients, surgical resection remains the standard of choice. Adjuvant radiotherapy seems to improve local control and survival. In more advanced disease, systemic therapy has been demonstrated to produce a 50 to 80% objective response rate. These observations have led to the development of multimodality strategy for the management of patients with thymoma.

References

Bernatz, P., Harrison, E., and Glagett, O. 1961. Thymoma. A clinico-pathological study. *J. Thorac. Cardiovasc. Surg. 42*:424–444.

Blumberg, D., Port, J.L., Weksler, B., Delgado, R., Rosai, J., Bains, M.S., Ginsberg, R.J., Martini, N., McCormack, P.M., and Rusch, V. 1995. Thymoma: a multivariate analysis of factor predicting survival. *Ann. Thoracic. Surg. 60*:908–913.

Bogot, N.R., and Quint, L.E. 2005. Imaging of thymic disorders. *Cancer Imag. 5*:130–149.

Bokemeyer, C., Nichols, C.R., Droz, J.P., Schmoll, H.J., Horwich, A., Gerl, A., Fossa, S.D., Beyer, J., Pont, J., Kanz, L., Einhorn, L., and Hartmann, J.T. 2002. Extragonadal germ cell tumors of the mediastinum and retroperitoneum: results from an international analysis. *J. Clin. Oncol. 20*:1864–1873.

Ciccone, A.M., and Rendina, E.A. 2005. Treatment of recurrent thymic tumors. *Semin. Thorac. Cardiovasc. Surg. 17*:27–31.

Ciernik, I.F., Meier, U., and Lutolf, U.M. 1994. Prognostic factors and outcome of incompletely resected invasive thymoma following radiation therapy. *J. Clin. Oncol. 12*:1484–1490.

Clark, P.B., Perrier, N.D., and Morton, K.A. 2005. Detection of an intrathymic parathyroid adenoma using single-photon emission CT 99mTc sestamibi scintigraphy and CT. *Am. J. Roentgenol. 184*:S16–18.

Detterbeck, F.C., and Parsons, A.M. 2004. Thymic tumors. *Ann. Thorac. Surg. 77*:1860–1869.

Drachman, D.B. 1994. Myasthenia gravis. *N. Engl. J. Med. 330*:1797–1810.

Duwe, D.V., Sterman, D.H., and Musani, A.I. 2005. Tumors of the mediastinum. *Chest 128*:2893–2909.

Eng, T.Y., and Thomas, C.R., Jr. 2005. Radiation therapy in the management of thymic tumors. *Semin. Thorac. Cardiovasc. Surg. 17*:32–40.

Engels, E.A., and Pfeiffer, R.M. 2003. Malignant thymoma in the United States: demographic patterns in incidence and associations with subsequent malignancies. *Int. J. Cancer 105*:546–551.

Evans, T.L., and Lynch, T.J. 2005. Role of chemotherapy in the management of advanced thymic tumors. *Semin. Thorac. Cardiovasc. Surg. 17*:41–50.

Fornasiero, A., Danilele, O., Ghiotto, C., Piazza, M., Fiore-Donati, L., Calabro, F., Rea, F., and Fiorentino, M.V. 1991. Chemotherapy for invasive thymoma: a 13 year experience. *Cancer 68*:30–33.

Giaccone, G., Ardizzoni, A., Kirkpatrick, A., Clerico, M., Sahmoud, T., and van Zandwijk, N. 1996. Cisplatin and etoposide combination chemotherapy for locally advanced or metastatic thymoma: a Phase II study of the European organization for research and treatment of lung cancer cooperative group. *J. Clin. Oncol. 14*:814–820.

Hasserjian, R.P., Ströbel, P., and Marx, A. 2005. Pathology of thymic tumors. *Semin. Thorac. Cardiovasc. Surg. 17*:2–11.

Hung, H.C., Lee, T., and Lee, S.K. 1999. Differential diagnosis of invasive thymoma and thymic carcinoma by CT findings. *Chin. J. Radiol. 24*:179–184.

Jeong, Y.J., Lee, K.S., Kim, J., Shim, Y.M., Han, J., and Kwon, O.J. 2004. Does CT of thymic epithelial tumors enable us to differentiate histologic subtypes and predict prognosis? *Am. J. Roentgenol. 183*:283–289.

Jung, K.J., Lee, K.S., Han, J., Kim, J., Kim, T.S., Kim, T.S., and Kim, E.A. 2001. Malignant thymic epithelial: CT-pathologic correlation. *Am. J. Roentgenol. 176*:433–439.

Kim, E.S., Putnam, J.B., Komaki, R., Walsh, G.L., Ro, J.Y., Shin, H.J., Truong, M., Moon, H., Swisher, S.G., Fossella, F.V., Khuri, F.R., Hong, W.K., and Shin, D.M. 2004. Phase II study of a multidisciplinary approach with induction chemotherapy, followed by surgical resection, radiation therapy and consolidation chemotherapy for unresectable malignant thymoma. *Lung Cancer 44*:369–379.

Kirkove, C., Berghmans, J., Noel, H., and Van de Merckt, J. 1992. Dramatic response of recurrent invasive thymoma to high doses of corticosteroids. *Clin. Oncol. 4*:64–66.

Koh, W.J., Loehrer, P.J., Sr., and Thomas, C.R., Jr. 1995. Thymoma: the role of radiation and chemotherapy. In: Wood, D.E., and Thomas, C.R., Jr. (Eds), *Mediastinal Tumors: Update 1995. Medical Radiology-Diagnostic Imaging and Radiation Oncology Volume*. Heidelberg, Germany: Springer-Verlag, pp. 19–25.

Kohman, L.J. 1997. Controversies in the management of malignant thymoma. *Chest 122*:S296–300.

Lara, P.N., Jr., Bonomi, P.D., and Faber, L.P. 1996. Retreatment of recurrent invasive thymoma with platinum, doxorubicin, and cyclophosphamide. *Chest 110*:1115–1117.

Levine, G.D., and Rosai, J. 1978. Thymic hyperplasia and neoplasia: a review of current concepts. *Hum. Pathol. 9*:495–515.

Loehrer, P.J., Sr., Kim, K.M., Aisner, S.C., Livingston, R., Einhorn, L.H., Johnson, D., and Blum, R. 1994. Cisplatin plus doxorubicin plus cyclophosphamide in metastatic or recurrent thymoma: final results of an intergroup trial. *J. Clin. Oncol. 12*:1164–1168.

Loehrer, P.J., Sr., Chen, M., Kim, K.M., Aisner, S.C., Einhorn, L.H., Livingston, R., and Johnson, D. 1997. Cisplatin, doxorubicin, and cyclophosphamide plus thoracic radiation therapy for limited-stage unresectable thymoma: an intergroup trial. *J. Clin. Oncol. 15*:3093–3099.

Loehrer, P.J., Sr., Wang, W., Aisner, S., Bonomi, P., Einhorn, L.H., Langer, C.J., Green, M.R., Livingston, R.B., Johnson, D.H., and Schiller, J. 2004a. Long-term follow-up of patients with locally advanced or metastatic thymic malignancies: the Eastern Cooperative Oncology Group (ECOG) experience. *J. Clin. Oncol. 23*:626 (Abstract 7050).

Loehrer, P.J., Sr., Wang, W., Johnson, D.H., and Ettinger, D.S. 2004b. Octreotide alone or with prednisone in patients with advanced thymoma and thymic carcinoma: an Eastern Cooperative Oncology Group Phase II trial. *J. Clin. Oncol. 22*:293–299.

Macchiarini, P., Chella, A., Ducci, F., Rossi, B., Testi, C., Bevilacqua, G., and Angeletti, C.A. 1991. Neoadjuvant chemotherapy, surgery and postoperative radiation therapy for invasive thymoma. *Cancer 68*:706–713.

Maggi, G., Casadio, C., Cavallo, A., Cianci, R., Molinatti, M., and Ruffini, E. 1991. Thymoma: results of 241 operated cases. *Ann. Thorac. Surg. 51*:152–156.

Maher, M.M., and Shepard, J.A. 2005. Imaging of thymoma. *Semin. Thorac. Cardiovasc. Surg. 17*:12–19.

Mangi, A.A., Wright, C.D., Allan, J.S., Wain, J.C., Donahue, D.M., Grillo, H.C., and Mathisen, D.J. 2002. Adjuvant radiation therapy for stage II thymoma. *Ann. Thorac. Surg. 74*:1033–1037.

Marino, M., and Muller-Hermelink, H.K. 1985. Thymoma and thymic carcinoma: relation of thymoma epithelial cells to the cortical and medullary differentiation of thymus. *Virchows Arch. A. Pathol. Anat. Histopathol. 407*:119–149.

Masaoka, A., Monden, Y., Nakahara, K., and Tanioka, T. 1981. Follow-up study of thymomas with special reference to their clinical stages. *Cancer 48*:2485–2492.

Morrissey, B., Adams, H., Gibbs, A.R., and Crane, M.D. 1993. Percutaneous needle biopsy of the mediastinum: review of 94 procedures. *Thorax 48*:623–637.

Naidich, D.P., Muller, N.L., Zerhouni, E.A., Webb, W.R., Krinsky, G.A., and Siegelman, S.S. 1999. In: *Computed Tomography and Magnetic Resonance of the Thorax*. Philadelphia, PA: Lippincot-Raven, pp. 70–76.

Okumura, M., Ohta, M., Tateyama, H., Nakagawa, K., Matsumura, A., Maeda, H., Tada, H., Eimoto, T., Matsuda, H., and Masaoka, A. 2002. The World Health Organization histologic classification system reflects the oncologic behavior of thymoma: a clinical study of 273 patients. *Cancer 94*:624–632.

Palmieri, G., Lastoria, S., Colao, A., Vergara, E., Varrella, P., Biondi, E., Selleri, C., Catalano, L., Lombardi, G., Bianco, A.R., and Salvatore, M. 1997. Successful treatment of a patient with a thymoma and pure red-cell aplasia with octreotide and prednisone. *N. Engl. J. Med. 336*:263–265.

Rea, F., Sartori, F., Loy, M., Calabro, F., Fornasiero, A., Daniele, O., and Altavilla, G. 1993. Chemotherapy and operation for invasive thymoma. *J. Cardiovasc. Surg. 106*:543–549.

Rosai, J., and Sobin, L.H.. 1999. Histological typing of tumours of the thymus. In Anonymous, *World Health Organisation, International Histological Classification of Tumours*. Heidelberg, Germany: Springer-Verlag, pp. 1–16.

Shin, D.M., Walsh, G.L., Komaki, R., Putnam, J.B., Nesbitt, J., Ro, J.Y., Shin, H.J., Ki, K.H., Wimberly, A., Pisters, K.M., Schrump, D., Gregurich, M.A., Cox, J.D., Roth, J.A., and Hong, W.K. 1998. A multidisciplinary approach to therapy for unresectable malignant thymoma. *Ann. Intern. Med. 129*:100–104.

Strobel, P., Bauer, A., Puppe, B., Kraushaar, T., Krein, A., Tokya, K., Gold, R., Semik, M., Kiefer, R., Nix, W., Scalke, B., Muller-Hermelink, H.K., and Marx, A. 2004. Tumor recurrence and survival in patients treated for thymomas and thymic squamous cell carcinomas: a retrospective analysis. *J. Clin. Oncol. 22*:1501–1509.

Strollo, D.C., and Rosado-de-Christenson, M.L. 2002. Primary mediastinal malignant germ cell neoplasms: imaging features. *Chest Surg. Clin. N. Am. 12*:645–658.

Termeer, A., Visser, F.J., and Mravunac, M. 2001. Regression of invasive thymoma following corticosteroid therapy. *Netherlands J. Med. 58*:181–184.

Therasse, P., Arbuck, S.G., Eisenhauer, E.A., Wanders, J., Kaplan, R.S., Rubinstein, L., Verweij, J., Van Glabbeke, M., van Oosterom, A.M., Christian, M.C., and Gwyther, S.G. 2000. New guidelines to evaluate the response to treatment in solid tumors. *J. Natl. Cancer Inst. 92*:205–216.

Thomas, C.R., Jr., Wright, C.D., and Loehrer, P.J., Sr. 1999. Thymoma: state of the art. *J. Clin. Oncol. 17*:2280–2289.

Tiseo, M., Monetti, F., Ferrarini, M., Serrano, J., Chiaramondia, M., and Ardizzoni, A. 2005. Complete remission to corticosteroids in an octreotide-refractory thymoma. *J. Clin. Oncol. 23*:1578–1579.

Tomiyama, N., Johkoh, T., Mihara, N., Honda, O., Kozuka, T., Koyama, M., Hamada, S., Okumura, M., Ohta, M., Eimoto, T., Miyagawa, M., Muller, N.L., Ikezoe, J., and Nakamura, H. 2002. Using the World Health Organization Classification of thymic epithelial neoplasms to describe CT findings. *Am. J. Roentgenol. 179*:881–886.

Venuta, F., Rendina, E.A., Pescarmona, E.O., De Giacomo, T., Vegna, M.L., Fazi, P., Flaishman, I., Guarino, E., and Ricci, C. 1997. Multimodality treatment of thymoma: a prospective study. *Ann. Thorac. Surg. 64*:1585–1591.

Venuta, F., Rendina, E.A., Longo, F., De Giacomo, T., Anile, M., Mercadante, E., Ventura, L., Osti, M.F., Francioni, F., and Coloni, G.F. 2003. Long-term outcome after multimodality treatment for stage III thymic tumors: a prospective study. *Ann. Thorac. Surg.* 76:1866–1872.

Wright, C.D., and Kessler, K.A. 2005. Surgical treatment of thymic tumors. *Semin. Thorac. Cardiovasc. Surg. 17*:20–26.

Yamakawa, Y., Masaoka, A., Hashimoto, T., Niwa, H., Mizuno, T., Fujii, Y., and Nakahara, K. 1991. A tentative tumor-node-metastasis classification of thymoma. *Cancer 68*:1984–1987.

53

Hemolymphangiomatosis of the Spleen: Conventional Diagnostic Imaging and Magnetic Resonance Imaging with Superparamagnetic Contrast Agent

Stefano Colagrande, Lucia Santoro, Simonetta Di Lollo, and Natale Villari

Introduction

Hemolymphangioma is a tumor composed of lymphatic and hematic cells. Several different localizations are described in the literature: orbit, tongue, esophagus, neck, heart, liver, pancreas, adrenal glands, uterine cervix, and lower extremity. Nevertheless, splenic localization is rare, and its imaging was illustrated many years ago. The splenic diffuse form, hemolymphangiomatosis, results even more rarely and to our best knowledge has been described only once (Santoro et al., 2005). Its etiopathogenesis is unclear, and perhaps this pathology may be a hamartoma. In fact, some authors considered this tumor a congenital malformation of the vascular system. In literature it was described as a case of hemolymphangioma of the pancreas and its development was explained by obstruction of the veno-lymphatic communication between dysembrioplastic vascular tissue and systemic circulation (Balderramo et al., 2003), although the splenic lymphatic system is really different from the pancreatic system.

Signs and symptoms of this tumor are poor; physical examination reveals splenomegaly; laboratory-hematic analysis shows mild thrombocytopenia without antiplatelet antibodies. The other peripheral blood tests are negative. Bone marrow biopsy/aspiration indicates normal hemopoiesis. We propose the finding of this splenic pathology also at magnetic resonance imaging after administration of a super-paramagnetic contrast agent. This contrast agent, adopted in study of the liver, is rarely used in splenic pathology (Wang et al., 2001). For our study, we have administered Resovist (SHU-555A, Schering, Berlin, Germany), a T2 dual-purpose contrast agent composed of superparamagnetic iron-oxide particles. After intravenous administration and consequent vascular phase, it is taken up exclusively by phagocytosis and deposited in the cells of the reticulo-endothelial system of the liver and spleen. Superparamagnetic iron-oxide particles have a strong effect on the shortening of both T1 and T2 relaxation times. In tissue, iron particles of this contrast agent determine local magnetic field inhomogeneities.

Diffusion of water molecules through these local field disturbances produces rapid proton dephasing, which results in preferential shortening of transverse relaxation time, T2, with less shortening effect on longitudinal relaxation time, T1. This T1 effect is more relevant when superparamagnetic iron-oxide particles are hydrated; therefore, they have also been used for T1-weighted imaging with vascular opacification. Its specific pharmacokinetic properties allow dynamic T1-weighted MR imaging after bolus infusion of SHU 555A, which gives signal changes (intravascular enhancement and then high signal intensity blood at T1-weighted images) quite similar but generally inferior to those determined by gadolinium chelates (Wang et al., 2001). Iron-oxide particles are used in particular as negative enhancers, because they have a large R_2/R_1 ratio, which means that the effect of T_2 shortening is greater than that of T_1 shortening (Chen et al., 1999). In fact, the more relevant superparamagnetic iron-oxide particles effect is represented by signal intensity loss in T2-weighted images of normal liver/splenic parenchyma and in benign masses, which have a well-represented reticulo-endothelial system. Conversely, malignant lesions have no phagocytic capabilities (due to the relative/absolute lack of a reticulo-endothelial system), and then they do not change their signal intensity in T2-weighted images, increasing conspicuity comparatively with surrounding normal liver/splenic parenchyma. As a consequence, superparamagnetic contrast agents are prevalently used to improve the detection rate for focal liver lesions. Moreover, because the signal decrease of benign lesions is proportional to the reticulo-endothelial system activity or tumor vascularity, some authors have utilized superparamagnetic iron-oxide particles for the purpose of improving focal liver lesions' characterization (Grazioli et al., 2003).

Pathology

Macroscopically, the spleen shows both bipolar diameter and weight increment, and the surface is even. The architecture is altered because of the presence of multiple cavities or lacunae in a limited residual normal parenchyma, conferring a "spongy" appearance to the spleen. Two types of lacunae can be found: some of these are in direct communication with vascular spaces and contain blood and/or clots; others are full of pink proteinaceous material with foamy macrophages, rare red blood cells, and crystals of cholesterol, and do not result directly linked to vessels. Microscopically, lacunae walls of both hematic and lymphatic spaces are lined by flat, and sometimes cuboid, endothelial cells, with rare papillary projections into the cystic lumen (Fig. 1).

Presently, two different types of endothelium cells that line hematic and lymphatic lacunae can be differentiated by immunohistochemical study. Hematic lacunae endothelium is anti-CD34 monoclonal antibody positive and anti-D2-40

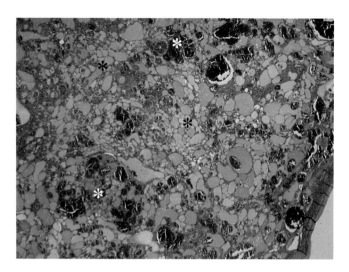

Figure 1 Hemolymphangiomatosis of the spleen. Photomicrograph (hematoxylin-eosin stain—10×) shows blood hematic (white asterisks) and serous liquid (black asterisks) interstitial lacunae.

monoclonal antibody negative. On the other hand, lymphatic lacunae endothelium are anti-CD34 monoclonal antibody negative and anti-D2-40 monoclonal antibody positive.

Imaging

Ultrasonography (US) was achieved by an Astro MP (Esa Ote-Ansaldo, Genoa, Italy) with a 3.5-MHz convex probe. Spiral computed tomography (CT) examination was performed using a Somatom Plus (Siemens, Erlangen, Germany) single-row scanner. After a direct scan and intravenous administration of 100 ml of iodinated contrast agent (Ultravist 370, Schering, Berlin, Germany), at a rate of 3 ml/s, four acquisitions were obtained (8-mm thickness; pitch = 1): hepatic arterial phase (30 s), portal venous phase (70 s), equilibrium phase (180 s), and very late phase (1 hr).

Magnetic resonance (MR) imaging examination was obtained by 1.5-T unit (Gyroscan ACS NT, Philips, Eindhoven, The Netherlands) with a body phased-array coil. Direct axial breath hold, fast field echo, T1-weighted (repetition time = 110 milliseconds, echo time = 1.8 milliseconds, flip angle = 80°, 7-mm slice thickness) and respiratory-gated free breath, turbo spin-echo, single-shot, T2-weighted (repetition time = 810–870 milliseconds, echo time = 80–210 milliseconds, turbo factor = 91–97, 4-mm slice thickness) sequences were performed; T2 sequences were also acquired with fat suppression. T1-weighted sequences were repeated 25, 70, and 180 seconds after administration of 1.4 ml of Resovist (SHU-555 A, Schering, Berlin, Germany), followed by a 20-ml saline solution flush; both T1- and T2-weighted sequences were performed again after 10 and 60 minutes.

Transabdominal US reveals splenomegaly with inhomogeneous echo texture, but without clear nodular masses;

this pattern is consistent with multiple hypo-hyperechoic confluent areas. CT at direct scan shows splenomegaly with inhomogeneous density because of diffuse hypodense areas, partially confluent, without clear edge, with variable diameters (from 1 mm to 4–5 cm). After intravenous administration of iodinated contrast agent, hypodense, variable shape, and partially confluent nodules become more evident due to the enhancement of the surrounding parenchyma. At very late scan (60 min), the spleen density was almost homogeneous for slow enhancement of the masses (Fig. 2).

MR examination shows inhomogeneous hypointense parenchyma, without evidence of clear masses at direct T1-weighted images and high-signal intensity confluent masses, with distorted structure at direct T2-weighted images. After Resovist administration, dynamic phases on T1-weighted images show a pattern similar to that described at computed tomography examination. At late scan on T1-weighted images (60 min), in contrast with CT, parenchymal homogeneity is absent, and only poor enhancement of some nodules can be observed. On T2-weighted scan there is no change in signal intensity of lesions, which appear hyperintense and surrounded by a thin layer of markedly hypointense enhanced parenchyma (Fig. 3). Hemolymphangiomatosis presents some of the characteristics of angiomas, such as high signal intensity on T2-weighted images and late homogeneous enhancement at CT study, but not the marked centripetal enhancement typical of liver hemangiomas. Moreover, late-phase images showed only slight T1 enhancement, without any T2 signal loss. This late contrastographic CT/MRI pattern

is probably related to the molecular dimensions of iodinated (1.5 nm) and iron-oxide contrast agent (62 nm) and to the dissimilar kinetics of these two contrast agents. The different type of described lacunae determines the diverse enhancement as well. The hematic lacunae are directly connected with the splenic vessels, while those containing serous proteinaceous liquid are not in direct connection with the hematic stream. As a consequence, on CT by 1 hr the iodinated contrast agent could be equilibrated through the extracellular fluid compartment, including the serous liquid lakes. Conversely, the superparamagnetic contrast agent, whose uptake is exclusively by phagocytosis, is not equilibrated through the extracellular fluid compartment, does not leave the vascular spaces, and does not demonstrate any negative enhancement of such interstitial lakes on T2 images.

Differential Diagnosis and Conclusions

Hemolymphangiomatosis must be differentiated from the other primary vascular neoplasms of the spleen. The benign primary vascular tumors comprise hemangioma, lymphangioma, and hamartoma, whereas those of intermediate biologic behavior include littoral cell angioma, hemangioendothelioma, and hemangiopericytomas (Abbott *et al.*, 2004). The primary malignant vascular neoplasm of the spleen is angiosarcoma, but the more common neoplastic disorder of the spleen is lymphoma. It is important to emphasize that the following pathologies are described on CT/MR imaging

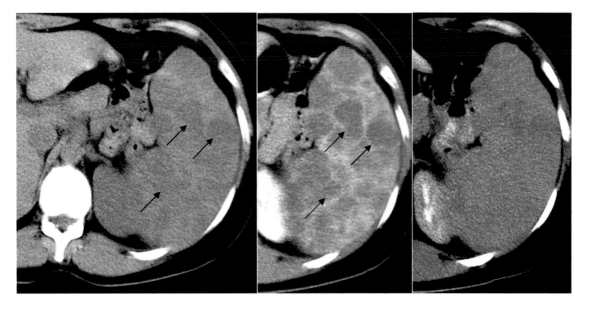

Figure 2 Hemolymphangiomatosis of the spleen. CT scans before (left) and after administration of iodinated contrast media during arterial perfusional phase (center) and very late phase (right). Direct and arterial phase scans show splenomegaly with multiple hypodense, partially confluent, and variable diameters nodules (black arrows). At very late scan, spleen parenchyma density becomes almost homogeneous due to slow enhancement of the masses.

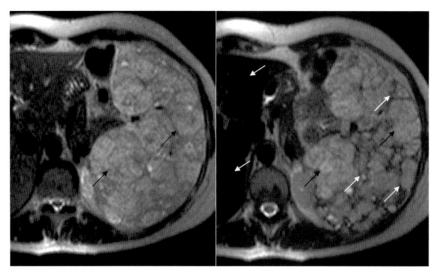

Figure 3 Hemolymphangiomatosis of the spleen. Axial MR T2-weighted scans before (left) and after administration of superparamagnetic contrast agent (right). Direct scan shows splenomegaly with high-signal intensity confluent masses (black arrows). After contrast media administration, there is no change in signal intensity of the lesions (black arrows), while liver and a thin layer of normal surrounding splenic parenchyma show signal intensity loss (white arrows).

only after using iodinated/paramagnetic contrast agents. To our knowledge, there are no data after superparamagnetic iron-oxide particle administration.

At first analysis, hemolymphangiomatosis may be considered to be the synthesis of two types of elementary lesions such as hemangioma/hemangiomatosis and lymphangioma/lymphangiomatosis. Hemangiomas consist of vascular channels of variable size, which are lined with a single layer of endothelium filled with red blood cells. In hemangiomatosis, sonography demonstrates echogenic masses with hypoanechoic vascular lacunae (cavernous forms). On CT scan, there are hypo- or isoattenuating masses, with homogeneous and marked enhancement. The enhancing peripheral nodules during the arterial phase are less evident than in liver hemangiomas, because splenic enhancement obscures them. During opacification, the mass never displays the typical marked centripetal enhancement seen in the liver, but shows discrete, mottled areas of heterogeneous density. On MRI, splenic hemangiomas, similar to liver hemangiomas, result as iso-low-T1 and high-T2 masses compared with surrounding normal parenchyma. After administration of the contrast agent, three patterns of enhancement have been described: immediate, homogeneous enhancement; early peripheral enhancement with uniform delayed enhancement; and peripheral enhancement with centripetal progression but persistent enhancement of a central fibrous scar (Abbott et al., 2004).

Lymphangiomatosis (in which multiple organs are usually involved), consists of a single layer of endothelium-lined spaces filled with eosinophilic proteinaceous material. Sonography shows well-defined hypoechoic lesions. On CT scan they appear as thin-walled low-attenuation nodules, without significant contrast enhancement. On MRI, lesions are hypointense to the surrounding parenchyma on T1-weighted images

and hyperintense on T2-weighted images, as cystic masses, without any enhancement after contrast agent administration.

It is emphasized that the lymphatic component of the lymphangiomatosis does not usually demonstrate any significant enhancement, whereas the lymphatic component of the hemolymphangiomatosis shows late enhancement with iodinated contrast agent (little molecules equilibrated through extracellular compartment). However, we must not forget that hemolymphangiomatosis data are few and that other patterns are possible.

Hamartomas are solid homogeneous masses almost exclusively of red pulp, but they can be heterogeneous, with rare cystic aspects and calcifications; they are also known as "splenoma." On sonograms they are hyperechoic relative to the normal splenic parenchyma. On CT scans, hamartomas may appear with various patterns (iso-hypoattenuating relative to the normal spleen before and after contrast agent; they can also appear as heterogeneous with contrast agent). These lesions have well-defined borders and a lack of any signs of infiltration of the surrounding parenchyma. On MR, hamartomas appear heterogeneously hyperintense on T2-weighted images and isointense to the normal spleen on T1-weighted images, with inhomogeneous diffuse enhancement after contrast agent administration. On delayed images, they show more uniform homogeneous enhancement.

Hemangioendothelioma is usually a large well-circumscribed, nonencapsulated solid splenic mass, with variable malignant potential; from a histopathological point of view, the main features are well-formed vascular channels with mild atypia and low mitotic rate of the endothelial line. On sonograms, hemangioendothelioma is a hypoechoic mass, well demarcated from the surrounding parenchyma. On CT, there is a low-attenuation mass that enhances after contrast agent, but is hypovascular relative to the surrounding parenchyma. On MR this mass may appear hypointense in T1- and T2-weighted images, due to the presence of hemosiderin (Abbott et al., 2004). At contrast-enhanced CT or MRI, the enhancement pattern may resemble that of a giant hemangioma, with nodular peripheral puddling of contrast material in the early phase, subsequent peripheral pooling, and central enhancement with variable delay. In larger tumors, to be considered with more malignant behavior, central enhancement is often lacking due to fibrosis, hemorrhage, or necrosis. These imaging features are not typical because hemangioendothelioma has an intermediate malignancy and a variable appearance.

Littoral cell angioma is a diffuse vascular neoplasm arising from littoral cells that normally line the splenic sinuses of the red pulp. These endothelial cells express both vascular and histiocytic antigens. Ultrasonography shows a diffuse heterogeneous echo texture of the spleen. On CT, there are multiple hypodense masses, which are hypoattenuated relative to the normal spleen. Such masses demonstrate, as hemangioma does, homogeneous contrast enhancement on delayed images and become isoattenuating relative to the remaining splenic parenchyma. On MRI, the presence of hemosiderin, due to the hematophagocytic capacity of the neoplastic cells, gives low signal intensity in both T1 and T2 images (Kinoshita et al., 2000).

Hemangiopericytomas is composed of spindle-shaped uniform tumor cells grouped around dilated vascular channels and have a relatively malignant potential. They appear as multiple hypoechoic nodules on sonograms. On CT, there is a large splenic mass, with polycyclic contours and smaller disseminated lesions throughout the spleen. After contrast agent administration, there is a discrete hyperattenuation of solid portions and septations. On MRI, lesions have low signal intensity at T1-weighted sequences and high signal intensity at T2-weighted pulse sequences

Angiosarcomas consist of disorganized anastomosing vascular channels lined by atypical endothelium cells that have nuclear pleomorphism and variable mitotic rate (with foci of extramedullar hematopoiesis). Angiosarcomas usually appear at US, CT, and MRI, as a large and dishomogeneous mass in enlarged spleen; there are also areas of necrosis, blood products, and extrasplenic tumor extension. In contrast to benign types, they always show heterogeneous enhancement after contrast agent administration.

Usually, malignancy and phlogosis are easily differentiable at imaging examination versus hemolymphangiomatosis due to, in both cases—with the exception of diffuse infiltration of lymphoma—there being no homogeneous enhancement during late-phase acquisition of CT. However, other possible radiologic differential diagnoses are given below.

Lymphoma, the most common splenic malignancy, has different appearances depending on the differing pathologic patterns: homogeneous enlargement without a discrete mass, solitary mass, multifocal lesions, and diffuse infiltration.

Multifocal lesions are hypodense nodules with variable enhancement on CT (Kinoshita et al., 2000).

The most common metastases that involve the spleen are from malignant melanoma and carcinoma of lung, breast, stomach, large bowel, and pancreas: they generally are hypoechoic at sonography, while the CT appearance depends on the degree of vascularization and necrosis.

Abdominal sarcoidosis is characterized by granulomatous lesions that involve lymph nodes, liver, and spleen. Sonography shows hyperechoic splenic parenchyma, with focal hypoechogenic lesions, and hypovascular at CT study. Finally, abscesses show central avascular hypodense regions with contrast-enhancing periphery at CT; infrequently, septations and/or gas can be demonstrated, at sonography, a homogeneously hypoechoic or bull's eye appearance can be found.

In conclusion, splenic hemolymphangiomatosis is a very rare pathology whose sonography, basal MRI, and late CT contrastographic features may resemble those of other diffuse benign vascular neoplasms described previously. On the other hand, it is not possible to demonstrate a real hemangioma-like enhancement during the vascular phase. Moreover, its late contrastographic pattern can be considered at least very indicative if CT and iron-oxide–enhanced MRI are applied as complementary diagnostic tools.

On the basis of this experience, the study of splenic parenchyma with superparamagnetic contrast agent could be interesting not only in detection but also in characterization of splenic focal lesions. Rationale is represented by the selective and active uptake by phagocytosis, without passive osmotic equilibrium through the extracellular fluid compartment, as interstitial contrast agents do, because of their small molecular dimensions. As a consequence, we can expect enhancement (relative signal improvement in T1-weighted and signal loss in T2 weighted late images, respectively) of all vascular neoplasm components directly linked with vascular spaces, due to trapping of the contrast agent in the hematic lacunae. Moreover, because of the lack of a reticulo-endothelial system, we can presume no signal change in malignancy, in particular no signal loss in T2-weighted late images, with important signal decrement of healthy surrounding parenchyma. Hereafter, if a greater series of cases confirm our suppositions, MRI with superparamagnetic contrast agent administration might become a diagnostic tool, complementary, for example, to PET in the diagnostic assessment of leukemia and lymphomas.

References

Abbott, R.M., Levy, A.D., Aguilera, N.S., Gorospe, L., and Thompson, W.M. 2004. From the archives of the AFIP: primary vascular neoplasms of the spleen: radiologic-pathologic correlation. *Radiographics 24*:1137–1163.

Balderramo, D.C., Di Tada, C., de Ditter, A.B., and Mondino, J.C. 2003. Hemolymphangioma of the pancreas: case report and review of the literature. *Pancreas 27*:197–199.

Chen, F., Ward, J., and Robinson, P.J. 1999. MR imaging of the liver and spleen: a comparison of the effects on signal intensity of two superparamagnetic iron oxide agents. *Magn. Reson. Imaging 17*:549–556.

Grazioli, L., Morana, G., Kirchin, M.A., Caccia, P., Romanini, L., Bondioni, M.P., Procacci, C., and Chiesa, A. 2003. MRI of focal nodular hyperplasia (FNH) with gadobenate dimeglumine (Gd-BOPTA) and SPIO (ferumoxides): an intra-individual comparison. *J. Magn. Reson. Imaging 17*:593–602.

Kinoshita, L.L., Yee, J., and Nash, S.R. 2000. Littoral cell angioma of the spleen: imaging features. *Am. J. Roentgenol. 174*:467–469.

Santoro, L., Santini, V., Di Lollo, S., Valeri, A., and Colagrande, S. 2005. Hemolymphangiomatosis of the spleen: imaging features. *J. Comput. Assist. Tomogr. 29*:831–833.

Wang, Y.X., Hussain, S.M., and Krestin, G.P. 2001. Superparamagnetic iron oxide contrast agents: physicochemical characteristics and applications in MR imaging. *Eur. Radiol. 11*:2319–2331.

54

Thyroid Cancer: ^{18}F-FDG-Positron Emission Tomography

Lioe-Fee de Geus-Oei, Martin Gotthardt, and Wim J.G. Oyen

Introduction

Primary treatment of differentiated thyroid carcinoma consists of total thyroidectomy followed by ablation of thyroid tissue remnants and possible metastases by means of radioactive iodine (iodine-131). After complete destruction of remnants, metastases of recurrence can be detected by measurement of the serum thyroglobulin level as well as by radionuclide imaging. The present chapter discusses the relevance of the application of ^{18}F-fluorodeoxyglucose (FDG) Positron Emission Tomography (PET) in the assessment of thyroid nodules and the relevance of the so-called thyroid PET incidentaloma. Information is provided on the current and future clinical use of FDG-PET for each type of thyroid cancer; differentiated thyroid carcinoma, Hürthle cell carcinoma, anaplastic thyroid carcinoma and medullary thyroid carcinoma. FDG-PET is diagnostic tool that recently became widely available. FDG is an analogue of glucose, reflecting cellular metabolic activity. The uptake of FDG in cells is related to the expression of the GLUTI transporter and hexokinase-I activity, both of which are upregulated.

Assessment of Thyroid Nodules

Solitary thyroid nodules are quite common, with a prevalence of 4 to 7% in the adult population of the United States.

Differentiated thyroid cancer, on the other hand, is uncommon, with an incidence of only 40 cases per million per year. Therefore, it is a major diagnostic challenge to select for surgery only those patients whose nodules are most likely malignant. The clinical findings that should raise the suspicion of malignancy include rapid growth, firm or hard nodules, regional lymphadenopathy, local invasion in the neck, and a family history of medullary thyroid carcinoma or multiple endocrine neoplasia or the combination of a thyroid nodule with paralysis of one or both vocal cords. Radionuclide scanning, using ^{123}I, ^{131}I, or ^{99m}Tc-pertechnetate is not routinely recommended, since thyroid scintigraphy does not significantly decrease the number of suspicious nodules (Hegedus, 2004), and most patients would also undergo a fine needle aspiration biopsy (FNAB) in such a diagnostic algorithm. Characteristics revealed by ultrasonography, such as hypoechogenicity, microcalcifications, irregular margins, increased nodular flow visualized by Doppler, and especially the evidence of invasion or regional lymphadenopathy, are associated with an increased risk of cancer. However, these features do not help to reliably distinguish between benign and malignant lesions (Rago *et al.*, 1998).

FNAB, preferably guided by ultrasonography, is the key investigation and initial diagnostic test in the evaluation of thyroid nodules. FNAB is safe, can be easily performed, without major complications, is cost-effective, and has a very high negative-predictive value of 98% (Kuma *et al.*, 1994). So, patients with nonmalignant cytology can be followed safely by sonography, as long as the size of the thyroid nodule remains constant. However, the recognized limitation of FNAB is that it shows inconclusive aspirates in up to 20% of cases. In patients with cytological findings suspicious for a follicular neoplasm, a Hürthle cell (oncocytic) neoplasm, or in the case of an atypical papillary cytology or a repeatedly insufficient sample ("nondiagnostic"), a hemithyroidectomy is necessary to allow a reliable histological diagnosis. Although routine FNAB clearly increases the relative number of cancers at operation, still 80 to 85% of hemithyroidectomized patients eventually turn out to have benign thyroid disease.

FDG-PET could be helpful in this situation. Several studies showed that FDG-PET provides a high negative-predictive value for thyroid malignancy, making this a potentially useful tool in the evaluation of thyroid nodules with inconclusive FNAB results (Kresnik *et al.*, 2003; de Geus-Oei *et al.*, 2006). Aspecific tumor-seeking agents, like FDG-PET, however, are not able to 100% differentiate benign from malignant thyroid nodules (Kresnik *et al.*, 2003; de Geus-Oei *et al.*, 2006). Most Hürthle cell adenomas and in some cases Hashimoto's thyroiditis, follicular adenomas, and hyperplastic nodules also accumulate FDG (Fig. 1). The use of semiquantitative data (standardized uptake values) in any individual case is not helpful in further differentiation, due to significant overlap

between benign and malignant lesions (Kresnik *et al.*, 2003; de Geus-Oei *et al.*, 2006). Nevertheless, FDG-PET has been shown to have a significant impact on patient management because it could be very helpful in the selection of patients who need surgery. The number of futile hemithyroidectomies in an algorithm that includes FDG-PET could be substantially reduced by ~ 66% (de Geus-Oei *et al.*, 2006).

Figure 2 shows a typical example of a patient with an inconclusive FNAB and FDG uptake in two nodules. In this patient histology revealed two malignancies in one lobe. Cumulative data from 8 studies showed that FDG-PET was able to detect 64 out of 65 malignancies. The only malignancy that was missed was from a study that did not use a modern dedicated PET-camera (Kresnik *et al.*, 2003; de Geus-Oei *et al.*, 2006). Another nuclear medicine technique, dual-phase ^{99m}Tc-sestamibi, did not provide such high negative-predictive value. Thirteen studies that reported on this issue included 210 thyroid carcinomas in total, of which 39 were missed with ^{99m}Tc-sestamibi scintigraphy (Demirel *et al.*, 2003; Hurtado-Lopez *et al.*, 2004). Like FDG-PET, ^{99m}Tc-sestamibi scintigraphy may also be positive in follicular adenomas, Hürthle cell adenomas, and Hashimoto's thyroiditis, and thus would not be helpful in raising the specificity. Also, other nuclear medicine methods, such as ^{99m}Tc-tetrofosmin, ^{201}Thallium, or ^{201}Thallium/^{99m}Tc-pertechnetate subtraction scan, have shown similar disappointing results.

A limitation of PET and other scintigraphic methods is the lack of anatomic information provided. More recently,

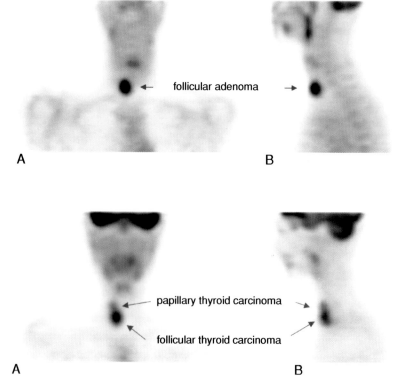

Figure 1 This 42 year-old woman had an inconclusive FNAB with many atypical Hürthle cells. FDG-PET showed intensely increased FDG uptake in the right thyroid lobe. Histology demonstrated a 2.7 cm follicular adenoma with focal Hürthle cell changes. (Reproduced with permission from de Geus-Oei LF, Pieters GF, Bonenkamp JJ, et al. *J. Nucl. Med.* 2006;47:770–775)

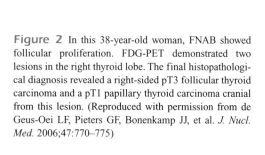

Figure 2 In this 38-year-old woman, FNAB showed follicular proliferation. FDG-PET demonstrated two lesions in the right thyroid lobe. The final histopathological diagnosis revealed a right-sided pT3 follicular thyroid carcinoma and a pT1 papillary thyroid carcinoma cranial from this lesion. (Reproduced with permission from de Geus-Oei LF, Pieters GF, Bonenkamp JJ, et al. *J. Nucl. Med.* 2006;47:770–775)

imaging with FDG-PET has been refined further with the development of combined PET and computed tomography scans (PET/CT), in which the PET images are fused with CT images. Integrated PET/CT combines the benefits of the two imaging modalities and provides the clinician with simultaneous metabolic and anatomic imaging information. It provides a detailed anatomic context for areas of increased uptake seen on PET scanning, allowing spatial localization of worrisome areas of increased metabolic activity, that can definitely be of help in the preoperative evaluation of thyroid nodules. Another concern that may arise from the limited spatial resolution of PET is that PET scanning will probably never be able to rule out microscopic disease. However, this is probably not a significant clinical problem, because it is generally supposed that thyroid carcinomas smaller than 1 cm in size are rarely of clinical significance. This is confirmed by a large autopsy series demonstrating a high prevalence of incidental and unrecognized minimal (occult) thyroid carcinomas.

Therefore, in case of an inconclusive cytology, FDG-PET seems the method of choice to decide whether surgery or a wait-and-watch strategy should be chosen. It is recommended that standardized uptake values (SUV) not be relied on in discriminating between malignant and benign thyroid lesions. Patients with a suspicious thyroid nodule with inconclusive FNAB in combination with any visible FDG-accumulation in the thyroid nodule should be taken to surgery. This advice, however, has not yet been implemented in official Nuclear Medicine Guidelines, since results from further studies with larger sample sizes are being awaited in order to determine the true efficacy and utility of FDG-PET for this indication.

Thyroid Positron Emission Tomography Incidentaloma

A thyroid PET incidentaloma, or a so-called thyroid metaboloma, is defined as a newly identified focus of increased FDG uptake in the thyroid in a patient investigated with FDG-PET for any other indication. Considering that the use of FDG-PET is rapidly increasing as an evaluating tool for various disease conditions, the incidence of thyroid FDG-PET incidentalomas is also increasing, and clinical meaning of the thyroid PET incidentaloma may become more relevant in interpreting FDG-PET scanning. Thyroid PET incidentalomas occur with a frequency of 1.2 to 4.0% in the total population that is referred for FDG-PET (Choi *et al.*, 2006). The risk of thyroid cancer in these incidentalomas of patients who underwent FDG-PET for alleged cancer or a previous history of cancer is very high, being 25–50% (Choi *et al.*, 2006). This is not surprising, because it is known that a previous history of cancer is a major risk factor for developing another cancer elsewhere in the body, especially when focal thyroid FDG uptake is found during the initial staging

of NSCLC (Yi *et al.*, 2005). In patients with NSCLC, second primaries are more frequently found than in patients with other cancer types (Even-Sapir *et al.*, 2006). Furthermore, it should be emphasized that thyroid PET incidentalomas seem to harbor a higher rate of malignancy than incidentalomas found on conventional imaging. Patients with thyroid incidentalomas detected with ultrasonography seem to belong to a totally different, less cancer-prone population. Therefore, the prevalence of thyroid ultrasound incidentalomas is much higher, ranging from 19 to 46%. The risk of cancer in these thyroid nodules, on the other hand, is very low, ranging from 1.5 to 10% (Burguera and Gharib, 2000). Furthermore, focal thyroid PET incidentalomas in particular carry a high risk of malignancy. The majority of patients with diffuse thyroid FDG uptake have chronic thyroiditis. Another important clinical issue is whether this focal uptake in the thyroid is due to a primary thyroid malignancy or to a metastasis from the underlying nonthyroidal cancer. It has been shown that metastases to the thyroid are not common, occurring in ~ 7% of all thyroid PET incidentalomas, mainly in patients with primary lung, breast, renal, gastrointestinal cancers, and melanoma (McDougall *et al.*, 2001). However, these percentages may differ owing to the varying incidence of benign and malignant thyroid diseases in different populations. Considering the high risk of malignancy, thyroid PET incidentalomas should not be overlooked and should prompt further investigation to rule out cancer, of course, only when the diagnosis of thyroid cancer would influence patient prognosis and management. From a palpable thyroid PET incidentaloma an FNAB should be obtained. Those patients with suspicious cytopathology should be referred for thyroidectomy. If no nodule is palpable, an ultrasound is advised, and when a nodule 1 cm or greater is imaged it should be sampled by ultrasound-guided FNAB.

Differentiated Thyroid Carcinoma

Differentiated thyroid carcinoma is the most common endocrine malignancy but is still rare (< 1% of all cases of cancer). In areas not associated with nuclear fallout, the annual incidence ranges between 2.0–3.8 cases/100,000 in women and 1.2–2.6/100,000 in men. Since the early 1950s, nuclear medicine has been one of the mainstays for management of differentiated thyroid carcinoma. Primary treatment of differentiated thyroid carcinoma consists of total thyroidectomy followed by ablation of thyroid tissue remnants and possible metastases by means of radioactive iodine (¹³¹I). After complete destruction of remnants, metastases or recurrence can be detected by measurement of the serum thyroglobulin level (Tg) as well as by radioiodine scintigraphy. Well-differentiated thyroid cancer is recognized as being one of the most curable of all neoplasms. After thyroidectomy and ¹³¹I ablative therapy, in the absence of widespread regional or distant disease, 10-year survival rates for papillary, follicular, and Hürthle cell carcinomas of 93, 85, and 76%, respectively, can be achieved (Hundahl *et al.*, 1998).

The degree of differentiation is associated with better patient survival. Furthermore, differentiated cancer cells not only produce Tg (a protein that can be assayed and used as a tumor marker), but also remain capable of accumulating iodine. Thus, post-total thyroidectomy remnants trap and organify iodide and perish in the process when a suitable beta emitter isotope such as ^{131}I is administered. Patients who present with ^{131}I-accumulating remnants or metastases receive ^{131}I treatment, which is curative in most cases. This iodine avidity can be used not only for treatment but also for tumor localization. Whole-body scintigraphy using ^{131}I or ^{123}I has been widely used for detection of residual disease or metastases of differentiated thyroid cancer. To minimize the impact of recurrences, early recognition and treatment are essential. Even with an estimated tendency of differentiated thyroid cancer to develop local or regional recurrences in 5–20% of cases, and distant metastases in 5–10% of cases, the combination of Tg measurement and radioiodine scintigraphy should alert the clinician with a sensitivity of 95% and specificity of close to 100%.

A considerable diagnostic dilemma occurs in ~ 15–20% of patients when dedifferentiation leads to a loss of the iodine concentrating ability of thyroid tumor cells (Baudin *et al.*, 2003). It is well known that dedifferentiation of thyroid cancer leads to the loss of the ability of thyroid cells to concentrate radioiodine, while the synthesis of Tg is maintained longer in the process of dedifferentiation (de Geus-Oei *et al.*, 2002). In these patients, detection of the (TSH-stimulated) circulating tumor marker Tg reveals that thyroid cancer tissue must be present; however, radioiodine imaging is negative. The reason for this false-negative ^{131}I whole-body scan may be insufficient TSH stimulation, iodine contamination, small tumor volume, or non-iodine-avid metastases. If the first and second reasons are excluded, and the patient truly has metastases that do not concentrate ^{131}I, even when it is given in high therapeutic doses, the patient should be scheduled for FDG-PET, which is now the method of choice to localize these iodine negative metastases. Whereas the role of FDG-PET in the preoperative assessment of thyroid nodules is not yet fully evaluated, use of this imaging modality in the follow-up of non-iodine-avid thyroid carcinoma belongs to the 1a indications for FDG-PET in oncology (Reske *et al.*, 2001).

Before the introduction of FDG-PET, localization of these iodine negative thyroid cancer recurrences/metastases was largely based on anatomical imaging such as ultrasonography, CT, and magnetic resonance imaging (MRI). These methods, however, are often of limited value in post-thyroidectomy patients owing to the difficulties in discriminating local recurrence from scar tissue in cases of altered anatomy, particularly after neck dissection (Ong *et al.*, 2005). However,

in patients with negative ^{131}I whole-body scan but detectable Tg, FDG-PET identifies the source of Tg production in up to 90% of cases (Schoder and Yeung, 2004). When detected early, it enables surgical treatment of accessible lesions, which is the only curative therapeutic option in patients with non-iodine-avid thyroid tumor tissue. Therefore, exact localization of these malignant thyroid tumor lesions is mandatory for successful resection (Figs. 3 and 4). The early use of FDG-PET in these patients changes the therapeutic strategy in up to 50% of patients (Wang *et al.*, 1999).

In contrast to functionally more differentiated thyroid carcinoma cells with a retained iodine-trapping mechanism and low glucose metabolism, dedifferentiated thyroid carcinoma cells have lost their iodine-trapping mechanism and have high glucose metabolism. This peculiar molecular behavior was first described by Feine *et al.* (1996) as the flip-flop phenomenon. "Flip-flop" describes the alternating uptake pattern of ^{131}I and FDG by differentiated thyroid carcinomas. High glucose consumption as reflected by high FDG uptake represents rapid tumor growth and poor differentiation, whereas most of the ^{131}I-positive metastases are FDG-negative. In some cases there might be a considerable overlap showing uptake of FDG as well as ^{131}I in the same lesion. This can be attributed to the coexistence of different tumor clones within the same tumor site. This suggests that the use of FDG-PET in differentiated thyroid cancer is not exclusively limited to I-131 negative/Tg positive patients.

The detection rate of metastases by FDG-PET varies for different organs, being highest in cervical lymph nodes and lowest in small pulmonary metastases (Dietlein *et al.*, 1997). Futhermore, the sensitivity of FDG-PET increases with increasing levels of serum Tg. FDG-PET seems to be most promising at Tg levels of > 10 microg/L (Schluter

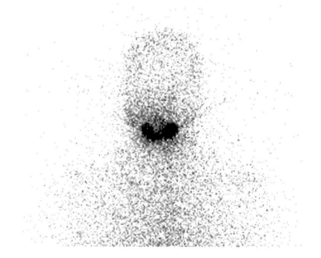

Figure 3 54-year-old female with a history of pT2N1Mx papillary thyroid carcinoma, for which she was twice treated with [131]I. The post-therapeutic ^{131}I scintigraphy did not show any pathologic uptake despite an elevated TSH-stimulated Tg (24.6 microg/L).

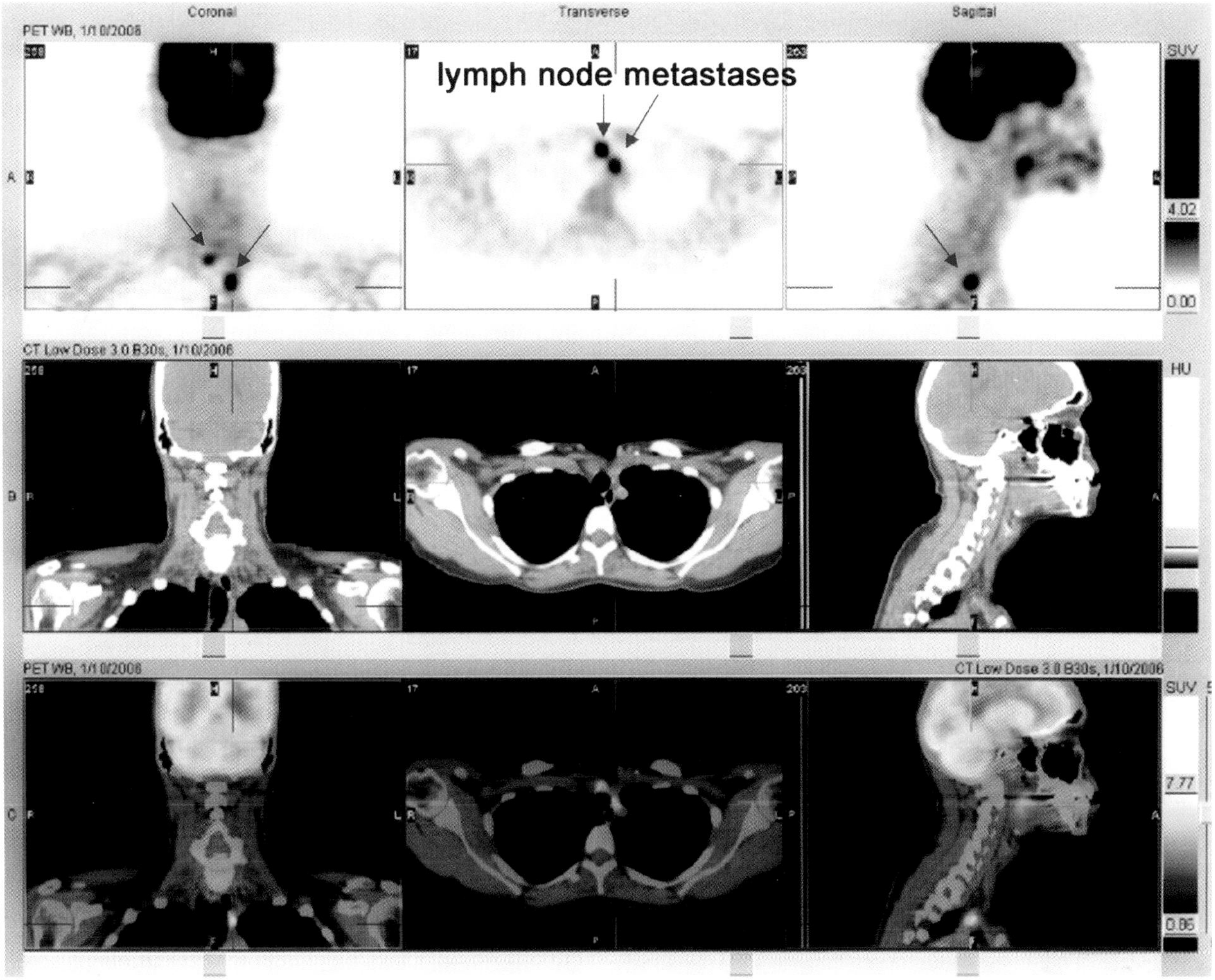

Figure 4 This FDG-PET/CT of the same patient demonstrated paratracheal pathologic uptake, according to lymph node metastases, which were confirmed after reoperation.

et al., 2001). In patients with elevated Tg levels, FDG-PET has a positive-predictive value of 92% (Wang *et al.*, 1999). However, also in case of Tg < 10 microg/L, it is justified to perform FDG-PET because detection of recurrence or metastases in an early stage is crucial with respect to both prognosis and survival. In these patients curative treatment can only be achieved when tumor tissues are completely resected before widespread metastatic disease occurs. Furthermore, a negative FDG-PET has a high negative-predictive value of 93% in patients with low Tg levels (Wang *et al.*, 1999).

Integrated PET/CT

In some conditions, FDG-PET is not able to adequately assess the non-iodine-avid disease. It is known that miliary lung metastases < 6 mm remain undetected by FDG-PET when FDG uptake is not very high (Palmedo *et al.*, 2006). Furthermore, FDG uptake can be seen in normal muscle due to muscle tension, in degenerative articulations, or in hypermetabolic brown fat in the region of the neck, mediastinum, and spine, thereby decreasing the specificity of the scan. In addition, intense FDG uptake by the thymus on FDG-PET does not necessarily indicate recurrence, and asymmetric increased FDG uptake in vocal cord paralysis must be interpreted with caution. Moreover, precise localization of iodine-negative/FDG-PET-positive disease is crucial to allow complete resection and cure of the patient. In all these cases, a combination of PET and CT seems to improve diagnostic accuracy in a therapeutically relevant way. The recent development of a hybrid spiral CT and PET scanner (integrated PET/CT) provides combined anatomic and functional imaging information, which allows tissue characterization as well as assessment of the exact localization and the extent of tumor tissue in one imaging procedure, without repositioning the patient. Integrated PET/CT can help to avoid pitfalls by precisely localizing the focal FDG uptake (e.g., by correction delineation of hypermetabolic brown fat). Diagnostic accuracy could be increased from 78 to 93% by integrated PET/CT in comparison to side-by-side interpretation of PET and CT (Palmedo *et al.*, 2006). PET/CT allows the detection of recurrent or metastatic thyroid cancer with added anatomic information, thereby directing surgical interventions (Fig. 4). Precise localization may aid the patient and surgeon by decreasing surgical time required to locate and remove a tumor, and also by decreasing the risk for false-negative results. Overall, the use of PET/CT leads to a change of therapy in ~ 48% of patients with non-iodine-avid but FDG-avid disease (Palmedo *et al.*, 2006).

Effect of Thyroid-Stimulating Hormone Levels on FDG Uptake

Recently, there has been debate over whether the sensitivity of FDG-PET could be further increased when scanning during elevated TSH levels. For radioiodine scanning of thyroid cancers, an elevated TSH level is essential because iodine uptake in the thyroid is largely driven by TSH. In contrast, cellular metabolism as reflected by the uptake of glucose is more closely related to the growth rate of a cell, which in the case of a dedifferentiated cancerous cell might be independent of TSH. The effect of TSH on glucose transporter activity and glucose metabolism is very complex and not yet fully understood. There is evidence that TSH can modulate glucose uptake and consumption in cultered human thyroid cells (Deichen *et al.*, 2004). TSH has been found to stimulate glucose transport and GLUT1 expression, while, on the other hand, high concentrations of peripheral hormones (in particular T3) appear to increase the Glut4 transport mechanism (Matthaei *et al.*, 1995). It is apparent that both an increase in TSH and an increase in peripheral hormone concentration do have stimulating effects on glucose transport and thus on FDG uptake by thyroid cancer cells.

Several clinical studies have shown that significantly more lesions could be identified after TSH stimulation than during TSH suppression (Fig. 5) (Chin *et al.*, 2004). TSH stimulation resulted in either detection of new lesions or classification of the FDG uptake pattern as typical for malignancy. For some patients this could alter clinical management of their disease. Furthermore, most thyroid tumor lesions exhibited a significant increase in FDG uptake during TSH stimulation, associated with an increase in the tumor-to-background ratio of 63% (Moog *et al.*, 2000). These findings suggested that there is at least partial dependency of FDG uptake in recurrent and metastatic thyroid carcinoma on the TSH level. However, other studies reported conflicting results (Wang *et al.*, 1999). It must be emphasized, however, that it is recommended that sequential PET examinations be performed under similar TSH conditions to prevent erroneous interpretation. Several studies examined the effects of recombinant human TSH (rTSH) on FDG uptake (Chin *et al.*, 2004).

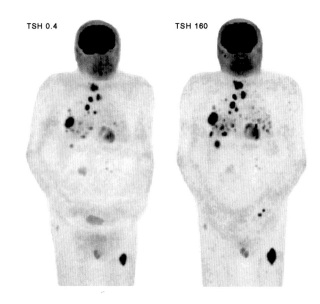

Figure 5 Widespread metastatic papillary thyroid carcinoma in a 60-year-old male. Compared to the FDG-PET during thyrotropin suppression (TSH 0.4), the FDG-PET during TSH stimulation (TSH 160) shows many more metastatic lesions. (Reproduced with permission from van Tol KM, Jager PL, Piers DA, et al. *Thyroid* 2002;12:381–387)

FDG-PET imaging after rTSH stimulation also revealed more lesions in a larger number of patients with a significant increase in tumor-to-background contrast compared to FDG-PET scanning in the same patients during TSH-suppressive T4 therapy (Chin *et al.*, 2004).

Prognostic Value of FDG-PET

The preservation of radioiodine uptake of metastatic thyroid lesions is generally considered to be a more differentiated phenotype. Metastatic lesions that do not concentrate radioiodine are associated with a more aggressive biological behavior. Prognosis in thyroid carcinoma is extremely variable, with 10-year overall survival rates for patients with papillary, follicular, Hürthle cell, and anaplastic carcinoma of 93%, 85%, 76%, and 14%, respectively (Hundahl *et al.*, 1998). Many formal prognostic systems, such as EORTC, TNM (Tumor Node Metastasis), AMES (age/metastases/extent/size), AGES (age/grade/extent/size), and MACIS (metastasis/age/completeness of resection/invasion/size), recognize that age, gender, histological type and grade, tumor size, extrathyroidal extension, and clinical stage at initial diagnosis are key predictors of survival (Sherman, 1999). The presence of distant metastases at initial diagnosis is a negative prognostic factor in virtually all of these models. There are no systems, however, to update the prognosis when metachronous metastases develop. About 26% of these individuals who eventually die of thyroid cancer live for more than 10 years with recurrent active disease; FDG-PET may provide prognostic information in this situation. FDG uptake seems to be restricted to more aggressive and high-grade tumors, whereas tumors with favorable prognosis demonstrate no significant tracer uptake (Schonberger *et al.*, 2002). A reduced survival in those patients with FDG-avid disease has been reported (Wang *et al.*, 2000). When integrating the results of FDG-PET in the TNM classification, it appeared that survival of stages I–III FDG-PET positive patients was very similar to that of patients with stage IV disease (Robbins *et al.*, 2006). On the other hand, the survival of stages I–III FDG-PET negative patients was excellent and significantly different from stages I–III FDG-PET positive patients. Patients with a positive FDG-PET have more than 7 times the risk of dying of thyroid cancer, compared to thyroid cancer survivors (with or without metastases) with a negative FDG-PET. Furthermore, the number and site of FDG-avid lesions are prognostically important. Patients with FDG-avid local recurrences have a much better prognosis than those with FDG-avid distant metastases (Robbins *et al.*, 2006). The accumulation of FDG may differ between different metastases of the same patient due to metabolic heterogeneity. Survival time has been shown to be inversely related to the degree of FDG uptake in the thyroid tumor lesion with the highest metabolic activity (e.g., lesion with the highest maximum SUV), suggesting that prognosis is determined by the tumor lesion with the most rapid growth potential c.q. the most aggressive behavior (Wang *et al.*, 2000). Two-year survival rates of 99% were reported in FDG-PET negative patients, compared to 52% in patients with the highest SUV$_{max}$.

Another strong predictor of survival is the volume of FDG-avid disease. A study with a large number of patients showed that the 3-year survival probability of patients with FDG-lesion volumes of 125 ml or less was 96% compared to 18% in patients with FDG-lesion volume greater than 125 ml (Wang *et al.*, 2000). Therefore, once distant metastases are diagnosed in patients with differentiated thyroid carcinoma, FDG-PET can identify high- and low-risk subsets. These findings were supported by an immunohistochemical study, which showed that glucose transporter 1 (GLUT1) gene expression is related to thyroid neoplasms with an unfavorable prognosis (Schonberger *et al.*, 2002). Microscopically, it was not possible to detect morphologic differences between the tumor cells expressing GLUT1 and those not expressing it. Therefore, assessment of GLUT1 expression may be a new prognostic marker *in vitro* and FDG a new prognostic marker *in vivo* to identify patients requiring more aggressive treatment. New therapeutic strategies are urgently needed for lesions that avidly accumulate FDG, as the survival of these patients is significantly reduced. When designing clinical trials for such high-risk patients, FDG-PET could be used as quantitative outcome measures. Major improvement in strategies that can affect redifferentiation, accompanied with restoration of iodine-avidity, are awaited (Coelho *et al.*, 2005).

Hürthle Cell Carcinoma

Hürthle cell carcinoma is a histologic subtype of differentiated thyroid carcinoma that is clinically more aggressive. It is a rare variant with an incidence of 3 to 6% of all thyroid malignancies, and it has unique histologic and pathophysiologic features that differentiate this subtype from other thyroid malignancies (Goldman *et al.*, 1996). The tumor is derived from follicular cells and is composed mostly of oncocytic, oxyphilic follicular cells. Despite preserved Tg expression and high differentiation, Hürthle cell carcinomas frequently do not incorporate radioiodine. Therefore, ^{131}I therapy is often not a good therapeutic option for treatment of recurrences and metastases, as indicated by the relatively low 10-year survival rate of 50–60%. In addition, the poorer prognosis may also be caused by its higher biologic aggressiveness compared to other differentiated thyroid carcinomas. In the follow-up of patients with Hürthle cell carcinomas, distant metastases occur in approximately 33% of cases, whereas in papillary and follicular thyroid cancer only 10% and 22% of patients suffer from metastatic disease (Lowe *et al.*, 2003). Local non–radioiodine-avid recurrence may require revision surgery and, potentially, external-beam radiation therapy. This makes exact localization of tumor tissue of great clinical importance.

Several functional imaging modalities have been proposed for imaging Hürthle cell cancer, using radiotracers such as ^{99m}Tc-sestamibi, ^{99m}Tc-dimercaptosuccinic acid, radiolabeled somatostatin analogs, radiolabeled anticarcinoembryonic antigen antibodies, and ^{201}Tl chloride (Forssell-Aronsson *et al.*, 2000). Although many of these modalities showed increased diagnostic sensitivity compared with radioiodine scintigraphy, none of them had very high sensitivity or specificity in detecting residual or recurrent disease.

Indeed, several reports have shown improved sensitivity using FDG-PET. Hürthle cell carcinoma demonstrated intense FDG uptake, and FDG-PET has been shown to be a powerful diagnostic technique for detecting radioiodine-negative recurrences and metastases of Hürthle cell carcinoma in patients with an elevated Tg level. A sensitivity of 92%, a specificity of 80%, a positive-predictive value of 92%, a negative-predictive value of 80%, and an accuracy of 89% have been reported (Plotkin *et al.*, 2002). FDG-PET can provide additional information on disease extent, leading to a change in patient management in approximately 50% of patients (Lowe *et al.*, 2003). Although only few results on the value of FDG-PET in the follow-up of Hürthle cell tumors have been published up to now, all authors rate FDG-PET as a powerful method superior to other diagnostic techniques in these non-iodine-avid recurrences. However, the usefulness of FDG-PET in patients with iodine-avid Hürthle cell carcinoma recurrence remains controversial. It is not expected that FDG-PET will demonstrate additional lesions in cases with ^{131}I-positive recurrences, and FDG-PET can even miss these iodine-avid recurrences, as is the case in papillary and follicular thyroid carcinoma (Plotkin *et al.*, 2002). Therefore, ^{131}I-scintigraphy should precede FDG-PET in all patients without iodine-negative recurrences. As in papillary and follicular thyroid cancer, the degree of FDG uptake in Hürthle cell tumor lesions provided significant prognostic information: the 5-year overall survival in patients with $SUV_{max} < 10$ was 92% and declined to 64% in those with $SUV_{max} > 10$ (Pryma *et al.*, 2006).

Anaplastic Thyroid Cancer

Anaplastic thyroid carcinoma accounts for 1 to 5% of all thyroid cancers and is characterized by poor outcome and extensive local invasion at the time of initial diagnosis. The diagnosis of anaplastic thyroid cancer is usually not difficult. Most of the time it occurs in elderly patients, and it is marked by rapid growth and extensive local invasion. An FNAB confirms the clinical impression, and regardless of the therapy the outcome is extremely bad, with survival beyond 1 year being uncommon. Thus, there is no real use for an elaborate staging procedure in these patients because almost all patients are classified as stage IV at diagnosis. Consequently, FDG-PET in anaplastic thyroid carcinoma has not been studied systemically. Also, no major publications have reported the use of other functional radionuclide imaging techniques in anaplastic thyroid carcinoma, which may be due to the lack of clinically relevant results. Imaging with ^{131}I scintigraphy and serum Tg measurements is not useful since these often do not adequately depict the disease status (McDougall *et al.*, 2001). However, in selected cases FDG-PET may be helpful in directing treatment and evaluating the efficacy of therapy. In some case reports and in some studies with limited numbers of patients, this malignancy showed intense FDG uptake (Schoder *et al.*, 2004), due perhaps to high levels of GLUT1 expression in the cytoplasm and on the cell membrane of anaplastic thyroid carcinoma. It has been shown that positive membranous staining was detected predominantly in thyroid neoplasms with an aggressive biological behavior, whereas low or no immunoreactivity could be seen in well-differentiated tumors or in normal thyroid epithelium (Schonberger *et al.*, 2002).

Medullary Thyroid Cancer

Medullary thyroid cancer is a relatively uncommon tumor and accounts for 4 to 10% of all thyroid malignancies. It originates from the calcitonin-producing parafollicular cells (C-cells) of the thyroid, and belongs to the group of neuroendocrine tumors. Cells are derived from the neural crest and secrete carcinoembryonic antigen (CEA) and calcitonin, as well as other polypeptides such as vasoactive intestinal polypeptide and somatostatin (Khan *et al.*, 2005). Medullary thyroid cancer

occurs sporadically or is hereditary, with an autosomal dominant pattern of inheritance. Genetic and biochemical testing allow early preclinical identification of familial forms. These familial forms account for 25% of all medullary thyroid cancers and include three well-defined syndromes: familial medullary thyroid cancer and multiple endocrine neoplasia (MEN) types 2A and 2B (Grauer *et al.*, 1990). Both sporadic and familial medullary thyroid cancers are characterized by relatively slow tumor growth but early lymphatic metastatic spread. In 71 to 80% of all patients, pathologically proven cervical lymph node metastases are already present at the time of initial diagnosis. The corresponding value for mediastinal involvement is 36%, whereas distant metastases have been reported in 20% of patients (Szakall *et al.*, 2002).

Complete surgical resection of all tumor manifestations still remains the only effective treatment with curative intent. The effect of external radiotherapy and chemotherapy remains disappointing (Orlandi *et al.*, 2001). Residual or recurrent disease is a frequently encountered problem, particularly in patients with advanced primary tumors, even after adequately performed dissection. These cases are difficult to manage and are clinically the most relevant group. Elevated serum calcitonin and CEA levels measured 8 to 12 weeks postoperatively suggest persistent tumor, while a progressive increase after previous normalization is indicative of relapse (Khan *et al.*, 2005). Measurement of these plasma markers is therefore the most frequently applied evaluation method in long-term follow-up. Early identification and treatment of recurrent, residual, or occult tumor are useful as reoperation is the only curative option that may also prevent the development of local symptoms or distant metastases, which is also important in patients who cannot be cured (Kebebew *et al.*, 2000). Locoregional control may prevent airway obstruction or invasion into great vessels. Patients with persistent hypercalcitoninemia after apparent curative primary surgery may have a good prognosis with a 10-year survival of up to 86%, underlining the clinical relevance of exact localization of tumor tissue in curable as well as in noncurable patients.

Localization of the site of disease is a major clinical problem, however, that has not been completely solved yet. Selective venous catheterization, with a correct localization rate of 89%, is the gold standard for identification of residual or recurrent lymph nodes (Abdelmoumene *et al.*, 1994). However, its invasiveness restricts general application, and it is only useful to be performed in the case of cervical lymph node metastases (Abdelmoumene *et al.*, 1994). Efforts are ongoing to develop reliable noninvasive methods to localize residual and distant metastases of medullary thyroid cancer. Up to now there is no single sensitive diagnostic imaging method to reveal all residual or metastatic medullary cancer lesions. Morphologic imaging techniques, such as ultrasonography, CT, MRI, and different scintigraphic procedures, are usually performed in patients who have elevated tumor marker levels for localizing the responsible tumor sites.

Despite high anatomical resolution, the morphologic imaging procedures are restricted to depiction of organ shape, tissue structure, and tissue size. Due to the smallness of most of the lymph node lesions, these investigations are often insufficient. Ultrasonography has shown a lymph node detection rate of 28–78%, compared with 38–70% for CT and 44–74% for MRI (Szakall et al., 2002). Various scintigraphic techniques, such as thallium chloride (^{201}Tl), ^{99m}Tc-sestamibi (MIBI) or ^{99m}Tc-tetrofosmin, pentavalent ^{99m}Tc-dimer-captosuccinic acid (^{99m}Tc(V)-DMSA), ^{111}In-pentetreotide (somatostatin receptor scintigraphy), radiolabeled anti-CEA antibodies, and radioiodinated meta-iodobenzylguanidine (^{123}I/^{131}I-MIBG), have been used for medullary thyroid tumor imaging during follow-up (Baudin et al., 1996). Furthermore, MIBG scintigraphy at tumor presentation is indicated when there are doubts regarding the existence of a concomitant pheochromocytoma (MEN syndrome) (Bombardieri et al., 2004). However, in all of the above-mentioned methods, the sensitivity is low, especially for small lesions. Due to variable tracer uptake and the lower spatial resolution, the diagnostic performance of all these tracers is unsatisfactory, and none of these tracers can be considered as the radiopharmaceutical of choice. Therefore, in many cases several anatomical and functional imaging modalities have to be performed consecutively in patients with elevated calcitonin levels until the tumor is localized.

FDG-PET has been shown to be a useful method in the staging and follow-up of medullary thyroid cancer. It appears that FDG-PET can identify metastatic disease more frequently than other functional imaging studies (Diehl et al., 2001). When comparing FDG-PET and CT, it is not unequivocally clear which imaging method performs better in localizing metastatic medullary thyroid cancer. Some studies show that CT is superior to FDG-PET, while other studies show the superiority of FDG-PET (Gotthardt et al., 2004). Nevertheless, the metabolic imaging findings may precede the morphologic changes evidenced by CT or MRI by several weeks. FDG-PET examination can be performed as early as 8 weeks after initial treatment when tumor markers may still be elevated and conventional imaging modalities are either negative or inconclusive to detect recurrent or metastatic disease due to postsurgical fibrotic changes (Khan et al., 2005). In patients with medullary thyroid cancer indicated by elevated calcitonin levels after complete thyroidectomy, FDG-PET has a sensitivity and specificity of 70–80% for localizing metastatic disease (Diehl et al., 2001; Schoder et al., 2004). One reason for this modest sensitivity of FDG-PET is the slow growth rate and low proliferation index of neuroendocrine tumors, resulting in a limited glucose consumption. This may also explain the inability to detect small foci of medullary thyroid cancer with FDG-PET in patients with only biochemical evidence of disease (de Groot et al., 2004). Nevertheless, FDG-PET was shown to be superior to all the scintigraphic imaging methods mentioned here in detecting occult medullary throid cancer lesions. FDG-PET was more sensitive in localizing lymph node involvement, especially in the cervical, supraclavicular, and mediastinal lymphatic regions (Szakall et al., 2002). Interestingly, there seems to be no correlation between the calcitonin level and the probability of lesion detection (Diehl et al., 2001; Schoder et al., 2004). However, it has been suggested that more undifferentiated tumors that secrete less calcitonin may show higher FDG uptake, in analogy to the situation in differentiated thyroid cancer. To avoid misinterpretation of PET due to FDG accumulation in inflammatory tissue and to allow better anatomical localization and determination of the extent of disease, additional information by CT or MRI is still needed (Gotthardt et al., 2004). Thus, a combination of CT and PET with integrated PET/CT seems to be the most appropriate noninvasive diagnostic approach in patients with medullary thyroid cancer (Gotthardt et al., 2004). Although recent reports indicate that novel, more specific radiotracers, such as 6-^{18}F-fluorodopamine or ^{18}F-DOPA or radiolabeled minigastrin, may be more appropriate for detecting recurrent or metastatic medullary thyroid cancer (Hoegerle et al., 2001; Gotthardt et al., 2006), presently combined FDG-PET and CT can be recommended in case of postoperative elevated plasma tumor marker levels to select patients for secondary surgical intervention.

Summary and Conclusions

1. FDG-PET could play an important role in the management of patients with inconclusive cytological findings of a thyroid nodule, because it has a high negative predictive value and is able to significantly reduce the number of futile hemithyroidectomies.

2. FDG-PET positive thyroid incidentalomas should not be overlooked and should prompt further investigation to rule out cancer, only when the diagnosis of thyroid cancer would influence patient outcome and management.

3. FDG-PET is a first-line investigation in patients with persistent or recurrent thyroid cancer as indicated by elevated serum thyroglobulin levels, but negative findings are found on ^{131}I whole-body scans after treatment.

4. FDG-PET should preferentially be performed on an integrated PET/CT system, because fusion of metabolic and anatomic information increases diagnostic accuracy, improves exact localization, reduces pitfalls, and changes therapeutic strategies in a considerable number of thyroid cancer patients.

5. FDG uptake under high TSH levels may be advantageous in increasing the sensitivity of FDG-PET. If available, the use of rhTSH instead of thyroid hormone withdrawal is advocated, because it avoids TSH-stimulated tumor growth, deep hypothyroidism-associated morbidity, and moreover it will result in the highest sensitivity and tumor-to-background contrast.

6. Besides localization of thyroid cancer lesions, FDG-PET provides prognostic information, which can be important

in patients with metachronous metastases in particular, and can be useful as a quantitative outcome measure in clinical trials.

7. FDG-PET is highly beneficial in Hürthle cell carcinoma patients with elevated Tg levels, but negative radioiodine scintigraphy, whereas its diagnostic impact on patients with radioiodine avid lesions remains limited.

8. FDG-PET in anaplastic thyroid carcinoma has not been studied systemically, because there is no definite clinical indication for elaborate staging procedures.

9. In medullary thyroid cancer, FDG-PET in combination with CT seems to be an accurate, noninvasive technique during follow-up for detecting tumoral spread in patients with postoperative persistently elevated or increasing CEA and/or calcitonin levels in order to identify the source of tumor marker production and to select patients for secondary surgical intervention.

References

Abdelmoumene, N., Schlumberger, M., Gardet, P., Roche, A., Travagli, J.P., Francese, C., and Parmentier, C. 1994. Selective venous sampling catheterisation for localisation of persisting medullary thyroid carcinoma. *Br. J. Cancer* 69:1141–1144.

Baudin, E., Do, C.C., Cailleux, A.F., Leboulleux, S., Travagli, J.P., and Schlumberger, M. 2003. Positive predictive value of serum thyroglobulin levels, measured during the first year of follow-up after thyroid hormone withdrawal, in thyroid cancer patients. *J. Clin. Endocrinol. Metab.* 88:1107–1111.

Baudin, E., Lumbroso, J., Schlumberger, M., Leclere, J., Giammarile, F., Gardet, P., Roche, A., Travagli, J.P., and Parmentier, C. 1996. Comparison of octreotide scintigraphy and conventional imaging in medullary thyroid carcinoma. *J. Nucl. Med.* 37:912–916.

Bombardieri, E., Seregni, E., Villano, C., Chiti, A., and Bajetta, E. 2004. Position of nuclear medicine techniques in the diagnostic work-up of neuroendocrine tumors. *Q. J. Nucl. Med. Mol. Imaging* 48:150–163.

Burguera, B., and Gharib, H., 2000. Thyroid incidentalomas. Prevalence, diagnosis, significance, and management. *Endocrinol. Metab. Clin. North Am.* 29:187–203.

Chin, B.B., Patel, P., Cohade, C., Ewertz, M., Wahl, R., and Ladenson, P. 2004. Recombinant human thyrotropin stimulation of fluoro-D-glucose positron emission tomography uptake in well-differentiated thyroid carcinoma. *J. Clin. Endocrinol. Metab.* 89:91–95.

Choi, J.Y., Lee, K.S., Kim, H.J., Shim, Y.M., Kwon, O.J., Park, K., Baek, C.H., Chung, J.H., Lee, K.H., and Kim, B.T. 2006. Focal thyroid lesions incidentally identified by integrated 18F-FDG PET/CT: clinical significance and improved characterization. *J. Nucl. Med.* 47:609–615.

Coelho, S.M., Vaisman, M., and Carvalho, D.P. 2005. Tumour re-differentiation effect of retinoic acid: a novel therapeutic approach for advanced thyroid cancer. *Curr. Pharm. Des.* 11:2525–2531.

de Geus-Oei, L.F., Oei, H.Y., Hennemann, G., and Krenning, E.P. 2002. Sensitivity of 123I whole-body scan and thyroglobulin in the detection of metastases or recurrent differentiated thyroid cancer. *Eur. J. Nucl. Med. Mol. Imag.* 29:768–774.

de Geus-Oei, L.F., Pieters, G.F., Bonenkamp, J.J., Mudde, A.H., Bleeker-Rovers, C.P., Corstens, F.H., and Oyen, W.J. 2006. 18F-FDG PET reduces unnecessary hemithyroidectomies for thyroid nodules with inconclusive cytologic results. *J. Nucl. Med.* 47:770–775.

de Groot, J.W., Links, T.P., Jager, P.L., Kahraman, T., and Plukker, J.T. 2004. Impact of 18F-fluoro-2-deoxy-D-glucose positron emission tomography (FDG-PET) in patients with biochemical evidence of recurrent or residual medullary thyroid cancer. *Ann. Surg. Oncol.* 11:786–794.

Deichen, J.T., Schmidt, C., Prante, O., Maschauer, S., Papadopoulos, T., and Kuwert, T. 2004. Influence of TSH on uptake of [18F]fluorodeoxyglucose in human thyroid cells *in vitro. Eur. J. Nucl. Med. Mol. Imag.* 31:507–512.

Demirel, K., Kapucu, O., Yucel, C., Ozdemir, H., Ayvaz, G., and Taneri, F., 2003. A comparison of radionuclide thyroid angiography, (99m)Tc-MIBI scintigraphy and power Doppler ultrasonography in the differential diagnosis of solitary cold thyroid nodules. *Eur. J. Nucl. Med. Mol. Imag.* 30:642–650.

Diehl, M., Risse, J.H., Brandt-Mainz, K., Dietlein, M., Bohuslavizki, K.H., Matheja, P., Lange, H., Bredow, J., Korber, C., and Grunwald, F., 2001. Fluorine-18 fluorodeoxyglucose positron emission tomography in medullary thyroid cancer: results of a multicentre study. *Eur. J. Nucl. Med.* 28:1671–1676.

Dietlein, M., Scheidhauer, K., Voth, E., Theissen, P., and Schicha, H. 1997. Fluorine-18 fluorodeoxyglucose positron emission tomography and iodine-131 whole-body scintigraphy in the follow-up of differentiated thyroid cancer. *Eur. J. Nucl. Med.* 24:1342–1348.

Even-Sapir, E., Lerman, H., Gutman, M., Lievshitz, G., Zuriel, L., Polliack, A., Inbar, M., and Metser, U. 2006. The presentation of malignant tumours and pre-malignant lesions incidentally found on PET-CT. *Eur. J. Nucl. Med. Mol. Imag.* 33:541–552.

Feine, U., Lietzenmayer, R., Hanke, J.P., Held, J., Wohrle, H., and Muller-Schauenburg, W. 1996. Fluorine-18-FDG and iodine-131-iodide uptake in thyroid cancer. *J. Nucl. Med.* 37:1468–1472.

Forssell-Aronsson, E.B., Nilsson, O., Bejegard, S.A., Kolby, L., Bernhardt, P., Molne, J., Hashemi, S.H., Wangberg, B., Tisell, L.E., and Ahlman, H. 2000. 111In-DTPA-D-Phe1-octreotide binding and somatostatin receptor subtypes in thyroid tumors. *J. Nucl. Med.* 41:636–642.

Goldman, N.D., Coniglio, J.U., and Falk, S.A. 1996. Thyroid cancers. I. Papillary, follicular, and Hürthle cell. *Otolaryngol. Clin. North Am.* 29:593–609.

Gotthardt, M., Battmann, A., Hoffken, H., Schurrat, T., Pollum, H., Beuter, D., Gratz, S., Behe, M., Bauhofer, A., Klose, K.J., and Behr, T.M. 2004. 18F-FDG PET, somatostatin receptor scintigraphy, and CT in metastatic medullary thyroid carcinoma: a clinical study and an analysis of the literature. *Nucl. Med. Commun.* 25:439–443.

Gotthardt, M., Dijkgraaf, I., Boerman, O.C., and Oyen, W.J., 2006. Nuclear medicine imaging and therapy of neuroendocrine tumours. *Cancer Imag.* 6:S178–S184.

Grauer, A., Raue, F., and Gagel, R.F. 1990. Changing concepts in the management of hereditary and sporadic medullary thyroid carcinoma. *Endocrinol. Metab Clin. North Am.* 19:613–635.

Hegedus, L. 2004. Clinical practice. The thyroid nodule. *N. Engl. J. Med.* 351:1764–1771.

Hoegerle, S., Altehoefer, C., Ghanem, N., Brink, I., Moser, E., and Nitzsche, E. 2001. 18F-DOPA positron emission tomography for tumour detection in patients with medullary thyroid carcinoma and elevated calcitonin levels. *Eur. J. Nucl. Med.* 28:64–71.

Hundahl, S.A., Fleming, I.D., Fremgen, A.M., and Menck, H.R. 1998. A National Cancer Data Base report on 53,856 cases of thyroid carcinoma treated in the U.S., 1985–1995 [see comments]. *Cancer* 83:2638–2648.

Hurtado-Lopez, L.M., Arellano-Montano, S., Torres-Acosta, E.M., Zaldivar-Ramirez, F.R., Duarte-Torres, R.M., Alonso-de-Ruiz, P., Martinez-Duncker, I., and Martinez-Duncker, C. 2004. Combined use of fine-needle aspiration biopsy, MIBI scans and frozen section biopsy offers the best diagnostic accuracy in the assessment of the hypofunctioning solitary thyroid nodule. *Eur. J. Nucl. Med. Mol. Imag.* 31:1273–1279.

Kebebew, E., Kikuchi, S., Duh, Q.Y., and Clark, O.H. 2000. Long-term results of reoperation and localizing studies in patients with persistent or recurrent medullary thyroid cancer. *Arch. Surg.* 135:895–901.

Khan, N., Oriuchi, N., Higuchi, T., and Endo, K. 2005. Review of fluorine-18-2-fluoro-2-deoxy-D-glucose positron emission tomography (FDG-PET) in the follow-up of medullary and anaplastic thyroid carcinomas. *Cancer Control 12*:254–260.

Kresnik, E., Gallowitsch, H.J., Mikosch, P., Stettner, H., Igerc, I., Gomez, I., Kumnig, G., and Lind, P. 2003. Fluorine-18-fluorodeoxyglucose positron emission tomography in the preoperative assessment of thyroid nodules in an endemic goiter area. *Surgery 133*:294–299.

Kuma, K., Matsuzuka, F., Yokozawa, T., Miyauchi, A., and Sugawara, M. 1994. Fate of untreated benign thyroid nodules: results of long-term follow-up. *World J. Surg. 18*:495–498.

Lowe, V.J., Mullan, B.P., Hay, I.D., McIver, B., and Kasperbauer, J.L. 2003. 18F-FDG PET of patients with Hürthle cell carcinoma. *J. Nucl. Med. 44*:1402–1406.

Matthaei, S., Trost, B., Hamann, A., Kausch, C., Benecke, H., Greten, H., Hoppner, W., and Klein, H.H. 1995. Effect of *in vivo* thyroid hormone status on insulin signalling and GLUT1 and GLUT4 glucose transport systems in rat adipocytes. *J. Endocrinol. 144*:347–357.

McDougall, I.R., Davidson, J., and Segall, G.M. 2001. Positron emission tomography of the thyroid, with an emphasis on thyroid cancer. *Nucl. Med. Commun. 22*:485–492.

Moog, F., Linke, R., Manthey, N., Tiling, R., Knesewitsch, P., Tatsch, K., and Hahn, K. 2000. Influence of thyroid-stimulating hormone levels on uptake of FDG in recurrent and metastatic differentiated thyroid carcinoma. *J. Nucl. Med. 41*:1989–1995.

Ong, S.C., Ng, D.C., and Sundram, F.X. 2005. Initial experience in use of fluorine-18-fluorodeoxyglucose positron emission tomography/computed tomography in thyroid carcinoma patients with elevated serum thyroglobulin but negative iodine-131 whole body scans. *Singapore Med. J. 46*:297–301.

Orlandi, F., Caraci, P., Mussa, A., Saggiorato, E., Pancani, G., and Angeli, A. 2001. Treatment of medullary thyroid carcinoma: an update. *Endocr. Relat. Cancer 8*:135–147.

Palmedo, H., Bucerius, J., Joe, A., Strunk, H., Hortling, N., Meyka, S., Roedel, R., Wolff, M., Wardelmann, E., Biersack, H.J., and Jaeger, U. 2006. Integrated PET/CT in differentiated thyroid cancer: diagnostic accuracy and impact on patient management. *J. Nucl. Med. 47*:616–624.

Plotkin, M., Hautzel, H., Krause, B.J., Schmidt, D., Larisch, R., Mottaghy, F.M., Boemer, A.R., Herzog, H., Vosberg, H., and Muller-Gartner, H.W. 2002. Implication of 2-18fluoro-2-deoxyglucose positron emission tomography in the follow-up of Hürthle cell thyroid cancer. *Thyroid 12*:155–161.

Pryma, D.A., Schoder, H., Gonen, M., Robbins, R.J., Larson, S.M., and Yeung, H.W. 2006. Diagnostic accuracy and prognostic value of 18F-FDG PET in Hürthle cell thyroid cancer patients. *J. Nucl. Med. 47*:1260–1266.

Rago, T., Vitti, P., Chiovato, L., Mazzeo, S., de Liperi A., Miccoli, P., Viacava, P., Bogazzi, F., Martino, E., and Pinchera, A. 1998. Role of conventional ultrasonography and color flow-Doppler sonography in predicting malignancy in "cold" thyroid nodules. *Eur. J. Endocrinol. 138*:41–46.

Reske, S.N., and Kotzerke, J. 2001. FDG-PET for clinical use. Results of the 3rd German Interdisciplinary Consensus Conference, "Onko-PET III," July 21 and September 19, 2000. *Eur. J. Nucl. Med. 28*:1707–1723.

Robbins, R.J., Wan, Q., Grewal, R.K., Reibke, R., Gonen, M., Strauss, H.W., Tuttle, R.M., Drucker, W., and Larson, S.M. 2006. Real-time prognosis for metastatic thyroid carcinoma based on 2-[18F]fluoro-2-deoxy-D-glucose-positron emission tomography scanning. *J. Clin. Endocrinol. Metab. 91*:498–505.

Schluter, B., Bohuslavizki, K.H., Beyer, W., Plotkin, M., Buchert, R., and Clausen, M. 2001. Impact of FDG PET on patients with differentiated thyroid cancer who present with elevated thyroglobulin and negative 131I scan. *J. Nucl. Med. 42*:71–76.

Schoder, H., and Yeung, H.W. 2004. Positron emission imaging of head and neck cancer, including thyroid carcinoma. *Semin. Nucl. Med. 34*:180–197.

Schonberger, J., Ruschoff, J., Grimm, D., Marienhagen, J., Rummele, P., Meyringer, R., Kossmehl, P., Hofstaedter, F., and Eilles, C. 2002. Glucose transporter 1 gene expression is related to thyroid neoplasms with an unfavorable prognosis: an immunohistochemical study. *Thyroid 12*:747–754.

Sherman, S.I. 1999. Toward a standard clinicopathologic staging approach for differentiated thyroid carcinoma. *Semin. Surg. Oncol. 16*:12–15.

Szakall, S, Jr., Esik, O., Bajzik, G., Repa, I., Dabasi, G., Sinkovics, I., Agoston, P., and Tron, L. 2002. 18F-FDG PET detection of lymph node metastases in medullary thyroid carcinoma. *J. Nucl. Med. 43*:66–71.

Wang, W., Larson, S.M., Fazzari, M., Tickoo, S.K., Kolbert, K., Sgouros, G., Yeung, H., Macapinlac, H., Rosai, J., and Robbins, R.J. 2000. Prognostic value of [18F]fluorodeoxyglucose positron emission tomographic scanning in patients with thyroid cancer. *J. Clin. Endocrinol. Metab. 85*:1107–1113.

Wang, W., Macapinlac, H., Larson, S.M., Yeh, S.D., Akhurst, T., Finn, R.D., Rosai, J., and Robbins, R.J. 1999. [18F]-2-fluoro-2-deoxy-D-glucose positron emission tomography localizes residual thyroid cancer in patients with negative diagnostic (131)I whole body scans and elevated serum thyroglobulin levels. *J. Clin. Endocrinol. Metab. 84*:2291–2302.

Yi, J.G., Marom, E.M., Munden, R.F., Truong, M.T., Macapinlac, H.A., Gladish, G.W., Sabloff, B.S., and Podoloff, D.A. 2005. Focal uptake of fluorodeoxyglucose by the thyroid in patients undergoing initial disease staging with combined PET/CT for non-small cell lung cancer. *Radiology 236*:271–275.

55

Thyroid Cancer: ^{18}F-Fluoro-2-Deoxy-D-Glucose Positron Emission Tomography (An Overview)

Kristoff Muylle and Patrick Flamen

Introduction

Thyroid carcinomas are fairly uncommon (±1% of new malignant disease) and include a broad range of disease types: 94% are differentiated thyroid carcinomas (DTC), 5% are medullary thyroid carcinoma (MTC), and the remaining 1% are anaplastic thyroid carcinoma (ATC).

Differentiated thyroid carcinomas (DTCs) are derived from the follicular epithelial cells and are either papillary thyroid carcinoma or follicular thyroid carcinoma. Patients with DTC have generally good prognosis, with a 10-year cancer-specific mortality of < 10%. Histological features, such as tumor size and extrathyroidal invasion, are of prognostic importance. Histological subtypes that are associated with adverse risk include tall-cell and columnar-cell variants of papillary-type carcinoma, oxyphilic (Hürthle) cells, and poorly differentiated and insular variants of the follicular type. Increased age and the presence of distant metastasis at initial diagnosis are associated with poor prognosis, independent of the type of cancer.

Medullary thyroid carcinoma (MTC) is a calcitonin and carcinoembryonic antigen (CEA) secreting neuroendocrine tumor of the parafollicular C-cells of the thyroid. This carcinoma occurs sporadically or is hereditary, and is characterized by early lymphatic metastatic spread; metastases are present in 35% of the patients at the time of initial diagnosis, predominantly in the cervical and mediastinal lymph nodes. The course of the disease is relatively slow, but characterized by high clinical recurrence rates.

Anaplastic thyroid carcinoma (ATC) is a very aggressive tumor with poor prognosis characterized by extended local invasion and high frequency of distant metastases at the time of initial diagnosis. The tumor occurs predominantly in older patients, and approximately half of the patients with ATC have a previous or coexistent DTC, with evidence of dedifferentiation (Sherman, 2003).

Diagnosis of Thyroid Cancer

Papillary, medullary, and anaplastic carcinoma can be readily diagnosed based on the cytological examination of a fine needle aspirate of the (usually solitary) thyroid nodule. Ultrasound guidance can augment the accuracy of this procedure. The presence of a photopenic or cold lesion on thyroid scintigraphy (with ^{99m}Tc-pertechnetate, ^{131}I or ^{123}I) increases the probability of malignancy, but this finding remains non-specific and nondiagnostic. Computed tomography (CT) and magnetic resonance imaging (MRI) have no role in the routine diagnostic assessment of most thyroid nodules.

Follicular carcinoma and benign follicular adenoma are usually cytologically indistinguishable. For those indeterminate, suspicious follicular lesions, the overall rate of carcinoma is ±20%, with high rates associated with large nodule size, increased age, and male sex. In order to confirm the diagnosis of follicular carcinoma, histological examination is needed to show either vascular invasion or invasion through the tumor capsule. Hürthle cell carcinoma (HCC) is an uncommon histological subtype of papillary and (more often) follicular thyroid cancer and is composed of at least 75% Hürthle cells, which are large mitochondrion-rich (oxyphilic) eosinophilic cells. Insular thyroid cancer is another rare subtype of follicular thyroid cancer and is characterized by early dedifferentiation.

Initial Treatment of Thyroid Cancer

Total thyroidectomy is the primary mode of therapy for patients with DTC if the primary tumor is 1 cm or more in diameter and, especially, if extrathyroidal extension or metastases are present. Central and ipsilateral neck dissections might reduce the frequency of regional recurrence, particularly when there is obvious nodal involvement from papillary carcinoma and the oxyphylic (Hürthle cell) variant of follicular carcinoma. Unilateral lobectomy might be sufficient if the tumor is < 1 cm in diameter and confined to one lobe.

Postoperative radioiodine (^{131}I) ablation is recommended by many experts for patients with a carcinoma of > 1–1.5 cm in diameter or of any size with obvious lymph node involvement, extrathyroidal extension, or multicentricity. It is carried out 4 weeks after total thyroidectomy, allowing the thyroid-stimulating hormone (TSH) level to increase (> 30 mU/l) and so optimizing iodine uptake by the remaining thyroid tissue. A postablation whole-body scintigraphy is performed 3 to 7 days later and is used as a highly specific method to visualize residual tumor tissue in DTC. Thyroid hormone replacement therapy is given 3 days after the ablative treatment.

Because surgical resection of all tumor tissue is the only curative treatment in patients with MTC, total thyroidectomy with central neck compartment dissection is indicated in all patients with MTC. This intervention is often associated by ipsi- or bilateral modified radical neck and/or mediastinal dissections, depending on the size, type (sporadic versus hereditary disease), and local disease extension (e.g., presence of central compartment disease) of the tumor. There is no role for postoperative radioiodine ^{131}I therapy in MTC. External beam radiotherapy should be considered for patients at high risk for local recurrence.

Treatment of ATC is usually palliative. In the minority of patients without extracervical or unresectable disease, surgical excision followed by adjuvant radiotherapy is indicated to prolong survival (Sherman, 2003).

Follow-Up of Thyroid Cancer

Serum thyroglobulin (Tg) measurement is the most sensitive tool in the follow-up of patients with DTC, treated with surgery and radioiodine ablation. Thyroglobulin is secreted by normal thyroid tissue and thyroid cancer cells. The production and secretion of Tg are TSH-dependent. Therefore, the sensitivity of the serum Tg assay for the detection of residual or recurrent thyroid carcinoma increases when serum TSH levels rise after discontinuation of thyroid hormone replacement or after administration of recombinant human TSH (rhTSH). An rhTSH stimulated rise of Tg above 2 ng/ml is a highly sensitive marker of DTC recurrence. Anti-Tg antibodies (TgAb) are present in as many as 25% of patients with DTC (compared with 10% in the general population). The presence of serum TgAb usually invalidates the serum Tg result. Therefore, any serum submitted for Tg measurement should be tested for the presence of TgAb.

Diagnostic radioiodine whole-body scanning, performed either after rhTSH administration or thyroid hormone withdrawal, is usually performed 6 to 12 months after the initial radioiodine ablation; if this first scan shows no abnormal radioiodine uptake, no further radioiodine scans are required. If significant tracer uptake is shown, a further ablative dose of radioiodine can be administered. A consensus report (Mazzaferri et al., 2003) advocated that rhTSH-stimulated Tg is sensitive enough to be the only test in the follow-up of low-risk DTC patients who have undergone total or near-total thyroidectomy and ^{131}I ablation showing no clinical evidence of tumor or detectable serum Tg levels during thyroxin therapy. The routine use of diagnostic whole-body scanning adds little information and should be discouraged in this (large) group of patients.

Ultrasonography of the neck is an accurate, and the preferred, anatomic imaging modality in patients with suspected residual or recurrent locoregional disease, especially for the identification of surgically removable lesions. Other conventional radiographic imaging tools such as CT and MRI are not routinely indicated in the assessment of recurrent thyroid carcinoma. CT is less operator dependent than ultrasonography, but the use of CT is restricted by the fact that it can only be performed without contrast enhancement to avoid iodine contamination, since further radioiodine administration might be necessary. For the detection of local recurrence, the interpretation of CT and MRI is often hampered by fibrosis or altered anatomy due to previous surgery.

Recurrent or occult disease is a frequently encountered problem in patients with MTC. Correct localization of resectable disease is very important, because surgical resection of all tumor tissue is the only effective treatment with curative intent for patients with MTC. Calcitonin and CEA serve as the tumor markers in the follow-up of MTC. No single diagnostic imaging modality is capable of depicting MTC with adequate diagnostic accuracy. Therefore, morphological and functional imaging modalities are performed consecutively to localize metastases.

Ultrasonography of the neck, CT, and MRI are used as morphological imaging tools. Computed tomography and MRI perform well for the detection of organ metastasis, but lack adequate diagnostic certainty for the assessment of local findings and lymph node staging. Functional scintigraphic imaging used in the follow-up of MTC includes imaging with nonspecific tracers such as ^{201}Tl-chloride, pentavalent ^{99m}Tc-dimercaptosuccinic acid ((V)-DMSA), and ^{99m}Tc-sestamibi (MIBI), and more specific tracers like ^{111}In-pentetreotide (somatostatin receptor scintigraphy, SRS), anti-CEA antibodies, or ^{123}I/^{131}I-meta-iodobenzylguanidine (MIBG). However, the diagnostic performance of these conventional nuclear medicine procedures is hampered by poor spatial resolution and variable tracer uptake. The reason for the low sensitivity of the actually used imaging procedures is the high prevalence of typically multiple, hypervascular, small (< 1 cm) hepatic metastases in patients with MTC and elevated calcitonin serum levels. A recent study (Szavcsur et al., 2005) including 60 patients with MTC reported liver involvement in 90% of the patients with MTC shown by liver angiography. Dynamic liver CT and MRI identified hepatic metastases with relatively low frequency (8/58 on MRI, and 7/60 on CT). Although selective venous catheterization is a powerful tool to identify small metastatic lesions, its invasiveness restricts its general use.

Patients with ATC are classified as stage IV at diagnosis and usually present with widespread local invasion and metastatic disease. Ultrasonography of the neck, CT, and MRI are commonly used in the initial staging of ATC, but further elaborate (functional) imaging procedures in the follow-up are not necessary, and have no or limited impact on patient management, because treatment of ATC is usually palliative.

[18]F-Fluoro-2-Deoxy-D-Glucose Positron Emission Tomography

Positron emission tomography (PET) using ^{18}F-fluoro-2-deoxy-D-glucose (FDG) as the radiotracer depicts cancer sites based on their increased glucose metabolism. More precisely, the increased FDG accumulation is based on an increased expression of glucose transporters (GLUT), together with an increase of hexokinase activity and a decreased activity of phosphatase seen in most types of tumors. The technique is increasingly used in cancer care because the molecular and metabolic mechanisms underlying the FDG uptake are completely independent of associated structural characteristics, resulting in a superior diagnostic specificity, and, because metabolic changes precede structural changes, increasing its sensitivity for early disease stages and its potential for early assessment of the post-therapeutic effects. Moreover, the

technique provides a quantitative assessment of the tumor metabolism, which is often needed (e.g., for the early assessment of a therapeutic response). For this, the most widely used index of FDG uptake is the standardized uptake value (SUV) corrected for body weight, calculated from the equation: $SUV = (Q \times W) / Q_{inj}$, where Q is the measured radiotracer concentration at the tumor site; Q_{inj} is the injected activity; and W is the body weight of the patient. Recent data have indicated that in well-standardized conditions the SUV is an excellent surrogate for the absolute FDG metabolic rate (expressed in mmoles/min/gr), as can be determined using complicated acquisition and processing methodology.

Another major advance in PET imaging has been the introduction of PET-CT allowing the quasisimultaneous acquisition of a whole-body CT and PET. The resulting co-registered whole-body PET-CT images allow the perfect integration of the metabolic with the structural and morphologic characteristics of the disease. This new modality has increasingly been used for clinical cancer imaging since 2001 and is rapidly establishing itself as the new standard of metabolic imaging in oncology.

Biological Mechanism of the Enhanced FDG-Uptake in Thyroid Cancer

The normal thyroid shows low avidity for FDG. The enhanced ability of thyroid cancers to transport and accumulate glucose is the basis for the use of FDG-PET to identify malignant tumors and metastases. Early clinical PET data indicated that the avidity of thyroid cancer for FDG is highly variable, often resulting in the nonvisualization of known recurrent or metastatic tumor sites. Fundamental research data, summarized here, have only recently demonstrated the underlying mechanisms responsible for this phenomenon.

Matsuzu et al. (2004) evaluated the differences in the expression of GLUT genes at the mRNA level between normal, diseased, and tumor-derived thyroid cells. They demonstrated GLUT1, 3, 4, and 10 mRNA expression in all thyroid tissues, regardless of histology. No difference was found in GLUT1 mRNA levels between normal thyroid tissue and benign thyroid disease, but GLUT1 mRNA level was significantly higher in tumor cells than in normal thyroid tissue and benign disease. No significant difference between normal and tumor-derived thyroid cells was observed for the expression of the other GLUT subtypes. Therefore, GLUT1 overexpression is most likely responsible for the observed enhanced uptake of glucose in thyroid carcinoma.

Matsuzu et al. (2005) investigated the effect of TSH stimulation on glucose uptake in human thyroid carcinoma cell lines. They showed a statistically significant increased glucose uptake in response to TSH. However, the expression of GLUT genes did not appear to be significantly affected by TSH, suggesting that TSH stimulation leads to an enhanced glucose uptake by increasing the number of preexisting GLUT units to the cell membrane rather than through an increased GLUT gene expression.

Hooft *et al.* (2005) compared FDG uptake in 19 patients with histologically proven recurrent thyroid cancer (13 papillary and 6 follicular tumors) with various biomarkers expected to be involved in the underlying biological mechanisms of FDG uptake in human thyroid cancer tissue. Thirteen of 19 recurrences were positive at PET. The statistical correlation between FDG uptake and the biomarkers revealed that FDG uptake was significantly correlated with hexokinase type I (HK I) and GLUT-1 cytoplasmic expression. The expression of Tg protein was negatively associated with a high FDG uptake, suggesting that FDG accumulation is more intense in poorly differentiated thyroid cancer, because a low level of Tg expression correlates with a poorly differentiated histological type. FDG uptake patterns were not related to age, gender, location of recurrent disease, histological tumor type, or tumor cell density.

In conclusion, the intensity of the accumulation of FDG of thyroid cancer seems to depend mainly on the GLUT1 expression, which is a function of the degree of cellular differentiation and the ambient TSH levels. Therefore, the staging accuracy of FDG-PET should be the highest in patients with dedifferentiating cancers studied in the presence of high TSH levels (hypothyroid state or stimulated by rhTSH).

FDG-PET in the Diagnostic Assessment of a Thyroid Nodule

As discussed earlier, the diagnostic work-up of a thyroid nodule remains problematic. A noninvasive test identifying a patient subgroup with a low cancer risk requiring only clinical follow-up without surgical exploration is lacking. Mitchell *et al.* (2005) recently evaluated the role of FDG-PET/CT in the preoperative assessment of a thyroid nodule in 31 patients with 48 thyroid lesions. They reported a sensitivity of 60% (9/15 malignant lesions were FDG-positive) and a specificity of 91% (30 of 33 benign lesions were FDG-negative), resulting in a positive and negative-predictive value of 75% and 83%, respectively. Based on these data, use of FDG-PET in a nonselected patient group should be discouraged.

Preliminary data indicate that FDG-PET could be clinically useful in patients with thyroid nodules with a follicular cytology in whom it is often impossible to differentiate adenoma from carcinoma (see Introduction). It has been reported (Kresnik *et al.*, 2003) that FDG-PET should be able to distinguish nodules with follicular cytology (Hürthle cell excluded) that need surgery (follicular carcinoma and follicular variant of papillary carcinoma) and patients that do not need surgery (multinodular goiter and follicular adenoma). Hürthle cell adenoma is a benign condition known to have

higher SUV, making a distinction between Hürthle cell adenoma and carcinoma based on FDG-PET impossible. In conclusion, FDG-PET is not recommended for the diagnostic assessment of thyroid lesions. Further studies are needed to define its utility in specific patient subgroups, such as those with follicular cytology.

FDG-PET in the Follow-Up of Differentiated Thyroid Cancer

FDG-PET in Differentiated Thyroid Cancer

Progressive dedifferentiation of thyroid cancer cells leads to a loss of iodine-concentrating ability, with resultant false-negative whole-body ^{131}I scintigraphy. The majority of these metastatic thyroid cancers still produce Tg, suggesting only partial dedifferentiation. The pattern of alternating ^{131}I and FDG uptake in metastatic thyroid cancer lesions has been described as the "flip-flop" phenomenon. This pattern was hypothesized to allow biochemical grading of thyroid cancer: FDG uptake seemed to be an indicator of poor functional differentiation (with the loss of iodine-transporting capacity), and possibly higher malignancy in thyroid cancer. Even in the same patient, FDG and iodine uptake may differ among the different metastatic sites, as is illustrated in the patient presented in Figure 1. Fundamental data, described earlier, have indicated that the loss of cellular differentiation leads to higher expression of GLUT, which itself is the important determinator of FDG accumulation. This offers the rationale for the clinical use of FDG-PET in recurrent or metastatic DTC.

Several studies have reported the utility of FDG-PET in thyroid cancer patients who present with an elevated Tg and a negative whole-body ^{131}I scintigraphy. Moreover, FDG-PET has been shown to have a considerable impact on the clinical management of these patients. The U.S. government has recently approved Medicare reimbursement for the use of FDG-PET in thyroid cancer patients who have a Tg > 10 ng/ml and a negative radioiodine whole-body scan in order to localize disease.

In a large multicenter study (Grünwald *et al.*, 1999), the clinical significance of FDG-PET was evaluated in 222 DTC patients (134 papillary, 80 follicular, 8 mixed-cell type tumors), previously treated with total thyroidectomy and a mean of three to four treatments with radioiodine. The overall sensitivity of FDG-PET for the detection of residual or metastatic DTC was 75%. In the group of patients with elevated Tg levels (≥ 5 ng/ml), the sensitivity (76%) was similar to that in the whole group. Considering patients with negative post-therapeutic ^{131}I scintigraphy, the sensitivity of FDG-PET was 85%. Specificity was 90% in the whole patient group. The sensitivity and specificity of the post-therapeutic whole-body

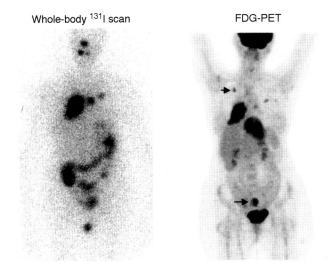

Whole-body ^{131}I scan   FDG-PET

Figure 1 The images show a whole-body ^{131}I scan and a maximum intensity projection (MIP) of an FDG-PET scan of a 64-year-old woman with known metastatic disease from a follicular carcinoma. The patient was previously treated by total thyroidectomy, several treatments with ^{131}I, external radiotherapy, chemotherapy, and surgery (inferior lobectomy of the right lung). Whole-body (+ tomography; not shown in the figure) ^{131}I imaging was performed 3 days after the administration of a therapeutic dose of ^{131}I (5920 MBq). It shows intense and extended ^{131}I uptake at the basis of the right lung and two smaller lesions at the left mediastinum and the left lung. FDG-PET performed one day before the therapeutic dose of ^{131}I shows besides the lesions seen on ^{131}I imaging, two additional significant lesions (arrows): a lesion at the apex of the right lung and an intense subcutaneous lesion localized posterior of the coccyx. The subcutaneous lesion posterior of the coccyx was surgically removed. Anatomopathology showed metastases of a poorly differentiated follicular thyroid tumor. Despite the treatment with ^{131}I and the surgical resection of the subcutaneous lesion, follow-up at 6 months showed a progressive disease with a minimal therapeutic effect at the FDG-avid lesions and the appearance of several new metastases in lungs, liver, lymph nodes, and soft tissue.

^{131}I scintigraphy (2–7 days after therapy with ^{131}I) were 50% and 99%, respectively. Tumor tissue was missed in only 7% when the results of FDG-PET and whole-body ^{131}I scintigraphy were combined.

FDG-PET In Hürthle Cell Carcinoma

Hürthle cell carcinoma (HCC) is a more aggressive, mostly follicular cancer variant with a higher risk of distant metastases and a poorer survival. Despite high differentiation and preserved Tg expression (allowing a follow-up for recurrent disease with Tg), HCC has a low or nonavidity for iodine. Therefore, in HCC the diagnostic and therapeutic use of iodine isotopes is mostly inadequate. FDG-PET is efficient for the detection of recurrent HCC. A meta-analysis (Plotkin et al., 2002) including data of 35 patients of two studies revealed an overall sensitivity of 92%, a specificity of 80%, and an overall accuracy of 89%. The same sensitivity was reported in another study (Lowe et al., 2003) including data of 14 FDG-PET scans (of 12 patients). Interestingly,

FDG-PET showed more extensive disease than the other imaging modalities. It was reported that 50% (7/14) of the FDG-PET scans lead to a change in patient management.

FDG-PET in Insular Thyroid Cancer

Insular thyroid cancer is a subtype of follicular thyroid carcinoma characterized by early dedifferentiation and hence unfavorable prognosis. Because insular thyroid cancer is rare, limited published data are available on its imaging with FDG-PET. Diehl et al. (2003) evaluated the use of FDG-PET for re-staging and follow-up in a limited series of 5 patients with increased Tg under TSH stimulation. All patients had been previously treated with ablative ^{131}I doses. Whole-body ^{131}I scintigraphy (performed within 10 days after the FDG-PET) was negative in 4 out of 5 patients, whereas FDG-PET depicted a total of 10 tumor sites (at least 1 in each patient) and had a direct impact on the further management in all 5 patients.

Prognosis for Differentiated Thyroid Cancer Based on FDG-PET

In addition to lesion detection accuracy, it has been shown that FDG-PET is an independent prognostic indicator in thyroid cancer. Robbins et al. (2006) evaluated the relationship between FDG-PET results and survival in patients with metastatic DTC. They analyzed the initial FDG-PET scans of 400 patients with follicular-cell derived DTC. A total of 221 (+/− 55%) of the PET scans were interpreted to be abnormal. Age (at the time of the FDG-PET scan), initial AJCC stage, histology, serum Tg (≤ or > 2 ng/ml on thyroxin suppression), radioiodine uptake, and FDG-PET outcomes all correlated with survival by univariate analysis. The site of the metastatic lesion was another important variable: patients with local recurrences on FDG-PET fared much better than those with distant metastases on FDG-PET. However, in a multivariate analysis, only age and PET results (namely, the FDG status, number of FDG-avid lesions, and the SUV of the most active lesion) continued to be strong predictors of survival. Patients with a positive FDG-PET had 7.3 times the risk of dying compared to patients (with or without metastases) with a negative FDG-PET. The median survival of the FDG-PET positive patients was only 53 months. At the end of the study, 89 (of 221) FDG positive patients had died, compared to only 4 (of 179) patients in the FDG negative cohort. The initial TNM stage correlated with survival on univariate analysis, but was not significant on multivariate analysis. In fact, the stage I–III patients with FDG-avid lesions had a survival very similar to all of the stage IV patients.

Based on the findings of this study, the authors recommended that an FDG-PET should be considered for all thyroid cancer patients who have a known or suspected metastatic lesion based on clinical findings, radiological imaging, or an elevated serum Tg (> 10 ng/ml on thyroxin suppression). The FDG-PET findings can be used to stratify these patients in terms of prognosis.

Impact of FDG-PET on Thyroid Cancer Management

Performing FDG-PET in MTC is likely to have a considerable impact on patient management. Wang *et al.* (2001), in a retrospective study, evaluated the ability of ^{131}I to destroy FDG-avid metastatic lesions in 25 MTC patients. All patients received at least one dose of ^{131}I treatment before a second FDG-PET was performed. The average interval between the two PET scans was 13 months and 10 months between the ^{131}I treatment and the follow-up FDG-PET. The follow-up FDG-PET showed a significant rise of the total volume of FDG-avid metastases and no significant changes in maximum SUV or serum Tg levels after ^{131}I therapy, while in a control group of FDG-PET-negative patients, the serum Tg significantly decreased to 38% of baseline after ^{131}I therapy.

Thus, the avidity of a lesion for FDG seems to indicate a certain resistance to radioiodine therapy. This is probably a consequence of a decreased iodine accumulation seen in the FDG positive lesions, leading to a decreased delivered absorbed dose per mCi ^{131}I administered, and thus to a decreased therapeutic effect. Further studies using PET-CT and [124]I (a positron emitter with a long half-life) are needed to establish dose-response curves in this type of lesion. In conclusion, the presence of FDG-avid lesions should lead the physician to consider other, often more aggressive therapeutic options (e.g., surgery, external radiation, chemotherapy, or redifferentiation therapy with retinoic acid) because high-dose ^{131}I therapy appears to have little or no effect on the viability of metastatic FDG-avid thyroid cancer lesions.

Influence of TSH Stimulation on FDG-PET in Thyroid Cancer

Similar to whole-body ^{131}I scintigraphy, FDG-PET imaging seems to be more accurate for the detection of recurrence or metastases of DTC when TSH levels are elevated, either due to withdrawal of thyroid hormone replacement therapy or due to administration of rhTSH (Petrich *et al.*, 2002; Chin *et al.*, 2004). Moreover, the use of rhTSH has the advantage of avoiding the morbidity of hypothyroidism and the risk of tumor progression associated with temporary withdrawal of thyroid hormone replacement therapy. Indication of whether or not to perform the PET study under TSH stimulation depends on the specific clinical problem setting. If a maximum FDG-PET sensitivity is recommended, for example, in a preoperative setting, then high TSH stimulation is needed. This is not necessary when, in the case of a patient with known metastatic disease, one is interested in evaluating

the residual metabolic activity of a known metastatic lesion under an adequate hormonal suppressive therapy.

FDG-PET in Medullary Thyroid Cancer

Despite the availability of numerous morphological and functional imaging tools (see Introduction), the localization of recurrent or metastatic disease often remains inadequate in patients with MTC. Several reports have shown encouraging results by FDG-PET imaging in patients with MTC. In a large retrospective multicenter study (Diehl *et al.*, 2001) including 100 FDG-PET scans in 85 patients, a comparative data analysis was performed between the findings obtained by SRS, (V)-DMSA, MIBI, CT, and MRI. The highest lesion detection probability (68%) was obtained by FDG-PET (versus 58% for MRI, 53% for CT, and less than 30% for all conventional nuclear medicine procedures. In that study, combining FDG-PET and MRI results raised the lesion detection probability to 90% (69% for FDG-PET and 58% for MRI alone). The lesion detection probability of FDG-PET was independent of the calcitonin level. The sensitivity and specificity of FDG-PET with respect to the histologically confirmed lesions were 78% and 79%, respectively. The sensitivity and specificity of the morphological imaging procedures were 82% and 67%, respectively, for MRI, and 50% and 20%, respectively, for CT. The sensitivity of conventional nuclear medicine procedures using single photon emitters (SRS, (V)-DMSA, and MIBI) was low (25%, 33%, and 25%, respectively), with a high specificity (92%, 78%, and 100%, respectively).

Another study (Szakall *et al.*, 2002) studied 40 patients with a postoperatively elevated plasma calcitonin level. They reported that compared to other imaging procedures, FDG-PET was more sensitive in localizing metastatic lymph node involvement especially in the cervical and mediastinal regions (which represent the first lymphatic levels of thyroid cancer). FDG-PET showed lymph node involvement in 95% (38/40) of the patients, compared to 65%, 54%, and 7%, respectively, for CT, MRI, and ^{131}I-MIBG. The positive FDG-PET findings were confirmed in 10 of 38 patients by histology and in 15 patients by subsequent radiological examinations. In the remaining 13 patients, the positive FDG-PET lesions were not validated, but clinical follow-up showed no contradictions with the FDG-PET findings. FDG-PET failed to detect several small pulmonary end hepatic lesions, partially due to the lack of iterative reconstruction and attenuation correction in this study.

In a recent prospective study (de Groot *et al.*, 2004), 26 patients were included with biochemical evidence (elevated calcitonin or CEA serum levels) of minimal residual or recurrent MTC after total thyroidectomy with central compartment dissection and additional selective neck dissection on indication. The FDG-PET findings were compared with conventional nuclear imaging (SRS and (V)-DMSA) and morphological imaging (CT, MRI, and ultrasonography, including bone scintigraphy) and validated by histology when possible. Lesions were detected in 50% of the patients by FDG-PET, in 19% and 21%, respectively, by SRS and (V)-DMSA, and in 40% of the patients by morphological imaging. The lesion-based analysis demonstrated a sensitivity of 96% for FDG-PET, compared to 41%, 57%, and 87%, respectively, for SRS, (V)-DMSA, and morphological imaging. In patients with a negative FDG-PET, no MTC was detected by any other imaging procedure. Positive FDG-PET findings led to surgery for resection of residual tumor or metastases in 9 of 26 patients (35%), and MTC was confirmed in 8 of 9 patients by histology. FDG-PET was false positive in one patient, where histology revealed normal thymus tissue without MTC. Postoperative serum calcitonin levels were reduced by an average of 58 ± 31% in all patients. One patient achieved disease-free status. The results of this study indicate that FDG-PET is the most feasible imaging procedure yet available in patients with postoperative elevated calcitonin or CEA serum levels for the detection of minimal residual or recurrent MTC. It has been shown that FDG-PET has a clinical impact on patient management and may be used for selecting patients who might benefit from surgery with curative intent and for guiding additional morphological imaging preoperatively.

In conclusion, compared to other noninvasive functional and morphological imaging tools, FDG-PET provides the highest lesion detection probability for MTC tissue, with a high sensitivity and specificity. However, FDG-PET alone does not provide an optimal sensitivity for the detection of all, particularly small, recurrences or metastases in patients with MTC. The reason for the relatively low lesion detection probability of FDG-PET, MRI, and CT is the high prevalence (up to 90%) of small infracentimetric hepatic metastases in these patients. Neuroendocrine tumors generally show a slow growth rate and low proliferation index, and hence a normal FDG metabolism. This is a limiting factor for the use of FDG PET in patients with MTC. However, the presence of FDG positive lesions in MTC might be a sign of dedifferentiation. Therefore, it can be hypothesized that FDG PET could depict patients with a more aggressive course of disease and hence might have a prognostic value in patients with MTC. Further studies are needed to clarify this point of interest.

FDG-PET in Anaplastic Thyroid Cancer

A limited number of reports (Jadvar and Fischman, 1999; Kresnik et al., 2003) indicate that ATC-derived lesions show intense FDG uptake. However, no major studies have evaluated the utility of FDG-PET in ATC. This is probably because ATC is relatively rare and FDG-PET has no clinical relevant impact on patient management, inasmuch as treatment of ATC is usually palliative at initial diagnosis.

Thyroid FDG-PET Incidentaloma

The normal thyroid is usually not visualized on FDG-PET because it shows low avidity for FDG. Occasionally, focal or diffuse increased FDG uptake in the thyroid is noted as an incidental finding when studying patients for another indication. A thyroid FDG-PET incidentaloma is defined as a newly identified thyroid lesion on FDG-PET imaging in a patient without a history of thyroid disease. Diffusely increased FDG uptake is generally benign and due to chronic thyroiditis, whereas focal thyroid FDG-PET incidentaloma carries a certain risk for malignancy. Three large retrospective studies (Cohen et al., 2001; Kang et al., 2003; Kim et al., 2005) including 4525, 1330, and 4136 patients, respectively, showed a similar prevalence of thyroid FDG-PET incidentaloma of 2.2–2.3% (0.6–1.1% with diffuse uptake and 1.1–1.6% with focal uptake). There was no significant difference between the prevalence of thyroid carcinoma in cancer patients and healthy individuals (Kang et al., 2003). In 27 to 50% of the patients with focal thyroid FDG uptake, histological diagnosis revealed the presence of thyroid malignancy. The majority (57–100%) of the malignant focal thyroid lesions were papillary carcinoma. Other types of thyroid cancer (e.g., HCC) were less frequently revealed. In one study, 2 of 4136 patients presented with metastasis to the thyroid from breast and esophagus carcinoma. The benign focal FDG-PET incidentalomas revealed mostly nodular hyperplasia, follicular adenoma, or indeterminate follicular lesions. In two out of three studies, the SUV was significantly higher in malignant lesions than in benign lesions. However, in the most recent study (Kim et al., 2005) and in accordance with our own experience, the SUV could not efficiently differentiate malignant from benign lesions in focal thyroid FDG-PET incidentalomas.

In conclusion, the high risk for thyroid malignancy (27–50%) in focal thyroid FDG-PET incidentaloma warrants further investigation by ultrasonography and cytological or histological examination if the nature of the thyroid disease has an impact on further patient management.

References

Chin, B.B., Patel, P., Cohade, C., Ewertz, M., Wahl, R., and Ladenson, P. 2004. Recombinant human thyrotropin stimulation of fluoro-D-glucose positron emission tomography uptake in well-differentiated thyroid carcinoma. *J. Clin. Endocrinol. Metab.* 89:91–95.

Cohen, M.S., Arslan, N., Dehdashti, F., Doherty, G.M., Lairmore, T.C., Brunt, L.M., and Moley, J.F. 2001. Risk of malignancy in thyroid incidentalomas identified by fluorodeoxyglucose-positron emission tomography. *Surgery* 130:941–946.

de Groot, J.W., Links, T.P., Jager, P.L., Kahraman, T., and Plukker, J.T. 2004. Impact of 18F-fluoro-2-deoxy-D-glucose positron emission tomography (FDG-PET) in patients with biochemical evidence of recurrent or residual medullary thyroid cancer. *Ann. Surg. Oncol.* 11:786–794.

Diehl, M., Graichen, S., Menzel, C., Lindhorst, E., and Grunwald, F. 2003. F-18 FDG PET in insular thyroid cancer. *Clin. Nucl. Med.* 28:728–731.

Diehl, M., Risse, J.H., Brandt-Mainz, K., Dietlein, M., Bohuslavizki, K.H., Matheja, P., Lange, H., Bredow, J., Korber, C., and Grunwald, F. 2001. Fluorine-18 fluorodeoxyglucose positron emission tomography in medullary thyroid cancer: results of a multicentre study. *Eur. J. Nucl. Med.* 28:1671–1676.

Grünwald, F., Kalicke, T., Feine, U., Lietzenmayer, R., Scheidhauer, K., Dietlein, M., Schober, O., Lerch, H., Brandt-Mainz, K., Burchert, W., Hiltermann, G., Cremerius, U., and Biersack, H.J. 1999. Fluorine-18 fluorodeoxyglucose positron emission tomography in thyroid cancer: results of a multicentre study. *Eur. J. Nucl. Med.* 26:1547–1552.

Hooft, L., van der Veldt, A.A., van Diest, P.J., Hoekstra, O.S., Berkhof, J., Teule, G.J., and Molthoff, C.F. 2005. [18F]fluorodeoxyglucose uptake in recurrent thyroid cancer is related to hexokinase I expression in the primary tumor. *J. Clin. Endocrinol. Metab.* 90:328–334.

Jadvar, H., and Fischman, A.J. 1999. Evaluation of rare tumors with [F-18]fluorodeoxyglucose positron emission tomography. *Clin. Positron Imaging* 2:153–158.

Kang, K.W., Kim, S.K., Kang, H.S., Lee, E.S., Sim, J.S., Lee, I.G., Jeong, S.Y., and Kim, S.W. 2003. Prevalence and risk of cancer of focal thyroid incidentaloma identified by 18F-fluorodeoxyglucose positron emission tomography for metastasis evaluation and cancer screening in healthy subjects. *J. Clin. Endocrinol. Metab.* 88:4100–4104.

Kim, T.Y., Kim, W.B., Ryu, J.S., Gong, G., Hong, S.J., and Shong, Y.K. 2005. 18F-fluorodeoxyglucose uptake in thyroid from positron emission tomogram (PET) for evaluation in cancer patients: high prevalence of malignancy in thyroid PET incidentaloma. *Laryngoscope* 115:1074–1078.

Kresnik, E., Gallowitsch, H.J., Mikosch, P., Stettner, H., Igerc, I., Gomez, I., Kumnig, G., and Lind, P. 2003. Fluorine-18-fluorodeoxyglucose positron emission tomography in the preoperative assessment of thyroid nodules in an endemic goiter area. *Surgery* 133:294–299.

Lowe, V.J., Mullan, B.P., Hay, I.D., McIver, B., and Kasperbauer J.L. 2003. 18F-FDG PET of patients with Hurthle cell carcinoma. *J. Nucl. Med.* 44:1402–1406.

Matsuzu, K., Segade, F., Matsuzu, U., Carter, A., Bowden, D.W., and Perrier, N.D. 2004. Differential expression of glucose transporters in normal and pathologic thyroid tissue. *Thyroid* 14:806–812.

Matsuzu, K., Segade, F., Wong, M., Clark, O.H., Perrier, N.D., and Bowden, D.W. 2005. Glucose transporters in the thyroid. *Thyroid* 15:545–550.

Mazzaferri, E.L., Robbins, R.J., Spencer, A., Braverman, L.E., Pacini, F., Wartofsky, L., Haugen, B.R., Sherman, S.I., Cooper, D.S., Braunstein, G.D., Lee, S., Davies, T.F., Arafah, B.M., Ladenson, P.W., and Pinchera, A. 2003. A consensus report of the role of serum thyroglobulin as a monitoring method for low-risk patients with papillary thyroid carcinoma. *J. Clin. Endocrinol. Metab.* 88:1433–1441.

Mitchell, J.C., Grant, F., Evenson, A.R., Parker, J.A., Hasselgren, P.O., and Parangi, S. 2005. Preoperative evaluation of thyroid nodules with 18FDG-PET/CT. *Surgery* 138:1166–1174.

Petrich, T., Borner, A.R., Otto, D., Hofmann, M., and Knapp, W.H. 2002. Influence of rhTSH on [(18)F]fluorodeoxyglucose uptake by differentiated thyroid carcinoma. *Eur. J. Nucl. Med. Mol. Imaging* 29:641–647.

Plotkin, M., Hautzel, H., Krause, B.J., Schmidt, D., Larisch, R., Mottaghy, F.M., Boemer, A.R., Herzog, H., Vosberg, H., and Muller-Gartner, H.W. 2002. Implication of 2-18fluoro-2-deoxyglucose positron emission tomography in the follow-up of Hürthle cell thyroid cancer. *Thyroid* 12:155–161.

Robbins, R.J., Wan, Q., Grewal, R.K., Reibke, R., Gonen, M., Strauss, H.W., Tuttle, R.M., Drucker, W., and Larson, S.M. 2006. Real-time prognosis for metastatic thyroid carcinoma based on 2-[18F]fluoro-2-deoxy-D-glucose-positron emission tomography scanning. *J. Clin. Endocrinol. Metab.* 91:498–505.

Sherman, S.I. 2003. Thyroid carcinoma. *Lancet* 361:501–511.

Szakall, S., Jr., Esik, O., Bajzik, G., Repa, I., Dabasi, G., Sinkovics, I., Agoston, P., and Tron, L. 2002. 18F-FDG PET detection of lymph node metastases in medullary thyroid carcinoma. *J. Nucl. Med.* 43:66–71.

Szavcsur, P., Godeny, M., Bajzik, G., Lengyel, E., Repa, I., Tron, L., Boer, A., Vincze, B., Poti, Z., Szabolcs, I., and Esik, O. 2005. Angiography-proven liver metastases explain low efficacy of lymph node dissections in medullary thyroid cancer patients. *Eur. J. Surg. Oncol.* 31:1051–1052.

Wang, W., Larson, S.M., Tuttle, R.M., Kalaigian, H., Kolbert, K., Sonenberg, M., and Robbins, R.J. 2001. Resistance of [18f]-fluorodeoxyglucose-avid metastatic thyroid cancer lesions to treatment with high-dose radioactive iodine. *Thyroid* 11:1169–1175.

56

Diagnosis of Thyroid Cancer in Children: Value of Power Doppler Ultrasound

Andrej Lyshchik and Valentina Drozd

Introduction

Thyroid nodules are relatively rare in children and have a prevalence ranging from 0.2 to 1.8% as compared to 4–7% in the general adult population (Raab *et al.*, 1995; Tan and Gharib, 1997). However, their real prevalence remains unknown because in most cases they are asymptomatic and detected incidentally by parents or by doctors during routine examinations for other purposes. In childhood and adolescence, the incidence of thyroid nodules may be influenced by dietary factors (iodine deficiency, goiterogens, iodine supplementation) and the type of investigation used to detect nodes. The first studies were based on neck palpation, and it is common knowledge that this is a very subjective method. More recent studies using ultrasound (US) examinations revealed significantly higher frequencies of thyroid nodules. However, at least in areas with sufficient iodine intake, the current prevalence of nodular thyroid disease in children has been estimated to be 5 to 10 times lower than that observed in adults.

In a random pediatric population, the majority of thyroid nodules are benign, hormonally inactive cysts, colloid nodules, or follicular adenomas. Autonomous toxic adenomas are capable of excessive amounts of thyroid hormone secretion, but they are exceedingly uncommon during the first two decades of life.

Thyroid nodules are more likely to be malignant in children than in adults. In the past, it was estimated that as many as half of them were carcinomas, but later studies indicated a lower fraction, an ~ 15–20% proved to be malignant, as opposed to 5% in adults. This decrease may reflect the decreasing exposure of children to radiation in recent years (Hung, 1999; Castro and Gharib, 2000). Therefore, pediatric thyroid nodules should be viewed with suspicion for cancer, and the diagnostic approach should be more aggressive than in adults.

U.S. National Cancer Institute statistics suggest that the annual incidence of thyroid cancer is 0.5 per 100,000 for patients younger than 20 years (Gorlin and Sallan, 1990). According to the data from the population-based Surveillance, Epidemiology, and End Results (SEER) program, this represents 1.4% of all pediatric malignancies in the United States with a steady rise in thyroid cancer incidence from the lowest rate at age 8–10 years throughout adolescence to adulthood (Gorlin and Sallan, 1990). Among 15–19-year-old patients, it is the eighth most commonly diagnosed cancer (7.5% of all cancers) and the second most common cancer among females in this age group (13.4% of all female cancers) (Wu *et al.*, 2005). Data from Germany showed that thyroid cancer totals about 0.5 to 1.5% of all malignancies in children and adolescents, which is comparable with SEER (Bucsky and Parlowsky, 1997).

Pathogenesis

Genetics and radiation exposure play important roles in thyroid cancer development in children. Five to 10% of cases of papillary thyroid carcinoma are familial and are usually inherited in an autosomal dominant manner. In addition, thyroid cancer is a well-known feature of patients with MEN II, Cowder, Gardner, and Pendred syndromes, Carney complex, and familial polyposis.

The thyroid gland of children is unusually sensitive to exposure to external radiation. As a result of the accident at the Chernobyl power station in April 1986, a very large population was exposed to high levels of isotopes of iodine (131-I, 133-I) and tellurium132, a precursor of 132-I. Accumulation of radioactive iodine by normal iodine-trapping mechanisms resulted in significant radiation doses to the thyroid gland (Kazakov *et al.*, 1992). As a result, a substantial increase in the incidence of childhood thyroid carcinoma was observed in Belarus and Ukraine. For example, in children younger than 15 years, exposed by radiation from the Chernobyl accident in April 1986, the relative incidence of thyroid cancer increased in Belarus from 0.1–0.3 per 100,000 before the accident to 3.3–13.5 per 100,000 in 1990–1996 (Reiners, 1998).

Another group of pediatric patients "at risk" are those who have received irradiation and chemotherapy for leukemia, Hodgkin's disease, and other malignancies of the head and neck, or those treated by radiation for head, neck, or mediastinal conditions (Ron, 1996; de Vathaire *et al.*, 1999). It is estimated that up to 50% of these children have elevated levels of thyroid-stimulating hormone (TSH) within the first year of therapy when no thyroid hormone supplementation is provided. Of these, 10 to 30% patients develop benign thyroid nodules and are considered at risk for thyroid cancer. The latent period between radiation exposure and thyroid cancer is at least 3 or 5 years, with the risk of thyroid cancer development persisting for 40 years (Ron *et al.*, 1995).

In such patients, systematic screening using US examination of the thyroid gland is used for the early detection of clinically undetectable nodules in high-risk groups/persons in an attempt to achieve the most effective treatment of thyroid cancer (Eden *et al.*, 2001; Drozd *et al.*, 1999). Unfortunately, the diagnostic accuracy of ultrasound criteria in differentiating between benign and malignant thyroid nodules in children is still controversial, and the question of whether detected thyroid nodules should undergo cytological and histological evaluation remains unresolved (Yip *et al.*, 1994; Bentley *et al.*, 2003; Koike *et al.*, 2001).

Clinical Presentation

The average age at diagnosis is 9 years, and in rare cases the onset may be as early as the first year of life. The ratio of girls to boys among children with thyroid cancer is 2:1, in contrast to the much higher predominance of girls with thyroid enlargement from other causes (Rudolph *et al.*, 2003). Thus, nodular enlargement is more likely to be cancerous in boys than in girls. Several studies showed that thyroid carcinoma in pediatric patients differs from that in adults with respect to its presentation and outcome. In children, it tends to present at a more advanced stage than in adults with a higher frequency of lymph node and pulmonary metastases (Grigsby *et al.*, 2002). Therefore, cancer diagnosis at an early stage is very important especially in a high-risk population because capsular invasion followed by distant spread or in some cases "dedifferentiation" can develop during the course of the disease (Pacini *et al.*, 1997). Therefore, some authors believe that all thyroid nodules that develop in children are potentially malignant and therefore should be excised as soon as possible (Desjardins *et al.*, 1987). Others believe that, because of the low incidence and degree of malignancy and the high level of suppressibility with L-T4 therapy, the risk of death and disability as a result of surgery is too high to justify a surgical approach (Van Vliet *et al.*, 1987). Consequently, most physicians adopt an intermediate approach and individualize the diagnosis and management of these patients.

Diagnostic Ultrasound Imaging

Ultrasound examination is a widely accepted imaging modality used to characterize thyroid nodules. It provides accurate estimation of thyroid size, gives a rough estimate of tissue structure, and aids in the accurate placement of needles for tissue biopsy or therapeutic purposes (Jarlov *et al.*, 1993; Naik and Bury, 1998). Reports on many studies on adult populations have been published assessing the ability to predict whether a thyroid nodule is benign or malignant on the basis of US findings. Several US features have been found to be associated with an increased risk of thyroid cancer, including presence of calcifications, hypoechogenicity, irregular margins, absence of a halo, and predominance of solid composition. However, the diagnostic accuracy for these criteria is extremely variable from study to study, and no US feature has both a high sensitivity and a high positive-predictive value for thyroid cancer (Frates *et al.*, 2005).

In the past decade, transducers with color Doppler capabilities have made it possible to display the speed and direction of blood flow. This methodology encodes the frequency of pulsed Doppler signals in color, which is overlaid on B-mode sonograms with their two-dimensional spatial information. Compared with conventional color flow Doppler imaging, power-mode Doppler uses the amplitude of the Doppler spectrum for signal processing since it is more dependent on the number of blood cells than on the flow rate. That makes power Doppler a more sensitive tool for assessing the low-speed blood flow within thyroid nodules.

Unlike conventional color flow Doppler, one characteristic of power-mode signal processing is that here the signals of opposing flow directions do not cancel out but add. This increases the sensitivity even for unfavorable angles of incidence. Modern Doppler technology allows blood flow imaging of vessels with very small diameter (less than 100 μm) and slow flow rates of only a few mm per second. Therefore, in many studies, power-mode Doppler sonography proved to be superior to color flow Doppler imaging with respect to thyroid imaging (Cerbone et al., 1999).

The most frequently used approach to evaluate the results of power Doppler sonography of thyroid tumors is to assess the intensity of perinodular or intranodular blood flow subjectively by comparing it with the surrounding thyroid tissue. In general, three types of nodule vascularization can be identified: type I, absence of flow signals; type II, increased perinodular vascularization; and type III, increased perinodular and intranodular vascularization (Figs. 1-3)

Benign Thyroid Lesions

Benign disorders that may present as solitary or multiple thyroid nodules include adenomas (e.g., follicular, embryo-nal, Hürthle cell), colloid (adenomatous) nodule, lymphocytic thyroiditis, thyroglossal duct cyst, ectopically located normal thyroid tissue, a single median thyroid, agenesis of one of the lateral thyroid lobes with hypertrophy of the contralateral lobe, thyroid cysts, and abscess. However, the vast majority of thyroid nodules in children are represented by cysts and nontoxic nonautoimmune nodular goiters and follicular adenomas. It should be noted that the presence of multiple nodules, as detected by ultrasonography or any other imaging procedure, does not exclude carcinoma. Indeed, it is just as likely to be present in a multinodular goiter as in a solitary nodule.

Thyroid cysts in pediatric patients are usually associated with nontoxic diffuse goiters. The majority of such cysts are localized colloid-filled follicles that appear as well-defined anechoic areas on B-mode on ultrasonograms and completely avascular on power Doppler ultrasonograms. On the other hand, some cysts, presumably those developed as a result of colloid nodule necrosis or hemorrhage, are complex, with both cystic and solid components, and these are as likely to be a carcinoma as is a solid nodule. Power Doppler US might be useful for evaluating mixed cystic and solid nodules and predominantly cystic nodules with a focal area that appears solid. This helps differentiate solid tissue, which will have blood flow, from an avascular blood clot or debris. When US-guided fine needle aspiration (FNA) is performed on such nodules, the needle should be directed toward the regions with visible flow to increase the likelihood of a diagnostic aspirate.

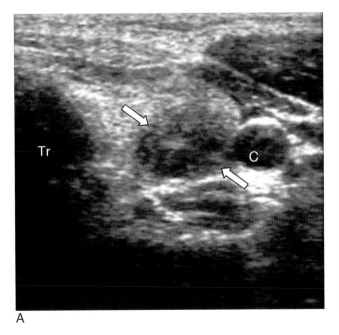

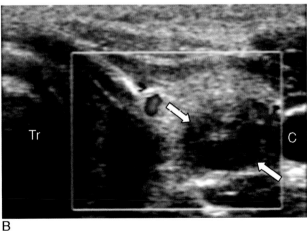

A   B

Figure 1 Absence of intranodular flow signals in thyroid papillary carcinoma (type I vascularization). (**A**) Transverse gray-scale image of a 15-year-old female demonstrates an 8-mm hypoechoic heterogeneous nodule with moderately irregular margin and absence of a "halo" sign (arrows). (**B**) Transverse power Doppler image of the same nodule in power Doppler mode demonstrates the absence of intranodular flow signals. C—carotid artery, T—thyroid gland, Tr—trachea.

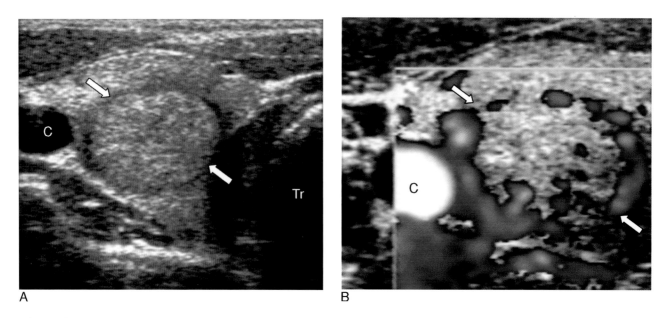

Figure 2 Increased perinodular vascularization in thyroid follicular adenoma (type II vascularization). (**A**) Transverse gray-scale image of a 13-year-old female demonstrates a 14-mm isoechoic homogeneous nodule with regular margin and "halo" sign (arrows). (**B**) Transverse power Doppler image of the same nodule (arrows) in power Doppler mode demonstrates substantially increased perinodular flow signals. C—carotid artery, Tr—trachea.

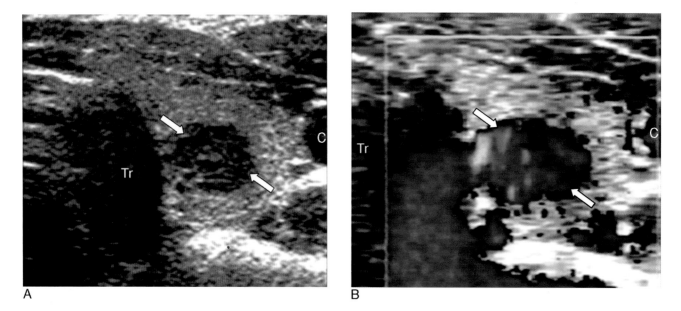

Figure 3 Increased intranodular vascularization of thyroid papillary carcinoma (type III vascularization). (**A**) Transverse gray-scale image of a 16-year-old female demonstrates a 7-mm hypoechoic, heterogeneous nodule with irregular margin and absence of "halo" sign (arrows). (**B**) Transverse power Doppler image of the same nodule in power Doppler mode demonstrates the noticeably increased intranodular vascularization. C—carotid artery, Tr—trachea.

Small solid lesions of nodular goiter and follicular adenoma often appear to be iso- or hypoechoic lesions with a relatively regular outline and absence of "halo" sign. The echogenic structure of benign thyroid nodules is usually heterogeneous. Small areas of cystic degeneration, hemorrhage, and necrosis may be seen in "old" nodules, especially in those larger then 15 mm in size.

Studies based on power Doppler examination of thyroid nodules in children as well as some well-documented studies in adults, reported significant size-dependency of the patterns of thyroid nodule vascularization (Lyshchik *et al.*, 2005; Rago *et al.*, 1998). Small benign nodules (less than 15 mm in diameter) are usually characterized by the absence of increased intranodular vascularization. However, with increase in nodule size, the increasing mass can develop a peripheral vascular rim, which is visualized as a Type II flow pattern on power Doppler ultrasonograms. With continued increase in nodule dimensions, the size of intranodular vessels and the speed of the blood flow in them increase, and those changes are usually detected by modern high-resolution ultrasound scanners. As a result, up to 50% of large (more than 15 mm in diameter) thyroid nodules in children might be characterized by Type III vascularization (Lyshchik *et al.*, 2005).

In iodine-deficient regions, benign thyroid nodules are often accompanied by endemic goiter, which on ultrasonography appears as diffusely enlarged thyroid lobes with a uniform or discretely irregular echo pattern. In some patients, benign thyroid nodules might be accompanied by goitrous autoimmune thyroiditis (Hashimoto's thyroiditis) or Graves' disease. In all patients with underlying diffuse thyroid diseases, power Doppler ultrasonography reveals rich vascularity and increased flow, which are correlated with the degree of thyroid inflammation and/or hyperfunction. Therefore, power Doppler assessment of thyroid nodules in patients with concomitant diffuse thyroid disease is challenging and in severe cases may be significantly affected by increased background Doppler signals from surrounding thyroid parenchyma leading to an increase in false-positive findings in patients with benign thyroid nodules. In some cases, power Doppler patterns may also be affected by the location of the lesion, as has been noted in superficially located timors, which may be a consequence of better signal reception from the superficial lesion. Therefore, in deeply located lesions, the absence of color signals could be due to an artifact rather than to poor vascularity (Mazzeo *et al.*, 1997).

Thyroid Cancer

Malignant thyroid disorders that present as thyroid nodules include tumors of follicular (papillary, follicular, and anaplastic) and nonfollicular origin (medullary carcinoma, metastatic tumors, teratoma, lymphoma, and others). Well-differentiated carcinomas of follicular origin account for over 60 to 90% of the malignant lesions in children. Papillary and follicular carcinoma rates vary by geographic location, perhaps because of differing iodine content in the soil and the diet. Follicular carcinoma has a greater prevalence in areas of iodine deficiency. On the other hand, in iodine-sufficient regions, the majority of thyroid cancer patients had a papillary type of the disease (Pizzo and Poplack, 1997). Characterization of the histopathologic type as follicular, papillary, or papillary-follicular carcinomas does not alter therapy. However, papillary and papillary-follicular cancers have higher recurrence rates than does follicular disease.

The ultrasonographic appearance of thyroid tumors of follicular origin in children has been studied in more depth than that of nonfollicular tumors. Malignant tumors often appear as hypoechoic, heterogeneous lesions with irregular outline and absence of a "halo" sign. Unlike in adult patients, calcifications are a rare finding in children with malignant thyroid tumors and have been reported in < 5% of malignant thyroid lesions. At power Doppler sonography, up to 72% of a malignant thyroid lesion may be characterized by a significant increase in intranodular vascularization.

Although the detection of intranodular vascularization may be considered a useful criterion for malignancy, a high rate of internal vascularization in large benign nodules substantially decreases the clinical value of this criterion. The combination of nodule hypoechogenicity or heterogeneity with Type III vascularization at power Doppler US can be helpful in thyroid cancer diagnosis. These criteria had very high specificity (98% and 95%, respectively). However, the sensitivity of these criteria is low (45% and 53%, respectively) (Lyshchik *et al.*, 2005).

The diagnostic accuracy of power Doppler ultrasonography depends on nodule size. Results of our previous study (Lyshchik *et al.*, 2005) showed, that in small thyroid lesions (less than 15 mm in diameter), the diagnostic value of power Doppler for thyroid cancer was higher than that among large lesions and showed 70% sensitivity and 88% specificity. A combination of outline irregularity or Type III vascularization with subcapsular location of small thyroid nodules could increase the specificity up to 97% and the overall accuracy up to 85%, with some decrease in the sensitivity (52%). On the other hand, in nodules larger than 15 mm in diameter, the diagnostic value of power Doppler US criteria for thyroid cancer was much lower than that for smaller nodules. In large lesions, Type III vascularization showed comparable sensitivity (73%) but low specificity (52%). Unfortunately, the combination of gray-scale and power Doppler US characteristics did not bring significant improvements to thyroid cancer diagnosis in nodules with a diameter larger than 15 mm.

In conclusion, power Doppler assessment of thyroid lesions in children is a useful addition to gray-scale US and may be helpful in selecting those patients who require future investigation. However, like other US features, Doppler US cannot be used to diagnose or exclude malignancy with a high degree of confidence. Rather, the Doppler US finding of predominantly internal or central blood flow appears to increase the chance that a small thyroid nodule is malignant. On the other hand, in the absence of flow, an otherwise suspicious lesion in a patient who is considered "at risk" for thyroid cancer development, a US-guided fine-needle biopsy is justified.

References

Bentley, A.A., Gillespie, C., and Malis, D. 2003. Evaluation and management of a solitary thyroid nodule in a child. *Otolaryngol. Clin. North Am. 36*:117–128.

Bucsky, P., and Parlowsky, T. 1997. Epidemiology and therapy of thyroid cancer in childhood and adolescence. *Exp. Clin. Endocrinol. Diabetes 105* (Suppl. 4):70–73.

Castro, M.R., and Gharib, H. 2000. Thyroid nodules and cancer: when to wait and watch when to refer. *Postgrad. Med. 107*:113–124.

Cerbone, G., Spiezia, S., Colao, A., Di Sarno, A., Assanti, A.P., Lucci, R., Siciliani, M., Lombardi, G., and Fenzi, G. 1999. Power Doppler improves the diagnostic accuracy of color Doppler ultrasonography in cold thyroid nodules: follow-up results. *Horm. Res. 52*:19–24.

de Vathaire, F., Hardiman, C., Shamsaldin, A., Campbell, S., Grimaud, E., Hawkins, M., Raquin, M., Oberlin, O., Diallo I., Zucker, J.M., Panis, X., Lagrange, J.L., Daly-Schveitzer, N., Lemerle, J., Chavaudra, J., Schlumberger, M., and Bonaiti, C. 1999. Thyroid carcinomas after irradiation for a first cancer during childhood. *Arch. Intern. Med. 159*:2713–2719.

Desjardins, J.G., Khan, A.H., Montupet, P., Collin, P.P., Leboeuf, G., Polychronakos, C., Simard, P., Boisvert, J., and Dube, L.J. 1987. Management of thyroid nodules in children: a 20-year experience. *J. Pediatr. Surg. 22*:736–739.

Drozd, V., Demidchik, E., Harabets, L., Lyshchik, A., and Reiners, C. 1999. Early diagnostics of radiation induced thyroid cancer in children of Belarus by ultrasound. In: Thomas, G., Karaoglou, A., and Williams, E.D. (Eds.), *Radiation and Thyroid Cancer. Proceedings of an International Seminar on Radiation and Thyroid Cancer.* World Scientific Publishing. 425–431.

Eden, K., Mahon, S., and Helfand, M. 2001. Screening high-risk populations for thyroid cancer. *Med. Pediatr. Oncol. 36*:583–591.

Frates, M.C., Benson, C.B., Charboneau, J.W., Cibas, E.S., Clark, O.H., Coleman, B.G., Cronan, J.J., Doubilet, P.M., Evans, D.B., Goellner, J.R., Hay, I.D., Hertzberg, B.S., Intenzo, C.M., Jeffrey, R.B., Langer, J.E., Larsen, P.R., Mandel, S.J., Middleton, W.D., Reading, C.C., Sherman, S.I., and Tessler, F.N. 2005. Society of Radiologists in Ultrasound. Management of thyroid nodules detected at US: Society of Radiologists in ultrasound consensus conference statement. *Radiology 237*:794–800.

Gorlin J.B., and Sallan, S. 1990. Thyroid cancer in childhood. *Endocrinol. Metab. Clin. North Am. 19*:649–662.

Grigsby, P.W., Galor, A., Michalski, J.M., and Doherty, G.M. 2002. Childhood and adolescent thyroid carcinoma. *Cancer 95*:724–729.

Hung, W. 1999. Solitary thyroid nodules in 93 children and adolescents. a 35-years experience. *Horm. Res. 52*:15–18.

Jarlov, A.E., Nygard, B., Hegedus, L., Karstrup, S., and Hansen, J.M. 1993. Observer variation in ultrasound assessment of the thyroid gland. *Br. J. Radiol. 66*:625–627.

Kazakov, V.S., Demidchik, E.P., and Astakhova, L.N. 1992. Thyroid cancer after Chernobyl. *Nature 359*:21.

Koike, E., Noguchi, S., Yamashita, H., Murakami, T., Ohshima, A., Kawamoto, H., and Yamashita, H. 2001. Ultrasonographic characteristics of thyroid nodules: prediction of malignancy. *Arch. Surg. 136*:334–337.

Lyshchik, A., Drozd, V., Demidchik, Y., and Reiners, C. 2005. Diagnosis of thyroid cancer in children: value of gray-scale and power doppler US. *Radiology 235*:604–613.

Mazzeo, S., Caramella, D., Lencioni, R., Viacava, P., De Liperi, A., Naccarato, A.G., Armillotta, N., Marcocci, C., Miccoli, P., and Bartolozzi, C. 1997. Usefulness of echo-color Doppler in differentiating parathyroid lesions from other cervical masses. *Eur. Radiol. 7*:90–95.

Naik, K.S., and Bury, R.F. 1998. Imaging the thyroid. *Clin. Radiol. 53*:630–636.

Pacini, F., Vorontsova, T., Demidchik, E.P., Molinaro, E., Agate, L., Romei, C., Shavrova, E., Cherstvoy, E.D., Ivashkevitch, Y., Kuchinskaya, E., Schlumberger, M., Ronga, G., Filesi, M., and Pinchera, A. 1997. Post-Chernobyl thyroid carcinoma in Belarus children and adolescents: comparison with naturally occurring thyroid carcinoma in Italy and France. *J. Clin. Endocrinol. Metab. 82*:3563–3569.

Pizzo, P.A., and Poplack, D.G. 1997. *Principles and Practice of Pediatric Oncology.* 3rd ed. Philadelphia: Lippincott-Raven, pp. 955–958.

Raab, S.S., Silverman, J.F., Elsheikh, T.M., Thomas, P.A., and Wakely, P.E. 1995. Pediatric thyroid nodules: disease demographics and clinical management as determined by fine needle aspiration biopsy. *Pediatrics 95*:46–49.

Rago, T., Vitti, P., Chiovato, L., Mazzeo, S., De Liperi, A., Miccoli, P., Viacava, P., Bogazzi, F., Martino, E., and Pinchera, A. 1998. Role of conventional ultrasonography and color flow-Doppler sonography in predicting malignancy in "cold" thyroid nodules. *Eur. J. Endocrinol 138*:41–46.

Reiners, C. 1998. Sequelae of Czernobyl. *Internist (Berl) 39*:592–593.

Ron, E. 1996. Thyroid cancer. In Schottenfeld, D., Fraumeni, J.F., Jr., (Eds.), *Cancer Epidemiology and Prevention.* 2nd ed. New York: Oxford University Press.

Ron, E., Lubin, J.H., Shore, R.E., Mabuchi, K., Modan, B., Pottern, L.M., Schneider, A.B., Tucker, M.A., and Boice, J.D., Jr. 1995. Thyroid cancer after exposure to external radiation: a pooled analysis of seven studies. *Radiat Res. 141*:259–277.

Rudolph, A.M., Hoffman, J.I.E., and Rudolph, C.D. 2003. *Rudolph's Pediatrics*, 21st ed. New York: McGraw-Hill, pp. 1770–1772.

Tan, G.H., and Gharib, H. 1997. Thyroid incidentalomas: management approaches to nonpalpable nodules discovered incidentally on thyroid imaging. *Ann. Intern. Med. 126*:226–231.

Van Vliet, G., Glinoer, D., Verelst, J., Spehl, M., Gompel, C., and Delange, F. 1987. Cold thyroid nodules in childhood: is surgery always necessary? *Eur. J. Pediatr. 146*:378–382.

Wu, X., Groves, F.D., McLaughlin, C.C., Jemal, A., Martin, J., and Chen, V.W. 2005. Cancer incidence patterns among adolescents and young adults in the United States. *Cancer Causes Control 16*:309–320.

Yip, F., Reeve, T., Poole, A., and Delbridge, L. 1994. Thyroid nodules in childhood and adolescence. *Austr. NZ. J. Sur. 64*:676–678.

Index

Note: Page numbers followed by "f" denote figures; "t" tables